QUICK REVIEW OF

PGMEE

for Various Post Graduate Medical Entrance Examinations

QUICK REVIEW OF

PGMEE

for Various Post Graduate Medical Entrance Examinations

(Including Medicine, Pediatrics, Dermatology and Venereal Diseases, Radiology, Psychiatry)

FOURTH EDITION

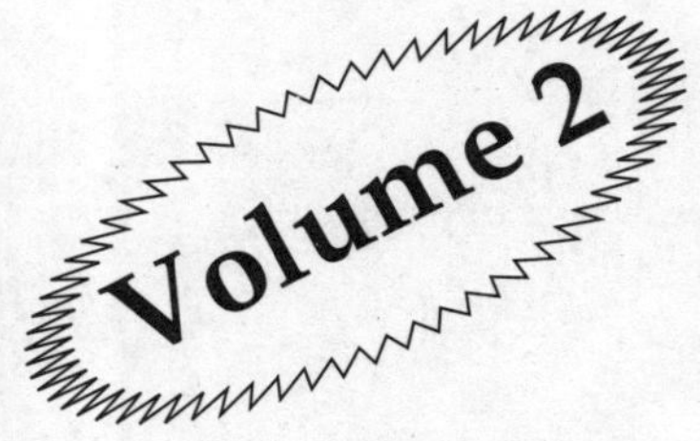

Sharad Chandra MBBS DCH

Editor and Compiler

Sangita Chandra MSc

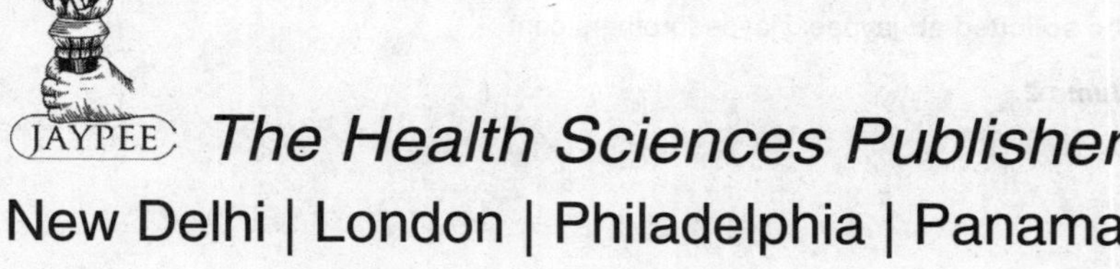

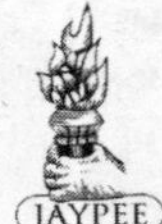

Jaypee Brothers Medical Publishers (P) Ltd

Headquarters

Jaypee Brothers Medical Publishers (P) Ltd
4838/24, Ansari Road, Daryaganj
New Delhi 110 002, India
Phone: +91-11-43574357
Fax: +91-11-43574314
Email: jaypee@jaypeebrothers.com

Overseas Offices

J.P. Medical Ltd
83 Victoria Street, London
SW1H 0HW (UK)
Phone: +44 20 3170 8910
Fax: +44 (0)20 3008 6180
Email: info@jpmedpub.com

Jaypee-Highlights Medical Publishers Inc
City of Knowledge, Bld. 235, 2nd Floor, Clayton
Panama City, Panama
Phone: +1 507-301-0496
Fax: +1 507-301-0499
Email: cservice@jphmedical.com

Jaypee Medical Inc
325 Chestnut Street
Suite 412, Philadelphia, PA 19106, USA
Phone: +1 267-519-9789
Email: support@jpmedus.com

Jaypee Brothers Medical Publishers (P) Ltd
17/1-B Babar Road, Block-B, Shaymali
Mohammadpur, Dhaka-1207
Bangladesh
Mobile: +08801912003485
Email: jaypeedhaka@gmail.com

Jaypee Brothers Medical Publishers (P) Ltd
Bhotahity, Kathmandu, Nepal
Phone +977-9741283608
Email: kathmandu@jaypeebrothers.com

Website: www.jaypeebrothers.com
Website: www.jaypeedigital.com

Inquiries for bulk sales may be solicited at: jaypee@jaypeebrothers.com

Quick Review of PGMEE, Volume 2

Fourth Edition: **2016**

ISBN 978-93-5090-648-4

Printed at Sanat Printers

This book is dedicated to
our illustrious readers
with best of luck and wishes

Preface to the Fourth Edition

Dear students,

It gives me immense pleasure and great honor in presenting the fourth edition, volume two of Quick Review Series, reloaded with latest questions. It follows essentially the pattern of earlier editions of this book. The study material provided in this book will help the medical students in meeting the challenges of All India, AIIMS, SGPGI, MAHE, JIPMER, and other PG entrance examinations conducted by various states/institutes.

This book is a compilation of previous years original question papers, which have been solved in a true sense. All questions are accompanied by a paragraph-length explanatory answer and specific reference. Whenever required, illustrations, tables, and X-ray films are added in conformity with textual descriptions to make the student fully understand the topic without consulting the standard textbook after each and every question. Questions on a topic have been clustered together in order to avoid unnecessary repetitions and to save the precious time of the readers. The answers are written after consulting standard textbooks, but sometimes the data in different books on a topic may vary. Sometimes the questions are framed in such a way that more than one choice is correct. In such a scenario the student should select the best choice. It has been my best endeavor to furnish accurate and maximum information, sufficient for the students, in simple language, obtained after sifting through several textbooks.

A compilation of this kind may not be complete in all respects. I am also conscious about the inept errors and misprints that might have crept in. In spite of these shortcomings, it is hoped, that the students will find this book comprehensive, helpful and inspiring. **Readers are requested to contribute by sending the question paper (Original or Photostat copy) of latest year in which they have appeared in order to enrich our questions bank**. All contributions will be duly acknowledged. I cordially invite all the readers to submit their comments, suggestions and criticism of the book. Useful suggestions for rectification and improvement would be gratefully acknowledged and incorporated in subsequent editions.

My obligations are indeed very great to Shri Jitendar P Vij (Group Chairman), Mr Ankit Vij (Group President) and Mr Tarun Duneja (Director-Publishing) and entire staff of M/s Jaypee Brothers Medical Publishers (P) Ltd, New Delhi, India for bringing out this book.

Sharad Chandra

Preface to the First Edition

My dear readers of Quick Review of PGMEE,

First of all I would like to thank you all for making the first edition a grand success. I was overwhelmed by the kind of response and appreciation I received by the letters of students from various parts of India. This second edition contains all the subject matter of Medicine, Pediatrics, Dermatology and Venereal Diseases, Radiology and Psychiatry and the number of questions have been increased. **The readers are requested to contribute the question papers of various state PGMEEs in which they appeared.** This will help to enhance our question bank. Each contribution will be duly acknowledged. As has been the experience of the past, most of the questions in various PG entrance examinations are repeated, therefore this book will be of immense help in successfully clearing the 'greatest hurdle' of the career of a medical student. The answers in this book are written after consulting various standard textbooks of respective fields. Medical knowledge changes constantly as a result of new research and clinical experience. Although I have made every effort to ensure that the information given is completely up-to-date but view of different authors may vary on certain matters. However, in case of any doubt the readers are welcome and encouraged to contact me on the e-mail address: **quickreview@yahoo.com** or by post at 288/30, Aryanagar, Lucknow-226004.

I am really thankful to Shri J.P. Vij, Chairman and Managing Director, Jaypee Brothers Medical Publishers (P) Ltd for taking personal interest in this book and for excellent quality of publication. The following readers deserve special words of acknowledgement and appreciation for their comments and contributions:

1. **Dr. Sujith Kumar 'Sushil'** — Netravathi Nagar, P.O. Kankanady, Garodi, Mangalore (Karnataka)
   - Contributed questions of CMC Vellore, 2002; PGMEE
2. **Dr. Sunita Singh** — ADMO, Central Railway Health Unit, Agra Cantt. (UP)
   - Contributed questions of MP 2001; PGMEE
3. **Dr. Paul Vincent** — Flat No. 6, Padma Flats, 20/1, Ist Cross Street, Kilpauk Garden Colony, Chennai (TN)
   - Contributed questions of AIIMS May 2002; PGMEE
4. **Dr. N.K. Kansal** — 569, Subhash Nagar, Lane No. 8, Meerut (UP)
5. **Dr. Apoorna Pandey** — LLRM College, Meerut (UP)

Sharad Chandra

Author strongly recommends following books for preparation of PGMEE:

1.	**Medicine**	**D**avidson's Principles and Practice of Medicine by Brian R. Walker
		Manual of Practical Medicine by R Alagappan
2.	**Pediatrics**	**T**he Short Textbook of Pediatrics by Suraj Gupte
		Ghai Essential Pediatrics by Vinod Kumar Paul
3.	**Dermatology and Venereal Diseases**	**R**oxburgh's Common Skin Diseases by R Marks
4.	**Radiology**	**T**extbook of Radiology and Imaging by David Sutton
		AIIMS-MAMC-PGI's Comprehensive Textbook of Diagnostic Radiology (3 Vols) by Niranjan Khandelwal
5.	**Psychiatry**	**A** Short Textbook of Psychiatry by Niraj Ahuja

Contents

PART I

Medicine *3*

PART II

Pediatrics *339*

PART III

Dermatology and Venereal Diseases *507*

PART IV

Radiology *579*

PART V

Psychiatry *643*

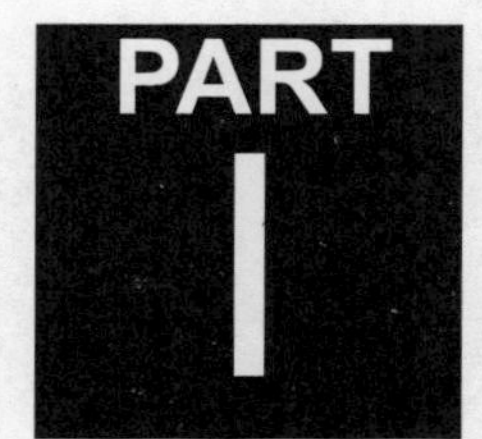

Medicine

Medicine

1. **In "tumor lysis syndrome" all the following are seen *except*:**
   A. Hyperuricemia **B.** Hyperkalemia
   C. Hyperphosphatemia **D.** Hypercalcemia *(PGI 1999, AIIMS May 2002, JIPMER 2002)*

2. **Hypercalcemia is seen in all *except*:**
   A. Sarcoidosis **B.** Tumor lysis syndrome
   C. Multiple myeloma **D.** Primary hyperparathyroidism *(AI 1997)*

3. ***Not* seen in tumor lysis syndrome:**
   A. Hyperphosphatemia **B.** Hypokalemia
   C. Hyperuricemia **D.** Hypocalcemia *(PGI 1997)*

Tumor lysis syndrome is characterized by various combinations of **hyperuricemia**, **hyperkalemia**, **hyperphosphatemia**, lactic acidosis, and **hypocalcemia** and is caused by the mass destruction of a large number of rapidly proliferating neoplastic cells. Frequently, ARF develops as a result of tumor lysis syndrome. It is most frequently associated with the treatment of Burkitt's lymphoma, acute lymphoblastic leukemia, and other high-grade lymphomas, but it also may be seen with chronic leukemias and, rarely, with solid tumors.

4. **Drug *not* used in prevention of rejection after transplantation:**
   A. Flucytosine **B.** Mycophenolate mofetil
   C. Rapamycin **D.** Azathioprine *(SGPGI 1999)*

Cyclosporine and tacrolimus are **calcineurin blockers**. *Although structurally different* they exert their immunosuppressive effect through the same pathway. Both of them bind within the 'T cell' to a particular cytoplasmic protein (immunophilin). The immunophilin for cyclosporine is cyclophilin while that for tacrolimus is FK binding protein. The resulting **immunophilin-drug complex** blocks the activity of calcineurin (a phosphatase) within the cytoplasm of the T cell. Calcineurin plays a critical role in facilitating the transcription of IL 2 (the main T cell growth factor) and other cytokines after T cell activation. Both agents are highly nephrotoxic. Various immunosuppressive agents and their mode of action are as under:

Azathioprine	Prevents lymphocyte proliferation
Mycophenolate mofetil	Prevents lymphocyte proliferation
Cyclosporine	Blocks interleukin (IL) 2 gene transcription
Tacrolimus	Blocks interleukin (IL) 2 gene transcription
Rapamycin	Blocks interleukin (IL) 2 receptor signal transduction
OKT3 monoclonal antibody	Depletion and blockade of T cells
ALG/ALS	Depletion and blockade of lymphocytes
Anti CD 25 monoclonal antibodies	Targets activated T cells
Corticosteroids	Widespread anti-inflammatory action

The introduction in 1980 of cyclosporine as an immunosuppressive agent contributed substantially to the improvement in survival after liver transplantation. Tacrolimus (FK 506) is a macrolide lactone antibiotic isolated from a Japanese soil fungus, *Streptomyces tsukubaensis*. It is 10 to 100 times more potent than cyclosporine.

5. ***Not* a clinical feature of normal pressure hydrocephalus:**
   A. Urinary incontinence
   B. Gait disturbance
   C. Aphasia
   D. Dementia *(AI 1991, 1992, 1997, UP 1997, PGI 1997)*

6. **Triad of normal pressure hydrocephalus is:**
   A. Gait disorder, urinary incontinence and lower cranial nerve palsy
   B. Gait disorder, urinary incontinence and dementia
   C. Ataxia, aphasia and gait disorder
   D. Tremor, aphasia and dementia *(AI 1999)*

In normal pressure hydrocephalus a triad of **memory loss**, **gait disturbance**, and **bladder incontinence** is *typical.*

7. **Which of the following is *not* used in acute asthma:**
   A. Ipratropium bromide **B.** Salbutamol
   C. Steroids **D.** Montelukast *(AIIMS May 2002)*

Montelukast sodium is a selective and orally active leukotriene receptor antagonist that inhibits the cysteinyl leukotriene CysL T_1 receptor. Montelukast is indicated for the prophylaxis and chronic treatment of asthma in patients' ages 2 years and older. **Montelukast should not be used as rescue medication to treat acute asthma episodes.** Patients should be advised to have appropriate rescue medication available. Use of montelukast may not eliminate the need for inhaled (ICS) or systemic corticosteroids. Safety and effectiveness of montelukast in patients younger than 2 years of age has not been established.

2 to 5 years of age	**6 to 14 years of age**	**15 years of age and older**
One 4 mg cherry chewable tablet daily in the evening	One 5 mg cherry chewable tablet daily in the evening	One 10 mg tablet daily in the evening

8. **Acute lung injury does *not* include which of the following conditions:**
   A. Cardiopulmonary bypass **B.** Aspiration
   C. Toxic gas injury **D.** Lung contusion *(AIIMS May 2002)*

Acute lung injury (ALI) develops rapidly after a predisposing condition triggers a systemic inflammatory response; often within 90 minutes. ALI is most strongly associated with conditions that produce direct alveolar injury or indirect injury via the pulmonary capillary bed. These are listed below:

Direct injury to alveolar epithelium	**Indirect lung injury**
• **Aspiration**	• Sepsis syndrome
• Diffuse infection	• Severe nonthoracic trauma
• Near drowning	• Hypertransfusion
• **Toxic inhalation**	• **Cardiopulmonary bypass**
• Airway contusion	

ALI is the consequence of an *unregulated over* expression of usual systemic inflammatory responses to infection and/or injury.

9. **Pseudofractures are seen in:**
   A. Hyperparathyroidism **B.** Osteoporosis
   C. Osteomalacia **D.** Hypoparathyroidism *(JIPMER 2002)*

The ***most specific*** **feature of osteomalacia is the presence of Looser transformation zones, also known as Milkman's pseudofractures or umbauzonen**. These zones appear as radiolucent defects several millimeters thick that extend perpendicular to the cortex and are frequently symmetrical. The defects are more prominent in the outer areas of the cortex but can extend to the endosteal surface. They frequently affect the scapula, femoral neck, ischium, and the ribs.

10. **A 25 years old girl presents with fever and weakness. There is *splenomegaly* of 3 cm below the costal margin. Hemoglobin is 8 mg/dL, TLC is 3000/mm, platelet count is 80,000/mm. *Least* likely diagnosis is:**
    A. Aplastic anemia
    B. Megaloblastic anemia
    C. Anemia of chronic disease
    D. ALL *(AIIMS 2000)*

11. In a young patient with aplastic anemia, the *treatment of choice* is:

A. ATG
B. Bone marrow transplantation
C. Danazol
D. G-CSF

(AI 2002)

Aplastic anemia is a disorder of hematopoiesis characterized by marked reduction or absence of erythroid, granulocytic, and megakaryocytic cells in the bone marrow with resultant pancytopenia. Most cases of aplastic anemia are acquired. In over 50% of patients, no cause can be determined (so-called **idiopathic aplastic anemia**). The onset of **aplastic anemia** is insidious and the *most common* presenting symptoms are those secondary to anemia and thrombocytopenia (progressive **weakness** and fatigue and **bleeding** from the skin, nose, gums, vagina, or GIT). Although the patient may be severely neutropenic, infection is *rarely* the presenting symptom. The *most frequent* physical findings are cutaneous and conjunctival **pallor** and **hemorrhages** (petechiae, ecchymoses, and gum bleeding). If anemia is severe, tachycardia and murmurs may be present. **Hepatosplenomegaly and lymphadenopathy are characteristically absent**. Confirmation of diagnosis requires morphologic and cytogenetic evaluation of the bone marrow. The pancytopenia of aplastic anemia is progressive and life-threatening and with transfusion support *alone*, up to 80% of patients with severe aplastic anemia are dead within 18 to 24 months. Allogeneic bone marrow transplantation and immunosuppressive therapy, have radically improved the prognosis of patients with severe forms of aplastic anemia. **Treatment with a human leukocyte antigen matched related marrow transplant is curative in 60 to 90% of patients. Transplantation from an HLA-compatible sibling is a 'curative' treatment for aplastic anemia.** Immunosuppressive therapy with antithymocyte or antithoracic duct lymphocyte globulin and/or cyclosporine can induce at least *partial* remission of disease in 60 to 80% of patients. Once the diagnosis of aplastic anemia is ascertained, family HLA typing should be done as soon as possible, particularly in *younger patients* (<45 years), since these patients are most likely to benefit from bone marrow transplantation from a histocompatible sibling.

12. *Investigation of choice* for invasive amebiasis is:

A. Indirect hemagglutination
B. ELISA
C. Counterimmunodiffusion assays
D. Microscopy

(AIIMS Nov 2001, AI 2002)

Serology is an important addition to the methods used for the parasitologic diagnosis of **invasive amebiasis**. Kits for the performance of **counterimmunodiffusion assays**, agar gel diffusion assays, and ELISAs are available, and the results of these tests are positive in more than 90% of patients with colitis, amebomas, or liver abscess.

13. Acute breathlessness is an important feature of:

A. Pericarditis
B. CHF
C. Pneumonia
D. Pulmonary embolism

(UP 2001)

14. *Most common symptom* of pulmonary embolism is:

A. Chest pain
B. Dyspnea
C. Hemoptysis
D. Cough

15. *Most common sign* of pulmonary embolism is:

A. Sweating
B. Tachypnea
C. Tachycardia
D. Cyanosis

Dyspnea is the *most frequent* symptom of pulmonary thromboembolism and tachypnea is its *most frequent* sign. Whereas dyspnea, syncope, hypotension, or cyanosis indicates a massive pulmonary thromboembolism, pleuritic pain, cough, or hemoptysis often suggest a small embolism located distally near the pleura. **A normal or *near* normal chest X-ray in a dyspneic patient suggests pulmonary thromboembolism**. Westermark's sign, Hampton's hump or an enlarged right descending pulmonary artery may also be seen. **Selective pulmonary angiography is the *most specific* examination available for establishing the definitive diagnosis of pulmonary thromboembolism** and can detect emboli as small as 1 to 2 mm.

16. Dose of digoxin is *not* altered in:

A. Hypomagnesemia
B. Renal failure
C. Hepatotoxicity
D. Hypokalemia

(AIIMS 1997)

17. *False* regarding digitalis is:
A. Lipid soluble
B. Actively metabolized in liver
C. Oral absorption
D. Renal excretion
(AI 1997)

18. Dose of digoxin is *not* reduced in which of the following condition:
A. Liver disease
B. Renal disease
C. Hypercalcemia
D. Hypoxia
(UP 1993, AIIMS 1996)

Digoxin is *not* metabolized by liver and is **excreted *as such* by kidney in urine**. *Hence* its dose is *not* reduced in hepatic failure *but* **dose should be reduced in renal failure** and in geriatric patients. Hypokalemia, hypercalcemia, quinidine and verapamil increase the toxicity of digitalis so its dose should be reduced.
- **Digitoxin is metabolized in liver, like all other 'toxins'.**

19. ECG finding in hypercalcemia is:
A. Prolonged PR interval
B. Paroxysmal atrial tachycardia
C. Short QT interval
D. Bundle branch blocks
(UP 1993, SGPGI 1996)

20. QT interval is shortened in:
A. Hyperkalemia
B. Hypercalcemia
C. Hypokalemia
D. Hypocalcemia
(AI 1993)

21. *Shortest* QT interval is seen in:
A. Hypocalcemia
B. Hypercalcemia
C. Hypokalemia
D. Hyperkalemia
(AI 1995)

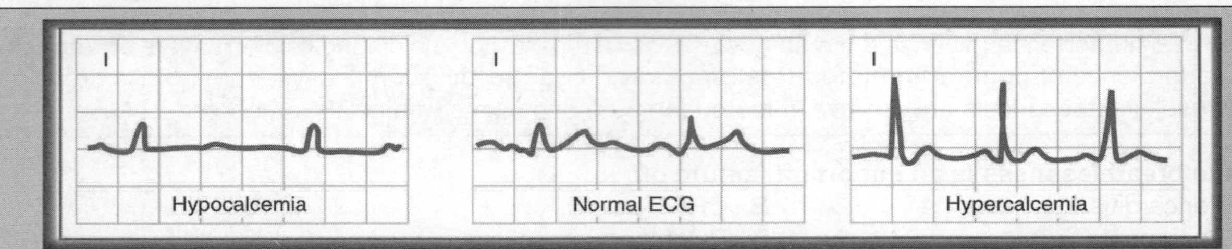

Conditions that prolong phase 2 such as amiodarone and hypocalcemia increase the QT interval. In contrast, shortening of ventricular repolarization (phase 2), as by digitalis or hypercalcemia, abbreviates the ST segment. **Hypocalcemia typically prolongs the QT interval (ST portion), while hypercalcemia shortens it.**

22. *False* regarding Reye's syndrome is:
A. Deep jaundice is present
B. Disease may be precipitated by salicylates
C. Prothrombin time is prolonged
D. It frequently complicates viral infection
(UP 1993, SGPGI 1996)

Fatty liver with encephalopathy or **Reye's syndrome is** an acute illness encountered exclusively in children below 15 years of age. It is characterized *clinically* by vomiting and signs of progressive central nervous system damage, signs of hepatic injury, and hypoglycemia. There is mitochondrial dysfunction with *decreased* activity of hepatic mitochondrial enzymes. Its cause is unknown, although **viruses** and drugs, particularly **salicylates**, have been implicated. The onset of disease follows an URTI, especially influenza or chickenpox and within 1 to 3 days, persistent vomiting occurs, together with stupor, which progresses rapidly to generalized convulsions and coma. **The liver is enlarged, but jaundice is characteristically absent or minimal. Elevations** in serum aminotransferases and **prothrombin time**, hypoglycemia, metabolic acidosis, and elevated serum ammonia levels are the major laboratory findings. The mortality rate in Reye's syndrome is approximately 50%. Treatment consists of infusions of glucose and fresh frozen plasma, as well as IV mannitol to reduce the cerebral edema. Chronic liver disease has *not* been reported.

23. *Not* a myeloproliferative disease:

A. Essential thrombocytosis **B.** CML
C. AML **D.** Polycythemia vera *(AIIMS 2000)*

24. *Not* an important feature of polycythemia vera:

A. Bone marrow hyperplasia **B.** Leukocyte alkaline phosphate increased
C. Splenomegaly **D.** Erythropoietin level increased *(UP 1993)*

25. In polycythemia vera all the following are seen *except*:

A. Thrombocytosis **B.** Increased B_{12} binding capacity
C. High erythropoietin level **D.** Splenomegaly *(AIIMS May 2001)*

26. *Not* seen in polycythemia vera:

A. Ocular congestion **B.** Increased RBC count
C. Increased erythropoietin level **D.** Increased vitamin B_{12} binding capacity *(AIIMS 1997)*

Polycythemia vera, idiopathic myelofibrosis, essential thrombocytosis, and chronic myelogenous leukemia are classified *together* under the heading **chronic myeloproliferative disorders**, because their pathophysiology involves the clonal expansion of a multipotent hematopoietic progenitor cell with the overproduction of 1 or more of the formed elements of the blood. These diseases may transform into acute leukemia naturally or as a consequence of mutagenic treatment. **Polycythemia vera** is the *most common* of the chronic myeloproliferative disorders, with a frequency of 29 per 100,000 and is a clonal disorder involving a multipotent hematopoietic progenitor cell in which there is *overproduction* of phenotypically *normal* red cells, granulocytes, and platelets in the *absence* of a recognizable physiologic stimulus. Its etiology is unknown. Uncontrolled erythrocytosis may lead to neurologic symptoms such as vertigo, tinnitus, headache, and visual disturbances.

Features of Polycythemia vera

- Elevated red cell mass
- Normal arterial oxygen saturation
- **Splenomegaly**
- *In the absence of splenomegaly:* Leukocytosis and thrombocytosis
- Plasma **erythropoietin level less than** 4 mU/ml

The **leukocyte alkaline phosphatase score** is *either* normal or **elevated**. **Elevated serum vitamin B_{12} or B_{12}-binding capacity** may be present. There is no correlation between **thrombocytosis** and thrombosis in polycythemia vera. Bone marrow biopsy usually reveals megakaryocyte hyperplasia and hypertrophy, as well as an **overall increase in marrow cellularity.**

27. *Not* seen in polycythemia rubra vera:

A. Increased platelets **B.** Leukocytosis
C. Decreased LAP score **D.** Increased vitamin B_{12} binding capacity *(AIIMS 2000)*

High LAP scores have been seen in **polycythemia vera**, myelofibrosis, aplastic anemia, mongolism, hairy cell leukemia, leukemoid reactions, and neutrophilia *either* physiological *or* secondary to infection.

28. Paradoxical pulse is seen in:

A. Severe AR + AS **B.** Severe AR
C. LVF **D.** Cardiac tamponade *(UP 1993)*

29. Pulsus paradoxus is seen in:

A. Adhesive pericarditis **B.** Rheumatic pericarditis
C. Uremic pericarditis **D.** Constrictive pericarditis *(AI 1992)*

30. Pulsus paradoxus is found in all *except*:

A. IPPV **B.** COPD
C. Constructive pericarditis **D.** Pericardial tamponade *(AIIMS 1998)*

31. Pulsus paradoxus is *not* seen in:

A. Cardiac tamponade
B. Severe bronchial asthma
C. Pregnancy
D. Constructive pericarditis

(KERALA 1999)

- **Paradoxical pulse** is a hallmark of cardiac tamponade and occurs in only approximately 1/3rd of patients with **constrictive pericarditis**. Paradoxical pulse is *not* pathognomonic of pericardial disease because it can be observed in restrictive cardiomyopathies and in some cases of hypovolemic shock, chronic obstructive airways disease, and severe bronchial asthma.
- **Pulsus alternans** is a pattern in which there is *regular* alteration of the pressure pulse amplitude, despite a regular rhythm. It is due to alternating left ventricular contractile force, **usually denotes severe impairment of left ventricular function**, and commonly occurs in patients who also have a loud 3rd heart sound. It may also occur during or following paroxysmal tachycardia or for several beats following a premature beat in patients *without* heart disease.
- In **pulsus bigeminus**, there is also a regular alteration of pressure pulse amplitude, but it is caused by a premature ventricular contraction that follows each regular beat.

32. Pulses bisferiens can occur in:

A. Has alternate high and low volume pulse
B. Has bifid anacrotic wave
C. Severe AR with good LV function
D. AS with AR

(KARNATAKA 2000)

The **pulses bisferiens**, which has 2 systolic peaks, is characteristic of **aortic regurgitation** (with or without accompanying **stenosis**) and of hypertrophic cardiomyopathy.

33. *Not* seen in acute severe asthma is:

A. Pulsus paradoxus
B. Hypercapnia
C. Acidosis
D. Cyanosis

(PGI 1999)

Hypoxia is a common finding during acute exacerbations, but frank ventilatory failure is relatively uncommon, being observed in 10 to 15% of patients. Most asthmatics have **hypocapnia** and a respiratory alkalosis. In acutely ill patients, the finding of a normal arterial carbon dioxide tension tends to be associated with quite severe levels of obstruction. The presence of **metabolic acidosis** in the setting of acute asthma signifies *severe* obstruction. **Cyanosis** is a very *late* sign.

34. *Bilateral* facial nerve palsy is *not* seen in:

A. Melkersson-Rosenthal syndrome
B. Ramsay Hunt syndrome
C. Guillain-Barré syndrome
D. Sarcoidosis

(UP 1993)

35. *Bilateral* facial paralysis is *not* seen in:

A. Ramsay Hunt syndrome
B. Melkersson-Rosenthal syndrome
C. Heerfordt's syndrome
D. Guillain-Barré syndrome

(AIIMS 1997)

36. Melkersson-Rosenthal syndrome consists of all *except*:

A. Deafness
B. Labial edema
C. Plication of the tongue
D. Recurrent facial paralysis

The *most common* form of facial paralysis is idiopathic, i.e. **Bell's palsy**. In **Ramsay Hunt syndrome**, pain and vesicles appear in the external auditory canal, and patients lose their sense of taste in the anterior 2/3rd of the tongue while developing **ipsilateral facial palsy**. The geniculate ganglion of the sensory branch of the facial nerve is involved. *Bilateral* facial paralysis (**facial diplegia**) occurs in acute inflammatory polyradiculoneuritis (**Guillain-Barré syndrome**) and in a variety of **sarcoidosis** known as uveoparotid fever (Heerfordt's syndrome). The **Melkersson-Rosenthal syndrome** consists of a *triad* of **recurrent facial paralysis**, recurrent and eventually permanent facial (particularly labial) **edema**, and less constantly, **plication** (a folding or being folded) of the tongue.

37. Bilateral LMN facial palsy is *not* seen in:
A. Transverse myelitis
B. Bilateral acoustic neuroma
C. Guillain-Barré syndrome
D. Sarcoidosis
(KARNATAKA 1994)

Transverse myelitis is an acute or subacute, generally monophasic, inflammatory disorder of the **spinal cord**.

38. *Not* a common cause of carpal tunnel syndrome:
A. Hypertension
B. Hypothyroidism
C. Rheumatoid arthritis
D. Pregnancy
(UP 1993)

The **carpal tunnel syndrome** is the compression neuropathy of the median nerve as it passes beneath the flexor retinaculum. Majority of patients are women in 50s or 60s and symptoms are bilateral in 50% of cases but are more *evident* in the dominant hand. Patient complains of progressive weakness or clumsiness due to impairment of the fine movements of the hand such as picking up a pin, knitting or sewing associated with *acroparesthesia* (attack of pain, tingling and numbness of the affected hand without involving ring and little finger).

IMPORTANT CAUSES OF CARPAL TUNNEL SYMDROME

- Idiopathic (*most common*)
- Excessive use of the wrist
- Tenosynovitis
- Local infiltration
- **Hypothyroidism**
- Colles' fracture
- Acromegaly
- Amyloidosis
- Mucopolysaccharidoses
- **Rheumatoid arthritis**
- Diabetes mellitus
- **Pregnancy**

In *wrist flexion test* (**Phalen's sign**) the patient is asked to flex both wrists and to keep them flexed for one minute. In more than 50% of patients of carpal tunnel syndrome there is prompt exacerbation of paresthesia in one or both hands and equally prompt relief from the symptoms when the flexion is discontinued. *Tourniquet test* is similar but in this test cuff of a sphygmomanometer is pumped up to the systolic blood pressure for the same time.

39. In which of the following, highly "selective" proteinuria is seen:
A. Focal sclerosis
B. Membranous glomerulonephritis
C. Mesangial proliferative glomerulonephritis
D. Minimal change disease
(UP 1993)

In children with **minimal change disease** (**MCD**), the **urine principally contains albumin** and *minimal* amounts of higher molecular weight proteins such as IgG and α2-macroglobulin. This **selective proteinuria** in conjunction with foot process effacement suggests injury to podocytes and loss of the fixed negative charge in the glomerular filtration "barrier" for protein. Proteinuria is typically *non*selective in adults, suggesting more *extensive* disturbance of membrane permeability.

40. Triad of glomerulonephritis, pulmonary hemorrhage and antibody to basement membrane is seen in:
A. Diabetic nephropathy
B. Mixed connective tissue disease
C. Systemic necrotizing vasculitis
D. Goodpasture's syndrome
(UP 1993)

Anti-GBM disease is an autoimmune disease in which auto-antibodies directed against type 4 collagen induce RPGN and crescentic glomerulonephritis. Between 50 and 70% of patients have lung hemorrhage; **the clinical complex of anti-GBM nephritis and lung hemorrhage is referred to as Goodpasture's syndrome.**

41. Tic douloureux is synonymous with:
A. Trigeminal neuralgia
B. Temporal lobe epilepsy
C. Glossopharyngeal neuralgia
D. Todd's paralysis

42. Trigeminal neuralgia is treated with:
A. Indomethacin
B. Chlorpromazine
C. Phenobarbitone
D. Carbamazepine
(UP 1993)

The most striking disorder of trigeminal nerve function is **tic douloureux** (paroxysmal facial pain or **trigeminal neuralgia**), a condition characterized by excruciating paroxysms of pain in the lips, gums, cheek, or chin and, very rarely, in the distribution of the ophthalmic division of the 5th nerve. **Carbamazepine is the drug of choice** and is effective initially in 75% of patients.

43. Increased serum iron and normal total iron binding capacity are seen in:
A. Anemia of chronic disease **B.** Iron deficiency anemia
C. Sideroblastic anemia **D.** Thalassemia *(UP 1993)*

44. Metal causing sideroblastic anemia is:
A. Selenium **B.** Cu
C. Hg **D.** Lead *(AIIMS 1991, UP 1997)*

45. Intracellular iron level is *not* decreased in:
A. Anemia due to gastric ulcer **B.** Sideroblastic anemia
C. Anemia due to chronic infection **D.** Hookworm anemia *(DELHI 1996)*

Sideroblastic anemias are a group of disorders of varying etiology in which the bone marrow demonstrates marked dyserythropoiesis and an abnormal intramitochondrial *accumulation* of iron in erythroid precursors. Hypochromic as well as normochromic RBCs are present in peripheral blood smear producing a *dimorphic* blood picture. Siderocytes are red blood cells containing granules of *non* heme iron which gives a positive Prussian blue reaction. Sideroblasts are erythroblasts with Prussian blue positive iron granules in their cytoplasm. The sideroblastic anemias may be **hereditary** (X-linked sideroblastic anemia (XLSA) results from the deficient activity of the erythroid form of ALA synthase and is associated with ineffective erythropoiesis, weakness, and pallor) or **acquired**. The causes of *acquired* sideroblastic anemia are as under:

Drug and chemicals	Blood disorders	Inflammations	Miscellaneous
• Chloramphenicol • Ethanol • Isoniazid • Cycloserine • **Lead**	• Myelofibrosis • Polycythemia vera • Myeloma • Acute leukemias • Hodgkin's lymphoma • Hemolytic anemia	• Rheumatoid arthritis • SLE	• Carcinoma • Myxoedema • Malabsorption

Differential Diagnosis of Microcytic Anemia

Tests	Sideroblastic Anemia	Iron Deficiency	Thalassemia
Smear	Variable	Micro/hypo	Micro/hypo with targeting
SI	Normal to high	Low	Normal to high
TIBC	**Normal**	High	Normal
Percent saturation	30-80	Less than 10	30-80
Ferritin (μg/L)	50-300	Less than 15	50-300
Hemoglobin pattern	Normal	Normal	Abnormal

46. Microcytic hypochromic anemia is *not* seen in:
A. Fanconi's anemia
B. Iron deficiency anemia
C. Lead poisoning
D. Thalassemia major *(AIIMS 1997)*

The general blood picture (GBP) in **Fanconi's aplastic anemia** reveals **normocytic and normochromic RBCs** along with leucopenia and thrombocytopenia.

47. Propranolol is *contraindicated* in:
A. Hypertension
B. CHF
C. Angina pectoris
D. Thyrotoxicosis
(UP 1993)

48. Drug used in angina that can cause CCF is:
A. Verapamil
B. Sorbitrate®
C. Propranolol
D. Nifedipine
(KERALA 1994)

49. Preoperative propranolol is *not* indicated in:
A. Hyperthyroidism
B. Migraine
C. CHF
D. Prolong QT syndrome
(UP 1998)

Absolute Contraindications of β-blockers	
• Congestive cardiac failure	• Cardiogenic shock
• 2nd- or 3rd-degree atrioventricular (AV) block	• Sinus bradycardia (heart rate less than 45 beats per minute)

50. All are seen in subacute thyroiditis *except*:
A. Increased radioiodine uptake
B. Pain
C. Raised ESR
D. Raised T_4 level
(UP 1993)

51. All are *true* about de Quervain's thyroiditis *except*:
A. Raised ESR
B. Subsides spontaneously
C. Autoimmune etiology
D. Pain and swelling of the thyroid occurs
(AI 2002)

Subacute thyroiditis is also known as *granulomatous, giant cell*, or **de Quervain's thyroiditis**. It is a disease of **viral** origin. Symptoms of thyroiditis usually start after an episode of upper respiratory infection and include asthenia, fever, malaise, and symptoms referable to stretching of the thyroid capsule, mainly **pain** over the thyroid or pain referred to the lower jaw, ear, or occiput. These symptoms may exist in a suppressed state for weeks before the diagnosis is suspected. Two laboratory findings are characteristic of this disease: a **high erythrocyte sedimentation rate** and a **depressed radioactive iodine uptake**. Early, many patients are mildly thyrotoxic due to leakage of hormone from the gland and the **serum T_4 and T_3 are high**; TSH is undetectable. Later, as glandular hormone is depleted, the patient may pass through a hypothyroid phase, in which serum T_4 and T_3 are low and TSH is increased. The disease is **usually self-limiting** and acute cases should be managed with oral prednisolone for 7 days and then it is gradually tapered off over the next month.

52. Nephrotic syndrome, which is *not* cured after eradicating malaria, is caused by:
A. *Plasmodium vivax*
B. *Plasmodium ovale*
C. *Plasmodium falciparum*
D. *Plasmodium malariae*

Glomerular Lesions Associated with Protozoan and Parasitic Infections

Plasmodium malariae	Nephrotic syndrome due to diffuse or focal proliferative glomerulonephritis, membranous glomerulopathy, and minimal change disease. **Remission is *not* induced by eradication of the malarial infection**.
Plasmodium falciparum	Transient proteinuria in 50% of cases Nephrotic syndrome in <1% of cases
Congenital toxoplasmosis	Induces immune-complex glomerulonephritis
Schistosoma mansoni	Nephrotic syndrome in 5 to 10% of cases
Loa loa	Membranous glomerulonephritis
Hydatid disease	Membranous glomerulopathy
Trichinosis	Proliferative glomerulonephritis.

53. Which of the following is a feature of *falciparum* malaria:
A. Black water fever **B.** Algid malaria
C. Cerebral malaria **D.** All of the above

Types of Complicated *falciparum* Malaria (Pernicious Malaria)

Cerebral malaria	Most dreaded complication of *Plasmodium falciparum* infection
Algid malaria	In this condition patient passes into shock associated with coma. Fever is usually absent
Black water fever	Waves of acute hemolysis occur resulting in hemoglobinemia and hemoglobinuria leading to passage of black urine
Dysenteric malaria	Patient passes loose stools mixed with blood and mucus
Choleraic malaria	Acute watery diarrhea and vomiting with dehydration
Bilious remittent fever	Fever with jaundice due to acute hepatic failure

- *Pernicious means = causing great injury, destruction; fatal; deadly.*

54. All are the features of cerebral malaria *except*:
A. Absent abdominal reflex **B.** Extensor planter reflex
C. Retinal hemorrhage **D.** *Focal* neurological deficit

Cerebral malaria is a potentially fatal disease caused by *Plasmodium falciparum*. Patient presents with sign and symptoms of **generalized** encephalopathy with high grade fever.

55. Which species commonly causes cerebral malaria:
A. *Plasmodium ovale* **B.** *Plasmodium malariae*
C. *Plasmodium falciparum* **D.** *Plasmodium vivax*

Types of Malaria

• *Plasmodium vivax*	Benign tertian malaria
• *Plasmodium falciparum*	Malignant tertian malaria (**cerebral**)
• *Plasmodium malariae*	Quartan malaria
• *Plasmodium ovale*	Ovale tertian malaria

- Tertian means every 2nd days and quartan means every 3rd days.

56. Genetically transmitted diseases which protect against malaria are all *except*:
A. Sickle cell anemia **B.** G6PD deficiency
C. Absence of Duffy blood group **D.** Hereditary spherocytosis

Diseases which Protect against Malaria

- Duffy-negative FyFy phenotype
- Glucose-6-phosphate dehydrogenase (G6PD) deficiency
- Sickle cell disease
- Melanesian ovalocytosis
- Thalassemia

57. *Radical* cure of *Plasmodium vivax* is by:
A. Chloroquine
B. Quinine
C. Primaquine
D. Tetracycline

58. Primaquine has *no role* in infection with:

A. *Plasmodium falciparum* **B.** *Plasmodium vivax*
C. *Plasmodium malariae* **D.** *Plasmodium ovale*

Primaquine is the only standard drug active against the intrahepatic **hypnozoite** forms of malarial species and is used for the **radical cure of *Plasmodium vivax* and *Plasmodium ovale* malaria** following schizonticidal therapy. Primaquine is also effective against the gametocytes of *Plasmodium falciparum*. Dose is 15 mg/day for 14 days in adults and 0.3 mg/kg/day for 14 days in children.

59. Malaria affects the following organs *except*:

A. Brain **B.** LIver
C. Heart **D.** Kidney

Renal impairment is common among adults suffering form severe *falciparum* malaria but rare among children .The childhood febrile convulsions may occur with any of the malarias but *Plasmodium falciparum* is responsible for **cerebral** malaria. Hypoglycemia in malaria occurs due to **failure of hepatic gluconeogenesis**.

60. Types of malaria *not* seen in India:

A. *Plasmodium falciparum* **B.** *Plasmodium vivax*
C. *Plasmodium malariae* **D.** *Plasmodium ovale*

Incidence of Malaria in India

• *Plasmodium vivax*	70%
• *Plasmodium falciparum*	25-30%
• *Plasmodium malariae*	< 1% (Tumkur and Hassan districts of Karnataka)

• *Plasmodium ovale* is a *very rare* parasite of man, mostly confined to tropical Africa and Vietnam.

61. In cerebral malaria the *drug of choice* is:

A. Tetracycline **B.** Primaquine
C. Chloroquine **D.** Quinine *(UP 1993)*

Quinine sulphate is the drug of choice in cerebral malaria and it should be given in the dose of 10 mg/kg/8 hourly in slow IV infusion in 10% dextrose (dissolved in a concentration of 1 mg/ ml to be infused over 4 hours).

62. Nephrocalcinosis is *common* in:

A. Type I renal tubular acidosis **B.** Type II renal tubular acidosis
C. Type III renal tubular acidosis **D.** Type IV renal tubular acidosis *(UP 1993)*

63. *Hyperkalemia* is characteristic of which type of RTA:

A. Type I **B.** Type II
C. Type III **D.** Type IV *(JIPMER 2002)*

Differential Diagnosis of Renal Tubular Acidosis

Feature	Type 1	Type 2	Type 4
Renal calculus/ nephrocalcinosis	**Yes**	No	No
Fanconi's syndrome	No	**Yes**	No
Serum potassium	Low	Low	**High**

Mnemonic: Renal st**one** are seen in type **one**..

64. Pseudotumor cerebri is *not* caused by:

A. Hypervitaminosis A **B.** Oral contraceptives
C. Tetracycline **D.** Gentamicin *(UP 1993)*

65. ***Not* a feature of pseudotumor cerebri:**
A. Normal sized ventricles on CT scan
B. Increased protein content in CSF
C. Absence of localizing neurological deficit
D. Papilledema *(AI 1991, SGPGI 1996, UP 1996)*

Pseudotumor cerebri: As the name itself indicates this condition produces clinical features that mimics those of brain tumor. Increased intracranial pressure is caused by diffuse cerebral edema. Common causes of pseudotumor cerebri are as under:

- Amiodarone
- Glucocorticoids
- Mineralocorticoids
- Hypoparathyroidism
- Idiopathic
- **Hypervitaminosis A**
- **Oral contraceptives**
- **Tetracycline**
- Galactosemia
- Obese adolescent girl

It is more common when glucocorticoids are being tapered off or after have been discontinued. **Clinical features are as under:**

- Headache
- Papilledema
- Morning vomiting
- 6th nerve palsy

It is important to note that the **signs of focal neurological disease are absent** and diagnosis should be suspected in a child with raised intracranial pressure in whom neither a mass lesion nor enlargement of ventricular system is found. **Lateral ventricles may be reduced in size** because of compression by edematous brain. **CSF is normal**. CT or MRI scan are required to *rule out* a focal mass lesion. If neuroradiologic studies are normal, the subarachnoid pressure should be measured by lumbar puncture to confirm that it is elevated. If it is elevated the diagnosis of pseudotumor cerebri (**idiopathic or benign intracranial hypertension**) is made by exclusion. No treatment is required in mild cases. Repeated removal of CSF via lumber puncture helps patients with severe increase in intracranial pressure. Corticosteroids are very effective but relapse occurs when therapy is discontinued. Weight reduction is useful in obese children. Treatment with a carbonic anhydrase inhibitor such as acetazolamide (**Diamox**® 50 mg/kg/day; 8 hourly) lowers intracranial pressure by reducing the production of cerebrospinal fluid.

66. In syringomyelia the sensation that is lost is:
A. Touch **B.** Pain and temperature
C. Pressure **D.** Two-point discrimination

67. Painless burn of hand is seen in:
A. Systemic lupus erythematosus **B.** Cord compression
C. Thalamic syndrome **D.** Syringomyelia *(AI 1999)*

68. Dissociated sensory loss is seen with:
A. Tabes dorsalis **B.** Syringomyelia
C. Cauda equina syndrome **D.** Multiple sclerosis *(AIIMS May 2001)*

69. Dissociated anesthesia is seen in:
A. Fredrick's ataxia **B.** Tabes dorsalis
C. Syringomyelia **D.** Motor neuron disease *(UP 1993)*

70. Dissociated sensory loss and balaclava helmet sensory loss is seen in:
A. Syringomyelia **B.** Extradural spinal tumor
C. Intradural extramedullary tumors **D.** None of the above

In **syringomyelia** the sensory loss is classically of **dissociated type**. In this type of sensory loss there is preservation of sense of light tough and proprioception but **sensations of pain and heat are lost**. Symptoms usually develop in one of the upper limbs and consist of wasting of hand muscles, weakness and sensory loss. This often results in **painless burns caused by cigarettes or cooking**. The sensory loss does not follow the distribution of the branches of trigeminal nerve but involve more peripheral areas of face sparing nose and mouth (**balaclava helmet sensory loss**).

- BALACLAVA HELMET is a knitted covering for the head and neck, with an opening for the nose and eyes, worn for protection against wind and extreme cold.

71. Systemic lupus erythematosus is *not* caused by which of the following drug:
A. Methotrexate
B. Phenytoin
C. Isoniazid
D. Hydralazine (UP 1993)

Drug-induced Lupus Erythematosus

- Acebutolol
- Asparaginase
- Barbiturates
- Bleomycin
- Cephalosporins
- **Hydralazine**
- Iodides
- **Isoniazid**
- Methyldopa
- Phenolphthalein
- **Phenytoin**
- Procainamide
- Quinidine
- Sulfonamides
- Thiouracil

72. Subarachnoid space ends at:
A. S_4 **B.** S_2
C. L_2 **D.** L_1 (UP 1993)

The subarachnoid space surrounds the brain and spinal cord and ends at the level of lower border of **S_2 vertebra**.

73. In diabetes joint commonly involved is:
A. Foot
B. Hip
C. Knee
D. Shoulder (AIIMS 1994)

74. Charcot's joint in diabetes affects:
A. Tarsal
B. Hip
C. Knee
D. Shoulder (UP 1993)

Neuropathic joint or Charcot's joint occurs in < 1% cases of diabetes mellitus yet *diabetes mellitus is the most common cause of Charcot's joint*. Leprosy and tertiary syphilis are other common causes seen in underdeveloped countries. ***Most common* joints to be involved are mid tarsal joints followed by metatarsophalangeal and ankle joints.** After a provocative incident such as a fracture or a twisting injury the joint collapses rather *painlessly*. X-rays demonstrate marked and rapid destruction of the joint. These changes may be mistaken as septic arthritis but the simultaneous involvement of several small joints and a lack of systemic signs should point to a neuropathic disorder. Joint aspiration will exclude the infection in doubtful cases. A rocker bottom deformity due to collapse of mid foot is *diagnostic.*

75. *Not* seen in botulism:
A. Ptosis **B.** Diplopia
C. Diarrhea **D.** Vomiting (UP 1993, 1997)

76. *Not* a clinical feature of botulism:
A. Descending paralysis
B. Bulbar palsy
C. Diarrhea
D. Nausea and vomiting (AI 1992)

77. *Not* a clinical manifestation of botulism:
A. Diplopia **B.** Diarrhea
C. Urinary retention **D.** No fever (AIIMS 1997)

Botulism is caused by potent protein neurotoxins elaborated by *Clostridium botulinum*. It is a paralytic disease that begins with cranial nerve involvement and progresses caudally to involve the extremities. The incubation period is usually 18 to 36 hours. Symmetric *descending paralysis* is characteristic and may lead to respiratory failure and death. *Cranial nerve involvement* produces **diplopia**, dysarthria, and/or dysphagia. Weakness progresses, *often rapidly*, from the head to involve the neck, arms, thorax, and legs; the weakness is occasionally asymmetric. **Nausea**, **vomiting**, and abdominal pain may occur before or after the onset of **paralysis**. Dizziness, blurred vision, dry mouth, and sore throat are common. Patients are generally alert and oriented, but they may be drowsy, agitated, and anxious. **Typically, they have no fever**. **Ptosis** is common; the pupillary reflexes may be depressed and fixed or dilated pupils are noted in 50% of patients. The gag reflex may be suppressed, and deep tendon reflexes may be normal or decreased. Paralytic ileus, **severe constipation**, and **urinary retention are common**.

78. Southern blot method is for analysis of:
- **A.** Carbohydrates
- **B.** Proteins
- **C.** RNA
- **D.** DNA

(UP 1993)

79. RNA fragments are sequenced by:
- **A.** Southern blot
- **B.** Northern blot
- **C.** Eastern blot
- **D.** Western blot

(AI 1999)

• **Northern blot**	Technique for analyzing mRNA
• **Southern blot**	Technique used in molecular genetics to analyze a small portion of DNA
• **Western blot**	Technique for analyzing protein antigen

80. Pin point pupils, loss of consciousness and hyperpyrexia is seen in:
- **A.** Subarachnoid hemorrhage
- **B.** Pontine hemorrhage
- **C.** Cerebral infarction
- **D.** Thalamic syndrome

81. A patient comes with sudden onset of hyperventilation, sweating and pinpoint pupils. *Most likely* diagnosis is:
- **A.** Cerebellar hemorrhage
- **B.** Pontine hemorrhage
- **C.** Thalamic hemorrhage
- **D.** Subarachnoid hemorrhage

(UP 1993)

Differential Diagnosis of Confusion and Coma

• **Basal ganglia & thalamic hemorrhage**	Acute but not instantaneous onset, vomiting, headache, hemiplegia, and characteristic eye signs
• **Subarachnoid hemorrhage**	Instantaneous onset, severe headache, neck stiffness, vomiting, third or sixth nerve lesions, transient loss of consciousness, or sudden coma with vigorous extensor posturing
• **Pontine hemorrhage**	Sudden onset, **pin point pupils**, loss of reflex eye movements and corneal responses, ocular bobbing, posturing, **hyperventilation**, and **sweating**
• **Cerebellar hemorrhage**	Occipital headache, vomiting, gaze paresis, and inability to stand
• **Basilar artery thrombosis**	Neurologic prodrome or warning spells, diplopia, dysarthria, vomiting, eye movement and corneal response abnormalities, and asymmetric limb paresis

82. Important role of renin is in:
- **A.** Malignant hypertension
- **B.** Renovascular hypertension
- **C.** Essential hypertension
- **D.** Coronary heart disease

(UP 1993)

Hypertension caused by renal disease is the result of *either*
- A derangement in the renal handling of sodium and fluids leading to volume expansion *or*
- An alteration in renal secretion of vasoactive materials resulting in a systemic or local change in arteriolar tone.

The main divisions of renal hypertension are **renovascular hypertension**, including pre-eclampsia and eclampsia, and **renal parenchymal hypertension**. The cause of renal vascular hypertension is that *decreased* perfusion of renal tissue due to stenosis of a main or branch renal artery **activates the renin-angiotensin system**. Circulating angiotensin II increases arterial pressure by directly causing vasoconstriction, by stimulating aldosterone secretion with resulting sodium retention, and/or by stimulating the adrenergic nervous system. Practically only about 50% of patients with renovascular hypertension have an absolute elevation in renin activity in peripheral plasma.

83. Horner's syndrome manifests as:
A. Miosis and ptosis **B.** Mydriasis
C. Ptosis and sweating **D.** Sweating *(AIIMS May 2002)*

84. *Not* a characteristic feature of Horner's syndrome:
A. Partial ptosis of the eyelid **B.** Anhydrosis
C. Exophthalmos **D.** Miosis *(UP 1993)*

Horner's syndrome (oculosympathetic paresis) is characterized by contraction of the pupil (**miosis**), partial ptosis of the eyelid, **en**ophthalmos, and sometimes **anhydrosis** over one side of the face. The syndrome is caused by paralysis of the *cervical sympathetic nerve trunk*.

- Ciliospinal reflex is the dilation of the pupil following stimulation of the skin of the neck by pinching or scratching.

85. *False* regarding hemolytic anemia is:
A. Hemosiderinuria **B.** Increased haptoglobin
C. Raised unconjugated bilirubin **D.** Raised LDH *(AI 1992, UP 1993)*

86. *Not* a clinical feature of hemolytic anemia:
A. Reticulocytosis **B.** Raised level of haptoglobin
C. Hemosiderinuria **D.** Unconjugated hyperbilirubinemia *(UP 1997)*

87. *False* regarding hemolytic anemia is:
A. Hemoglobinuria **B.** Hemosiderinuria
C. Raised unconjugated bilirubin **D.** Increased haptoglobin *(AIIMS 1991)*

88. *Not* seen in hemolytic anemia:
A. Increased haptoglobin **B.** Spherocytosis
C. Reticulocytosis **D.** Hemosiderinuria *(AI 1991)*

Haptoglobin is an α globulin which is present in high concentration (~1.0 g/L) in the plasma. It binds specifically and tightly to the protein (globin) in hemoglobin and the hemoglobin-haptoglobin complex is cleared within minutes by the mononuclear phagocyte system. Thus **patients with significant hemolysis, either intravascular or extravascular, have low or absent levels of serum haptoglobin.** Laboratory evaluation of hemolysis can be done as under:

Test	Extravascular	Intravascular
Routine blood film	Polychromatophilia	Polychromatophilia
Reticulocyte count	Raised	Raised
Bone marrow examination	Erythroid hyperplasia	Erythroid hyperplasia
Plasma bilirubin	Raised unconjugated	Raised unconjugated
Plasma haptoglobin	Low, absent	Absent
Plasma hemoglobin	Normal or raised	High
Lactate dehydrogenase	Raised (variable)	High (variable)
Urine bilirubin	0	0
Urine hemosiderin	0	+
Urine hemoglobin	0	+ in severe cases

89. Painless effusion in joints of congenital syphilis is known as:
- **A.** Synovitis
- **B.** Clutton's joint
- **C.** Charcot's joint
- **D.** Barton's joint

(UP 1994)

Clutton's joint is a late manifestation of **congenital syphilis** that *typically* develops between the ages of 8 and 15 years. It is caused by chronic **painless** synovitis with **effusions** of large joints, particularly the knees and elbows.

90. Beriberi disease is due to deficiency of:
- **A.** Vitamin C
- **B.** Vitamin B
- **C.** Vitamin A
- **D.** Vitamin D

(UP 1994)

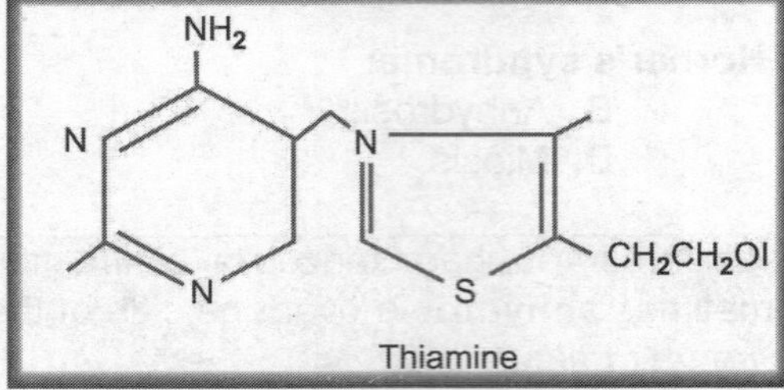

Thiamine

The two major manifestations of thiamine (**vitamin B_1**) deficiency involve the cardiovascular (**wet beriberi**) and nervous systems (**dry beriberi** and the Wernicke-Korsakoff syndrome).

91. Palmar erythema is seen in:
- **A.** Respiratory failure
- **B.** ARF
- **C.** CHF
- **D.** Hepatic failure

(UP 1994)

Signs and Symptoms of Hepatocellular Failure

- Ascites
- Jaundice
- Spider nevi
- Gynecomastia
- Testicular atrophy
- Sensitivity to drugs (morphine, barbiturates)
- Flapping tremors
- Generalized edema
- Bleeding tendency
- **Palmar erythema**
- Loss of body hair
- Encephalopathy

92. The *treatment of choice* for chronic partial and tonic clonic seizures is:
- **A.** Trimethadione
- **B.** Phenytoin
- **C.** Diazepam
- **D.** Ethosuximide

(SGPGI 2002)

93. Drug *not* used in *maintenance* therapy of epilepsy is:
- **A.** Carbamazepine
- **B.** Phenytoin
- **C.** Phenobarbitone
- **D.** Diazepam

(UP 1994)

Antiepileptic Drugs Used in Maintenance Therapy

Focal-Onset Seizures	Generalized Tonic-Clonic	Absence	Myoclonic	Atonic
FIRST-LINE				
Carbamazepine Phenytoin Valproic acid	Valproic acid Carbamazepine Phenytoin	Ethosuximide Valproic acid	Valproic acid	Valproic acid
ALTERNATIVES				
Lamotrigine Gabapentin Phenobarbital Primidone	Phenobarbital Primidone	Acetazolamide Clonazepam Phenobarbital	Clonazepam Acetazolamide	Clonazepam

94. Drug useful in both absence seizures (Petit Mal) and generalized, tonic-clonic seizures (Grand Mal) is:

A. Carbamazepine
B. Phenytoin
C. Sodium valproate
D. All of the above

(KERALA 1999)

95. Which antiepileptic drug acts by potentiating the action of GABA:

A. Phenobarbitone
B. Phenytoin
C. Valproic acid
D. Carbamazepine

Valproic acid or **sodium valproate** is a **broad spectrum anticonvulsant** which **acts by potentiating the inhibitory neurotransmitter GABA**. It should be started in the dose of 15 mg/kg/day and may be increased in steps of 5 mg/kg/day until a clinical effect is seen or a maximum dose of 30 mg/kg/day has been achieved.

96. Meningitis is caused by:

A. *Neisseria meningitidis*
B. *Haemophilus influenzae*
C. *Streptococcus pneumoniae*
D. All of the above

(UP 1994)

Organism causing meningitis	Incidence in adults
Streptococcus pneumoniae	30-50%
Neisseria meningitidis	10-35%
Staphylococcus aureus	5-15%
Gram-negative bacilli	1-10%
Streptococci	5%
Listeria monocytogenes	5%
Haemophilus influenzae	1-3%

97. Secondary hyperparathyroidism is caused by:

A. Solitary adenoma
B. Wermer's syndrome
C. Cardiac failure
D. CRF

(UP 1994)

Secondary hyperparathyroidism occurs when partial resistance to the *metabolic actions* of the hormone leads to excessive PTH production. *Secondary* hyperparathyroidism occurs in patients with **renal failure**, **osteomalacia** (vitamin D deficiency), and **pseudohypoparathyroidism** (deficient response to PTH at the level of the receptor). The clinical manifestations of secondary hyperparathyroidism vary in these states but *hypocalcemia* seems to be the *common denominator* in secondary hyperparathyroidism.

98. Basal ganglion tremors are:

A. Flapping tremor
B. Resting tremor
C. Intension tremor
D. Action tremor

(UP 1994)

Resting tremor with stooped posture, bradykinesia, and mask facies suggests Parkinson's disease. Parkinsonism is an example of a degenerative process affecting the **basal ganglia** (corpus striatum).

99. Cannon waves are seen in:

A. AF
B. Pulmonary stenosis
C. Complete heart block
D. Sinus bradycardia

(KARNATAKA 1994)

100. Cannon 'a' waves are seen in:

A. Atrial flutter
B. Atrial fibrillation
C. Complete heart block
D. Cardiac tamponade

(UP 1994)

- The normal jugular venous pulse (JVP) reflects phasic pressure changes in the right atrium and consists of 2 or sometimes 3 positive waves and 2 negative troughs.

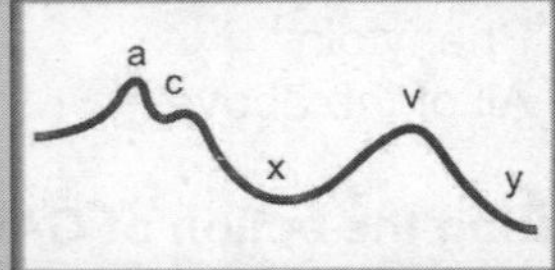

Positive presystolic *a* wave is produced by venous distention due to right atrial contraction and is the dominant wave in the JVP. **Large *a* waves indicate that the right atrium is contracting against an increased resistance**, such as occurs with *tricuspid stenosis* or with increased resistance to right ventricular filling (*pulmonary hypertension* or *pulmonic stenosis*). Large '*a*' waves also occur during arrhythmias whenever the right atrium contracts when the tricuspid valve is closed by right ventricular systole. Such "**cannon**" *a* waves may occur regularly (*junctional rhythm*) or irregularly (*atrioventricular dissociation with ventricular tachycardia* or *complete heart block*).
- **Severe tricuspid stenosis** is associated with marked hepatic congestion, often resulting in cirrhosis, jaundice, serious malnutrition, anasarca, and ascites. Congestive hepatomegaly and, in cases of severe tricuspid valve disease, splenomegaly are present. The jugular veins are distended, and in patients with sinus rhythm there may be **"giant" *a* waves**.

101. All are seen with hyperkalemia *except*:

A. High T wave
B. Prolonged PR interval
C. Depressed ST segment
D. Prolonged QT interval

The *most important* changes seen in hyperkalemia are cardiac arrhythmias with high-peaked T waves (**'tented' T waves**). The QT interval in the ECG is *not* prolonged. Treatment should be started and depends on serum potassium level.

• Serum potassium level < 6.5 mEq/L or mild ECG changes such as tall T wave.	7.5% $NaHCO_3$ 2 ml/kg slow diluted IV.
• Serum potassium level > 6.5 mEq/L or ominous ECG changes such as wide QRS complex	10% calcium gluconate 0.5 ml/kg over 10 minutes slow diluted IV under cardiac monitoring followed by 1 gm/kg of 50% glucose and 0.1 unit/kg of insulin.

Note: Inhaled salbutamol also lowers serum potassium levels.

102. *First* change in ECG seen in hyperkalemia is:

A. Absent P waves
B. Increased QRS interval
C. Tall tented T wave
D. Increased PQ interval

(UP 1994, KERALA 1994)

103. 'Sinewave' pattern in ECG is seen in:

A. Hypokalemia
B. Hyperkalemia
C. Hyponatremia
D. Hypernatremia

104. In hyperkalemia, ECG change shows:
- **A.** U wave
- **B.** Tall T wave
- **C.** Decreased PR interval
- **D.** Short ST segment

(AIIMS 1992, MP 2001)

- **Hyperkalemia** is defined as a plasma K^+ concentration > 5.0 mmol/L and it occurs as a result of either K^+ release from cells or decreased renal loss. Most serious effect of hyperkalemia is cardiac toxicity, which *does not* correlate well with the plasma K^+ concentration. The **earliest ECG changes include increased T wave amplitude, or peaked T waves**. More severe degrees of hyperkalemia result in a **prolonged PR interval and QRS duration**, atrioventricular conduction delay, and loss of P waves. Progressive widening of the QRS complex and merging with the T wave produces a **'sinewave pattern'**. The terminal event is ventricular fibrillation or asystole.
- *Pseudohyperkalemia* is *artificially* elevated plasma K^+ concentration due to K^+ movement out of cells immediately prior to or following venipuncture. Contributing factors of pseudohyperkalemia are prolonged use of a tourniquet with or without repeated fist clenching, hemolysis, and marked leukocytosis or thrombocytosis. Metabolic acidosis can be associated with mild hyperkalemia resulting from intracellular buffering of H^+.

105. Following are causes of pseudohyperkalemia *except*:
- **A.** Thrombocytosis
- **B.** Hemolysis
- **C.** Leukocytosis
- **D.** Eosinophilia

(UP 1997)

Pseudohyperkalemia represents a *falsely* raised plasma K^+ concentration due to K^+ movement out of cells immediately prior to venipuncture. Contributing factors are:
- Prolonged use of a tourniquet
- Repeated fist clenching
- Hemolysis
- Leukocytosis
- Thrombocytosis.

106. *Not* a treatment of hyperkalemia:
- **A.** Sodium bicarbonate
- **B.** Calcium gluconate
- **C.** Insulin
- **D.** Steroid

(AI 1995)

Serum potassium level	Management plan
• **If the serum K^+ level is less than 6.5 mEq/L**	1-2 ml/kg of 7.5% $NaHCO_3$ over 15 minutes
• **If the serum K^+ level is more than 6.5 mEq/L**	0.5 ml/kg of 10% calcium gluconate over 10 minutes under cardiac monitoring followed by 0.5-1 gm/kg of 50% dextrose + 0.1-0.2 units/kg of insulin. Inhaled β_2 agonists (salbutamol) also reduce serum K^+ level.

107. Risus sardonicus is seen in:
- **A.** Leprosy
- **B.** Tetanus
- **C.** Strychnine poisoning
- **D.** TMJ ankylosis

(UP 1994)

In **tetanus**, *typically*, the patient **1st notices** increased tone in the masseter muscles (trismus, or **lockjaw**). Sustained contraction of the facial muscles results in a grimace or sneer (**risus sardonicus**), and contraction of the back muscles produces an arched back (opisthotonos).

108. An intelligent dwarf child with square fingers and palms and backache has:
- **A.** Nutritional dwarfism
- **B.** Hypothyroidism
- **C.** Marion dwarf
- **D.** Achondroplasia

(UP 1994)

109. Achondroplasia is inherited as:
- **A.** Autosomal dominant
- **B.** Autosomal recessive
- **C.** X-linked dominant
- **D.** X-linked recessive

Achondroplasia is the *most common* genetic skeletal dysplasia. It is an *autosomal dominant* disorder in which there is marked shortening of the limbs. It may also arise from a fresh gene mutation (80%). There is failure of normal ossification in long bone which may be only 50% of their normal length. Growth of the trunk is only slightly impaired therefore the dwarfism is *disproportionate* and the shortening is specially marked in the proximal segments in the limbs (*rhizomelic limb shortening*). Achondroplasia is usually apparent at birth as the newborn is strikingly dwarfed with very short limbs that are out of proportion to the trunk. Adult patients are seldom more than 4 feet 3 inches (130 cm) in height. The **hands are short and broad** and the **central three digits are almost equal in length and divergent** (**trident hand**). Head is larger than normal with depressed nasal bridge and bulging forehead. There is marked lumbar lordosis and thoracic kyphosis. The life expectancy is usually normal and there is **no mental retardation**. Achondroplasia may be complicated by hydrocephalus due to obstruction at foramen magnum and by lumber cord and nerve root compression syndromes, hearing impairment due to repeated otitis media, strabismus and dental malocclusion.

110. A 6 months old infant has multiple fractures with trivial trauma. The diagnosis is:

A. Rickets
B. Osteogenesis imperfecta
C. Achondroplasia
D. Battered baby syndrome *(UP 1994)*

111. Multiple fractures in children with joint laxity and deafness are seen in:

A. Osteomalacia
B. Osteochondromatosis
C. Osteogenesis imperfecta
D. Ehlers-Danlos syndrome *(UP 1998)*

112. *Not* a feature of osteogenesis imperfecta:

A. Blue sclera
B. Cataract
C. Multiple fractures
D. Hearing loss *(AIIMS 1997)*

Osteogenesis imperfecta is a hereditary disorder that causes a generalized decrease in bone mass (*osteopenia*) and makes the bones brittle. The disorder is often associated with **blue sclerae**, dental abnormalities (dentinogenesis imperfecta), **hearing loss**, and a positive family history. There is excessive **hyperlaxity of ligaments** mainly at the small joints of hand, feet, and knee. Some have **multiple fractures in infancy and childhood**, improve after puberty, and fracture more frequently later in life.

113. Oculocutaneous albinism is:

A. X-linked recessive
B. X-linked dominant
C. Autosomal recessive
D. Autosomal dominant *(UP 1994)*

Albinism is a group of genetically inherited conditions caused by defective melanin production. The biosynthesis of melanin by melanocytes requires the *oxidative enzyme* **tyrosinase**. In albinism the tyrosinase system is *supposed* to be defective. The disorder may be generalized effecting the skin, eyes and hair (oculocutaneous albinism) or localized affecting *primarily* the eyes (ocular albinism). The oculocutaneous albinism may be further subclassified as *tyrosinase negative* or *tyrosinase positive* depending on the ability of a hair bulb plucked from the patient and incubated in tyrosine solution to synthesize melanin. This test is not accurate until a child is 3-5 years old. There are 10 different types of oculocutaneous albinism (OCA) and 4 types of ocular albinism (OA). **Tyrosinase positive OCA is the most common form of albinism having normal tyrosinase activity.** Worldwide prevalence of albinism (all types) is 1 in 20,000. **OCA is inherited as an autosomal recessive trait** *except* for a *rare* type that is dominantly inherited. **OA is inherited as an X-linked or autosomal recessive trait.** Partial albinism (piabaldism) is inherited as an autosomal dominant trait. Clinical manifestations common in all forms are depigmentation of skin, iris and retina. Nystagmus, strabismus, photophobia, decreased visual acuity and presence of red reflex are common ocular findings. Blindness and skin cancer are the 2 major sequelae of albinism.

114. Mediastinal shift occurs in:

A. Pneumothorax
B. Cryptogenic fibrosing alveolitis
C. Bronchitis emphysema
D. Lobar pneumonia *(UP 1994)*

Classic radiographic findings of **tension pneumothorax**, such as inversion of the diaphragm and **contralateral shift of the mediastinum**, are present when large volumes of air accumulate in the pleural space.

115. Streptokinase therapy in myocardial infarction is *most effective* when given within:

A. < 2 hours **B.** > 24 hours
C. 4-6 hours **D.** 2-4 hours *(UP 1994)*

The thrombolytic agents' tissue plasminogen activator, **streptokinase**, and anisoylated plasminogen streptokinase activator complex (APSAC) have been approved by the FDA for IV use in acute myocardial infarction. All these drugs act by promoting the conversion of plasminogen to plasmin, which subsequently lyses fibrin thrombi. The principal goal of thrombolysis is prompt restoration of coronary arterial patency. Thrombolytic therapy can reduce the relative risk of in-hospital death by up to 50% when administered within the 1st hour of the onset of symptoms of myocardial infarction. Since myocardium can be rescued *only* before it has been irreversibly injured, the timing of thrombolytic therapy is of extreme importance in achieving maximum benefit. It is clear that "**every minute counts**" and that **patients treated within 1 to 3 hours of the onset of symptoms generally benefit most.** Streptokinase is administered as 1.5 million units IV over 1 hour. ***Clear* contraindications** to the use of thrombolytic agents include a history of cerebrovascular bleed at any time, a non-hemorrhagic stroke or other cerebrovascular event within the past year, marked hypertension at any time during the acute presentation, suspicion of aortic dissection, and active internal bleeding (excluding menses). ***Relative* contraindications** to thrombolytic therapy, which require careful assessment of the risk & benefit ratio, include *current use of anticoagulants*, a *recent* (within 2 weeks) *invasive or surgical procedure* or *prolonged (>10 min) cardiopulmonary resuscitation*, known *bleeding diasthesis, pregnancy*, a hemorrhagic ophthalmic condition (*hemorrhagic diabetic retinopathy*), *active peptic ulcer disease*, and a *history of severe hypertension* that is currently adequately controlled. Because of the risk of an allergic reaction, patients should not receive streptokinase if that agent had been received within the *preceding* 5 days to 2 years. *Hemorrhage is the most frequent and potentially the most serious complication.*

116. *Drug of choice* for pain in myocardial infarction is:

A. Morphine **B.** Diazepam
C. Fortwin **D.** NSAID

117. *Not* used in treatment of MI:

A. Pentazocine **B.** Vasodilators
C. Platelet function inhibitors **D.** Fibrinolytic agent *(PGI 1997)*

Morphine is an extremely effective analgesic for the pain associated with myocardial infarction. **Pentazocine is less desirable than morphine** or other opioid agonist analgesics for relief of pain due to acute myocardial infarction because of CVS effects that tend to **increase cardiac work.**

118. Duchenne pseudomuscular dystrophy is inherited as:

A. Autosomal recessive **B.** X-linked dominant
C. X-linked recessive **D.** Autosomal dominant

119. *False* regarding Duchenne muscular dystrophy:

A. *Congenital* hypotonia **B.** Respiratory failure in 2nd decade of life
C. Cardiomyopathy **D.** X-linked recessive *(AI 1996)*

120. Most *characteristic* feature of Duchenne muscular dystrophy is:

A. Early involvement of respiratory muscle
B. Wasting of distal muscle
C. Association with sensory deficit
D. Pseudohypertrophy of muscle *(UP 1996)*

121. Creatine phosphokinase (CPK) is increased in:

A. Hepatocellular carcinoma
B. Renal cell carcinoma
C. Cirrhosis
D. Pseudohypertrophic muscular dystrophy *(UP 1994)*

Duchenne muscular dystrophy (DMD) or **pseudohypertrophic muscular dystrophy** is an **X-linked recessive** disorder and it occurs with an incidence of about 30 per 100,000 live-born males. **Disorder becomes apparent between ages 3 and 5 years.** The boys fall frequently and have difficulty in keeping up with their friends when playing. Running, jumping, and hopping are abnormal. By the age of 5 years muscle weakness is obvious on muscle testing. On getting up from the floor, the boy uses his hands to climb upon himself (**Gowers' maneuver**). In younger children, the calf muscles are usually enlarged from true muscle hypertrophy but later calf enlargement is *appropriately* called **pseudohypertrophy** since muscle is replaced by fat and connective tissue. A cardiac cause of death is *un*common despite the presence of a **cardiomyopathy** in *almost all* patients. Intellectual impairment is common; the average IQ is approximately 1 SD below the mean. **Serum creatine phosphokinase (CK) levels are invariably elevated up to 20 and 100 times normal.** The muscle biopsy demonstrates **muscle fibers of "varying" size** as well as small groups of necrotic and regenerating fibers; connective tissue and fat replace lost muscle fibers. A *definitive diagnosis* of DMD can be made on the basis of **dystrophin deficiency** in biopsied muscle tissue or mutation analysis on peripheral blood leukocytes. *Prednisone* in a dose of 0.75 mg/kg per day has been shown to significantly alter the progression of DMD for up to 3 years. By age 16 to 18, patients are predisposed to serious, sometimes **fatal pulmonary infections.**

122. Muscle *not* involved in Duchenne muscular dystrophy:
- **A.** Infraspinatus
- **B.** Brachioradialis
- **C.** Gastrocnemius
- **D.** Vastus medialis

(AIIMS 1997)

In DMD loss of muscle strength is progressive, with predilection for **proximal limb muscles** and the neck flexors; leg involvement is more severe than arm involvement.

123. Hypercalcemia is *not* seen in:
- **A.** Sarcoidosis
- **B.** Milk alkali syndrome
- **C.** Squamous cell carcinoma of lung
- **D.** Pseudohypoparathyroidism

(UP 1994)

Classification of Causes of Hypercalcemia

Parathyroid-related	**Malignancy**	**Vitamin D-related**	**High bone turnover**	**Renal failure**
Primary hyperparathyroidism	Breast	Vitamin D intoxication	Hyperthyroidism	Severe secondary hyperparathyroidism
Solitary adenomas	**Lung**	Sarcoidosis	Immobilization	Aluminum intoxication
Multiple endocrine neoplasia	Kidney	Idiopathic hypercalcemia of infancy	Thiazides	Milk-alkali syndrome
Lithium	Multiple myeloma		Vitamin A intoxication	
Familial hypocalciuric hypercalcemia	Leukemia			
	Lymphoma			

124. *Not* a feature of primary hyperaldosteronism:
- **A.** Increase in Na^+ retention
- **B.** Increase intravascular volume
- **C.** Edema
- **D.** Hypertension

(UP 1994)

125. In Conn's syndrome, all the following are seen *except*:
- **A.** Hypokalemia
- **B.** Hypernatremia
- **C.** Hypertension
- **D.** Edema

(AI 2002)

126. *False* regarding Conn's syndrome:
- **A.** Generalized edema
- **B.** Raised blood pressure
- **C.** Low renin levels
- **D.** Hypokalemia

(AIIMS 1992)

127. Excess aldosterone is *not* associated with:

A. Hypertension
B. Water retention
C. Hyperkalemia
D. Hypokalemia
(AI 1993)

128. A 25 years old man presents with hypertension. His serum sodium is 145 mEq/L, potassium is 1.3 mEq/L and serum creatinine is 1.2 mg. *Most likely* diagnosis is:

A. Renal parenchymal disease
B. Cushing syndrome
C. Conn's syndrome
D. Pheochromocytoma
(PGI 1996)

In primary hyperaldosteronism, or **Conn's syndrome**, neuromuscular complications are due to K^+ depletion. Primary aldosteronism is also termed pseudoprimary aldosteronism, **idiopathic hyperaldosteronism**, and nodular hyperplasia. Hypersecretion of aldosterone increases the renal distal tubular exchange of intratubular Na^+ for secreted K^+ and H^+, with progressive depletion of body potassium and development of hypokalemia. Most patients have diastolic **hypertension**, and headaches. The hypertension is due to the *increased Na^+ reabsorption* and **extracellular volume expansion**. **K^+ depletion** is responsible for the muscle weakness and fatigue and is due to the effect of K^+ depletion on the muscle cell membrane. The *polyuria* results from impairment of urinary concentrating ability and is often associated with *polydipsia*. In the absence of associated CHF, renal disease, or preexisting abnormalities (*thrombophlebitis*), **edema is characteristically absent.** Patients with primary aldosteronism characteristically *do not have edema*, since they exhibit an "**escape**" phenomenon from the sodium-retaining aspects of mineralocorticoids. In cases of long duration, nephropathy with azotemia may be associated with CHF and edema. The diagnosis is suggested by persistent *hypo*kalemia in a *non*edematous patient with a normal Na^+ intake who is *not* receiving potassium-*wasting* diuretics such as furosemide, ethacrynic acid and thiazides.

The criteria for the diagnosis of primary aldosteronism are as under:

(1) Diastolic hypertension without edema;

(2) Hyposecretion of renin (as judged by **low plasma renin activity levels**) that fails to increase appropriately during volume depletion (upright posture, sodium depletion);

(3) Hypersecretion of aldosterone that does not suppress appropriately in response to volume expansion (salt loading).

129. Cushing's syndrome is commonly caused by:

A. Adrenal carcinoma
B. Ectopic adrenal tissue
C. Adrenal hyperplasia
D. Adrenal adenoma
(UP 1994)

Cushing's syndrome or post pubertal or adult hypercorticism is due to excessive endogenous production of glucocorticoids mainly hydrocortisone. **In most cases the cause is *bilateral adrenal hyperplasia* due to hypersecretion of pituitary ACTH or production of ACTH by a nonendocrine tumor.** Pituitary dependent Cushing's syndrome is the *most common* cause and accounts for 66% of all cases, while adrenal adenoma accounts for 20% and carcinoma—which may be bilateral-account for 5% of cases. Remaining cases are due to ectopic production of ACTH like *substances* from benign tumors such as bronchial carcinoids or malignant tumors of pancreas, mediastinum or bronchus. A lemon on match stick appearance is characteristic of this disease.

130. Pernicious anemia is due to deficiency of:

A. Pyridoxine
B. Folic acid
C. Vitamin B_{12}
D. Vitamin D
(UP 1994)

131. *False* regarding pernicious anemia:

A. Parenteral vitamin B_{12} is therapeutic
B. Premature graying of hair
C. Hyperchlorhydria
D. Autoimmune disease
(AI 1992)

132. In which of the following condition increased gastrin levels with decreased HCl level is seen:

A. Stomach carcinoma
B. Atrophic gastritis
C. Pernicious anemia
D. Zollinger-Ellison syndrome
(AIIMS 1994)

Pernicious anemia is a chronic disorder of middle and old age and the *basic pathological lesion* is gastric atrophy resulting in **vitamin B_{12} deficiency**. The clinical features are those of the vitamin B_{12} deficiency viz. macrocytic anemia, glossitis and CNS involvement. There is considerable evidence for **immunologic abnormalities** in pernicious anemia. Laboratory examination will reveal **hypergastrinemia** and pentagastrin-fast **achlorhydria** as well as the hematologic and other laboratory abnormalities. With *adequate* treatment the prognosis is excellent. The mainstay of treatment for **cobalamin** deficiency is **replacement** therapy. As the defect often is one of absorption, replacement should be administered parenterally, specifically in the form of intramuscular cyanocobalamin (vitamin B_{12}).

- *Pernicious* means causing great injury, destruction, or ruin; fatal; deadly.

133. *Decreased* protein content in pleural effusion is seen in:

A. Bacterial pneumonia | **B.** Malignancy
C. Tuberculosis | **D.** Cirrhosis *(UP 1994)*

When a patient is diagnosed to have a **pleural effusion**, every effort should be made to determine the cause. The 1st step is to determine whether the effusion is a **transudate** or an **exudate**. A **transudative pleural effusion** occurs when **systemic factors** that influence the formation and absorption of pleural fluid are changed and the leading causes are left ventricular failure, pulmonary embolism, and *cirrhosis*. An **exudative pleural effusion** occurs when **local factors** that influence the formation and absorption of pleural fluid are changed and the leading causes are bacterial pneumonia, malignancy, viral infection, and pulmonary embolism. **Exudative pleural effusions** meet at least 1 of the following criteria, whereas transudative pleural effusions meet *none*.

- Pleural fluid protein/serum protein >0.5
- Pleural fluid LDH/serum LDH >0.6
- Pleural fluid LDH more than two-thirds normal upper limit for serum

134. In which of the following conditions does hyperglycemia occur:

A. Addison's disease | **B.** Uremia
C. Acromegaly | **D.** Starvation *(AI 2002)*

Growth hormone excess results in **acromegaly**, an insidious, chronic, debilitating disease associated with bony and soft tissue overgrowth. Insulin resistance is found in 80% of patients, although **abnormal glucose tolerance** (20 to 40%) and clinical diabetes mellitus (13 to 20%) are *less* common.

135. In antiphospholipid antibody syndrome all the following are seen *except*:

A. Recurrent fetal loss | **B.** Neurological symptoms
C. Thrombocytosis | **D.** Prolonged aPTT *(AI 2002)*

136. A young lady with spontaneous abortions has a history of joint pains and fever. She currently presents with thrombosis of her leg vein. Her aPTT is prolonged. The diagnosis is *most likely* to be:

A. Inherited protein C and S deficit | **B.** Factor XII deficiency
C. Antiphospholipid antibody syndrome | **D.** Increased antithrombin III levels *(AI 2002)*

Antiphospholipid antibodies (APLA) are antibodies directed against *certain* phospholipids. There are found in variety of clinical situations. APLA are important to detect because in certain patients they are associated with a syndrome that includes a **hypercoagulable state**, **thrombocytopenia**, **fetal loss**, dementia, **strokes**, optic changes, Addison's disease, and skin rashes. APLA react with phospholipid. Phospholipids are used in coagulation tests to provide a surface for the coagulation reaction to occur. The basis for all these tests is that if there are antibodies binding to the phospholipid, it will interfere with the coagulation reaction and prolong the clotting time. Once **an elevated aPTT** is found one *must* verify it is due to an inhibitor by demonstrating it does not correct with a 50:50 mix. This is done by making a mixture of the patient's and normal pool plasma and performing an aPTT on it. Then the mixture is incubated for 30, 60 and 120 minutes and aPTT's are performed at various times.

137. Medullary cystic disease of the kidney is *best* diagnosed by:

A. Ultrasound | **B.** Nuclear scan
C. Urography | **D.** Biopsy *(AI 2002)*

Medullary cystic disease (MCD) appears to be an autosomal dominant disease. The kidneys tend to be small, with cysts throughout the medulla; the cortex and papilla rarely have cysts. MCD presents in the 3rd or 4th decade, though some cases may be diagnosed in the elderly population. CT scan is more sensitive than ultrasound in making the diagnosis. **Open renal biopsy**, including medullary tissue, **may be required for diagnosis** in some cases.

138. A patient presents with hypertension and dizziness. The X-ray shows anterior "rib notching". The diagnosis is most likely to be:

A. Pheochromocytoma
B. Coarctation of the aorta
C. Neurofibromatosis
D. Marfan syndrome

(AI 2002)

Narrowing or constriction of the lumen of the aorta may occur anywhere along its length but is **most common distal to the origin of the left subclavian artery** near the insertion of the ligamentum arteriosum. **Coarctation of the aorta** is a congenital malformation in which a segment of the aorta is constricted, narrowed, or obliterated. In the majority of cases, an abrupt, short, segmental membranous stenosis, formed by media, intima, and fibromuscular tissue, is present in the region of the aortic isthmus and ductus arteriosus. Headache, epistaxis, cold extremities, and claudication with exercise may occur, and attention is usually directed to the CVS when a heart murmur or **hypertension** in the upper extremities and absence, marked diminution, or delayed pulsations in the femoral arteries are detected on physical examination. On plain X-rays, obscuration of the superior margin of the aortic arch together with widening of the left side of the mediastinum may suggest a *superior mediastinal mass*. Additional radiographic findings include left ventricular hypertrophy and/or dilatation; prominence of the ascending aorta; other abnormalities of the aortic arch such as the **classic "3" sign**; prominence of the left subclavian artery; enlargement of the internal mammary arteries; **rib notching**; notching of the lateral scapular margin, and the *reverse* "3" sign on barium esophagram. Contrast-enhanced CT may identify the aortic narrowing and deformity and the poststenotic dilatation associated with coarctation, but **definitive assessment require aortograpy** for pressure measurements and complete delineation of collateral pathways.

139. Renal vein thrombosis is *most likely* in which of the following conditions:

A. Membranous glomerulonephritis
B. Membranoproliferative glomerulonephritis
C. Rapidly progressive glomerulonephritis
D. Minimal change disease

(AI 2002)

Renal vein thrombosis is particularly common (40%) in patients with nephrotic syndrome due to **membranous glomerulopathy**, membranoproliferative glomerulonephritis, and amyloidosis.

140. Renal osteodystrophy differs from nutritional and metabolic rickets due to the presence of:

A. Hyperphosphatemia
B. Hypercalcemia
C. Hypophosphatemia
D. Hypocalcemia

(AI 2002)

The bone disease in patients with secondary hyperparathyroidism and renal failure is usually termed **renal osteodystrophy**. In addition to hypercalcemia and ***hyperphosphatemia***, patients with secondary hyperparathyroidism may develop bone pain, ectopic calcification, and pruritus. In vitamin D deficiency (**rickets**), whether due to dietary lack, inadequate sunlight exposure, or intestinal malabsorption, serum calcium levels are normal or low, **whereas phosphorus and 25(OH)D levels are consistently low**, the latter usually < 8 ng/mL.

141. A 10 years old child presents with anemia and recurrent fractures. The X-ray shows diffuse *hyperdensity* of bone. The diagnosis is *most likely* to be:

A. Osteogenesis imperfecta
B. Osteopetrosis
C. Osteochondroma
D. Hyperparathyroidism

(AI 2002)

Osteopetrosis is also called **marble bone disease** and **Albers-Schönberg disease**; this is a rare idiopathic condition of bone. Infantile osteopetrosis is an autosomal recessive trait that is manifested in utero and progresses after birth with **anemia**, hepatosplenomegaly, hydrocephalus, cranial nerve involvement, and death, often due to infections. Roentgenograms reveal **uniformly dense**, sclerotic bone, often with no distinction between the cortical and cancellous regions. Fractures may occur with trivial trauma. Healing of such **fractures** is usually slow *but* satisfactory.

142. While inserting a central venous catheter, a patient develops respiratory distress. The *most likely* cause is:
- **A.** Hemothorax
- **B.** Pneumothorax
- **C.** Pleural effusion
- **D.** Hypovolemia

(AI 2002)

143. While undergoing central venous catheterization through internal jugular vein, the patient suddenly developed respiratory distress and hypoxemia. *Most likely* cause is:
- **A.** Septicemia
- **B.** Carotid artery injury
- **C.** Tamponade
- **D.** Pneumothorax

(AIIMS 2000)

The insertion of a **central venous catheter** should always be done *only* by trained personnel under aseptic techniques. **Major mechanical complications include pneumothorax**; hemothorax from laceration of the subclavian artery or vein; brachial plexus injury; and malpositioning of the catheter in a cerebral vein, the azygos vein, or the right ventricle. The correct catheter position *must* be confirmed by X-ray before hypertonic nutrient solution is infused.

144. The systeme international d'unites (SI) unit for blood pressure is:
- **A.** Torr
- **B.** mm Hg
- **C.** Pa
- **D.** cm H_2O

(AI 2002)

SI (Systeme International d'unites) derived units

Quantity	Name of unit	Symbol of unit
• **Area**	Square meter	M^2
• **Force**	Newton	N
• **Pressure**	Pascal	Pa
• **Work, energy**	Joule	J
• **Celsius temperature**	Degree Celsius	°C

145. Which of the following is *not* seen in atrial myxoma:
- **A.** Fever
- **B.** Increased ESR
- **C.** Hypertension
- **D.** Embolic phenomenon

(AI 2002)

146. Lentigines and blue nevus are associated with which of the following cardiac lesion:
- **A.** Cardiomyopathy
- **B.** Pericarditis
- **C.** Atrial myxoma
- **D.** Cardiac arrhythmia

(JIPMER 2002)

147. Prolonged fever is seen in:
- **A.** Liposarcoma
- **B.** Neurofibromatosis
- **C.** Exostosis
- **D.** Atrial myxoma

(AI 1992)

148. *False* regarding atrial myxoma is:
- **A.** No sex preference
- **B.** Stimulates mitral stenosis
- **C.** Occur at right atrium
- **D.** Most common benign tumor of heart

(AI 1995)

149. *True* regarding cardiac myxoma is:
- **A.** Common in females
- **B.** Distant metastasis is seen
- **C.** Rarely reoccurs after excision
- **D.** Most common site is left atrium

(AI 1999)

150. Which is *not* true of sporadic myxoma:
- **A.** Diagnosed by 2D echocardiography
- **B.** Female preponderance
- **C.** Occur at all ages
- **D.** Most common type of primary cardiac tumor

151. Left atrial myxoma is *best* diagnosed by:
- **A.** ECG
- **B.** Cardiac catheterization
- **C.** Echocardiogram
- **D.** Chest X-ray

152. The *most common* intracavitary benign cardiac tumor is:

A. Leiomyoma
B. Myxoma
C. Neuroma
D. Sarcoid

Myxomas are the *most common* primary cardiac tumor for all age groups, accounting for 50% of all cases at postmortem. They occur at all ages and **show no sex preference**. Although the large majority of myxomas are sporadic, some are familial with autosomal dominant transmission or are part of a syndrome. The large majority of sporadic myxomas are solitary and located in the atria, particularly the **left**, where they arise from the interatrial septum in the neighborhood of the fossa ovalis. The symptoms and signs of atrial myxomas are dependent on position. A characteristic low-pitched sound, termed a "*tumor plop*," is audible during early or middiastole and is due to the tumor abruptly *stopping* as it strikes the ventricular wall. They may also present with peripheral or **pulmonary emboli** or any of several *non-cardiac* signs and symptoms including **fever**, weight loss, cachexia, malaise, arthralgia, rash, clubbing, Raynaud's phenomenon, hypergammaglobulinemia, anemia, polycythemia, leukocytosis, **elevated ESR**, thrombocytopenia, or thrombocytosis. Left atrial myxoma may obstruct left atrial emptying, causing dyspnea, a diastolic murmur, and hemodynamic changes *resembling* those of **mitral stenosis**. Certain constellations of findings are known as the **NAME syndrome** (nevi, atrial myxoma, myxoid neurofibroma, and ephelides) or the **LAMB syndrome** (**lentigines**, atrial myxoma, and **blue nevi**). Myxomas are frequently misdiagnosed as endocarditis, collagen vascular disease, or non-cardiac tumor. **Two-dimensional echocardiography is the investigation of choice.** Surgical excision utilizing cardiopulmonary bypass is indicated and is generally curative.

153. A patient with nephrotic syndrome with *longstanding* corticosteroid therapy may develop all of the following *except*:

A. Hyperglycemia
B. Hypertrophy of muscle
C. Neuropsychiatric symptoms
D. Suppression of the pituitary adrenal axis *(AI 2002)*

Side Effects of Glucocorticoids

- Cushing's habitus
- Hyperglycemia
- Susceptibility to infection
- Peptic ulceration
- Posterior subcapsular cataract
- Growth retardation
- Suppression of hypothalamic pituitary adrenal axis
- Fragile skin, purple striae
- Muscular weakness
- Delayed wound healing
- Osteoporosis
- Glaucoma
- Psychiatric disturbances

154. Roth's spots are seen in the:

A. Pharynx
B. Heart
C. Fundus
D. Palms

155. Roth's spots are seen in:

A. Subacute bacteria endocarditis
B. Rheumatic fever
C. Thrombocytopenic purpura
D. Malaria

156. *Not* a clinical feature of SABE:

A. Osler's node
B. Janeway lesion
C. Erythema nodosum
D. Roth's spot *(UP 1995)*

157. Osler's nodes are seen in:

A. Finger or toe pads in infective endocarditis
B. DIP joints in rheumatoid arthritis
C. DIP joints in rheumatoid osteoarthritis
D. PIP joints in rheumatoid osteoarthritis *(AIIMS 1998)*

Splenomegaly and petechiae tend to occur in **infective endocarditis** of long duration. Splinter hemorrhages are subungual, linear, dark-red streaks that may appear in endocarditis but also commonly result from trauma. **Roth's spots** are oval, **retinal hemorrhages** with a clear, pale center; they may also occur in connective tissue disease and severe anemia. **Osler's nodes** (small, tender nodules, usually on the finger or toe pads, which persist for hours to days may also develop in other diseases. **Janeway lesions** are small hemorrhages with a slightly nodular character on the palms and soles and are most commonly seen in acute endocarditis.

158. Isolated hematuria is *not* seen in:

- **A.** Hereditary nephritis
- **B.** Thin basement membrane disease
- **C.** Lead nephropathy
- **D.** Burger's disease

(UP 1995)

159. In a patient with raised IgA levels, the *most common* finding is:

- **A.** Proteinuria
- **B.** GI bleed
- **C.** Hematuria
- **D.** Hypertension

(AIIMS May 2001)

Isolated hematuria without proteinuria, other cells, or casts is indicative of bleeding from the urinary tract. Hematuria is defined as 2 to 5 red blood cells per high-power field and can be detected by dipstick. Common causes of isolated hematuria include stones, neoplasms, tuberculosis, trauma, and prostatitis. *Isolated microscopic hematuria* can be a manifestation of glomerular diseases. **The most common etiologies of isolated glomerular hematuria are IgA nephropathy (Burger's disease)**, hereditary nephritis, and thin basement membrane disease. *Alport's syndrome is the most common form of hereditary nephritis which is usually transmitted as an X-linked dominant trait, and is associated with sensorineural deafness, ophthalmologic abnormalities, and progressive renal insufficiency*

160. *Not* commonly seen in hemochromatosis:

- **A.** Hypogonadism
- **B.** Neuropathy
- **C.** Cirrhosis
- **D.** Diabetes

(UP 1995)

161. A diabetic patient presents with arthritis, skin hyperpigmentation and hypogonadism. *Most probably* he has:

- **A.** Systemic lupus erythematosus
- **B.** Wilson's disease
- **C.** Hemochromatosis
- **D.** Rheumatoid arthritis

(AI 2001)

Hemochromatosis is a disorder of iron storage in which inappropriate increase in intestinal iron absorption causes deposition of excessive amounts of iron in parenchymal cells with eventual tissue damage and impaired function of organs, *especially* the liver, pancreas, heart, and pituitary. **Cirrhosis** of the liver, **diabetes mellitus**, **arthritis**, **cardiomyopathy**, and hypogonadotrophic **hypogonadism** are *common* manifestations. Initial symptoms include weakness, lassitude, weight loss, **change in skin color**, abdominal pain, loss of libido, and symptoms of diabetes mellitus. Hepatomegaly, pigmentation, spider angiomas, splenomegaly, arthropathy, ascites, cardiac arrhythmias, CHF, loss of body hair, testicular atrophy, and jaundice are prominent in advanced disease. *Liver* is the first organ to be affected and hepatocellular *carcinoma* develops in about 30% of patients with cirrhosis.

162. Macula ceruleae is seen in:

- **A.** *Phthirus pubis*
- **B.** *Pediculosis humanis corporis*
- **C.** *Pediculosis capitis*
- **D.** *Pediculosis canis*

(JIPMER 2000)

The 'cosmopolitan crab' or 'pubic louse' (*Phthirus pubis*) is transmitted by sexual contact but can infest eyelashes, axillary hair, and hair in other sites as well as pubic hair. Intensely 'pruritic' lesions and 2 to 3 mm blue macules (**maculae ceruleae**) develop at the site of bites. Blepharitis commonly accompanies infestations of the eyelashes.

163. Organ *least* involved in primary hemochromatosis is:

- **A.** Heart
- **B.** Testes
- **C.** Pancreas
- **D.** Pituitary

(AIIMS 1994)

Hemochromatosis is a common disorder of iron storage in which *inappropriate* increase in intestinal iron absorption leads to deposition of *excessive* amounts of iron in parenchymal cells with eventual tissue damage and impaired function of organs, mainly the **liver**, **pancreas**, heart, and **pituitary**. Iron is increased in amount in many organs, particularly in the liver, heart, and pancreas and to a lesser extent in the endocrine glands.

164. ***Most common*** **type of lung carcinoma is:**
- **A.** Anaplastic
- **B.** Small cell
- **C.** Adenocarcinoma
- **D.** Squamous cell

(UP 1995)

Type of lung cancer	Incidence (%)
• Adenocarcinoma (and all subtypes)	32
• Squamous cell (epidermoid) carcinoma	29
• Small cell carcinoma	18
• Large cell carcinoma	9
• Bronchioloalveolar carcinoma	3
• Carcinoid	1.0
• Mucoepidermoid carcinoma	0.1
• Sarcoma and other soft tissue tumors	0.1
• Adenoid cystic carcinoma	< 0.1
• All others and unspecified carcinomas	11.0

* As per Harrison's *Principles of Internal Medicine 14th edition.*

According to Bailey and Love's SHORT PRACTICE OF SURGERY; 23rd edition; the **squamous cell carcinoma accounts for the majority of lung cancers** (60%) and adenocarcinoma is less common (15%) than squamous cell carcinoma in the United Kingdom *although the incidence may vary in different countries.*

165. Decreased serum iron and total iron binding capacity is seen in:
- **A.** Sideroblastic anemia
- **B.** Thalassemia
- **C.** Anemia of chronic disease
- **D.** Iron deficiency

(UP 1995)

166. A 7 years old anemic child has decreased serum iron level and low serum iron binding capacity. The anemia is:
- **A.** Sideroblastic
- **B.** Beta thalassemia
- **C.** Iron deficiency
- **D.** Chronic infection

(SGPGI 1996))

While a majority of patients demonstrate a normocytic, normochromic anemia, some will appear to have a more severe defect in iron supply and will develop a mild microcytosis and hypochromia. Various laboratory findings in '**inflammatory anemia**' are as under:

• **Anemia**	Mild
• **MCV (fL)**	80-90
• **Morphology**	Normocytic
• **SI**	< **50**
• **TIBC**	< **300**
• **Saturation (%)**	10–20
• **Serum ferritin (μg/L)**	30-200
• **Iron stores**	2–4+

167. ***Best*** **treatment for hairy cell leukemia is:**
- **A.** Pentostatin
- **B.** Splenectomy
- **C.** Corticosteroid
- **D.** Alkylating agent

(AI 1993, UP 1995)

168. *Treatment of choice* in hairy cell leukemia is:

A. α interferon **B.** Splenectomy
C. Cyclophosphamide **D.** Chlorambucil *(UP 1998)*

169. *Not* used in the treatment of hairy cell leukemia:

A. interferon α **B.** Splenectomy
C. Steroid **D.** Pentostatin *(AIIMS 1997)*

Hairy cell leukemia is a rare disorder with characteristics of activated B cells, with expression of interleukin (IL) 2 receptors (CD25) and specific adhesion molecules involved in localizing cells to the spleen and marrow. The standard treatment for cytopenias due to hairy cell leukemia *used to be* **splenectomy** *but* its treatment has been revolutionized by the purine analogues, specifically **cladribine**. Cladribine induces a high complete response rate (>80%) often with single course of treatment. Cladribine is very active in patients *previously treated with* **pentostatin** or **interferon** α. It remains unknown if these patients will be 'cured', since minimal residual disease can be detected in patients in long clinical remissions.

170. *Not* present in cardiac tamponade:

A. Depression of ST segment **B.** Paradoxical pulse
C. Increased vein pressure **D.** Shock *(UP 1995)*

The accumulation of fluid in the pericardium in an amount sufficient to cause serious obstruction to the inflow of blood to the ventricles is known as **cardiac tamponade** and this grave complication may be fatal if it is not recognized and treated promptly. The 3 *most common* causes of tamponade are neoplastic disease, idiopathic pericarditis, and uremia, but it can also result from bleeding into the pericardial space either following cardiac operations and trauma (including cardiac perforation during diagnostic procedures) or from tuberculosis. The 3 main *features* of tamponade are elevation of intracardiac pressures, limitation of ventricular filling, and **reduction of cardiac output**. The *classic* findings of falling arterial pressure, **rising venous pressure**, and faint heart sounds usually are seen *only* with severe, acute tamponade, as occurs with cardiac trauma or rupture. Widening of the area of flatness to percussion across the anterior aspect of the chest wall, a **paradoxical pulse**, relatively clear lung fields, diminished pulsations of heart on fluoroscopy, enlargement of the cardiac silhouette, reduction in amplitude of the QRS complexes, and *electrical alternans* of the P, QRS, and T waves should raise the suspicion of cardiac tamponade. Diagnosis is established by echocardiography.

171. Finding in cardiac tamponade is:

A. 3rd heart sound **B.** Pericardial knock
C. Positive Kussmaul sign **D.** Prominent X, absent Y wave in JVP *(UP 1999)*

Cardiac tamponade should be suspected in any patient with hypotension and elevation of jugular venous pressure with a **prominent *X* descent**, often the ***Y* descent is diminutive or absent. A positive Kussmaul sign and pericardial knock is *rare* in cardiac tamponade**.

172. Long QT interval is *not* seen in:

A. Intracranial bleed **B.** Hypothermia
C. Hypercalcemia **D.** Hypokalemia *(UP 1995)*

Hypocalcemia typically prolongs the **QT interval** (ST portion), while ***hypercalcemia* shortens it**. *Hypokalemia* prolongs ventricular repolarization, often with prominent U waves. Prolongation of the QT interval is also seen with drugs such as *quinidine, disopyramide, procainamide, tricyclic antidepressants, phenothiazines, amiodarone* and *sotalol*. Marked QT prolongation, sometimes with deep, wide T wave inversions, may occur with *intracranial bleeds*, particularly subarachnoid hemorrhage. *Hypothermia* also prolongs repolarization, usually with a distinctive convex elevation of the J point (**Osborn wave**).

173. Hypokalemia causes:

A. GI bleeding
B. Intestinal colic
C. Muscle weakness
D. Hypertonia

174. *Not* seen in hypokalemia:

A. Muscular weakness **B.** Fatigue
C. *Increased* peristalsis **D.** Abdominal distention *(KERALA 1994)*

Hypokalemia is defined as a plasma K^+ concentration < 3.5 mmol/L. Symptoms rarely occur unless the plasma K^+ concentration is < 3 mmol/L. **Fatigue**, myalgia, and **muscular weakness** of the lower extremities are common features. More severe hypokalemia may lead to progressive weakness, hypoventilation and eventually complete paralysis. Smooth-muscle function may also be affected and manifest as **paralytic ileus**.

175. Blue-green pus is seen in infection of:

A. *Klebsiella* **B.** *Streptococcus*
C. *Staphylococcus* **D.** *Pseudomonas* *(UP 1995)*

Pseudomonas aeruginosa is a small, aerobic gram-negative rod belonging to the family Pseudomonadaceae. It is motile by virtue of its single polar flagellum. More than half of all clinical isolates produce the **blue-green pigment pyocyanin**.

176. Which of the following is *true* regarding human plague:

A. Penicillin is the drug of choice
B. Streptomycin is the drug of choice
C. Bubo rarely recedes without incision and drainage
D. Vector is rat

177. Incubation period of plague is...........days:

A. 16-21 **B.** 10-15
C. 7-10 **D.** 2-7 *(UP 1995)*

Plague is an acute, febrile, zoonosis caused by infection with *Yersinia pestis*. Plague is one of the most virulent and potentially lethal infectious diseases known. Bubonic plague usually has an **incubation period of 2 to 6 days**. **Streptomycin is the drug of choice.**

178. Conjugated hyperbilirubinemia is seen in:

A. Physiological jaundice **B.** Choledocholithiasis
C. Extravascular hemolysis **D.** Intravascular hemolysis *(UP 1995)*

Passage of gallstones into the common bile duct (**choledocholithiasis**) occurs in about 10 to 15% of patients with cholelithiasis. Gradual obstruction of the CBD over a period of weeks or months usually leads to initial manifestations of jaundice or pruritus (**obstructive jaundice**) *without* associated symptoms of biliary colic or cholangitis. *Painless* jaundice may occur in patients with choledocholithiasis, but this manifestation is more characteristic of biliary obstruction secondary to malignancy of the head of pancreas, bile ducts, or ampulla of Vater.

179. *Not* seen in scurvy in adults:

A. Hemarthrosis **B.** Purpura
C. Scurvy rosary **D.** Perifollicular hyperkeratosis *(UP 1995, SGPGI 1999)*

In adults, the features of **scurvy** include **perifollicular hyperkeratotic** papules in which hairs become fragmented and buried; perifollicular hemorrhages; **purpura**; hemorrhage into the muscles of the arms and legs with secondary phlebothromboses; **hemarthrosis**; splinter hemorrhages in the nail beds; gum involvement that includes swelling, friability, bleeding, secondary infection, and loosening of the teeth; poor wound healing and breakdown of recently healed wounds; petechial hemorrhages in the viscera; and emotional changes. Terminally, icterus, edema, and fever are common, and convulsions, hypotension, and death may occur abruptly.

180. *Not* a clinical manifestation of scurvy in children:

A. Retrobulbar hemorrhage **B.** Intracerebral hemorrhage
C. Perifollicular hemorrhage **D.** Hemorrhage into the periosteum of long bone *(AIIMS 1997)*

In infancy and childhood scurvy, **hemorrhage into the periosteum of long bones** leads to painful swellings and may result in epiphyseal separation. Pain results in *pseudo* paralysis and legs assume the typical **frog leg position.** The sternum may sink inward, leaving a sharp elevation at the rib margins so called *scorbutic rosary*. Purpura and ecchymoses may develop in the skin, and gum lesions occur. **Retrobulbar**, subarachnoid, and **intracerebral hemorrhages** rapidly conclude in death if treatment is delayed. Administration of 3 to 4 ounces of orange or tomato juice per day will produce quick healing but ascorbic acid is preferred. The daily *therapeutic* dose is 100-200 mg or more (orally or parenterally).

181. Clubbing and hemoptysis is seen in:

A. Pneumonia
B. Empyema
C. Crohn's disease
D. Bronchiectasis *(UP 1995)*

Bronchiectasis is an abnormal and permanent dilatation of bronchi which is associated with destructive and inflammatory changes in the walls of medium-sized airways, often at the level of segmental or subsegmental bronchi. Patients *typically* present with persistent or recurrent cough and purulent sputum production. **Hemoptysis** occurs in 50 to 70% of cases and as with other types of chronic intrathoracic infection, **clubbing** may be present.

182. *False* regarding Zollinger-Ellison syndrome is:

A. Ca^{++} provocative test is *best*
B. Serum gastrin level is high
C. Associated with MEN I
D. Usually multiple ulcers *(UP 1995)*

Zollinger-Ellison syndrome consists of ulcer disease of the upper gastrointestinal tract, marked increase in gastric acid secretion, and non-beta islet cell tumors of the pancreas. These tumors are known as gastrinomas because they contain **gastrin, which circulates in large amounts**. The diagnosis of Zollinger-Ellison syndrome should be suspected in every patient of recurrent peptic ulceration, especially when **multiple ulcers** are present or when they are present in unusual site in GI tract. In an estimated 20 to 60% of patients with ZES, the gastrinoma is a component of the **multiple endocrine neoplasia type 1** (MEN 1) syndrome. Zollinger-Ellison syndrome type 1 is a rare condition characterized by antral G cell hyperplasia, hypergastrinemia and chronic peptic ulceration. Zollinger-Ellison syndrome type II may be due to an ulcerogenic non beta cell tumor or diffuse hyperplasia of the islet cells. The tumor secretes gastrin and is generally situated in the tail of pancreas. 50% of these tumors are malignant. There is intractable peptic ulceration (often in jejunum), hypergastrinemia with massive acid hypersecretion (up to 500 ml/hour), diarrhea, and sometimes steatorrhea or hypokalemia. Diarrhea occurs in about 40% of patients of Zollinger-Ellison syndrome due to the outpouring of large amounts of hydrochloric acid into the proximal duodenum. Acid secretion studies and estimation of circulating gastrin will establish the diagnosis and in type I disease the plasma gastrin levels are further increased by meat extracts while in type II disease 2 mg/kg Ca^{++} in 1 minute will do the same. The *secretin injection test* is the *most valuable* provocative test in identifying patients with ZES. **The diagnosis of gastrinoma in a patient with clinical features consistent with ZES depends on the demonstration of increased serum gastrin levels by radioimmunoassay.** Treatment consists of partial gastrectomy to remove the G cell bearing area in type 1, while total gastrectomy with removal of the tumor should be done in type II disease. The *proton pump blockers* omeprazole and lansoprazole are the agents of choice in reducing gastric acid secretion and healing ulcers in patients with Zollinger-Ellison syndrome. The initial daily dose of omeprazole or lansoprazole is 60 mg in a single dose administered in the morning before breakfast.

183. *Not* seen in asthma:

A. Paradoxical pulse
B. pCO_2 = 40 mmHg
C. Accessory muscles becomes active
D. Expiratory rhonchi *only* *(UP 1995)*

184. Definite diagnosis of bronchial asthma is made by:

A. Decreased FEV_1/ FVC ratio on spirometry
B. Relief of symptoms after bronchodilators
C. *Reversible* responsiveness of bronchial musculature
D. Methacholine challenge *(UP 1998)*

The symptoms of asthma consist of a triad of *dyspnea*, *cough*, and *wheezing*. In its most typical form, asthma is an episodic disease, and all 3 symptoms coexist. Respiration becomes audibly harsh, **wheezing in both phases of respiration becomes prominent**, expiration becomes prolonged, and patients frequently have tachypnea, tachycardia, and mild systolic hypertension. The **accessory muscles become visibly active**, and a **paradoxical pulse often develops**. **The diagnosis of asthma is established by demonstrating reversible airway obstruction.** *Reversibility* is traditionally defined as a 15% or greater increase in FEV_1 following 2 puffs of a β adrenergic agonist (inhaler Ventolin® or Asthalin ®). Once the diagnosis is established, the course of the illness and the effectiveness of therapy can be followed by measuring peak expiratory flow rates (PEFRs) at home and/or the FEV_1 in the laboratory.

185. *Most common* presentation of unilateral renal artery stenosis is:

A. Polycythemia
B. Peripheral edema
C. Hypertension
D. Uremia

(UP 1995)

Stenosis of the main renal artery and/or its major branches accounts for 2 to 5% of hypertension. Bilateral involvement was found in 50% of cases. Angiotensin converting enzyme (ACE) inhibitors are *contraindicated* in patients with *bilateral* renal artery stenosis but are the **drugs of choice in patients with *unilateral* renal artery stenosis** and a normally functioning contralateral kidney. They are also drug of choice in patients with chronic renal failure with or without diabetes mellitus.

186. In tension pneumothorax, drainage tube is inserted through:

A. 6th ICS in axillary line
B. 2nd ICS in axillary line
C. 2nd ICS in midclavicular line
D. 6th ICS in midclavicular line

(UP 1995)

Tension pneumothorax usually occurs during mechanical ventilation or *resuscitative efforts*. The positive pleural pressure is life-threatening as ventilation is severely compromised and because the positive pressure is transmitted to the mediastinum, which results in decreased venous return to the heart and reduced cardiac output. It should be treated as a medical emergency because if the tension in the pleural space is not relieved, the patient will die due to inadequate cardiac output or marked hypoxemia. **A large-bore needle should be inserted into the pleural space through the 2nd anterior intercostal space** and if large amounts of gas escape from the needle after insertion, the diagnosis is established. The needle should be left in place until a thoracostomy tube is inserted.

187. Recurrent hematuria in a deaf-mute is seen in:

A. Nephrotic syndrome
B. Renal cyst
C. Fanconi anemia
D. Alport's syndrome

(JIPMER 1998)

188. *True* regarding classic Alport's syndrome is:

A. Hematuria
B. Autosomal recessive
C. Conductive deafness
D. All of the above

(UP 1995)

Alport's syndrome (AS) is an inherited disorder characterized by *hematuria*. 4 forms of the disease are now recognized:

(1) Classic AS, which is inherited as an **X-linked disorder** with **hematuria**, *sensorineural* **deafness**, and conical deformation of the anterior surface of the lens (lenticonus);
(2) A 2nd X-linked form associated with diffuse leiomyomatosis;
(3) An autosomal recessive form;
(4) An autosomal dominant form.

The 2 autosomal forms can cause renal disease without deafness or lenticonus.

189. *Initial* sign of Alport's syndrome is:

A. Sensorineural high frequency deafness
B. Oliguria
C. Proteinuria
D. Microscopic hematuria

(AIIMS 1997)

190. Characteristic *initial* manifestation of Alport's syndrome is:

A. Nephrotic syndrome
B. Hypertension
C. Deafness
D. Microscopic hematuria

(SGPGI 1999)

The diagnosis of *classic* Alport's syndrome is based on X-linked inheritance of hematuria, sensorineural deafness, and lenticonus. The **mean age for onset of renal disease is 6 years** but **it has been noted as early as 1st few months of life. Hematuria is the most common manifestation**; initially it is **microscopic** but episodes of gross hematuria do occur, sometimes in relation to exercise and respiratory tract infection. About 50% of patients have sensorineural high frequency deafness which usually has its onset in the 1st decade of life. Deafness is more severe in males and is usually progressive. Ocular abnormalities occur in 10% of patients; most frequent are cataracts, myopia, lenticonus, keratoconus, nystagmus and microspherophakia.

191. *Best* investigation for hypothyroidism is:

A. ELISA
B. T_4
C. T_3
D. Serum TSH

(UP 1995)

192. Most diagnostic test for primary hypothyroidism is:

A. Ca^{++}
B. TSH
C. T_3
D. T_4

(AIIMS 1998)

The ***single most useful* measurement is the serum thyroid stimulating hormone (TSH),** which is increased in the thyroprivic and goitrous varieties and is usually normal or undetectable in pituitary or hypothalamic hypothyroidism.

193. In hypothyroidism, treatment response is monitored by:

A. TSH
B. FT_4
C. T_4
D. T_3

(AI 1996)

In treatment of hypothyroidism although the serum T_3 may be superior to the serum T_4 as an indicator of the metabolic state in patients receiving levothyroxine, **the optimal dose is *best determined* by clinical criteria and measurement of TSH** by an ultrasensitive assay.

194. In subclavian steal syndrome the blood flow in vertebral artery is:

A. Reversed
B. Increased
C. Diminished
D. Absent

(UP 1996)

If the first part of the subclavian artery is obstructed, the **direction of blood flow in vertebral artery may be reversed** to provide a collateral circulation to the arm. This may result in periods of cerebral ischemia known as **"subclavian steal syndrome".** The syndrome consists of syncopal attack and visual disturbance associated with arm exercise and a diminished blood pressure in the affected limb is occasionally seen.

195. Polyuria with low fixed specific gravity is seen in:

A. Competitive water drinking
B. CRF
C. Diabetes insipidus
D. Diabetes mellitus

(UP 1996)

Diabetes insipidus *refers* to the passage of a large quantity of dilute urine. This state of excessive water intake and hypotonic polyuria may be due to failure of AVP release in response to normal physiologic stimuli (**central or neurogenic diabetes insipidus**) or failure of the kidney to respond to AVP (**nephrogenic diabetes insipidus**). **Polyuria,** excessive thirst, and polydipsia are invariably present in diabetes insipidus. Urinary concentration of < 290 mmol/kg (**specific gravity less than 1.010**) is usual.

196. Bone marrow leukocytosis is *not* seen in:

A. Aplastic anemia
B. Gaucher's disease
C. Kala azar
D. All of the above

(UP 1996)

- Parasitologic diagnosis of visceral leishmaniasis (**kala azar**) is done by demonstration of the parasite on stained slides or in cultures of a tissue aspirate or a biopsy specimen (e.g., of spleen, liver, bone marrow, or lymph node). The **diagnostic yield is highest for splenic aspiration** (98% for splenic aspirates vs. < 90% for other specimens), but this procedure can cause hemorrhage. Phagocytic cells crowds the bone marrow and may also be found in the lungs, GI tract, kidneys, pancreas, testes and other organs.
- In **Gaucher's disease** the distended phagocytic cells known as Gaucher's cells accumulate in the bone marrow producing small focal areas of bone erosion.
- In **aplastic anemia** the bone marrow aspirate typically shows numerous spicules with empty fatty spaces and few hematopoietic cells. The *hypocellularity* is secondary to a marked decrease in megakaryocytes, granulocytes, and erythroid cells.

197. In a case of kala azar aldehyde test becomes positive after:

A. 2 weeks
B. 4 weeks
C. 8 weeks
D. 12 weeks

Aldehyde test or **Napier test** is a serological test for kala azar and depends upon increase in serum gamma globulins. Kala azar is characterized by hypergammaglobulinemia and hypoalbuminemia. **Aldehyde test is not positive until the disease has been of 3 months (12 wks) of duration.** In this test 2 ml of serum is taken in a small test tube and 2 drops of 40% formalin is added to it. If the test is positive a jelly like milky white opacity appears in 2-20 minutes.

198. *Most common* cause of intracerebral bleeding is:

A. Tumor
B. Trauma
C. Hypertension
D. Rupture of aneurysm *(AI 1993, AIIMS 1995, UP 1996)*

199. The *most common* site of cerebral hemorrhage in hypertension is:

A. Pons
B. Cerebrum
C. Putamen
D. Thalamus

Intracerebral hemorrhage is the *most common* type of non-traumatic intracranial hemorrhage. It is an important cause of stroke, especially in Asians and blacks. **Hypertension** and cerebral amyloid angiopathy cause the majority of these hemorrhages. **Intracerebral hemorrhage** usually results from spontaneous rupture of a small penetrating artery deep in the brain. The ***most common* sites** are the basal ganglia (**putamen**, thalamus, and adjacent deep white matter), the deep cerebellum, and the pons. **The putamen is the *most common* site for hypertensive hemorrhage** and the adjacent internal capsule is invariably damaged.

200. Specific diagnostic investigation in DIC is:

A. Thrombocytopenia and schistocytes
B. Fibrin degradation product assay
C. Raised PTT and PT
D. Increased bleeding time *(AIIMS 1998)*

201. Diagnosis of disseminated intravascular coagulation is *best* confirmed by:

A. Defective platelet function
B. Prolongation of prothrombin time
C. Fibrin degradation products in serum
D. Fragmented red cells in the PBS *(UP 1996)*

202. *Not* a laboratory finding of DIC:

A. Low FDP
B. High aPTT
C. High PT
D. Thrombocytopenia *(AI 1996)*

203. *Not* a feature of DIC:

A. Thrombocytopenia
B. Normal aPTT
C. Prolonged PT
D. Hypofibrinogenemia *(AI 1995, 2001)*

204. *False* regarding DIC:

A. Hypofibrinogenemia
B. Increased PT and aPTT
C. Thrombocytosis
D. Increase in fibrin degradation products *(AI 1992)*

205. Disseminated intravascular coagulation is *not* seen in:

A. Post partum hemorrhage
B. Accidental hemorrhage
C. Amniotic fluid embolism
D. Diabetes mellitus *(AI 1992)*

Disseminated intravascular coagulation can be either an explosive and life-threatening bleeding disorder or a relatively mild or *sub* clinical disorder. There is a long list of diseases complicated by disseminated intravascular coagulation *but* it is **most frequently associated with obstetrical catastrophes**, metastatic malignancy, massive trauma, and bacterial *sepsis*. Most patients have *extensive* skin and mucous membrane bleeding and hemorrhage from multiple sites, usually surgical incisions or venipuncture or catheter sites. Laboratory findings include **thrombocytopenia** and the presence of *schistocytes* or **fragmented RBCs** ; **prolonged prothrombin time (PT)** and **aPTT** and thrombin time and a **reduced fibrinogen level** from depletion of coagulation proteins; and **elevated fibrin degradation products (FDP)** from *intense* secondary fibrinolysis. The *D dimer immunoassay* is a more specific FDP assay. The cardinal manifestation of DIC **which correlates most closely with bleeding** is the **plasma fibrinogen level** i.e. *low fibrinogen levels are associated with more bleeding*.

206. *Not* included in the treatment of disseminated intravascular coagulation:

A. ε-aminocaproic acid (EACA)
B. Fresh frozen plasma
C. Heparin
D. Platelet transfusion *(KARNATAKA 2000)*

Patients with bleeding as a major symptom should receive **fresh frozen plasma** to replace depleted clotting factors and **platelet concentrates** to correct thrombocytopenia. Those with acrocyanosis and incipient gangrene or other thrombotic problems need immediate anticoagulation with intravenous **heparin**. ε-aminocaproic acid (EACA) may promote thrombus formation in patients with disseminated intravascular coagulation and must *not* be used unless heparin is administered *concurrently*.

207. Fanconi syndrome is associated with:

A. Fructose intolerance
B. Hypophosphatemia
C. Generalized aminoaciduria
D. All of the above *(UP 1996)*

Fanconi syndrome is a *generalized* defect in *proximal* tubule transport involving **amino acids**, glucose, **phosphate**, uric acid, Na^+, K^+, HCO_3^-, and proteins. A variety of *inherited* disorders are also *associated* with Fanconi syndrome including Wilson's disease, galactosemia, tyrosinemia, cystinosis, **fructose intolerance**, and Lowe's oculocerebral syndrome and the syndrome may be *acquired* in multiple myeloma, amyloid, and heavy metal toxicity. The patients may present with a wide collection of laboratory abnormalities including proximal renal tubular acidosis, glucosuria with a normal serum glucose, **hypophosphatemia**, hypouricemia, hypokalemia, **generalized aminoaciduria**, and low-molecular-weight proteinuria. Rickets and osteomalacia are common findings secondary to the hypophosphatemia. Polyuria, salt wasting, and hypokalemia may be quite severe. *Treatment* includes phosphate supplements and calcitriol along with liberal intake of salt and water. Aminoaciduria, glucosuria, hypouricemia, and proteinuria *do not* require treatment.

208. Regarding Fanconi syndrome all are correct *except*:

A. Usually presents by 6 months, but may present later
B. Linear growth is impaired
C. Polyuria and polydipsia are the features
D. None of the above

Fanconi syndrome or de Toni-Debré -Fanconi syndrome is characterized by glycosuria, aminoaciduria and phosphaturia *(mnemonic GAP)*. Aminoaciduria is generalized and other associated abnormalities may be bicarbonaturia, hyperkaliuria, **uricosuria** and sodium wasting. Clinical features are **linear growth failure** and vitamin D deficiency rickets. Symptoms typically appear in **1st six months of life** and consist of vomiting, **polydipsia**, **polyuria** and constipation.

209. Drug *not* used in thyrotoxic crisis is:

A. Corticosteroid **B.** Iodine
C. Carbimazole **D.** Propranolol *(UP 1996)*

Thyrotoxic crisis, or storm, is a fulminating increase in the signs and symptoms of thyrotoxicosis and this disturbance usually occurr*ed* postoperatively in patients *poorly* prepared for surgery. *Treatment* consists of supportive therapy while undertaking procedures to lessen thyrotoxicosis *as rapidly as possible*. Supportive therapy includes treatment of dehydration and the IV administration of glucose and saline, vitamin B complex, and **glucocorticoids**. Digitalization is required to control ventricular rate in those with atrial fibrillation. If shock exists, intravenous pressor agents (dopamine) should be used. Therapy of the hyperthyroidism consists of blockade of hormone synthesis by the immediate and continued administration of large doses of an antithyroid agent (e.g., 100 mg **propylthiouracil** every 2 h). Hormone release is inhibited through the administration of **large doses of iodine** intravenously or by mouth. Adrenergic antagonists are an important and critical part of the therapeutic regimen in the *absence* of cardiac failure. **Propranolol** can be administered in doses of 40 to 80 mg Q 6 hourly.

210. *Most important* drug used in acute MI with multiple *ectopic*:

A. Streptokinase **B.** β-adrenoceptor blocking agents
C. Procainamide **D.** Digoxin *(UP 1996)*

211. *Most* of the death in myocardial infarction results in the........day:

A. First **B.** Second
C. Fifth **D.** Seventh

The prognosis in acute myocardial infarction is largely dependent on 2 general classes of complications viz. electrical complications (*arrhythmias*) and mechanical problems (*pump failure*). **Most deaths from myocardial infarction are due to the sudden development of ventricular fibrillation** and vast majority of deaths due to ventricular fibrillation occur **within the first 24 hours** of the onset of symptoms, and, of these, **over 50% occur in the 1st hour**. Prophylactic antiarrhythmic therapy (either intravenous lidocaine early or oral agents later) is *contraindicated* for ventricular premature beats in the absence of clinically important ventricular tachyarrhythmias. **β-adrenoceptor blocking agents** are effective in abolishing **ventricular ectopic activity** in infarction patients and in the prevention of ventricular fibrillation. Pacing does appear to be helpful in patients with inferoposterior infarction who have complete heart block associated with heart failure, hypotension, marked bradycardia, or *significant* ventricular ectopic activity.

212. ATT used in patients of renal failure is:

A. Pyrazinamide **B.** Isoniazid
C. Rifampicin **D.** Ethambutol *(UP 1996)*

- **R**ifampicin is safe in **r**enal disease.
- Streptomycin and ethambutol are safe in liver disease.

213. In acute respiratory failure, *most frequent* abnormality seen in ECG is:

A. Right ventricular hypertrophy **B.** Ventricular arrhythmia
C. AV block **D.** Supra ventricular arrhythmia *(UP 1996)*

Complications arising in the course of treatment for **acute respiratory failure** are cardiac arrhythmias (**most often multifocal supraventricular tachycardias**), LVF, pulmonary emboli, and GI hemorrhage from *stress* ulceration.

214. Psychiatric manifestations are common in:

A. Hepatic porphyria **B.** Porphyria cutanea tarda
C. Congenital erythropoietic porphyria **D.** Acute intermittent porphyria *(KERALA 1994)*

215. *Not* a feature of acute intermittent porphyria:

A. Hematuria **B.** Abdominal pain
C. Leukocytosis **D.** Fever *(UP 1996)*

Abdominal pain is the *most common* symptom of acute intermittent porphyria. Ileus, abdominal distention, and decreased bowel sounds are common. Abdominal tenderness, **fever**, and **leukocytosis** are *usually* absent or **mild** because the symptoms are neurologic *rather* than inflammatory. Nausea, vomiting, constipation, tachycardia, hypertension, mental symptoms, pain in the limbs, head, neck, or chest, muscle weakness, sensory loss, dysuria, and urinary retention are *characteristic* and tachycardia, hypertension, restlessness, tremors, and excess sweating are due to sympathetic over activity. **Psychiatric symptoms** such as anxiety, insomnia, depression, disorientation, hallucinations, and paranoia may occur in acute attacks.

216. *Not* a clinical feature of SLE:
- **A.** Psychosis
- **B.** Coombs' positive hemolytic anemia
- **C.** Sterility
- **D.** Recurrent abortion

(UP 1996, AI 1998)

Fertility rates are normal in patients with SLE, *but* **spontaneous abortion** and stillbirths are frequent (10 to 30%), especially in women with lupus anticoagulant and/or antibodies to cardiolipin. The lupus anticoagulant (LA) belongs to a family of 'antiphospholipid antibodies'. *Clinical manifestations* of LA and antibodies to cardiolipin include thrombocytopenia, recurrent venous or arterial clotting, *recurrent fetal loss*, and valvular heart disease. Anemia of chronic disease occurs in most patients when lupus is active. **Hemolysis** occurs in a small proportion of those with **positive Coombs' tests**. *Less* frequent manifestations include **psychosis**, organic brain syndromes, focal infarcts, extra pyramidal disorders, cerebellar dysfunction, hypothalamic dysfunction with inappropriate antidiuretic hormone secretion, *pseudotumor* cerebri, subarachnoid hemorrhage, aseptic meningitis, transverse myelitis, optic neuritis, cranial nerve palsies, and peripheral sensorimotor neuropathy.

217. Bronchiectasis, eosinophilia and asthma are seen in:
- **A.** Aspergillosis
- **B.** Histoplasmosis
- **C.** Nocardiosis
- **D.** Mucormycosis

218. In which of the following condition, allergic bronchopulmonary aspergillosis is seen:
- **A.** Tubercular cavity
- **B.** Bronchitis
- **C.** Bronchiectasis
- **D.** Bronchus carcinoma

(AIIMS 1991)

219. *False* regarding allergic aspergillosis is:
- **A.** Pleural effusion
- **B.** Pulmonary infiltrates
- **C.** Central bronchiectasis
- **D.** Asthma

(UP 1995)

220. *False* regarding allergic bronchopulmonary aspergillosis is:
- **A.** Eosinophilia
- **B.** Asthma
- **C.** Pleural effusion
- **D.** Central bronchiectasis

(AI 1993)

Allergic bronchopulmonary aspergillosis (**ABPA**) is the *most common* example of the allergic bronchopulmonary mycoses. **Diagnostic features ABPA are as under:**

MAIN CRITERIA

- **Bronchial asthma**
- **Pulmonary infiltrates**
- **Peripheral eosinophilia** (>1000/μL)
- Immediate wheal-and-flare response to *Aspergillus fumigatus*
- Serum precipitins to *Aspergillus fumigatus*
- Elevated serum IgE
- **Central bronchiectasis**

OTHER FEATURES

- History of brownish plugs in sputum
- Culture of *Aspergillus fumigatus* from sputum
- Elevated IgE (and IgG) class antibodies specific for *Aspergillus fumigatus*

221. Megaloblastic anemia is *not* caused by:

A. Folic acid deficiency
B. Lead poisoning
C. Vitamin B_{12} deficiency
D. Orotic aciduria

(UP 1995)

- Lead-associated anemia is usually **normocytic** and normochromic and may be accompanied by basophilic stippling.
- Megaloblastic anemias are disorders caused by impaired DNA synthesis. *Most* megaloblastic anemias are due to a deficiency of cobalamin (**vitamin B_{12}**) and/or **folic acid**.
- Megaloblastic anemia is a *regular* feature of **orotic aciduria** in which there is a deficiency of orotidylic decarboxylase and phosphorylase leading to a defect in pyrimidine metabolism and characterized by *retarded growth and development* as well as by the *excretion of large amounts of orotic acid*.

222. In pre-excitation syndrome ECG shows:

A. Q waves
B. Delta waves
C. Long PR interval
D. Tall T waves

The basic abnormality in Wolff-Parkinson-White syndrome or **pre-excitation syndrome** is an extra AV bypass tract that conducts the impulse in an antegrade direction producing a *typical* ECG pattern of a **short PR interval** (less than 0.12 s), a slurred upstroke of the QRS complex (**delta wave**), and a wide QRS complex.

- **Normal PR interval** 0.12 to 0.2 s
- **Normal QRS duration** 0.1 s
- **Normal QT interval** 0.4 s

Delta wave

223. Drug of choice in WPW syndrome with atrial fibrillation is:

A. Procainamide
B. Disopyramide
C. Adenosine
D. Verapamil

(UP 1995, 1998)

In patients with the Wolff-Parkinson-White syndrome and atrial fibrillation, DC *cardioversion* should be carried out if there is a life-threatening, rapid ventricular response. Otherwise, *lidocaine* (3 to 5 mg/kg) or **procainamide** (15 mg/kg) administered IV over 15 to 20 minutes will usually slow the ventricular response.

224. The *best* treatment for Wolf-Parkinson White syndrome is:

A. Carotid massage
B. IV verapamil
C. Cardioversion
D. Surgical excision of the tract

In WPW **surgical ablation of bypass tracts** offers a permanent cure of supraventricular tachycardia (SVT) and most atrial fibrillations associated with supraventricular tachycardia. The arrival of radiofrequency catheter ablation has virtually eliminated the need for surgery.

225. Paroxysmal nocturnal hemoglobinuria is due to:

A. Acquired hemoglobin defect
B. Complement mediated RBC lysis
C. Autoimmune disorder
D. Congenital membrane defect

(KERALA 1994)

The *fundamental* abnormality in **paroxysmal nocturnal hemoglobinuria** is an **acquired defect of a red blood cell membrane** which renders it unusually **sensitive to lysis by the complement of normal serum.**

226. Troglitazone is the drug used in the treatment of:

A. Type 2 diabetes mellitus
B. Petit mal epilepsy
C. Hyperlipidemia
D. Candidiasis

(JIPMER 2000)

Troglitazone is used as an *adjunct to insulin* in **NIDDM** patients whose hyperglycemia is inadequately controlled (glycosylated hemoglobin concentrations > 8.5%) by an insulin dose of more > 30 USP insulin units per day.

227. ***Not*** **an important feature of paroxysmal nocturnal hemoglobinuria:**

A. High leukocyte alkaline phosphatase **B.** Hemosiderinuria
C. Hypocellular marrow **D.** Pancytopenia *(AIIMS 1993, UP 1997, AIIMS 2000)*

228. ***Not*** **a feature of paroxysmal nocturnal hemoglobinuria is:**

A. High leukocyte alkaline phosphate (LAP)
B. Thrombocytopenia
C. Hemosiderinuria
D. Venous thrombosis *(AIIMS 1997)*

- **Paroxysmal nocturnal hemoglobinuria** (PNH) is a clonal hemopathy caused by a defect in the PIG-A gene. It is characterized by *partial* or *complete* inability to construct a glycosylphosphatidylinositol (**GPI**) *anchor* for the attachment of membrane proteins such as CD55, CD59, and others. There are 3 common manifestations of PNH viz. hemolytic anemia, **venous thrombosis**, and deficient hematopoiesis. Red blood cells are normochromic and normocytic *unless* iron deficiency has occurred due to the chronic loss of iron in the urine. Mild **granulocytopenia** and **thrombocytopenia** are commonly present and are manifestations of deficient hematopoiesis. Clinical hemoglobinuria is present only *intermittently* in most patients and never occurs in some, but **hemosiderinuria** is usually present in all patients. **Marrow aplasia** may also occur during the course of classical hemolytic PNH. **Aplastic anemia** can be the initial hematologic manifestation of this disease. Therapy with androgens frequently results in a rise in hemoglobin level. Glucocorticoids also may be effective in reducing the rate of hemolysis but should be given in moderate doses (15 to 30 mg prednisone) *only on alternate days.* Transfusion therapy is useful in PNH not *only* for raising the hemoglobin level but *also* for suppressing the marrow production of red blood cells during episodes of sustained hemoglobinuria.
- **Low scores** (LAP) have been associated with CML, **PNH**, thrombocytopenic purpura, and hereditary hypophosphatasia.

229. Folic acid deficiency in megaloblastic anemia is due to:

A. Methylcobalamin is *co*factor **B.** Inhibit purine synthesis
C. Intrinsic factor deficiency **D.** Folate trap mechanism *(UP 1997)*

Methylcobalamin is an essential *co*factor in the conversion of homocysteine to methionine. When this reaction is impaired, folate metabolism is deranged. This leads to defect in DNA synthesis and the megaloblastic maturation pattern in patients who are deficient in cobalamin. In cobalamin deficiency, the unconjugated N^5-methyltetrahydrofolate newly taken from the bloodstream cannot be converted to other forms of tetrahydrofolate by methyl transfer. This is the called **folate trap** hypothesis.

230. ***Not*** **a clinical feature of Henoch-Schönlein purpura:**

A. Thrombocytopenia **B.** Increased serum IgA
C. Glomerulonephritis **D.** Arthralgia *(UP 1997)*

231. ***False*** **regarding Henoch-Schönlein purpura is:**

A. Nephritis **B.** Arthritis
C. Centrifugal rash **D.** Thrombocytopenia *(AIIMS 1991)*

232. ***Not*** **a feature of Henoch-Schönlein purpura:**

A. Renal failure may cause death **B.** IgA deposition in mesangium
C. Hematuria **D.** Thrombocytopenia *(AI 2000)*

233. ***Not*** **a characteristic feature of Henoch-Schönlein purpura:**

A. Abdominal pain **B.** Arthralgia
C. Thrombocytopenia **D.** Glomerulonephritis *(AI 1994)*

234. Important feature of Henoch-Schönlein purpura is:

A. Aneurysm of branching point **B.** Absent radial pulse
C. Membranous glomerulonephritis **D.** Raised IgA *(AI 1992)*

235. Thrombocytopenia is seen in all *except*:

A. Thrombocytopenic purpura **B.** Immunogenic thrombocytopenia
C. Henoch-Schönlein purpura **D.** Hemolytic uremic syndrome *(AIIMS 1998)*

Henoch-Schönlein purpura is also known as **anaphylactoid purpura**. It is a *distinct* 'systemic vasculitis syndrome' that is characterized by palpable purpura (most commonly distributed over the buttocks and lower extremities), **arthralgias**, **gastrointestinal signs** and symptoms, and **glomerulonephritis**. It is a small vessel vasculitis. There is mild leukocytosis, a **normal platelet count**, and *occasionally* eosinophilia. Serum complement components are normal, and **IgA levels are elevated** in about 50% of patients. The prognosis is excellent and most patients recover completely, and some do not require therapy. When therapy is required, prednisone in doses of 1 mg/kg per day is the drug of choice.

236. *Not* a clinical feature of pancreatic cholera:

A. Metabolic acidosis **B.** Hypocalcemia
C. Hypochlorhydria **D.** Hypokalemia *(UP 1997)*

The Verner-Morrison or watery diarrhea syndrome or **pancreatic cholera** consists of watery diarrhea, **hypokalemia**, **hypochlorhydria**, and **metabolic acidosis.** This syndrome is believed to be due to overproduction of vasoactive intestinal peptide (VIP), although plasma VIP levels may not be elevated. **Hypercalcemia** is caused by the effects of VIP on bone.

237. *Single* drug used in prophylaxis of tuberculosis is:

A. Pyrazinamide **B.** Isoniazid
C. Rifampicin **D.** Ethambutol *(UP 1997)*

When supervised prophylaxis is required, **isoniazid** may be given at a dose of 15 mg/kg (up to 900 mg) twice weekly.

238. *Not* a cause of hypokalemia:

A. K^+ *sparing* diuretic **B.** Licorice ingestion
C. Liddle's syndrome **D.** Bartter's syndrome *(UP 1997)*

239. All the following are features of Bartter's syndrome *except*:

A. Hypokalemia **B.** Hypertension
C. Alkalosis **D.** Increased rennin and aldosterone *(JIPMER 2002)*

Some Causes of Hypokalemia

Excessive renal loss	Nonrenal loss	Shift from ECF to ICF
• Tubular diseases (drugs, cystinosis) • Aldosterone, glucocorticoids • Diuretics • Non-reabsorbable anions (penicillin, bicarbonate)	• Vomiting • Diarrhea • Laxative abuse • Licorice ingestion	• Insulin • β_2 catecholamines • Alkalosis

- **Bartter's syndrome** is characterized by **hypokalemia**, metabolic **alkalosis**, **hyperreninemic hyperaldosteronism** secondary to ECF volume contraction, and juxtaglomerular apparatus hyperplasia.
- **Liddle's syndrome** is a rare familial (autosomal dominant) disease characterized by hypertension, hypokalemic metabolic alkalosis, renal K^+ wasting, and suppressed renin and aldosterone secretion.
- Limited intake

240. Sensory involvement is *not* seen in:

A. Wilson's disease **B.** Acute intermittent porphyria
C. Guillain-Barré syndrome **D.** Infectious mononucleosis *(AI 2001)*

241. All are seen in Wilson's disease *except*:

A. Positive Babinski sign **B.** Rigidity
C. Spasticity **D.** Sensory symptoms *(UP 1997)*

242. *Not* a feature of Wilson's disease:

A. Sensor changes
B. Spasticity
C. Rigidity
D. Intention tremors (*AI 1992*)

243. *Not* a feature of Wilson's disease:

A. Features of chronic active hepatitis
B. Mental changes
C. Increased ceruloplasmin
D. Increased copper content in liver (*AI 1991*)

244. All of the following are *true* about Wilson's disease *except*:

A. Increased liver copper
B. Increased serum ceruloplasmin level
C. Chronic active hepatitis
D. Hemolysis (*SGPGI 2002*)

245. Wilson's disease is due to deposition of:

A. Arsenic
B. Copper
C. Iron
D. Zinc (*MP 2001*)

246. *Not* seen in Wilson's disease:

A. Chorea
B. Dysphagia
C. Peripheral neuropathy
D. Dysarthria (*AI 2001*)

247. All are the features of Wilson's disease *except*:

A. Manic depressive psychosis
B. Chorea
C. Testicular atrophy
D. Chronic active hepatitis (*AIIMS 1997*)

248. *Not* a recognized feature of Wilson's disease:

A. Histopathological features of chronic active hepatitis
B. Increased copper content of liver
C. Increased serum ceruloplasmin levels
D. Psychological disturbance (*SGPGI 1996)*)

249. Characteristics of Wilson's disease include:

A. Kayser-Fleischer ring in the cornea
B. Ceruloplasmin deficiency
C. Psychiatric symptoms preceding neurological symptoms
D. All of the above

Wilson's disease is an inherited disorder of copper metabolism in which there is impairment of the normal excretion of hepatic copper resulting in **toxic accumulations of the metal in liver**, brain, and other organs. In about 50% of patients any of the 4 types of hepatic disturbances may herald the clinical onset. In most other patients neurologic or **psychiatric disturbances** are the *first* clinical signs and are always accompanied by Kayser-Fleischer rings. The neurologic manifestations include resting and intention tremors, **spasticity**, **rigidity**, **chorea**, drooling, **dysphagia**, and **dysarthria**. Babinski sign may be positive, and abdominal reflexes are often absent. **Sensory changes, *except* headache, never occur**. Schizophrenia, **manic-depressive psychoses**, and **classic neuroses** may occur, but the most common disturbances are bizarre behavioral patterns that defy classification. In about 50% of patients any of 4 types of hepatic disturbances may herald the clinical onset viz. acute hepatitis, **parenchymal liver disease** (chronic active hepatitis), cirrhosis and fulminant hepatitis which are generally fatal. The diagnosis is confirmed by the demonstration of either:

- A serum ceruloplasmin level **less than** 200 mg/L *and* Kayser-Fleischer rings or
- A serum ceruloplasmin level less than 200 mg/L *and* a concentration of copper in liver biopsy greater than 250 μg/g dry weight.

Most symptomatic patients excrete more than 100 μg copper per day in urine and have histologic abnormalities on liver biopsy. Penicillamine is administered orally in an initial dose of 1 gram daily in single or divided doses at least 30 minutes before and 2 hour after eating. Because penicillamine has an *anti*pyridoxine effect, 25 mg/d of pyridoxine is also given.

250. The term "crossed aphasia" means:
- **A.** Right hemispherical lesion in right handed person
- **B.** Right hemispherical lesion in left handed person
- **C.** Left hemispherical lesion in left handed person
- **D.** Left hemispherical lesion in right handed person *(JIPMER 2002)*

A language disturbance occurring after a **right hemisphere lesion** in a **right hander** is called **crossed aphasia**.

251. Glucagonoma is characterized by which of the following skin disorders:
- **A.** Necrolytic migratory erythema
- **B.** Erythema chronicum migrans
- **C.** Erythema gyratum repens
- **D.** Acrodermatitis enteropathica *(JIPMER 2002)*

A rare syndrome of diabetes mellitus and **necrolytic migratory erythema** in association with a pancreatic islet cell tumor was described by *McGovern* in 1966. The characteristic **glucagonoma** skin rash (**necrolytic migratory erythema**) is erythematous, raised, scaly, sometimes bullous, psoriatic, and ultimately crusted which is located primarily on the face, abdomen, perineum, and distal extremities.

252. Hypophosphatemia is *not* caused by:
- **A.** Glucocorticoid administration
- **B.** Salicylate poisoning
- **C.** Diabetic ketoacidosis
- **D.** Familial hypophosphatemia *(UP 1998)*

Causes of Hypophosphatemia

- Aldosteronism
- Licorice ingestion
- Volume expansion
- Inappropriate secretion of vasopressin
- Mineralocorticoid administration
- **Glucocorticoid administration**
- Diuretic therapy
- Polyostotic fibrous dysplasia
- Metaphyseal chondrodysplasia
- After kidney transplantation
- Oncogenic osteomalacia
- Recovery from hemolytic uremic syndrome
- Following parathyroidectomy
- Acute leukemia
- Insulin
- Glucagon
- Epinephrine
- Androgens
- Glucocorticoids
- Oral contraceptives
- Vitamin D deficiency
- Malabsorption
- Steatorrhea
- Secretory diarrhea
- Vomiting
- PO_4-binding antacids
- Renal rickets
- Fanconi syndrome
- **Familial hypophosphatemia**
- Hyperparathyroidism
- Renal tubular defects
- Recovery from hypothermia
- Burkitt's lymphoma
- Histiocytic lymphoma
- Acute myelomonocytic leukemia
- Acute myelogenous leukemia
- Treatment of pernicious anemia
- "Hungry bone" syndrome
- Glucose
- Fructose
- Glycerol
- Lactate
- Amino acids
- Xylitol
- Sepsis
- Alcohol withdrawal
- Heat stroke
- Neuroleptic malignant syndrome
- Hepatic coma
- **Salicylate poisoning**
- Gout
- Panic attacks
- Psychiatric depression

253. Reticulocyte count is *not* increased in which of the following:
- **A.** Hemorrhage
- **B.** Hemolytic anemia
- **C.** Myeloid metaplasia
- **D.** Treated iron deficiency anemia *(UP 1998)*

Idiopathic myelofibrosis (**agnogenic myeloid metaplasia** or **myelofibrosis with myeloid metaplasia**) is a clonal disorder of a multipotent hematopoietic progenitor cell of unknown etiology. It is characterized by **marrow fibrosis**, myeloid metaplasia with extramedullary hematopoiesis, and splenomegaly.

254. *True* regarding Anton syndrome is:
- **A.** Cortical blindness
- **B.** Patient denies that he is blind
- **C.** Both
- **D.** None

(UP 1998)

Visual anosognosia is also known as **Anton's syndrome** after Sir. Gabriel Anton, great German psychiatrist. It is a neurological syndrome in which **patients who cannot see deny that they are blind**. Excuses such as "It's too dark" or "my glass number is not correct" are often offered. **The lesion is in the visual area of the cortex of the brain**

255. In giardiasis, malabsorption is due to:
- **A.** Hypogammaglobulinemia
- **B.** Lactose intolerance
- **C.** Bacterial overgrowth
- **D.** Adherence of trophozoites

(UP 1998)

Giardia lamblia is a cosmopolitan protozoal parasite that inhabits the small intestines of humans and other mammals and giardiasis is one of the *most common* parasitic diseases worldwide. **Trophozoites adhere to the epithelium** but they *do not* cause invasive or locally destructive alterations. The development of lactose intolerance and significant malabsorption in a minority of infected adults and children are clinical signs of the loss of brush border enzyme activities. In most infections the morphology of the bowel is *un*altered.

256. All of the following are effective in giardiasis *except*:
- **A.** Furazolidone
- **B.** Metronidazole
- **C.** Tinidazole
- **D.** Cotrimoxazole

Drugs Useful in Giardiasis

- Metronidazole
- Tinidazole
- Furazolidone
- Quinacrine

257. All are seen in hepatorenal syndrome *except*:
- **A.** Normal renal biopsy
- **B.** Low Na^+ in urine
- **C.** Normal urinary sediments
- **D.** Normal GFR

(UP 1998)

Hepatorenal syndrome is a serious complication in the patient with cirrhosis and ascites. It is characterized by *worsening* azotemia with Na^+ retention and oliguria in the *absence* of identifiable specific causes of renal dysfunction. The kidneys are structurally intact; **urinalysis** and pyelography are **usually normal**. **Renal biopsy is also normal**. The diagnosis is supported by the demonstration of avid urinary Na^+ retention. *Typically,* **the urine sodium concentration is < 5 mmol/L**. The **urinary sediment is unremarkable**.

258. *Most common* congenital heart disease (CHD) is:
- **A.** ASD
- **B.** VSD
- **C.** TOF
- **D.** PDA

259. A patent ductus is necessary for survival for all the following conditions *except*:
- **A.** Underdeveloped aortic arch
- **B.** TGV
- **C.** Left ventricular hypoplasia
- **D.** Truncus arteriosus

(AIIMS May 2002)

Congenital heart disease (CHD) occurs in 8 per 1000 live births. **Ventricular septal defects comprise 25-30% (most common CHD)** while ASD and PDA comprise 6-8% each. Coarctation of aorta, tetralogy of fallot and pulmonary and aortic valve stenosis each account for 5-7% of CHD. Transposition of great vessels (TGV) is the *2nd most common* (TOF is the *most common* cyanotic CHD) cyanotic lesion accounting for 3-5% of all cardiac lesions. CHDs may be classified as under:

• Duct dependent *systemic* blood flow (left sided obstructive lesions)	Aortic stenosis, coarctation of aorta, interrupted aortic arch, hypoplastic left heart syndrome (HLHS).
• Duct dependent *pulmonary* blood flow	Pulmonary stenosis, pulmonary atresia with intact ventricular septum (hypoplastic right heart syndrome), tricuspid atresia, TOF, Ebstein's anomaly.
• Parallel circulation / transposition of great vessels	50% cases are associated with VSD.
• Lesions with complete intracardiac mixing of blood	Truncus arteriosus, total anomalous pulmonary venous connection, complex single ventricle.
• Left to right shunt lesions	Patent ductus arteriosus, complete atrioventricular canal, VSD.

- **Hypoplastic left heart syndrome** (HLHS) includes a number of cardiac lesions in which there is **underdevelopment of the left ventricle** and the **ascending aortic arch**. The oxygenated pulmonary *venous* blood "returns" to the left atrium and thereafter passes through an *obligatory* atrial communication (ASD or PDA) into the right side of the heart and pulmonary artery. *Systemic blood flow* is due to *retrograde* flow of blood through a patent foramen ovale (PFO). Newborns with HLHS *typically* are full term and 'well' in the nursery (they may be discharged without suspicion of a cardiac disease). Symptoms start as the *ductus arteriosus* begins to close and the child becomes gray and limp; there is poor perfusion of the body and tachypnea is due to pulmonary *over* circulation. Medical palliation for HLHS includes **PGE_1 infusion in an effort to maintain the systemic blood flow through PDA.**

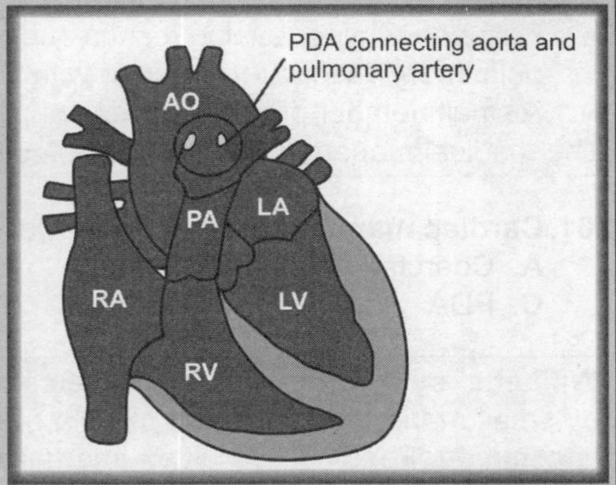

- In **transposition of great vessels** (TGV) the aorta arises from right ventricle and pulmonary artery from left ventricle. 50% of patients have an associated VSD (leading to ejection systolic murmur). In patients with an intact inter-ventricular septum a communication is *must* either as PDA or as patent foramen ovale. The *newborn is clinically cyanosed within few hours of life* due to mixing of oxygenated and deoxygenated blood. Initial management consists of:
  1. Make certain that there is adequate mixing between 2 parallel circuits by **maintaining the patency of PDA through PGE_1.**
  2. Maximization of mixed venous oxygen saturation.

  If the patient does *not* respond to the above measures foramen ovale should be enlarged by balloon atrial septostomy (*Rashkind procedure*). In this procedure a deflated balloon is inserted into a vein, passed through the foramen ovale, and then inflated and pulled vigorously through the atrial septum to enlarge the opening and improve oxygenation of the blood. Definitive management consists of surgical correction with an 'arterial switch' operation (*Jatene operation*) in *early* neonatal period.
- In **truncus arteriosus** there is a single trunk arising from the 2 ventricles which are *typically* connected via a VSD. *Typically* there is no obstruction to the pulmonary blood flow and the lungs are 'flooded'. There is tachypnea and congestive cardiac failure (CCF). Cyanosis is minimal or mild. Precordium is hyperdynamic and an ejection systolic murmur is often present. CXR demonstrates cardiomegaly with increased pulmonary vascular markings. Treatment is *surgical* closure of the VSD and creation of a right ventricle to pulmonary artery homograft.

Remembering the names of common *cyanotic* congenital heart diseases is as easy as remembering 1, 2, 3, 4 & 5.

	Common *cyanotic* congenital heart diseases (the infamous 5 Ts)
1	**T**runcus Arteriosus (1 vessel)
2	**T**ransposition of the Great Vessels (2 vessels transposed)
3	**T**ricuspid **Atresia** (3 means Tri); and pulmonary **atresia**
4	**T**etralogy of Fallot (4 means Tetra)
5	**T**otal Anomalous Pulmonary Venous Return (5=5 words)

260. All are *false* regarding VSD *except*:

A. Pulmonary oligemia in CXR
B. Small hole closes spontaneously
C. Defect is usually in muscular part
D. Endocarditis is the *most common* complication *(AIIMS 1997)*

VSD is the *most common* cardiac malformation accounting for about 25% of CHD. The **majority of defects are of the membranous portion** in a posteroinferior location, anterior to the septal leaflet of tricuspid valve. The clinical features vary according to the size of defect and the pulmonary blood flow and pressure. *Typically* there is a loud, harsh or blowing left parasternal pansystolic murmur heard best over the *lower* left sternal border and frequently accompanied by a thrill. The LR shunt is limited in the neonates and the systolic murmur may not be audible during the first few days of life. CXR is usually normal although minimal cardiomegaly and borderline **increase in pulmonary vasculature** may be observed. The natural course of VSD includes the following:

- 50% of *small* defects close spontaneously, most frequently during the first year of life. It is unusual for moderate or large defects to close spontaneously.
- A majority of children remain asymptomatic without any evidence of increase in heart size, pulmonary arterial pressure or resistance.
- Infective endocarditis occurs in **< 1% of cases.**
- Pulmonary hypertension results due to high pulmonary blood flow (PBF). A few patients will develop elevated pulmonary vascular resistance with time if the defect is not repaired.
- A small number of patients *acquire* pulmonary stenosis which "protects" the pulmonary circulation.

The medical management of *large* defects is aimed at the control of CHF.

261. Cardiac manifestation of Williams' syndrome is:

A. Coarctation of aorta
B. Endocardial cushion defect
C. PDA
D. Supravalvular aortic stenosis *(AIIMS 1998)*

Williams' syndrome (infantile hypercalcemia, elfin facies, and supravalvular aortic stenosis) is characterized by small mandible, prominent maxilla and a sharp upturned nose. The upper lip is prominent and malocclusion is common. Feeding difficulties and failure to thrive (FTT) are common during the 1st year of life. Mild mental retardation is present. **Majority of patients have supravalvular aortic stenosis** while some has mild stenosis of peripheral pulmonary arteries, hypoplasia of aorta, ASD or VSD. Some patients develop nephrocalcinosis with impaired renal function.

262. *False* regarding thymoma:

A. Hypergammaglobulinemia
B. Superior mediastinal compression syndrome
C. Pure red cell aplasia
D. Myasthenia gravis *(AI 1997)*

263. In thymoma, all are seen *except*:

A. Red cell aplasia
B. Hypoalbuminemia
C. Hypogammaglobulinemia
D. Myasthenia gravis *(AIIMS 1995, AIIMS May 2001)*

264. *Not* associated with thymoma:

A. Myasthenia gravis
B. Pure red cell aplasia
C. Hypergammaglobulinemia
D. Pemphigus *(UP 1997)*

265. Thymoma is *not* associated with:

A. Myasthenia gravis
B. Hypergammaglobulinemia
C. Isaac's syndrome
D. Pure red cell aplasia *(AI 1992, 1994, 1995, 2001)*

266. Thymoma is associated with:

A. Esophageal stricture
B. Hypergammaglobulinemia
C. Scleroderma
D. Myasthenia gravis *(AI 2000)*

267. Thymoma is *not* associated with:

A. Isaac's syndrome
B. Hypergammaglobulinemia
C. Pure red cell aplasia
D. Myasthenia gravis *(AIIMS 1994)*

Thymoma Associated Paraneoplastic Syndromes

- Myasthenia gravis: 30% of thymomas
- Encephalopathy
- Morvan's fibrillary chorea
- CRMP-5
- Pseudo-obstruction
- Cushing syndrome
- Pure red cell aplasia
- Rippling muscle syndrome
- Cerebellar: CV2 syndrome
- Pemphigus
- Hypercalcemia
- Autonomic neuropathy
- Alopecia
- Hypogammaglobulinemia
- Granulomatous myositis
- Isaac's syndrome

268. *Not* a clinical feature of tabes dorsalis:

A. Hyper-reflexia
B. Bladder incontinence
C. Argyll Robertson pupil
D. Ataxia *(AI 1995, UP 1997)*

269. *False* regarding tabes dorsalis is:

A. Posterior column involvement
B. Hyper-reflexia
C. Urinary bladder incontinence
D. Ataxia *(AI 1992)*

Tabes dorsalis is also known as **locomotor ataxia**. In this condition these is **sclerosis of the posterior columns of the spinal cord** due to infection of the CNS with *Treponema pallidum*. Inability to maintain posture when the eyes are closed and a wide-base gait are characteristic of this condition (locomotor ataxia). Sharp, stabbing pain and paresthesias are common features. **Ankle and knee jerks are diminished or lost.** Other features are pupillary changes, optic atrophy, **bladder disturbances**, and trophic ulcers, especially on the feet. The small, irregular **Argyll Robertson pupil** is a feature of *both* tabes dorsalis and paresis. Argyll Robertson pupil reacts to accommodation but not to light.

Mnemonic: In **A**rgyll **R**obertson **P**upil **A**ccommodation **R**eflex is **P**resent.

270. *False* regarding tabes dorsalis is:

A. Bilateral Argyll Robertson pupil
B. Hyper-reflexia
C. Bladder disturbance
D. Romberg's sign *(AIIMS 1997)*

The *most common* symptoms of tabes are characteristic fleeting and repetitive, lancinating pains, which occur mostly in the legs and sometimes in the back, thorax, abdomen, arms, and face. Ataxia of the legs and gait due to loss of position sense occurs in 50% of patients. Paresthesia, **bladder disturbances**, and acute abdominal pain with vomiting (**visceral crisis**) occur in 15 to 30%. The cardinal signs of tabes are **loss of reflexes** in the legs, impaired position and vibratory sense, **Romberg's sign**, and **bilateral Argyll Robertson pupils**, which fail to constrict to light but react with accommodation.

271. *Not* a clinical feature of hypertrophic cardiomyopathy:

A. Digoxin is useful
B. Irregular thickness of septum
C. Dynamic obstruction
D. Double apical impulse *(AI 1992, UP 1997)*

272. *False* regarding hypertrophic cardiomyopathy is:

A. Treatment by digoxin
B. Diastolic dysfunction
C. Sub-aortic narrowing
D. Asymmetrical septal hypertrophy *(AIIMS 1996)*

273. *False* regarding hypertrophic obstructive cardiomyopathy:

A. Asymmetrical septal hypertrophy
B. Forward flow obstruction
C. Digoxin is useful
D. Anterior motion of mitral valve *(AIIMS 1991)*

274. ***False*** **regarding hypertrophic cardiomyopathy is:**
- **A.** Digoxin is the treatment of choice
- **B.** Hallmark of obstructive HCMP is a systolic murmur
- **C.** Symptoms are not related to the presence of severity of an outflow gradient
- **D.** Most common compliant is dyspnea *(AIIMS 1997)*

Hypertrophic cardiomyopathy is characterized by left ventricular hypertrophy, typically of a *non*-dilated chamber, without obvious cause such as hypertension or aortic stenosis. The first clinical manifestation of the disease may be sudden death, *frequently* occurring in children and young adults, often during or after physical exertion. In symptomatic patients, the ***most common*** **complaint is dyspnea**. The hallmark of obstructive hypertrophic cardiomyopathy is a **systolic murmur**, which is harsh, diamond-shaped, and begins well after the 1st heart sound, since ejection is unimpeded early in systole. The murmur is best heard at the lower left sternal border as well as at the apex, where it is often more holosystolic and blowing in quality, no doubt due to the mitral regurgitation that usually accompanies obstructive **hypertrophic cardiomyopathy**. Symptoms are *not* related to the presence or severity of an outflow gradient. Competitive sports and probably strenuous activity should be prohibited. **β-adrenergic blockers often are used and may improve angina pectoris and syncope in 50% of patients. Digitalis, diuretics, nitrates, and β-adrenergic agonists are best avoided.**

275. ***False*** **regarding renal tubular acidosis is:**
- **A.** Hypokalemia
- **B.** Increased anion gap
- **C.** Acidosis
- **D.** Defective bicarbonate reabsorption *(UP 1997)*

276. ***False*** **regarding renal tubular acidosis is:**
- **A.** High urinary pH
- **B.** Hyperchloremia
- **C.** Bicarbonaturia
- **D.** Increased anion gap *(AI 1992)*

277. ***False*** **regarding renal tubular acidosis:**
- **A.** HCO_3 increases in urine
- **B.** Urine pH more than 6
- **C.** Hyperchloremic acidosis
- **D.** Reduced anion gap *(AIIMS 1991)*

In comparison to the glomerular diseases the renal tubular diseases are *rare* and due to there *non* specific and vague clinical features they are *frequently* missed by the pediatrician or detected late. RTA comprises a group of 'tubular' defects characterized by an inability to appropriately acidify the urine resulting in metabolic acidosis. The underlying abnormality consists of an **impairment of HCO_3^- reabsorption** or **excretion of H^+** or a *combination* of both. 2 major varieties of RTA are seen in children viz. distal RTA (type 1) and proximal RTA (type 2). **RTA type 1** is characterized by severe rachitic deformities, failure to thrive and features of hypokalemia. There is *persistent severe hyperchloremic metabolic acidosis* due to impaired capacity of the distal tubule to secrete H^+. The urine is alkaline with continuous bicarbonaturia. This persistent acidosis results in *buffering* of H^+ in the bones with release of Ca^{++} resulting in hypercalciuria and nephrocalcinosis. Blood pH is below 7.2; bicarbonate < 15 mmol/L; serum K^+ below 2.5 mEq/L and urine pH > 6. **Serum anion gap is normal** Hypokalemia should be corrected before correction of acidosis which is treated by administration of alkali solutions. Alkali therapy is to be continued life long.

278. Anion gap is *not* increased in:
- **A.** Diabetic ketoacidosis
- **B.** Salicylates
- **C.** Renal tubular acidosis
- **D.** Starvation *(AIIMS 1992, UP 1993)*

279. Widened anion gap is *not* seen in:
- **A.** Diabetic ketoacidosis
- **B.** Lactic acidosis
- **C.** Diarrhea
- **D.** Acute renal failure *(AI 1991, AIIMS May 2002)*

280. Normal anion gap in humans is (in mmol/L):
- **A.** 5-6
- **B.** 10-12
- **C.** 20-30
- **D.** 14-20 *(SGPGI 2002)*

288. ***Most common* malignancy of oral cavity is:**

A. Columnar cell carcinoma
B. Transitional cell carcinoma
C. Squamous cell carcinoma
D. Adenocarcinoma *(AI 1992)*

As in other regions of the upper aerodigestive system, the **majority of malignancies of the oral cavity and oropharynx are squamous cell carcinomas.**

289. Malignant transformation is *most common* in:

A. Postbulbar ulcer
B. Stromal ulcer
C. Gastric ulcer
D. Chronic duodenal ulcer *(AIIMS 1991)*

Malignant changes *only* occur in the **gastric ulcers** therefore endoscopy and biopsy is essential before starting medical treatment for an *apparently* benign gastric ulcer.

290. In hemolytic anemia, gallstones are:

A. Oxalate stone
B. Mixed stone
C. Cholesterol stone
D. Pigment stone *(UP 1993)*

Chronic hemolytic states or alcoholic liver disease are associated with an *increased incidence of pigment stones.*

291. In keloid, best treatment is:

A. Wide excision
B. Wide excision and radiotherapy
C. Intralesional steroid
D. Intralesional excision *(AIIMS 1994)*

292. ***True* regarding keloid is:**

A. Common in old people
B. Continues to get worse even after 1 year
C. Appears few days after surgery
D. Appears immediately after surgery *(JIPMER 1995)*

True keloid in white people is a *rare* condition and the *only* common site is **over the sternum.** True keloid spreads into the normal tissue not affected by original injury or operation however in many scars it is very difficult to determine with certainty that whether it is hypertrophic scar or keloid. **Hypertrophic scar never get worse after 6 months but a true keloid continues to get worse even after a year or sometimes up to 10 years.** Many keloids are untreatable and *only* surgical treatment is generally unsuccessful. Some keloids improve by pressure application and in some intralesional injections of steroids such as triamcinolone may be helpful. However, **the best cure rate is achieved by a combination of surgery and postoperative interstitial radiotherapy.**

293. What percent of patients with perforated peptic ulcer will show free gas under the diaphragm:

A. 100
B. 70
C. 50
D. 90

294. In peptic ulcer perforation the *investigation of choice* is:

A. CT scan
B. Ultrasonography
C. X-ray abdomen
D. Paracentesis *(KERALA 1994)*

Perforation of peptic ulcer is 8 times more common in men than in women and *most often* the ulcer that perforates is situated on the **anterior surface of duodenum. Plain X ray of abdomen** in erect position will reveal a translucent area under the right cupola of diaphragm in 70% of cases.

295. ***Not* a treatment modality of carcinoma prostate:**

A. Flutamide
B. Leuprolide
C. Bicalutamide
D. Somatostatin analogue *(PGI 1997)*

RBC counts are raised in 2 conditions:
- Traumatic lumbar puncture
- Subarachnoid hemorrhage

* Low chloride is seen in tubercular meningitis due to chloride loss as a result of protracted vomiting and is *not specific* for tubercular meningitis.

287. *Not* a characteristic CSF change in acute pyogenic meningitis:
A. Reduction of C reactive protein
B. Polymorphonuclear leukocytes
C. Marked fall in sugar content
D. Rise in protein content
(UP 1997)

288. In pyogenic meningitis the CSF finding is:
A. Increased chloride and increased glucose
B. Increased protein and increased glucose
C. Less glucose and more protein
D. CSF contains no organism
(AI 1993, 1996, 1998)

CSF Findings

	Appearance	Pressure	Cells	Protein	Sugar
Normal	Watery	100-180 mm of CSF	0-5 all lymphocytes	20-40 mg%	40-80 mg%
Acute bacterial meningitis	Turbid	Raised	100-5000 **Neutrophil** predominant	**100-400mg%**	**Low Organism may be seen**
Tubercular meningitis	Clear or cloudy	Raised	10-500 Lymphocyte predominant	80-400 mg% or more	Low Organism may be seen
Viral encephalitis	Clear	Normal	20-2000 Lymphocyte predominant	150 mg%	Normal C/S sterile

289. The *most common* cause of Addison's disease is:
A. Autoimmune etiology
B. Tuberculosis
C. Metastatic carcinoma
D. Meningococcal septicemia
(AIIMS May 2002)

290. Feature of Addison's disease is:
A. Hypoglycemia
B. Hypokalemia
C. Hypernatremia
D. Decreased serum bicarbonates
(UP 1997)

291. *Characteristic* feature of Addison's disease is:
A. Hypernatremia
B. Hypokalemia
C. Hypoglycemia
D. Hypertension
(AI 1993)

Primary adrenocortical deficiency or **Addison's disease** results from progressive destruction of the adrenals, which must involve more than 90% of the glands before adrenal insufficiency appears. ***Now* the most frequent cause is idiopathic atrophy, and an autoimmune mechanism is probably responsible.** It is characterized by an insidious onset of fatigability, weakness, anorexia, nausea and vomiting, weight loss, cutaneous and mucosal pigmentation, **hypotension**, and occasionally **hypoglycemia. Serum Na^+, Cl^-, and HCO_3^- levels are reduced, and the serum K^+ level is elevated.** All patients with adrenal insufficiency should receive specific hormone replacement. *Hydrocortisone* is the mainstay of treatment and the dose for most adults is 20 to 30 mg/day. As the replacement dosage of hydrocortisone *does not* replace the mineralocorticoid component of the adrenal hormones, mineralocorticoid supplementation is also needed. This is usually done by the administration of 0.05 to 0.1 mg *fludrocortisone* per day by mouth. Patients also should be instructed to maintain a generous intake of sodium (3 to 4 g/ day).

292. ***Most common* presentation of primary hyperparathyroidism is:**
A. Myopathy
B. Asymptomatic hypocalcemia
C. Asymptomatic hypercalcemia
D. Nephrolithiasis
(UP 1998)

Primary hyperparathyroidism is a generalized disorder of calcium, phosphate, and bone metabolism due to an increased secretion of parathyroid hormone which usually leads to hypercalcemia and hypophosphatemia. **The diagnosis is frequently made in patients who have no symptoms (asymptomatic)** and minimal, *if any*, signs of the disease other than **hypercalcemia** and elevated levels of PTH.

293. ***False* regarding Ménétrier's disease is:**
A. Hypergastrinemia
B. Protein losing gastropathy
C. Foveolar hypertrophy
D. Most common symptom is epigastric pain
(UP 1998)

Ménétrier's disease is a clinical entity characterized by large, tortuous gastric mucosal folds, which may be localized or may involve the whole stomach. The mucosal thickening is due to **massive foveolar hyperplasia** (hyperplasia of surface and glandular mucous cells). The *most common* symptom is **epigastric pain**. Patients often develop a **protein-losing gastropathy** resulting in hypoalbuminemia and edema.

294. ***Not* a presenting feature of Ménétrier's disease:**
A. Anorexia
B. Constipation
C. Edema
D. Weight loss
(KARNATAKA 2000)

The most common symptom of **Ménétrier's disease** is epigastric pain. **Anorexia**, nausea, vomiting, and **weight loss** are less frequent. Patients often develop a protein-losing gastropathy resulting in hypoalbuminemia and **edema**.

295. Fatal familial insomnia is associated with:
A. Vascular disease
B. Neoplastic disease
C. Degenerative disease
D. Prion disease
(AI 1999)

296. Creutzfeldt-Jakob disease is caused by:
A. Riluzole used for treatment
B. Prion
C. JC virus
D. Nonspongiform change
(PGI 1999)

297. Kuru is caused by:
A. Chlamydia
B. Virus
C. Protozoan
D. Prion
(UP 1998)

Human Prion Diseases

- Kuru
- Creutzfeldt-Jakob disease (CJD)
- Gerstmann-Sträussler-Scheinker (GSS) syndrome
- Fatal familial insomnia

298. ***Most common* malignancy seen in AIDS patients is:**
A. Renal cell carcinoma
B. Colon carcinoma
C. Lymphoma
D. Kaposi's sarcoma
(AI 1992, UP 1998)

299. All are HIV associated malignancies *except*:
A. Kaposi's sarcoma
B. Lung carcinoma
C. Non-Hodgkin Lymphoma
D. Anogenital carcinoma
(PGI May 2001)

A variety of neoplastic and premalignant diseases occur with increased frequency in HIV-infected patients (**Kaposi's sarcoma**, lymphoma, and intraepithelial dysplasia of the cervix and anus).

300. ***Drug of choice* in acute migraine is:**
A. Pizotifen
B. Methysergide
C. Clonidine
D. Ergotamine

306. *Earliest* manifestation of upper limb ischemia is:

A. Rest pain
B. Gangrene of fingers
C. Claudication
D. Pain in the passive hyperextension of finger *(UP 1998)*

The high risk injuries for **Volkmann's ischemia** are fractures of the elbow, forearm bones, and proximal 1/3rd of tibia. *Classical features of ischemia are 5 Ps viz. Pain, Paresthesia, Pallor, Paralysis and Pulselessness.* The **earliest of these classical features to appear is pain** and it is *criminal* to wait for all of them to be present without intervention. The ischemic muscle is highly sensitive to stretch therefore if the limb is unduly painful, swollen or tense the muscle should be tested by stretching (*when toes or fingers are* ***passively hyperextended*** *there is increased pain in the forearm or calf*). It should be kept in mind that *the presence of pulse* ***does not*** *exclude the diagnosis of Volkmann's ischemia*.

307. Fournier's gangrene occurs in the:

A. Toes **B.** Scrotum
C. Fingers **D.** Muscles

Necrotizing fasciitis caused by mixed aerobic-anaerobic bacteria is responsible for Fournier's gangrene. Leakage into the perineal area results in a so called **Fournier's gangrene**, which is characterized by massive swelling of the **scrotum** and penis extending into the perineum or the abdominal wall and legs.

308. Paget's disease of nipple should be treated with:

A. Irradiation **B.** Mastectomy
C. 5 FU **D.** Antibiotic cream *(AIIMS 1991)*

Treatment of Paget's disease of the nipple is **mastectomy** and in the absence of a palpable lump in the breast the prognosis is good.

309. Definitive operation for transposition of great vessels was:

A. Rashkind procedure **B.** Mustard's procedure
C. Aortic pulmonary window **D.** Tausig Blalock procedure

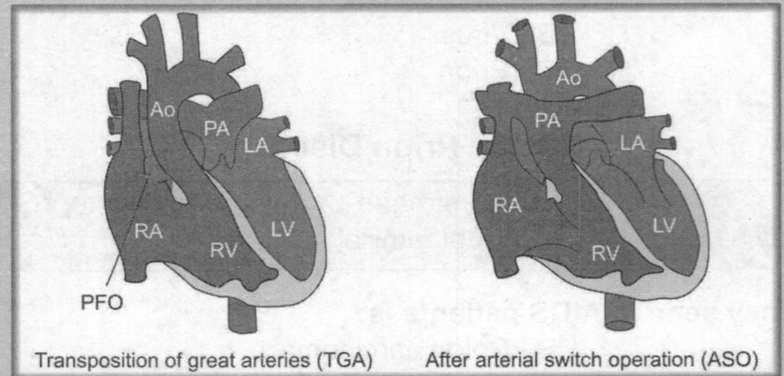

Transposition of great arteries (TGA) After arterial switch operation (ASO)

In **transposition of great arteries** (TGA) the aorta arises from right ventricle and pulmonary artery from left ventricle. 50% of patients have an associated VSD (leading to *ejection systolic murmur*). In patients with an intact interventricular septum a communication is *must* either as PDA or as patent foramen ovale (PFO). The **newborn is clinically cyanosed within few hours of life** due to mixing of oxygenated and deoxygenated blood. Initial management consists of:

1. Make certain that there is adequate mixing between two parallel circuits.
2. Maximization of mixed venous oxygen saturation.

If the patient does not respond to the above measures foramen ovale should be enlarged by balloon atrial septostomy (*Rashkind procedure*). In this procedure a deflated balloon is inserted into a vein, passed through the foramen ovale, and then inflated and pulled vigorously through the atrial septum to enlarge the opening and improve oxygenation of the blood. **Definitive management consists of surgical correction with an arterial switch operation (ASO) in early neonatal period.** Mustard's procedure was previously used.

310. *Not* a feature of bulbar urethra injury:

A. Fracture of pelvic | **B.** Retention of urine
C. Urethral hemorrhage | **D.** Perineal hematoma *(UP 1997)*

Rupture of urethra can be divided into 2 varieties namely rupture of bulbous urethra and rupture of membranous (intrapelvic) urethra. Each variety is again subdivided into *complete and incomplete forms* (which refer to circumference of the urethral wall) and *total and partial* (which refer to thickness of the urethral walls). **Rupture of bulbous urethra** is the more common injury and in *each and every case* there is history of fall on a projecting object. The classical **triad of signs** includes **retention of urine, urethral hemorrhage, and a perineal hematoma**. The *most common* cause of rupture of membranous (intrapelvic) urethra in civilian life is **pelvic fracture.**

311. Deficiency of which of the following element is *not* seen with hyperalimentation:

A. Magnesium | **B.** Potassium
C. Calcium | **D.** Phosphate *(JIPMER 1993)*

Biochemical Complications of Parenteral Nutrition

- Hyponatremia
- Hypokalemia
- Hypomagnesemia
- Hypophosphatemia
- Hypoglycemia
- Azotemia
- Hyperammonemia
- Hyper-osmolar dehydration
- Hyperglycemia

312. Tietze's syndrome usually develops at which of the following costal cartilage:

A. 2nd | **B.** 6th
C. 8th | **D.** 4th

Tietze's syndrome is a common, painful and nonsuppurative swelling of the **2nd or 3rd costal cartilages.** This is a self-limiting disease for which no cause is known. The pain may be confused with that of MI. There is no specific therapy, but some relief is provided by injecting the area with local anesthetics and corticosteroids.

313. Virchow's lymph nodes are:

A. Mediastinal | **B.** Axillary
C. Right supraclavicular | **D.** Left supraclavicular *(UP 1994)*

Virchow's node is an enlarged **left supraclavicular node** which is infiltrated with metastatic cancer from a gastrointestinal primary.

314. In which of the following condition, "strawberry gallbladder" is seen:

A. Cholesterolosis | **B.** Adenomyomatosis
C. Porcelain gallbladder | **D.** Gangrene of gallbladder *(JIPMER 1991)*

Cholesterolosis is a condition characterized by abnormal deposition of lipid, mainly cholesterol esters, in the lamina propria of the gallbladder wall. When the deposition is diffused the gallbladder is known as "**strawberry gallbladder**"; the gallbladder mucosa is brick red and speckled with bright yellow flecks of lipid. The localized variety demonstrates solitary or multiple "cholesterol polyps" studding the gallbladder wall. Cholesterol stones of the gallbladder are found in 50% of case.

315. Burst abdomen *most commonly* occurs on the:

A. 2nd day | **B.** 5th day
C. 7th day | **D.** 9th day

Burst abdomen or abdominal dehiscence is seen in 1-2% of laparotomy wounds mostly between the **6th and 8th day** of the operation. A serosanguineous (pink) discharge from the wound is a predecessor of disruption. It is the most *pathognomic* sign of impending wound disruption and it signifies that intraperitoneal contents are lying extraperitoneally.

311. Ranson criterion is used in:
- **A.** Gallstone ileus
- **B.** Acute appendicitis
- **C.** Acute cholecystitis
- **D.** Acute pancreatitis

(UP 2001)

312. *Not* included in the Ranson criteria for the prognosis of acute pancreatitis:
- **A.** Serum amylase > 350 IU
- **B.** AST > 250 IU/L
- **C.** Age > 55 years
- **D.** WBC > 16,000 cells/mm^3

(AI 1998)

313. *Not* a prognostic marker in acute pancreatitis:
- **A.** Hypocalcemia
- **B.** Increased LDH
- **C.** Leukocytosis
- **D.** Decreased serum lipase

(AIIMS May 2001)

It is important to identify patients with **acute pancreatitis** who have an increased risk of mortality. **Ranson** and Imrie have used multiple prognostic criteria and have established that there is an increased mortality rate when 3 or more risk factors are present either at the time of admission to the hospital or during the initial 48 hours of hospitalization.

RANSON - IMRIE CRITERIA
At admission or diagnosis
• Age > 55 years • Leukocytosis more than 16,000/μL • Hyperglycemia more than 200 mg/dL • Serum LDH more than 400 IU/L • Serum AST more than 250 IU/L
During initial 48 hours
• Fall in hematocrit by more than 10% • Fluid deficit of more than 4000 mL • Hypocalcemia [calcium concentration **less than** 8.0 mg/dL] • Hypoxemia (PO_2 less than 60 mmHg) • Increase in blood urea nitrogen to more than 5 mg/dL after IV fluid administration • Hypoalbuminemia (albumin level less than 3.2 g/dL)

314. Acute pancreatitis *cannot* occur in:
- **A.** Hypocalcemia
- **B.** Alcoholism
- **C.** Hereditary pancreatitis
- **D.** Hypercalcemia

(UP 2001)

315. *Not* a cause of acute pancreatitis:
- **A.** Hypercalcemia
- **B.** Hemochromatosis
- **C.** Gallstone
- **D.** Alcohol

(AI 1994)

316. Causes of pancreatitis are all the following *except*:
- **A.** Cystic fibrosis
- **B.** Chronic alcoholism
- **C.** Hypocalcemia
- **D.** CBD stone

(SGPGI 2002)

Some Causes of Acute Pancreatitis

Alcohol ingestion	Trauma
Biliary tract disease (**gallstones**)	Hypertriglyceridemia
Postoperative state (after abdominal or nonabdominal operation)	Apolipoprotein CII deficiency syndrome
Endoscopic retrograde cholangiopancreatography (ERCP)	**Hypercalcemia** (e.g., hyperparathyroidism), drug-induced
Hereditary pancreatitis	Renal failure
Mumps	After renal transplantation
Viral hepatitis	Acute fatty liver of pregnancy
Ascariasis	Coxsackievirus
Mycobacterium avium complex (MAC)	Echovirus
Infections with *Mycoplasma, Campylobacter,* other bacteria	Cytomegalovirus
Azathioprine, 6-mercaptopurine	Ischemic-hypoperfusion state (after cardiac surgery)
Sulfonamides	Atherosclerotic emboli
Thiazide diuretics	Systemic lupus erythematosus
Furosemide	Necrotizing angiitis
Estrogens (oral contraceptives)	Thrombotic thrombocytopenic purpura
Tetracycline	Penetrating peptic ulcer
Valproic acid	Obstruction of the ampulla of Vater
Pentamidine	Regional enteritis
Dideoxyinosine	Duodenal diverticulum
Hypertriglyceridemia	Pancreatic cancer
Sphincter of Oddi dysfunction	**Cystic fibrosis**
Truly idiopathic	Pancreas divisum

317. Organism which causes pancreatitis:

A. Measles **B.** Mumps
C. Influenza **D.** Herpes

Infectious Causes of Acute Pancreatitis

- *Mumps*
- Viral hepatitis
- Coxsackievirus, echovirus, cytomegalovirus
- Ascariasis
- *Mycoplasma*, *Campylobacter*, *Mycobacterium avium* complex.

318. All are *false* regarding Klinefelter's syndrome *except*:

A. Subnormal intelligence
B. Subluxation of lens
C. Cataract
D. Short stature *(AIIMS 1991)*

319. *Not* a clinical feature of Klinefelter's syndrome:

A. *Oligospermia* **B.** Gynecomastia
C. Diabetes mellitus **D.** 47 X X Y *(UP 2001)*

329. In a patient of fracture of 10–12th ribs, the cause of hypotension is:
A. Intercostal artery damage **B.** Aortic damage
C. Pulmonary contusion **D.** Abdominal viscera injury *(AIIMS 1999)*

330. *Not* a radiological sign of splenic rupture:
A. Elevated left dome of diaphragm **B.** Obliteration of splenic shadow
C. Obliteration of psoas shadow **D.** Upper rib fracture *(UP 2001)*

Weight of normal adult spleen is 150 gm. **Absence of spleen** is a rare condition but when it occurs it is often associated with congenital heart disease (**Ivemask syndrome**). **Splenunculi** are single or multiple accessory spleens found near the **hilum of spleen (50% cases)**, related to splenic vessels and behind the tail of pancreas (30%) or in the splenic ligament and mesocolon. *Essential lesion in Hereditary spherocytosis is an increase in permeability of the RBC membrane to the Na^+ and chronic ulcers of the leg can occur.* **The standard treatment of hereditary spherocytosis is splenectomy** *which should ideally be done at the age of 7 years.* **Kehr's sign** is pain referred to the **left shoulder** associated with hyperesthesia in that region (*seen in splenic rupture*). **Ballance's sign** is positive in 25% of cases. The radiological signs of splenic rupture are as under:

• Obliteration of the splenic outline	• Obliteration of the psoas shadow
• Indentation of the left side of the gastric air bubble	• **Fracture of lower rib or ribs** on left side (27% cases)
• Elevation of left side of diaphragm	• Free fluid between gas filled intestinal coils

Immediate laparotomy and splenectomy along with blood transfusion is the treatment of choice.

331. *False* regarding malignant melanoma is:
A. Most common type is superficial spreading melanoma
B. Stage IIB has satellite deposits
C. Acral-lentiginous melanoma has good prognosis
D. Lentigo maligna melanoma is least common *(AI 1997)*

332. Which of the following is the *most severe* form of malignant melanoma:
A. Those in choroid **B.** Those arising in lower limb
C. Nodular infiltrating type **D.** Superficially spreading *(KERALA 1994)*

• **Superficial spreading melanomas**	Most common variety (64%); can occur on any part of body and are usually > 0.5 mm in diameter; usually palpable
• **Nodular melanoma**	**Most malignant form** (12%); common in younger age groups
• **Lentigo maligna melanoma**	Also known as Hutchinson's melanotic freckle; least common type (7–15%); common on the face of old people.
• **Acral-lentiginous melanoma**	Found on palms and soles; most common type of melanoma found in Japanese population; **prognosis is poor** like that of nodular melanoma.
• **Amelanotic melanoma**	Pink in color; worse prognosis than nodular; may present with lymph node metastasis.

STAGING OF MALIGNANT MELANOMA

Primary	Breslow thickness	Clark's level
$_pT_{is}$	Melanoma *in situ*	I
$_pT_1$	Melanoma < 0.75 mm	II
$_pT_2$	Melanoma 0.76–1.5 mm	III
$_pT_3$	Melanoma 1.51–4.0 mm	And/or IV
$_pT_4$	Melanoma 4 mm and/or satellites within 2 cm of primary	And/or V

326. *False* regarding tricuspid atresia is:

A. *Decreased* pulmonary blood supply is seen in PA view of CXR
B. Right ventricular hypoplasia
C. Fixed split S_2
D. Left axis deviation *(AIIMS 1998, UP 2000)*

Tricuspid atresia is characterized by atresia of the tricuspid valve, patent foramen ovale (PFO), and **hypoplasia of the right ventricle** and pulmonary artery. The patient has **severe cyanosis** due to *compulsory* mixing of systemic and pulmonary venous blood in the left ventricle. CXR shows pulmonary under-circulation. The ECG *characteristically* shows right atrial enlargement, **left axis deviation**, and **left ventricular hypertrophy**. *Atrial septostomy* and palliative operations to increase pulmonary blood flow may allow survival to the 2nd or 3rd decade. A *Fontan atriopulmonary* connection may then allow "functional" correction.

327. Major criteria for AIDS *does not* includes:

A. Weight loss > 10%
B. Persistent diarrhea
C. Persistent cough
D. Persistent fever *(UP 2001)*

For the purposes of AIDS surveillance an adult or adolescent (>12 years of age) is considered to have AIDS if at least 2 of the following major signs are present in combination with at least 1 of the minor signs:

Major signs	Minor signs
• Weight loss >/= 10% of body weight • Chronic diarrhea for more than 1 month • Prolonged fever for more than 1 month (intermittent or constant)	• Persistent cough for more than 1 month [a,b] • Generalized pruritic dermatitis • History of herpes zoster [b] • Oropharyngeal candidiasis • Chronic progressive or disseminated herpes simplex infection • Generalized lymphadenopathy

[a] For patients with tuberculosis, persistent cough for more than 1 month should *not* be considered as minor sign.

[b] Indicates changes from the 1985 provisional WHO clinical case definition for AIDS.

328. Diameter of normal mitral valve orifice is:

A. 6-8 cm^2
B. 4-6 cm^2
C. 1 cm^2
D. 2-4 cm^2 *(AIIMS 1994)*

329. Left ventricular dysfunction is seen in:

A. Aortic regurgitation
B. Aortic stenosis
C. Mitral regurgitation
D. Mitral stenosis *(UP 1999)*

330. Left ventricular hypertrophy is *not* seen in:

A. MS
B. AS
C. Aortic incompetence
D. Essential hypertension *(KARNATAKA 2000)*

Mitral stenosis is generally rheumatic in origin and only *rarely*, it is congenital. 66% of all patients with mitral stenosis are females. **In normal adults the mitral valve orifice is 4 to 6 cm^2**. In the presence of significant obstruction, i.e., when the orifice is less than approximately 2 cm^2, blood can flow from the left atrium to the left ventricle only if propelled by an abnormally elevated left atrioventricular pressure gradient; the hemodynamic hallmark of mitral stenosis. **Left ventricular dysfunction**, as reflected in reduced ejection fraction, occurs in about 25% of patients with severe, chronic mitral stenosis. When the ECG shows **left ventricular hypertrophy**, it indicates that an additional lesion which places a significant burden on the left ventricle, such as **mitral regurgitation**, **aortic valve disease**, or **hypertension**, is present.

331. Lung carcinoma with *worst* prognosis is:

A. Large cell carcinoma
B. Small cell carcinoma
C. Adenocarcinoma
D. Epidermoid *(UP 1999)*

Histologic type of thoracic malignancy	5-year survival rate
• Adenocarcinoma (and all subtypes)	17
• Bronchioloalveolar carcinoma	42
• Squamous cell (epidermoid) carcinoma	15
• **Small cell carcinoma**	**5**
• Large cell carcinoma	11
• Carcinoid	83
• Mucoepidermoid carcinoma	39
• Adenoid cystic carcinoma	48
• Sarcoma and other soft tissue tumors	30
Total	**14**

332. ***False*** **regarding Gaucher's disease is:**

A. Hepatomegaly
B. Autosomal dominant inheritance
C. No neurological symptoms in adult form
D. β-glucosidase deficiency *(UP 1999)*

Gaucher's disease is a multisystemic lipidosis characterized by hematologic troubles, organomegaly, and skeletal involvement. It usually manifests as bone pain and pathologic fractures. It is the *most common* lysosomal storage disease. The 3 clinical subtypes are divided on the basis of *absence or presence and progression of neurologic manifestations* viz. **type 1, the adult, non-neuronopathic form**; type 2, the infantile or acute neuronopathic form; and type 3, the juvenile or Norrbotten form. All 3 are inherited as **autosomal recessive traits**. It results from deficiency of the lysosomal hydrolase, **acid β-glucosidase**, encoded by a gene on chromosome 1 (q21 to q31). Most patients of type 1 disease are symptomatic by adolescence. Features include easy bruisability due to thrombocytopenia, chronic fatigue due to anemia, **hepatomegaly** with or without elevated LFT, splenomegaly, bone pain, and occasional lung involvement. Bone involvement, which occurs in > 20% of patients, can cause pain or pathologic fractures or be manifested only by radiologic findings, including Erlenmeyer flask deformities of the distal femur. The **pathologic hallmark of the disease is the Gaucher's cell** in the RE system, particularly in the bone marrow.

333. ***False*** **regarding Kawasaki's disease is:**

A. Generally benign and self limiting **B.** Coronary artery aneurysm
C. Occurs > 5 years of age **D.** Fever *(UP 1999)*

334. ***Not*** **a characteristic feature of Kawasaki's disease:**

A. Desquamation of skin of finger and toes
B. Cervical lymphadenopathy
C. Thrombocytopenia
D. Conjunctival effusion *(UP 2000)*

335. ***Not*** **a feature of Kawasaki's disease:**

A. Desquamation of skin of finger and toes
B. Coronary artery aneurysm
C. Thrombocytopenia
D. Conjunctival effusion *(AIIMS 1997)*

336. Kawasaki's disease is treated with:

A. Chemotherapy
B. IV glucocorticoids
C. Oral glucocorticoids
D. Immunotherapy *(AI 2001)*

Mucocutaneous lymph node syndrome or **Kawasaki's disease** is an acute, **febrile**, multi-system disease of **children under 5 years of age**, characterized by *un*responsiveness to antibiotics, nonsuppurative **cervical adenitis**, and changes in the skin and mucous membranes such as edema, **congested conjunctivae**, erythema of the oral cavity, lips, and palms, and **desquamation of the skin of the fingertips**. **Disease is generally benign and self-limiting** but it is associated with **coronary artery aneurysms** (between the 3rd and 4th weeks of illness) in about 25% of cases, with an overall case fatality rate (CFR) of 0.5 to 2.8%. There is polymorphonuclear leukocytosis, thrombo*cytosis* and elevated CRP and ESR. **Aspirin** (100 mg/kg/day qid) is used for control of fever and acute symptom. *Later on* aspirin should be continued in a dose of 5 mg/kg/day OD as an antithrombotic agent for 6 to 8 weeks. IV **γ-globulin** within the 1st 10 days of illness reduces the occurrence of coronary artery aneurysm.

337. Sudden pain in thyroid nodule indicates:

A. Malignant change
B. Hemorrhage
C. Infarction
D. Necrosis

(UP 1999)

Sudden hemorrhage into a **nodule** may lead to an acute, **painful swelling** in the neck and may produce or enhance compressive symptoms.

338. Kussmaul's breathing is due to presence of:

A. Bicarbonate
B. H^+ ions (*acidosis*)
C. Chloride ions
D. K^+ ions

339. Kussmaul's breathing is seen in:

A. Metabolic acidosis
B. Metabolic alkalosis
C. Respiratory alkalosis
D. Respiratory acidosis

(UP 1999)

Metabolic acidosis can occur due to an increase in endogenous acid production (such as lactate and ketoacids), loss of HCO_3^- (as in diarrhea), or accumulation of endogenous acids (as in renal failure). Metabolic acidosis has profound effects on the respiratory system, CVS, and CNS. The fall in blood pH is associated with a characteristic increase in ventilation, especially tidal volume (**Kussmaul's respiration**).

340. Initial treatment of Shy-Drager syndrome is:

A. β-blockers
B. Prazosin
C. Fludrocortisone
D. None of the above

(UP 1999)

Shy-Drager syndrome is a well-characterized severe form of **multiple system atrophy** that is accompanied by *autonomic failure*. Most patients present with autonomic dysfunction *alone*, and other neurologic manifestations usually develop within 5 years. Chronic orthostatic hypotension results due to primary autonomic nervous system insufficiency. Most patients require drug therapy for management of hypotension. **Fludrocortisone**, which enhances renal Na^+ conservation and increases the sensitivity of arterioles to norepinephrine, is **the initial drug of choice.** Other drugs have been used with variable success to elevate blood pressure. These include β-blockers (propranolol, pindolol, and xamoterol), sympathomimetics (ephedrine, midodrine), dopamine antagonists (metoclopramide), and venoconstrictors (dihydroergotamine).

341. Cardiomyopathy is seen in:

A. Rheumatoid arthritis
B. Holt-Oram syndrome
C. Friedreich's ataxia
D. Refsum's disease

(UP 1999)

342. *Most common* cardiac anomaly in Friedreich's ataxia is:

A. Cardiomyopathy
B. Conduction defect
C. Mitral stenosis
D. Patent ductus arteriosus

(UP 1999)

343. Bilateral absent ankle jerk with extensor planter reflex is seen in:

A. Ataxia telangiectasia
B. Syringomyelia
C. Upper motor neuron lesion
D. Friedreich's ataxia

(AIIMS 1998)

Friedreich's ataxia is the most common form of inherited ataxia, comprising one-half of all hereditary ataxias. It presents before 25 years of age with progressive staggering gait, frequent falling, and titubation (a coarse and backward tremor of the trunk). The lower extremities are more severely affected than the upper ones. Dysarthria may be the presenting symptom, and rarely progressive scoliosis, foot deformity, nystagmus, or **cardiopathy** is *initial* signs. **Extensor plantar responses** (with *normal* tone in trunk and extremities), **absent deep tendon reflexes**, and weakness (greater distally than proximally) are frequently found. Loss of vibratory and proprioceptive sensation is seen.

344. Titubation is characteristic of lesion in:

A. Basal ganglia
B. Motor cortex
C. Cerebellum
D. ARAS

Titubation (Latin: *titubatio*, staggering) may be defined as a coarse and backward tremor of the trunk. In patients with **cerebellar disease**, standing provokes this tremor.

345. Hallmark of polymorphic ventricular tachycardia is:

A. Short QT interval
B. Prolonged QT interval
C. Short PR interval
D. Prolonged PR interval

(KARNATAKA 2000)

Terfenadine, astemizole, and cisapride can cause **polymorphic ventricular tachycardia** (**torsade de pointes**) when their metabolism is blocked by inhibitors of CYP3A, such as ketoconazole, itraconazole, and erythromycin.

346. Torsades de pointes are seen in:

A. Metabolic acidosis
B. Hypomagnesemia/hypokalemia
C. Hypermagnesemia
D. Metabolic alkalosis

(UP 1999)

347. In Torsades de pointes the ECG finding is:

A. Short QT interval
B. Short QRS interval
C. Prolonged QT interval
D. Prolonged QRS interval

(AIIMS 1997)

Torsades de pointes (*twisting of the points*) or **polymorphic ventricular tachycardia** is ventricular tachycardia characterized by polymorphic QRS complexes that change in amplitude and cycle length, giving the impression of oscillations around the baseline. **This rhythm is always associated with QT prolongation**. QT prolongation may result from electrolyte disturbances (such as **hypokalemia** and **hypomagnesemia**), use of antiarrhythmic drugs (mainly quinidine), phenothiazines and tricyclic antidepressants, liquid protein diets, intracranial events, and bradyarrhythmias, mainly 3rd-degree AV block. It also may occur as an isolated *idiopathic* congenital or acquired anomaly.

348. *Not* a blood borne disease:

A. Hepatitis E
B. Hepatitis D
C. Hepatitis C
D. Hepatitis B

(UP 1999)

349. *False* regarding hepatitis E is:

A. No carrier state
B. High mortality in pregnant women
C. May produce chronic hepatic disease
D. Fecal-oral transmission

(UP 2001)

350. *Most common* route of spread in hepatitis E is:

A. IV injection
B. Intercourse
C. Fecal oral
D. Blood transfusion

(AI 1993)

351. Most dangerous hepatitis in pregnancy is:

A. Hepatitis E
B. Hepatitis C
C. Hepatitis A
D. Hepatitis B

(AIIMS 1995)

352. ***True* regarding hepatitis E is:**

A. Seen in post-transfusion cases
B. Increase mortality in pregnancy
C. Alpha interferon given for carriers
D. Associated with hepatitis B *(AIIMS 1998)*

- All cases of acute viral hepatitis are caused by 1 of 5 viral agents' viz. hepatitis A virus, hepatitis B virus, hepatitis C virus, the HBV-associated delta agent or hepatitis D virus, and **hepatitis E** virus. A 6th agent, hepatitis G virus, has been discovered in 1996 but its role in acute viral hepatitis is still to be established. **All these human hepatitis viruses are RNA viruses, *except* for hepatitis B, which is a DNA virus.** All types of viral hepatitis produce clinically similar diseases which range from asymptomatic and inapparent to fulminant and fatal acute infections. **Bloodborne types (HBV, HCV, and HDV)** may also present with sub-clinical *persistent infections* to rapidly progressive chronic liver disease with cirrhosis and even hepatocellular carcinoma.
- **Hepatitis E virus is an enterically transmitted virus** that occurs primarily in India, Asia, Africa, and Central America. No case of chronic disease has been reported so far. **HEV has a propensity to induce a fulminating form of acute disease particularly in pregnant women; up to 20% of whom may develop fulminating hepatitis.**

353. Dane particle pertains to:

A. HAV
B. HNAB
C. HBV
D. None

The hepatitis B virus is a DNA virus. It is also known as Dane particle.

354. ***Best* means of giving hepatitis B vaccine is:**

A. Subcutaneous
B. Intradermal
C. Intramuscular gluteal
D. Intramuscular deltoid

For *pre*exposure prophylaxis against hepatitis B, 3 **intramuscular** injection of hepatitis B vaccine in **deltoid region** should be given on 0, 1, and 6 months.

355. Incubation period of hepatitis B is:

A. 4 weeks to 6 months
B. 6 days to 6weeks
C. 6 months to 6years
D. > 6 years

Incubation Period of Hepatitis

• **Hepatitis A**	15 to 45 days
• **Hepatitis B**	30 to 180 days
• **Hepatitis D**	30 to 180 days
• **Hepatitis C**	15 to 160 days
• **Hepatitis E**	14 to 60 days

356. Korsakoff's psychosis is due to involvement of:

A. Nondominant cerebral hemispheres
B. Dominant hemispheres
C. Both A and B
D. Either of temporal lobe *(UP 1999)*

Korsakoff's psychosis is frequently persistent and the residual mental state and is characterized by gaps in memory, confabulation, and disordered **temporal sequencing**.

357. Unconjugated hyperbilirubinemia is seen in all the following *except*:

A. Crigler-Najjar syndrome
B. Dubin-Johnson syndrome
C. Breast milk jaundice
D. Gilbert's syndrome *(SGPGI 2002)*

358. *Most severe* hyperbilirubinemia occurs in:
A. Dubin-Johnson syndrome
B. Crigler-Najjar syndrome type I
C. Crigler-Najjar syndrome type II
D. Gilbert's syndrome *(UP 1999)*

Syndrome		Enzyme deficient	Bilirubin
Crigler-Najjar-1	AR	*Absent* glucuronyl transferase	Unconjugated **> 20 mg/dL**
Crigler-Najjar-2	AD	Decreased glucuronyl transferase	Unconjugated < 20 mg/dL
Gilbert's syndrome	AD	Decreased glucuronyl transferase with decreased hepatic uptake	Unconjugated < 6 mg/dL
Dubin-Johnson syndrome	AR	Impaired biliary secretion **(dark grey discoloration of liver)**	Conjugated < 5 mg/dL
Rotor syndrome	AR	Decreased hepatic uptake, storage and secretion	Conjugated < 5 mg/dL

359. Autosomal dominant inheritance is seen in:
A. Hemophilia
B. Huntington's chorea
C. Hunter's syndrome
D. Hurler syndrome *(UP 1999)*

360. Disorder genetically transmitted by single autosomal dominant gene is:
A. Huntington's disease
B. CJD
C. PKU
D. Catatonic schizophrenia *(KARNATAKA 1996)*

Autosomal dominant disorders	Autosomal recessive disorders
• Familial hypercholesterolemia	• Deafness
• Hereditary nonpolyposis colon cancer	• Albinism
• Polyposis of the colon	• Wilson's disease
• $BRCA_1$ and $BRCA_2$ breast cancer	• Hemochromatosis
• Hereditary hemorrhagic telangiectasia	• Sickle cell anemia
• Marfan's syndrome	• β-thalassemia
• Hereditary spherocytosis	• Cystic fibrosis
• Adult polycystic kidney disease	• Hereditary emphysema (α_1 antitrypsin deficiency)
• **Huntington's chorea**	• Homocystinuria
• Acute intermittent porphyria	• Friedreich's ataxia
• Osteogenesis imperfecta tarda	• Phenylketonuria
• von Willebrand's disease	
• Myotonic dystrophy	
• Familial hypertrophic cardiomyopathy	
• Neurofibromatosis	
• Tuberous sclerosis	

361. Chvostek's sign and Trousseau's sign is seen in:
A. Hyperparathyroidism
B. Hypoparathyroidism
C. Hyperthyroidism
D. Hyperthyroidism *(UP 2001)*

Neuromuscular and neurologic manifestations of **chronic hypocalcemia** include muscle spasms, carpopedal spasm, facial grimacing, and, in extreme cases, laryngeal spasm and convulsions. Respiratory arrest may occur. **Chvostek's** or **Trousseau**'s **sign** can be used to confirm latent tetany.

Classification of hypocalcemia (*excluding* neonatal hypocalcemia)

PTH absent	PTH ineffective	PTH overwhelmed
• Hereditary **hypoparathyroidism** • Hypomagnesemia • Acquired hypoparathyroidism	• Chronic renal failure • Decreased dietary intake or sunlight • Anticonvulsant therapy • Vitamin D-dependent rickets type I • Intestinal malabsorption • Vitamin D-dependent rickets type II • Pseudohypoparathyroidism	• Severe, acute hyperphosphatemia • Tumor lysis • Acute renal failure • Rhabdomyolysis • Osteitis fibrosa after parathyroidectomy

362. HLA matching is *not* necessary in which of the following organ transplantation:

A. Liver
B. Bone marrow
C. Pancreas
D. Kidney

(JIPMER 2002)

Donor 'livers' for **liver transplantation** are procured mainly from the victims of the head injury and organs from brain dead donors up to 60 years of age are acceptable. Compatibility in ABO blood group and organ size between donor and recipient are important considerations in donor selection. *However*, **tissue typing for HLA matching is not required.**

363. Lyme disease is caused by:

A. *Borrelia burgdorferi*
B. *Borrelia falciparum*
C. *Borrelia turicatae*
D. *Borrelia recurrentis*

364. All the following diseases are transmitted by flea bites *except*:

A. Plague
B. Murine typhus
C. Chiggerosis
D. Lyme disease

(JIPMER 2002)

Lyme borreliosis is a **tick-transmitted** spirochetal illness which begins with a characteristic expanding skin lesion known as erythema migrans. *Borrelia burgdorferi* is the causative agent of the disease.

365. In temporal lobe epilepsy treatment is:

A. Ethosuximide
B. Carbamazepine
C. Clobazam
D. Valproic acid

(UP 1999)

Mesial temporal lobe epilepsy is the *most common* syndrome associated with *complex-partial seizures* and is an example of symptomatic, partial epilepsy. **Carbamazepine is a first-choice anticonvulsant** because of its relatively low behavioral and psychological toxicity and the rarity of serious adverse effects. It is indicated for the treatment of partial seizures with simple or *complex* symptomatology (psychomotor, temporal lobe); generalized tonic-clonic seizures (grand mal); mixed seizure patterns.

366. Chronic inflammatory bowel disease is associated with which of the following:

A. Primary sclerosing cholangitis
B. Cholangiosarcoma
C. Fibrosis
D. Chronic hepatitis

(UP 1999)

367. Ulcerative colitis is *not* accompanied by:

A. Interstitial nephritis
B. Pyoderma gangrenosum
C. Iridis
D. Arthritis

(SGPGI 1996))

Complications of Ulcerative Colitis

General complications	Local complications
• Abnormal liver function test	• Pseudopolyposis
• Cirrhosis	• Carcinoma
• Pyoderma gangrenosum	• Fibrous strictures
• Erythema nodosum	• Toxic megacolon
• Arthritis	• Massive hemorrhage
• Iridis	• Rectovaginal fistula
• Ankylosing spondylitis	• Fistula in ano
• Stomatitis	• Ischio-rectal abscess
• Renal disease	• Hemorrhoids
• Anemia	
• **Sclerosing cholangitis**	
• Carcinoma of bile duct	

368. In diabetes mellitus 'hypoglycemia unawareness' is due to:

A. Necrobiosis lipoidica
B. Insulin resistance
C. Diabetic neuropathy
D. Switch over insulin to oral drugs *(UP 2000)*

369. Hypoglycemia unawareness in diabetes mellitus is because of:

A. Lipodystrophy
B. Insulin resistance
C. Autonomic neuropathy
D. Switch over insulin to oral hypoglycemic drugs *(AI 2000)*

Because the initial clinical signals of hypoglycemia are dependent on adrenaline, the loss of the catecholamine response results in the syndrome of **hypoglycemia unawareness**. This phenomenon originally was thought to be *solely* due to **autonomic neuropathy** in patients with *long-standing* diabetes but now it is recognized that the syndrome may be caused by low blood glucose in the *absence* of neuropathy.

370. Insulin resistance is due to:

A. IgD
B. IgA
C. IgG
D. IgM *(PGI 1997)*

Insulin resistance is defined as the requirement of 200 or more units of insulin per day to control hyperglycemia and prevent ketosis. Anti-insulin antibodies of the **IgG class** are present in most subjects within 60 days of the initiation of insulin therapy.

371. Weight loss is seen in:

A. Hypothyroidism
B. Insulin secreting tumor
C. Pheochromocytoma
D. Cushing syndrome *(AIIMS 1996, 1999, AI 1996, 1998, UP 2000)*

In patients of **pheochromocytoma** symptoms and signs of an increased metabolic rate, such as profuse sweating and mild to moderate **weight loss**, are common.

372. *Not* a characteristic feature of Turner's syndrome:

A. Polycystic kidney
B. Short neck
C. Coarctation of aorta
D. Ovarian dysgenesis *(AIIMS 1998, UP 2000)*

373. 45, XO chromosomal anomaly, short stature and genital infantilism are seen in:

A. Gonadal agenesis
B. Klinefelter's syndrome
C. Down's syndrome
D. Turner's syndrome *(AIIMS 2000)*

Gonadal dysgenesis or **Turner's syndrome** is characterized by primary amenorrhea, sexual infantilism, short stature, multiple congenital anomalies, and bilateral streak gonads in phenotypic women with any of several defects of the X chromosome. Incidence is 1 in 3000 newborn females. 50% of patients have a **45, XO karyotype**. Gonadal dysgenesis is the most common cause of primary amenorrhea, accounting for 33% of such patients. External genitalia are unambiguously female but remain immature, and there is no breast development *unless* exogenous estrogen is given. The fallopian tubes and uterus are immature, and bilateral streak gonads are present in the broad ligaments. Lymphedema of the hands and feet, **webbing of the neck**, low hairline, redundant skin folds on the back of the neck, a shieldlike chest with widely spaced nipples, and growth retardation are other features. Micrognathia, epicanthal folds, prominent low-set or deformed ears, a fishlike mouth, and ptosis may be seen. Short 4th metacarpals are present in 50%, and 10 to 20% have **coarctation of the aorta**. Renal malformations (**horse shoe kidney**), pigmented nevi, hypoplastic nails, tendency to keloid formation, perceptive hearing loss, unexplained hypertension, glucose intolerance, and autoimmune thyroid disease are associated features.

374. HbA_1 is:

A. A result of enzymatic degradation of glucose
B. Indicative of level of glucose in diabetic patient
C. Mutant of hemoglobin
D. Absent in normal people *(AI 1995)*

375. Significance of glycosylated hemoglobin is:

A. Useful in fetal damage
B. Indicates abnormal hemoglobin
C. Long-term measurement of blood sugar
D. Useful in fetal lung maturity *(AIIMS 1999, UP 2000, AI 2001)*

376. Glycosylated hemoglobin which indicates *good* control of diabetes is:

A. 8% **B.** 10%
C. 15% **D.** 20%

Glycosylated hemoglobin (HbA_1) is a *reliable* index of **long-term control of blood sugar**. The mean blood glucose concentration over the previous few months is represented by the concentration of glycosylated hemoglobin.

Value in percent	Inference
• 6-9%	Very good metabolic control
• 9-12%	Fair control
• 12%	Poor control

377. Increased cardiac silhouette is *not* seen in:

A. CHF
B. Pericardial effusion
C. Multi-valvular rheumatic heart disease
D. Uncomplicated tetralogy of Fallot *(UP 2000)*

378. Boot shaped heart with pulmonary oligemia is seen in:

A. TGA **B.** TOF
C. ASD **D.** PDA *(SGPGI 2002)*

Four components of the **tetralogy of Fallot** are **VSD**, **pulmonary stenosis**, **aortic override** of the VSD, and **right ventricular hypertrophy**. X-ray examination *characteristically* reveals a **normal-sized, boot-shaped heart** (coeur en sabot) with prominence of the right ventricle and a concavity in the region of the pulmonary conus. The pulmonary vascular markings are *typically* diminished.

379. Drug *essential* in Sheehan's syndrome is:

A. Gonadotropins **B.** Cortisone
C. Thyroxin **D.** Estrogen *(AI 1991)*

If systemic hypotension develops, as with **postpartum hemorrhage**, the pituitary may undergo infarction (**Sheehan's syndrome or post partum pituitary necrosis**). The management of the patients who have already developed Sheehan's syndrome should be done by endocrinology department and consists of "maintenance régime" of thyroxin, **adrenal cortical hormone** and possibly gonadotropin.

380. Poor prognostic factor in scleroderma is:

A. Telangiectasia **B.** Dysphagia
C. Renal involvement **D.** Cutaneous calcification *(AI 1991)*

In scleroderma death occurs most often from cardiac, **renal**, or pulmonary involvement.

381. Virus implicated in hepatocellular carcinoma is:

A. HCV **B.** HEV
C. HDV **D.** HAV *(PGI 1998)*

382. *Most common* predisposing factor for hepatocellular carcinoma in India is:

A. Mixed micronodular cirrhosis **B.** Hepatitis B
C. Non A, non B hepatitis **D.** Alcoholic cirrhosis *(AIIMS 1992)*

Primary **hepatocellular carcinoma** is 1 of the most common tumors in the world. It is especially found in regions of Asia and sub-Saharan Africa. **The main reason for the high incidence of hepatocellular carcinoma in parts of Asia and Africa is the frequency of chronic infection with hepatitis B virus (HBV) and hepatitis C virus (HCV).** These chronic infections often lead to cirrhosis, which itself is an important risk factor for hepatocellular carcinoma.

383. *Small* intestine biopsy is diagnostic in:

A. Whipple's disease **B.** Tropical sprue
C. Hirschsprung's disease **D.** Amyloidosis *(PGI 1998)*

Whipple's Disease is a rare disorder characterized by arthralgia, abdominal pain, and diarrhea, progressive weight loss, dilated lacteals in the bowel wall, and impaired intestinal absorption. The diagnosis of Whipple's disease is made by **demonstrating the presence in the mucosa of macrophages** containing large cytoplasmic granules that stain brilliant magenta with the periodic acid Schiff (PAS) reagent. In addition to the PAS-positive macrophages, **jejunal biopsy** specimens frequently show dilated lymphatics and some degree of blunting of the intestinal mucosal villi.

384. Electrical alternans in ECG is seen in:

A. Dilated cardiomyopathy **B.** Pericardial effusion
C. Hypertrophic cardiomyopathy **D.** Hypertension *(PGI 1998)*

385. Electrical alternans is seen in:

A. COPD **B.** Left atrial myxoma
C. Restrictive cardiomyopathy **D.** Cardiac tamponade *(AI 1993)*

Electrical alternans is a beat-to-beat alternation in 1 or more components of the ECG signal and it is a common type of nonlinear cardiovascular response to a variety of disturbances. **Total electrical alternans (P-QRS-T) with sinus tachycardia is a *relatively* specific sign of pericardial effusion, often with cardiac tamponade.**

386. *Most common* age of presentation of gastric ulcer is:

A. 6th decade of life **B.** 3rd decade of life
C. 4th decade of life **D.** 5th decade of life *(KERALA 1999)*

The incidence of gastric ulcer peaks in the **6th decade** of life. Slightly more than half of gastric ulcers occur in males.

387. *Most common* cardiac manifestation of sarcoidosis is:

A. PAT **B.** Atrial fibrillation
C. Heart block **D.** Cor pulmonale *(KERALA 1999)*

About 5% of patients of **sarcoidosis** have heart involvement. Left ventricular wall involvement is common while arrhythmias are frequent. **Serious conduction disturbances, including complete heart block, may occur.** Papillary muscle dysfunction, pericarditis, and congestive heart failure are also seen. Cor pulmonale secondary to chronic pulmonary fibrosis may occur but is *un*common.

388. Romberg's sign indicates *dys*function of:

A. Cerebellum
B. Sensory cortex
C. Lateral spinothalamic tracts
D. Anteiror column

(SGPGI 1999)

Romberg's sign is the inability to maintain body balance when the eyes are shut and the feet are close together. The sign is said to be positive if the patient sways and falls when the eyes are closed. This is seen in **sensory ataxia**. Sensory ataxia is caused by lesions that affect the peripheral sensory fibers, dorsal root ganglia cells, posterior columns of the spinal cord, lemniscal system in the brainstem, thalamus, or parietal cortex.

389. HLA B-27 is *not* associated with:

A. Rheumatoid arthritis
B. Psoriatic arthritis
C. Reiter's syndrome
D. Ankylosing spondylitis

(SGPGI 1999)

390. HLA B-27 is *not* associated with:

A. Psoriatic arthritis
B. Behçet's syndrome
C. Ankylosing spondylitis
D. Reiter's disease

(AI 2000)

391. Ankylosing spondylitis is associated with:

A. HLA B-27
B. HLA DR-4
C. HLA B-8
D. HLA A-3

(AI 1999)

392. Rheumatoid arthritis is associated with:

A. DR-2
B. DR-3
C. DR-4
D. DR-5
E. HLA B-27

(PGI May 2001)

HLA Association of Common Rheumatic Disorders

Disorder	HLA
• Ankylosing spondylitis	B-27
• Reiter's syndrome	B-27
• Acute anterior uveitis	B-27
• Reactive arthritis	B-27
• Psoriatic arthritis	B-27
• Juvenile rheumatoid arthritis	B-27
• Rheumatoid arthritis	Dw-4/DR-4
• Sjögren's syndrome	Dw-3

393. Palatal myoclonus is seen in:

A. Guillain-Barré syndrome
B. Cerebellar infarction
C. Multiple sclerosis
D. Epilepsy

(SGPGI 1999)

Occlusion of superior cerebellar artery results in severe ipsilateral cerebellar ataxia, nausea and vomiting, dysarthria, and contralateral loss of pain and temperature sensation over the extremities, body, and face. Partial deafness, ataxic tremor of the ipsilateral upper extremity, Horner's syndrome, and **palatal myoclonus** may also occur.

394. Progressive multifocal leukoencephalopathy is caused by:

A. HHV-8
B. Parvovirus
C. JC virus
D. Hanta virus

(PGI 1996, 1999)

Progressive multifocal leukoencephalopathy is a progressive disorder characterized by widespread demyelinating lesions of the brain, brainstem, and cerebellum and it is caused by the **JC virus**. It is associated with chronic neoplastic diseases including Hodgkin's disease, chronic lymphocytic leukemia, and lymphosarcoma. It may also occur as a complication of AIDS and in immunocompromised patients. *Clinically* there is paralysis, blindness, aphasia, ataxia, dysarthria, dementia, confusional states, and coma. There is no treatment till date and death occurs 3 to 6 months after onset of neurological symptoms.

395. Malarial relapse is due to:

A. Trophozoites
B. Merozoites
C. Hypnozoites
D. Sporozoites

(JIPMER 1995)

In *Plasmodium vivax* and *Plasmodium ovale* infections, a proportion of the intrahepatic forms do not divide *immediately* but remain 'dormant' for months to years before replication begins. These dormant forms (**hypnozoites**) are the cause of the relapses that characterize infection with these 2 species.

396. *Not* seen in Dressler's syndrome:

A. Usually in 1st or subsequent week after infarction
B. Ventricular tachycardia
C. Fever
D. Pericarditis

(DELHI 1990)

Post-myocardial infarction syndrome or **Dressler's syndrome** characterized by **fever** and pleuropericardial chest pain, is due to an autoimmune **pericarditis**, pleuritis, and/or pneumonitis. It may begin from **a few days to 6 weeks after myocardial infarction** and usually responds promptly to treatment with aspirin.

397. Herpes-zoster *most commonly* affects:

A. Spinal cord medulla
B. Dorsal root ganglia
C. Sympathetic ganglia
D. Anterior horn cells

(PGI 1993)

398. Zoster recurrence occurs after infection with:

A. Smallpox
B. HSV 1
C. Varicella
D. HSV 2

(MP 2001)

Varicella-zoster virus cause 2 distinct clinical entities viz. varicella, or chickenpox, and herpes zoster, or shingles. With reactivation of latent VZV (which is most common after the 6th decade of life), herpes zoster presents as a dermatomal vesicular rash, frequently associated with severe pain. **Herpes zoster** is a sporadic disease due to *reactivation* of *latent* varicella-zoster virus from the **dorsal root ganglia**.

399. Sézary syndrome is:

A. Locke's disease
B. Merck's disease
C. T-cell lymphoma
D. B-cell lymphoma

(PGI 1997)

Sézary syndrome is a form of cutaneous **T-cell lymphoma** in which there is cutaneous and systemic involvement.

400. Mallory-Weiss syndrome is:

A. Rectosigmoid junction tear
B. Duodenojejunal junction tear
C. Gastroesophageal junction tear
D. Gastroduodenal junction tear

(PGI 1997, AIIMS 1999)

In **Mallory-Weiss syndrome** there is hemorrhage from the upper GIT due to a **tear in the mucosa of the esophagus or gastroesophageal junction**. This syndrome is associated with chronic alcoholism and is usually *preceded* by severe vomiting.

401. In phenothiazines induced dystonia the *drug of choice* is:

A. Metoclopramide **B.** Diphenhydramine
C. Pimozide **D.** Trifluoperazine *(AI 1991)*

Chlorpromazine, fluphenazine, mesoridazine, perphenazine, prochlorperazine, promazine, promethazine, thioridazine, and trifluoperazine derivatives are known as phenothiazines. Haloperidol, loxapine, pimozide, and thiothixene differ *structurally* but have similar pharmacologic activity. The **main mode of action of these agents is *inhibition* of dopaminergic neurotransmission** in the central nervous system, but they also block some α adrenergic, histaminergic, muscarinic, and serotonergic actions. Acute dystonic reactions produced by them respond rapidly to IV **diphenhydramine** (1 mg/kg body weight given over 2 min) or *benztropine* (1 to 2 mg).

402. Metabolic alkalosis is *not* seen in:

A. Cushing disease
B. Ureterosigmoidostomy
C. Prolonged vomiting
D. Thiazide diuretic *(AI 1991)*

Ureterosigmoidostomy is a method of **urinary diversion** and was first used *Henri Chaput* in 1894. The procedure was subsequently modified *Coffey* and *Grey Turner*. In this procedure the ureters are cut obliquely and pulled into the gut by a stitch. The typical biochemical changes are **hyperchloremic acidosis** with **potassium depletion** and are seen in *every* patient. These changes are due to a combination of **reabsorption of urea** and chloride and progressively diminishing renal function due to chronic pyelonephritis.

403. Toxoplasmosis in pregnancy is treated with:

A. Nifurtimox **B.** Pyrimethamine
C. Spiramycin **D.** Suramin *(KARANTAKA 1994)*

Spiramycin is used as an alternative drug in the treatment of toxoplasmosis during pregnancy. Pyrimethamine and sulfadiazine combination is considered to be more effective than spiramycin. *However*, because spiramycin has not been found to be teratogenic and has been found to be safe in the pregnant woman, fetus, and newborn, it is often used to treat toxoplasmosis during pregnancy and congenital toxoplasmosis. Spiramycin reduces the transmission of toxoplasmosis from the pregnant woman to the fetus; however, it will not affect the severity of disease in an already infected fetus.

404. Drug of *choice* for ocular toxoplasmosis is:

A. Riboflavin **B.** Ganciclovir
C. Tetracycline **D.** Pyrimethamine

Patients with **ocular toxoplasmosis** are treated for 4 weeks with **pyrimethamine + sulfadiazine/clindamycin.**

405. In what percentage of patients with anorexia nervosa, amenorrhea is present:

A. 100% **B.** 50%
C. 25% **D.** 80% *(PGI 1996)*

406. *Not* a feature of anorexia nervosa:

A. Avoidance of high caloric foods
B. Amenorrhea is rare
C. Loss of weight at time of presentation
D. Predominantly seen in females *(AI 1994)*

The weight criterion for diagnosis of anorexia nervosa is 85% or less than expected ideal weight. A body mass index of <18 is considered the threshold level for diagnosis. **Amenorrhea is an invariable feature**. Anorexia nervosa is thus the only psychiatric illness including a mandatory endocrine component. An expressed intense fear of gaining weight or becoming fat, even when underweight, and a disturbance of body image (the way the body is perceived by the patient) complete the diagnostic tetrad.

	Anorexia Nervosa	Bulimia
Predominant sex	**Female**	Female
Method of weight control	Reduction of intake	Vomiting
Binge eating	Uncommon	Invariant
Weight at diagnosis	**Markedly decreased**	Near normal
Ritualized exercise	Usual	Rare
Amenorrhea	**100%**	**50%**
Other endocrine changes	Common	Uncommon
Antisocial behavior	Rare	Frequent
CVS changes (bradycardia, hypotension)	Common	Uncommon
Skin changes (hirsutism, dryness, carotenemia)	Usual	Rare
Hypothermia	Usual	Rare
Edema	Present or absent	Present or absent
Medical complications	Hypokalemia, cardiac arrhythmias	Hypokalemia, cardiac arrhythmias, aspiration of gastric contents, esophageal or gastric rupture

407. Drug of choice in anorexia nervosa is:

A. Fluoxetine　**B.** Phenytoin
C. Haloperidol　**D.** Cyproheptadine

Drug of choice of anorexia nervosa is **fluoxetine**.

408. Sturge-Weber syndrome is associated with:

A. Hemangiosarcoma　**B.** Lymphangioma
C. Cavernous hemangioma　**D.** Port-wine stain　*(DELHI 1996)*

409. *False* regarding Sturge-Weber syndrome is:

A. Focal seizure on same side　**B.** Capillary hemangioma
C. Sensory motor paralysis　**D.** Cerebral cortex atrophy　*(AIIMS 1996)*

Sturge-Weber syndrome or encephalotrigeminal angiomatosis was first described in 1879 by *W Allen Sturge*, who described a child with sensorimotor seizures **contralateral** to a facial "**port-wine stain**". *Weber* provided the first radiographic demonstration of an important component of the disorder- intracerebral meningeal angiomatous calcification (characteristic **tram line calcification** seen in simple X-ray) ipsilateral to a trigeminal nevus.

• **Port**- after *Oporto*, city in Portugal (a sweet, usually **dark-red**, fortified wine).

410. All of the following are *anterior* mediastinal masses *except*:

A. Thymomas　**B.** Teratoma
C. Thyroid masses　**D.** Gastroenteric cysts

411. *Most common* anterior mediastinum tumor is:

A. Vascular cyst　**B.** Neurogenic tumor
C. Thymoma　**D.** Lymphoma　*(AI 1999)*

412. *Not* an anterior mediastinal tumor:

A. Teratoma　**B.** Lymphoma
C. Neurofibroma　**D.** Thymoma　*(AIIMS 1991)*

413. *Not* a middle mediastinal mass:
- **A.** Pleuropericardial cyst
- **B.** Gastroenteric cyst
- **C.** Bronchogenic cyst
- **D.** Vascular masses

(AIIMS 1995, SGPGI 1999)

414. *Most common* lesion of *middle* mediastinum is:
- **A.** Neurogenic tumor
- **B.** Aneurysm
- **C.** Congenital cyst
- **D.** Germ cell tumor

(AIIMS 1996, AI 1998)

415. *Most common* tumor of *posterior* mediastinum:
- **A.** Teratoma
- **B.** Neurogenic
- **C.** Lymphoma
- **D.** Thymoma

(AI 1992, 1995)

416. *Most common* tumor of posterior mediastinum is:
- **A.** Cyst
- **B.** Lymphoma
- **C.** Neurofibroma
- **D.** Thymoma

(AIIMS 1998)

Differential Diagnosis of Mediastinal Masses in Descending Order of Frequency

Anterior mediastinum	Middle mediastinum	Posterior mediastinum
• Thymomas • Lymphomas • Teratoma • Thyroid masses	• Vascular masses • Lymph node enlargement from metastases or granulomatous disease • Pleuropericardial cyst • Bronchogenic cysts	• Neurogenic tumors • Meningoceles • Meningomyeloceles • Gastroenteric cysts • Esophageal diverticula

417. Inherited disorder of *metabolism* is:
- **A.** Patau's syndrome
- **B.** Down syndrome
- **C.** Maple syrup urine disease
- **D.** Duchenne's muscular dystrophy

(AI 1992)

Decarboxylation of branched chain amino acids (leucine, isoleucine and valine) is carried out by a complex enzyme system (**branched chain ketoacids dehydrogenase**) using thiamine pyrophosphate as a co-enzyme. **Deficiency of this enzyme system results in an inborn error of metabolism known as maple syrup urine disease (MSUD).** The designation comes from the sweet odor of 'maple syrup' found in body fluids especially urine. Several forms of this disease are known. The *classical* form presents in the neonatal period with lethargy, poor feeding, hypertonicity, convulsions, *resistant* hypoglycemia, metabolic acidosis and coma. Death occurs in a few weeks to few months in untreated or ill-treated cases. The diagnosis can be established by noting the *peculiar* odor of urine and demonstrating elevated levels of branched chain amino acids in urine and plasma. Acute management consists of providing high calories by parenteral route and performing peritoneal dialysis to remove excess amount of branched chain amino acids from the circulation. The diet should be low in these amino acids and synthetic formulas are available in the market. Some forms of MSUD respond to thiamine.

418. *Not* associated with microcytic hypochromic anemia:
- **A.** Liver disease
- **B.** Thalassemia
- **C.** Pyridoxine deficiency
- **D.** ARF

(AI 1992)

Patients with **chronic liver disease** (CLD) from nearly any cause often develop a **mild normocytic anemia**.

419. *Most common* cause of death in acute poliomyelitis is:
- **A.** Intercostal muscle paralysis
- **B.** Respiratory failure
- **C.** Convulsions
- **D.** Cardiac arrest

(AI 1992)

In 2-20% of cases of **acute poliomyelitis** the outcome may be **fatal due to involvement of the muscles affecting the vital functions especially respiration.**

420. *Most common* presentation of craniopharyngioma is:

A. Cardiac disturbance
B. Endocrinal disturbance
C. Visual complaints
D. Nausea and vomiting *(AI 1992)*

421. *Most common* clinical feature of craniopharyngioma is:

A. Headache
B. Convulsions
C. Field defect
D. Optic atrophy *(AIIMS 1993)*

Craniopharyngioma arise from remnants of Rathke's pouch and comprise 3 to 5% of all intracranial neoplasms. Most of these tumors are suprasellar in location, but about 15% are intrasellar. Presenting complaints in *adult* patients are as under:

Visual complaints	80%
Headaches	40%
Hypogonadism	35%
Mental deterioration or personality change	26%
Diabetes insipidus	15%
Weight gain	15%
Panhypopituitarism	7%

Craniopharyngiomas may enlarge and become symptomatic during pregnancy. **Suprasellar calcification** in a flocculent, granular, or curvilinear pattern is seen on skull X-rays in most children and in *some* adults with craniopharyngioma. *Treatment* of craniopharyngiomas is often *un*satisfactory.

422. *Not* a clinical feature of Eaton-Lambert syndrome:

A. Associated with lung carcinoma
B. Female predominant
C. Affects pelvic muscle first
D. Proximal muscle weakness *(AI 1992, UP 1997)*

The **Lambert-Eaton myasthenic syndrome** is a presynaptic disorder of the neuromuscular junction which can cause weakness like that of myasthenia gravis. The **proximal muscles of the lower limbs are most commonly affected**, but other muscles may also be involved. Cranial nerve involvement causes ptosis of the eyelids and diplopia which occur in up to 70% of patients and resemble features of myasthenia gravis. A great majority of patients have an associated malignancy, **most commonly small cell carcinoma of the lung**, which is thought to trigger the autoimmune response. *Treatment* of the neuromuscular disorder involves plasmapheresis and immunosuppression.

423. Nephrocalcinosis is seen in all *except*:

A. Hyperparathyroidism
B. Vitamin D intoxication
C. Medullary sponge kidney
D. Cystic disease of kidney *(AI 1992)*

Calcification in the kidney can be classified broadly into 2 categories based on its location:
1. **Calcification within the pyelocalyceal lumina or nephrolithiasis;**
2. **Intraparenchymal calcification or nephrocalcinosis.**

Calcium salts may be deposited in areas of diseased tissue (*dystrophic calcification*) as in renal infection, neoplasm, or vascular disease, or laid down in basically normal tissue (*metastatic calcification*), the reason for and mechanism of such deposition being unknown in many cases. Nephrocalcinosis can also be categorized with respect to its predominant location. A limited group of diseases may produce calcification confined to, or predominantly located in, the renal cortex — *cortical nephrocalcinosis.* Other conditions spare the cortex and cause calcium salt deposition in the medullary interstitium or lumina of the nephrons — *medullary nephrocalcinosis.*

Stricture of CBD → Benign → Postoperative (80%)
Stricture of CBD → Benign → Inflammatory conditions (20%)
Stricture of CBD → Malignant

Stricture of the common bile duct may be benign or malignant. 80% of benign strictures are postoperative and rest 20% are inflammatory. Postoperative strictures are a result of *preventable* errors in technique of cholecystectomy. Postoperative strictures may involve either the common bile duct or the common hepatic duct. In 85% of cases the injury *declares itself* in the postoperative period by a profuse and persistent discharge of bile if the drainage has been provided or by bile peritonitis if drainage has not been provided or worsening obstructive jaundice.

406. Femoral hernia is *differentiated* from inguinal hernia by which of the following:

A. Mid inguinal ligament **B.** Inferior epigastric artery
C. Femoral artery **D.** Pubic tubercle *(AIIMS 1998)*

407. Femoral hernia in comparison to pubic tubercle is:

A. Inferolateral **B.** Inferomedial
C. Superomedial **D.** Superolateral *(UP 1998)*

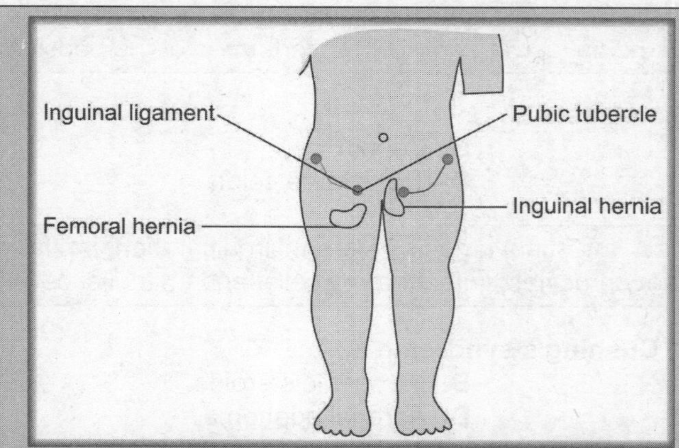

An inguinal hernia is present **above and medial** to the medial end of the inguinal ligament at its attachment to the **pubic tubercle** while the femoral hernia is present **below this**.

408. *False* regarding dentate line in anal canal is:

A. Haustral folds one cm below **B.** Anal mucous glands open
C. 2 cm from anal verge **D.** Transitional epithelium above line *(AIIMS 1998)*

The dentate line is morphologically and surgically most important landmark in the anal canal. It represents the fusion of proctodaeum and post-allantoic gut and the position of anal membrane, the remnants of which may be seen as anal papillae, situated on the free margins of the anal walls. It separates the following structures:

Above	Below
Portal venous system	Systemic venous system
Insensitive autonomic nerves	Very sensitive spinal nerves
Cubical epithelium	Squamous epithelium

409. *Most common* site of lymphoma of GI tract is:

A. Ileum **B.** Colon
C. Stomach **D.** Duodenum *(AIIMS 1998)*

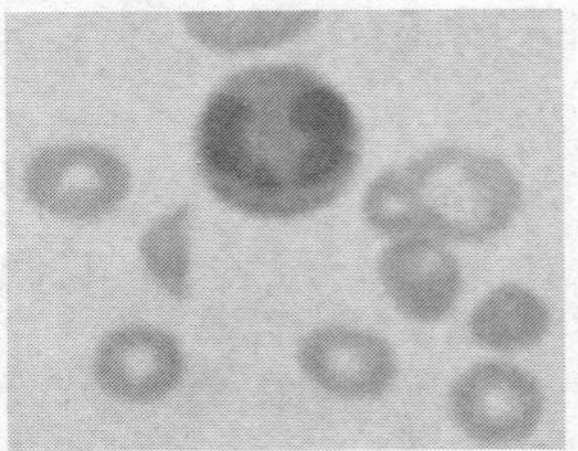

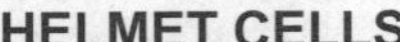

HELMET CELLS

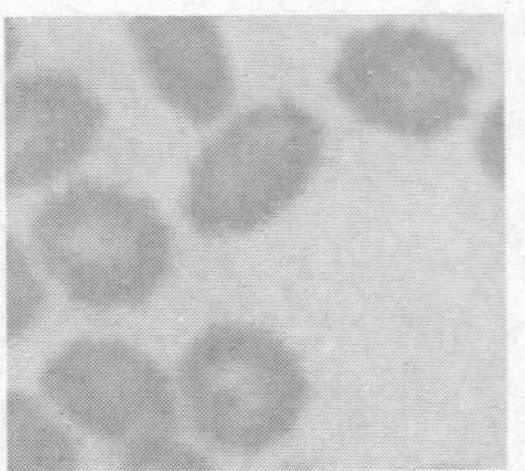

BURR CELLS

Clinical features: Onset is acute with extreme pallor, **purpura** or bruising, irritability, lethargy and reduced urine output. Hypertension, edema, splenomegaly, mild jaundice, **seizures** and signs of congestive cardiac failure such as hepatomegaly, cardiomegaly, pulmonary edema, tachycardia, gallop rhythm and venous distention may develop. About 90% of patients now survive the acute phase.

Laboratory data: Hemoglobin level of 5-7 gm% is common and is associated with reticulocytosis and thrombocytopenia. TLC of 15 to 20000/cubic mm with predominance of polymorphs is a common finding. An unexplained significant hypokalemia is sometimes seen. This is a *paradoxical finding* in a patient of ARF and hemolytic anemia.

429. *Minimum* pericardial fluid is *best* detected by:

A. Echocardiography **B.** ECG
C. CT **D.** CXR *(AI 1992)*

Echocardiography is the **most effective** diagnostic laboratory technique available for **pericardial effusion**, since it is sensitive, specific, simple, noninvasive, and may be performed at the bedside.

430. *Most common* site for amebiasis is:

A. Hepatic flexure **B.** Cecum
C. Sigmoid colon **D.** Transverse colon *(AI 1993)*

The **earliest** intestinal lesions of intestinal amebiasis are microulcerations of the mucosa of the **cecum**, sigmoid colon, or rectum that release erythrocytes, inflammatory cells, and epithelial cells.

431. *Most common* cause of Cushing's syndrome is:

A. Ectopic ACTH **B.** Iatrogenic steroids
C. Pituitary adenoma **D.** Adrenal adenoma *(AIIMS 1991, AI 1993)*

The *most common* cause of **Cushing's syndrome** is **iatrogenic administration of steroids** for a variety of reasons.

432. Fasciculations are seen in:

A. Duchenne muscular dystrophy **B.** Polymyositis
C. Poliomyelitis **D.** Motor neuron disease *(AI 1993, MP 2001)*

433. Motor neuron disease is characterized by:

A. Sensory loss **B.** Rigidity
C. Fasciculation **D.** Focal seizure *(AIIMS 1995)*

Amyotrophic lateral sclerosis is the *most common* form of progressive **motor neuron disease**. Motor neuron degenerative disorders involve both lower motor neurons and upper *or* corticospinal motor neurons. Although *at its onset* amyotrophic lateral sclerosis may cause selective loss of function of only upper or lower motor neurons, it *ultimately* causes progressive loss of both categories of motor neurons. The 1st evidence of the disease typically is insidiously developing asymmetric weakness, usually 1st evident distally in 1 of the limbs. Weakness caused by denervation is associated with progressive wasting and atrophy of muscles and, particularly early in the illness, spontaneous twitching of motor units (**fasciculations**). There is no treatment available but recently, the drug *riluzole* has been approved for use.

434. All are paraneoplastic syndromes *except*:
- **A.** Cerebellar degeneration
- **B.** Lambert-Eaton myasthenic syndrome
- **C.** Amyotrophic lateral sclerosis
- **D.** Opsoclonus myoclonus

(AIIMS May 2001)

Some Paraneoplastic Syndromes

- Photoreceptor, retinal degeneration
- Limbic encephalitis
- Brainstem encephalitis
- Subacute cortical *cerebellar degeneration*
- *Opsoclonus-myoclonus*
- *Lambert-Eaton myasthenic syndrome*
- Myasthenia gravis
- Polymyositis
- Necrotizing myelopathy
- Subacute motor neuronopathy
- Acute demyelinating polyneuropathy (Guillain-Barré syndrome)
- Chronic demyelinating polyneuropathy
- Neuropathy with paraproteinemia
- Subacute sensory neuronopathy
- Sensorimotor neuropathy
- Necrotizing myopathy

435. In cryptococcal meningitis the *drug of choice* is:
- **A.** Zidovudine
- **B.** Clotrimazole
- **C.** Amphotericin B
- **D.** Pentostatin

(AI 1993)

Treatment Protocol of Cryptococcal Meningitis

• **Patients with AIDS and cryptococcosis**	Start with IV amphotericin B (with or without flucytosine) and followed by Fluconazole-400mg OD during active infection then 200mg OD indefinitely.
• **Patients without AIDS**	**Amphotericin B** alone or combined with flucytosine. Dose of amphotericin B is 0.5 to 0.7 mg/kg per day when it is used alone and 0.3 to 0.5 mg/kg per day when it is used in combination with flucytosine.

436. Which of the following is *not* a feature of digitalis toxicity:
- **A.** Xanthopsia
- **B.** Paroxysmal atrial tachycardia
- **C.** ST depression
- **D.** Nausea

Features of Digitalis Toxicity

Extracardiac manifestations	Cardiac manifestations
• Anorexia	• Bradycardia
• Nausea	• Multiple ventricular ectopic
• Vomiting	• Ventricular bigeminy (*alternate* ventricular ectopic)
• Diarrhea	• Paroxysmal atrial tachycardia
• Xanthopsia—altered color vision	• Ventricular tachycardia
	• Ventricular fibrillation

437. *Not* used in treatment of digitalis toxicity:
- **A.** Lignocaine
- **B.** Fab particle
- **C.** Atropine
- **D.** Peritoneal dialysis

(AI 1993, AIIMS 1996)

438. Treatment of digoxin overdose *does not* include:
- **A.** Hemodialysis
- **B.** Phenytoin
- **C.** Potassium
- **D.** Lignocaine

(AI 1997)

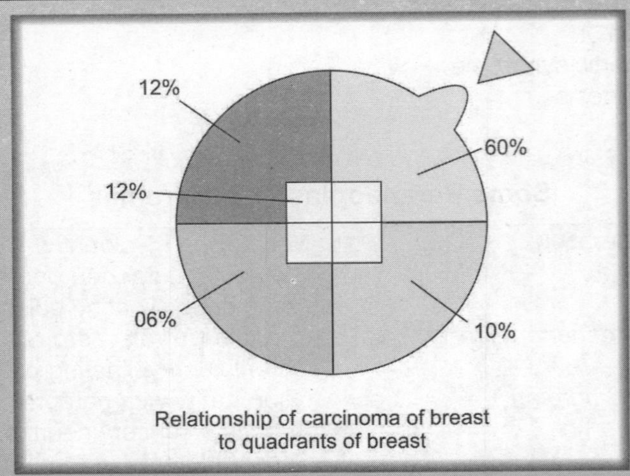

Relationship of carcinoma of breast to quadrants of breast

While any portion of the breast, including the axillary tail, may be involved, **breast cancer commences most frequently in the upper, outer quadrant.**

422. Which of the following is *not* a *pre*malignant ulcer:

A. Radiodermatitis
B. Marjolin's ulcer
C. Bazin's disease
D. Paget's disease of nipple

(KERALA 1994)

Premalignant Conditions of Skin

- Bowen's disease
- Leukoplakia
- Radiodermatitis
- Paget's disease of nipple
- Senile (solar) keratosis
- Chronic scars

Bazin's disease (**erythema induratum**) is a chronic disease of skin seen in young adult females and is characterized by hard cutaneous nodules that break down to form necrotic ulcers and leave atrophic scars. The disease is invariably preceded by tuberculosis.

Marjolin's ulcer is a carcinoma which develops in a scar. It grows slowly because the scars are relatively avascular, is painless because the scars contain no nerve, no secondary deposit occur in regional lymph nodes because the lymphatic vessels have been already destroyed.

423. Correct daily replacement dose of thyroxine in an adult is:

A. 1-2 mg
B. 0.1-0.2 mg
C. 4-5 mg
D. 6-7 mg

(AI 1993)

Hypothyroidism is a preventable cause of mental retardation. Sodium-L-thyroxine is the treatment of choice in hypothyroidism. The goal is to maintain T4 and TSH in normal range. It is available as 100 μg tablet (Tab. Eltroxin) and the dosages are as under:

• **Newborns**	**10-15 μg/ kg/day**
• **Children**	**4 μg/ kg/day**
• **Adults**	**2 μg/ kg/day**

424. Witzelsucht syndrome (Pathological joking) is seen in:

A. Frontal lobe tumors
B. Parietal lobe tumors
C. Temporal lobe tumors
D. IV ventricular tumor

Witzelsucht syndrome is a condition produced by **frontal lobe lesions** characterized by self-amusement from poor jokes and puns.

425. ***Treatment of choice*** **of umbilical adenoma in a newborn is:**

A. Occlusion with a coin
B. Ligature
C. Surgery
D. Cyst of epididymi

- **Umbilical adenoma or raspberry tumor** is commonly seen in infants. It is due to a partially or occasionally completely unobliterated vitellointestinal duct. Mucosa prolapsing from umbilicus gives rise to a "raspberry" like tumor which is moist with mucus and tends to bleed. If tumor is pedunculated, a **ligature** is tied around it and in a few days the polypus drops off; sometimes it reappears then *umbilectomy* is indicated. It should be differentiated from umbilical granuloma which is chronic infection of umbilical stump. There is no certain means to differentiate it with umbilical adenoma except that one application of silver nitrate stick destroys granuloma but adenoma soon reappears.
- **Umbilical granuloma is a chronic infection of the umbilical cicatrix.** There is no *certain* way to distinguish it from umbilical adenoma and *usually* a granuloma can be destroyed by a *single* application of $AgNO_3$ stick followed by dry dressing but the adenoma soon reoccurs in spite of these measures.

426. Posterior urethral valves are ***most commonly*** **situated:**

A. Above verumontanum
B. At verumontanum
C. Below verumontanum
D. Bladder neck

Congenital valves of posterior urethra are often symmetrical and occur **usually just below**, but *occasionally* above **the verumontanum**. They allow the ingress of a catheter but obstruct the outflow of urine.

* Verumontanum is an elevation on the *floor of the prostatic portion of the urethra* where the seminal ducts enter.

427. ***Most common*** **benign tumor of stomach is:**

A. Adenoma
B. Lipoma
C. Hamartoma
D. Leiomyoma

Benign Tumors of Stomach

Leiomyoma	**Most common benign neoplasm**
Neurofibroma	Arise from nerve, symptoms same as leiomyoma
Adenomatous polypus	Usually multiple, as a rule are situated in distal half of stomach
Aberrant pancreas	Sometimes found in wall of stomach
Ménétrier's disease	There is giant hypertrophy of mucosa of gastric fundus, may predispose to carcinoma associated with protein loss and may require partial gastrectomy

428. Idiopathic retroperitoneal fibrosis involves first:

A. Ureter
B. Kidney
C. Stomach
D. Duodenum *(AIIMS 1993)*

429. Ormond's disease is:

A. Idiopathic lymphadenopathy
B. Retractile testis
C. Retroperitoneal fibrosis
D. Idiopathic mediastinitis

Retroperitoneal fibrosis or Ormond's disease is a condition in which there is development of a mass of fibrotic tissue in the retroperitoneal space. **This may lead to physical compression of the ureters**, and even the vena cava and aorta. **Most patients present with ureteric obstruction and often renal failure.** This disease may be associated with taking *methysergide* for migraine, and with some other drugs.

430. Lateral aberrant thyroid is:

A. Metastatic carcinoma
B. Anatomic abnormality
C. Lingual thyroid
D. Developmental abnormality *(AIIMS May 2002)*

451. *Most common* cause of hyperparathyroidism:

A. Werner's syndrome **B.** Multiple adenomas
C. Chief cell hyperplasia **D.** Solitary adenoma *(AI 1997)*

452. *Most common* cause of primary hyperparathyroidism is:

A. Parathyroid carcinoma **B.** Parathyroid adenoma
C. Chronic renal disease **D.** Hyperplasia of parathyroid glands *(SGPGI 1999)*

The cause of hyperparathyroidism is 1 or more *hyper* functioning glands. **A single abnormal gland is the cause in approximately 80% of patients**; which is usually a benign neoplasm or **adenoma** and *rarely* a parathyroid carcinoma.

453. Retinopathy in diabetes mellitus depends upon:

A. Duration of disease **B.** Age of patient
C. Blood sugar level **D.** Severity of disease *(AI 1995)*

The frequency of incidence of **diabetic retinopathy** increases with the **length of time** the patient has had diabetes. Frequency is not altered by level of hyperglycemia and has no relation with the control of diabetes. Diabetic neuropathy and retinopathy are primarily due to activation of the polyol pathway.

454. Tumor metastasis spread through CSF is:

A. Craniopharyngioma **B.** Glioblastoma
C. Medulloblastoma **D.** Ependymoma *(AI 1996)*

455. Brain tumor associated with CSF invasion is:

A. Oligodendroglioma **B.** Glioblastoma multiforme
C. Medulloblastoma **D.** Ependymoma *(AI 1995)*

456. Craniospinal irradiation is useful in which of the following conditions:

A. Astrocytoma **B.** Oligodendroglioma
C. Medulloblastoma **D.** Oncocytoma *(AI 2002)*

Medulloblastomas frequently disseminate along CSF pathways. In adults, surgical excision should be followed by chemotherapy and **irradiation of the entire neuraxis**, with a boost in radiation dose to the primary tumor.

457. Sickle cell anemia is due to:

A. Point mutation **B.** Translocation
C. Trisomy **D.** Monosomy *(PGI May 2001)*

Sickle cell anemia (SCA) is the *most common* inherited blood disorder in the United States, affecting about 72,000 Americans or 1 in 500 African Americans. SCA is characterized by episodes of pain, chronic hemolytic anemia and severe infections, usually beginning in early childhood. SCA is an autosomal recessive disease **caused by a point mutation** in the hemoglobin β gene found on chromosome 11p15.4.

458. *Most common* cause of osteomyelitis in sickle cell anemia is:

A. *Salmonella* **B.** *Staphylococci*
C. *Pseudomonas* **D.** *Escherichia coli* *(AI 1995, SGPGI 2002)*

Patients with **sickle cell disease** have an increased susceptibility to infection and **salmonella osteomyelitis** is 1 such infection that is *rarely* seen in patients without sickling disorders.

459. *Most common* tumor to metastasize in heart is:

A. Hodgkin's lymphoma **B.** Renal cell carcinoma
C. Bronchogenic carcinoma **D.** Malignant melanoma *(AI 1995, UP 1997)*

Tumors metastatic to the heart are many times more common than primary tumors. Although cardiac metastases occur in 1 to 20% of *all* tumor types, the incidence is particularly high in *malignant melanoma* and, to a somewhat lesser extent, in leukemia and lymphoma. In *absolute numbers*, **cardiac metastases are most common in carcinoma of the breast and lung**, due to high incidence of these cancers.

460. In SABE diagnosis is made by:

A. Anti streptolysin
B. ASLO titer
C. Anti DNAase
D. Serial blood culture *(AI 1995)*

Criteria for diagnosis of SABE depend heavily on **blood culture** and cardiac echocardiography.

461. In anemia of chronic disease there is:

A. Raised serum iron
B. Low serum ferritin
C. Low TIBC
D. Low HBA_2 *(AIIMS 1994, AI 1995)*

The common diagnostic problem in IDA is the confusion between iron deficiency and an inflammatory **'block'** in iron *delivery* from the RE system to the erythroid progenitors (**the anemia of chronic disease**). Inflammatory **cytokines**, such as *tumor necrosis factor*, *interleukin* (IL) 1, *interferon* (IFN) β, and IFNγ are capable of suppressing erythropoietin secretion, erythroid precursor proliferation, and the *delivery of iron to the marrow*. **Both the serum iron (SI) and TIBC decline in patients with inflammatory anemias (anemia of chronic disease).**

Differential Diagnosis of Hypoproliferative Anemia

Tests	Iron Deficiency	Inflammation	Renal Disease	Hypometabolic States
Anemia	Mild to severe	Mild	Mild to severe	Mild
MCV (fL)	70-90	80-90	90	90
Morphology	Normocytic or microcytic	Normocytic	Normocytic	Normocytic
SI	Less than 30	Less than 50	Normal	Normal
TIBC	More than 360	Less than 300	Normal	Normal
Saturation (%)	Less than 10	10-20	Normal	Normal
Serum ferritin (μg/L)	Less than 15	30-200	115-150	Normal
Iron stores	0	2-4+	1-4+	Normal

462. Prominent 'V' wave in JVP suggests:

A. Mitral stenosis
B. Pulmonary hypertension
C. Tricuspid regurgitation
D. Pulmonary stenosis *(AI 1995)*

Tricuspid regurgitation (TR) is frequently seen in 20-50% of all patients with rheumatic heart disease (RHD). Most of the time TR is associated either with MS or MR. If TR is associated with *severe* MS then it is mostly 'functional' due to associated pulmonary hypertension. But if it is associated with pure or dominant MR then TR is *probably* 'organic' in origin because severe pulmonary hypertension *does not* develop *only* due to MR. Clinical features of TR result mainly from 'systemic venous congestion' and reduction of cardiac output. With the onset of TR in patients with pulmonary hypertension, symptoms of pulmonary congestion diminish, but the clinical manifestations of right-sided heart failure become prominent. The neck veins are distended with **prominent *v* waves**, and marked hepatomegaly, ascites, pleural effusions, edema, systolic pulsations of the liver and positive hepatojugular reflux are common. A prominent right ventricular pulsation along the left parasternal region and a blowing holosystolic murmur along the lower left sternal margin, which may be intensified during inspiration and reduced during expiration or the valsalva maneuver, are *characteristic* findings; atrial fibrillation is frequently present.

463. Bromocriptine is used to treat:

A. Myxedema
B. Parkinsonism
C. Medullary carcinoma thyroid
D. Obesity

443. *Most common* form of anthrax is:

A. Wool sorter's disease
B. Alimentary type
C. Cutaneous type
D. None

Anthrax is an acute bacterial infection which is caused by *Bacillus anthracis*. It occurs frequently in herbivorous animals. In man, the **most common form is cutaneous anthrax**, which is characterized by the development of a localized skin lesion with a central eschar surrounded by marked nonpitting edema.

444. Nerve lying close to Wharton's duct is:

A. Hypoglossal
B. Alveolar
C. Facial
D. Lingual

(PGI 1991)

Wharton's duct is the duct of the submandibular salivary gland and opens into the mouth at the side of the frenulum linguae. The **lingual nerve** is attached to the upper pole of the submandibular gland by the facial sheath of the gland. **The nerve passes forwards and downwards between the Wharton's duct and the deep part of the gland before passing medially under the duct opposite the first lower molar.**

445. *True* regarding von Graefe's sign:

A. Lagging behind of the upper eyelid
B. Retraction of the upper eyelid with infrequent wrinkling
C. Absence of wrinkling of the fore head
D. Convergence of the eyes is difficult

(DELHI 1993)

Some Clinical Signs of Thyrotoxicosis

• **Dalrymple's sign**	Unnatural degree of separation between the margins of two lids.
• **Möbius's sign**	Imperfect power of convergence.
• **Stellwag's sign**	Diminished frequency of blinking and imperfect closure of lids during the act.
• **von Graefe's sign**	The failure of the eyelid to move downward promptly with the eyeball and the lid moves tardily and jerkily.

446. Carotid sheath does *not* contain:

A. Carotid artery
B. Internal jugular vein
C. Vagus nerve
D. Phrenic nerve

Carotid sheath is the portion of cervical or pretracheal fascia enclosing the **carotid artery**, **interior jugular vein**, and **vagus nerve**.

447. Musculoskeletal abnormality in neurofibromatosis is:

A. Pseudoarthrosis
B. Scoliosis
C. Café au lait spots
D. All of the above

Neurofibromatosis Type 1 (von Reckling-Hausen's Disease)

- Benign tumors of the peripheral nerves called neurofibromas
- Hamartomas of the iris (Lisch nodules)
- Pseudoarthrosis of the tibia
- Scoliosis
- Hypertension
- Mental retardation
- Pigmented lesions of the skin called cafe au lait spots
- Axillary freckling
- Hydrocephalus from aqueductal stenosis
- Short stature
- Epilepsy

- Presence of at least six café au lait spots of *more* than 1.5 cm in diameter is diagnostic of NF1.

471. In multiple myeloma *best* indicator of prognosis is:
A. Serum alkaline phosphate
B. Number of plasma cells in marrow
C. Serum β_2 microglobulin
D. Serum level of Ca^{++} *(AI 1995)*

472. *Best* marker for prognosis of multiple myeloma is:
A. β_1 microglobulin
B. β_2 microglobulin
C. Serum Ca^{++}
D. Bone marrow plasma cells *(AIIMS 1999, 2000)*

Serum β_2 **microglobulin** is the **single most powerful** predictor of survival in patients of multiple myeloma and can substitute for staging.

473. Serum alkaline phosphate is *not* raised in:
A. Hyperparathyroidism
B. Osteomalacia
C. Paget's disease
D. Multiple myeloma *(AIIMS 1994)*

474. *False* regarding multiple myeloma is:
A. Increased alkaline phosphatase
B. Casts
C. Increased uric acid
D. Increased Ca^{++} *(PGI 1998)*

In multiple myeloma serum alkaline phosphatase is usually **normal** even with extensive bone involvement because of the absence of osteoblastic activity.

475. In which of the following condition γ glutamyl transpeptidase is elevated:
A. Secondaries in liver
B. Alcoholic liver disease
C. Viral disease
D. Liver disease *(AI 1995)*

476. Specific enzyme elevated in alcoholism is:
A. Gamma glutamyl transferase
B. Alkaline phosphate
C. AST
D. ALT *(AIIMS 1994)*

477. Alcoholism is *best* marked by:
A. GGT
B. Macrocytosis
C. SGOT
D. SGPT

Laboratory Tests in Alcoholics

• MCV	91 fL or higher
• **γ glutamyl transferase (GGT)**	**30 or more units**
• Serum uric acid	Greater than 7 mg/dL
• Carbohydrate-deficient transferrin	20 g/L or more
• Triglycerides	180 mg/dL or more

478. Angina pectoris and syncope are *most likely* to be associated with:
A. Tricuspid stenosis
B. Mitral regurgitation
C. Mitral stenosis
D. Aortic stenosis *(AI 1994)*

479. Recurrent chest pain and syncope is commonly seen in:
A. Mitral stenosis
B. Aortic regurgitation
C. MVP
D. Aortic stenosis *(KERALA 1991)*

480. Sudden death is common in:
A. Patent ductus arteriosus
B. Aortic stenosis
C. Mitral stenosis
D. Arterial VSD *(JIPMER 1990)*

Most patients with pure or predominant aortic stenosis have gradually increasing obstruction for years but do not become symptomatic until the 5th to 7th decades of life. **Exertional dyspnea, angina pectoris, and syncope are the 3 cardinal symptoms.** Among adults dying with valvular aortic stenosis, **sudden death**, which most probably results from an arrhythmia, occurred in 10 to 20% and at an average age of 60 years.

481. *Not* a feature of Behçet's syndrome:

A. Common in youngsters
B. Seen only in tropics
C. Multisystem involvement
D. Recurrent aphthous stomatitis *(AI 1994)*

Behçet's syndrome is a multisystem disorder with recurrent oral and genital ulcerations as well as ocular involvement.
Internationally agreed diagnostic criteria of Behçet's syndrome
Recurrent oral ulceration + 2 of the following: • Recurrent genital ulceration • Eye lesions • Skin lesions • Pathergy test
Behçet's syndrome affects mainly young adults, with males having *more severe* disease than females.

482. In Behçet's syndrome:

A. There is a strong association with HLAB-5
B. There may be recurrent deep venous thrombosis
C. The skin may be hyperactive to minor injury
D. All of the above

Behçet's syndrome appears to be linked to **HLA-B5 and -DR5 alloantigens**. Peripheral vein **thrombosis** is seen in 25% of the patients which may affect superficial as well as **deep veins**. Pulmonary thromboembolism is a rare complication. **Nonspecific skin inflammatory reactivity** to any scratches or intradermal saline injection (pathergy test) is a common and specific manifestation of this syndrome.

483. Which of the following is a feature of Behçet's syndrome:

A. A strong association with HLAB-5
B. Recurrent deep venous thrombosis
C. Skin may be hyperactive
D. All of the above

Feature of Behçet's Syndrome

• Autoimmune disease	• Linked to HLA-B5 and -DR5
• Recurrent aphthous ulcerations	• Folliculitis
• Erythema nodosum	• Vasculitis
• Positive pathergy test	• Iritis
• Posterior uveitis	• Retinal vessel occlusions
• Optic neuritis	• Hypopyon uveitis
• Arthritis	• Superficial or deep peripheral vein thrombosis
• Benign intracranial hypertension	• Psychiatric disturbances
• Pyramidal involvement	• Multiple sclerosis-like picture
• Mucosal ulcerations of the gut	• Pulmonary emboli

- **Pathergy test** consists of nonspecific skin inflammatory reactivity to any scratches or intradermal saline injection.

484. Hemiplegia is commonly associated with infarction of area of distribution in..........artery:

A. Anterior communicating artery
B. Posterior cerebral artery
C. Middle cerebral artery
D. Anterior cerebral artery *(AI 1994)*

The clinical features of an ischemic stroke vary depending on the site of the occlusion and the extent of the spared collateral flow. The characteristic presentation is the **abrupt onset of a hemiparesis in an individual in the atherosclerotic age group**. Almost any symptom of brain dysfunction may occur. **Symptoms and signs of carotid system disease most commonly affect the distribution of the middle cerebral artery** and the patient may exhibit a contralateral hemiparesis, hemisensory deficit, and hemianopia. If the 'dominant' hemisphere is involved, there is some degree of aphasia.

485. Normal portal venous pressure is:

A. 20-25
B. 22-25
C. 8-12
D. 3-5

(AI 1994, MP 2001)

Normal pressure in the portal vein is low (**10 to 15 cm saline**) because vascular resistance in the hepatic sinusoids is minimal.

486. Characteristic feature of frontal lobe tumor is:

A. Antisocial behavior
B. Distractibility
C. Abnormal gait
D. Aphasia

(AI 1994)

487. Frontal lobe lesion causes:

A. Side determination
B. Visual defect
C. Urinary incontinence
D. Personality change

(AIIMS 1997)

Frontal lobe tumors may present with personality change or depression.

488. *Most common* manifestation of osteoporosis is:

A. Loss of weight
B. Bowing of legs
C. Backache
D. Compression fracture of spine

(AI 1994)

In **osteoporosis** the **most frequent symptoms from vertebral body fractures are pain in the back** and deformity of the spine which usually results from collapse of the vertebrae, especially in the dorsal and lumbar regions, is typically acute in onset, and often radiates around the flank into the abdomen.

489. In thyrotoxicosis β blockers *do not* control:

A. Oxygen consumption
B. Tachycardia
C. Anxiety
D. Tremors

(AI 1994)

In hyperthyroidism propranolol reduces the following

- Sweating
- Tachycardia
- Anxiety
- Tremor
- Conversion of T_4 to T_3

490. Marker of *acute* hepatitis B is:

A. HBeAg
B. HBcAg
C. HBsAg
D. IgM anti HBc

(MP 2001)

491. Acute infection of hepatitis B virus is characterized by:

A. Anti HBeAg
B. IgM anti-HBc + HBsAg
C. Anti HBsAg
D. HBsAg

(AI 1999)

492. A donor for blood transfusion is screened for hepatitis B. All are safe *except*:

A. Anti HBeAg positive
B. HBsAg + IgM anti-HBc positive
C. Anti HBsAg + HBeAg
D. Anti HBsAg positive

(AI 2000)

493. Hepatitis B *infectivity* is indicated by:
- **A.** HBeAg + Anti HBsAg
- **B.** HBsAg + HBeAg
- **C.** Anti HBcAg + Anti HBeAg
- **D.** HBeAg + Anti HBcAg

(AI 1994)

- A **diagnosis of hepatitis B virus infection can usually be made by detection of HBsAg in serum**. Sometimes, levels of HBsAg are too low to be detected during acute HBV infection, even with the current generation of highly sensitive immunoassays and in such cases; the diagnosis can be established by the presence of **IgM anti-HBc**.
- Another serologic marker that can be of value in patients with hepatitis B is **HBeAg**. Its **principal clinical usefulness is as an indicator of relative infectivity.**

494. '*a*' wave in JVP is absent in:
- **A.** Sick sinus syndrome
- **B.** Tricuspid atresia
- **C.** Atrial fibrillation
- **D.** Mitral stenosis

(AI 1994)

The **'*a*' wave is absent in patients with atrial fibrillation**, and there is an increased delay between the '*a*' wave and the carotid arterial pulse in patients with 1st-degree atrioventricular block.

495. *Not* a feature of Marfan's syndrome:
- **A.** High arched foot
- **B.** High palate
- **C.** Arachnodactyly
- **D.** Short stature

(AI 1994)

496. *Not* a clinical feature of Marfan's syndrome:
- **A.** Aortic regurgitation
- **B.** Genu valgum
- **C.** Ectopia lentis
- **D.** Hyperelasticity of joints

(AIIMS 1995)

Some Features of Marfan's Syndrome

Ocular signs and conditions	**Musculoskeletal signs and conditions**
Upward **ectopia lentis**	**Arachnodactyly** (Spider fingers)
Myopia	Pectus deformity (pigeon breast or funnel breast)
Iridodenesis	**High narrow palate**
Glaucoma	Arm span exceeds height
Retinal detachment	Leg length exceeds trunk length
Cardiovascular signs and conditions	**Hyperextensible joints and ligaments**
Mitral valve prolapse	Pes plantus
Aortic root dilatation	Hammer toes
Myocardial infarction	Vertebral column deformities (Kyphoscoliosis)
Aortic insufficiency	Inguinal hernia
Congestive heart failure	Striae distensae
Subacute bacterial endocarditis	**Body habitus**
Aortic dissection	**Tall** (Height exceeds 95th percentile for age)
	Extremely slender build

497. Gas gangrene is *most commonly* due to:
- **A.** *Clostridium tetani*
- **B.** *Clostridium welchii*
- **C.** *Clostridium difficile*
- **D.** *Clostridium botulinum*

(MP 2001)

Clostridium perfringens (Clostridium welchii) possesses 17 possible virulence factors, including 12 active tissue toxins and enterotoxins. This species has been divided into 5 types (A to E) on the basis of 4 major toxins: alpha, beta, epsilon, and iota. The α toxin is a phospholipase C (lecithinase) which splits lecithin into phosphorylcholine and diglyceride. This α **toxin has been associated with gas gangrene** and is known to be hemolytic, to destroy platelets and polymorphonuclear leukocytes, and to cause widespread capillary damage.

498. Food poisoning is caused by all *except*:
A. *Bacillus anthrax*
B. *Shigella*
C. *Escherichia coli*
D. *Vibrio parahaemolyticus*
(AIIMS 1997)

499. Food poisoning with incubation period of *less than* 6 hours and which is *not* fatal is:
A. *Salmonella*
B. *Clostridium*
C. *Vibrio cholerae*
D. *Bacillus*
(MP 2001)

Classification of Food Poisoning According to Incubation Period

1 to 6 hours	8 to 16 hours	More than 16 hours
• *Staphylococcus aureus* • *Bacillus cereus*	• *Clostridium perfringens* • *Bacillus cereus*	• *Vibrio cholerae* • Enterotoxigenic *Escherichia coli* • *Salmonella typhimurium* and other species • *Shigella* spp. • *Vibrio parahaemolyticus*

Food poisoning produced by *Bacillus cereus* is mild and self-limiting requiring no specific treatment.

500. Dose of mercaptopurine requires reduction with:
A. Allopurinol
B. Thiazide
C. Spironolactone
D. Methotrexate
(MP 2001)

Azathioprine and 6-mercaptopurine are metabolized by the enzyme xanthine oxidase. *Logically* there metabolism is inhibited by allopurinol (allopurinol and its metabolite, oxipurinol decrease the production of uric acid by *inhibiting the action of xanthine oxidase*) and dose has to be reduced by 25-50% if allopurinol is given concurrently.

501. *Most common* enzyme deficiency is:
A. G6PD
B. Glucose 1, 6 diphosphatase
C. Hexokinase
D. Glucose-6-phosphatase
(MP 2001)

Enzyme deficiency states in order of prevalence: **glucose-6-phosphate dehydrogenase** (G6PD) >>> pyruvate kinase > glucose-6-phosphate isomerase > rare deficiencies of other enzymes in the pathway.

502. Hemophilia is associated with all *except*:
A. Males more commonly affected
B. Increased PT
C. Increased aPTT
D. X-linked recessive
(MP 2001)

503. *Not* a feature of hemophilia:
A. Decreased factor VIII level
B. Bleeding into tissue and joints
C. Increased aPTT
D. Increased PT
(AIIMS 1992)

504. *Not* a characteristic feature of hemophilia A:
A. Prolonged prothrombin time
B. Prolonged partial thromboplastin time
C. Low factor VIII level
D. Bleeding into soft tissue, muscles and joints
(SGPGI 1996)

505. *Least* likely cause of a prolonged bleeding time is:
A. Scurvy
B. Hemophilia A
C. von Willebrand's disease
D. Thrombocytopenia
(KARNATAKA 2000)

Most of the *inherited* plasma coagulation disorders are due to defects in single coagulation proteins, with the **2 X-linked disorders, factors VIII and IX deficiency**, accounting for the majority of the congenital coagulation disorders. 1 in 10,000 male children is born with deficiency or dysfunction of the factor VIII molecule. The resulting disorder, hemophilia A, is characterized by bleeding into soft tissues, muscles, and weight-bearing joints. Normal hemostasis requires at *least* 25% factor VIII activity, *symptomatic* patients have factor VIII levels < 5%. Patients with <1% factor VIII activity have *severe* disease, i.e. they bleed frequently even *without* discernible trauma. Patients with levels between 1 and 5% have *moderate* disease with less frequent bleeding episodes. Those with levels > 5% have *mild* disease with infrequent bleeding that is usually secondary to trauma. Patients suspected of having hemophilia should be advised to have a platelet count, bleeding time, PT, and aPTT. *Typically*, the patient will have **a prolonged aPTT with all other tests normal**. Each unit of factor VIII infused (defined as the amount present in 1 mL normal plasma) will raise the plasma level of the recipient by 2% per kg of body weight. **Factor VIII has a half-life of 8 to 12 hour**. Desmopressin (DDAVP) can *transiently* increase the factor VIII level (2-3 fold).

506. A patient presented with ecchymoses and petechiae all over body with *increased bleeding time* and normal clotting time. All of the following points to the diagnosis *except*:

A. Decreased platelet in blood
B. Bleeding into the joints and muscle
C. Hypersplenism
D. Increased megakaryocytes in marrow *(AIIMS 1999)*

Most important *screening* tests of the primary hemostatic system are

- A bleeding time (a sensitive measure of platelet function);
- A platelet count;
- A prothrombin time;
- aPTT

1 in 10,000 males is born with deficiency or dysfunction of the factor VIII and the resulting disorder, **hemophilia A**, is characterized by bleeding into soft tissues, muscles, and weight-bearing joints. Typically, the patient will have a prolonged aPTT with all other tests *normal*. The patient in question has all the features of thrombocytopenia except bleeding into joints and muscle which is a feature of hemophilia.

507. Acute bronchiolitis is *most commonly* caused by:

A. Mycoplasma
B. Parainfluenza type III
C. RSV
D. Adenovirus *(MP 2001)*

Acute bronchiolitis is cause by respiratory syncytial virus (RSV) in 50-60% of cases. Other viruses responsible for acute bronchiolitis are parainfluenza virus 1, parainfluenza virus 2, adenovirus, influenza virus and rhinovirus. Rarely *Mycoplasma* and *Chlamydia* may also cause this disease.

508. For diagnosis of acute rheumatic fever, the essential feature is:

A. Erythema marginatum
B. One major and two minor Jones' criteria
C. Recent sore throat infection
D. Prior history of rheumatic fever *(MP 2001)*

The Jones' Criteria for Rheumatic Fever

Major criteria	**Minor criteria**	
	Clinical	**Laboratory**
Carditis		
Migratory polyarthritis	Fever	Elevated ESR
Sydenham's chorea	Arthralgia	Elevated CRP
Subcutaneous nodules		Prolonged PR interval
Erythema marginatum		

PLUS (ESSENTIAL CRITERIA)
Supporting evidence of a **recent group A streptococcal infection** which includes any one of the following:
• Positive throat culture for *Streptococcus*
• Rapid antigen detection test
• Elevated or increasing streptococcal antibody test (**ASO titer** > 200 Todd's unit in adults or > 300 Todd's unit children).

*Diagnosis of rheumatic fever is highly probable if **2 major or 1 major** and 2 minor criteria are present along with the evidence of previous streptococcus infection.

509. *Most common* cause of mediastinitis is:
- **A.** Idiopathic
- **B.** Drugs
- **C.** Esophageal rupture
- **D.** Tracheal rupture

(AI 1997)

Most cases of **acute mediastinitis** are either due to **esophageal perforation** or occur after median sternotomy for *cardiac surgery*.

510. *Not* a malignant tumor:
- **A.** Ependymoma
- **B.** Hemangioblastoma
- **C.** Astrocytoma
- **D.** Glioma

(AI 1997)

Hemangioblastomas are benign lesions that are most frequently seen in young and middle-aged patients, with a peak age incidence in the 4th and 5th decades. These tumors comprise about 7% of primary posterior fossa tumors and about 1% of all intracranial neoplasms. They are frequently located in the cerebellar hemispheres. Rarely, these tumors may be found in the brainstem or spinal cord and hardly ever in the supratentorial region. Hemangioblastomas may be seen in association with retinal angiomas and visceral tumors as part of von Hippel-Lindau disease. In these cases there may be multiple hemangioblastomas.

511. Coarctation of aorta is *not* associated with:
- **A.** PDA
- **B.** Renal artery stenosis
- **C.** Turner syndrome
- **D.** Bicuspid aortic valve

(AIIMS 1995, AI 1997)

512. *Not* a feature of coarctation of aorta:
- **A.** Right ventricular failure
- **B.** Infective endocarditis
- **C.** Bicuspid aortic valve
- **D.** Cerebral aneurysm

(AIIMS 1998)

Coarctation of the aorta is a condition in which a segment of the aorta is constricted, narrowed, or obliterated. In the majority of cases, an abrupt, short segment membranous stenosis, formed by media, intima, and fibromuscular tissue, is present in the region of the aortic isthmus and ductus arteriosus. Coarctation of the aorta is associated with other congenital anomalies such as **bicuspid aortic valve** (70%), **patent ductus arteriosus**, ventricular septal defect, tricuspid atresia, and transposition of the great vessels. Noncardiac associations include berry aneurysms in the circle of Willis and **Turner's syndrome**. Diagnosing coarctation early is important to prevent associated complications including aortic aneurysm, dissection, and **bacterial endocarditis** at the coarctation site or bicuspid aortic valve. **Cerebral aneurysms** and, in particular, berry aneurysms may be associated with polycystic kidney disease, Ehlers-Danlos syndrome, **coarctation of the aorta**, moyamoya disease, fibromuscular dysplasia, and arteriovenous malformations of the brain.

OTHER CONDITIONS ASSOCIATED WITH COARCTATION OF AORTA		
• Turner's syndrome (XO)	• Bicuspid aortic valve	• Parachute mitral valve
• Supravalvar mitral ring	• Subaortic stenosis	• Shone complex

513. In mitral stenosis:
- **A.** QRS are widened
- **B.** Left axis deviation
- **C.** Left ventricular hypertrophy
- **D.** Right ventricular hypertrophy

(AI 1997)

In mitral stenosis with severe pulmonary hypertension, **right axis deviation** and **right ventricular hypertrophy are often present**.

514. Bilateral hilar lymphadenopathy and noncaseating granuloma is seen in:
- **A.** Stein Leventhal syndrome
- **B.** Systemic lupus erythematosus
- **C.** Sarcoidosis
- **D.** Scleroderma

(AI 1997)

Sarcoidosis is a 'disease' of unknown etiology that is difficult to define. It is characterized *pathologically* by widespread **noncaseating granulomas**. Such granulomas are *not* exclusive to sarcoidosis and have been seen in many other conditions, such as tuberculosis, fungal disease, berylliosis, and in association with carcinoma and lymphoma. The CXR is abnormal in more than 90% of patients with sarcoidosis. Lymph node enlargement, parenchymal abnormalities, or a combination of the 2 constitute the major radiographic changes. **Bilateral hilar adenopathy is the most frequent finding and occurs in up to 98% of cases of nodal enlargement.**

515. Spinal segment in knee jerk is:
- **A.** L_1
- **B.** L_3
- **C.** L_4
- **D.** B and C

(AI 1997)

Deep reflexes		Superficial reflexes	
Jerk	**Segmental level**	**Reflex**	**Segmental level**
Ankle jerk	$S_{1,2}$	Plantar reflex	$S_{1,2}$
Knee jerk	$L_{3,4}$	Abdominal reflexes	T_{7-11}
Biceps jerk	$C_{5,6}$	Cremasteric reflex	L_1
Triceps jerk	$C_{7,8}$		
Radial jerk	C_6		
Jaw jerk	Pons		

- Variations of these levels are given by different authors.

516. Adult polycystic kidney is:
- **A.** X-linked dominant
- **B.** Autosomal recessive
- **C.** Autosomal dominant
- **D.** X-linked recessive

(AIIMS 1993, AI 1997)

517. In adult polycystic kidney, all are *true except*:
- **A.** Cysts are seen in the liver, lung and the pancreas
- **B.** Hematuria occurs
- **C.** Hypertension is *rare*
- **D.** Autosomal dominant transmission is seen

(AIIMS May 2001, AIIMS Nov 2001)

518. *Not* a manifestation of polycystic kidney:
- **A.** Hematuria
- **B.** Renal failure
- **C.** Acute retention
- **D.** Renal hypertension

(PGI 1996)

Autosomal dominant polycystic kidney (*syn.* congenital cystic kidneys) disease has a prevalence of 1:300 to 1:1000 and accounts for approximately 10% cases of end-stage renal disease in the USA. 90% of cases are inherited as an autosomal dominant trait, and approximately 10% are spontaneous mutations. **In 18% of cases there is an associated congenital cystic liver** and occasionally the pancreas and lung are also affected. It is slightly more common in women and 6 important clinical features are as under:

- Renal enlargement
- Hematuria **(25%)**
- Hypertension **(75%)**
- Pain
- Infection (*most common complication*)
- Uremia

Patients pass abundant urine of low specific gravity (1.010 or less) which neither contains cast nor cells. One kidney is larger than the other. Severe anemia is common. Ultrasonography and CT scan demonstrate multiple cysts in both kidneys. Typical **spider leg appearance** is seen in excretory urography. Rovsing's operation is done for polycystic kidney. **Renal transplant** is done if renal failure occurs.

Infantile polycystic kidney is an unrelated, *autosomal recessive* and rare condition in which the kidneys are large and many cases are stillborn, rest of the patient die of renal failure in early life.

- Mnemonic : *"Adults are dominant so are their polycystic kidneys"*

519. *False* regarding clozapine is:

A. Extrapyramidal side effect
B. Agranulocytosis
C. Precipitates seizure
D. Used in schizophrenia *(AI 1997)*

Clozapine is an atypical antipsychotic drug. It is indicated *only* in the management of severely ill **schizophrenic patients** who have *failed* to respond to other neuroleptic agents or who cannot tolerate the adverse effects produced by those agents. Because of the significant risk of **agranulocytosis** and **seizures** with clozapine, the patient should be given an adequate trial with at least 2 different standard antipsychotic medications before clozapine therapy is initiated.

520. *Most common* cause of amebic lung abscess is:

A. Hematogenous spread from gut
B. Hematogenous spread from liver
C. Direct spread from liver
D. Aspiration *(AI 1997)*

Amebic pleuropulmonary disease is usually secondary to liver abscess. The *clinical manifestations* of amebic pleuropulmonary disease are those of liver and lung abscess *combined*. Patients have right upper quadrant pain, weight loss, fever, and, *rarely*, jaundice. The liver is usually enlarged and tender and pleuritic chest pain is a frequent symptom. The cough is usually dry at first but may subsequently become productive of sputum that has been characterized as "**chocolate sauce**" or "liver paste." Leukocytosis is generally present; eosinophilia may be present. Diagnosis is made by identification of amebae in the stool and occasionally in the sputum. Serologic tests, the best of which is an *indirect hemagglutination test*, can be of considerable value. Demonstration of the presence of a liver abscess by CT scan, ultrasound, or radionuclide liver scans is useful. Treatment is the same as for intestinal amebiasis, using metronidazole or other antiamebic drugs.

521. Warm autoimmune hemolytic anemia is *not* seen in:

A. Mycoplasma pneumonia
B. Non Hodgkin's lymphoma
C. α methyldopa therapy
D. Systemic lupus erythematosus *(AI 1997)*

522. Cold antibodies are seen in all *except*:

A. Syphilis
B. Mycoplasma
C. Infectious mononucleosis
D. Lymphoma

COMMON CAUSES OF WARM-ANTIBODY ASSOCIATED HEMOLYTIC ANEMIA

Drugs	Lymphomas	Miscellaneous
• Quinidine	• CLL	• SLE
• Penicillin	• Non-Hodgkin's lymphomas	• Viral infections
• Alpha-methyldopa	• Hodgkin's disease	• Idiopathic

COMMON CAUSES OF COLD-ANTIBODY IMMUNOHEMOLYTIC ANEMIA

- Infectious mononucleosis
- Mycoplasma infection
- Lymphoma
- Paroxysmal cold hemoglobinuria
- Idiopathic

523. Donath-Landsteiner antibody is seen in which of the following condition:

A. PNH
B. Paroxysmal cold hemoglobinuria
C. Chronic lymphocytic leukemia
D. Systemic lupus erythematosus *(PGI 1999)*

Antibodies that react with polysaccharide antigens are usually of IgM class and react better at temperatures < 37°C (cold-reactive antibodies). Uncommonly, the antibody is of IgG class such as the **Donath-Landsteiner antibody of paroxysmal cold hemoglobinuria**.

524. Hyperprolactinemia is caused by all *except*:

A. Metoclopramide B. Bromocriptine
C. Methyldopa D. Phenothiazines *(AI 1997)*

Causes of Hyperprolactinemia

Physiological states	Drugs	Diseases
• Pregnancy • Nursing (early) • "Stress" • Sleep • Nipple stimulation • Food ingestion	• Phenothiazines • Butyrophenones • Thioxanthenes • Metoclopramide • Sulpiride • Respiradone • Methyldopa • Reserpine • Estrogens • Antiandrogens • Opiates • Verapamil	• Prolactinomas • Adenomas secreting GH and prolactin • Adenomas secreting ACTH and prolactin (Nelson's syndrome and Cushing's disease) • Nonfunctioning chromophobe adenomas with pituitary stalk compression • Granulomatous diseases, especially sarcoidosis • Craniopharyngiomas and other tumors • Cranial irradiation • Stalk section • Empty sella • Vascular abnormalities, including aneurysm • Lymphocytic hypophysitis • Metastatic carcinoma • Primary hypothyroidism • Chronic renal failure • Cirrhosis • Chest wall trauma (including surgery, herpes zoster) • Seizures

525. Budd-Chiari syndrome is due to:

A. IVC obstruction B. Congenital portal hypertension
C. Acute portal hypertension D. Hepatic vein obstruction *(AI 1999, 2001)*

526. *Most common* cause of Budd-Chiari syndrome is:

A. Renal cell carcinoma B. Paroxysmal nocturnal hemoglobinuria
C. Hepatocellular carcinoma D. Valve in hepatic vein *(AI 1997, AIIMS 1994, 2000)*

527. Budd-Chiari syndrome is *not* caused by:

A. Oral contraceptive B. PNH
C. Dilantin D. Polycythemia *(SGPGI 1999)*

The ***most common* cause of Budd-Chiari syndrome is thrombosis of the hepatic veins**, often in the setting of polycythemia rubra vera, myeloproliferative syndromes, *paroxysmal nocturnal hemoglobinuria*, oral contraceptive use, or other hypercoagulable states; it also may result from invasion of the inferior vena cava by tumor, such as renal cell or primary hepatocellular carcinoma. However, idiopathic membranous obstruction of the inferior vena cava is the most common cause of this syndrome in *Japan*.

528. ***False* regarding Budd-Chiari syndrome:**
- **A.** Seen in hypercoagulable states
- **B.** Ascites is minimal
- **C.** Liver transplantation may be required *(KARNATAKA 2000)*
- **D.** It is due to obstruction of hepatic venous outflow secondary to spontaneous thrombosis of hepatic veins

Budd-Chiari syndrome is the clinical manifestation of hepatic venous 'outflow' obstruction. Acute and chronic forms exist, both resulting in severe centrilobular congestion and hepatocellular necrosis and atrophy. The acute form occur secondary to thrombosis of the supra-hepatic or intrahepatic inferior vena cava or main hepatic veins. The thrombosis may be secondary to **hypercoagulable states**, such as are seen with polycythemia vera, pregnancy, and with oral contraceptive use. Thrombosis can also result from tumor involvement, particularly from hepatocellular carcinoma, renal cell carcinoma, or adrenal carcinoma. *Additionally*, **intravascular webs or membranes and right atrial or vena cava anomalies can cause significant hepatic outflow obstruction**. In the chronic form of Budd-Chiari syndrome, fibrosis of the intra-hepatic veins occurs, presumably related to inflammation. **Symptoms are:**
- Right-sided abdominal pain and a large liver
- Jaundice (yellowing of the skin)
- **Ascites** (swelling of the abdomen due to the development of fluid in the abdomen)
- Vomiting of blood

Hepatic venography or liver biopsy showing centrilobular congestion and sinusoidal dilatation in the absence of right-sided heart failure establishes the diagnosis of Budd-Chiari syndrome. Treatment varies and includes medical therapy for symptoms and possibly anticoagulation, surgical intervention, and radiological procedures. In patients who undergo **transplantation** for *hepatic vein thrombosis (Budd-Chiari syndrome)*, postoperative anticoagulation is essential; underlying myeloproliferative disorders may have to be treated but are not a contraindication to liver transplantation.

529. Drug *not* used in anthrax is:
- **A.** Tetracycline
- **B.** Erythromycin
- **C.** Gentamicin
- **D.** Ciprofloxacin
- **E.** Penicillin

(CMC VELLORE 2002)

Viable *Bacillus anthracis* organisms disappear from the lesions of cutaneous **anthrax** within 5 hours of the initiation of treatment with parenteral **penicillin G**. For penicillin-*sensitive* adults, treatment with **ciprofloxacin**, **erythromycin**, **tetracycline**, or chloramphenicol may be substituted.

530. Drug of choice for anthrax is:
- **A.** Erythromycin
- **B.** Streptomycin
- **C.** Penicillin
- **D.** Tetracycline

Penicillin G	20 lakh international units of penicillin G QID IV until edema subsides and when the edema subsides 10 day course should be completed with oral penicillin.

531. Cysticercosis in brain is caused by:
- **A.** *Schistosoma mansoni*
- **B.** *Echinococcus*
- **C.** *Taenia solium*
- **D.** *Taenia saginata*

(CMC VELLORE 2002)

Humans are the *only* definitive hosts for *Taenia solium*; pigs are the usual intermediate hosts, although dogs, cats, and sheep may harbor the larval forms. The pork tapeworm *Taenia solium* can cause 2 distinct forms of infection. The form that develops depends on whether humans are infected with adult tapeworms in the intestine or with larval forms in the tissues (**cysticercosis**).

532. Graham Steell murmur is heard in:
- **A.** Aortic incompetence
- **B.** Aortic stenosis
- **C.** Pulmonary incompetence
- **D.** Tricuspid stenosis

533. Austin Flint murmur is seen in:
- **A.** Mitral regurgitation
- **B.** Aortic regurgitation
- **C.** Tricuspid stenosis
- **D.** Pulmonary regurgitation

534. Murmur in Eisenmenger's complex is:

A. Graham Steell murmur
B. Austin Flint murmur
C. Carey-Coombs' murmur
D. None

(UP 1997, CMC VELLORE 2002)

Eisenmenger syndrome is a term used to designate a condition in which there is a *large* communication between the 2 circulations at the aortopulmonary, ventricular, or atrial levels and bidirectional or **predominantly right-to-left shunts** because of high-resistance and obstructive pulmonary hypertension. It is a progressive, cyanotic, heart condition named after Dr Victor Eisenmenger who first described it in 1897. *The principal physiological abnormality is an elevation of pulmonary vascular resistance.* In VSD the pulmonary hypertension occurs as a result of high pulmonary blood flow due to **left to right shunt**. A few patients may develop elevated pulmonary vascular resistance (**pulmonary hypertension**) if the defect is *not* repaired in time. This pulmonary hypertension is responsible for 'reversal' of shunt (**right to left shunt**), a condition known as *Eisenmenger syndrome.* Symptoms may *not* occur till 2nd or 3rd decade of life. Cyanosis, dyspnea, fatigue and tendency to develop dysrhythmias begin to occur. CHF, chest pain, syncope and hemoptysis are features of *late* stage of disease. *On examination* there is a right ventricular heave and a loud narrowly split 2nd heart sound. A soft ejection systolic murmur may be audible along the left sternal border. **Functional incompetence of pulmonary valve produces** a blowing diastolic murmur along the left sternal border (**Graham Steell murmur**).

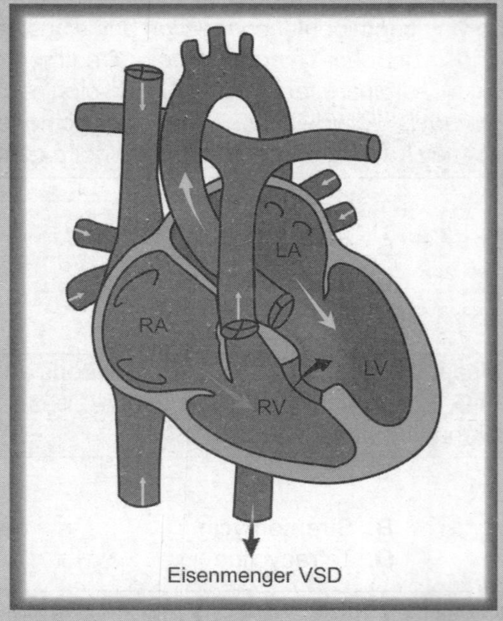

Eisenmenger VSD

- **Carey-Coombs' murmur** is a soft mid-diastolic murmur sometimes heard in patients with **acute rheumatic fever.**
- **Austin Flint murmur** is heard in severe, chronic **aortic regurgitation**, and it may be either mid-diastolic or pre-systolic.

535. *Not* included in treatment of *Helicobacter pylori*:

A. Cisapride
B. Omeprazole
C. Clarithromycin
D. Metronidazole

(AIIMS 1997)

536. Drug *not* effective against *Helicobacter pylori* is:

A. Erythromycin
B. Amoxycillin
C. Metronidazole
D. Colloidal bismuth

(AI 1993)

537. Which of the following drug is *not* used to eradicate *Helicobacter pylori*:

A. Bismuth
B. Ranitidine
C. Tetracycline
D. Metronidazole

(PGI Dec 2000)

Drugs Effective against *Helicobacter pylori*

- Amoxicillin
- Tetracycline
- Clarithromycin
- Omeprazole
- Bismuth chelate
- Metronidazole

538. *Not* used for diagnosing *Helicobacter pylori*:

A. SAFA test
B. Gastric biopsy
C. Rapid urease test
D. Urea breath test *(AI 1999)*

539. *Correct* statement regarding *Helicobacter pylori* is:

A. It invades the gastric mucosa
B. Serology differentiates between active and remote infection
C. Indirect transmission
D. Rapid urease test of gastric biopsy is diagnostic *(AIIMS 1997)*

Invasive tests	Noninvasive tests
• Biopsy urease • Histology • Culture	• Serology • Urea breath test

540. Regimen used for eradication of *Helicobacter pylori* gastritis is:

A. Metronidazole + bismuth + ranitidine
B. Amoxycillin + omeprazole + clarithromycin
C. Clarithromycin + ranitidine + metronidazole
D. Ampicillin + omeprazole + tinidazole *(CMC VELLORE 2002)*

Recommended Regimens for Eradication of *Helicobacter pylori* Infection

Drug 1	Drug 2	Drug 3	Duration
STANDARD TRIPLE-THERAPY REGIMEN			
Bismuth subsalicylate (2 tabs 6 hourly)	Tetracycline HCl (500 mg 6 hourly)	Metronidazole (250 mg 8 hourly)	2 weeks
TRIPLE-THERAPY REGIMENS WITH ACID REDUCTION			
Omeprazole (20 mg 12 hourly)	Clarithromycin (250 mg 12 hourly)	Metronidazole (500 mg 12 hourly)	1 week
Omeprazole (20 mg 12 hourly)	Clarithromycin (500 mg 12 hourly)	Amoxycillin (1 g 12 hourly)	1 week

541. *Not* caused by *Helicobacter pylori*:

A. Fundal gastritis
B. Gastric lymphoma
C. Gastric ulcer
D. Duodenal ulcer *(AI 1999)*

Diseases Caused by *Helicobacter pylori*

- Peptic ulcer disease
- Adenocarcinomas of the stomach *except* those arising in the gastric cardia
- Primary gastric non Hodgkin's lymphoma

542. Drug *not* useful in management of *acute* attack of asthma is:

A. Sodium cromoglycate
B. Inhaled salbutamol
C. Injection hydrocortisone
D. Subcutaneous adrenaline *(CMC VELLORE 2002)*

543. All of the following are useful for treating *acute* bronchial asthma in children *except*:

A. 100% oxygen
B. IV Hydrocortisone
C. Nebulization with salbutamol liquid
D. Sodium cromoglycate inhalation

ACUTE EXACERBATIONS OF BRONCHIAL ASTHMA MAY BE CLASSIFIED AS UNDER:

Parameter	**Mild**	**Moderate**	**Severe**	**Imminent respiratory arrest**
Breathlessness	Walking; Can lie down	Talking Infant-softer shorter cry; difficulty feeding Prefers sitting	Infant-stops feeding Hunched forward	
Talks in	Sentences	Phrases	Words	
Alertness	May be agitated	Usually agitated	Usually agitated	Drowsy or confused
Respiratory rate	Increased	Increased	Often >30/min	
Use of accessory muscles and supra-sternal retractions	Usually not	Usually present	Usually present	Paradoxical thoraco-abdominal movement

NORMAL RESPIRATORY RATE AT DIFFERENT AGE

Age	**Normal rate**
• **<2 months**	<60/min
• **2-12 months**	<50/min
• **1-5 years**	<40/min
• **6-8 years**	<30/min

Management protocol of acute exacerbation of bronchial asthma

1. Oxygen by mask @ 5 liter / minute to achieve oxygen saturation of > 90%.
2. Nebulization with **salbutamol** 0.15 mg / kg / dose (minimum 2.5 mg); diluted in normal saline with oxygen @ 6 liter / minute, every 20 minutes for 3 doses. Asthalin® respirator solution contains 5 mg salbutamol / ml.

Or

Injection **adrenaline** (1 in 1000 dilution) 0.01 ml per kg subcutaneous up to maximum 3 doses at 20 minutes interval.

3. **Hydrocortisone** 10 mg / kg (IV) stat followed by oral prednisolone 2 mg / kg / day.

- **Sodium cromoglycate is useful in prevention and long-term management of asthma. It has got no role in acute exacerbation of asthma.**

544. Smoking is *not* associated with malignancies of:

A. Pancreas
B. Kidney
C. Liver
D. Bladder

(AIIMS 1992)

545. Smoking predisposes to all *except*:

A. Lymphoma
B. Carcinoma pancreas
C. Larynx carcinoma
D. Bladder carcinoma

(AI 1999)

Diseases Caused by Smoking

- **Carcinoma lung**
- Carcinoma larynx and oral cavity
- Carcinoma esophagus
- Carcinoma kidney
- Carcinoma pancreas
- Carcinoma urinary bladder
- **COPD**
- Peptic ulcer
- **Myocardial infarction**
- **Systemic atherosclerosis**

*More common diseases are shown in **bold letters**.

546. Upper motor neuron lesion cause:

A. Localized muscle atrophy **B.** Rigidity
C. Fasciculation **D.** Weakness and spasticity *(AI 1999)*

Motor 'unit' consists of an *upper motor neuron* (UMN) and a *lower motor neuron* (LMN) and the muscle fibers supplied by it. Upper motor neuron originates in the cerebral cortex descends into corona radiata crosses the internal capsule then travels through the brainstem where it may terminate if it is that of a cranial nerve or may descend into the spinal cord. Here it synapses with the lower motor neuron which finally innervates the muscle fibers. **Any lesion affecting the UMN is associated with spasticity of the muscles which it used to innervate**. Lesions associated with LMN injury result in flaccid paralysis.

Clasp-knife phenomenon: Increased muscle resistance to passive movement of a joint followed by a sudden release of the muscle; commonly seen in patients with spasticity.

Clonus: Spasmodic alternation of muscular contractions between antagonistic muscle groups caused by a hyperactive stretch reflex from an *upper motor neuron lesion*.

Spastic Quadriplegia: Paralysis of all 4 extremities. There is usually associated mental defect. Pseudobulbar palsy is prominent and convulsions are common.

547. Myotonic dystrophy gene is coded at chromosome:

A. 24 **B.** 21
C. 19 **D.** 20 *(AI 1999)*

Myotonic dystrophy is an autosomal dominant disorder. It is transmitted by a mutation consisting of an unstable expansion of a CTG trinucleotide repeat sequence in a gene at **19**q13.3.

548. *Not* seen in Laurence-Moon-Biedl syndrome:

A. Polydactyly **B.** Obesity
C. Retinal detachment **D.** Retinitis pigmentosa
E. Hypogonadism *(CMC VELLORE 2002)*

Feature of Laurence-Moon-Bardet-Biedl Syndrome (LMBBS)

• **Inheritance**	Autosomal recessive
• **Stature**	Normal; infrequently short
• **Obesity**	Generalized Early onset, 1-2 yrs
• **Cranofacies**	Not distinctive
• **Limbs**	**Polydactyly**
• **Reproductive status**	**Hypogonadism**
• **Other features**	**Obesity**
• **Mental retardation**	Present

The earliest formal description of LMBBS was provided in a paper published by John Zachariah Laurence (1829-1870), an eminent 19th century ophthalmic surgeon based in London and his then House-surgeon, Robert Moon (1844-1914) who was in fact an American. In this report they described 4 out of 8 siblings with retinitis pigmentosa, lack of intelligence, short stature for their age and hypogenitalism in the *males*. A few years later the same family was re-examined and some noted to have spastic paraparesis. There was no further mention of the syndrome until 1920, when George Bardet submitted his MD thesis on hypothalamic obesity. Bardet was at that time working with Louis Pasteur in Paris and recognized that a number of his cases had unusual features in particular hexadactyly, retinitis pigmentosa and obesity. In 1922 Artur Biedl, an Austrian professor of pathology and endocrinology published a short independent account of 2 siblings with "congenital deformations (retinitis pigmentosa and polydactyly) and an intellectual torpidity (slow and dull; apathetic)". **Retinitis pigmentosa** is commonly cited in LMBBS, however the preferred term rod-cone dystrophy should be used as it more accurately describes the pathological process and in early disease there may be no pigmentary changes seen despite significant visual disturbance.

549. Diethylcarbamazine citrate acts on:

A. Adult filarial parasite
B. Microfilariae and kills them
C. Does not allow multiplication of adult forms
D. Paralyze adult worms *(CMC VELLORE 2002)*

Diethylcarbamazine citrate (DEC) is the *only* drug available for filariasis. It has a highly **selective effect on microfilariae** (Mf). In a dose of 6 mg/kg/day 8 hourly in divided doses it clears the Mf of *Wuchereria bancrofti* and *Brugia malayi* from the peripheral blood in 7 days. Most important action of DEC is alteration of Mf membrane so that they are readily phagocytosed by tissue fixed macrophages but not be circulating macrophages.

550. Hand-foot and mouth disease is caused by:

A. Coxsackievirus A16 **B.** CMV
C. Enterovirus **D.** Arbovirus *(CMC VELLORE 2002)*

Most cases of Hand-foot and mouth disease are due to coxsackievirus A16.

551. Hand-foot syndrome is seen in:

A. Sickle cell disease **B.** Thalassemia major
C. ALL **D.** Fanconi's anemia

Sickle cell dactylitis or **hand-foot syndrome** is seen in sickle cell disease and sickle cell thalassemia.

552. *Not* a bactericidal drug:

A. Penicillins **B.** Cephalosporins
C. Sulfonamides **D.** Quinolones *(CMC VELLORE 2002)*

Sulphonamides are **primarily bacteriostatic** against many gram-positive and gram-negative bacteria.

553. IgA induced vasculitis is seen in:

A. Glomerulonephritis **B.** Henoch-Schönlein purpura
C. Nephrotic syndrome **D.** Hemolytic uremic syndrome *(CMC VELLORE 2002)*

Nephritis is seen in 80% of cases of **Henoch-Schönlein purpura** and manifests as a nephritic urine sediment and moderate proteinuria. The *sine qua non* for diagnosis of the disease is the presence of mesangial **IgA deposition** on immunofluorescence microscopy. Biopsy of involved skin reveals dermal IgA deposition and leukocytoclastic **vasculitis**. **IgA** deposition is also seen in areas of uninvolved skin.

554. Digitalis is *contraindicated* in cardiac failure caused by following:

A. Valvular heart disease **B.** Myocardial infarction
C. Thyrotoxicosis **D.** Anemia *(CMC VELLORE 2002)*

Digitalis is contraindicated in ischemic heart disease including acute myocardial infarction.

555. *True* regarding right ventricular infarction:

A. Volume expanders **B.** Digoxin
C. Diuretics **D.** Pacing *(AIIMS 1991)*

556. Acute right ventricular infarct is treated with:

A. IV fluids **B.** Diuretics
C. Vasodilators **D.** Digoxin *(AI 2001)*

Therapy for **right ventricular infarction** consists of **volume expansion** to maintain adequate right ventricular preload and efforts to improve left ventricular performance with attendant reduction in pulmonary capillary wedge and pulmonary arterial pressures.

557. Ascarbose used in diabetes mellitus acts by:

A. Increasing secretion of insulin
B. Increases sensitive of tissue to insulin
C. Reduces blood glucose levels
D. Reduces absorption of glucose from the gut wall *(CMC VELLORE 2002)*

It should be noted that the **inhibitors of α glucosidases** (ascarbose or Glucor®) act by inhibiting the enzymes of the small intestine which degrade the starch in small molecules. This involves a deceleration of the digestion of the carbohydrates. This results in lowering of the peak blood sugar concentration after meals.

558. Prosopagnosia is:

A. Inability to speak **B.** Inability to read
C. Inability to identify faces **D.** Inability to write *(AI 1999)*

A patient with prosopagnosia is unable to recognize familiar faces; rarely even his/her own face in mirror.

559. Hepatic encephalopathy is *not* precipitated by:

A. Superimposed acute liver disease **B.** GI bleeding
C. Barbiturates **D.** Hyperkalemia *(AI 1999)*

560. Acute hepatocellular failure is *most likely* to be precipitated by:

A. Oral lactulose **B.** Upper GI bleeding
C. Large carbohydrate meal **D.** Large IV albumin infusion *(AIIMS 1992)*

Common Precipitants of Hepatic Encephalopathy

Increased nitrogen load	Electrolyte and metabolic imbalance	Drugs	Miscellaneous
GI bleeding	Hypokalemia	Narcotics	Infection
Excess dietary protein	Alkalosis	Tranquilizers	Surgery
Azotemia	Hypoxia	Sedatives	Superimposed acute liver disease
Constipation	Hyponatremia	Diuretics	Progressive liver disease

* The *most common* predisposing factor is gastrointestinal bleeding.

561. *Most common* cause of subarachnoid hemorrhage is:

A. Trauma **B.** Berry aneurysm
C. AV malformation **D.** Hypertension *(AIIMS 1998, AI 1999)*

562. A 25-year-old man develops *sudden* severe headache with loss of consciousness. CSF is blood stained. Most *likely* diagnosis is:

A. Encephalopathy
B. Embolic stroke
C. Thrombotic CVA
D. Ruptured cerebral aneurysm

(AIIMS 1994)

563. Subarachnoid hemorrhage is caused by:

A. Dural sinuses
B. Venae comitantes of corpus striatum
C. Rupture of vertebral artery aneurysm
D. Rupture of circle of Willis aneurysm

(AI 1998, AIIMS May 2001)

The **most common cause of spontaneous subarachnoid hemorrhage is a ruptured saccular aneurysm**. Other causes are bleeding from an arteriovenous malformation or extension into the subarachnoid space from a primary intracerebral hemorrhage. Saccular aneurysms are found at the bifurcations of the large arteries at the base of the brain and rupture into the subarachnoid space in the basal cisterns. About 85% of aneurysms occur on the anterior circulation, mostly on the circle of Willis. The common sites are the junction of the anterior communicating artery with the anterior cerebral artery, the junction of the posterior communicating artery with the internal carotid artery, and the bifurcation of the middle cerebral artery. Most aneurysms present without warning as sudden subarachnoid hemorrhage. Sudden unexplained headache at *any location* should be viewed with suspicion as it may be due to subarachnoid hemorrhage and be investigated because a *major* hemorrhage may be impending. **Sudden loss of consciousness** may be preceded by a brief moment of agonizing (**the worst headache of life!**) headache, but most patients 1st complain of headache upon regaining consciousness. The **hallmark of rupture of aneurysm is blood in the CSF**. Approximately 80% of patients have enough blood to be visualized on a CT scan obtained within 72 hours but a small hemorrhage may not be seen. If the CT scan *neither* establishes the diagnosis of SAH *nor* demonstrates a mass lesion or obstructive hydrocephalus, a lumbar puncture (LP) should be performed to establish the presence of subarachnoid blood.

564. LVH is seen in:

A. Carcinoid syndrome
B. Aortic regurgitation
C. ASD with fossa ovalis
D. Pure mitral stenosis

(AI 1999)

Aortic regurgitation is less common than MR. The precordium is hyperkinetic with laterally displaced apical impulse. There is a wide pulse pressure and a bounding 'waterhammer' pulse is present. *On auscultation* the heart sounds are diminished in intensity and a high pitched soft **diastolic murmur** is present. The longer the murmur the more severe the AR. **Cardiomegaly with dilated left ventricle** is a common finding in CXR. A salt restricted diet should be given and if CHF develops it should be managed by digoxin (20 µgm/kg stat; 10 µgm/kg after 8 hours; 10 µgm/kg again after 8 hours; 10 µgm/kg ones daily as maintenance dose), *diuretic* (spironolactone) and ACE inhibitors.

565. Primaquine causes hemolysis in:

A. G6PD deficiency
B. Malaria
C. Methemoglobin reductase deficiency
D. NADP deficiency

(AI 1998)

Some Drugs Causing Hemolytic Anemia in G6PD Deficiency

- Aminosalicylic acid
- Antimalarials, e.g. primaquine
- Aspirin
- Chloramphenicol
- Septran®
- Dapsone
- Nalidixic acid
- Nitrofurantoin
- Phenacetin
- Probenecid
- Procainamide
- Quinidine
- Sulfonamides
- Vitamin C
- Vitamin K

566. Splenectomy is most useful in:

A. Sickle cell anemia
B. Henoch-Schönlein purpura
C. Hereditary spherocytosis
D. Thrombocytopenia

(AI 1998)

Splenectomy reliably corrects the anemia in **hereditary spherocytosis**, although the RBC defect and its consequent morphology persist. Polyvalent pneumococcal vaccine should be administered to all patients before they undergo splenectomy.

567. In PSVT the *drug of choice* is:

A. Adenosine **B.** Lignocaine
C. Quinidine **D.** Amiodarone *(AIIMS 1998, AI 1996, 1998)*

If carotid sinus massage is unsuccessful to terminate the attack of **PSVT**, verapamil (2.5 to 10 mg intravenously) or **adenosine** (6 to 12 mg intravenously) is the agent of choice. Adenosine is preferred because of its extremely short half-life, lessening the consequences of any side effects.

568. Hypoglycemia is seen in:

A. Acromegaly **B.** Cushing's syndrome
C. Hypothyroidism **D.** Hypopituitarism *(AIIMS May 2001)*

Hypopituitarism means deficiency of 1 or more pituitary hormones. It has got many causes. Pituitary hormone deficiency may be congenital or acquired and isolated growth hormone or gonadotropin deficiency is common. *Temporary* ACTH deficiency due to long-term glucocorticoid therapy is also common, but *permanent* isolated deficiency of ACTH or TSH is rare. The features of hypopituitarism depend on the specific pituitary hormones that are lacking. Children with combined GH and cortisol deficiency often develop **hypoglycemia**.

569. *False* regarding chronic bronchitis is:

A. Hemoptysis **B.** > 2 consecutive years
C. Productive cough **D.** Cough for 3 months *(KERALA 1995)*

Chronic bronchitis is a condition associated with *excessive* tracheobronchial mucus production sufficient to cause cough with expectoration for at least 3 months of the year for > 2 consecutive years.

570. Nasal allergy is *most often* due to:

A. Automobile dust **B.** Pollen grains
C. Animal dust **D.** House dust *(PGI 1993)*

Allergic rhinitis is characterized by rhinorrhea; sneezing; obstruction of the nasal passages; conjunctival, nasal, and pharyngeal itching; and lacrimation, all occurring in relationship to allergen exposure. Although commonly *seasonal* due to elicitation by **airborne pollens**, it can be perennial in an environment of chronic exposure.

571. Loud S_3 is a feature of:

A. Severe MR **B.** Mitral stenosis
C. ASD **D.** Old age *(JIPMER 1993)*

A low-pitched 3rd heart sound occurring 0.12 to 0.17 second after the aortic valve closure sound is caused by the sudden tensing of the papillary muscles, chordae tendineae, and valve leaflets and is **an important auscultatory feature of severe mitral regurgitation.**

572. *Most common* cause of organic amnestic syndrome is:

A. Vitamin deficiency **B.** Hypoxia
C. Alzheimer's disease **D.** Concussion *(KARNATAKA 1995)*

Prolonged untreated thiamine deficiency can result in an irreversible dementia/amnestic syndrome (Korsakoff's psychosis) or even death.

573. Chemical transmitter in REM sleep is:

A. Acetylcholine **B.** Serotonin
C. GABA **D.** Dopamine *(PGI 1996)*

Early studies implicate serotonin as the primary sleep-promoting neurotransmitter, while catecholamines were considered to be responsible for wakefulness. **Cholinergic neurotransmission is known to play a role in REM sleep generation.**

574. Legionnaires' disease causes:
- **A.** Acute respiratory infection
- **B.** Congenital malformations
- **C.** Neoplastic disease
- **D.** Urinary tract infection

575. Pontiac fever is caused by:
- **A.** Marburg virus
- **B.** Legionella
- **C.** Tuberculosis bacilli
- **D.** Sindbis virus

576. A 28-year-old lady presented with *diarrhea, confusion* and high grade *fever* and *headache* with *bilateral pneumonitis*. The causative agent is:
- **A.** *Pseudomonas*
- **B.** *Streptococcus pneumonia*
- **C.** *Neisseria meningitidis*
- **D.** *Legionella* *(AI 2000)*

Legionellosis refers to the 2 clinical syndromes caused by bacteria of the genus *Legionella*.
- **Pontiac fever** is an acute, febrile, self-limited illness. Malaise, fatigue, and myalgias are the most frequent symptoms of Pontiac fever, occurring in 97% of cases. Fever (generally with chills) develops in 80 to 90% of cases and headache in 80%. Other symptoms (seen in less than half of the cases) include arthralgias, nausea, cough, abdominal pain, and diarrhea.
- **Legionnaires' disease** is the designation for **pneumonia** caused by these species. The incubation period for Legionnaires' disease is 2 to 10 days. The clinical features may range from a mild cough and a slight fever to stupor with widespread **pulmonary infiltrates** and multisystem failure. Nonspecific symptoms such as malaise, fatigue, anorexia, and **headache** are seen early in the illness. Watery **diarrhea** is reported in 25 to 50% of cases. The most common neurologic abnormalities are **confusion** or changes in mental status. **A temperature in excess of 40.5°C is** seen in 20% of the cases.

577. In hepatic encephalopathy the antibiotic which retards NH_3 formation and absorption is:
- **A.** Ceftriaxone
- **B.** Chloramphenicol
- **C.** Cefixime
- **D.** Neomycin *(AI 2000)*

578. Drug *not* used in hepatic encephalopathy is:
- **A.** Phenobarbitone
- **B.** Lactulose
- **C.** Mannitol
- **D.** Metronidazole *(KARNATAKA 1996)*

Hepatic encephalopathy is a state of disordered CNS function associated with severe acute or chronic liver disease. Encephalopathy may be *acute* and reversible or *chronic* and progressive. In severe cases, irreversible coma and death may occur. The *most common* predisposing factor is **gastrointestinal bleeding**, which leads to an increase in the production of NH_3 and other nitrogenous substances which are then absorbed.

Stage	Mental status	Asterixis	EEG
I	Euphoria or depression, mild confusion, slurred speech, disordered sleep	+/–	Usually normal
II	Lethargy, moderate confusion	+	Abnormal
III	Marked confusion, incoherent speech, sleeping but arousable	+	Abnormal
IV	Coma; initially responsive to noxious stimuli, later unresponsive	–	Abnormal

Management guidelines
• Nil orally • RT for suction • Syrup lactulose (Duphalac®) 1 mg/kg/dose 6 hourly (2 liquid stools per day) • High bowel wash 6 hourly • 20% mannitol-5 ml/kg/dose to reduce cerebral edema • 10% dextrose to prevent hypoglycemia • Vitamin K (0.2 mg/kg; maximum 10 mg IV stat) • Fresh frozen plasma or blood may be required to control bleeding • IV ranitidine (Aciloc®) 12 hourly • Intestinal NH_3 production by bacteria can also be decreased by oral administration of a "nonabsorbable" antibiotic such as **neomycin** (3 gm/M^2 per day in 4 divided doses). Equal benefits may be achieved with broad-spectrum antibiotics such as tetracycline, ampicillin, or metronidazole. • If convulsions occur half the dose of diazepam (0.15 mg/kg) should be used. • Correction of fluid and electrolyte imbalance • IV systemic antibiotics in stage 3 and 4.

579. A patient presents with hyperpigmented lesion on mucosa of lip and oral cavity. She has melena and her elder sister also has similar complains. *Most likely* diagnosis is:

A. Familial polyposis coli
B. Gardener's syndrome
C. Villous adenoma
D. Peutz-Jeghers syndrome *(AI 2000, AIIMS 2000)*

580. A female patient presents with pigmentation of the lips and oral mucosa and colonic polyps. Her sister also has the same history. The diagnosis is:

A. Peutz-Jeghers syndrome
B. Carcinoid
C. Melanoma
D. Villous adenoma *(AIIMS May 2001)*

Peutz-Jeghers syndrome is an autosomal dominant condition consisting of **GI polyposis** and **mucocutaneous melanotic pigmentation**. It is the *most frequent* of the polyposis syndromes to involve the small bowel. About **50% of the reported cases have a family history** of the disease while the remainders of the cases are considered secondary to sporadic mutations. **The characteristic pigmented mucosal lesions appear on the lips and buccal mucosa.** This pigmentation usually occurs early in infancy or early childhood. Other pigmented areas affect the face, fingers, toes, palms of the hands, and soles of the feet. Interestingly, the skin pigmentation may fade or disappear with age. Gastrointestinal polyps are invariably part of the disease. The small bowel is involved with benign hamartomatous polyps in 95% of cases. Adenomatous polyps are present in the colon in approximately 30% of cases, whereas the stomach has adenomatous polyps in approximately 25% of patients. Esophageal polyps are rarely seen. Importantly, despite the benign course of the small bowel hamartomas, there is a higher incidence of gastrointestinal malignancy, particularly of the colon and stomach, than in the general population at large. Rarely, polyps may be identified in the urinary or respiratory tracts. There is also an increased incidence of ovarian neoplasms in women with the syndrome. The common presenting complaints are abdominal pain, obstruction, **rectal bleeding**, anemia, and extrusion of a polyp. Intussusception occurs in 47% of patients and is an important presenting obstructive symptom.

581. Drug used in prophylaxis of meningococcal meningitis is:

A. Penicillin **B.** Ampicillin
C. Rifampicin **D.** Erythromycin *(SGPGI 1999, AI 2000)*

582. Drug *not* used in prophylaxis of meningococcal meningitis:

A. Penicillin **B.** Ofloxacin
C. Rifampicin **D.** Ceftriaxone *(AIIMS 1993)*

Neisseria meningitidis can cause a variety of infections but bacteremia and meningitis are by far the most common. Penicillin G remains the drug of choice for meningococcal disease. The recommended regimen for *prophylaxis* of meningococcal meningitis is as under:
• **Rifampin** at a dosage of 10 mg/kg (up to 600 mg) every 12 h for 2 days for adults and children over 1 year of age and 5 mg/kg every 12 hour for 2 days for children < 1 year old. • **Ciprofloxacin** or **ofloxacin** (a single oral dose of 500 or 400 mg, respectively) is a suitable alternative for adults but is not recommended for children or pregnant women. • A single 250-mg intramuscular dose of **ceftriaxone** is recommended for pregnant contacts; for children < 12 years of age, 125 mg of ceftriaxone can be given.
Vaccines are available against 4 serogroups of meningococci: A, C, W-135, and Y. **No effective serogroup B vaccine as yet available.**

583. Palpable purpura is seen in all *except*:

A. ITP
B. Henoch-Schönlein purpura
C. Polyarteritis nodosa
D. Acute meningococcemia

(PGI 1997)

584. Palpable purpura is seen in all *except*:

A. Drug induced vasculitis
B. Henoch-Schönlein purpura
C. Essential mixed cryoglobulinemia
D. Giant cell arteritis

(AIIMS 1999, AI 2000)

585. *Non* palpable purpura is seen in:

A. Temporal arteritis
B. Drug induced vasculitis
C. Cryoglobulinemia
D. Henoch-Schönlein purpura

(UP 2000)

Some Causes of Palpable Purpura

Vasculitis	Emboli
• Leukocytoclastic vasculitis • Polyarteritis nodosa • Henoch-Schönlein purpura	• Acute meningococcemia • Disseminated gonococcal infection • Rocky Mountain spotted fever • Ecthyma gangrenosum
Most patients of **essential mixed cryoglobulinemia** present with a variable combination of **leukocytoclastic vasculitis**, skin ulcerations, arthralgias, fatigue, and Raynaud's phenomenon. Renal disease complicates 50% of cases and generally develops after 1 to 2 years.	
Vasculitis associated with **drug reactions** usually presents as **palpable purpura** which may be generalized or limited to the lower extremities or other dependent areas; however, urticarial lesions, ulcers, and hemorrhagic blisters may also occur.	

586. A 35-year-old man has carcinoma bronchus with decreased pulmonary functions. Which of the following drug should *not* be given to him:

A. Vinblastine
B. Mithramycin
C. Bleomycin
D. Adriamycin

(AI 2000)

Pulmonary toxicity occurs in 10 to 40% of patients treated with bleomycin, usually 4 to 10 weeks after initiation of treatment. Approximately 1% of treated patients have died of pulmonary fibrosis.

587. Hepatitis C is associated with:

A. Scleroderma
B. Cryoglobulinemia
C. Anti LKM antibodies
D. Polyarteritis nodosa

(AI 2000)

In hepatitis C and D, antibodies to liver-kidney microsomes (LKM) may be found but the *species* of LKM antibodies in the 2 types of hepatitis are different from each other.

588. Autosomal dominant inheritance is seen in:

A. Hemophilia **B.** Bloom's syndrome
C. Retinoblastoma **D.** Ataxia telangiectasia *(AI 2000)*

- **Retinoblastoma is the most common intraocular malignancy of childhood** and nearly 66% of cases appear before the third birthday. Retinoblastoma was previously known as *glioma retinae*. Now it is *better* termed as retinoblastoma because the malignant growth consists of proliferation of neural cells which have failed to evolve normally. Retinoblastoma is confined to the infants and is always congenital. The 2nd eye is affected independently and not by metastasis in 30% of cases. Several children of the same family may be affected as the inheritance pattern is **autosomal dominant** with variable gene penetrance.
- **Bloom's syndrome** is characterized by small body size, immunodeficiency, light-sensitive facial erythema, and a major predisposition to cancer.
- **Ataxia-telangiectasia** is associated with increased numbers of translocations, particularly involving the T cell receptor loci.

589. A 28-year-old male comes with history of exposure 3 weeks back, having cervical lymphadenopathy, hepatosplenomegaly. The early diagnosis of HIV is done by:

A. Lymph node biopsy **B.** ELISA
C. p24 antigen **D.** Western blot *(AI 2000, 2001)*

Throughout the course of HIV infection, equilibrium exists between p24 antigen and anti-p24 antibodies. **During the 1st few weeks of infection, before an immune response develops, there is a brisk rise in p24 antigen levels.** After the development of anti-p24 antibodies, these levels decline.

590. A 65-year-old female Meena gives the history of severe unilateral headache on the right side and complains of blindness since 2 days. On examination there is a thick cord like structure on the lateral side of the head. The ESR is 80 mm/hr in the first hour. The *most likely* diagnosis is:

A. Temporal arteritis **B.** Migraine
C. Cluster headache **D.** Sinusitis *(AIIMS May 2001)*

591. *False* regarding temporal arteritis is:

A. Sudden blindness is a complication **B.** Low ESR
C. Anemia **D.** Polymyalgia rheumatica *(AIIMS 1995)*

Temporal arteritis (cranial or giant cell arteritis) is an inflammation of medium- and large-sized arteries which characteristically involves 1 or more branches of the carotid artery, mainly the **temporal artery**, hence the name. It is characterized *clinically* by the classic complex of fever, anemia, **high ESR**, and headaches in an **elderly** patient. Other manifestations include malaise, fatigue, anorexia, weight loss, sweats, and arthralgias. **Headache** is the predominant symptom and may be associated with a tender, **thickened, or nodular artery**. A dreaded complication of temporal arteritis is ocular involvement primarily due to ischemic optic neuritis, which may lead to serious visual symptoms, even **sudden blindness** in some patients. The disease is closely associated with **polymyalgia rheumatica.** *Characteristic laboratory findings* in addition to the elevated ESR include a normochromic or slightly hypochromic **anemia**. Liver function abnormalities are common, particularly increased alkaline phosphatase levels. **Temporal arteritis** is elegantly sensitive to glucocorticoid therapy. Treatment should start with prednisone, 40 to 60 mg per day for about 1 month, followed by a gradual tapering to a maintenance dose of 7.5 to 10 mg per day.

592. A HIV positive patient has intractable seizures and cerebral calcification. *Most likely* organism is:

A. *Isospora belli*
B. Neurocysticercosis
C. *Toxoplasma gondii*
D. *Cryptococcus neoformans* *(AIIMS May 2001)*

Toxoplasma gondii is the *most common* cause of *secondary* central nervous system infection in patients with AIDS, accounting for 38% of all such infections. It accounts for 50 to 60% of all mass lesions in the CNS of patients with HIV infection and is responsible for 28% of 1st seizures.

593. An 8-year-old child suffering from *recurrent attacks of polyuria* since childhood presents to the pediatric OPD. On examination, the child has *short stature*, vitals and BP is normal. Serum creatinine is 6 mg%, HCO_3^{--} 16 mEq, Na^+ 134, K^+ 4.2 on USG bilateral small kidneys are seen. The *most likely* diagnosis is:

A. Polycystic kidney disease **B.** Medullary cystic kidney disease
C. Nephronophthisis **D.** Reflux nephropathy *(AIIMS May 2001)*

Patients with *juvenile nephronophthisis* present during **childhood** with symptoms of **polyuria**, **growth retardation**, anemia, and **progressive renal failure**. Most patients develop end stage renal disease prior to the age of 20 years. Juvenile nephronophthisis accounts for 2 to 10% cases of renal failure in children. Features of tubule damage are often found, including **hyperkalemia** and hyperchloremic metabolic acidosis. Radiographic studies demonstrate **small kidneys**, loss of the corticomedullary junction, and multiple cysts in the medulla. Treatment is mainly supportive, as there is no specific therapy to prevent loss of renal function.

594. *Right* sided infective endocarditis *cannot* occur in:

A. Puerperal sepsis **B.** ASD
C. Tetralogy of Fallot **D.** IV drug abusers *(KARNATAKA 2000)*

595. Infective endocarditis is *least* likely to occur in:

A. MVP **B.** Small VSD
C. TOF **D.** ASD *(AIIMS May 2001)*

Patients of **congenital heart disease** (CHD) having a high velocity of blood ejected through a hole or stenotic orifice are more susceptible to endocarditis. Therefore children with VSD, *left* sided valvular disease and systemic pulmonary arterial communication (including palliative shunts) are at the highest risk. Tetralogy of Fallot (**TOF**), **VSD**, AS, PDA, TGV and palliative shunts are the most frequent structural lesions associated with endocarditis. In older children congenital bicuspid aortic valves and mitral valve prolapse (**MVP**) pose additional risks for endocarditis. Surgical 'repair' of CHD *may reduce* but *does not eliminate* the risk of endocarditis except the repair of a simple ASD or PDA.

596. Mycosis fungoides is *best* treated by:

A. IV doxorubicin (Adriamycin) **B.** Surgery
C. 5 GU cream **D.** Electron beam therapy *(AIIMS 1991)*

Local and systemic therapies are used in the treatment of mycosis fungoides. Patients with disease limited to the skin may be *cured* with **electron beam radiation therapy**.

597. Dopamine is preferred in shock because:

A. Rapid action **B.** Renal vasodilatation
C. Cardiac stimulation **D.** Potent vasoconstriction *(AIIMS 1991)*

Dose Dependent Actions of Dopamine

Dose	Action
• **0.5-2 μg/kg/minute**	Increases renal and splanchnic blood flow (perfusion) and mild vasodilation;
• **3.0-10 μg /kg/minute**	Increased renal blood flow with positive ionotropic effect on heart and mild vasoconstriction;
• **10-20 μg /kg/minute**	Tachycardia and vasoconstriction.

598. The most frequent cause of *peripheral* cyanosis is:

A. Interatrial septal defect
B. Interstitial pulmonary fibrosis
C. Slowed circulation through skin
D. Methemoglobinemia

599. Cyanosis is *not* seen in patient with severe anemia because:

A. RBCs are defective **B.** Capillary dilatation occurs
C. Hypoxia is rare **D.** Minimum 5 gm hemoglobin is required *(AIIMS 1991)*

Cyanosis occurs when there is excess of *desaturated* hemoglobin or *abnormal* hemoglobin in the capillaries. **Deoxygenated hemoglobin level above 5 gm% leads to cyanosis**. Therefore presence or absence of cyanosis depends upon the *absolute* value of deoxygenated hemoglobin. **In cases of anemia, when the hemoglobin concentration is already low (may be less than 5 gm% in severe cases), cyanosis is *not* commonly seen.**
Cyanosis can be of 3 types:

1. **Peripheral cyanosis** which is due to slow capillary blood flow which allows more time for extraction of oxygen from blood to the tissues. It can be due to 2 conditions:
   A) *Reduced cardiac output* such as in **shock**, **mitral stenosis,** etc
   B) *Local vasoconstriction* due to **cold**
2. **Central cyanosis** which occurs due to excess deoxygenated hemoglobin in blood leaving aorta. It can be of 3 types:
   A) *Due to inadequate oxygenation* of blood which may be due to inadequate oxygen supplied to the lungs as occurs in **pneumonia** or **chronic bronchitis** or **poliomyelitis** or **fibrosing alveolitis**.
   B) *Due to shunting* of blood from *right to left* side of heart as it occurs in **tetralogy of Fallot**.
   C) *Due to an absolute excess of desaturated hemoglobin*, the percentage saturation being normal. This occurs in **primary polycythemia**.
3. **Entrogenous cyanosis** (due to abnormal hemoglobin) due to presence of excess **sulfhemoglobin** or **methemoglobin**.

600. Cyanosis is *not* caused by:
A. Cirrhosis with portal hypertension
B. Carboxyhemoglobinemia
C. Sulfhemoglobinemia
D. Methemoglobinemia *(AIIMS 1994)*

601. About central cyanosis *true* is:
A. Hb< 5 gm/dl
B. Hb< 2 gm/dl
C. Methemoglobin less than 2.5 gm/dl
D. Sulfhemoglobin more than 0.5 gm/dl *(PGI May 2001)*

Cyanosis is a bluish color of the skin and mucous membranes due to an increased amount of reduced hemoglobin, or of hemoglobin derivatives, in the small blood vessels. It is most marked in the lips, nailbeds, ears, and malar eminences. Cyanosis becomes obvious when the mean capillary concentration of reduced hemoglobin exceeds 5 g/dL. Hemoglobin has an affinity for carbon monoxide that is about 200 times higher than its affinity for oxygen. *A cherry-colored flush, rather than cyanosis, is caused by carboxyhemoglobin.* Cyanosis also is observed when nonfunctional hemoglobin such as **methemoglobin** or **sulfhemoglobin** is present in blood.

Abnormal hemoglobin	Minimal level required to produce cyanosis
• **Deoxyhemoglobin**	5 gm/dL
• **Methemoglobin**	1.5 gm/dL
• **Sulfhemoglobin**	0.5 gm/dL

602. A 20-year-old girl with UTI on treatment develops blue lips and nails with normal vitals:
A. Cardiac right to left shunt
B. Sickle cell disease
C. Sideroblastic anemia
D. Methemoglobinemia *(UP 1999)*

Methemoglobinemia occurs due to exposure to chemicals that oxidize the iron in hemoglobin from its ferrous (Fe^{++}) to its ferric (Fe^{+++}) state. Methemoglobin (**ferric hemoglobin**) *cannot* carry oxygen and results in a 'functional' anemia. It also shifts the oxygen-dissociation curve towards the left, limiting the release of oxygen to tissues. Symptoms are due to hypoxia and anaerobic metabolism. **Cyanosis** that is unresponsive to O_2 and may have a gray-brown hue occurs with methemoglobin levels > 15% (**1.5 g/dL absolute methemoglobin**). **Patients are asymptomatic** until methemoglobin levels exceed 20 to 30%. Clinical features vary according to the level of methemoglobin:

20 to 30%	>45%	>70%
• Headache • Tachycardia • Dizziness • Fatigue	• Dyspnea • Bradycardia • Hypoxia • Acidosis • Seizures • Coma • Cardiac arrhythmias	• Fatal

Oxidizing agents include local anesthetics such as benzocaine, nitrites, nitrates, naphthalene, nitrobenzene and related chemicals, oxides of nitrogen, phenazopyridine, primaquine and related antimalarials, and **sulfonamides**.

Most oxidizing agents are eliminated by metabolism therefore diuresis is ineffective. Supplemental O_2 should be administered. Methylene blue is indicated for methemoglobin levels above 30%. Methylene blue is given at a dose of 1 to 2 mg/kg body weight as a 1% solution over 5 minutes and if a clinical response is not observed within 1 hour, the dose may be repeated.

603. All of the following are *true* about primary CNS lymphoma *except*:

A. Causes focal signs
B. Most are of T-cell origin
C. Multicentric location
D. Associated with latent Epstein-Barr virus infection *(SGPGI 2002)*

Primary CNS lymphoma presents within the neuraxis without evidence of systemic lymphoma. They are **B cell malignancies** of intermediate to high grade and occur most frequently in immunosuppressed individuals, such as organ transplant recipients or AIDS patients. In these settings, CNS lymphomas are *always* associated with latent **Epstein-Barr virus** infection of the tumor cells. In immunocompetent patients, CT or MRI scan *most often* reveal a uniformly enhancing **mass lesion** while in immunosuppressed patients, primary CNS lymphoma is likely to be **multicentric** and exhibit ring enhancement or to arise in the meninges. Prognosis is poor. *Radiotherapy is the mainstay of treatment*, although systemic combination chemotherapy can provide additional benefit.

604. *Drug of choice* for acute gout is:

A. Probenicid
B. Allopurinol
C. Sulphonamide
D. Indomethacin *(SGPGI 2002)*

NSAIDs are the agents of choice for management of acute gout and it is important to start the treatment as early as possible; to use adequate doses and to avoid salicylates and diuretics. **Indomethacin** 50 mg 6 hourly or naproxen 250 mg 8 hourly should be given until the acute attack subsides. Treatment is then continued with a lower dose for next 10 days. Colchicine is *highly effective* but may cause vomiting and diarrhea in *many* patients.

605. The *treatment of choice* for intestinal and extraintestinal amebiasis is:

A. Diloxanide furoate
B. Chloroquine
C. Metronidazole
D. Tetracycline *(SGPGI 2002)*

Metronidazole is the drug of choice for amebic liver abscess. 2nd-line therapeutic agents' emetine and chloroquine should be avoided if possible because of the potential cardiovascular and gastrointestinal side effects of the former and the higher relapse rates with the latter.

Asymptomatic patients (luminal agents)		**Acute colitis**	
Iodoquinol	650 mg tid for 20 days	Metronidazole + Luminal agent	750 mg PO or IV tid for 5 to 10 days
Diloxanide furoate	500 mg tid for 10 days		
Paromomycin	500 mg tid for 10 days		

Amebic liver abscess	
Metronidazole	750 mg PO or IV tid for 5 to 10 days
Tinidazole	2 g PO
Ornidazole	2 g PO
+ Luminal agent as above	

606. All the following are used in the treatment of hypertensive emergencies *except*:
A. Prazosin
B. Nitroglycerin
C. Sodium nitroprusside
D. Nifedipine
(SGPGI 2002)

Drugs used to Treat Hypertensive Emergencies

Immediate onset	**Delayed onset**
• Nitroprusside	• Enalaprilat
• Trimethaphan	• Hydralazine
• Nitroglycerin	• Labetalol
• Diazoxide	• Nifedipine

607. The histological finding in acute rheumatic fever which would best aid in diagnosis is:
A. Increased vascularity of myocardial valves
B. Osler's nodule
C. Aschoff bodies
D. Vegetations over mitral valve
(SGPGI 2002)

In **acute rheumatic fever** focal, inflammatory and widely disseminated lesions are found in various organs. In the heart they are known as **Aschoff bodies**. They are foci of fibrinoid necrosis surrounded by lymphocyte, macrophages and occasional plasma cells. Aschoff bodies are pathognomic of rheumatic fever.

608. All the following are seen in nephrotic syndrome *except*:
A. Albuminuria
B. Hypoalbuminemia
C. Edema
D. Hypocomplementemia
(SGPGI 2002)

609. Which of the following is/are *true* about nephrotic syndrome:
A. Hematuria
B. Azotemia
C. Proteinuria
D. All the above
(SGPGI 2002)

610. Nephrotic syndrome is *not* associated with:
A. Hypertension
B. Massive proteinuria
C. Marked edema
D. Hypoproteinemia
(AIIMS 1993)

611. A 2-year-old boy developed generalized pitting edema in 7 days and significant decreased in urinary output. His blood pressure is 104/70 mmHg, urine examination shows hyaline cast +; proteinuria +++; no WBC and RBC. Most likely diagnosis is:
A. Increase in blood volume
B. Increase in blood urea
C. Selective proteinuria
D. Low serum complement level
(AIIMS 1999)

612. *Not* seen in nephrotic syndrome:
A. Hypoalbuminemia
B. Increased α_2 globulin
C. Hyperlipidemia
D. Hypercalcemia
(PGI 1999)

Nephrotic syndrome is characterized by heavy proteinurea (>40 mg / M^2 / hour), **hypoproteinemia**, edema and **hyperlipidemia**. More than 90% of children with nephrotic syndrome have some form of *idiopathic nephrotic syndrome* of which 85% show *minimal change disease* as renal pathology while the incidence of focal sclerosis is 10% and that of mesangial proliferation is 5%. In remaining 10% of cases nephrotic syndrome is due to some form of glomerulonephritis of which membranous and membranoproliferative are more common. The basic pathological abnormality in nephrotic syndrome is **heavy proteinurea** due to increased glomerular capillary wall permeability. The protein loss generally exceeds 2gm/day and is composed *mainly* of albumin. *Thus* it may be said that hypoproteinemia is essentially hypoalbuminemia. **Edema** appears when the serum albumin level falls below 2.5 gm/dL due to decrease in plasma oncotic pressure. Almost all serum lipids (cholesterol and triglyceride) and lipoprotein levels are elevated. Laboratory findings are as under:

• Proteinuria	3+ or 4+ (> 2gm/24 hours)
• Serum cholesterol	Elevated
• Serum triglyceride	Elevated
• Serum albumin	< 2gm/dL
• Total serum calcium	Reduced
• C3 level	Normal
• Renal function	Generally normal but may be reduced

If the age of child is *between 1-8 years* it is most likely that the child is having minimal change disease and oral steroid therapy should be started as *prednisolone* 2 mg/kg/day or 60 mg/m²/day (maximum 60 mg/kg/day) in 3 divided doses *without* further investigation. **Renal biopsy is indicated if the age of child is <1 years or >8 years.** A combination of Furosemide (1-2 mg/kg/day) and spironolactone is useful in reducing edema. *Average* time required for response of prednisolone is about 2 weeks and response is defined as the point at which the urine becomes free of protein. If the child continues to have proteinuria of 2+ or more after one month prednisolone therapy then the nephrotic syndrome is termed as *steroid resistant* and is an indication of renal biopsy. 5 days after the urine becomes 'free' of protein (-ve, trace or 1+) the total dose of prednisolone is given as a *single* dose with breakfast on alternate day for 3-6 months. After such a period prednisolone is discontinued *abruptly*.
A relapse is defined as recurrence of edema and *not merely proteinuria* which occurs *intermittently* and resolves *spontaneously*. Repeated relapse and severe corticosteroid toxicity are indication of cyclophosphamide therapy (3 mg/kg/day OD) along with alternate day prednisolone for 3 months. TLC must be monitored during cyclophosphamide therapy and it should be with held if TLC falls below 5000.

* In children with MCD the urine contains albumin principally and *minimal* amounts of higher molecular weight proteins such as IgG and α_2 macroglobulin.

613. In nephrotic syndrome, levels of all serum proteins decrease *except*:

A. Transferrin
B. Albumin
C. Ceruloplasmin
D. Fibrinogen

In nephrotic syndrome hyperfibrinogenemia occurs due to increased hepatic synthesis of fibrinogen.

614. A young child had nephrotic syndrome and was started on steroids. He was responding to steroid therapy. If a biopsy were to be done, what would the light microscopy have shown:

A. Endothelial thickening
B. Split basement membrane
C. Loss of foot processes
D. No abnormality

(AIIMS Nov 2001)

615. In nephrotic syndrome due to minimal change disease, the pathology is:

A. Loss of foot process and loss of the fixed *negative charge* in the glomerular filtration barrier for protein
B. Loss of foot processes only
C. Deposition of antigen antibody complex
D. Destruction of glomerulus alone

(AIIMS Nov 2001)

Kidneys, ureters and bladder (KUB) are retroperitoneal structures and kidneys lie at the level of L_1-L_4 vertebrae. Each kidney has 8 to 12 pyramid-shaped lobes. The functional unit of kidney is nephrons and there are about 1 million of them in each kidney. **Minimal change disease** (also called nil disease, lipoid nephrosis, or foot process disease) is so named because glomerular size and architecture are **normal by light microscopy**. *Electron microscopy* reveals **diffuse fusion of epithelial foot processes** and hyperactivity of mesangial area. *Selective proteinuria* in combination with foot process effacement suggests injury to podocytes and loss of the fixed *negative charge* in the glomerular filtration barrier for protein.

616. Neurotransmitter involved in nigrostriatal pathway is:

A. Serotonin
B. Dopamine
C. Cholinergic
D. Adrenergic

(SGPGI 2002)

617. The pathology in Parkinsonism lies in:

A. Substantia nigra **B.** Hippocampus
C. Red nucleus **D.** Hypothalamus

There is a system of dopaminergic neurons in nigrostriatal dopaminergic system with cell bodies in substantia nigra and axon endings in caudate nucleus. In Parkinson's disease there is loss of dopaminergic cells in the substantia nigra which leads to striatal dopamine *depletion*. As dopamine activates excitatory D_1 receptors in the direct pathway and represses inhibitory D_2 receptors in the indirect pathway, this depletion leads to decreased activity of the direct pathway and increased activity of the indirect pathway.

618. Which of the following complications of diabetes *cannot* be prevented by strict control of blood sugar:

A. Nerve conduction velocity **B.** Amyotrophy
C. Fluorescein leak **D.** Microalbuminuria *(AIIMS 1991)*

Thorough control with insulin infusion pumps has been reported to **decrease microalbuminuria**, **improve motor nerve conduction velocity**, lower plasma lipoproteins, and **decrease capillary leakage of fluorescein** in the retina. **Firm evidence fails to show that late complications can be reversed by long-term return of the plasma glucose to *near*-normal levels.** Retinopathy may progress despite successful reversal of diabetes by pancreatic transplantation and the progression of diabetic complications after the return of the plasma glucose level to normal or near normal has been termed hyperglycemic memory. Diabetic amyotrophy is a form of neuropathy, *although* atrophy and weakness of the large muscles in the upper leg and pelvic girdle resemble primary muscle disease. Anorexia and depression may be associated with amyotrophy.

619. *False* regarding CRF:

A. Decreased half-life of insulin **B.** Serum vitamin D is increased
C. Hypocalcemia **D.** Hyperphosphatemia *(AIIMS 1991)*

- Plasma levels of many polypeptide hormones (parathyroid hormone, **insulin**, glucagon, luteinizing hormone, and prolactin) **rise with renal failure**, often markedly, not only because of impaired renal catabolism but also because of enhanced glandular secretion. Uremic patients are also resistant to the action of insulin. As insulin is removed from the plasma largely by renal cells, which degrade it intracellularly, circulating insulin levels in plasma are slightly or moderately increased in most fasting uremic subjects and levels in excess of normal are usually demonstrable after a glucose load. The glucose intolerance of uremia results mainly from this peripheral resistance to the action of insulin.
- Vigorous use of phosphate-*binding* agents, calcium supplements, and vitamin D to maintain the serum levels of calcium (9.5 to 10.5 mg/dL) and phosphorus (4.5 to 6.0 mg/dL) are frequently effective in suppressing parathyroid levels and preventing osteitis fibrosa and osteomalacia.

620. *Not* common in alcoholism:

A. Polycythemia **B.** Dementia
C. Polyneuritis **D.** Hypomagnesemia *(AIIMS 1991)*

- Permanent CNS impairment (**alcohol induced *persisting* dementia**) can develop and accounts for up to 20% of chronically demented patients.
- Chronic intake of high doses of ethanol causes peripheral neuropathy in 5 to 15% of alcoholics, which is possibly related to thiamine deficiency.
- Low blood levels of K^+, Mg^+, Ca^{++}, Zn, and phosphorus can occur as a consequence of dietary deficiency and acid-base imbalances during excess alcohol ingestion or withdrawal.

621. *False* regarding cholera is:

A. Infectivity
B. Denudation of jejunal mucosa
C. Watery stool
D. Stool HCO_3^- is twice plasma HCO_3 *(AIIMS 1991)*

Cholera is an acute diarrheal disease (**ADD**) which can, in a matter of hours, result in severe, rapidly progressive dehydration and death. The term cholera generally refers to disease caused by *Vibrio cholerae* serogroup O_1. *Vibrio cholerae* O_1 exists in two biotypes viz. *classic* and *El Tor* that are distinguished on the basis of a number of characteristics including phage susceptibility and hemolysin production. Cholera is predominantly a pediatric disease in endemic areas. Cholera is a toxin-mediated disease and its characteristic **watery diarrhea** is due to the action of cholera toxin (CTX). CTX is a potent protein enterotoxin elaborated by the organism in the small intestine. After a 24 to 48 hours incubation period, cholera begins with the sudden *painless* watery diarrhea that may quickly become voluminous and often is followed by vomiting. The stool has a characteristic "rice-water". Laboratory investigation reveal an elevated hematocrit in nonanemic patients; normal Na^+, K^+, and Cl^- levels; a markedly **reduced HCO_3^- level** (<15 mmol/L); and an elevated anion gap (due to increases in serum lactate, protein, and phosphate). Arterial pH is usually *low* (7.2). **Only the rapid and adequate replacement of fluids, electrolytes, and base is required. Ringer's lactate is the best choice**. Although *not necessary for cure*, the use of an antibiotic to which the organism is susceptible will reduce the duration and volume of fluid loss and will speed up the clearance of organism from the stool. **Single-dose tetracycline (2 g) or doxycycline (300 mg) is effective in adults but is not recommended for children under 8 years of age**. For *children*, **furazolidone (5 mg/kg/day in 4 divided doses for 3 days) is the drug of choice** and Septran® (TMP 5 mg/kg and SMX 25 mg/kg in 2 divided doses for 3 days) the 2nd choice.

622. Diagnostic of thiamine deficiency is:

A. FIGLU test
B. Microcytic anemia
C. Low RBC transketolase
D. Low RBC acetylcholine *(AIIMS 1991)*

The most reliable test to detect thiamine deficiency is the measurement of whole-blood or RBC transketolase activity.

623. *Not* seen in Brown-Séquard's syndrome:

A. Ipsilateral loss of joint sense
B. Contralateral loss of pain sense
C. Ipsilateral monoplegia
D. Ipsilateral loss of temperature *(AIIMS 1991)*

Brown-Séquard's hemicord syndrome consists of **ipsilateral weakness (pyramidal tract) and loss of joint position and vibratory sense (involvement of posterior column),** with **contralateral loss of pain and temperature sense (involvement of spinothalamic tract)** below the lesion. The sensory level for pain and temperature is 1 or 2 levels below the lesion.

624. *Not* used in treatment of hypercalcemia:

A. Riluzole
B. Risedronate
C. Plicamycin
D. Gallium nitrate *(AIIMS 1997)*

625. *Not* used in the treatment of hypercalcemia:

A. Biphosphonate
B. Penicillamine
C. Mithramycin
D. Steroid *(AIIMS 1996)*

626. *Not* a treatment of hypercalcemia:

A. Ketoconazole
B. Frusemide
C. Plicamycin
D. Oral phosphate *(AIIMS 1991)*

Therapies for Severe Hypercalcemia

- Hydration with saline
- Forced diuresis; saline + **loop diuretic**
- Gallium nitrate
- **Plicamycin (Mithramycin)**
- **Phosphate** (oral or IV)
- First generation bisphosphonates-etidronate
- Second generation bisphosphonates- (tiludronate, pamidronate, alendronate, and risedronate)
- Calcitonin
- Glucocorticoids
- Dialysis

627. *Not* a feature of magnesium deficiency:

A. Delirium
B. Raised serum calcium
C. Convulsions
D. Athetoid tetany *(AIIMS 1991)*

Symptoms of severe Mg^{++} deficiency, including paresthesia, muscular cramps, irritability, decreased attention span, and **mental confusion**, may require months to appear. The physical findings are mainly due to the *associated **hypo**calcemia* and include positive Trousseau and Chvostek signs, peculiar movements of the fingers (athetoid tetany) and occasionally **convulsions**.

628. Dawn phenomenon is:

A. Postprandial coma
B. Breakfast hypoglycemia
C. Early morning hyperglycemia
D. Early morning hypoglycemia *(AIIMS 1991)*

The Somogyi effect	The Dawn phenomenon
It may be defined as rebound **hyperglycemia** which occurs after an episode of hypoglycemia due to release of counter regulatory hormones.	It is **early morning** rise in plasma glucose (**hyperglycemia**) due to increased insulin requirement.

629. Colchicine is *not* used in:

A. Adrenal adenoma
B. Amyloidosis
C. Familial Mediterranean fever
D. Cirrhosis of liver *(AIIMS 1991)*

Indications of Colchicine

• Gouty arthritis	• Familial Mediterranean fever
• Primary amyloidosis	• Primary biliary cirrhosis

630. Shrinking lung syndrome is seen in:

A. Dermatomyositis
B. Polymyositis
C. Systemic lupus erythematosus
D. Systemic sclerosis *(AIIMS 1991, PGI 1997)*

Shrinking lung syndrome results from respiratory and diaphragmatic muscle dysfunction and can be found in up to **25% of patients of systemic lupus erythematosus**. Lack of appropriate diaphragmatic excursion results in generalized atelectasis and reduced lung compliance. With assisted ventilation the lungs will re-expand. The CXR findings include low lung volumes and basilar atelectasis.

631. Lesion of caudate nucleus produces:

A. Athetosis
B. Chorea
C. Hemiballismus
D. All of the above

632. *Semi*-purposive movements in a boy are generally seen in:

A. Encephalitis
B. Brain abscess
C. Rheumatic fever
D. Systemic lupus erythematosus *(AIIMS 1992)*

Chorea	It is defined as recurrent, jerky and semi-purposive movements of limbs, face and trunk. **C**horea is usually associated with degeneration of **C**audate nucleus.
Athetosis	It is a slow writhing, movement that occurs almost continuously in distal muscles. It occurs due to lesion in extrapyramidal system and its cortical connection.
Hemiballismus	It is a sudden and violent flinging movement of a proximal limb, usually an arm. It occurs due to lesion of the glutamatergic neurons in the subthalamic nucleus
Sydenham's chorea occurs in less than 10% of patients with rheumatic fever. The period between the onset of the initiating streptococcal infection and the onset of Sydenham's chorea may be as long as several months. This CNS disorder is a part of the rheumatic fever complex and should be managed as such. Patients with Sydenham's chorea should be given secondary prophylaxis for prevention of recurrent attacks, even if they *do not* appear to have rheumatic heart disease.	

633. Hypersensitive pneumonitis is associated with which of the following:

A. Raised serum precipitins | **B.** Hilar lymphadenopathy
C. Increased eosinophils | **D.** Raised IgE *(AIIMS 1992)*

Precipitins indicate adequate exposure to the suspected causative agent for generation of an immunologic response. The diagnosis of **hypersensitivity pneumonitis** should not be established *only* by the presence of precipitins but they are powerful *supporting* evidence to the diagnosis.

634. Site of action of blocking immunoglobulins in myasthenia gravis is:

A. Motor end plate | **B.** Presynaptic vesicles
C. Synapse | **D.** Cell body

635. *Not* a characteristic feature of myasthenia gravis:

A. Sometimes spontaneous regression | **B.** Proximal muscle involvement
C. Absent deep reflexes | **D.** Fatigue with exertion *(AIIMS 1997)*

In **myasthenia gravis** (MG) the *fundamental defect* is a decrease in the number of available acetylcholine receptors (AChRs) at the *post*synaptic muscle membrane. The neuromuscular abnormalities in MG are brought about by an autoimmune response mediated by specific anti-AChR *antibodies*. The cardinal features are weakness and **fatigability** of muscles. The weakness increases during repeated use (fatigue) and may improve following rest or sleep. Exacerbations and **remissions** may occur. The cranial muscles, particularly the lids and extraocular muscles, are often involved early, and diplopia and ptosis are common initial complaints. In about 85% of patients, the weakness becomes generalized, affecting the limb muscles as well. The limb weakness in MG is often **proximal** and may be asymmetric. **Despite the muscle weakness, deep tendon reflexes are preserved.**

636. *Not* an indication for thymectomy in myasthenia gravis:

A. Thymic hyperplasia | **B.** Thymoma
C. Young female | **D.** Males > 66 years *(AIIMS 1992)*

Thymectomy should be carried out in all patients with generalized myasthenia gravis between the ages of puberty and at least 55 years. Whether **thymectomy** should be recommended in children, in adults over 55 years of age and in patients with weakness limited to the ocular muscles is still a *matter of debate*.

637. *Characteristic* feature of idiopathic hypoparathyroidism is:

A. Candidiasis | **B.** Subcutaneous calcification
C. Nephrocalcinosis | **D.** Bilateral cataract *(AIIMS 1992)*

Hypoparathyroidism may occur in association with other various developmental defects or as part of a complex hereditary autoimmune syndrome involving failure of the adrenals, the ovaries, and the parathyroids in association with **recurrent mucocutaneous candidiasis**, alopecia, vitiligo, and pernicious anemia.

638. Myasthenia gravis is diagnosed by using:

A. Gallamine | **B.** Edrophonium
C. Succinylcholine | **D.** Atropine *(AIIMS 1992)*

639. Best diagnostic aid to myasthenia gravis is:

A. History | **B.** EMG
C. Chest X-ray | **D.** Response to IV edrophonium

The suspected diagnosis of **myasthenia gravis** must *always* be confirmed definitively before treatment is undertaken; this is important because (1) other treatable conditions may closely resemble MG and (2) the treatment of MG may involve surgery and the prolonged use of drugs with adverse side effects. Drugs which inhibit the enzyme acetylcholine esterase allow acetylcholine to interact repeatedly with the limited number of acetylcholine receptors, producing improvement in the strength of myasthenic muscles. **Edrophonium** is used most commonly, because of the rapid onset (30 s) and short duration (about 5 min) of its effect.

640. In *Pneumocystis carinii* pneumonia the *treatment of choice* is:
A. Zidovudine
B. Ciprofloxacin
C. Cotrimoxazole
D. Pentamidine
(AIIMS 1992)

641. In severe *Pneumocystis carinii* pneumonia, the *drug of choice* is:
A. Penicillin
B. Cefoperazone
C. Cefotaxime
D. Trimethoprim + sulphamethoxazole
(KERALA 1999)

Cotrimoxazole or trimethoprim-sulfamethoxazole (Septran®) which acts by inhibiting folic acid synthesis is considered the drug of choice for *all forms* of **pneumocystosis**.

642. In hypokalemia the ECG finding is:
A. RSR pattern
B. Tall T-wave
C. ST depression
D. Prominent U-wave
(AIIMS 1992)

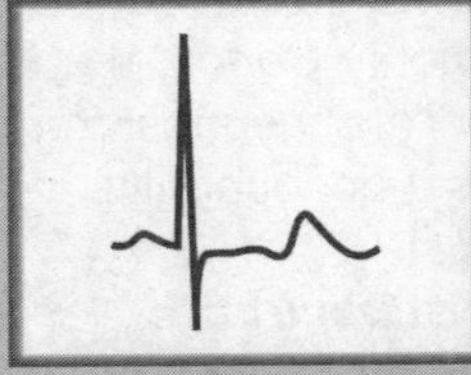

An abnormal **increase in U-wave amplitude** is *most commonly* due to drugs (quinidine, procainamide, disopyramide) or **hypokalemia**.

643. HBsAg carrier status is associated with all *except*:
A. Infectious mononucleosis
B. Down syndrome
C. Chronic renal failure
D. Polyarthritis nodosa
(AIIMS 1992)

For *unknown* reasons, people with **Down syndrome** are more susceptible to **hepatitis B** infection. A proportion of patients with chronic persistent hepatitis or chronic active hepatitis develop manifestations of immune-complex disease; systemic necrotizing vasculitis (**polyarteritis nodosa**) and **membranoproliferative glomerulonephritis** being the most common.

644. *Most common* complication of prosthetic valve is:
A. Embolism
B. Subacute bacterial endocarditis
C. Rejection
D. Infarction

The *most common* complication of prosthetic valve is **prosthetic valve endocarditis**.

645. In drug addicts endocarditis is common due to:
A. *Pseudomonas*
B. *Staphylococcus aureus*
C. *Streptococcus viridans*
D. Group D streptococcus
(AIIMS 1992)

646. Prosthetic valve endocarditis is *most commonly* caused by:
A. *Coxiella burnetii*
B. *Candida*
C. *Streptococcus epidermidis*
D. *Staphylococcus aureus*
(AIIMS 1997)

Endocarditis can be classified in 3 categories viz. **native valve endocarditis**, **endocarditis in intravenous drug abusers**, and **prosthetic valve endocarditis**.

- Streptococci cause about 55% of cases of **native valve endocarditis** in patients who do not abuse IV drugs. Viridans streptococci (most commonly *Streptococcus sanguis*, *Streptococcus mutans*, *Streptococcus mitis* or *Streptococcus milleri*) account for about 75% of these cases; *Streptococcus bovis* and other streptococci cause 20 and 5%, respectively.
- The skin is most common the source of microorganisms responsible for endocarditis in **IV drug abusers**. ***Staphylococcus aureus* causes > 50% of cases**, streptococci and enterococci about 20%, and fungi (mainly *Candida*) and gram-negative bacilli (usually *Pseudomonas* species) about 6% each.
- Early onset **prosthetic valve endocarditis** (onset of symptoms within 60 days of surgery) is a consequence of valve contamination *during* the procedure or of perioperative bacteremia. Late onset prosthetic valve endocarditis (onset of symptoms after 60 days) may have the same pathogenesis as early endocarditis (especially during the 1st year) but with a long incubation period; it may also result from transient bacteremia. 50% of all episodes of early-onset endocarditis and 33% of all episodes of late-onset endocarditis are caused by staphylococci, and ***Staphylococcus epidermidis* is more frequently involved than *Staphylococcus aureus***. Gram-negative bacilli cause up to 15%, and fungi (most commonly *Candida*) up to 10%, of early-onset cases; they are less common in late-onset endocarditis. Streptococci are the *most frequent* single cause of late-onset endocarditis (40% of cases) but are *un*common in early-onset endocarditis.

Endocarditis can *also* be classified as *acute* or *subacute*:

- **Acute endocarditis is most frequently caused by *Staphylococcus aureus***; occurs on a *normal* heart valve; is rapidly destructive; is fatal in less than 6 weeks.
- **Subacute endocarditis is caused by viridans streptococci**; occurs on damaged valves; takes > 6 weeks, perhaps as long as a year, to be fatal.

Simplified table of etiological agents of various types of endocarditis

• Native valve endocarditis	Viridans streptococci
• IV drug abusers	*Staphylococcus aureus*
• Prosthetic valve endocarditis (early onset)	*Staphylococcus epidermidis*
• Prosthetic valve endocarditis (late onset)	Streptococci
• Acute endocarditis	*Staphylococcus aureus*
• Subacute endocarditis	Viridans streptococci

647. In IV drug users, *most common* heart valve involved is:

A. Tricuspid valve
B. Pulmonary valve
C. Mitral valve
D. Aortic valve

(AIIMS 1997)

In IV drug abusers the tricuspid valve is infected in about 50% of cases, the aortic valve in 25%, the mitral valve in 20%, and multiple valves in the remaining. More than 75% of patients with *Staphylococcus aureus* infection and a much lower percentage of those infected with other organisms have tricuspid valve endocarditis.

648. Bronchial asthma is associated with raised levels of:

A. Thromboxane
B. Leukotriene
C. PGI_2
D. PGE_8

(AIIMS 1992)

The cells which play important roles in the **pathogenesis of bronchial asthma** are mast cells, eosinophils, macrophages, neutrophils, and lymphocytes. The mediators released (histamine; bradykinin; the **leukotrienes** C, D, and E; platelet-activating factor; and prostaglandins E_2, F_{2a}, and D_2) produce an intense, immediate inflammatory reaction producing bronchoconstriction, vascular congestion, and edema formation. **Leukotrienes** also account for some of the other pathophysiologic features of asthma, such as increased mucus production and impaired mucociliary transport. *Montelukast* sodium (Romilast®) is a selective and orally active *leukotriene receptor antagonist* that inhibits the cysteinyl leukotriene CysL T_1 receptor. Montelukast is indicated for the *prophylaxis* and chronic treatment of asthma in patients of ages 2 years and older.

649. Asymmetrical radial pulse is seen in which of the following:
- **A.** Takayasu's disease
- **B.** Aortic regurgitation
- **C.** Coarctation of aorta
- **D.** Dissecting aneurysm of aorta *(AIIMS 1992)*

Takayasu's arteritis (aortic arch syndrome) is an inflammatory and stenotic disease of medium and large sized arteries characterized by a strong 'liking' for the aortic arch and its branches. The generalized symptoms include malaise, fever, night sweats, arthralgias, anorexia, and weight loss which may occur months before vessel involvement is apparent. **Pulses are commonly absent in the involved vessels**, particularly the subclavian artery. Death occurs from congestive heart failure or cerebrovascular accidents. Typical laboratory findings include an elevated ESR, mild anemia, and elevated immunoglobulin levels.

650. Vaccine *not* recommended in symptomatic patient of HIV is:
- **A.** DPT
- **B.** Hib conjugate
- **C.** BCG
- **D.** Measles *(AIIMS 1992)*

HIV infected children are recommended to take DPT, OPV or IPV, measles, MMR, Hib conjugate and hepatitis B vaccines. *However*, OPV and BCG in *symptomatic* children need to be withheld *although* these *may be given* in asymptomatic children.

651. In HIV patient the *most common* form of tuberculosis is seen in:
- **A.** Genitourinary tract
- **B.** Intestine
- **C.** Lungs
- **D.** Lymph nodes *(KERALA 1999)*

Mycobacterium tuberculosis experienced a resurgence associated with the HIV epidemic. Approximately **60 to 80% of patients have pulmonary tuberculosis**, and 30 to 40% have extrapulmonary tuberculosis.

652. PUO in a farmer dealing with goat's milk is likely due to:
- **A.** *Bacillus anthracis*
- **B.** *Histoplasma*
- **C.** *Brucella*
- **D.** *Mycobacterium* *(AIIMS 1992)*

Human brucellosis can be caused by any of 4 species viz. *Brucella melitensis* (the *most common* cause worldwide) is acquired mainly from **goats**, sheep, and camels; *Brucella abortus* from cattle; *Brucella suis* from hogs (*Sus scrofa)*; and *Brucella canis* from dogs. The *most common* symptoms are **fever**, chills, diaphoresis, headaches, myalgia, fatigue, anorexia, joint and low-back pain, weight loss, constipation, sore throat, and dry cough. Combination of doxycycline and an aminoglycoside (streptomycin, gentamicin, or netilmicin) for 28 days followed by the combination of doxycycline and rifampin for 4 to 8 weeks is the most effective regimen.

653. *Not* seen in CRF:
- **A.** Metabolic acidosis
- **B.** Increased Mg^{++}
- **C.** Increased phosphate
- **D.** Decreased sodium *(AIIMS 1992)*

654. Which of the following changes of chronic renal failure is *not* improved by dialysis:
- **A.** Volume expansion and contraction
- **B.** Hypernatremia and hyponatremia
- **C.** Hyperkalemia and hypokalemia
- **D.** Decreased high-density lipoprotein level

IMPROVE AFTER DIALYSIS	DEVELOP AFTER DIALYSIS
Volume expansion and contraction	• Aluminum-induced osteomalacia
• Hypernatremia and hyponatremia	• Muscle cramps
• Hyperkalemia and hypokalemia	• Dialysis disequilibrium syndrome
• Metabolic acidosis	• Dialysis dementia
• Hyperphosphatemia	• Hypotension and arrhythmias
• Hypocalcemia	• Hepatitis
• Vitamin D-deficient osteomalacia	• Idiopathic ascites
• Carbohydrate intolerance	• Peritonitis
• Hypothermia	• Microcytic (aluminum-induced) anemia
• Fatigue*	• Leukopenia
• Impaired mentation*	• Hypocomplementemia
• Lethargy	
• Asterixis	
• Muscular irritability	
• Myoclonus	
• Coma	
• Congestive heart failure or pulmonary edema	
• Pericarditis	
• Uremic lung	
• Pallor*	
• Ecchymoses	
• Uremic frost	
• Nausea and vomiting	
• Uremic fetor	
• Gastroenteritis	
• Normocytic, normochromic anemia*	
DEVELOP OR PERSIST AFTER DIALYSIS	
• Myopathy	
• Accelerated atherosclerosis	
IMPROVE, DEVELOP OR PERSIST AFTER DIALYSIS	
• Hyperpigmentation	
• Gastrointestinal bleeding	
IMPROVE OR DEVELOP AFTER DIALYSIS	
• Bleeding diathesis*	

***Improves with dialysis and erythropoietin therapy.**

655. Bleeding time is prolonged in:

A. Hemolytic telangiectasia
B. Henoch-Schönlein purpura
C. von Willebrand's disease
D. Hemophilia

(AIIMS 1992, 1993)

656. *False* regarding von Willebrand's disease:

A. Impaired clot aggregation on glass surface
B. Ristocetin cofactor assay
C. Factor VIII deficiency
D. Increased bleeding time

(AIIMS 1997)

von Willebrand's disease (vWD) is the *most common* inherited bleeding disorder (1 in 800 to 1000 individuals). The *most diagnostic* pattern is the combination of:

- A prolonged bleeding time;
- A reduction in plasma von Willebrand's factor concentration;
- A parallel reduction in biologic activity as measured with the ristocetin cofactor assay;
- Reduced factor VIII activity.

657. *Most common* mode of inheritance of von Willebrand's disease is:

A. Co-dominant
B. X-linked recessive
C. Autosomal dominant
D. Autosomal recessive *(AIIMS 2000)*

All forms of von Willebrand's disease are inherited as autosomal dominant traits *except* type III.

658. Murmur of idiopathic hypertrophic cardiomyopathy is increased by all *except*:

A. Valsalva maneuver **B.** Exercise
C. Digoxin **D.** Squatting *(AIIMS 1992)*

659. Murmur of HOCM is decreased in:

A. Amyl nitrate inhalation **B.** Valsalva maneuver
C. Standing position **D.** Supine position *(AIIMS 2000)*

Conditions that increase myocardial contractility, such as **exercise**, isoproterenol, and **digitalis**, and those that *reduce* ventricular volume, such as the **Valsalva maneuver**, **sudden standing**, nitroglycerin, **amyl nitrite**, or tachycardia, all may cause an **increase** in the gradient and the **murmur**. *On the other hand*, elevation of arterial pressure by phenylephrine, squatting, sustained handgrip, augmentation of venous return by passive leg raising, and expansion of the blood volume all increase ventricular volume and ameliorate the gradient and murmur.

660. 100% HLA association is seen with:

A. Narcolepsy **B.** Schizophrenia
C. Myasthenia gravis **D.** Multiple sclerosis

661. Histocompatibility complex associated with narcolepsy is:

A. B_4 **B.** DR_4
C. DR_2 **D.** DR_3 *(JIPMER 1995)*

Narcolepsy is a chronic ailment consisting of recurrent attacks of drowsiness and sleep during daytime. The *most common* symptoms are excessive daytime sleepiness with involuntary daytime sleep episodes, disturbed nocturnal sleep, and cataplexy (sudden weakness or loss of muscle tone without loss of consciousness that is elicited by emotion). Narcolepsy is *virtually* 100% associated with DR2 in both Japanese and Caucasians.

662. In immunocompromised patients the intestinal parasitic disease is:

A. Trichuriasis **B.** Hookworm
C. Strongyloidiasis **D.** Ascariasis *(AIIMS 1993)*

Strongyloides stercoralis is distinguished by a capacity to *replicate* in the human host. This power permits ongoing cycles of *auto*infection due to internal production of infective larvae. **Strongyloidiasis** can thus persist for decades without further exposure of the host to exogenous infective larvae. In immunocompromised hosts, large numbers of invasive *Strongyloides* larvae can disseminate widely and can be fatal.

Common opportunistic infections in HIV patients

Parasitic	Bacteria	Fungal
• *Strongyloides stercoralis* • *Toxoplasma gondii* • *Pneumocystis carinii* • *Cryptosporidium* • *Isospora belli*	• *Mycobacterium tuberculosis* • *Mycobacterium avium intracellulare* (MAC) • *Salmonella* • *Campylobacter* • *Nocardia* • *Actinomycetes* • *Legionella*	• *Candida* • *Cryptococcus* • *Aspergillus* • *Histoplasma*
Malignancy		**Viral**
• Kaposi's sarcoma and lymphomas		• *Cytomegalovirus* • *Herpes simplex virus*

663. Anterior uveitis is seen in:

A. Pauci articular JRA
B. Polyarticular JRA
C. Still's disease
D. Rheumatoid arthritis

(AIIMS May 2002)

Anterior uveitis develops in sarcoidosis, ankylosing spondylitis, juvenile rheumatoid arthritis, inflammatory bowel disease, psoriasis, Reiter's syndrome, and Behcet's disease. It is also associated with herpes infections, syphilis, Lyme disease, onchocerciasis, tuberculosis, and leprosy.

JRA	Systemic	Polyarticular RF -ve	Polyarticular RF +ve	Pauciarticular Type I	Pauciarticular Type II
Percentage	20%	25%	10%	30%	15%
Sacroiliitis	No	No	Rare	No	Common
Iridocyclitis	No	Rare	No	50% chronic	20% acute
Rheumatoid factor	Negative	Negative	100%	Negative	Negative
ANA	Negative	25%	75%	60%	Negative
Boys/girls	60% boys	90% girls	80% girls	80% girls	90% boys

664. Kussmaul's sign is *not* seen in:

A. Left ventricular failure
B. Right ventricular failure
C. Cardiac tamponade
D. Constrictive pericarditis

(AI 2001)

- Clinically significant right ventricular infarction causes signs of severe **right ventricular failure** (jugular venous distention, **Kussmaul's sign**, and hepatomegaly) with or without hypotension. ST-segment elevations of the right-sided precordial ECG leads, particularly lead V_4R, are frequently present in the first 24 hours in patients with right ventricular infarction.
- Weakness, fatigue, weight loss, and anorexia are common in patients of chronic **constrictive pericarditis**. The cervical veins are distended and may remain so even after intensive diuretic treatment, and venous pressure may fail to decline during inspiration (**Kussmaul's sign**).
- A positive **Kussmaul's sign** is *rare* in **cardiac tamponade.**

665. *Not* included in the triad of Huntington's disease:

A. Early onset of memory loss
B. Cog wheel rigidity
C. Cognitive symptoms
D. Chorea

(AI 2001)

Huntington's disease is a genetic, autosomal dominant, degenerative brain disease. The 2 clinical hallmarks of the disease are **chorea** and **behavioral disturbance**. **Memory is frequently *not* impaired until late in the disease**, but attention, judgment, and executive functions may be seriously deficient at an early stage. Early onset before the age of 20 is associated with **rigidity**, ataxia, cognitive decline, and more rapid progression, with a typical duration of about 8 years.

666. A 40-year-old patient has 2 episodes of headache daily for last 2-3 weeks, and no previous history of similar disease. Headache wakes him from sleep and remains for one hours associated with *lacrimation*, and *nasal stuffiness*. The pain is deep *excruciating* and *limited to the right side* of head with no neurological abnormality. *Most likely* diagnosis is:

A. Brain tumor
B. Cluster headache
C. Tension headache
D. Migraine

(AIIMS 1999, AI 2001)

667. *Drug of choice* to prevent cluster headache is:

A. Lithium
B. Aspirin
C. Phenytoin
D. Methysergide

In **cluster headache** periorbital, or temporal, pain begins without warning and reaches a climax within 5 minutes. Pain is **strictly unilateral** and usually affects the same side in subsequent months. It is often **excruciating** in intensity and is deep, non-fluctuating, and explosive in quality; only rarely is it pulsatile. Attacks last from 30 min to 2 h; there are often associated symptoms of homolateral **lacrimation**, reddening of the eye, **nasal stuffiness**, lid ptosis, and nausea. Alcohol provokes attacks in about 3/4th of patients but ceases to be provocative when the bout remits. This on-off vulnerability to alcohol is pathognomonic of cluster headache. Only *rarely* do foods or emotional factors precipitate pain, in *contrast* to migraine. Most suitable treatment is the administration of drugs to *prevent* cluster attacks until the bout is over. Helpful prophylactic drugs are prednisone, lithium, methysergide, ergotamine, and verapamil. **Lithium** (600 to 900 mg daily) is particularly useful for the chronic form of the disorder.

668. A young patient presents with jaundice, his bilirubin is 21mg%; direct is 9.6mg%, alkaline phosphate is 84 KA units. *Most likely* diagnosis is:

A. Obstructive jaundice
B. Chronic active hepatitis
C. Viral hepatitis
D. Hemolytic jaundice *(AIIMS 1999, AI 2001)*

In **acute viral hepatitis** the serum bilirubin typically rises to levels ranging from **5 to 20 mg/dL**. Peak levels of SGPT vary from 400 to 4000 IU or more. In most cases, the total serum bilirubin (TSB) is *equally divided* between the conjugated and unconjugated fractions. Serum alkaline phosphatase may be normal or only mildly elevated.

669. A young male with gallbladder stone, has serum bilirubin 2.5, hemoglobin 6 gm%, urine shows urobilinogen *positive*. Most likely diagnosis is:

A. Protoporphyria
B. Hepatocellular jaundice
C. Obstructive jaundice
D. Hemolytic jaundice *(AIIMS 1999, AI 2001)*

Congenital hemolytic jaundice: Jaundice may be intermittent and tends to be less pronounced in early childhood. Because of the increased bile pigment production, **gallstones** of pigment type are common, even in childhood. Under normal circumstances, the daily urinary excretion of urobilinogen does not exceed 4 mg. When the hepatic uptake and excretion of **urobilinogen** is impaired (hepatocellular disease) or the production of bilirubin is greatly increased (hemolysis), daily urinary urobilinogen excretion may increase significantly.

670. *Not* seen in Steele-Richardson-Olszewski syndrome:

A. Convulsions
B. Gaze palsy progressive supranuclear
C. Dementia
D. None of the above *(PGI 1997)*

671. A 45-year-old man has history of dementia, ataxia and difficulty in downward gaze. *Most likely* diagnosis is:

A. Progressive supranuclear palsy
B. Alzheimer's disease
C. Parkinson's disease
D. Normal pressure hydrocephalus *(AIIMS 2000, AI 2001)*

672. A 60-year-old man has repeated fall and develops rigidity and ophthalmoplegia. *Most likely* diagnosis is:

A. Parkinsonism
B. Huntington's chorea
C. Shy-Drager syndrome
D. Supranuclear palsy *(AIIMS 2000)*

Progressive supranuclear palsy or Steele-Richardson-Olszewski syndrome is a degenerative disorder characterized *pathologically* by neuronal loss, gliosis, and neurofibrillary tangles in the midbrain, pons, basal ganglia, and dentate nuclei of the cerebellum. The disease generally begins between the ages of 45 and 75 years; it affects men twice as frequently as women. Supranuclear ophthalmoplegia is characteristic. Axial dystonia in extension is common and is frequently accompanied by limb **rigidity** and bradykinesia. The combination of supranuclear ophthalmoplegia and axial rigidity results in common presenting complaint of **'frequent falls'**. A **global impairment of intellectual function** is common. This disease should be considered whenever a middle-aged or elderly person with repeated falls has an extrapyramidal syndrome accompanied by nuchal dystonia and **paralysis of voluntary downgaze**. Seizures and sleep apnea may occur. There is only a *limited* response to Levo dopa, and there is no other effective treatment. Patient usually dies within 5 to 10 years.

673. Chromosomal anomaly associated with Alzheimer's dementia is:
- **A.** Turner syndrome
- **B.** Trisomy 21
- **C.** Trisomy 18
- **D.** Patau syndrome

(AI 2001)

Several genetic factors play important roles in the pathogenesis of at least some cases of Alzheimer's disease. 1 is the amyloid precursor protein gene on chromosome 21. Adults with trisomy 21 (**Down syndrome**) *always* develop the typical neuropathologic hallmarks of AD if they survive beyond age 40.

674. Alzheimer's disease typically affects:
- **A.** Nucleus basalis of Meynert
- **B.** Amygdala
- **C.** Parietal cortex
- **D.** Basal ganglion

In Alzheimer's disease there is reduction of acetylcholine due to degeneration of cholinergic neurons in the **nucleus basalis of Meynert** that project to many areas of cortex.

675. A 48-year-old *obese* patient presents with random blood sugar 400 mg%, urine sugar and ketones positive. Most appropriate drug in this scenario is:
- **A.** Insulin
- **B.** Metformin
- **C.** Glibenclamide
- **D.** Troglitazone

(AI 2001)

Diabetic ketoacidosis cannot be reversed without insulin. For several years 50 or more units of insulin was given per hour until ketosis was reversed, but now most patients are treated by "low-dose" insulin schedules in which 8 to 10 units of insulin are infused intravenously each hour.

676. *Not* seen in hemoglobin electrophoresis in sickle cell anemia:
- **A.** Hb S
- **B.** Hb F
- **C.** Hb A
- **D.** B and C

(AI 2001)

Condition	Hemoglobin Electrophoresis
• Sickle cell trait	Hb S/A:40/60
• Sickle cell anemia	**Hb S/A:100/0** **Hb F**:2-25%
• S/β^{o} thalassemia	Hb S/A:100/0 Hb F:1-10%
• S/β^{+} thalassemia	Hb S/A:60/40
• Hemoglobin SC	Hb S/A:50/0 Hb C:50%

677. A 50-year-old chronic smoker presented with history of hemoptysis. He was having truncal obesity and hypertension, an elevated ACTH level which was not suppressible with high dose dexamethasone. *Most likely* diagnosis is:
- **A.** Ectopic ACTH producing lung cancer
- **B.** Pituitary tumor
- **C.** Adrenal adenoma
- **D.** Bilateral adrenal hyperplasia

(AI 2001)

Paraneoplastic Syndromes

Syndrome	Hormones	Associated tumors
Hypercalcemia of malignancy	Parathyroid hormone-related peptide Parathyroid hormone	Head and neck cancer Bladder cancer Myeloma *Non* small cell lung cancer Breast cancer Renal cell carcinoma
Syndrome of inappropriate vasopressin secretion	Arginine vasopressin Atrial natriuretic peptide	Small cell lung cancer Head and neck cancer Non-small cell lung cancer
Cushing's syndrome	Adrenocorticotropic hormone Corticotropin-releasing hormone	Small cell lung cancer Carcinoid tumors
Acromegaly	Growth hormone-releasing hormone Growth hormone	Carcinoid Small cell lung cancer Pancreatic islet cell tumors
Gynecomastia	Human chorionic gonadotropin	Testicular cancer Lung cancer Carcinoid tumors of the lung and GIT
Non-islet cell tumor hypoglycemia	Insulin-like growth factor-2	Sarcomas

678. Hypercalcemia is common in:

A. Large cell carcinoma **B.** Oat cell carcinoma
C. Adenocarcinoma **D.** Squamous cell carcinoma *(PGI 1997)*

679. Hypercalcemia occurs in which type of lung cancer:

A. Oat cell **B.** Giant cell
C. Squamous cell **D.** Alveolar cell

Hypercalcemia of malignancy is the *most common* paraneoplastic endocrine syndrome and is responsible for about 40% of all hypercalcemia. Hypercalcemia with cancer is classified as humoral hypercalcemia of malignancy (**HHM**), which is caused by circulating hormones, or local osteolytic hypercalcemia (**LOH**), which is caused by local paracrine factors secreted by cancers within bone. Parathyroid hormone-related peptide causes nearly all cases of humoral hypercalcemia of malignancy. The cancers responsible for HHM in patients are *non*-small cell lung cancer and cancers of the breast, kidney, head and neck, and bladder. **HHM** is **particularly common in patients with cancers of squamous cell histology.**

680. A 26-year-old man presented with hemoglobin 6 gm%, WBC 2000/cu mm, normal differential count *except* for having 6% *blast cells*, platelet count is 80,000.Examination revealed spleen is moderately enlarged. Most likely diagnosis is:

A. Hemolysis **B.** ITP
C. Leukemia **D.** Aplastic anemia *(AI 2001)*

Fever, **splenomegaly**, hepatomegaly, lymphadenopathy, sternal tenderness, and evidence of infection and hemorrhagic tendencies are often present at diagnosis of **AML**. **Anemia** is usually present at diagnosis and can be *severe*. 25 to 40% of patients will have TLC < 5000/μL, and 20% will have counts > 100,000/μL. The **majority of leukocytes are usually blast cells**. **Platelet counts under 100,000/μL** are found at diagnosis in about 75% of patients, and about 25% of patients will have < 25,000/μL.

681. *Most common* type of ASD is:

A. Ostium primum **B.** Sinus venosus type
C. Endocardial cushion defect **D.** Ostium secundum

The *most common* atrial septal defect involves the fossa ovalis and is of the **ostium secundum** type.

682. *False* regarding ASD is:

A. Pulmonary hypertension
B. Right ventricular hypertrophy
C. Left atrial hypertrophy
D. Right atrial hypertrophy *(AI 2001)*

The physiology of an **atrial septal defect** (ASD) of the foramen ovale type (ostium secundum) is similar to that of the ostium primum-type ASD when the latter exists without physiologically significant incompetency of either atrioventricular (A-V) valve. The shunted blood passes from the left atrium to the right atrium and courses through the right heart and pulmonary vascular bed. These structures dilate to accommodate the added volume. Thus, the right atrium, right ventricle, pulmonary artery, and pulmonary vascular bed enlarge. **The left atrium, although it carries extra blood, does not enlarge, because the aperture in the atrial septum allows the blood to escape easily during both phases of the cardiac cycle.** With such a ready escape hatch, there is no stimulus for the left atrium to enlarge.

683. *Not* a clinical feature of ostium secundum type ASD:

A. Mid diastolic rumble along the left sternal border
B. Wide and fixed splitting of 2nd heart sound
C. Surgery is advised even in asymptomatic patients
D. Frequent occurrence of congestive cardiac failure in childhood *(SGPGI 1996)*

A child with an **ostium secundum type ASD** is *often* asymptomatic and the lesion is discovered during a routine physical examination. **It only rarely produces CHF in infancy.** The heart may be normal in size or may be enlarged. A right ventricular systolic 'lift' is palpable from the left border to the midclavicular line. A soft ejection systolic murmur is best heard in the upper left sternal border and is produced by increased blood flow in pulmonary artery. **The 2nd heart sound at the upper left sternal edge is widely split and fixed in all phases of respiration.** This is a characteristic finding of ASD. A **mid diastolic 'rumbling' murmur** due to high flow across the tricuspid valve is sometimes audible at the lower left sternal edge. The lesion is well tolerated during childhood and symptoms usually appear in 3rd decade of life or later. Open heart surgery with cardiopulmonary bypass allows accurate closure and the mortality rate is < 1%. **The surgery is advised even in asymptomatic patients prior to entry into school.** The results are gratifying in most of the cases with prompt disappearance of the symptoms.

684. Wide splitting of S_2 is seen in:

A. Cardiomyopathy
B. VSD
C. PDA
D. ASD

685. *Reversed* splitting of S_2 is seen in all *except*:

A. Left bundle branch block
B. Systemic hypertension
C. Aortic stenosis
D. Atrial septal defect

Different Types of Splitting of S_2

Normal	Reversed	Wide and fixed	Wide and mobile
• Children • Young adults	• Left bundle branch block • Aortic stenosis • Hypertension • Hypertrophic cardiomyopathy	• Atrial septal defect	• Right bundle branch block • Pulmonary stenosis

686. *Most common* fungal infection seen in febrile neutropenic patient is:

A. *Aspergillus fumigatus*
B. Mucormycosis
C. *Aspergillus niger*
D. *Candida* spp. *(AI 2001)*

Neutropenic patients are predisposed to invasive fungal infections, ***most commonly* those due to *Candida*** and *Aspergillus* species and occasionally those caused by *Fusarium*, *Trichosporon*, and *Bipolaris*.

687. Treatment of choice of a patient of CLL *with* systemic symptoms is:
- **A.** No treatment required
- **B.** Chlorambucil
- **C.** Radiotherapy
- **D.** Doxorubicin

No treatment is required in initial stages of CLL because the disease has a very long course. The indications for treating patients are:
- **Symptomatic lymphadenopathy**
- **Organ involvement**
- **Cytopenia due to progressive disease or autoimmune phenomena**
- **Systemic symptoms**

Chlorambucil is as effective as combination therapy with cyclophosphamide, vincristine, and prednisone (CVP).

688. Leukemia associated with autoimmune hemolytic anemia is:
- **A.** ALL
- **B.** CML
- **C.** CLL
- **D.** AML

(AIIMS 1993, 1994, AI 2001)

Autoimmune phenomena are seen in up to 20% of patients of CLL, *most commonly* **hemolytic anemia** and less frequently thrombocytopenia or pure red cell aplasia.

689. Amylase is increased in pleural effusion in following condition:
- **A.** Pancreatic disease
- **B.** Esophageal rupture
- **C.** Both
- **D.** None

(AI 2001)

If the pleural fluid amylase level is elevated, the diagnosis of esophageal rupture or pancreatic disease is likely.

690. Which of the following is *false* regarding neurocysticercosis:
- **A.** Calcification on X-ray skull
- **B.** Meningoencephalitic variety is most common
- **C.** Convulsions
- **D.** Mimics cerebral tumor

Neurocysticercosis generally occurs in a previously healthy and normal child. Seizures are the **most common** mode of presentation (90%); partial seizure being more frequent than generalized. It may also mimic cerebral tumor and present by features of raised intracranial tension (15%). It may also be detected accidentally in plain X-ray skull or CT scan where calcification may be seen. Neurocysticercosis is of the following types depending upon the site of the cyst.
- Parenchymal
- Racemose
- Meningoencephalitic
- Disseminated
- Intra-ventricular

Of these, **the parenchymal variety is *most common* and found in 95% of cases**. It consists of single or few-isolated lesion in parenchyma of brain.

691. Neurocysticercosis is diagnosed by:
- **A.** Pneumoencephalography
- **B.** EEG
- **C.** Angiography
- **D.** CT scan

Neuroimaging using a CT scan or MRI scan is the only diagnostic modality which can satisfactorily demonstrate a cyst of neurocysticercosis. Scan will show a ring enhancing lesion with surrounding cerebral edema if present. The only important differential diagnosis in India is a tuberculoma. The two can be differentiated by serological tests such as ELISA.

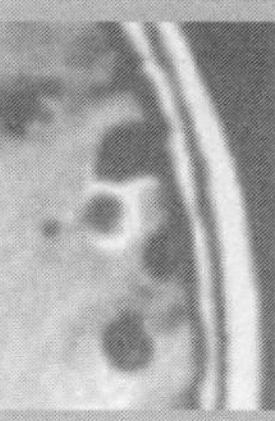

692. *True* regarding neurocysticercosis is:

A. Steroids are used in management of hydrocephalus
B. Usually presents with 6th nerve palsy and hemiparesis
C. Albendazole is *more effective* than praziquantel
D. Usually present with seizure *resistant* to antiepileptic drugs *(AI 2001)*

For *symptomatic* patients with **neurocysticercosis (NCC)**, both praziquantel (50 mg/kg per day in 3 doses for 15 days) and albendazole (15 mg/kg per day in 3 doses for 28 days) are effective. A clinical comparison between praziquantel and albendazole reveals utility of **albendazole as a better choice**. Because both drugs provoke strong inflammatory responses around dying cysticerci and patients receiving *either* drug should be hospitalized and given high doses of glucocorticoids during treatment. The efficacy of therapy can be monitored by CT or MRI scanning.

693. *Not* used in the treatment of cysticercosis:

A. Niclosamide
B. Flubendazole
C. Praziquantel
D. Albendazole *(AIIMS 1996)*

Neurocysticercosis is a pleomorphic disease that causes several neurological syndromes and pathological lesions. Therapies include a combination of symptomatic drugs, cysticidal drugs, surgical resection of lesions, and placement of ventricular shunts. The first cysticidal drug used in humans was *metrifonate*. *However*, the presence of severe cholinergic side effects limited its use. Thereafter, **praziquantel**, a drug that was originally used in veterinary medicine, proved to be effective in human cysticercosis. Some imidazoles have also been used to treat parenchymal brain cysticerci. **Flubendazole** was administered to 13 patients with neurocysticercosis at daily doses of 40 mg/kg for 10 days, and showed promising results. However, problems related to poor intestinal absorption of the drug has limited its use. Thereafter, **albendazole** appeared as an excellent alternative to praziquantel.

694. *Not* caused by hypervitaminosis A:

A. Hypotension
B. Bony swelling
C. Loss of hair
D. Anorexia *(AIIMS 1993)*

Features of Vitamin A Toxicity

Acute toxicity	Chronic toxicity
• ABDOMINAL PAIN	• BONE AND JOINT PAIN
• NAUSEA	• HYPEROSTOSES
• VOMITING	• HAIR LOSS
• PAPILLEDEMA	• DRYNESS AND FISSURES OF THE LIPS
• HEADACHE	• ANOREXIA
• DIZZINESS	• BENIGN INTRACRANIAL HYPERTENSION
• SLUGGISHNESS	• LOW-GRADE FEVER
• BULGING FONTANEL	• PRURITUS
	• WEIGHT LOSS
	• HEPATOSPLENOMEGALY

695. Mononeuritis multiplex is seen in:

A. Bronchus carcinoma
B. Guillain-Barré syndrome
C. Leprosy
D. Syphilis *(AIIMS 1993)*

696. Mononeuritis multiplex is a feature of:

A. Polyarteritis nodosa
B. Hypersensitive vasculitis
C. Leprosy
D. All of the above

Peripheral nerve disorders are divided into 2 categories:

- Lesions of isolated peripheral nerves or nerve roots (MONONEUROPATHY)
- Multiple isolated lesions of peripheral nerves (MONONEURITIS MULTIPLEX)

CAUSES OF MONONEUROPATHY MULTIPLEX	
COMMON CAUSES	**RARE CAUSES**
• Polyarteritis nodosa	• Mixed cryoglobulinemia
• Vasculitis syndrome	• Sjögren's syndrome
• Rheumatoid arthritis	• Wegener's granulomatosis
• Systemic lupus erythematosus	• Progressive systemic sclerosis
• Mixed connective tissue disease	• Churg-Strauss allergic granulomatosis
	• Hypersensitivity angiitides
	• Leprosy
	• Sarcoidosis
	• Amyloidosis
	• Hypereosinophilic syndrome
	• Cryoglobulinemia
	• Diabetic neuropathy

697. Episodic muscle weakness *does not* occur in:

A. Eaton Lambert's syndrome
B. Hyperglycemia
C. Hyperkalemia
D. Hypocalcemia

(AIIMS 1993)

698. Episodic generalized weakness is *not* caused by:

A. Hyperkalemia
B. Hypernatremia
C. Hypermagnesemia
D. Hypercalcemia

Causes of Episodic Generalized Weakness

• Hypokalemia*	• Myasthenia gravis
• Hyperkalemia**	• Lambert-Eaton syndrome
• Hypercalcemia	• Sodium channelopathies
• Hypocalcemic tetany	• Chloride channelopathies
• Hyponatremia	• Periodic paralyses and myotonias
• Hypophosphatemia	• Cataplexy and sleep paralysis associated with narcolepsy
• Hypermagnesemia	• Multiple sclerosis
• Hyperventilation	• Transient ischemic attacks
• Hypoglycemia	• Metabolic defects of muscle
***Hypokalemia**	****Hyperkalemia**
• Primary aldosteronism (Conn's syndrome)	• Addison's disease
• Barium poisoning	• Chronic renal failure
• Renal tubular acidosis	• Hyporeninemic hypoaldosteronism
• Juxtaglomerular apparatus hyperplasia (Bartter's syndrome)	
• Villous adenoma of colon	
• Alcoholism	
• Diuretics	
• Licorice	
• Glucocorticoids	
• Para aminosalicylic acid	

699. Flapping tremors are seen in all *except*:

A. Thyrotoxicosis
B. Uremia
C. Liver failure
D. CO_2 narcosis

(AIIMS 1993)

- Abnormal involuntary movements are divided into those that are *rhythmical* and those that are *irregular*. **Rhythmical abnormal involuntary movements are termed as tremors.** Tremors are divided into 3 types' viz. rest tremor, postural tremor, and intention tremor. **Rest tremor** is characteristic of Parkinsonism, a hypokinetic movement disorder, and is therefore commonly associated with bradykinesia and cogwheel rigidity. A **postural tremor** that develops acutely is usually due to toxic or metabolic factors (*hyperthyroidism*) or stress. **Intention tremor** is a sign of cerebellar disease.
- *Asterixis* is an intermittent inhibition of muscle contraction that occurs with metabolic encephalopathy such as **uremia**, **CO_2 narcosis**, **hepatic failure** etc. When due to hepatic coma, asterixis is called 'liver flap' or 'liver tremor'.

700. Asterixis (flapping tremor) is seen in:

A. Thyrotoxicosis
B. β_2 stimulant therapy
C. Parkinsonism
D. CO_2 narcosis *(UP 1997)*

701. Flapping tremor is *not* seen in:

A. Thyrotoxicosis
B. Uremic patient
C. CO_2 necrosis
D. Wilson disease *(UP 1996)*

Asterixis is an intermittent inhibition of muscle contraction that occurs with *metabolic* encephalopathy.

702. In hyperprolactinemia the *investigation of choice* is:

A. Steroid assay
B. Prolactin estimation
C. LH estimation
D. TRH estimation *(AIIMS 1993)*

Serum prolactin levels should be measured in all patients with unexplained hypogonadism, galactorrhea, or infertility. If a random prolactin concentration is elevated, further evaluation is necessary after it is established that the observed elevations are not simply normal minimal elevations (< 30 μg/L) due to stress or food intake.

703. *Best* diagnostic test for bronchiectasis is:

A. CXR
B. Bronchography
C. Bronchoscopy
D. CT scan *(AIIMS 1993)*

Plain X-rays usually suffice to define pulmonary processes, but in difficult cases the lungs can be shown exquisitely by high-resolution computed tomography (CT), which is particularly useful for interstitial processes and in generalized pulmonary illnesses. **CT has also superseded bronchography in the study of bronchiectasis.**

704. Hyperkalemia does *not* occur in:

A. Cushing's syndrome
B. ARF
C. 21-hydroxylase deficiency
D. Pentamidine *(AIIMS 1993)*

Some Causes of Hyperkalemia

- Renal failure
- Gordon's syndrome
- Cyclosporine
- Hyporeninemia
- ACE inhibitors
- NSAIDs
- Adrenal insufficiency
- Pseudohypoaldosteronism
- Tubulointerstitial disease
- K^+ sparing diuretics
- Trimethoprim
- Pentamidine
- Heparin
- Adrenal enzyme deficiency (21-hydroxylase, 3β-hydroxysteroid dehydrogenase, corticosterone methyl oxidase)

705. Rhinocerebral mucormycosis can occur in all *except*:

A. Organ transplantation
B. Uncontrolled diabetes mellitus
C. CRF
D. Deferoxamine therapy *(AIIMS 1993)*

Rhinocerebral mucormycosis is a rare fungal infection that usually develops during or following an episode of **diabetic ketoacidosis**. Other conditions most commonly associated with mucormycosis include chronic steroid use, metabolic acidosis, **organ transplantation**, leukemia/lymphoma, treatment with **deferoxamine** and AIDS.

706. Which of the following does *not* change with age:

A. Hematocrit **B.** Glucose tolerance test
C. GFR **D.** FEV_1 *(AIIMS 1993)*

Anemia is a frequent finding among the elderly. This is often erroneously referred to as anemia of old age. The Framingham study and others, however, have shown that **healthy elderly do not demonstrate a change in hematocrit with aging**. *In addition*, there is no evidence that the totipotential stem cell responsible for red cell production is deranged or damaged, neither is the ability of the bone marrow to respond to erythropoietin under basal conditions. *Therefore*, anemia in the elderly is *always* due to a pathologic condition or represents a response to a pathologic condition.

707. Idiopathic orthostatic hypotension is also known as:

A. Shy-Drager syndrome **B.** Von Hippel-Lindau disease
C. Kugelberg-Welander disease **D.** Louis-Bar syndrome

Diseases	Synonym
• Shy-Drager syndrome	Idiopathic orthostatic hypotension
• Von Hippel-Lindau disease	Cerebello-retinal hemangioblastoma
• Kugelberg-Welander disease	Hereditary proximal spinal muscular atrophy
• Louis-Bar syndrome	Ataxia telangiectasia

708. Which of the following is *true* about maladie de Roger:

A. Small VSD **B.** Harsh pan-systolic murmur
C. Most defect close spontaneously **D.** All of the above

maladie de Roger or Roger's disease is synonym for a *small VSD*. As the defect is small, it gives rise to turbulent blood flow across the defect producing *harsh pansystolic murmur*. Spontaneous closure occurs in 30 to 40% of cases by the age of 2 years.

709. White patch in the throat may be due to:

A. *Candida*
B. Smoker's leukoplakia
C. Nicotinic stomatitis
D. All of the above

Differential Diagnosis of White Lesions of Oral Mucosa

• Lichen planus	• Frictional keratosis
• White sponge nevus	• Candidiasis (oral thrush)
• Smoker's leukoplakia and smokeless tobacco lesions	• Hairy leukoplakia
• Nicotinic stomatitis	• Chemical burns

710. Turner's sign is seen in:

A. Myocarditis
B. Cholecystitis
C. Pancreatitis
D. Pleural effusion

Signs of Acute Pancreatitis

Cullen's sign	A faint blue discoloration around the umbilicus may occur as the result of hemoperitoneum.
Turner's sign	A blue-red-purple or green-brown discoloration of the flanks reflects tissue catabolism of hemoglobin.

711. Hemoptysis is seen in:

A. Aortic stenosis
B. Pulmonary stenosis
C. Mitral stenosis
D. Tricuspid stenosis

In **mitral stenosis**, hemoptysis occurs due to rupture of pulmonary-bronchial venous connections that is secondary to pulmonary venous hypertension. It occurs commonly in cases that have raised left atrial pressures without markedly elevated pulmonary vascular resistances and is almost never fatal.

712. Reticulocytosis is *not* seen in:

A. Anemia in CRF
B. Hereditary spherocytosis
C. Following acute bleeding
D. Paroxysmal nocturnal hemoglobinuria *(AIIMS 1994)*

Reticulocyte count increases in the conditions in which there is enhanced destruction or loss of RBCs such as in acute hemorrhage, congenital hemolytic anemias and autoimmune hemolytic anemias such as paroxysmal nocturnal hemoglobinuria. **Anemia of chronic renal failure** is classified under the heading anemia of chronic disease in which there is *under utilization* of iron reserves, **hence there is no reticulocytosis**. The anemia associated with acute infections and chronic inflammatory diseases results from the release of inflammatory cytokines.

713. Which of the following drugs cause diarrhea:

A. Morphine
B. Atropine
C. Magnesium sulphate
D. Guanethidine

Magnesium sulphate is an osmotic *purgative* that is not absorbed in the intestine and retains water osmotically. Mg^{++} also releases cholecystokinin, which may supplement the purgative action.

714. In methemoglobinemia:

A. Methane is present in hemoglobin
B. Methane is present in the beta globulin chain
C. Oxidized hemoglobin contains ferrous iron
D. Oxidized hemoglobin contains ferric iron

Methemoglobinemia	Oxidized hemoglobin contains ferric *rather than* ferrous iron
Sulfhemoglobinemia	Sulfur is present in the porphyrin ring and alters its ability to bind oxygen
Carboxyhemoglobinemia	Carbon monoxide bound to the heme iron

715. *Isolated* 3rd nerve palsy is seen in:

A. Frontal lobe tumor
B. Weber's syndrome
C. Diabetes mellitus
D. Lateral medullary syndrome

In diabetes mellitus *mono*neuropathy may occur rarely. There is a sudden wrist drop, foot drop, or paralysis of the 3rd, 4th, or 6th cranial nerves. Other single nerves, including the recurrent laryngeal, may also be involved. Mononeuropathy is usually resolved spontaneously over a few-week period.

716. Which carcinoma of lung responds *best* to chemotherapy:

A. Squamous cell type
B. Oat cell type
C. Clara cell type
D. Small cell type

Small cell carcinomas **are managed mainly by chemotherapy with or without radiotherapy. In contrast, non-small cell cancers that are found to be localized at the time of presentation should be subjected to either surgery or radiotherapy.**

717. Mee's lines in the nails are characteristic of which poisoning:
A. Lead **B.** Arsenic
C. Mercury **D.** Nicotine

Typical findings of chronic arsenic poisoning are skin and nail changes, such as:
- Hyperkeratosis
- Hyperpigmentation
- Exfoliative dermatitis
- **Mee's lines** (transverse white striae of the fingernails)
- Sensory and motor polyneuritis manifested by numbness and tingling in a "stocking-glove" distribution, distal weakness, and quadriplegia
- Inflammation of the respiratory mucosa.

718. Myocardial rupture as a result of myocardial infarction occurs usually during the:
A. 1st week **B.** 2nd week
C. 3rd week **D.** 5th week

719. A patient of inferior wall infarction develops shock on 3rd day. *Most common* cause is:
A. Right ventricular infarction **B.** Ventricular aneurysm
C. Cardiac rupture **D.** Atrial fibrillation *(AIIMS 1999)*

Myocardial rupture is a serious complication of myocardial infarction, which usually occurs during the 1st week after the onset of symptoms of myocardial infarction. Its frequency increases with the age of the patient.

720. Chemoprophylaxis is used in all *except*:
A. Malaria **B.** Typhoid
C. Meningococcal meningitis **D.** Pertussis

Chemoprophylaxis

Malaria	Mefloquine, doxycycline, chloroquine.
Meningococcal meningitis	Rifampin in a dosage of 10 mg/kg (up to 600 mg) 12 hourly for 2 days for adults and children over 1 year **and** 5 mg/kg 12 hourly for 2 days for children less than 1 year.
Pertussis	Erythromycin (preferably the estolate) at 40 to 50 mg/kg per day in four divided doses (maximum, 2 gram per day) for 14 days.

721. Hypersegmented neutrophils are seen in:
A. CML **B.** Alcoholism
C. Iron deficiency anemia **D.** Myelodysplasia

If **heavy drinking** is associated with folic acid deficiency, it leads to hypersegmented neutrophils, reticulocytopenia, and hyperplastic bone marrow.

722. *Not* a feature of rheumatic heart disease in our country:
A. School going population is most often affected
B. Aortic valve is most commonly affected
C. Affects younger age group
D. CHF and cardiomegaly is seen in most of the cases *(AIIMS 1994)*

723. In rheumatic fever, *earliest* valvular lesion is:
A. AR **B.** AS
C. MR **D.** MS *(AIIMS 1995)*

Mitral regurgitation is the *most common* valvular involvement in children with rheumatic heart disease. AR is less common than MR. Other lesions are MS and TR.

724. The *most common* heart valve abnormality in acute MI is:

A. MR **B.** AR
C. MS **D.** AS *(AIIMS May 2002)*

The incidence of apical systolic murmurs of **mitral regurgitation** during the 1st few days after the onset of a myocardial infarction varies from **10 to 50%**.

725. Routine screening for Down syndrome is done if maternal age is above:

A. 45 years **B.** 35 years
C. 40 years **D.** 30 years *(AIIMS 1994)*

Advanced maternal age (**35 years or greater** at the time of delivery) is an indication for screening of autosomal trisomy.

726. *True* regarding Barrett's esophagus is:

A. Asymptomatic
B. Dilated tortuous esophagus
C. Premalignant
D. Squamous metaplasia of esophagus *(AIIMS 1994)*

727. Adenocarcinoma is commonly found in:

A. Chronic smoking **B.** Plummer-Vinson syndrome
C. Barrett's esophagus **D.** Achalasia cardia *(AIIMS 1996)*

728. Barrett's esophagus may lead to:

A. Stricture formation **B.** Squamous cell carcinoma
C. Reflux esophagitis **D.** Peptic ulcer *(AIIMS 1998)*

In patients with *persistent* gastroesophageal reflux (GER) the distal esophagus becomes lined with **columnar secretory epithelium** instead of the *usual* stratified squamous epithelium. This condition is known as **Barrett's esophagus** because it was described by Barrett in 1957. Esophagitis may progress to scarring and stricture formation. **Adenocarcinoma is the most ominous complication of Barrett's esophagus** because it has been proved *beyond doubts* that person with this condition are 40 times more prone to develop this malignancy than the health population.

729. In *non*smokers the *most common* type of bronchogenic carcinoma is:

A. Large cell **B.** Small cell
C. Squamous cell **D.** Adenocarcinoma *(AIIMS 1994)*

The *most common* form of lung cancer arising in lifetime **nonsmokers**, in women, and in young patients (less than 45 years old) is **adenocarcinoma**.

730. Recovery of myocardium after myocardial infarction occurs in about...........weeks:

A. 12 **B.** 8
C. 6 **D.** 2 *(AIIMS 1994)*

A maximal (symptom-limited) exercise stress test may be carried out **4 to 6 weeks** after infarction.

731. Hyperbaric oxygen is used in:

A. Anemia **B.** Anaerobic infection
C. CO poisoning **D.** Ventilatory failure *(AIIMS 1994)*

Hyperbaric oxygen therapy has been advocated by some experts for treatment of anaerobic infections but is of no proven value.

732. *Not* associated with EBV:

A. Burkitt's lymphoma
B. Bell's palsy
C. Guillain-Barré syndrome
D. Hepatitis *(AIIMS 1994)*

Epstein-Barr virus is the cause of infectious mononucleosis, which is characterized by fever, sore throat, lymphadenopathy, and atypical lymphocytosis. EBV is also associated with several human cancers, including nasopharyngeal carcinoma, **Burkitt's lymphoma**, Hodgkin's disease, and B-cell lymphoma. Acute EBV infection has also been associated with cranial nerve palsies (especially 7th), **Guillain-Barré syndrome**, acute transverse myelitis, and peripheral neuritis. *Rare* complications associated with acute EBV infection include **hepatitis**, myocarditis or pericarditis with ECG changes, pneumonia with pleural effusion, interstitial nephritis, and vasculitis.

733. In Noonan's syndrome the cardiac anomaly is:

A. Coarctation of aorta
B. Pulmonary stenosis
C. ASD
D. VSD *(AIIMS 1995)*

Noonan's syndrome (XY Turner phenotype) is an autosomal dominant disorder seen in both sexes. It is characterized by webbed neck, short stature, *congenital heart disease*, cubitus valgus, and other congenital defects despite normal karyotypes and normal gonads. The cardiac defect is *most often* the **pulmonary valvular stenosis** or atrial septal defect, whereas, coarctation of aorta is rare; the reverse is true for 'true' Turner syndrome.

734. *False* regarding fibrolamellar carcinoma of liver is:

A. Common in females
B. Nests of cell with fibrous stroma
C. Worse prognosis
D. Diffuse involvement of liver *(AIIMS 1994)*

735. *False* regarding fibrolamellar carcinoma of liver:

A. Younger age of onset
B. Alpha fetoproteins are > 1000 units/ml
C. Better prognosis than hepatocellular carcinoma
D. More common in women *(AI 2001)*

736. *Best* prognosis is of:

A. Angiosarcoma of liver
B. Hepatoblastoma
C. Fibrolamellar carcinoma of liver
D. Hepatocellular carcinoma of liver *(AIIMS 1998)*

Fibrolamellar carcinoma is a distinct *variant* of hepatocellular carcinoma with characteristic morphology of malignant hepatocytes enmeshed in lamellar fibrous tissue. This tumor is non-encapsulated but well circumscribed and contains fibrous lamellae. It usually **occurs in young adults** and has no association with preexisting cirrhosis, HBV or HCV, or other known risk factors. **α-Fetoprotein levels are only uncommonly elevated**. **The prognosis is better than for hepatocellular carcinoma** and some patients survive several years after tumor resection.

737. *True* regarding rabies is:

A. Local wound care is of no use
B. Vaccine is given intramuscularly
C. HDVC is live attenuated
D. Fluorescent antibody is the treatment of choice *(AI 1991)*

Rabies is an acute viral disease of the central nervous system that affects all mammals and that is transmitted by infected secretions, usually saliva. The rabies virus is a bullet-shaped, enveloped, single-stranded RNA virus that is 75 to 80 nm in diameter and belongs to the rhabdovirus family.

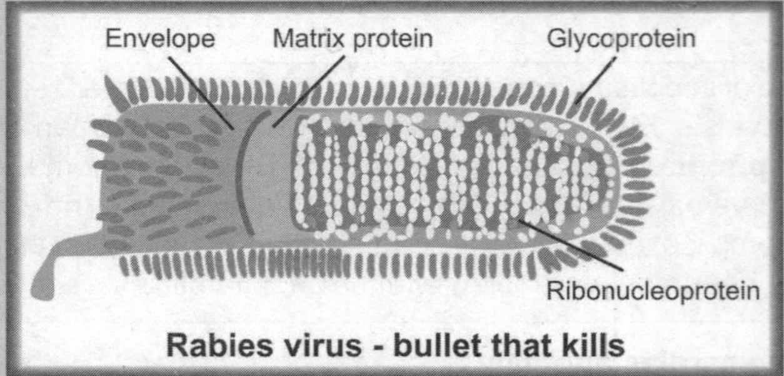

Rabies virus - bullet that kills

- Local treatment of the bite wound is an important component of rabies prevention. The wound should be scrubbed with soap and then flushed with water.
- 50% of the total dose of 20 units per kilogram for *human rabies immune globulin* is given by local infiltration of the wound, and the rest is administered intramuscularly into the gluteal region.
- Five 1-mL doses of HDCV are given intramuscularly, preferably in the deltoid or anterolateral thigh area; days 0, 3, 7, 14, and 28.

738. The characteristic feature of rabies is:

A. Brainstem encephalitis
B. Peripheral neuropathy
C. Patchy meningitis
D. Ventriculitis

The clinical manifestations of rabies can be divided into 4 stages:
- A nonspecific prodrome
- An acute encephalitis similar to other viral encephalitides,
- Profound dysfunction of brainstem (**brainstem encephalitis**) centers that produces the classic features of rabies encephalitis
- Death or in rare cases recovery.

739. Human bite infection is commonly caused by:

A. Staphylococcus
B. Anaerobic bacilli
C. Anaerobic streptococci
D. Spirochete *(AIIMS 1996)*

Human bites more frequently become infected than do bites inflicted by other animals. Common aerobic isolates include viridans streptococci, *Staphylococcus aureus*, *Eikenella corrodens* and *Haemophilus influenzae*. **Anaerobic species, including *Fusobacterium nucleatum* and *Prevotella*, *Porphyromonas*, *Peptococcus*, and *Peptostreptococcus* species, are isolated from 50% of human-bite wound infections**; many of these isolates produce β-lactamases.

740. *False* regarding thoracic outlet syndrome:

A. Resection of 1st rib is the treatment
B. Physiotherapy and position relieves the symptoms
C. Most common radial nerve involvement
D. Neurological signs and symptoms are common *(AIIMS 1996, 1998)*

Thoracic outlet compression syndrome is a 'symptom complex' which results from compression of the neurovascular bundle (artery, vein, or nerves) at the thoracic outlet as it courses through the neck and shoulder. Patients may develop shoulder and arm pain, weakness, paresthesia, claudication, Raynaud's phenomenon, and even ischemic tissue loss and gangrene. Most patients can be managed by conservative methods. They should be instructed to **avoid the positions that cause symptoms** and **many patients benefit from shoulder girdle exercises**. Surgical procedures such as **removal of the 1st rib** or resection of the scalenus anticus muscle are occasionally necessary for relief of symptoms or treatment of ischemia.

741. Zenker's diverticulum presents with:

A. Found in stomach **B.** Dysphagia
C. Dysphonia **D.** Reflux esophagitis *(AIIMS 1996)*

Zenker's diverticulum is a herniation of the mucous membrane of the esophagus through a defect in the wall of the esophagus. A **Zenker's diverticulum** arises in the natural zone of weakness in the posterior hypopharyngeal wall and causes **halitosis and regurgitation of saliva and food particles consumed several days back**. When it becomes large and filled with food, such a diverticulum may compress the esophagus and cause **dysphagia** or complete obstruction. *Symptomatic* Zenker's diverticula are treated by cricopharyngeal myotomy with or without diverticulectomy.

742. Macrocytic anemia is seen in all *except*:

A. Thiamine deficiency **B.** Copper deficiency
C. Orotic aciduria **D.** Liver disease *(AIIMS 1996)*

A morphological classification of anemia is often used in which the RBCs are characterized by their mean corpuscular volume (MCV).

Type of anemia	MCV
• **Microcytic**	< 75 fL
• **Normocytic**	75-100 fL
• **Macrocytic**	> 100 fL

Megaloblastic anemia may be seen in a number of conditions but almost all cases in children result from a deficiency of folic acid or vitamin B_{12}. **Orotic aciduria** is a genetically determined defect in pyrimidine biosynthesis associated with a severe megaloblastic anemia, neutropenia and crystalluria due to excretion of orotic acid. Physical and mental retardation are frequently present. Megaloblastic anemia can also occur in Lesch-Nyhan syndrome. 2 instances of **thiamine responsive and thiamine dependent megaloblastic anemia** have been reported in which the administration of thiamine (100 mg/day) produces a brisk reticulocytosis and a sustained increase in hemoglobin. Sensorineural deafness and diabetes mellitus were associated and pathogenesis is unclear. A pathogenesis of **anemia due to liver diseases** *per se* is not fully understood. *Most commonly* the morphologically abnormal RBCs are macrocytes and target cells. MCV is about 110 fL.

743. *False* regarding hepatocellular carcinoma is:

A. Aflatoxins are the etiological agent
B. Fibrolamellar type has best prognosis
C. Marker's are increased
D. Uncommon among Asians *(AIIMS 1996)*

The most common type of primary liver cancer is **hepatocellular carcinoma**. Fibrolamellar carcinoma, cholangiocarcinoma, hepatoblastoma, and angiosarcoma are *uncommon* to rare. Although much less common than metastatic liver cancer in most areas of the world, hepatocellular carcinoma is the most common internal malignancy and an important cause of death in certain areas of Africa and **Southeast Asia**. Chronic hepatitis B virus (HBV) infection is largely responsible for the high prevalence of the tumor in endemic areas. Chronic hepatitis C virus (HCV) infection has been recognized as an important factor in the genesis of hepatocellular carcinoma. Environmental carcinogens may also play a role; e.g. ingestion of food contaminated with **fungal aflatoxins** is believed to contribute to the high incidence of hepatocellular carcinoma in subtropical regions. Abdominal pain, weight loss, a right upper quadrant mass, and unexplained deterioration in a previously stable patient with cirrhosis are the most common clinical presentations. Fever is relatively common and may simulate infection. Except for the presence of α-fetoprotein in serum, biochemical tests are of little diagnostic help. Elevated serum des-γ-carboxyprothrombin, a prothrombin precursor, can also be a biochemical marker for hepatocellular carcinoma, but more data are needed to establish its clinical value. Abdominal US, CT, and MRI are important diagnostic aids and can sometimes detect sub-clinical carcinomas. The prognosis for hepatocellular carcinoma is usually grim, and treatment is generally unsatisfactory. The prognosis of **fibrolamellar carcinoma is better than for hepatocellular carcinoma**, and some patients survive several years after tumor resection.

744. Aflatoxin may cause:

A. Botulism
B. Cholangiocarcinoma
C. Lathyrism
D. Hepatoma

(KERALA 1994)

HBV and aflatoxin B_1 have been implicated in the pathogenesis of hepatocellular carcinoma in regions of Africa and southern China where *both* agents are prevalent.

745. In rheumatoid arthritis (RA) the characteristic joint involvement is:

A. Hip joint
B. Metacarpophalangeal joint
C. Knee joint
D. Spine

(AIIMS 1996)

Although inflammation can affect any diarthrodial joint, **rheumatoid arthritis** most often causes symmetric arthritis with characteristic involvement of certain specific joints such as the proximal interphalangeal and **metacarpophalangeal joints**. The distal interphalangeal joints are *rarely* involved.

746. In rheumatoid arthritis, part of spine involved is:

A. Sacral
B. Lumbar
C. Cervical
D. Thoracic

(AIIMS 1997)

Axial involvement in **rheumatoid arthritis** is usually limited to the **upper cervical spine**. Involvement of the lumbar spine is *not* seen, and lower back pain cannot be attributed to rheumatoid inflammation.

747. All are caused by lupus anticoagulant *except*:

A. Valvular heart disease
B. Increased prothrombin time
C. Arterial thrombosis
D. Recurrent abortion

(AIIMS 1996)

Clinical manifestations of **lupus anticoagulant** (LA) include thrombocytopenia, recurrent venous or arterial clotting, recurrent fetal loss, and valvular heart disease.

748. Leukocyte alkaline phosphatase is *not* increased in:

A. Polycythemia vera
B. CML
C. Myelofibrosis
D. None of the above

(AIIMS 1995)

Low scores (LAP) have been associated with **CML**, PNH, thrombocytopenic purpura, and hereditary hypophosphatasia. **In CML regardless of the total white count, the score remains low. High scores** have been seen in **polycythemia vera**, **myelofibrosis**, aplastic anemia, mongolism, hairy cell leukemia, leukemoid reactions, and neutrophilia *either* physiological *or* secondary to infection. It is also increased in Hodgkin disease. Serial LAP activity can be a useful adjunct in evaluating the activity of Hodgkin disease as well as its response to therapy. Increase in LAP does not occur in cases of sickle cell crisis, possibly due to zinc deficiency (leukocyte alkaline phosphatase is a zinc metalloenzyme) but more likely relating to a mild defect in the hypothalamic-pituitary-adrenal axis with decreased plasma cortisol response in patients in sickle cell crisis.

749. *Not* a manifestation of insulinoma:

A. Psychological alteration
B. Visual disturbance
C. Weight loss
D. Fasting hypoglycemia

(AIIMS 1995)

750. *Not* a characteristic feature of insulinoma:

A. Weight loss
B. Fasting hypoglycemia
C. Majority are solitary tumors
D. Majority are benign tumors

(SGPGI 1999)

Whipple's triad is the classic presentation of **insulinoma**. It consists of fasting hypoglycemia, *symptoms* of hypoglycemia, and immediate relief after IV glucose administration. **Weight gain** may result from increased food ingested to combat symptoms of hypoglycemia. Symptoms due to the hypoglycemia include headache, slurred speech, **psychological alterations**, **visual disturbances**, confusion, and, ultimately, coma and death. *Multiple* primary tumors are found in around 10% of patients and 10% of patients have *malignant* disease, with spread to the local lymph nodes and the liver.

751. In acute myocardial infarction, *earliest* finding of ECG is:

A. Prominent U wave
B. Widened QRS complex
C. ST depression
D. ST elevation *(AIIMS 1995)*

The ECG is a basis in the diagnosis of acute and chronic ischemic heart disease and ischemia exerts complex time-dependent effects on the electrical properties of myocardial cells. When the acute ischemia is transmural, the ST segment is shifted in the direction of the outer (epicardial) layers, **producing ST elevations** and sometimes, in the earliest stages of ischemia, tall, positive so-called hyperacute T waves over the ischemic zone.

752. *Most common* cause of lactic acidosis during the treatment of diabetes is:

A. Oral hypoglycemics
B. Phenformin
C. Diet restriction
D. Insulin *(AIIMS 1995)*

Metformin is a biguanide useful in NIDDM patients who are not responsive to diet and exercise and it may be prescribed as monotherapy in obese diabetics. The main action of metformin is the inhibition of hepatic gluconeogenesis, and it also may increase glucose disposal in muscle and adipose tissue. In contrast to sulfonylureas, metformin does not cause hypoglycemia. **Metformin can cause lactic acidosis, like the earlier biguanides**. To avoid lactic acidosis, the drug should not be given to patients with renal disease. It should be stopped at once if nausea, vomiting, diarrhea, or intercurrent illness appears.

Drugs producing metabolic acidosis

- Acetazolamide
- Metformin
- Paraldehyde (degraded)
- Phenformin
- Salicylates
- Spironolactone

753. Piecemeal necrosis on liver biopsy is seen in:

A. Chronic active hepatitis
B. Indian childhood cirrhosis
C. Alcoholic hepatitis
D. Primary alcoholic cirrhosis *(AIIMS 1995)*

Chronic active hepatitis is characterized by continuing hepatic necrosis, portal/periportal and, to a lesser extent, lobular inflammation, and fibrosis. **Piecemeal necrosis is the minimal histologic requirement to ascertain a diagnosis of chronic active hepatitis**, but this change is seen even in mild, relatively non-progressive forms of chronic active hepatitis. Destruction of the hepatocytes at the periphery of the lobule, with erosion of the limiting plate of hepatocytes surrounding the portal triads is known as piecemeal necrosis.

754. *Most common* malignant change seen in renal transplant is:

A. Renal cell carcinoma
B. Cervix carcinoma
C. Skin and lip carcinoma
D. Lymphoma *(AIIMS 1995)*

The incidence of tumors in patients on immunosuppressive therapy is about 100 times greater than that in the general population. The ***most common* lesions are cancer of the skin and lips** and carcinoma *in situ* of the cervix, as well as lymphomas, such as non-Hodgkin's lymphomas.

755. In ulcerative colitis the *drug of choice* is:

A. Aminosalicylic acid
B. Sulfasalazine
C. Prednisolone
D. Salazopyrin *(AIIMS 1995)*

The principal drugs used in the treatment of **ulcerative colitis** are the anti-inflammatory agents—**sulfasalazine** and glucocorticoids.

756. Heberden's nodes are seen in:

A. Proximal interphalangeal joint of RA
B. Proximal interphalangeal joint of osteoarthritis
C. Distal interphalangeal joint of osteoarthritis
D. Proximal distal interphalangeal joint of RA *(AIIMS 1995)*

Heberden's node

Bouchard's node

The *most common* form of idiopathic osteoarthritis is the **Heberden's nodes which are the bony enlargements of the distal interphalangeal (DIP) joints**. Heberden's nodes develop gradually, with little or no discomfort. But sometimes they may present with acute pain, redness, and swelling, which may be triggered by minor trauma. A similar process at the proximal interphalangeal joints leads to Bouchard's nodes.

757. Paradoxical breathing is characteristic of:
- **A.** Pneumonia
- **B.** Pneumothorax
- **C.** Atelectasis
- **D.** Diaphragmatic paralysis

758. *False* regarding diaphragmatic paralysis:
- **A.** Diaphragmatic pacing is useful if any nerve is intact
- **B.** Causes normocapnic failure
- **C.** Sniff test is positive in unilateral diaphragmatic paralysis
- **D.** None

(AIIMS 1995)

759. In which of the following condition, paradoxical respiration is seen:
- **A.** Severe asthma
- **B.** Bulbar polio
- **C.** Diaphragmatic palsy
- **D.** Multiple fracture of rib

((KERALA 1990))

- Most patients with severe *bilateral* diaphragmatic weakness present with **hypercapnic respiratory failure**, frequently complicated by cor pulmonale and right ventricular failure, atelectasis, and pneumonia. The most common causes are *high* spinal cord injury, thoracic trauma (including cardiac surgery), multiple sclerosis, anterior horn disease, and muscular dystrophy. The degree of diaphragmatic weakness is best quantitated by measuring trans-diaphragmatic pressures. The treatment of choice is assisted ventilation and if the nerve to the diaphragm is intact, **diaphragmatic pacing** may be a viable alternative.
- *Unilateral* paralysis of the diaphragm is much more common than is bilateral paralysis and the most common cause is nerve invasion from malignancy, usually a bronchogenic carcinoma. Patients with a unilateral paralyzed diaphragm are usually asymptomatic. The diagnosis is suspected by finding an elevated hemidiaphragm on the CXR and the confirmation is best established with the "**sniff test**." In sniff test the patient is observed with fluoroscopy while sniffing. The **paralyzed diaphragm will move paradoxically upward due to the negative intrathoracic pressure.**

760. Hirsutism is caused by all of the following drugs *except*:
- **A.** Phenobarbitone
- **B.** Phenytoin
- **C.** Minoxidil
- **D.** Cyclosporine

(AIIMS 1995)

Hirsutism can be caused by drugs that exert their effects independent of androgens and do not produce defeminization or virilization (**phenytoin**, **minoxidil**, diazoxide, **cyclosporine**, and hexachlorobenzene).

761. Brain tumor associated with CNS invasion is:
- **A.** Oligodendroglioma
- **B.** Glioblastoma multiforme
- **C.** Medulloblastoma
- **D.** Ependymoma

(AIIMS 1995)

Medulloblastoma occurs in young children and affects the vermis of the cerebellum. It is a rapidly growing tumor and **produces seedling metastasis in the CSF pathway** and 4th ventricle. It is a radiosensitive tumor.

762. ***Not* a cause of osteoporosis:**

A. Osteogenesis imperfecta **B.** Hypophosphatasia
C. Hypogonadism **D.** Hypoparathyroidism *(AIIMS 1995, AI 1998)*

763. Osteoporosis is *not* seen in:

A. Cushing's disease **B.** Hyperthyroidism
C. Hypoparathyroidism **D.** Hyperparathyroidism *(AI 1996, 1998)*

764. Osteoporosis is *not* seen in:

A. Steroid therapy **B.** Hypoparathyroidism
C. Rheumatoid arthritis **D.** Thyrotoxicosis *(AI 1994)*

765. Osteoporosis is *not* seen in:

A. Thyrotoxicosis **B.** Hypoparathyroidism
C. Rheumatoid arthritis **D.** Chronic heparin administration *(AIIMS 1996, UP 2000, AI 2000)*

766. Osteoporosis is *not* seen in:

A. Steroid therapy **B.** Hypoparathyroidism
C. Scurvy **D.** Old age *(AI 1991)*

767. ***Not* a cause of osteoporosis:**

A. Scurvy **B.** Methotrexate
C. Osteogenesis imperfecta **D.** Heparin administration *(AIIMS 1998)*

Conditions Associated with Osteoporosis

- Idiopathic osteoporosis (juvenile and adult)
- Type I & II osteoporosis
- Hypogonadism
- Hyperadrenocorticism
- Chronic glucocorticoid administration
- **Hyper**parathyroidism
- Thyrotoxicosis
- Malabsorption
- Scurvy
- Calcium deficiency
- Immobilization
- Chronic heparin administration
- Systemic mastocytosis
- Osteogenesis imperfecta
- Homocystinuria due to cystathionine synthase deficiency
- Ehlers-Danlos syndrome
- Marfan's syndrome
- Rheumatoid arthritis
- Malnutrition
- Alcoholism
- Epilepsy
- Primary biliary cirrhosis
- Chronic obstructive pulmonary disease
- Menkes' syndrome
- Adult hypophosphatasia
- Other metabolic bone diseases

768. Familial hypercholesterolemia is because of:

A. Dysbetalipoproteinemia **B.** Familial apoprotein C II deficiency
C. Lipoprotein deficiency **D.** Mutation in gene for LDL receptors *(AIIMS 1997)*

769. Tendon xanthomas are seen in:

A. Familial lipoprotein lipase deficiency **B.** Familial hypertriglyceridemia
C. Dysbetalipoproteinemia **D.** Familial hypercholesterolemia *(AIIMS 1998)*

Familial hypercholesterolemia (FH) is a co-dominant genetic disorder that occurs in the heterozygous form in approximately 1 in 500 individuals. **FH is due to mutations in the gene for the LDL receptor.** Plasma levels of total and LDL cholesterol are *elevated at birth* and remain so throughout life. In adults, total cholesterol levels range from 275 to 500 mg/dL. Plasma triglyceride (TG) levels are *typically* normal, and HDL cholesterol levels are normal or reduced. *Tendon xanthomas* most commonly involve the Achilles tendons and the extensor tendons of the knuckles and are found in about 75% of adults with FH.

770. Zinc deficiency causes:
- **A.** Hypogonadism
- **B.** Diarrhea
- **C.** Alopecia
- **D.** All of the above

771. *Not* a manifestation of Zinc deficiency:
- **A.** Hypogonadism
- **B.** Cardiomyopathy
- **C.** Growth retardation
- **D.** Alopecia

(AIIMS 1997)

Features of Zinc Deficiency

- Growth retardation
- Dermatitis
- Immunologic dysfunction
- Psychological disturbances
- Impaired spermatogenesis
- Alopecia
- Diarrhea
- Failure to thrive
- Gonadal atrophy
- Congenital malformations

772. Blood culture is indicated in all *except*:
- **A.** Malaria
- **B.** Septicemia
- **C.** SABE
- **D.** Enteric fever

(AIIMS 1997)

- Specific diagnosis of typhoid depends on the isolation of salmonellae from stool, **blood**, or tissue fluids.
- The critical diagnostic finding in endocarditis is bacteremia. Blood cultures are positive in more than 95% of patients.
- Blood cultures yield bacteria or fungi in about 20 to 40% of cases of severe sepsis and 40 to 70% of cases of septic shock.
- The diagnosis of **malaria** rests on the demonstration of asexual forms of the parasite in **peripheral blood smears**.

773. *Not* seen in hyponatremia:
- **A.** Periodic muscle paralysis
- **B.** Convulsions
- **C.** Raised ICT
- **D.** Headache

(AIIMS 1997)

774. *Earliest* indicator of sodium loss is:
- **A.** Orthostatic hypertension
- **B.** Arrhythmia
- **C.** Altered sensorium
- **D.** Reduced skin turgidity

(JIPMER 1995)

A plasma Na^+ concentration less than 135 mmol/L is known as hyponatremia. The clinical manifestations of hyponatremia are due to osmotic water shift leading **cerebral edema**. The symptoms are primarily *neurologic*, and their severity is dependent on the rapidity of onset and absolute decrease in plasma Na^+ concentration. Patients may be asymptomatic, or complain of nausea and malaise. As the plasma Na^+ concentration falls, the symptoms progress to include **headache**, lethargy, confusion, and obtundation. Stupor, **seizures**, and coma do not occur unless the plasma Na^+ concentration falls acutely below 120 mmol/L or decreases rapidly.

775. In rheumatoid arthritis, common type of anemia is:
- **A.** Macrocytic hypochromic
- **B.** Hypochromic, normocytic
- **C.** Hyperchromic, normocytic
- **D.** Normocytic, normochromic

(AIIMS 1997)

776. *Not* a complication of rheumatoid arthritis:
- **A.** Polycythemia
- **B.** Splenic infarct
- **C.** Endocarditis
- **D.** Pericarditis

(PGI 1993)

Normochromic, **normocytic** anemia is frequently present in *active* **rheumatoid arthritis**. It is due to ineffective erythropoiesis because large stores of iron are found in the bone marrow.

777. *Most common* site of iatrogenic rupture of esophagus is:
- **A.** Abdominal
- **B.** Thoracic region above aortic arch
- **C.** Thoracic region below aortic arch
- **D.** Cervical esophagus

(AIIMS 1997)

Instrumental perforation usually occurs in the **pharynx** or lower esophagus, often just above the diaphragm in the posterolateral wall.

778. Spontaneous rupture of spleen is seen in:

A. Hereditary spherocytosis
B. Infectious mononucleosis
C. Polycythemia rubra vera
D. CML *(AIIMS 1997)*

The **spleen rupture** is seen in < 0.5% of cases of **infectious mononucleosis** and is more common among males than among females. It may be manifest as abdominal pain, referred shoulder pain, or hemodynamic compromise.

779. *Not* a characteristic feature of Plummer-Vinson syndrome:

A. Dysphagia
B. Common in elderly male
C. Esophageal webs
D. Premalignant *(AIIMS 1997)*

The combination of symptomatic hypopharyngeal webs and iron-deficiency anemia in middle-aged **female** constitute **Plummer-Vinson syndrome or Paterson-Brown-Kelly syndrome**. A curious radiological finding seen in this syndrome is the presence of a **web in postcricoid region**. It produces **dysphagia**. Hemoglobin is low and there is a hypochromic microcytic anemia. All cases will have a low serum iron and consequently a high iron binding capacity. A small but significant proportion of patients develop **postcricoid carcinoma**. Iron should be given orally until hemoglobin comes to normal level.

780. Inappropriate ADH secretion (SIADH) is *not* seen in:

A. Head injury
B. Small cell carcinoma of lung
C. Acute encephalitis
D. Chromophobe adenoma

781. SIADH is associated with which of the following:

A. Small cell carcinoma of lung
B. Squamous cell carcinoma of lung
C. Adenocarcinoma of lung
D. Large cell carcinoma of lung *(AIIMS 1997)*

782. SIADH occurs in all *except*:

A. Migraine
B. Chronic meningitis
C. Guillain-Barré syndrome
D. Acute intermittent porphyria *(KERALA 1999)*

Causes of SIADH

Malignant neoplasms with autonomous AVP release	Nonmalignant pulmonary diseases	CNS disorders
• Small cell carcinoma of lung • Carcinoma of pancreas • Lymphoma, lymphocytic lymphoma, Hodgkin's disease • Carcinoma of duodenum • Thymoma	• Tuberculosis • Lung abscess • Pneumonia • Viral pneumonitis • Empyema • Chronic obstructive airways disease	• Skull fracture • Subdural hematoma • Subarachnoid hemorrhage • Cerebral vascular thrombosis • Cerebral atrophy • Acute encephalitis • Tuberculous meningitis • Purulent meningitis • Guillain-Barré syndrome • Lupus erythematosus • Acute intermittent porphyria
Drugs	**Other causes**	
• Chlorpropamide • Vincristine • Vinblastine • Cyclophosphamide • Carbamazepine • Oxytocin • General anesthesia • Narcotics • Tricyclic antidepressants	• Hypothyroidism • Positive pressure ventilation	

783. Lateral medullary syndrome is caused by thrombosis of:
- **A.** Posterior inferior cerebellar artery
- **B.** Anterior inferior cerebellar artery
- **C.** Superior cerebellar artery
- **D.** Posterior communicating branch of middle cerebral artery

784. *Not* a feature of Wallenberg's syndrome:
- **A.** Ipsilateral involvement of lower cranial nerve
- **B.** Ipsilateral involvement of sympathetic tract
- **C.** Ipsilateral loss of taste
- **D.** *Ipsilateral* loss of pain and temperature *(AIIMS 1997)*

785. *Not* a characteristic feature of lateral medullary syndrome:
- **A.** Crossed hemi-anesthesia
- **B.** Horners's syndrome is *rare*
- **C.** Dysphagia
- **D.** Numbness *(AIIMS 1997)*

786. *Not* a feature of lateral medullary syndrome:
- **A.** Impairment of pain over contralateral half of the body
- **B.** Impairment of sensation over ipsilateral face
- **C.** Falling to the side opposite to the lesion
- **D.** Ipsilateral Horner's syndrome *(SGPGI 1999)*

Lateral medullary syndrome of Wallenberg (occlusion of any of 5 vessels may be responsible viz. vertebral, posterior inferior cerebellar, superior, middle, or inferior lateral medullary arteries).	
On side of lesion	
Pain, numbness, impaired sensation over half the face	Descending tract and nucleus 5th nerve
Ataxia of limbs, falling to side of lesion	Uncertain restiform body, cerebellar hemisphere, cerebellar fibers, spinocerebellar tract (?)
Nystagmus, diplopia, oscillopsia, vertigo, nausea, vomiting	Vestibular nucleus
Horner's syndrome (miosis, ptosis, decreased sweating)	Descending sympathetic tract
Dysphagia, hoarseness, paralysis of palate, paralysis of vocal cord, diminished gag reflex	Issuing fibers 9th and 10th nerves
Loss of taste	Nucleus and tractus solitarius
Numbness of ipsilateral arm, trunk, or leg	Cuneate and gracile nuclei
On side opposite to the lesion	
Impaired pain and thermal sense over half the body, sometimes face	Spinothalamic tract

787. Tumor *common* in AIDS is:
- **A.** Uterus carcinoma
- **B.** Urinary bladder carcinoma
- **C.** B-cell lymphoma
- **D.** Lung carcinoma *(UP 1997)*

788. In patients of AIDS, *least* common tumor is:
- **A.** Primary CNS lymphoma
- **B.** Astrocytoma
- **C.** Burkitt's lymphoma
- **D.** Kaposi's sarcoma *(AIIMS 1997)*

A variety of neoplastic and premalignant diseases occur with increased frequency in HIV-infected patients. Among them are **Kaposi's sarcoma**, **lymphoma**, and intraepithelial dysplasia of the cervix and anus. 3 main categories of lymphoma are seen in patients with HIV infection: grade 3 or 4 immunoblastic lymphoma, Burkitt's lymphoma, and primary CNS lymphoma.

789. In which of the following condition, concentric hypertrophy of left ventricle is seen:
A. Hypertrophic cardiomyopathy
B. Mitral stenosis
C. Mitral regurgitation
D. Essential hypertension *(AIIMS 1997)*

The **concentric hypertrophy** associated with **chronic hypertension** can also impair ventricular filling but rarely causes overt heart failure.

790. The following conditions predispose to leukemias:
A. Bloom syndrome
B. Down syndrome
C. Fanconi anemia
D. All of the above

791. AML is seen with increased frequency in all *except*:
A. Fanconi anemia
B. Bloom syndrome
C. Fragile X syndrome
D. Down syndrome *(AIIMS 1997)*

Conditions Associated with an Increased Incidence of AML

- Down syndrome (trisomy of chromosome 21)
- Patau syndrome (trisomy of chromosome 13)
- Klinefelter syndrome (XXY and variants)
- Fanconi anemia
- Bloom syndrome
- Ataxia telangiectasia
- Kostmann syndrome

792. Galactorrhea is *not* seen with the use of:
A. Reserpine
B. Phenothiazines
C. Bromocriptine
D. Metoclopramide *(AIIMS 1997)*

Drugs Causing Galactorrhea

- Phenothiazines
- Butyrophenones
- Methyldopa
- Verapamil
- Metoclopramide
- Tricyclic antidepressants
- Opiates
- Reserpine
- Domperidone

793. Disorder of language of cerebral origin is:
A. Aphasia **B.** Dysarthria
C. Stuttering **D.** Echolalia

794. Lesion in inferior frontal gyrus causes:
A. Motor aphasia
B. Incomprehension of spoken language
C. Incomprehension of written language
D. Defect in articulation *(AIIMS 1997)*

Language is used for communication and reshaping of thoughts and experiences by linking them to arbitrary symbols known as '**words**'. The neural substrate of language is made up of a distributed network centered in the perisylvian region of the **left** hemisphere. The posterior pole of this 'network' is called **Wernicke's area** and includes the *posterior third of the superior temporal gyrus* and a surrounding *rim of the inferior parietal lobule*. An *important function of Wernicke's area is to transform sensory inputs into their neural word representations*. The anterior pole of the language 'network' is known as **Broca's area**. Broca's area includes the *posterior part of the inferior frontal gyrus* and a surrounding *rim of prefrontal heteromodal cortex*. An essential function of Broca's area is to *transform neural word representations into their articulatory sequences so that the words can be uttered in the form of spoken language*. Wernicke's and Broca's areas are *interconnected* with each other and with additional perisylvian, temporal, prefrontal, and posterior parietal regions, making up a 'neural network' performing the various aspects of language function. Damage to any 1 of these components or to their interconnections can give rise to language disturbances known as **aphasia**. If this sensory appreciation of the words appears normal and the articulatory apparatus is unharmed, yet the patient is unable to speak words which have a meaning both to him and to the listener, the condition is known as **motor aphasia**. One of the earliest changes is the loss of names (nominal aphasia) so that the patient circumvents the use of the name by a phrase (as one does with a limited knowledge of a foreign language). The faculty of writing is also lost (*agraphia*). **Motor aphasia is commonly associated with a right hemiplegia due to left middle cerebral artery thrombosis involving the Broca's area of the left inferior frontal gyrus (area 44).** In **sensory aphasia** *impression upon which the speech is based becomes meaningless*. The patient may hear words which convey nothing to him (word deafness) or may seen written words which convey nothing to him (word blindness). Simple commands such as "raise your hand" will not be executed as the patient does not grasp the meaning of the words. Sensory aphasia arises from lesions in the left superior temporal gyrus (area 42).

795. *Most common* type of aphasia in AD is seen in:

A. Trans cortical motor **B.** Trans cortical sensory
C. Anomic aphasia **D.** Broca's aphasia *(AIIMS 1999)*

Anomic aphasia is the single most common language disturbance seen in head trauma and metabolic encephalopathy. This is also the *most common* aphasia seen in Alzheimer's disease (AD).

796. Recurrent giardiasis is common in:

A. C_1 esterase inhibitors deficiency
B. DiGeorge syndrome
C. C_8 deficiency
D. Common variable immunodeficiency *(AIIMS 1997, 2000)*

Diagnosis of **common variable immunodeficiency** should be considered in adults with chronic pulmonary infections, some of whom will present with unexplained bronchiectasis. Intestinal diseases, including **chronic giardiasis**, intestinal malabsorption, and atrophic gastritis with pernicious anemia, are common in these patients.

797. Viral meningitis is *most commonly* caused by:

A. Echovirus **B.** Coxsackievirus
C. Poliovirus **D.** Enteroviruses *(AIIMS 1997)*

At least 2/3rd of the cases of CSF culture-negative aseptic meningitis are due to enteroviruses, making this viral group by far the most important cause of viral meningitis. Viruses causing aseptic meningitis are listed below:

Common	Less Common	Rare
• Enteroviruses	• Herpes simplex virus- 1	• Adenoviruses
• Arboviruses	• Lymphocytic choriomeningitis virus	• Cytomegalovirus
• Human immunodeficiency virus	• Mumps virus	• Epstein-Barr virus
• Herpes simplex virus- 2		• Influenza A, B
		• Measles
		• Parainfluenza
		• Rubella
		• Varicella zoster virus

798. Sjögren's syndrome is *not* associated with:

A. Primary biliary cirrhosis
B. Rheumatoid arthritis
C. Chronic active hepatitis
D. Mid line granuloma *(AIIMS 1997)*

Sjögren's syndrome is the association of xerostomia, keratoconjunctivitis sicca with a *connective tissue disorder*. Most often the associated connective tissue disorder is rheumatoid arthritis but several other disorders may be associated and are listed below:

- Systemic lupus erythematosus
- Primary biliary cirrhosis
- Myasthenia gravis
- Thyroiditis
- Progressive systemic sclerosis
- Chronic active hepatitis
- Polymyositis

Primary Sjögren's syndrome or **sicca syndrome** is the term used when severe keratoconjunctivitis sicca and xerostomia occur in the *absence* of an associated connective tissue disorder.

799. Alkaline phosphatase is *not* increased in:

A. Paget's disease
B. Hypophosphatasia
C. Osteomalacia
D. Hyperparathyroidism *(AIIMS 1997)*

Rickets is a feature of a *deficiency* of alkaline phosphatase in infants and children termed **hypophosphatasia.**

800. Alkaline phosphatase is raised in:

A. Osteoporosis
B. CRF
C. Primary hyperparathyroidism
D. Multiple myeloma *(AI 1999)*

Raised levels of alkaline phosphatase	Reduced levels of alkaline phosphatase
• Hyperparathyroidism • Paget's disease • Osteomalacia • Rickets • Caffey disease • Osteoblastic bone tumors (metastatic or osteogenic sarcoma) • Pregnancy • Childhood • Liver disease such as biliary obstruction • Total parenteral nutrition (TPN) • Sepsis • Thyrotoxicosis • Chronic inflammatory bowel disease	• Malnutrition • Excess vitamin D ingestion • Hypophosphatasia

Normal value in adults is 45-125 U/L and in children 20-150 U/L.

801. *Pure* motor neuropathy *does not* occur in:

A. Guillain-Barré syndrome
B. Porphyria
C. Dapsone intoxication
D. Lead intoxication *(AIIMS 1997)*

Lesions affecting at any level of the motor unit (anterior horn cell, motor axon, or neuromuscular junction) may result in a *purely* lower motor syndrome without sensory disturbance. Examples of motor neuronopathies include the lower-motor form of amyotrophic lateral sclerosis, poliomyelitis, hereditary spinal muscular atrophies, and adult variant of hexosaminidase A deficiency. Motor neuropathies may be due to **lead or dapsone intoxication**, occasionally with **porphyria**, and also with multifocal motor neuropathy.

802. In primary idiopathic polymyositis, which of the following group of muscles are never involved:
A. Ocular muscle
B. Extensor neck muscle
C. Pharyngeal muscles
D. Proximal limb girdle
(SGPGI 1996))

803. In polymyositis which of the following muscle is *not* involved:
A. Muscles of pharynx
B. Muscles of trunk
C. Neck muscle
D. Ocular muscle
(AIIMS 1997)

804. In polymyositis, which of the following muscle is *not* involved:
A. Thigh
B. Girdle
C. Ocular
D. Neck
(AI 1996)

Dermatomyositis and **polymyositis** are diseases of autoimmune etiology in which the skeletal muscle is damaged by a nonsuppurative inflammatory process. The term **polymyositis** is used when the condition *spares* the skin and the term **dermatomyositis** when polymyositis is *associated* with a characteristic skin rash. Patients 1st notice the weakness of the proximal limb muscles, especially the hips and thighs, and find difficulty in arising from the squatting or kneeling position and in climbing or descending stairs. Early symptoms of **dysphagia** and weakness of flexor muscles of the neck in a patient with a chronic myopathy indicate the diagnosis of polymyositis. **Ocular muscles are almost never affected** *except* in a rare association with myasthenia gravis. Corticosteroids in high dosage are the accepted treatment for severe dermatomyositis-polymyositis, though there is no controlled trial to prove its effectiveness.

805. 4th heart sound is heard in all *except*:
A. Ventricular aneurysm
B. MR
C. Cardiomyopathy
D. Hypertension
(AIIMS 1995)

4th heart sound is frequently present in patients with systemic **hypertension**, aortic stenosis, hypertrophic **cardiomyopathy**, ischemic heart disease, and acute **mitral regurgitation**.

806. In 1998, Noble prize for research in medicine was given for:
A. NO
B. Super oxide
C. N_2O
D. H_2O_2
(AIIMS 1998)

Ferid Murad was an American physician, pharmacologist, and Nobel laureate who **shared the 1998 Nobel Prize in physiology or medicine with colleagues Louis Ignarro and Robert Furchgott. Murad determined that NO is a signaling molecule**—a molecule that transmits messages from one cell to another. Murad investigated the action of NO in the blood vessels of the cardiovascular system.

807. *Not* associated with hypercoagulable state:
A. Weber Christian disease
B. Protein S deficiency
C. Protein C deficiency
D. Antiphospholipid antibody
(AIIMS 1998)

Hypercoagulable state may be induced by **antiphospholipid antibodies**, factor V mutations, **protein C deficiency**, **protein S deficiency**, antithrombin III deficiency, systemic neoplasm, and traumatic and surgical tissue injury.

808. A patient of AIDS with *Pneumocystis carinii* infection is treated with aerosol pentamidine. He may develop all of the following *except*:
A. Extra-thoracic infection
B. Cavitation
C. Pneumothorax
D. Lower lobe infiltration
(AIIMS 1998)

The classic findings on CXR in *Pneumocystis carinii* pneumonia (PCP) consist of bilateral diffuse infiltrates starting in the perihilar regions, but a variety of atypical manifestations (nodular densities, **cavitary lesions**) have also been found. **Patients who receive aerosolized pentamidine have an increased frequency of upper-lobe infiltrates and pneumothorax.** However, early in the course of pneumocystosis, the CXR may be normal. Frequency of **extrapulmonary pneumocystosis** is between <1 to 3%. A risk factor in HIV-infected patients is the administration of aerosolized pentamidine and the most common sites of extrapulmonary involvement are the lymph nodes (40 to 50%); next in frequency are the spleen, liver, and bone marrow (30 to 40%).

809. An HIV patient with perihilar infiltrates and *without* pleural effusion in the X-ray is most likely to have:

- **A.** *Pneumocystis carinii* pneumonia
- **B.** Kaposi's sarcoma
- **C.** Tuberculosis
- **D.** Lymphoma

(AIIMS May 2002)

While CXR may reveal a variety of patterns in patients of *Pneumocystis carinii* pneumonia (PCP), the most common finding is either a normal film or a faint bilateral interstitial infiltrate. **The classic finding of a dense, perihilar infiltrate described in patients with non-HIV-associated PCP is *rarely* seen in patients with AIDS.**

810. Non-synchronized DC shock is given in:

- **A.** Ventricular fibrillation
- **B.** Ventricular tachycardia
- **C.** Atrial fibrillation
- **D.** Atrial flutter

(AIIMS 1998)

Electrical cardioversion and defibrillation is the *most reliable* methods for terminating arrhythmias. External cardioversion is performed by placing 2 paddles, 12 cm in diameter, in firm contact with the chest wall, with 1 paddle located to the right of the sternum at the level of the 2nd rib and the other in the left anterior axillary line in the 5th intercostal space. **Energy is delivered synchronously with the QRS complex for all arrhythmias *except ventricular flutter and ventricular fibrillation*, because asynchronous shocks can produce ventricular fibrillation.**

811. Vaccine prescribed to a child with nephrotic syndrome is:

- **A.** *Bordetella pertussis*
- **B.** Hepatitis B virus
- **C.** Pneumococcal
- **D.** *Haemophilus influenzae*

(PGI 1998)

812. Pneumococcal vaccine is *not* indicated in:

- **A.** Diabetes mellitus
- **B.** Cystic fibrosis
- **C.** Renal failure
- **D.** Sickle cell anemia

(AIIMS 1998)

Recommendations for Pneumococcal Vaccination

Immunocompetent group	Immunocompromised group
• Chronic pulmonary disease	• HIV infection
• Chronic cardiovascular disease	• Leukemia
• Chronic liver disease	• Lymphoma
• Alcoholism	• Hodgkin's lymphoma
• Diabetes mellitus	• Multiple myeloma
• Cerebrospinal fluid leak	• Generalized malignancy
• Asplenia	• Chronic renal failure
• Residents of health care facilities	• *Nephrotic syndrome*
• Sickle cell disease	• Organ or bone marrow transplant
	• Immunosuppressive/steroids

813. A patient presents with history of low grade fever 10 days back, which decreased with some antipyretics. Now he is again having fever and peripheral smear examination showed gametocytes of *Plasmodium falciparum*. Which of the following drugs will you give for him:

- **A.** Artemether
- **B.** Quinine
- **C.** Ciprofloxacin
- **D.** Primaquine
- **E.** Cephalosporins

(PGI Dec 2000)

Quinine has reemerged as **1st line drugs for the treatment of falciparum malaria** because of widespread chloroquine resistance. Quinine in combination with a 2nd active drug is recommended as oral therapy for *Plasmodium falciparum* malaria.

814. A 50-year-old asymptomatic man on routine investigation was found to have 3 times increased alkaline phosphatase with normal serum calcium and phosphorus. *Most likely* diagnosis is:

- **A.** Metastasis form primary carcinoma
- **B.** Primary hyperparathyroidism
- **C.** Paget's disease of bone
- **D.** Osteoporosis

(AIIMS 1999)

Many patients of **Paget's disease** are **asymptomatic** and the disorder is discovered accidentally during radiologic examination of the pelvis or spine for an *un*related problem or because of the finding of **an elevated level of plasma alkaline phosphatase**. Although increased bone resorption enhances release of calcium and phosphate ions from bone, utilization of these ions for new bone formation and feedback control of PTH secretion usually maintain the concentration of **calcium ions in the plasma at normal levels.** The **concentration of phosphate in the plasma is normal or slightly elevated**.

815. Interferon is *not* used in:

A. Myelomonocytic leukemia
B. Chronic hepatitis B
C. CML
D. Hairy cell leukemia *(JIPMER 1993)*

816. Interferon is *not* useful in:

A. Polymyositis
B. Hepatitis C
C. CML
D. Hairy cell leukemia *(AIIMS 1998)*

Indications of α interferon

- Hairy cell leukemia
- Condylomata acuminata
- Chronic active hepatitis
- Renal carcinoma
- Laryngeal papillomatosis
- Malignant melanoma
- Mycosis fungoides
- AIDS-associated Kaposi's sarcoma
- Carcinoma, bladder
- Cervical carcinoma
- Chronic myelocytic leukemia
- Non-Hodgkin's lymphomas
- Multiple myeloma

Chronic granulomatous disease is an indication for use of γ interferon.

817. Insulin resistance is *not* seen in:

A. Excess growth hormone
B. Obesity
C. Lipodystrophy
D. Addison's disease *(AIIMS 1998)*

Causes of Insulin Resistance

- Obesity (*most common*)
- Generalized and partial lipodystrophies
- Alstrom syndrome
- Rabson-Mendenhall syndrome
- Acromegaly
- Myotonic dystrophy
- Werner syndrome
- Insulin receptor abnormalities
- Pineal hypertrophy syndrome
- Ataxia-telangiectasia
- Leprechaunism
- Cushing's syndrome
- Thalassemia major

818. Gonadectomy is done in:

A. Mixed gonadal dysgenesis
B. Klinefelter syndrome
C. Kallmann syndrome
D. Down syndrome *(AIIMS 1998)*

Mosaicism for a Y-bearing cell line, usually the 45, X/46, XY karyotype, is responsible for most cases of **mixed gonadal dysgenesis**. When the diagnosis is established in phenotypic females, prophylactic **gonadectomy** should be performed as gonadal tumors may occur in childhood and because the testes secrete androgen at puberty and thus cause virilization.

819. Complication of sickle cell anemia is:

A. Splenomegaly
B. Predispose to bladder tumor
C. Urolithiasis
D. Priapism *(AIIMS 1998)*

Patients with sickle cell disease manifest the clinical features of chronic anemia with pallor of the mucous membranes, fatigue, and decreased exercise tolerance. Other features include leg ulcers, **priapism**, repeated episodes of pulmonary infarction, and "acute chest syndrome" characterized by fever, chest pain, and pulmonary infiltrates.

820. Clubbing is *not* seen in:
A. Cyanotic heart disease
B. Cryptogenic fibrosing alveolitis
C. Primary biliary cirrhosis
D. Chronic bronchitis *(AIIMS 1998)*

821. Clubbing is *not* seen in:
A. Mesothelioma
B. Left to right shunt
C. Empyema
D. Cirrhosis *(AIIMS 1992)*

Some Causes of Clubbing

CVS disorders	**Pulmonary diseases**
• *Cyanotic* congenital heart disease • Infective endocarditis	• Primary lung cancer • Metastatic lung cancer • Lung abscess • Bronchiectasis • Fibrosing alveolitis • Cystic fibrosis • Mesothelioma
GI diseases	
• Hepatic cirrhosis • Ulcerative colitis • Regional enteritis (Crohn's disease) • Celiac disease	
Miscellaneous	
• Hereditary (birth defects) • Idiopathic	

Mnemonic causes of **CLUBBING**
Cyanotic congenital heart disease
Lung disease (hypoxia, lung cancer, bronchiectasis, cystic fibrosis)
Ulcerative colitis/Crohn's disease
Biliary cirrhosis
Birth defect (harmless)
Infective endocarditis
Neoplasm
GI malabsorption

822. Gardner's syndrome has all of the following *except*:
A. Skull osteomas
B. Polyposis coli
C. Dental defect
D. Xanthomas *(PGI May 2001)*

823. *False* regarding Gardner's syndrome is:
A. Dental abnormality
B. Osteoma
C. CNS tumor
D. Desmoid tumor *(PGI 2000)*

Gardner's syndrome is a variant of familial adenomatous polyposis (FAP). It is an autosomal dominant disease characterized by **gastrointestinal polyps**, multiple **osteomas**, and skin and soft tissue tumors. Cutaneous findings include epidermoid cysts, **desmoid tumors**, and other benign tumors. Polyps have a 100% risk of undergoing malignant transformation; consequently, early identification of the disease is critical. **Dental abnormalities** (un-erupted teeth, supernumerary teeth) may occur.

824. *Not* a cause of CNS vasculitis:
A. PAN
B. Behçet's disease
C. Whipple's disease
D. Systemic lupus erythematosus *(PGI 2000)*

Many forms of vasculitis may involve the central nervous system (CNS), including **Behçet's disease**, **polyarteritis nodosa**, vasculitis associated with connective tissue diseases such as lupus (**systemic lupus erythematosus**), and others.

825. Which of the following is the single recessive gene inherited disease:

A. Parkinsonism
B. Schizophrenia
C. Tuberous sclerosis
D. Wilson's disease *(PGI 2000)*

> **Wilson's disease** is an **autosomal recessive** hyperkinetic movement disorder in which decrease in ceruloplasmin levels result in the deposition of copper in the liver and in the globus pallidus and putamen. In advanced cases, these neural structures atrophy, and there is associated cortical injury. Clinically, it is characterized by dementia, psychiatric disorders, and tremor (classically, a "wing-beating" tremor of the upper extremities).

826. Bronchial adenoma *commonly* presents as:

A. Chest pain
B. Dyspnea
C. Recurrent hemoptysis
D. Wheezing *(AI 1996, 1998)*

> **Bronchial adenomas** are slow-growing, endobronchial lesions which represent 50% of all benign pulmonary neoplasms. Patients may have a chronic cough, **recurrent hemoptysis**, or obstruction with atelectasis, lobar collapse, or pneumonitis and abscess formation.

827. *Most common* trisomy among the following is:

A. Trisomy 5
B. Trisomy 18
C. Trisomy 21
D. Trisomy 13 *(AI 1998)*

> One in every 150 newborn babies has an abnormality in the *number* or *structure* of the normally 46 chromosomes in a karyotype. **Trisomy 21 (Down syndrome) is the most frequent autosomal syndrome.**

828. In cerebral aneurysm rupture which of the following nerve is involved:

A. Oculomotor
B. VII
C. VIII
D. Trochlear *(AI 1998)*

> The clinical spectrum of cerebral aneurysm rupture includes nonspecific symptoms such as headache, dizziness, motor or sensory disturbances, more specific clinical signs such as **oculomotor nerve palsy**, and "the warning leak" syndrome or the typical presentation of acute intracranial pressure and meningeal syndrome resulting from a substantial intracranial bleed.

829. All of the following metastatic tumors compress spinal cord *except*:

A. Meningioma
B. Breast carcinoma
C. Lymphoma
D. Lung carcinoma *(AI 1998)*

> Almost any malignant tumor is able to metastasize to the spinal canal, although **breast**, **lung**, prostate, kidney, **lymphoma**, and plasma cell dyscrasia are particularly *frequent*.

830. Nosocomial pneumonia is caused by which of the following organism:

A. Mycoplasma
B. Gram negative cocci
C. Gram positive bacilli
D. Gram negative bacilli *(AI 1998)*

> The production of chromosomally encoded, inducible β-lactamases by some aerobic **gram-negative bacilli** (*Serratia marcescens*, *Enterobacter cloacae*, *Citrobacter freundii*, *Morganella morganii*, *Pseudomonas aeruginosa*, and *Acinetobacter calcoaceticus*) has important implications for the management of **nosocomial pneumonia** in hospitals where these organisms are common nosocomial pathogens.

831. *Not* a predisposing factor of Alzheimer's disease:

A. Smoking
B. Head injury
C. Low education level
D. Down syndrome *(AI 1999)*

Predisposing Factors for Alzheimer's Disease

• Old age	• Positive family history	• Female gender
• NSAIDs	• Lower educational level	• Head trauma
• Amyloid angiopathy	• Down's syndrome	• Environmental factors

832. ***False*** **regarding subacute combined degeneration:**
- **A.** Brisk ankle reflexes
- **B.** Corticospinal involvement
- **C.** Posterior column involvement
- **D.** Due to vitamin B_{12} deficiency

(AI 1999)

833. Pyramidal tract involvement with absent ankle jerk is seen in:
- **A.** Frederick's ataxia
- **B.** Subacute combined degeneration of the spinal cord
- **C.** Lathyrism
- **D.** Tabes dorsalis

(AIIMS May 2001)

Subacute combined degeneration due to vitamin B_{12} deficiency is a 'treatable' myelopathy which presents with paresthesia in the hands and feet, early loss of vibration and position sensation, and a progressive spastic and ataxic weakness. **Loss of reflexes** due to a superimposed peripheral neuropathy is present in many cases.

834. Blood of a patient is ***anti*** **HBsAg (HBsAb) positive** ***but*** **all other tests are** ***negative*****. This may be due to:**
- **A.** Chronic active hepatitis
- **B.** Carrier state
- **C.** Vaccine given
- **D.** Acute infection

(AIIMS 2000)

Serological Markers of HBV Infection

Clinical condition	**HBsAg**	**HBsAb**	**HBcAb Total**	**HBcAb IgM**	**HBeAg**	**HBeAg**	**HBV DNA**
Acute infection	+	–	+	Strong +	+ to –	– to +	+
Resolving infection	+	–	+	+	–	+	–
Immune status (exposure)	–	+	+	–	–	+	–
Immune status (vaccination)	–	+	–	–	–	–	–
Chronic infection or carrier	+	–	+	+ or –	+ or –	+ or –	+ or –

Serological Tests to be done for HBV Infections

Infection type	**Tests to order**	**Abbreviation**
Acute infection	Hepatitis B core antibody Hepatitis B surface antigen Hepatitis Be antibody	HBcAb HBsAg HBeAb
Resolving infection	Hepatitis B core antibody Hepatitis B surface antigen Hepatitis B surface antibody	HBcAb HBsAg HBsAb
Immune status (exposure)	Hepatitis B core antibody	HBcAb
Immune status (vaccination)	Hepatitis B surface antibody	HBsAb
Chronic infection or carrier	Hepatitis B surface antigen Hepatitis Be antigen	HBsAg HBeAg

835. ***Most important*** **prognostic factor in an infarct case is:**
- **A.** Ejection fraction
- **B.** CPK
- **C.** Ventricular tachycardia
- **D.** Left main coronary artery obstruction

(AIIMS 2000)

Many clinical factors have been found to be associated with an increase in cardiovascular risk following initial recovery from a MI. The most important factors include persistent ischemia (spontaneous or provoked), **depressed left ventricular ejection fraction** (< 40%), rales above the lung bases on examination or congestion on CXR, and symptomatic ventricular arrhythmias.

836. *Not* associated with carpal tunnel syndrome:

A. Acromegaly
B. Hypertension
C. Myxedema
D. Pregnancy
(AIIMS 1994)

837. *Not* a cause of carpal tunnel syndrome:

A. Hypertension
B. Rheumatoid arthritis
C. Hypothyroidism
D. Pregnancy
(AI 1996)

Important Causes of Carpal Tunnel Syndrome

- Idiopathic (most common)
- Excessive use of the wrist
- Tenosynovitis
- Local infiltration
- Hypothyroidism
- Colles' fracture
- Acromegaly
- Amyloid
- Mucopolysaccharidoses
- Rheumatoid arthritis
- Diabetes mellitus
- Pregnancy

838. A 60-year-old man, who is a known case of liver cirrhosis, presents with increased levels of AFP, hepatomegaly 3 cm below costal margin. USG showed lesions involving the right lobe of liver. *Most likely* diagnosis is:

A. Metastasis
B. Hepatic adenoma
C. Hepatocellular carcinoma
D. Focal nodular hyperplasia
(AIIMS 2000)

Hepatocellular carcinoma is up to 4 times more common in men than in women and usually arises in a **cirrhotic liver**. The most common presenting features are abdominal *pain* with detection of an abdominal mass in the right upper quadrant. Serum elevations of alkaline phosphatase and α fetoprotein (AFP) are common. *Imaging methods* used to detect liver tumors include ultrasound, CT scan, MRI scan, hepatic artery angiography and radionuclide scans with ^{99m}Tc. Ultrasound should be the first procedure if hepatocellular carcinoma is suspected because it is less costly than scanning procedures, is relatively sensitive, and can detect most tumors > **3 cm**. AFP levels greater than 500 µg/L are found in about 70 to 80% of patients with hepatocellular carcinoma.

839. Which among the following resembles calcivirus:

A. HAV
B. HBV
C. HCV
D. HEV
(AIIMS Nov 2001)

There is no genomic or antigenic homology between HEV and HAV or other picornaviruses, and **HEV**, although *resembling* **calciviruses** appears to be sufficiently distinct from any known agent to merit a new classification of its own within the α virus group.

840. A patient with a bee-sting developed itching and subcutaneous edema, which progressed to involve the face. There was laryngeal edema with difficulty in breathing. The immune mechanism implicated in the causation of these manifestations is:

A. Immune complexes
B. IgE antibodies
C. IgG antibodies
D. Cytotoxic T cells
(AIIMS Nov 2001)

The fixation of **IgE** to human mast cells and basophils, a process termed *sensitization*, prepares these cells for subsequent antigen-specific activation. The life-threatening anaphylactic response of a sensitized human appears within minutes after administration of specific antigen (**such as bee-sting**) and is manifested by respiratory distress often followed by vascular collapse or by shock without antecedent respiratory difficulty. **Laryngeal edema** may be experienced as a "lump" in the throat, hoarseness, or stridor, while bronchial obstruction is associated with a feeling of tightness in the chest and/or audible wheezing.

841. Joint *least commonly* involved in ankylosing spondylitis is:

A. Lesser femoral trochanter
B. Spine
C. Wrist and hand
D. Sacroiliac joint
(AI 1996)

Virtually in all cases of **ankylosing spondylitis**, the **sacroiliac joints are the first site of involvement**, which is almost always bilaterally symmetrical from the onset of the disease. Generally other **spinal segments** are sooner or later affected. Other frequent sites include attachments of the sacroiliac ligaments and **greater and lesser femoral trochanters**.

842. Eosinophilia is seen in all *except*:
- **A.** Hodgkin's lymphoma
- **B.** Glucocorticoids
- **C.** Rheumatoid arthritis
- **D.** NSAID therapy

843. Eosinophilia is *not* caused by:
- **A.** Babesiosis
- **B.** Paragonimus
- **C.** Filariasis
- **D.** Ascariasis

(AI 1996)

Eosinophilia is defined as the presence of more than 500 eosinophils/μL of blood and is common in many conditions.

Causes of Eosinophilia	
Drugs	**Allergies**
• Iodides • Aspirin • Sulfonamides • Nitrofurantoin • Penicillins • Cephalosporins • Chlorpropamide • Erythromycin estolate • Imipramine • L-Tryptophan • Methotrexate • Procarbazine	• Hay fever • Asthma • Eczema • Serum sickness • Allergic vasculitis • Pemphigus
Collagen vascular diseases	**Malignancies**
• Rheumatoid arthritis • Eosinophilic fasciitis • Allergic angiitis • Periarteritis nodosa	• Hodgkin's disease • Mycosis fungoides • CML • Carcinoma lung • Carcinoma stomach • Carcinoma pancreas • Carcinoma ovary • Carcinoma uterus
Others	
• Job's syndrome • Chronic granulomatous disease • Helminthic infestation • Loeffler's endocarditis • Eosinophilic leukemia • Idiopathic hypereosinophilic syndrome	

- Babesiosis is a *protozoan* disease of animals that is transmitted by ticks.

844. Bilateral parotid gland enlargement is *not* seen in:
- **A.** Sjögren's syndrome
- **B.** Systemic lupus erythematosus
- **C.** Chronic pancreatitis
- **D.** Sarcoidosis

(AIIMS 1996, AI 1998)

Differential Diagnosis of Bilateral Parotid Gland Enlargement

- Mumps
- Influenza
- Epstein-Barr virus
- Coxsackievirus A
- Cytomegalovirus
- HIV
- Sarcoidosis
- Amyloidosis
- Sjögren's syndrome
- Diabetes mellitus
- Hyperlipoproteinemias
- Chronic pancreatitis
- Hepatic cirrhosis
- Acromegaly
- Gonadal hypofunction

845. To qualify as a solitary pulmonary nodule in chest X-ray the size should *not* exceed:

A. 3 cm **B.** 8 cm
C. 9 cm **D.** 6 cm

Solitary pulmonary nodule is defined as a radiological density completely surrounded by normal lung, with circumscribed margins **not more than 6 cm** in greatest diameter.

846. The *investigation of choice* for a solitary pulmonary nodule is:

A. CT
B. MRI
C. FNAC guided by imaging
D. USG

(AIIMS May 2002)

Nonsmoking patients under 35 years with **solitary pulmonary nodule** (SPN) should be followed with serial CXR every 3 months for 1 year and then yearly. If any significant growth is found, a histologic diagnosis is required. *For patients over age 35* and *all patients with a history of smoking*, **a histologic diagnosis must be made.** The sample can be obtained either at the time of nodule resection or, if the patient is a poor operative risk, via transthoracic fine-needle biopsy (**FNAC**).

847. Risk of transmission of HIV following single needle stick injury is:

A. 100% **B.** 90%
C. 0.3% **D.** 50%

(PGI 1999)

The risk of HIV transmission following skin puncture from a needle or a sharp object that was contaminated with blood from a person with documented HIV infection is just about 0.3%.

848. A doctor, while drawing blood for an HIV positive patient felt a needle stick injury. The prophylaxis which is to be given is:

A. AZT + lamivudine for 4 weeks
B. AZT + lamivudine + indinavir for 4 weeks
C. AZT + lamivudine + nevirapine for 4 weeks
D. AZT + stavudine + nevirapine for 4 weeks

(AIIMS May 2002)

A surgeon who has been *contaminated* with HIV infected blood should immediately clean the contaminated area by washing under running water and when the source patient comes form a high-risk group and HIV status is not known, it is important that **postexposure prophylaxis (PEP)** should be offered. PEP should be started *within* 1 hour of injury and consists of **zidovudine (AZT)** 250 mg 12 hourly, **lamivudine** 150 mg12 hourly and **indinavir** 800 mg 8 hourly; **for 1 month**. An HIV test should be repeated 12 weeks after the 'baseline' HIV test which is carried out immediately.

849. About medullary sponge kidney *false* is:

A. Autosomal dominant
B. Nephrocalcinosis
C. Normal serum calcium
D. Nephrotic syndrome

(PGI May 2001)

Although some cases of **medullary sponge kidney (MSK)** have *apparent* autosomal dominant inheritance, most are sporadic. The pathologic lesion is cystic dilation of the inner medullary and papillary collecting ducts (CDs), with collecting diameters ranging from 1 to 5 mm. Bilateral renal involvement is present in 70% of cases. Stones are frequently found in the dilated collecting ducts. Patients generally present in the 3rd or 4th decade with kidney stones, infection, or recurrent hematuria. There is normocalcemic hypercalciuria and mildly diminished urine-concentrating ability. However, up to 10% of patients may develop advanced renal failure in the long-term.

850. *Left* sided pleural effusion is seen in:

A. Pancreatitis **B.** CHF
C. Both **D.** None *(PGI May 2001)*

- Congestive heart failure (CHF) is the *most common* cause of pleural effusion. Between 58 and 72% of patients with CHF can have pleural effusions larger than 250 ml; 88% have bilateral effusions, 8% have unilateral right-sided effusion, and 4% have unilateral left-sided effusion.
- Corroborative findings on CXR in chronic pancreatitis include elevation of the left hemidiaphragm, linear at-electasis in the lower lobes, and the presence of a left-sided pleural effusion.

851. Hypocomplementemia is found in:

A. Poststreptococcal glomerulonephritis
B. MCD
C. Both
D. None *(PGI May 2001)*

Serum C3 levels and CH_{50} are *depressed* within 2 weeks in about 90% of cases of poststreptococcal glomerulo-nephritis. Complement levels usually return to normal within 6 to 8 weeks.

852. Rubella in fetus is diagnosed by:

A. IgG antibody in mother
B. IgM antibody in mother
C. IgA antibody in fetus
D. IgM antibody in fetus *(AIIMS May 2002)*

Rubella can cause severe outcomes in the fetus, including fetal death and premature delivery, if the mother is infected during *early* pregnancy. A variety of congenital defects are caused by rubella, viz. cataracts, cardiac abnormalities, deafness, and mental retardation. Fetal abnormalities are greatest when maternal rubella occurs during the 1st trimester, with 80% of children affected; the percentage falls to about 25% when infection occurs at the end of the 2nd trimester. Congenital infection can be diagnosed *prenatally* by detecting rubella **IgM antibody** in **fetal blood** obtained under USG guidance.

853. A pregnant lady is detected to be HBsAg positive at 22 weeks of pregnancy. The treatment of the baby includes:

A. HBV vaccination
B. HBV vaccination + HBV immunoglobulin
C. Immunoglobulin alone
D. Immunoglobulins followed by vaccine after 1 month if HBsAg negative *(AIIMS May 2002)*

Newborn of HBsAg positive mother should be managed with hepatitis B active and passive immunization. The **1st immunization and HBIG** (0.5ml) should be given **within 1st 12 hours of life** and the vaccine should be repeated at the age of 1 and 6 months.

854. Danazol is given in the treatment of:

A. Cyclical mastalgia
B. Non-cyclical mastalgia
C. Mastitis
D. Fibrocystic breast disease *(AIIMS May 2002)*

Indications of Danazol

- Endometriosis
- Menorrhagia
- Gynecomastia
- Fibrocystic breast disease
- Precocious puberty
- *Prophylactic* treatment of hereditary angioedema

855. A newborn baby is affected from encephalitis with skin lesion. The agent is likely to be:

A. HSV-1 **B.** HSV-2
C. Japanese encephalitis B **D.** Meningococci *(AIIMS May 2002)*

Herpes simplex viruses (HSV-1, HSV-2; *Herpesvirus hominis*) cause a variety of infections involving mucocutaneous surfaces, the central nervous system and occasionally visceral organs. **HSV-2 is the usual cause of meningo-encephalitis in newborns** while HSV-1 is common in older patients.

856. *Not* seen in Goodpasture's syndrome:

A. Diffuse alveolar involvement **B.** Anti-GBM antibody
C. Hemorrhage **D.** Crescentic glomerulonephritis *(PGI 1999)*

The clinical complex of **anti-GBM nephritis** and **pulmonary hemorrhage** is known as **Goodpasture's syndrome.** Renal biopsy is the 'gold standard' for diagnosis of anti-GBM nephritis. The *typical* morphologic pattern on light microscopy is diffuse proliferative glomerulonephritis, with focal necrotizing lesions and crescents in more than 50% of glomeruli (**crescentic glomerulonephritis**).

857. *Apart from* hereditary spherocytosis, spherocytes are seen in:

A. Immune hemolytic anemia **B.** PNH
C. Thalassemia **D.** Iron deficiency *(PGI 1999)*

Autoimmune acquired hemolytic anemia (AIHA) is the term used to describe a group of hemolytic anemias which result from the development of antibodies directed against antigens present on the surface of patients own RBCs. The antibodies are generally of IgG class or less frequently of IgM or IgA class. The typical blood picture is one with anemia, reticulocytosis and **spherocytosis**.

858. Rheumatoid factor is:

A. IgE against Fc of IgG **B.** IgM against Fc of IgG
C. IgG against Fc of IgM **D.** IgA against Fc of IgM *(PGI 1999)*

859. Rheumatoid factor in rheumatoid arthritis is important because:

A. RA factor is associated with bad prognosis
B. Absent RA factor rules out the diagnosis of rheumatoid arthritis
C. It is very common in childhood rheumatoid arthritis
D. It correlates with disease activity very well *(AI 2002)*

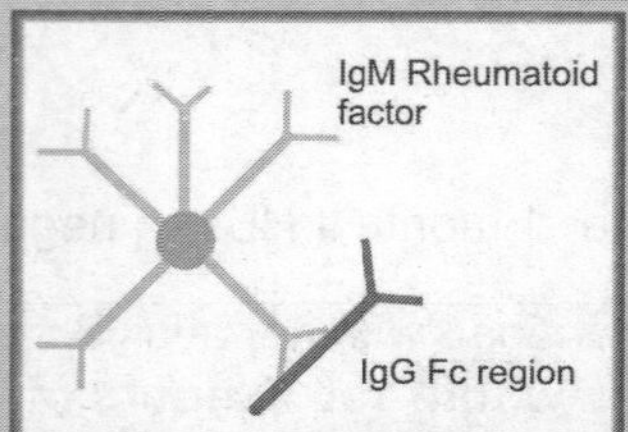

Most assays of **rheumatoid factor** detect an **IgM antibody that is directed against the Fc portion of IgG**. ELISA testing is capable of detecting other classes of rheumatoid factors (IgG, IgA) but these are not widely used clinically. Rheumatoid factor is *neither* sensitive *nor* specific enough to rule in or out rheumatoid arthritis. The rheumatoid factor is present in 70-80% of patients who have RA. This means that 20-30% of patients with RA are sero*negative* for rheumatoid factor. It is most useful as a 'prognostic' indicator in patients with RA. **People with RA who are rheumatoid factor positive typically have a more 'aggressive' disease.** It is also useful in confirming one's clinical impression that a polyarthritis that looks like RA is even more likely to be RA.

Rheumatological diseases	• Rheumatoid arthritis • SLE • Sjögren's syndrome • Mixed connective tissue disease • Myositis • Cryoglobulinemia
Infectious diseases	• SBE • Tuberculosis • Syphilis • Chronic hepatitis — especially hepatitis C • Leprosy • Kala-azar
Other	• Normal aging individuals • Idiopathic pulmonary fibrosis • Cirrhosis • Sarcoidosis • Waldenstrom's macroglobulinemia

860. *Not* a cause of cor pulmonale:

A. Chronic bronchitis **B.** Emphysema
C. Lung abscess **D.** Chronic asthma *(KARNATAKA 2000)*

Some Causes of Cor Pulmonale

Obstructive lung disease (OLD)	**Restrictive lung disease (RLD)**
• Chronic bronchitis • Emphysema • Chronic asthma **Secondary to pulmonary vascular disease** • Repeated pulmonary emboli • Pulmonary vasculitis • Congenital heart disease with left-to-right shunting (ASD, VSD, PDA) • Pulmonary venoocclusive disease	• Interstitial fibrosis • Lung resection • Obesity • Myxedema • Muscle weakness • Kyphoscoliosis • Upper airway obstruction • Diminished respiratory drive • Vasoconstriction secondary to high altitude

861. In herpes simplex encephalitis the CT and EEG findings are confined to which of the following lobe:

A. Occipital **B.** Temporal
C. Frontal **D.** parietal *(KARNATAKA 2000)*

There is a significant mortality from herpes simplex encephalitis, which is the *most common* form of sporadic encephalitis in the USA. **Temporal lobe involvement is *most common***, though frontal and parietal lobe infection occurs. In the early stages CT is less sensitive (79%) than radionuclide imaging (90%).

862. *Most common* cause of spontaneous pneumothorax is:

A. Rupture of sub-pleural bleb **B.** Tuberculosis
C. Trauma **D.** Asthma

863. Spontaneous pneumothorax is *not* common in:

A. Radiation pneumonitis
B. Cryptogenic fibrosing alveolitis
C. Histiocytosis
D. Lymphangioleiomyomatosis *(KARNATAKA 2000)*

Spontaneous pneumothorax has a predisposition for otherwise healthy men during the 3rd or 4th decade of life. **It is *most frequent* due to an apical bleb** that is a gas pocket within the visceral pleura; it forms as a result of rupture and centrifugal dissection of air from perforated subpleural alveoli. Chronic obstructive pulmonary disease (COPD) accounts for a 2nd peak in the incidence of spontaneous pneumothorax in the 6th and 7th decades. Recurrent pneumothorax can occur with chronic infiltrative lung disease, including idiopathic pulmonary fibrosis, sarcoidosis, **eosinophilic granuloma**, **lymphangioleiomyomatosis**, **radiation pneumonitis,** silicosis, and tuberous sclerosis.

864. Primary spontaneous pneumothorax is often associated with:

A. Smoking
B. Female sex
C. Exercise
D. Short stature *(PGI May 2001)*

Primary spontaneous pneumothoraces are generally due to rupture of apical pleural blebs, small cystic spaces that lie within or immediately under the visceral pleura. **Primary spontaneous pneumothoraces occur almost exclusively in smokers**, suggesting that the patients indeed do have subclinical lung disease.

865. Spontaneous pneumothorax is *not* seen in:

A. Positive end pressure ventilation
B. Bronchopulmonary aspergillosis
C. Eosinophilic granuloma
D. Marfan's syndrome *(AI 1991)*

866. Pneumothorax is *not* a feature of:

A. Bronchopulmonary aspergillosis
B. Assisted ventilation
C. Eosinophilic granuloma
D. Marfan's syndrome *(AIIMS 1994)*

Spontaneous pneumothorax has been seen in the wake of infection pulmonary infarcts, lung abscesses, and septic emboli. Pneumothorax can complicate **Marfan's syndrome**. Pneumothorax as a manifestation of barotrauma is a complication of **mechanical ventilation** in the intubated patient and occurs in 15 to 20%. In **eosinophilic granuloma** of the lung, a spontaneous pneumothorax can ensue in 15 to 50% of affected patients.

867. Following infection associated with AIDS can cause retinal involvement *except*:

A. Varicella-zoster virus
B. HSV
C. HPV
D. CMV *(KARNATAKA 2000)*

In HIV patients both **herpes simplex virus** and **varicella-zoster virus** *rarely* cause a widespread, bilateral necrotizing retinitis known as the *acute retinal necrosis syndrome*. This syndrome, in contrast to **cytomegalovirus** retinitis, is associated with pain, keratitis, and iritis.

868. *False* regarding hypokalemic periodic paralysis is:

A. *Sodium* channel defect
B. Affects proximal limb muscles more
C. Decrease serum K^+ level
D. Autosomal dominant *(KARNATAKA 2000)*

Hypokalemic periodic paralysis causes episodic weakness, which affects proximal limb muscles more than distal ones. Rarely ocular, bulbar, or respiratory muscles are affected. Respiratory muscle weakness may lead to death. *Diagnosis* is confirmed by demonstrating a **low serum K^+ level** during a paralytic attack and by excluding secondary causes of hypokalemia. The molecular defect is in the **calcium channel**. It is transmitted in a dominant manner.

869. Thrombin time is prolonged in which of the following:

A. ITP
B. Factor II deficiency
C. Dysfibrinogenemia
D. von Willebrand's disease *(KARNATAKA 2000)*

Dysfibrinogenemias are almost always inherited as autosomal dominant traits. Patients with dysfibrinogenemia have a slightly prolonged PT and PTT, a **prolonged thrombin time**.

870. Serum CPK levels are *low* in myopathy associated with which of the following:

A. Hypoparathyroidism
B. Hyperparathyroidism
C. Hypothyroidism
D. Hyperthyroidism *(KARNATAKA 2000)*

Thyrotoxic patients commonly have proximal muscle weakness and atrophy. Other neuromuscular disorders associated with hyperthyroidism are periodic paralysis, myasthenia gravis, and a progressive ocular myopathy associated with proptosis (Graves' ophthalmopathy). **Serum creatine phosphokinase (CPK) levels are low in thyrotoxic myopathy.**

871. Example of a *single* gene disorder is:

A. Hypertension
B. Diabetes mellitus
C. Glycogen storage disease
D. Marfan's syndrome

(KERALA 1994)

Single gene disorders are those disorders in which 1 gene plays a predominant role in determining disease. Common examples are as under:

- Neurofibromatosis
- Familial hypercholesterolemia
- Myotonic dystrophy
- Familial polyposis of the colon
- Adult polycystic kidney disease
- Globin disorders
- Marfan's syndrome
- Osteogenesis imperfecta
- Achondroplasia
- Huntington's disease
- Cystic fibrosis

872. Dominant trait express in:

A. Males only
B. Both homozygous and heterozygous states
C. Heterozygous state
D. Homozygous state

(KERALA 1994)

- The life providing material in the nucleus of every cell is **deoxyribonucleic acid** (DNA). Each of the 46 chromosomes in the human cell is made up of **a single molecule of DNA.** *DNA is a double stranded chain* along which thousands of segments are defined and demarcated as **genes**. Genes are the basic unit of inherited biological information and each gene codes for the synthesis of a specific protein. Each gene occurs at a specific point known as **locus** on the chromosome. A set of genes is known as **genome**. In a pair of chromosomes there are 2 forms known as **alleles** of each gene. Full genetic make up of an individual is known as **genotype** and a finished person (a product of genotype and environmental factors) is known as **phenotype**.
- Monogenic disorders ordinarily exhibit 1 of 3 patterns of inheritance viz. autosomal dominant, autosomal recessive and X-linked. The overall frequency of monogenic disorders is approximately 10 per 1000 live births, comprising about 7 in 1000 dominant, about 2.5 in 1000 recessive, and about 0.4 in 1000 X-linked conditions (*except* color blindness).
- The terms *dominant* and *recessive* refer to the clinical phenotype associated with a particular allele.
- Dominant means a trait or characteristic that is expressed in the offspring although it is carried on *only* 1 of the homologous chromosomes.

873. Waddling gait is most frequently seen in:

A. Cushing disease
B. Common peroneal nerve injury
C. Bilateral dislocation of hip
D. Myopathy

(TN 1995)

Waddling gait results from *proximal lower limb weakness*, **most often from myopathy** but infrequently from neuromuscular junction disease or a proximal symmetric spinal muscular atrophy.

874. Decreased melanin pigmentation is seen in:

A. Whipple's disease
B. PKU
C. Polyostotic fibrous dysplasia
D. None of the above

(PGI 1993)

Phenylalanine is a competitive inhibitor of tyrosinase which is a key enzyme in the pathway of melanin synthesis. In PKU this block and reduced availability of the melanin precursor tyrosine, accounts for the hypopigmentation of hair and skin.

875. Gait in Parkinsonism is:

A. Dancing gait
B. High stepping gait
C. Festinate gait
D. Ataxic gait

(KERALA 1994)

In patients of **Parkinsonism** walking is often difficult to 'initiate'. They walk with small, shuffling steps, have no arm-swing, are unsteady and may have difficulty in stopping. Some patients walk with a **festinating gait** (at an increasing speed to prevent themselves from falling because of their abnormal center of gravity).

876. The defect in thrombasthenia is in:

A. Platelet contraction **B.** ADP secretion
C. Platelet aggregation **D.** Platelet adhesion *(KARNATAKA 1994)*

Platelets of patients with Glanzmann's disease or **thrombasthenia** are deficient in or have a defect in the glycoprotein IIb-IIIa complex. Their platelets do not bind fibrinogen and **cannot form aggregates**.

877. Edema is a feature of:

A. Vitamin B_{12} deficiency **B.** Protein deficiency
C. Cushing syndrome **D.** Hyperthyroidism *(KERALA 1994)*

Edema is defined as a clinically apparent increase in the interstitial fluid volume, which may expand by several liters before the anomaly is obvious. The colloid oncotic pressure of the plasma may be reduced resulting in edema, due to any factor that may induce **severe hypoalbuminemia** (malnutrition, liver disease, loss of protein into the urine or into the GIT, or a severe catabolic state).

878. *Not* included in the differential diagnosis of chylous ascites:

A. CHF **B.** Tuberculosis
C. Filariasis **D.** Nephrotic syndrome *(KERALA 1994)*

Chylous ascites is a term used for a turbid, milky, or creamy peritoneal fluid due to the presence of thoracic or intestinal lymph. Chylous ascites is *most often* the result of lymphatic obstruction from trauma, tumor, **nephrotic syndrome**, **tuberculosis**, **filariasis**, or congenital abnormalities.

879. Pleural calcification is *commonly* seen in:

A. Bronchogenic carcinoma **B.** Hyperparathyroidism
C. Asbestosis **D.** Silicosis *(DELHI 1996)*

Although **calcifications within plaques associated with the pneumoconiosis are usually due to asbestos dust inhalation**, other rare and doubtful causes of localized pleural calcifications due to dust inhalation have been reported, such as with calcimine, bakelite, and muscovite mica. Old tuberculosis or empyema and hemothorax can result in calcifications. *Rare* causes of localized pleural calcification that may simulate plaques include radiation, mineral oil aspiration, pulmonary infarction, pancreatitis, chronic renal failure, and scleroderma (both with secondary hyperparathyroidism). In general, it is best to consider calcified plaques as the result of asbestos fiber inhalation *until proven otherwise*.

880. *Investigation of choice* to diagnose epilepsy is:

A. EEG **B.** Angiogram
C. CT scan **D.** MRI *(KERALA 1994)*

All patients who have a possible seizure disorder should be evaluated with an EEG as soon as possible. The EEG may help to establish the diagnosis of epilepsy, classify the seizure type, and provide proof for the existence of a particular epilepsy syndrome.

881. *Not* an indication for bone marrow transplant:

A. Myelofibrosis **B.** Hypoplastic anemia
C. CML **D.** Thalassemia major *(KARNATAKA 1995)*

882. Bone marrow transplant is the *indicated* in:

A. Aplastic anemia **B.** Myelodysplastic syndrome
C. Acute leukemia **D.** All of the above

Indications of Bone Marrow Transplant

Malignant conditions	Nonmalignant conditions
• **Acute leukemia** (ALL and AML)	• **Aplastic anemia**
• **CML**	• Pure red cell aplasia
• **Myelodysplastic syndrome**	• Paroxysmal nocturnal hemoglobinuria
• Lymphoma	• Fanconi's anemia
• Testicular cancer	• Sickle cell anemia
• Ovarian cancer	• **Thalassemia**
• Neuroblastoma	• Severe combined immunodeficiency
• Peripheral neuroepithelial tumors	• Leukocyte adhesion defects
• Wilms' tumor	• Glanzmann's thrombasthenia
• Hodgkin's disease	• Gaucher's disease
• Multiple myeloma	• Adrenoleukodystrophy
• Chronic lymphocytic leukemia	• Lesch-Nyhan syndrome
• **Myelofibrosis**	• Type IIa glycogen storage disease
• Breast cancer	• Osteopetrosis
• Ewing's sarcoma	• Radiation injury
	• Chronic granulomatous disease
	• Chédiak-Higashi syndrome
	• Hurler's syndrome
	• Hunter's syndrome
	• Metachromatic leukodystrophy

883. Senile plaques in brain are a feature of:

A. Multiple sclerosis **B.** Parkinsonism
C. Alzheimer's disease **D.** Motor neuron disease *(JIPMER 2000)*

The *most important* microscopic findings in **Alzheimer's disease** are neuritic **senile plaques** and neurofibrillary tangles. These 2 lesions accumulate in small numbers during normal aging of the brain but occur in quantitative excess in the dementia of Alzheimer's disease.

884. Downbeat nystagmus is characteristic of:

A. Cerebellar lesions **B.** Labyrinthine lesions
C. Posterior fossa lesions **D.** Vestibular lesions

Causes of Downbeat Nystagmus

- Lesions near the craniocervical junction
- Basilar invagination
- Chiari malformation
- Brainstem or cerebellar stroke
- Anticonvulsant intoxication
- Lithium toxicity
- Multiple sclerosis

885. Caplan's syndrome is seen in:

A. Rheumatoid arthritis
B. Pulmonary edema
C. COPD
D. Hypercalcemia *(KERALA 1994)*

886. Rheumatoid arthritis associated with pneumoconiosis is known as:

A. Middle lobe syndrome **B.** Black lung syndrome
C. Caplan's syndrome **D.** Hamman-Rich syndrome

In 1953 Caplan first described **rheumatoid nodules** in the lungs in coal miners, and the condition has been referred to as **Caplan's syndrome** or **rheumatoid pneumoconiosis**. Only patients with a classic appearance of Caplan's syndrome are found to have rheumatoid factor in their serum. The term *rheumatoid lung* is more accurate than Caplan's syndrome in describing rheumatoid nodular changes in the lung because they occur just as commonly in silicosis.

887. Generalized lymphadenopathy is seen in all *except*:
A. CLL
B. Tertiary syphilis
C. ALL
D. Infectious mononucleosis
(KARNATAKA 1994)

Generalized lymphadenopathy is often associated with *non*malignant disorders such as **infectious mononucleosis** (Epstein-Barr virus or cytomegalovirus), toxoplasmosis, AIDS, other viral infections, systemic lupus erythematosus, and mixed connective tissue disease. **Acute** and **chronic lymphocytic leukemias** and malignant lymphomas also produce generalized lymphadenopathy in adults.

888. Oral anti-diabetic *drug of choice* in renal failure is:
A. Metformin
B. Glipizide
C. Tolbutamide
D. Chlorpropamide
(KARNATAKA 1994)

In patients with **significant renal disease**, it is wise to use **tolbutamide** or tolazamide, because these agents are metabolized and inactivated *exclusively* by the liver.

889. Mode of action of atrial natriuretic peptide is:
A. Increasing blood volume
B. Decreasing cardiac output
C. Increasing venous pressure
D. Increasing renin secretion
(PGI 1993)

890. Atrial natriuretic peptide acts by:
A. Increasing renin secretion
B. Increasing venous pressure
C. Inhibiting sodium reabsorption in distal tubules
D. Increasing blood volume

Atrial natriuretic peptide is a peptide, which is *secreted by the atrial tissue of the heart* in response to an increase in blood pressure. It affects blood pressure, blood volume, and cardiac output. It increases the excretion of sodium and water in urine, thus **reducing** blood volume and blood pressure and **cardiac output**. It acts by **inhibiting sodium reabsorption in distal tubules**. These actions reduce the workload on the heart.

891. *Absolute* indication for hemodialysis is:
A. Hyperkalemia > 6.5 mEq/L
B. Pericarditis
C. GI bleeding
D. Convulsion
(DELHI 1993)

Indication for Hemodialysis or Peritoneal Dialysis

Absolute dialysis indications	Relative dialysis indications
• Uremic symptoms • Pericarditis	• Hypervolemia • Hyperkalemia or other electrolyte abnormalities • Metabolic acidosis

892. Uncinate fits are seen in tumors of ....lobe:
A. Occipital
B. Parietal
C. Temporal
D. Frontal
(SGPGI 1996)

Uncinate fit is an episodic attack characterized by olfactory and gustatory hallucinations, usually disagreeable and sometimes convulsions and temporary loss of senses of taste and smell. This is associated with lesions of the **uncinate gyrus of the brain**. Uncinate gyrus is a gyrus of the **temporal lobe of the brain** consisting of the recurved rostral portion of the hippocampal gyrus.

893. Best treatment modality for CML is:

A. Radiotherapy **B.** Allogeneic bone marrow transplantation
C. Hydroxyurea **D.** Interferon *(PGI 1998)*

The diagnosis of chronic myeloid leukemia is established by identifying cytogenetically or molecularly a clonal expansion of a hematopoietic stem cell possessing a reciprocal translocation between chromosomes 9 and 22. The disease is characterized by the inevitable transition from a chronic phase to an accelerated phase and on to 'blast crisis'. **Allogeneic bone marrow transplantation is the only curative therapy for CML** and, when feasible, is the treatment of *choice*.

894. Blast crisis in CML is *not* indicated by:

A. Bleeding tendencies **B.** *Sudden* enlargement of spleen
C. High fever **D.** Lymphadenopathy *(MP 1998)*

Blast crisis or 'blast transformation' may be suspected clinically because it is commonly associated with malaise, fatigue, anorexia, night sweats, bone pain and splenic discomfort. The patient may feel markedly unwell before any overt changes appear in the GBP or even bone marrow. The important physical signs are weight loss, pallor, **pyrexia**, sternal tenderness, **progressively increasing splenomegaly** and the appearance of **lymphadenopathy** which is *typically* absent in the chronic phase of CML. If the disease is unresponsive to treatment, **death usually results from hemorrhage or infection** or a combination of both. The *most common* change in the GBP is a rapidly rising WBC count, a falling hemoglobin level, development of thrombocytopenia and appearance of a large proportion of blast cells. The *spectrum* WBC precursors characteristic of chronic phase of disease is lost and a cell distribution typical of *acute* leukemias occur. In majority of cases the blast cells are of myeloid series but in 30% of cases they show lymphoblastic features. The bone marrow aspirate reveals up to 80% or more of blast cells.

895. In CML the *drug of choice* is:

A. Hydroxyurea **B.** 5 FU
C. Busulphan **D.** Chlorambucil *(AI 1995)*

Allogeneic bone marrow transplant is the only 'curative' therapy for CML and, *whenever feasible*, is the treatment of choice. **Hydroxyurea** (*ribonucleotide reductase* inhibitor) induces rapid disease control. Busulphan, an alkylating agent that acts on early progenitor cells, has a more prolonged effect but its use is not recommended because of its serious side effects.

896. Increased C peptide is seen in:

A. Hepatoma **B.** Insulinoma
C. Glucagonoma **D.** Gastrinoma *(AP 1997)*

Suppression of the release of endogenous insulin and **C peptide** during insulin infusion is *impaired* in persons with **insulinomas**.

897. Anterior uveitis and parotid enlargement is seen in:

A. Rheumatoid arthritis **B.** Sjögren's syndrome
C. Lupus erythematosus **D.** Sarcoidosis *(AP 1997)*

The *Heerfordt-Waldenstrom syndrome* describes individuals with fever, **parotid enlargement**, **anterior uveitis**, and facial nerve palsy and is a feature of **sarcoidosis**.

898. Pellagra like dermatitis is seen in:

A. Lymphoma **B.** Systemic lupus erythematosus
C. Dermatomyositis **D.** Carcinoid syndrome *(JIPMER 1995)*

Serotonin is the *most common* secretory 'product' of **carcinoid tumors**. Upto 50% of the dietary intake of tryptophan can be converted to serotonin by these cells, which may leave inadequate substrate for incorporation into proteins and conversion to niacin. Due to this, patients with widely metastatic carcinoid tumors may suffer symptoms of protein malnutrition or mild **pellagra**.

899. Part of heart *most commonly* affected in carcinoid syndrome is:

A. Inflow tract of right ventricle **B.** Outflow tract of right ventricle
C. Outflow tract of left ventricle **D.** Inflow tract of left ventricle

900. *Not* a recognized feature of carcinoid syndrome:

A. Increased urinary excretion of vanillylmandelic acid
B. Skin changes of pellagra
C. Bronchospasm
D. Flushing *(SGPGI 1996)*

Manifestations of the **carcinoid syndrome** include the triad of cutaneous flushing, diarrhea, and valvular heart disease and, less commonly, telangiectasias, wheezing, and paroxysmal hypotension. Endocardial fibrosis may cause valvular heart disease, usually affecting the **proximal side of the tricuspid** and pulmonary valves and leading to tricuspid insufficiency, pulmonary stenosis, and secondary right-sided heart failure.

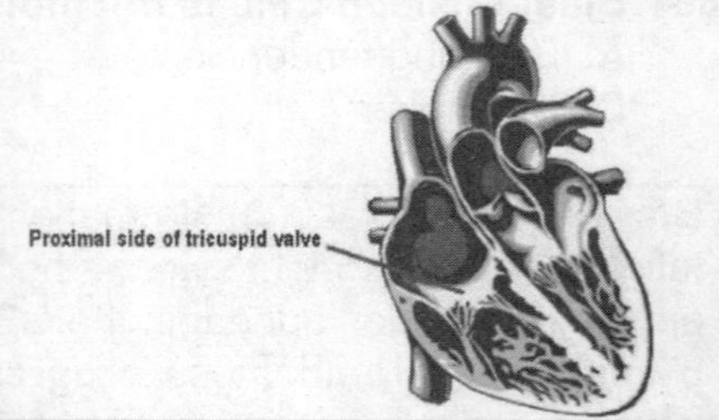

901. 'Giant cell' pneumonia is seen in:

A. Epstein-Barr virus **B.** Cytomegalovirus
C. Measles **D.** Varicella *(PGI 1998)*

Patients with defects in cell-mediated immunity (patients with congenital cellular immune defects or malignancy, recipients of immunosuppressive therapy, or persons infected with human immunodeficiency virus) are at risk for severe protracted and *fatal* **measles**. In these immunosuppressed patients, measles may *not* be accompanied by a rash. Complications are primary measles or **giant cell pneumonia**, progressive encephalitis, and in HIV-infected patients progression to AIDS.

902. Myoclonic jerk is typically seen in:

A. Tricyclic antidepressant poisoning **B.** BSE
C. SSPE **D.** Steele-Richardson syndrome *(PGI 1998)*

Subacute sclerosing pan encephalitis (SSPE) is a *rare* disease with nonspecific symptoms which give way to progressive intellectual deterioration, focal and/or generalized seizures, **myoclonus**, ataxia, and visual disturbances.

903. *Not* seen in histiocytosis X:

A. Langerhans' cells are *pathognomic* **B.** Letterer-Siwe disease
C. Hand-Schüller-Christian disease **D.** Eosinophilic granuloma *(PGI 1997)*

The term **histiocytosis "X"** implies to the condition which is caused by a reactive histiocytosis to an unknown infectious agent "X". 3 varieties have been described which share the common histological feature of an infiltrating histiocytosis but have widely varied clinical manifestations. The Langerhans' cell is considered today to be the main element in active lesions of histiocytosis X and its presence is *sine qua non* (absolute prerequisite) for the diagnosis of this disorder. It was, therefore, appropriate that the *Writing Group* of the 'Histiocyte Society' recently proposed that histiocytosis X be now referred to as **Langerhans' cell histiocytosis**.

• **Eosinophilic granuloma**	Older child with only 1 or more bone lesions.
• **Hand-Schüller-Christian disease**	Child with bone and soft tissue involvement.
• **Letterer-Siwe disease**	Infant and younger child with *only* soft tissue involvement.

Skeleton is the *most commonly* involved tissue in histiocytosis "X" and in a child over 5 years of age may be the only site of involvement. The **lesions** may be single or multiple and are **most commonly found in the skull**, long bones, spine, and pelvis. *Radiologically* the lesions appear as **"punched out"** areas. Cyclophosphamide, vinca alkaloids, methotrexate, 6 mercaptopurine, chlorambucil or prednisone may be used as single agents for patients with disseminated and progressive disease. For solitary bone lesions curettage may be sufficient.

904. The histologic 'hallmark' of Langerhans' cells granulomatosis is:
A. Dendritic cell processes
B. Giant mitochondria
C. Birbeck granules
D. Eosinophilic granules

In Langerhans' cell granulomatosis (eosinophilic granuloma or histiocytosis X) intra-cytoplasmic organelles known as X bodies or **Birbeck granules** are seen in electron microscopy.

905. Macrocytic anemia is seen in all *except*:
A. Thalassemia
B. Acute blood loss
C. Alcoholism
D. Aplastic anemia *(PGI 1997)*

Severe iron deficiency and the inherited defects in globin chain synthesis, the *thalassemias*, produce a moderate to marked *micro*cytic, hypochromic anemia.

906. Carey-Coombs' murmur is found in:
A. TAPVC
B. Tetralogy of Fallot
C. TR
D. Acute rheumatic fever *(PGI 1997)*

A soft mid-diastolic murmur may sometimes be heard in patients with **acute rheumatic fever (Carey-Coombs' murmur**). It is due to inflammation of the mitral valve cusps or excessive left atrial blood flow as a result of mitral regurgitation.

907. *Most common* cause of death in *adults* due to PDA is:
A. Rupture of the ductus
B. Aneurysmal dilatation
C. Infective endocarditis
D. Cardiac failure *(PGI 1997)*

The ***most important* causes of death in adults with patent ductus are cardiac failure** and infective endocarditis; occasionally severe pulmonary vascular obstruction may cause aneurysmal dilatation, calcification, and rupture of the ductus.

908. *Most common* cause of chronic recurrent diarrhea in HIV patient is:
A. *Campylobacter*
B. *Entamoeba histolytica*
C. *Cryptosporidium*
D. *Giardia lamblia* *(KERALA 1999)*

Cryptosporidia, microsporidia, and *Isospora belli* are the *most common* opportunistic protozoa that infect the GIT and cause diarrhea in HIV-infected patients.

909. *Not* used to treat raised ICT:
A. Tetracycline
B. Repeated lumber tapping
C. Corticosteroids
D. Diuretics *(KERALA 1999)*

The **normal intracranial pressure (ICP) is 10-15 mmHg** and it varies slightly with heart beat and respiration. ICP can be measured by an intraventricular catheter, a subdural or extradural transducer. All of them are inserted via a *burr hole*. Raised ICP may be due to *physiological* processes such as *coughing, sneezing, and straining, etc.* Or it may be due to *pathological processes* such as *craniostenosis, space occupying lesions (SOL) such as hematoma, abscess or neoplasm, hydrocephalus, venous obstruction, arterial dilatation (high* $PaCO_2$*), cerebral edema and head down position*. Raised ICP manifests with headache, vomiting, **drowsiness**, **bradycardia**, **hypertension** and **papilledema**. *Neurogenic* pulmonary edema may occur. When the ICP equals arterial blood pressure the cerebral blood flow (CBF) stops. ICP may be *decreased* due to dehydration; blood loss and removal of SOL. Methods of reducing the ICP are as under:

- **Hyperventilation:** Is of value for at least 24 hours.
- **Diuretics:** Mannitol ($C_6H_{12}O_6$) is a hyperosmotic agent which is an isomer of *sorbitol*. **It is a hexahydric alcohol related to hexose sugars.** Dose is 0.5-1.5 gm/kg/dose intravenous over 10-20 minutes. A 20% solution is most commonly used. **It starts to lower the ICP in 5 minutes and the maximum affect is at 45 minutes. The affect lasts for 4-6 hours**. *It may precipitate CHF*. **It is often combined with a loop diuretic such as frusemide** (0.5-1 mg/kg/dose). Urea and oral glycerol are also effective.
- **Removal of CSF:** Up to 150 ml of CSF may be removed via a needle or catheter. Spinal drainage is useful for aneurysm surgery but may precipitate *tonsillar herniation* in the presence of SOL.
- **Steroids:** Dexamethasone (4 mg 6 hourly) gives a rapid *although temporary* clinical improvement by reducing the edema around tumors. It is of no value in head injury.
- **Hypothermia:** Reduces ICP and provide some protection against brain ischemia.
- **Lignocaine:** Causes cerebral vasoconstriction.
- **Control of arterial and venous pressure:** Hypotensive agents and head up tilt.

910. *Most common* cause of dementia in people more than 65 years of age is:

A. Turner syndrome **B.** Parkinson's disease
C. Alzheimer's disease **D.** Huntington's chorea *(KERALA 1999)*

Alzheimer's disease (AD) is the most common cause of dementia. About 10% of all persons over the age of 70 have significant memory loss, and more than 50% is the result of AD.

911. Holiday heart syndrome is commonly associated with:

A. PAT **B.** Ventricular premature complexes
C. Atrial premature complexes **D.** Atrial fibrillation *(KERALA 1999)*

Individuals who consume large quantities of alcohol over many years may develop a clinical picture similar to idiopathic dilated cardiomyopathy and **alcoholic cardiomyopathy** is the major form of secondary dilated cardiomyopathy. Key to the treatment of alcoholic cardiomyopathy is *total* and *permanent* abstinence. A second presentation of alcoholic cardiotoxicity is **holiday heart syndrome.** It appears after a drinking spree; **atrial fibrillation is seen most frequently**, followed by atrial flutter and ventricular premature depolarizations. Other patients develop left ventricular hypertrophy, perhaps related to concomitant systemic hypertension; they may present with symptoms of pulmonary congestion due to diminished compliance of the left ventricle.

912. Which is *not true* regarding alcoholic cardiomyopathy:

A. Low cardiac output **B.** Ventricular arrhythmias
C. Systemic vasodilatation **D.** Atrial fibrillation

Alcoholic Cardiomyopathy

- Atrial fibrillation
- Ventricular premature depolarizations
- Low cardiac output
- Atrial flutter
- Left ventricular hypertrophy
- Pulmonary edema

913. Extradural hemorrhage is due to rupture of which of the following artery:

A. Middle meningeal
B. Anterior meningeal
C. Posterior meningeal
D. Middle cerebral

(AIIMS 1998, UP 2000)

The *classical* syndrome of **acute extradural hemorrhage** results from injury to the anterior and posterior branches of **middle meningeal artery**.

914. In hemoptysis, blood usually comes from:

A. Pulmonary arteries
B. Pulmonary veins
C. Bronchial arteries
D. Bronchial veins

(KERALA 1995)

The **bronchial arteries** originate either from the aorta or from intercostal arteries and are the **source of bleeding** in bronchitis or bronchiectasis or with endobronchial tumors.

915. *Not* seen in emphysema:

A. Damage to alveoli
B. Rhonchi
C. Decreased vital capacity
D. Hyperinflation

(KERALA 1995)

Emphysema is defined as the permanent, abnormal distention of the air spaces distal to the terminal bronchiole with **destruction of alveolar septa**. Patients often give a long history of exertional dyspnea with minimal cough that is productive of only small amounts of mucoid sputum. The total lung capacity and residual volume are invariably increased, the **vital capacity is low**, and the maximal expiratory flow rates are diminished. On CXR the diaphragms are low and flattened the bronchovascular shadows do not extend to the periphery of the lung. The cardiac shadow is lengthened and narrowed. These findings in association with a large retrosternal translucency on lateral CXR are interpreted as **hyperinflation**, which correlates well with increases in total lung capacity and loss of elastic recoil.

916. *Best* method for decreasing blood cholesterol level is:

A. High fiber diet with low cholesterol
B. Unsaturated fatty acid with high fiber diet and low cholesterol diet
C. High fiber diet with saturated fatty acids and low cholesterol diet
D. Low fiber diet with restricted dietary cholesterol

(KERALA 1995)

Individuals with hyperlipidemia should be encouraged to eat a diet **lower** in *cholesterol* and *saturated fat*.

917. Diabetes mellitus is *not* seen in:

A. Myotonic dystrophy
B. Ataxia telangiectasia
C. Noonan syndrome
D. Acromegaly

(JIPMER 1995)

Secondary Forms of Diabetes

- Chronic pancreatitis in alcoholics
- Pheochromocytoma
- **Acromegaly**
- Administration of steroid hormones
- Cushing's syndrome
- Severe burns
- Acute myocardial infarctions
- Lipodystrophies
- **Myotonic dystrophy**
- **Ataxia telangiectasia**

918. Lasègue's sign is seen in:

A. Sciatica
B. Myasthenia gravis
C. Intracranial lesions
D. Transaction of spinal cord

Lasègue's sign consists of pain and discomfort in the back when the fully extended leg of the supine patient is gently raised. This is seen in **sciatica**.

919. Neuropathic joint is *not* seen in:

A. Fredrick's ataxia
B. Syringomyelia
C. Tabes dorsalis
D. Diabetes mellitus

(KERALA 1994)

920. Neuropathic joints are *not* seen in:

A. Tabes dorsalis
B. Leprosy
C. Diabetes mellitus
D. Myopathy

(KERALA 1990)

Disorders Associated with Neuropathic Joint Disease

- Diabetes mellitus
- Tabes dorsalis
- Leprosy
- Meningomyelocele
- Syringomyelia
- Amyloidosis
- Congenital indifference to pain

921. *True* regarding Korsakoff's psychosis is:

A. Anterograde amnesia
B. Delirium
C. Coarse tremor
D. Disorientation

(PGI 1998)

Korsakoff's syndrome presents with profound **anterograde amnesia,** i.e. inability to learn new material; and a milder retrograde amnesia, along with impairment in visuospatial, abstract, and conceptual reasoning but with a normal intelligence quotient.

922. Botulinum toxin is used in the treatment of:

A. Trigeminal neuralgia
B. Torticollis
C. Focal dystonia
D. Amyotrophic lateral sclerosis

(PGI 1998)

Writer's cramp is a task-specific **focal dystonia** in which abnormal posturing of the hand and forearm occurs when the hand is used for writing. Other task-specific dystonias include *violinist's cramp*, *barber's cramp*, and *telegrapher's cramp*, in each of which dystonic posturing occurs when the hand is used for a skilled, *occupationally* related function. Drug treatment is usually unsatisfactory. Injections of **botulinum toxin** into the involved muscles are sometimes helpful, but function usually remains impaired.

923. *Pneumocystis carinii* pneumonia is:

A. Interstitial
B. Hemorrhagic
C. Eosinophilic
D. Alveolar pneumonia

(PGI 1998)

***Pneumocystis carinii* pneumonia** (PCP) occurs in premature, malnourished infants; children with primary immunodeficiency diseases; patients receiving immunosuppressive therapy (glucocorticoids) for cancer, organ transplantation, and other disorders; and patients of AIDS. The frequency of pneumocystosis among patients infected with human immunodeficiency virus far exceeds that among other immunocompromised hosts. On microscopic examination of pulmonary sections stained with H and E, the alveoli are filled with a typical foamy, vacuolated exudate. Severe disease may include **interstitial edema**, fibrosis, and hyaline membrane formation.

924. *Not* seen in diphtheria:

A. Polyneuropathy
B. Endotoxemia
C. Cardiomyopathy
D. Pseudomembrane formation

(JIPMER 1998)

Diphtheria is a *localized* infection of mucous membranes or skin caused by *Corynebacterium diphtheriae*. A characteristic **pseudomembrane** may be present at the site of infection and some strains of *Corynebacterium diphtheriae* produce diphtheria toxin (DT). DT is a protein that can cause **myocarditis**, **polyneuritis**, and other systemic toxic effects.

925. Wenckebach's phenomenon is defined as:

A. Shortened ST interval
B. Irregular heart rate and premature ventricular beats
C. Slurred QRS complex
D. Progressive lengthening of PR interval till a beat is dropped

(DELHI 1996)

Wenckebach's period or **Wenckebach's phenomenon** is a form of incomplete heart block in which there is **progressive lengthening of the P-R interval until there is no ventricular response**; and then the cycle of increasing P-R intervals begins again.

926. ***False*** **regarding** ***Klebsiella pneumoniae*****:**

A. It is also known as Friedlander's pneumonia
B. Ampicillin is the drug of choice
C. Bulging fissure sign
D. Upper lobe involvement *(KARNATAKA 1996)*

927. Which of the following is ***false*** **regarding** ***Klebsiella pneumoniae*****:**

A. Chocolate colored sputum
B. Seen in alcoholics
C. Seen in older age group
D. Penicillin is the drug of choice

Klebsiella pneumoniae or **Friedländer's pneumonia** is a cause of lobar pneumonia found typically in **alcoholic men over 40 years** of age with underlying diseases such as diabetes mellitus and COPD. Other common features are:

- High mortality
- Upper lobe more frequently involved
- Expectoration of large amount of **chocolate colored sputum**
- **Gentamicin** along with a **third generation cephalosporin** (ceftazidime) is the drug of choice.

928. Bulging fissure sign in X-ray is seen in infection with:

A. Loeffler's bacillus
B. *Klebsiella pneumoniae*
C. *Staphylococcus aureus*
D. *Haemophilus influenzae* *(PGI 1999)*

Bulging fissure sign is seen in infection with ***Klebsiella pneumoniae***

929. Which of the following drug causes diarrhea:

A. Methyldopa
B. Purgatives
C. Cocaine
D. All of the above

Drug Causing Diarrhea

- Broad spectrum antibiotics
- Clindamycin
- Cocaine
- Colchicine
- Digitalis
- Guanethidine
- Lactose excipients
- Lincomycin
- Magnesium in antacids
- Methyldopa
- Misoprostol
- Oral contraceptives
- Purgatives
- Reserpine
- Ticlopidine

930. ***True*** **about sickle cell anemia is:**

A. In β chain valine is present in place of glutamic acid as 6th amino acid
B. In β chain glutamic acid is present in place valine of as 6th amino acid
C. In α chain valine is present in place of glutamic acid as 6th amino acid
D. In α chain glutamic acid is present in place of valine as 6th amino acid

Sickle cell anemia is characterized by formation of hemoglobin S. In this hemoglobin **valine is present in place of glutamic acid as the 6th amino acid in the β globin chain.**

Mnemonic: **G**lutamic acid **G**oes when **V**aline **V**isits.

SOME ABNORMAL HEMOGLOBINS

Name	Mutation	Main clinical features
Sickle or S	$\beta^{6Glu \rightarrow Val}$	Anemia, ischemic infarcts
C	$\beta^{6Glu \rightarrow Lys}$	Mild anemia
E	$\beta^{26Glu \rightarrow Lys}$	Microcytic anemia, splenomegaly
Köln	$\beta^{98Val \rightarrow Met}$	Hemolytic anemia or Heinz bodies
Yakima	$\beta^{99Asp \rightarrow His}$	Polycythemia
Kansas	$\beta^{102Asn \rightarrow Lys}$	Mild anemia

931. *Not* a good risk factor in multiple myeloma:

A. IgG spike < 5 gm/dL
B. Hematocrit > 40%
C. Hypocalcemia
D. Azotemia *(PGI 1999)*

Serum creatinine level	Stage	Median survival in months
A < 2 mg/dL	IA	61
B > 2 mg/dL	IIA,B	55
	IIIA	30
	IIIB	15

932. Pigment gallstones are *not* seen in:

A. Hemolytic anemia
B. TPN
C. *Clonorchis* infestation
D. Alcoholic cirrhosis *(PGI 1999)*

In USA, chronic hemolytic states (with increased conjugated bilirubin in bile) or alcoholic liver disease are associated with an increased incidence of pigment stones. Pigment stone formation is especially prominent in Asians and is often associated with infections in the biliary tree. **Risk factors for pigment stones are as under:**

- Demographic/genetic factors: Asia, rural setting
- Chronic hemolysis
- Alcoholic cirrhosis
- Chronic biliary tract infection, *parasite* infestation
- Increasing age

933. In congenital erythropoietic porphyria the enzyme deficient is:

A. UPG decarboxylase
B. PBG deaminase
C. Uroporphyrinogen III synthase
D. Ferrochelatase *(PGI 1999)*

934. *False* regarding congenital erythropoietic porphyria:

A. Autosomal recessive
B. BMT is the treatment of choice
C. Due to deficiency of URO synthase
D. Hypertrichosis of face and extremities are common *(SGPGI 1996))*

Congenital erythropoietic porphyria (*Gunther's disease*) is an autosomal recessive condition due to deficiency of uroporphyrinogen III synthase activity and is associated with hemolytic anemia and cutaneous lesions. Skin thickening, focal hypo- and hyperpigmentation, and hypertrichosis of the face and extremities are characteristic. The transfusion of sufficient blood to suppress erythropoiesis is effective but results in iron overload. **Bone marrow transplantation was tried in 1 patient, who died from transplant complications.**

935. Differential cyanosis is seen in:

A. Tetralogy of Fallot
B. TGA
C. PDA
D. TAPVC

(PGI 1999)

In **PDA** with severe pulmonary vascular disease there is reversal of flow through the ductus, unoxygenated blood is shunted to the descending aorta, and the toes (*but not the fingers*) which become cyanotic and clubbed (**differential cyanosis**).

936. Pituitary tumor which is *most* responsive to 'medical' therapy is:

A. Thyrotropin secreting tumors
B. Prolactinoma
C. ACTH secreting tumor
D. Growth hormone secreting tumor

(SGPGI 1999)

Prolactinomas are the most common *functional* pituitary adenomas. Microprolactinomas are more common than macroprolactinomas, and 90% of patients with microprolactinomas are women while 60% of patients with macroprolactinomas are men. Irregular menses, amenorrhea, and galactorrhea are likely to result in early diagnosis, and this fact may partially explain the predominance of microadenomas in women. **The treatment of choice is medical therapy.** Dopamine agonist drugs lower prolactin concentrations in almost all hyperprolactinemic patients. **Bromocriptine**, an ergot derivative with dopamine agonist actions, is the only effective prolactin lowering agent approved for this purpose in the USA.

937. HTLV-I is associated with:

A. Huntington's chorea
B. Hodgkin's lymphoma
C. AIDS
D. Tropical spastic paraparesis

(SGPGI 1999)

HTLV-I is the cause of at least 2 important diseases viz. **adult T cell leukemia/lymphoma** and **tropical spastic paraparesis**, also called HTLV-I-associated myelopathy (HAM).

938. SLE like syndrome is *not* caused by:

A. Levamisole
B. Oral contraceptives
C. D-penicillamine
D. Methyldopa

(SGPGI 1999)

939. SLE like syndrome may be caused by:

A. Practolol
B. Metoprolol
C. Alprenolol
D. Timolol

Some Drugs Causing Systemic Lupus Erythematosus

- Procainamide
- Hydralazine
- Isoniazid
- Chlorpromazine
- D-penicillamine
- Ethosuximide
- Practolol
- Methyldopa
- Quinidine
- Interferon α
- Hydantoin
- Oral contraceptives

940. *Not* seen in Waldenstrom's macroglobulinemia:

A. IgM spike on SPE
B. Hyperviscosity
C. Hypercalcemia
D. Positive Coombs' test

(PGI 1999)

A malignancy of lymphoplasmacytoid cells which secreted **IgM** was described by Waldenstrom in 1948. Contrary to myeloma, the disease was associated with lymphadenopathy and hepatosplenomegaly, but the major clinical manifestation was the **hyperviscosity syndrome**. Like myeloma, the disease involves the bone marrow, but unlike myeloma, **it does not cause bone lesions or hypercalcemia.** Patients may have a normocytic, normochromic anemia, but rouleaux formation and a positive Coombs' test are much more common than in myeloma.

941. Erythema chronicum migrans is seen in:

A. Glucagonoma **B.** Lyme disease

C. Diabetes mellitus **D.** Bronchus carcinoma *(PGI 1998)*

Erythema chronicum migrans is the rash of Lyme disease and it typically manifests as singular or multiple annular plaques.

942. All of the following drugs precipitate hypertensive crisis in pheochromocytoma *except*:

A. Opiates **B.** Saralasin

C. Phenoxybenzamine **D.** Methyldopa *(AIIMS May 2002)*

Pheochromocytoma occurs at all ages but is *most common* in young to midadult life. Most patients come to attention as a result of **hypertensive crisis**, paroxysmal symptoms suggestive of seizure disorder or anxiety attacks, or hypertension that responds poorly to conventional treatment. Hypertension is the most common manifestation.

Opiates	Histamine
Saralasin	Adrenocorticotropin
Glucagon	Methyldopa
Tricyclic antidepressants	Guanethidine

943. *Drug of choice* for very high circulatory catecholamine in pheochromocytoma is:

A. Propranolol **B.** Doxazosin

C. Prazosin **D.** Phenoxybenzamine *(KARNATAKA 2000)*

The induction of stable α adrenergic blockade is the basis of preoperative management of pheochromocytoma and provides the foundation for successful surgical treatment. Once the diagnosis is established, the patient should be placed on **phenoxybenzamine** to induce a long-lived, noncompetitive α receptor blockade.

944. Drug *not* used alone in pheochromocytoma is:

A. Metyrosine **B.** Atenolol

C. Calcium channel blockers **D.** Sodium nitroprusside *(AIIMS 1999)*

Nitroprusside, calcium channel blocking agents, and *maybe* ACE inhibitors reduce blood pressure in patients with pheochromocytoma. In cases of metastatic or locally invasive pheochromocytoma or in patients with intercurrent illness when the surgery is not feasible, long-term *medical* management is required. When the manifestations cannot be adequately controlled by adrenergic blocking agents, the concomitant administration of **metyrosine** may be required. β **adrenergic receptor blocking agents should be given only after** α **blockade has been induced.**

945. Lupus pernio is characteristic of:

A. Amyloidosis **B.** Coccidioidomycosis

C. Sarcoidosis **D.** Histoplasmosis *(PGI 1996, KARNATAKA 2000)*

The most common skin lesions in **sarcoidosis** are erythema nodosum, plaques, maculopapular eruptions, subcutaneous nodules, and **lupus pernio**.

946. *Not* a characteristic lab finding of Wegener's granulomatosis:

A. Reduced levels of hemoglobin **B.** Reduced levels of complement

C. Elevated levels of IgA **D.** Elevated ESR *(KARNATAKA 2000)*

Typical laboratory findings of Wegener's granulomatosis include a markedly **elevated ESR**, **mild anemia** and leukocytosis, **mild hypergammaglobulinemia (particularly of the IgA class)**, and mildly elevated rheumatoid factor. Thrombocytosis may be seen as an acute-phase reactant; **hypocomplementemia is not seen** despite the presence of circulating immune complexes in some patients.

947. Extraparenchymal *restrictive* lung disease does *not* occur in:

A. Congenital kyphoscoliosis
B. Emphysema
C. Myasthenia gravis
D. Obesity

(KARNATAKA 2000)

Obstructive lung disease (OLD)	Restrictive lung disease (RLD)
• Chronic bronchitis • Emphysema • Chronic asthma	• Interstitial fibrosis • Lung resection • Obesity • Myxedema • Muscle weakness • Kyphoscoliosis • Upper airway obstruction • Diminished respiratory drive • Vasoconstriction secondary to high altitude

948. Hand-foot syndrome is seen with the use of:

A. Bleomycin
B. Adriamycin
C. Busulphan
D. 5 FU

Hand-foot syndrome is also known as palmar-plantar erythrodysesthesia syndrome. It is a side effect of **5 fluorouracil**. It starts with tingling sensations in hands and feet and progresses over the next few days to pain while holding objects or walking. Symmetrical swelling and erythema of palms and soles, with tenderness of the distal phalanges, occurs rapidly, accompanied by desquamation. Symptoms usually resolve over 5 to 7 days following withdrawal of fluorouracil. The drug of choice is oral pyridoxine.

949. Human liver transplant was pioneered by:

A. Halstead
B. Christian Barnard
C. Starzl
D. Alexis carrel

(KARNATAKA 2000)

Liver transplant was pioneered in the 1960s by Starzl at the University of Colorado.

950. Gottron's papule is seen in:

A. Systemic lupus erythematosus
B. Systemic sclerosis
C. Dermatomyositis
D. Dermatitis herpetiformis

(KARNATAKA 2000)

Approximately 33% of patients have violaceous, flat-topped papules over the dorsal interphalangeal joints that are pathognomonic of *dermatomyositis* (**Gottron's sign or Gottron's papules**).

951. Penicillamine is *not* used in............ poisoning:

A. Lead
B. Copper
C. Arsenic
D. Mercury

952. D-penicillamine is useful in all *except*:

A. Rheumatoid arthritis
B. Mercury poisoning
C. Wilson's disease
D. Hemochromatosis

953. D-penicillamine is used in treating:

A. Systemic sclerosis
B. Systemic lupus erythematosus
C. Systemic infection
D. DLE

(KARNATAKA 2000)

Many drugs have been used in the treatment of **systemic sclerosis** without any consistent or prolonged benefit. In uncontrolled studies, D-penicillamine has been reported to reduce skin thickening and prevent development of significant organ involvement.

Common indications of D- penicillamine	
• Wilson's disease	• **C**opper poisoning
• Scleroderma	• **M**ercury poisoning
• Rheumatoid arthritis	• **L**ead poisoning
• Cystinuria	• Cystine stones

☺ *Mnemonic :* ***CML***

954. Wrist drop, punctate basophilia and encephalopathy occur in:
- **A.** Lead poisoning
- **B.** Arsenic poisoning
- **C.** Iron poisoning
- **D.** Copper poisoning

(AIIMS May 2002)

Symptoms of Chronic Lead Poisoning

- Abdominal colic and constipation;
- Lead line which is a stripped blue line on the junction of gums to the teeth;
- Hypochromic anemia;
- **Punctate** (marked with dots or tiny spots) **basophilia** in RBCs;
- Paralysis affecting extensor muscles of finger and wrist causing **wrist drop** and claw-shaped hand;
- **Encephalopathy**, hypertension, interstitial nephritis.

955. A boy presents with ascending paralysis followed by increasing respiratory muscle involvement. CSF examination shows albuminocytologic dissociation. Which of the following is the best treatment:
- **A.** Prednisolone IV
- **B.** Immunoglobulins IV
- **C.** Corticosteroids
- **D.** Oral prednisolone

(AIIMS May 2002)

956. *Not* used in the treatment of Guillain-Barré syndrome:
- **A.** IV gamma globulin
- **B.** IV methyl prednisolone
- **C.** Plasmapheresis
- **D.** Ventilatory support

(KARNATAKA 1996)

Clinical features of Guillain-Barré syndrome include areflexic motor paralysis with or without sensory disturbance together with an acellular rise of total protein in the cerebrospinal fluid (**albuminocytologic dissociation**) by the end of the 1st week of symptoms. **Intravenous administration of high-dose immunoglobulin** (2 g/kg body weight given over 5 days) is as effective as **plasmapheresis**, and is more easily administered. In contrast, **glucocorticoid treatment has not been shown to be effective**.

957. Lesion of the Meyer's loop of the optic radiation causes:
- **A.** Bitemporal hemianopia
- **B.** Superior quadrantic hemianopia
- **C.** Central scotoma
- **D.** Homonymous hemianopia

(AIIMS May 2002)

Damage to the optic radiations in the temporal lobe (**Meyer's loop**) produces a **superior quadrantic homonymous hemianopia**.

958. Wernicke's encephalopathy is due to deficiency of:
- **A.** Thiamine
- **B.** Riboflavin
- **C.** Pyridoxine
- **D.** Niacin

959. *Not* a feature of Wernicke's encephalopathy:
- **A.** Dementia
- **B.** Global confusion
- **C.** Ophthalmoplegia
- **D.** Ataxia

(PGI 1997)

Wernicke's encephalopathy is due to a deficiency of **thiamine**. The characteristic clinical triad is:
- Global confusion
- Ophthalmoplegia
- Ataxia

Mnemonic: **GOA**

960. An alcoholic patient presented with complaints of confusion. He was administered IV glucose and suddenly developed Wernicke's encephalopathy. The treatment is:

A. IV vitamin B_1
B. IV 5% dextrose
C. IV 50% dextrose
D. IV normal saline *(AIIMS May 2002)*

Wernicke's disease is a medical emergency that requires **immediate administration of thiamine**, in a dose of 50 mg either IV or IM. The dose should be given daily until the patient resumes a normal diet and should be begun *prior* to treatment with IV glucose solutions because such infusions may precipitate Wernicke's disease or acute cardiovascular beriberi in a previously unaffected patient or cause a rapid worsening of an early form of the disease. That's why; thiamine should be administered to all alcoholic patients requiring parenteral glucose.

961. ABG of a patient reveals pH 7.2; HCO_3^- 36 mmol/L; pCO_2 60 mmHg. *Most likely* diagnosis is:

A. Repository alkalosis
B. Metabolic alkalosis
C. Metabolic acidosis
D. Repository acidosis *(AIIMS 1999)*

962. Blood examination of a patient with *head injury* reveals pH 7.2, $PaCO_2$ 65 mmHg and bicarbonate 30. He has:

A. Metabolic alkalosis
B. Metabolic acidosis
C. Respiratory alkalosis
D. Respiratory acidosis *(AIIMS 1999)*

Term	Definition
Proton or H^+	A hydrogen atom whose neutralizing electron has been removed.
pH	Negative logarithm of hydrogen ion concentration
Acid	Proton or H^+ donor
Base	Proton or H^+ acceptor
Buffer	A substance which *reduces* the change in hydrogen ion concentration of a solution on addition of an acid or base.

The pH of the body fluids is maintained in a relatively narrow range (between **7.35 and 7.45**) by the presence of 'buffers' which are the *first line of defense* against such changes. However, buffers cannot *maintain* acid base balance without *compensatory* physiological changes in *lungs* followed by *corrective* physiological changes in *kidneys*. The major buffer systems of body are as under:

Bicarbonate-carbonic acid	Extracellular fluid
Protein-organic phosphates	Intracellular fluid
Mono-di hydrogen phosphate	Urine

SIMPLE DISORDERS

	pH	pCO_2	Bicarbonate
Metabolic acidosis	Reduced	Reduced	Reduced
Metabolic alkalosis	Increased	Increased	Increased
Respiratory acidosis	*Reduced*	*Increased*	*Increased*
Respiratory alkalosis	Increased	Reduced	Reduced

NORMAL VALUES

Arterial O_2 tension	PaO_2	95 ± 5 mmHg
Arterial CO_2 tension	$PaCO_2$	40 ± 2 mmHg
Arterial O_2 saturation	SaO_2	$97 \pm 2\%$
Arterial blood pH	pH	7.40 ± 0.02
Arterial bicarbonate	HCO_3^-	24 ± 2 mEq/L

Systemic arterial blood pH is maintained between 7.35 and 7.45 by extracellular and intracellular chemical buffering together with respiratory and renal 'regulatory' mechanisms. Under most circumstances, CO_2 production and excretion are matched, and the usual steady-state **$PaCO_2$ is maintained at 40 mmHg**. The $PaCO_2$ is regulated mainly by neural respiratory factors and is *not* subject to regulation by the rate of CO_2 production i.e. **hypercapnia is usually the result of hypoventilation** *rather* than of increased CO_2 production. Increases or decreases in $PaCO_2$ represent derangements of neural respiratory control or are due to compensatory changes in response to a primary alteration in the plasma (HCO_3^-). **Changes in $PaCO_2$ can cause acidosis or alkalosis, depending on whether $PaCO_2$ is above or below the normal value of 40 mmHg** (*respiratory* acidosis or alkalosis).

963. Respiratory alkalosis is seen in:

A. Morphine poisoning
B. Ethanol poisoning
C. Salicylate poisoning
D. Barbiturate poisoning

Acute salicylate poisoning is more common in children. Serious toxicity occurs when the serum salicylate level is more than 50 mg/dl. As salicylic acid is an acid it produces metabolic acidosis and it directly stimulates the respiratory centers to produce hyperventilation leading to **respiratory alkalosis**. **Other causes of respiratory alkalosis are as under:**

Toxic stimulation of respiratory centers	**Lack of oxygen**	**Central neurogenic hyperventilation**
• Hepatic coma • Septicemia • Water intoxication	• Pulmonary disease • Cardiac failure • Blood loss • Alveolar capillary block • CO poisoning	• Pontine hemorrhage • Pontine lesion due to infection • Pontine lesion due to malignancy
Hysterical over breathing	**Stimulation of respiratory centers by drugs**	**Excessive artificial respiration**
	• Salicylate poisoning • Atropine poisoning	• Intermittent positive pressure ventilation

964. Respiratory acidosis is caused by:

A. Morphine
B. Asthma
C. Emphysema
D. All of the above

Causes of Respiratory Acidosis

Central	**Airway**	**Parenchyma**	**Neuromuscular**	**Miscellaneous**
Sedatives Stroke Infection Anesthetics Morphine	Obstruction Asthma	Emphysema Pneumoconiosis Bronchitis Adult respiratory distress syndrome Barotrauma	Muscular dystrophies Poliomyelitis Kyphoscoliosis Myasthenia	Obesity Hypoventilation

965. Cataract, mental retardation and short 4th metacarpal are the features of:

A. Hypothyroidism
B. Pseudohypoparathyroidism
C. Hyperthyroidism
D. Hyperparathyroidism *(PGI 1999)*

Pseudohypoparathyroidism is a hereditary disorder characterized by symptoms and signs of hypoparathyroidism, in association with distinctive skeletal and developmental defects. The hypoparathyroidism is due to a *deficient end-organ response* to PTH. Most patients demonstrate a characteristic 'phenotype' termed **Albright's hereditary osteodystrophy** (AHO), consisting of short stature, round face, skeletal anomalies (brachydactyly), and heterotopic calcification. **Brachydactyly most often affects the 1st, 4th and the 5th metacarpals**. 1st and 5th metatarsals are also involved. As a result the index finger may be *longer* than the middle finger. **Mental retardation** is common as are calcifications of the basal ganglia and **lenticular cataracts**. The error in *Albright's hereditary osteodystrophy* (pseudohypoparathyroidism) is the 'opposite' of that found in the *McCune-Albright syndrome* (fibrous dysplasia). In the AHO, inactivating mutations in Gαs proteins result in *deficient* activity and decreased responsiveness to hormones that function through cyclic AMP-mediated signal transduction pathways.

966. C-reactive protein is raised in:

A. Infections
B. Inflammatory arthritis
C. Autoimmune disorders
D. All of the above

C-reactive protein (CRP) is a protein *usually* not found in the blood. It is present in many acute inflammatory conditions. CRP appears within 24 to 48 hours after inflammation begins and disappears when inflammation is suppressed by salicylates or steroids. It is *non*specific acute phase reactant, which increases, in a number of **infectious, inflammatory or autoimmune conditions**.

967. C-reactive protein is significantly increased in all the following *except*:

A. Rheumatic fever
B. Rheumatoid arthritis
C. Systemic vasculitis
D. Systemic sclerosis *(JIPMER 2002)*

Conditions Associated with Raised CRP

General inflammatory conditions	**Inflammatory disease**
• Inflammatory disease • Infections • Neoplastic disease	• Rheumatoid arthritis • Rheumatic fever • Inflammatory bowel disease • Seronegative arthritis (Reiter's syndrome) • Vasculitis (e.g. hypersensitivity vasculitis)
Detection and monitoring of infection	**Detection of tissue injury**
• Bacterial infection in SLE • Neonatal infection • Postoperative infection • Intercurrent infection in leukemia • Pyelonephritis	• Myocardial infarction • Transplant rejection • Neoplasia (e.g. Burkitt's lymphoma)
Cardiovascular disease risk	**Normal conditions with elevated CRP**
• Increased CRP predictive of CAD	• Medications (e.g. oral contraceptives) • Third trimester of pregnancy

968. *Most common* Mendelian disorder among the following is:

A. Autosomal dominant
B. Autosomal recessive
C. X-linked dominant
D. X-linked recessive

Relative Frequency of Mendelian Disorders

• **Monogenic disorders**	10 in 1000
• **Autosomal dominant**	7 in 1000
• **Autosomal recessive**	2.5 in 1000
• **X-linked conditions**	0.4 in 1000

❖ Monogenic disorders consist of AD, AR and X-linked conditions

969. Which of the following is the *most common* cause of female pseudohermaphroditism:

A. PCOD **B.** CAH
C. Ovarian agenesis **D.** Turner syndrome *(AIIMS May 2002)*

Congenital adrenal hyperplasia due to *classic* 21-hydroxylase deficiency is the *most common* cause of ambiguous genitalia in the newborn.

970. Which of the following is the scale used in comparing the grade of pain:

A. McGill's pain chart **B.** Visual Analogue Scale
C. Numerical charts **D.** CHEOPES *(AIIMS May 2002)*

There are many situations in clinical practice when it is necessary to assess the degree of pain in a patient. This may be either to ascertain how painful a clinical procedure is or to compare the pain relief or pain inflicted by a treatment. Pain is an unpleasant sensory and emotional experience associated with actual or potential tissue damage or described in terms of such damage. Pain is thus a subjective experience and therefore impossible to measure directly, but a quantitative estimation of pain can be obtained. However, there are only few available tests to quantify separate aspects of pain. The validity and reliability of the different methods have been questioned. The **Visual Analogue Scale** (VAS) is commonly used to assess for example the degree of muscle pain. VAS consists of a 100 mm horizontal or vertical line with the two endpoint labeled "no pain" and "worst pain ever experienced".

Instructions for Health Distress Index Visual Analogue Scale

Mark an "▯" on the line which indicates a range of feelings. For instance, if you were feeling "Moderately High Discomfort" you would indicate it on the line below as such:

No discomfort |————————————————▯————| Extreme Discomfort

However, if you were feeling only "Somewhat Low Discomfort" you would indicate it on the line below as such:

No Discomfort |—————▯————————————————| Extreme Discomfort

Visual Analogue Scale

Name or ID:____________ Date:__________ Time:__________

Pain Area # 1: ____________ Symptom Area # 2: ____________

1. No Pain in Area # 1 |————————————————| Very High Level of Pain in Area # 1
2. No Pain or Symptom in Area # 2 |————————————————| Very High Level of Pain or Symptom in Area # 2
3. Very Relaxed |————————————————| Very Tense

[For Office Use Only:] Clinic ID: __________ Practitioner ID: __________

971. ST depression is seen in all the following *except*:

A. Coronary vasospasm **B.** Acute MI
C. Ventricular aneurysm **D.** LBBB *(AIIMS May 2002)*

- ST segment depression demonstrates myocardial subendocardial injury. Etiology of these changes could be **non-Q wave infarction** or **angina** (ischemia). It is important to correlate clinical findings, and cardiac enzyme results with the ECG to differentiate the significance of the ECG changes.
- Left bundle branch block demonstrates ST segment depression and T wave inversion on leads I, aVL, V_{4-6} as a normal variant.
- Digitalis effect demonstrates ST segment depression with a "scooped out" look particular to this condition.
- In **ventricular aneurysm** there is persistent ST segment *elevation* following a myocardial infarction. Changes are localized to leads reflecting myocardial injury, and may be permanent.

972. The shape of RBC is maintained by:

A. Spectrin
B. Ankyrin
C. Fibrin
D. Alpha glycoprotein

(AIIMS May 2002)

Spectrin is an important protein for maintaining erythrocyte shape—it helps organize integral proteins in the plasma membrane, anchor other important structural proteins to a cytoskeleton, and its interaction with other proteins gives erythrocytes robust deformable properties that contribute to their long-life.

973. Vitamin E deficiency is associated with:

A. Pseudotumor cerebri
B. Hyperkeratosis
C. Ataxia
D. Cholestasis

(PGI 1993)

Vitamin E deficiency may be associated with a discrete syndrome, as when deficiency is due to a selective malabsorption of the vitamin or when an autosomal recessive mutation causes vitamin E deficiency and **ataxia**.

974. Acute leukemia phase is seen in all *except*:

A. Hodgkin's lymphoma
B. CLL
C. CML
D. PNH

(PGI 1996)

Chronic lymphocytic leukemia (**CLL**) is the *most common* type of indolent leukemia.

975. Antihypertensive drug which should *not* be given to a truck driver is:

A. Propranolol
B. Aldomet®
C. Clonidine
D. Hydralazine

(PGI 1995)

Clonidine should be used with caution when driving or doing things requiring alertness, because of possible drowsiness.

976. *Not* seen in SIADH:

A. Hyperuricemia
B. Concentrated urine
C. Lethargy
D. Hyponatremia

(JIPMER 1995)

SIADH should be suspected in patients who have **hyponatremia** and **concentrated urine** (osmolality >300 mmol/kg) associated with **lethargy** and in the absence of edema, orthostatic hypotension, and features of dehydration. The diagnosis is 'supported' by the finding of blood urea nitrogen, *serum uric acid*, creatinine, and albumin concentrations in the *low-normal or subnormal range*.

977. Reactive arthritis is commonly caused by:

A. *Shigella sonnei*
B. *Shigella flexneri*
C. *Shigella boydii*
D. *Shigella dysenteriae*

(KERALA 1995)

Less common *extra*intestinal manifestations of shigellosis include seizures in some patients and **reactive arthritis** in others; both of these manifestations are usually due to infection with ***Shigella flexneri*** strains.

978. Virus *most commonly* causing aplastic crisis in hemolytic anemia is:

A. HTLV
B. Parvovirus
C. HIV
D. Herpes virus

(DELHI 1996)

The major clinical features of *hereditary spherocytosis* are anemia, splenomegaly, and jaundice. Compensatory erythroid hyperplasia of the bone marrow occurs. Compensation may be temporarily interrupted by episodes of **erythroid hypoplasia** precipitated by infections, particularly **parvovirus**.

979. Dementia in a patient of CRF with chronic hemodialysis is due to:

A. Hypertensive encephalopathy
B. Hypokalemia
C. Uremia
D. Aluminum toxicity

(PGI 1996)

Aluminum toxicity has been *best* documented with the **dialysis dementia** syndrome in which water used during renal dialysis was contaminated with **excessive amounts of aluminum** resulting in a progressive encephalopathy associated with confusion, memory loss, agitation, and, later, lethargy and stupor.

980. Calcification of basal ganglion is *least* likely in:
A. Hypoparathyroidism
B. Pseudohypoparathyroidism
C. Idiopathic
D. Berry's aneurysm
(AIIMS 1997)

Basal ganglia calcification is seen in patients with **hypoparathyroidism** and in patients with **pseudohypoparathyroidism**. However, most frequently the calcification is **idiopathic** (? physiologic) and is not associated with any known disease process. It usually is symmetrical and involves the globus pallidus and sometimes also the dentate nuclei of the cerebellum.

981. In morphine poisoning, type of respiration is:
A. Diaphragmatic
B. Slow
C. Deep rapid
D. Rapid shallow
(AIIMS 1997)

The typical syndrome of *morphine* poisoning includes **shallow respirations at a rate of 2 to 4 per minute**, pupillary miosis, bradycardia, hypothermia, and absence of responsiveness to external stimulation.

982. Kala azar is transmitted by:
A. Droplet infection
B. Sandflies
C. Anopheles
D. Black fly

Kala azar or Leishmaniasis is transmitted by the bite of female sandflies –*Phlebotomus.*

983. *Not* a clinical manifestation of kala azar:
A. Dysphagia and chest pain
B. Pancytopenia
C. Fever and cough
D. Splenomegaly
(AIIMS 1999)

Kala azar conjures up the classic image of profoundly cachectic, **febrile** patients who are heavily parasitized and have life-threatening disease. **Splenomegaly** *typically* is more 'impressive' than hepatomegaly. The abnormal laboratory findings associated with advanced disease include **pancytopenia**, hypergammaglobulinemia (chiefly involving IgG, from polyclonal B cell activation) and hypoalbuminemia. Sodium antimony gluconate is the drug of choice and should be given in a dose of 20 mg/kg/day IM OD for 28 days.

984. If kala azar is *not* responding to the primary treatment, then which of the following should be used:
A. Splenectomy
B. Ketoconazole
C. Amphotericin B
D. Double dose of antimony
(AI 1997)

985. Drug *not* used in treatment of kala azar:
A. Pentamidine
B. Amphotericin
C. Clindamycin
D. Sodium stibogluconate
(SGPGI 1996))

Pentavalent antimonial agent (20 mg of **sodium antimony gluconate**/kg given intravenously or intramuscularly once daily for 28 days) still constitutes 1st-line therapy of **kala azar**. In *our* country, where unresponsiveness to sodium antimony gluconate therapy is becoming increasingly problematic, **amphotericin B** (0.5 to 1.0 mg/kg daily or every other day, given IV for a total dose (TD) of 7 to 20 mg/kg has been found to be a highly effective, *though* potentially toxic, alternative. **Pentamidine** (2 to 4 mg/kg daily or every other day, given IV or IM for at least 15 doses) is also reasonably effective.

986. A continuous machinery murmur is heard in:
A. PDA
B. VSD
C. ASD
D. TOF

A thrill and continuous **"machinery" murmur** with a late systolic accentuation at the upper left sternal edge is characteristic of PDA.

987. Curschmann's spirals in sputum are seen in:
A. Tuberculosis
B. Asthma
C. Bronchitis
D. Bronchiectasis

The most striking macroscopic finding in **bronchial asthma** is occlusion of bronchi and bronchioles with thick mucous plugs. Microscopically the mucous plugs contain whorls of epithelium giving rise to characteristic **Curschmann's spirals**. Numerous eosinophils and Charcot-Leyden crystals may also be present.

988. Enzyme deficient in diabetes mellitus is:
A. Glucokinase
B. Hexokinase
C. Phosphorylase
D. Pyrophosphate dehydrogenase

Maturity onset diabetes of young type 2 is due to mutations in the **glucokinase gene** which is located on the short arm of chromosome 7.

989. Which of the following enzyme is deficient in MODY type 2:
A. Glucokinase
B. Hexokinase
C. Phosphorylase
D. Pyrophosphate dehydrogenase

Disease	Site of mutation
MODY 1	Long arm of chromosome 20
MODY 2	Glucokinase gene located on the short arm of chromosome 7
MODY 3	Long arm of chromosome 12

- MODY stands for maturity-onset diabetes of the young.

990. Which antitubercular drug is used in a patient of renal failure:
A. Isoniazid
B. Rifampicin
C. Ethambutol
D. Pyrazinamide

991. Which one of the following therapies would be safe in a patient with pulmonary tuberculosis having markedly abnormal liver function:
A. Streptomycin + Isoniazid
B. Streptomycin + Ethambutol
C. Ethambutol + Isoniazid
D. Rifampicin + Isoniazid

Drugs	Renal disease	Hepatic disease
• **Ethambutol**	Decrease dose	No change
• **Streptomycin**	Decrease dose and frequency	No change
• **Isoniazid**	Decrease dose	Avoid use or decrease dose
• **Pyrazinamide**	Decrease dose	Avoid use or decrease dose
• **Rifampicin**	No change	Avoid use or decrease dose

MNEMONIC: **R**ifampicin is safe in **R**enal disease.

992. Deposition in alkaptonuria is *not* seen in:
A. Pinna
B. Eye
C. Nose
D. Cartilage

(AIIMS May 2002)

The hallmark of **alkaptonuria** is passage of urine that becomes black upon standing. The defect lies in the *catabolic* pathway of tyrosine. The earliest sign of the disorder is the tendency for diapers to stain black. Throughout childhood and most of early adulthood, an asymptomatic, **slowly progressive deposition of pigment like polymer material into collagenous tissues occurs**. In the 4th decade, external signs of pigment deposition, called *ochronosis*, begin to appear. The **slate blue, gray, or black discoloration of sclerae and ear cartilage** is indicative of widespread staining of the body tissues, particularly **cartilage**. The hips, knees, and intervertebral joints are affected most commonly and show clinical symptoms resembling rheumatoid arthritis.

993. Drug *not* causing cholestatic liver injury is:

A. Ciprofloxacin
B. Erythromycin estolate
C. Clavulanic acid/amoxicillin
D. Chlorpromazine *(SGPGI 1999)*

Some Drugs Causing Cholestatic Jaundice

- Acetohexamide
- Anabolic steroids
- Androgens
- **Chlorpromazine**
- Chlorpropamide
- **Clavulanic acid/amoxicillin**
- Cyclosporine
- **Erythromycin estolate**
- Flucloxacillin
- Gold salts
- Methimazole
- Nitrofurantoin
- Oral contraceptives
- Phenothiazines

994. Drug *very* effective in renal involvement in scleroderma is:

A. Nifedipine
B. Captopril
C. D-penicillamine
D. Prednisolone *(SGPGI 1999)*

Renal involvement in scleroderma is often accompanied by hypertension and mild to moderate proteinuria. Antihypertensive agents are often effective in lowering BP and stabilizing or *reversing* renal failure. These drugs include propranolol, clonidine, and minoxidil. ***Particularly* effective are the ACE inhibitors, which include captopril, enalapril, and lisinopril.**

995. *Treatment of choice* of pseudomembranous colitis is:

A. Amikacin **B.** Bacitracin
C. Vancomycin **D.** Ampicillin *(SGPGI 2002)*

996. *Not* used in the treatment of pseudomembranous colitis:

A. Vancomycin **B.** Cholestyramine
C. Ampicillin **D.** Metronidazole *(SGPGI 1999)*

The most characteristic form of antibiotic-associated colitis caused by *Clostridium difficile* is **pseudomembranous colitis** (PMC). Diarrhea is the key feature and is usually watery, voluminous, without gross blood or mucus and is often associated with abdominal cramps and tenderness, fever, and leukocytosis. Given *orally* (a route by which it is *not* absorbed), **vancomycin** (Vancocin CP®) can be used to treat antibiotic-associated pseudomembranous colitis in patients who have failed to respond to **metronidazole**, the *drug of choice*. The resin **cholestyramine** binds the cytotoxin of *Clostridium difficile* and has been used with some success to treat severe cases. Because cholestyramine also binds vancomycin, the 2 drugs should not be used in combination.

997. Idiopathic ulcerative colitis *most commonly* involves:

A. Cecum and ascending colon **B.** Colon and rectum
C. Cecum and decending colon **D.** Rectum *(SGPGI 1999)*

The *etiology* of **ulcerative colitis** remains obscure till date and in spite of intensive bacteriological study no organism has been incriminated. **In 95% of cases the disease starts in the rectum to spread proximally.** In the presence of an *incompetent* ileocaecal valve retrograde ("**backwash**") ileitis involves the last 30 cm of ileum. It is a nonspecific inflammatory disease primarily affecting the mucosa and the superficial part of submucosa and the deeper layers are involved only in severe disease. The disease is characterized by multiple minute ulcers which may be discrete or numerous. In chronic cases numerous *inflammatory* polyps (**pseudopolyps**) occur in 20% of cases. In fulminant cases a portion of colon, usually the transverse colon, may become acutely dilated and the wall of colon may become extremely thin and may perforate (**toxic megacolon**). With time the chronic inflammation may lead to severed dysplasia or carcinoma *in situ*. The disease is more common in females in their third decade of life and *watery diarrhea* occurring day and night in a person of previously normal bowel habits is the **first symptom.** There may be a rectal discharge of mucus which may be purulent or blood stained. The ***earliest*** **radiological sign is the loss of haustration, mainly in the distal colon.** Other features include a narrow contracted *"pipe stem"* colon, alteration in mucosal outline and *pseudopolyposis.* Corticosteroids are very useful drugs and can be used locally or systemically. **Sulphasalazine** or other derivatives of 5 aminosalicylic acid (5 ASA) such as *mesalazine* and *olsalazine* can be given topically or systemically and their main function is maintaining a remission rather than treating an acute attack. Nonspecific antidiarrheal agents have no place *whatsoever* in the management of ulcerative colitis.

998. Heparin's major mode of action is:

A. Inhibits synthesis of thrombin
B. Inhibits factor VII synthesis
C. Not easily controlled
D. Activates plasmin

999. Efficiency of anticoagulant heparin is *best* monitored by:

A. Clotting time **B.** FDP
C. PT **D.** aPTT *(KERALA 1999)*

Heparin is a naturally occurring mucopolysaccharide polymer with tetrasaccharide sequences that **bind to and activate antithrombin III**. It is an extremely potent anticoagulant that can dramatically **reduce thrombin generation** and fibrin formation. Heparin is administered to patients with acute thrombosis or embolism by continuous IV infusion at a rate sufficient to raise the activated partial thromboplastin time (aPTT) to 1.5 to 2 times the patient's preheparin aPTT. Heparin's anticoagulant effect can be rapidly *reversed* by the administration of protamine sulfate.

1000. Late systolic murmur is seen in which of the following condition:

A. Large VSD
B. Small VSD
C. MVP
D. Tricuspid valve endocarditis *(KERALA 1999)*

Nonejection or midsystolic clicks, occurring with or without a **late systolic murmur**, often denote **prolapse of one or both leaflets of the mitral valve**. They also may be caused by tricuspid valve prolapse.

1001. *Most common* cause of osteomyelitis in drug addicts is:

A. *Haemophilus influenzae* **B.** *Escherichia coli*
C. *Staphylococcus aureus* **D.** *Salmonella* *(PGI 1997)*

Staphylococcus aureus, *Pseudomonas aeruginosa*, and *Serratia* infections are associated with IV drug use in some parts of the USA and may involve the sacroiliac, sternoclavicular, or pubic joints as well as the spine.

1002. *True* regarding Lesch-Nyhan syndrome is:

A. Adenine phosphoribosyl transferase deficiency
B. Myoadenylate deaminase deficiency
C. Partial HPRT deficiency
D. Total HPRT deficiency *(PGI 1997)*

A **complete deficiency of hypoxanthine phosphoribosyltransferase** (**HPRT**), the Lesch-Nyhan syndrome, is characterized by hyperuricemia, self-mutilative behavior, choreoathetosis, spasticity, and mental retardation. A partial deficiency of **HPRT**, the *Kelley-Seegmiller syndrome*, is associated with hyperuricemia but no central nervous system manifestations. In the **Lesch-Nyhan syndrome** (juvenile gout), enzymatic overproduction of purine and consequently of uric acid occurs. Affected children show growth and mental retardation, a tendency to self-mutilation often manifested by amputation of the fingertips and phalanges, and multiple radiolucent uric acid calculi. The disorder has an X-linked recessive type of inheritance.

1003. *Most specific* for systemic lupus erythematosus is:

A. Antinuclear antibody
B. Anti-Sm
C. Anti-Ro
D. Anti-RNA *(PGI 1997)*

Antibodies of Systemic Lupus Erythematosus

Antibody	%	Important features
Antinuclear antibodies	98	
Anti-DNA	70	Anti-dsDNA is *relatively* disease-specific; anti-ss DNA is not.
Anti-Sm	30	Specific for SLE.
Anti-RNP	40	
Anti-Ro (SS-A)	30	
Anti-La (SS-B)	10	
Antihistone	70	More frequent in drug-induced LE (95%) than in spontaneous SLE.
Antiphospholipid	50	

Mnemonic: Anti-**Sm** is **s**pecific **m**ost.

1004. *Most common* cause of hemobilia is:

A. Hepatoma
B. Liver hemangioma
C. Liver trauma
D. Portal infection *(SGPGI 1996)*

1005. All of the following suggest hemobilia *except*:

A. *Lower* GI bleeding
B. Upper abdominal trauma
C. Jaundice
D. Intermittent colicky abdominal pain

Hemobilia may occur after traumatic or operative injury to the liver or bile ducts, intraductal rupture of a hepatic abscess or aneurysm of the hepatic artery, biliary or hepatic tumor hemorrhage, or mechanical complications of choledocholithiasis or hepatobiliary parasitism. Patients present with a classic triad of **biliary colic**, **obstructive jaundice**, and **melena** or occult blood in the stools. Melena or black terry stool is characteristic of upper GI hemorrhage and is due to reaction of blood with HCl secreted from stomach. It occurs when there is bleeding above the ligamentum teres, hence upper GI bleeding.

1006. Spastic paraplegia is seen in all *except*:

A. Lead poisoning
B. Motor neuron disease
C. Cervical spondylosis
D. Lathyrism

Lead produces demyelination of peripheral nerves which leads to **flaccid paralysis** because the lower motor neuron is involved.

1007. *Not* a recognized tumor marker:

A. AFP
B. Acid phosphate
C. β hCG
D. Neuron-specific enolase *(SGPGI 1996)*

Some Tumor Markers

Hormones	Oncofetal antigens
• Human chorionic gonadotropin • Calcitonin • Catecholamines	• Alfa-fetoprotein (AFP) • Carcinoembryonic antigen (CEA)
Tumor associated proteins	**Enzymes**
• Prostate specific antigen • Monoclonal immunoglobulin • CA-125 • CA 19-9 • CD30 • CD25	• Prostatic acid phosphatase • Neuron specific enolase • Lactate dehydrogenase

1008. Acanthosis is *not* associated with:

A. GI malignancy
B. Gout
C. Cushing's syndrome
D. Diabetes mellitus

(SGPGI 1996)

Acanthosis nigricans also can be a reflection of an internal malignancy, most commonly of the gastrointestinal tract. Acanthosis nigricans is associated with obesity, but it may be a reflection of an endocrinopathy such as acromegaly, Cushing's syndrome, the Stein-Leventhal syndrome, or insulin-resistant diabetes mellitus (type A, type B, and lipoatrophic forms).

1009. Water bottle configuration of the heart on chest X-ray is seen in:

A. Hypothyroidism
B. Carcinoid syndrome
C. Beriberi
D. Obesity

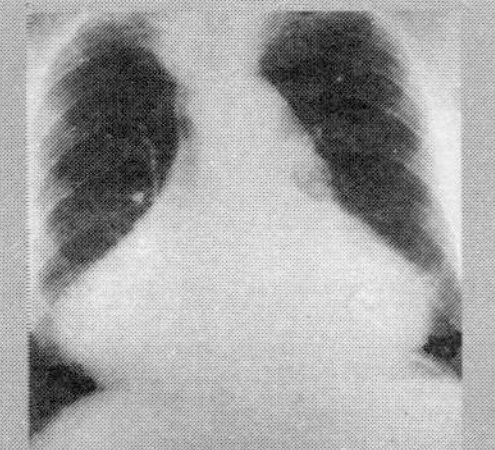

"Water bottle" configuration

In **hypothyroidism** the CRX show cardiomegaly, often with a "**water bottle" configuration**, pleural effusions, and evidence of congestive heart failure.

1010. Radiation nephritis is characterized by all *except*:

A. *Mild* hypertension
B. Massive proteinuria
C. Rapidly developing azotemia
D. Anemia

Radiation nephritis: Renal dysfunction can occur if both kidneys are exposed to 2300 rad or more of X-ray during a period of 1 month or less. Clinical presentations consist of:

- Rapidly progressive azotemia,
- Moderate to malignant hypertension
- Anemia
- Proteinuria
- Ultimately CRF develops in 50% of cases

1011. Carbamazepine toxicity is precipitated by:
- **A.** Valproic acid
- **B.** Erythromycin
- **C.** Theophylline
- **D.** Vitamin K

(JIPMER 2000)

Concurrent use of **erythromycin** or troleandomycin with **carbamazepine** may inhibit carbamazepine metabolism, resulting in **increased** plasma concentrations and **toxicity.**

1012. Monday chest tightness is a symptom classically seen in:
- **A.** Bagassosis
- **B.** Silicosis
- **C.** Berylliosis
- **D.** Byssinosis

Byssinosis is characterized by chest tightness at the end of the 1st day of the workweek ("Monday chest tightness").

1013. Normal mean Reid index is:
- **A.** 0.22
- **B.** 0.35
- **C.** 0.44
- **D.** 0.66

Reid index is based on the ratio of the thickness of the submucosal glands to that of the bronchial wall. In normal people it is **0.44 +/- 0.09**, whereas in patients of chronic bronchitis it is 0.52 +/- 0.08.

1014. Which of the following is *not* a feature of Addison's disease:
- **A.** Hypertension
- **B.** Weight loss
- **C.** Pigmentation of skin
- **D.** Weakness

FEATURES OF PRIMARY ADRENOCORTICAL DEFICIENCY (ADDISON'S DISEASE)

- Weakness
- Pigmentation of skin
- Weight loss
- Anorexia, nausea, and vomiting
- *Hypo*tension (<110/70)
- Pigmentation of mucous membranes
- Abdominal pain
- Salt craving
- Diarrhea
- Constipation
- Syncope
- Vitiligo

1015. Drugs causing metabolic acidosis are all *except*:
- **A.** Metformin
- **B.** Spironolactone
- **C.** Phenformin
- **D.** Albendazole

Some Drugs Causing Metabolic Acidosis

- Acetazolamide
- Metformin
- Paraldehyde
- Phenformin
- Salicylates
- Spironolactone

1016. Digoxin toxicity is *not* accentuated by:
- **A.** Hepatic dysfunction
- **B.** Hypokalemia
- **C.** Renal disease
- **D.** Quinidine

Digoxin is excreted unchanged by kidney, so liver disease has no effect on its metabolism. Phenytoin and lignocaine are useful in digoxin induced arrhythmias.

Factors and drugs increasing digoxin toxicity

- Hypokalemia
- Renal disease
- Verapamil and amiodarone
- Hypercalcemia
- Quinidine
- Potassium sparing diuretics

1017. Which of the following is *not* a feature of Felty's syndrome:

A. Rheumatoid arthritis
B. Splenomegaly
C. Neutropenia
D. Osteoarthritis

Features of Felty's Syndrome

- Chronic rheumatoid arthritis
- Splenomegaly
- Neutropenia
- Anemia
- Thrombocytopenia

1018. In aortic regurgitation, the left ventricle is:

A. Hypertrophic
B. Dilated
C. Small
D. Atrophic

In severe and long-standing aortic regurgitation stroke volume may be 2 or 3 times the normal thus exposing the left ventricle to volume overload. This volume overload leads to **left ventricular hypertrophy.**

1019. The human parathormone:

A. Increases bone reabsorption
B. Lowers serum calcium
C. Increases renal tubular reabsorption of phosphate
D. Causes reabsorption of calcium in the kidney

Parathyroid hormone is secreted by 4 parathyroid glands present on the posterior surface of thyroid gland. Human parathyroid hormone is a linear polypeptide containing 84 amino acid residues. Important functions are as under:

- **Increased resorption of bone**
- Increasing plasma calcium ions
- Reducing plasma phosphate
- Increasing urinary excretion of phosphates by decreasing the reabsorption of phosphate in proximal convoluted tubules of kidney.

1020. *True* about Huntington's disease is:

A. Autosomal dominant
B. Usually onset is in childhood
C. Associates with rheumatic fever
D. Disappears with rest and sedation

"**Huntington's disease** is defined as a relentlessly progressive *disease of middle* life characterized by chorea and dementia which is transmitted as an *autosomal dominant* fashion". It has an incidence of 1/10,000. The two important features of the disease are **chorea and behavioral disturbance**. **Onset is usually in the 4th decade of life**, but there is a wide range in age of onset, from childhood to greater than 70 years.

1021. Broad cast in the urine are *typically* seen in:

A. Acute glomerulonephritis
B. Acute renal failure
C. Chronic renal failure
D. Nephrotic syndrome

Different Types of Urinary Casts

• **WBC casts with bacteria**	Pyelonephritis
• **WBC and/or WBC casts**	Interstitial nephritis, SLE and transplant rejection
• **Degenerated cellular casts (*waxy casts)***	Chronic renal diseases
• **Broad casts**	CRF
• **Broad casts + cellular casts + RBC**	Chronic glomerulonephritis with persistent active glomerulitis
• **Broad casts** are formed in distal tubules of enlarged nephrons. Enlargement of nephrons occur due to 'compensatory hypertrophy' which is seen in conditions in which the renal mass is reduced such as **chronic renal failure**.	

1022. RBC casts in urine are seen in:

A. Nephrotic syndrome
B. Renal amyloidosis
C. CRF
D. Acute nephritis

Features of Acute Nephritis

- Hematuria
- RBC casts
- Azotemia
- Oliguria
- Edema
- Hypertension

1023. Prophylactic dose of tetanus immune globulin is:

A. 250 international units
B. 500 international units
C. 1000 international units
D. 1500 international units

The *prophylactic* dose of **tetanus immune globulin is 250 international units.** It should be given if risk of tetanus is there in any injury along with an injection of tetanus toxoid to build active immunity. Tetanus immune globulin produces a protective antibody level in the serum for at least 4 to 6 weeks.

1024. The treatment of acute cardiac tamponade is:

A. Emergency paracentesis
B. Emergency thoracotomy
C. IV digitalis
D. Wait and watch

Acute cardiac tamponade is a life-threatening situation and **paracentesis** should be performed at once to decompress the heart.

1025. Amyl nitrate is used in the poisoning of:

A. Carbon monoxide
B. Cyanide
C. Salicylates
D. Morphine

- **Cyanide** is a poison that **inhibits mitochondrial enzyme cytochrome oxidase**. This results in blocking of the electron transport leading to reduced oxidative metabolism and oxygen utilization.
- Antidotal therapy consists of **amyl nitrite**, sodium nitrite, and sodium thiosulfate. These 3 substances act as under:

1. Nitrites produce methemoglobinemia.
2. The affinity of cyanide is *greater* for methemoglobin than the affinity for cytochrome oxidase. This promotes the dissociation of cyanide from cytochrome oxidase.
3. Thiosulfate reacts with the cyanide, which is slowly released from cyanomethemoglobin, forming the relatively *non*toxic thiocyanate.
4. Thiocyanate is excreted in the urine.

1026. Zieve's syndrome is seen in:

A. Portal cirrhosis
B. Hepatocellular carcinoma
C. Hereditary spherocytosis
D. Chronic alcoholism

Zieve's syndrome is the association of hemolytic anemia with cirrhosis, hyperlipidemia and jaundice in **chronic alcoholics**. Spherocytes are present in peripheral blood. Osmotic fragility of RBCs is increased unlike other liver disorders in which osmotic fragility is reduced.

1027. Relatively specific test for pheochromocytoma is:
- **A.** Ultrasound
- **B.** Estimation of urinary metanephrines
- **C.** Estimation of urinary vanillylmandelic acid
- **D.** Phentolamine test

The following 3 assays may be employed to diagnose pheochromocytoma:
- Vanillylmandelic acid (VMA)
- Metanephrines
- Unconjugated or "free" catecholamines.

The assays of **metanephrines** or catecholamines are both more sensitive and more specific than VMA assay.

1028. Bloody mucoid diarrhea is *not* seen in infection with:
- **A.** *Shigella* spp.
- **B.** *Vibrio cholerae*
- **C.** *Salmonella* spp.
- **D.** *Campylobacter jejuni*

Cholera begins with the sudden onset of painless watery diarrhea, which consists of grey, cloudy, sweet "rice water stool" **not containing bile, blood** or offensive odor. **Causes of bloody diarrhea or dysentery are as under:**
- *Shigella*
- *Campylobacter jejuni*
- *Aeromonas hydrophilia*
- *Giardia lamblia*
- *Salmonella*
- *Yersinia enterocolitica*
- *Entamoeba histolytica*

❖ *Shigella and Salmonella* spp. account for majority of cases of dysentery.

1029. ASO titers are useful in the diagnosis of:
- **A.** Acute rheumatoid arthritis
- **B.** Acute rheumatic fever
- **C.** Ankylosing spondylitis
- **D.** Osteoarthritis

1030. In the Jones criteria for rheumatic heart disease the major criteria are all *except*:
- **A.** Carditis
- **B.** Fever
- **C.** Erythema marginatum
- **D.** Subcutaneous nodule

1031. The major criteria for rheumatic fever are the following *except*:
- **A.** Carditis
- **B.** Polyarthritis
- **C.** Erythema marginatum
- **D.** ESR above 20 mm/hour

1032. Migrating polyarthritis is characteristically seen in:
- **A.** Syphilitic arthritis
- **B.** Rheumatoid arthritis
- **C.** Psoriatic arthritis
- **D.** Rheumatic fever

ASO titer is elevated in 80% of patients of acute rheumatic fever but low ASO titer does not exclude rheumatic fever. If antideoxyribonuclease B, antistreptokinase and antihyaluronidase antibody tests are also done at least 1 antibody titer is elevated in 95% of patients. Diagnosis of acute rheumatic fever is highly probable when either 2 major criteria **or** 1 major and 2 minor criteria are present **along with** evidence of antecedent streptococcal infection.

THE JONES CRITERIA FOR RHEUMATIC FEVER		
Major criteria	**Minor criteria**	
	Clinical	**Laboratory**
Carditis		
Migratory polyarthritis	Fever	Elevated ESR
Sydenham's chorea	Arthralgia	Elevated CRP
Subcutaneous nodules		Prolonged PR interval
Erythema marginatum		
PLUS (ESSENTIAL CRITERIA)		
Supporting evidence of a recent group A streptococcal infection which includes any one of the following:		
• Positive throat culture for *Streptococcus*		
• Rapid antigen detection test		
• Elevated or increasing streptococcal antibody test (**ASO titer** > 200 Todd's unit in adults or > 300 Todd's unit children).		

1033. Which of the following is *false* regarding rheumatic nodules:

A. Found over extensor surface
B. Tender on palpation
C. Coincides with subsidence of rheumatic process
D. Pea size nodules

Features of Rheumatic Nodules

- Found almost exclusively in children;
- Found in 10-20% patients with active disease;
- Generally are a few millimeters in diameter:
- Persist for several days;
- Most numerous over bony prominences and extensor surfaces of large and small joints, scalp, ulnar border of forearm and spine;
- Their appearance usually coincides with subsidence of rheumatic process;
- They are hard, painless, **nontender**, nonpruritic and freely mobile.

1034. Which of the following is *not* a feature of classical migraine:

A. Hallucinations
B. No aura
C. Fortification spectrum
D. Scotomas

Migraine is defined as recurrent headache intercepted by symptom free intervals along with at least 3 of the following:

1. Abdominal pain
2. Nausea or vomiting
3. Throbbing headache
4. Unilateral headache
5. Aura (visual/sensory or motor)
6. Relieved by sleep
7. Positive family history

Migraine may be further classified into 4 categories:

- **Classical migraine** (Migraine *with* **aura**)-Aura precedes or accompany headache and **scotomas** and/or **hallucinations** occur in about 33% of patients. **Fortification spectrum** is a highly characteristic syndrome that occurs in about 10% of patients of classical migraine. It begins as a small para-central scotoma. This scotoma slowly expands into a "C" shape and luminous angles appear at the enlarging outer edge. These angles become colored as the scintillating scotoma expands and moves toward the periphery of the involved half of the visual field. It finally disappears over the horizon of peripheral vision and the entire process takes about 20 to 25 minutes. This phenomenon never occurs during the headache phase and is pathognomonic for migraine.

- **Common migraine** (Migraine *without* aura)-Manifested by headache, nausea, vomiting and photophobia.
- **Hemiplegic migraine**-Prolonged headache lasting for hours or days followed by hemiparesis, which resolves spontaneously.
- **Basilar migraine**-Occipital headache.

1035. Differential diagnosis of mitral stenosis includes:
A. Left atrial myxoma
B. Ebstein's anomaly
C. Aortico pulmonary window
D. All of the above

Differential Diagnosis of Mitral Stenosis

- Left atrial myxoma
- Austin Flint murmur
- Pulmonary venoocclusive disease
- Cor triatriatum
- Ostium secundum atrial septal defect

1036. Differential diagnosis of aortic stenosis includes all *except*:
A. Hypertrophic cardiomyopathy
B. Congestive cardiomyopathy
C. Left atrial myxoma
D. Heart block

Differential Diagnosis of Aortic Stenosis

- Hypertrophic cardiomyopathy
- Congestive cardiomyopathy
- Fixed subaortic stenosis
- Heart block

1037. Convulsions are commonly precipitated in chronic renal failure by:
A. Hyperkalemia
B. Hypokalemia
C. Hyponatremia
D. Hypomagnesemia

Neurological Features of CRF

Symptoms	Signs
• Drowsiness	• Intellectual deterioration
• Loss of concentration	• Hyperreflexia
• Tremor	• Loss of ankle jerk
• Convulsions	• Foot drop
• Restless and cramps in legs	• Deafness
• Paresthesia	• Sensory loss
• Wasting and weakness of legs and hands	• Coma

Hyponatremia or water intoxication lowers the osmolality of extracellular fluid, thus forcing the water to enter the neurons producing cerebral edema, which leads to convulsions. Stupor, seizures, and coma usually do not occur *unless* the plasma Na^+ concentration falls acutely below 120 mmol/L.

1038. In *adults* jaundice is clinically detectable in the sclera when the serum bilirubin concentration exceeds:
A. 1 mg%
B. 2 mg%
C. 5 mg%
D. 7 mg%

Jaundice can be clinically detected in adults when the serum bilirubin level exceeds 2.0 mg/dL and in newborn babies when the serum bilirubin level exceeds 7 mg/dL. Scleral tissue is rich in elastin and has a high affinity for bilirubin; therefore scleral icterus is a more sensitive sign of hyperbilirubinemia than generalized jaundice.

1039. Hamman-Rich syndrome is treated with:
A. Vitamin B_6
B. Vitamin B_{12}
C. Isoniazid
D. Steroids

Hamman-Rich syndrome or **idiopathic pulmonary fibrosis** is a diffuse inflammatory disease involving the gas exchanging tissue of lung leading to thickening and fibrosis of alveolar walls. **Oral corticosteroids are the drug of choice for this condition.** Oral prednisone is started in a dose of 1 mg/kg daily and given for about 8 weeks. If the condition improves then the dose is reduced to 0.25 mg/kg/day and given for 6 months. If condition does not responds to prednisone oral cyclophosphamide is an alternative.

1040. Which of the following is the *best* diagnostic method of confirming tuberculous peritonitis:

A. Culture of peritoneal fluid
B. Mantoux
C. Peritoneal biopsy
D. Upper GI contrast films

Tuberculous peritonitis: As the yield of direct smear and culture is low; a large volume of ascitic fluid should be cultured to increase the yield. **Peritoneal biopsy is the best method to establish the diagnosis**.

1041. Important toxicity of ethambutol is:

A. Jaundice
B. Epigastric pain
C. Retrobulbar neuritis
D. Skin rash

(UP 1997)

1042. Optic neuritis is a side effect of:

A. Rifampicin
B. Pyrazinamide
C. Ethambutol
D. PAS

Retrobulbar optic neuritis is the *only serious* side effect of this tuberculostatic drug. It occurs most frequently with daily doses of 25 mg per kg of body weight and after 2 months of therapy.

1043. Metyrapone inhibits:

A. 11b-hydroxylase
B. 21 B hydroxylase
C. Both
D. None

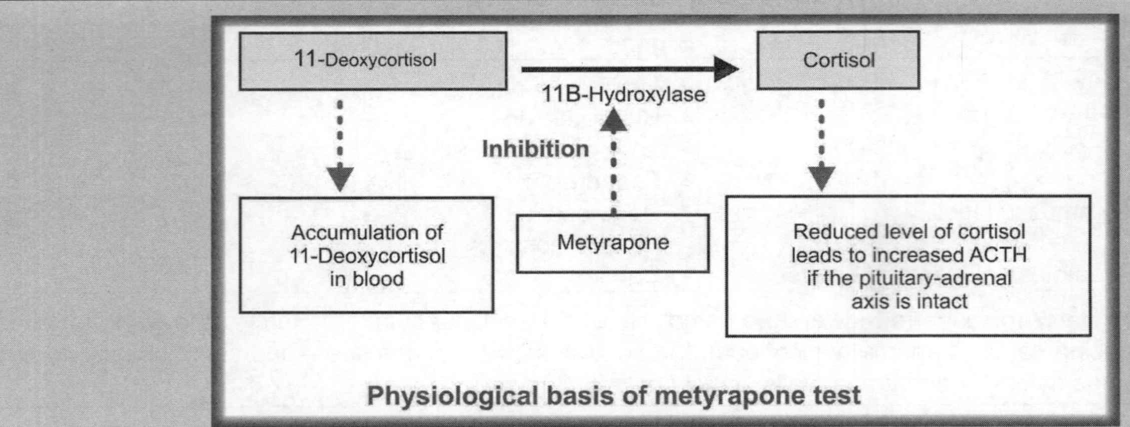

Physiological basis of metyrapone test

Metyrapone inhibits 11b-hydroxylase in the adrenal. It is used to test the integrity of the pituitary-adrenal axis in the "**metyrapone test**". As the enzyme 11b-hydroxylase is inhibited, conversion of 11-deoxycortisol to cortisol is impaired. This leads to accumulation of 11-deoxycortisol in blood and decline in blood levels of cortisol. The hypothalamic pituitary axis responds to decreased cortisol blood level by releasing more ACTH.

1044. Which of the following drugs *commonly* cause aplastic anemia:

A. Prednisolone
B. Penicillin
C. Minocycline
D. Chloramphenicol

Drugs and Chemicals Causing Aplastic Anemia

• Carbamazepine	• Phenylbutazone
• Carbimazole	• Phenytoin
• **Chloramphenicol**	• Potassium perchlorate
• Cytotoxics	• Quinacrine
• Felbamate	• Sulfonamides
• Gold salts	• Thiouracils
• Mepacrine	• Trimethadione
• Mephenytoin	• Zidovudine (AZT)
• Oxyphenbutazone	• Benzene
• Solvents	• Insecticides

1045. Renal papillary necrosis can be caused by:

A. Phenacetin **B.** Sulphonamides
C. Gentamicin **D.** Penicillin

Interstitial nephritis	Renal papillary necrosis
• Cephalosporins	• Phenacetin
• Ciprofloxacin	• Acetaminophen (paracetamol)
• Allopurinol	
• Furosemide	
• NSAID	
• Penicillins *especially* methicillin	
• Phenindione	
• Rifampicin	
• Sulphonamides	
• Thiazides	

1046. Which of the following is a form of dyskinesia:

A. Torsion dystonia **B.** Tics
C. Chorea **D.** All of the above

Different Types of Dyskinesia

• Tremor	• Chorea	• Myoclonus
• Tics	• Torsion dystonia	

Abnormal involuntary movements (dyskinesias) are of 5 types as shown in the table above. Each type of dyskinesia is caused by a variety of diseases. All dystonias disappear during sleep, made worse by anxiety and stress and improved by relaxation.

1047. Determination of FIGLU in urine demonstrates deficiency of:

A. Iron
B. Vitamin B_{12}
C. Folic acid
D. Pyridoxine *(UP 1997)*

FIGLU excretion is a test for folic acid deficiency. In this test, if histidine is administered to a patient with folic acid deficiency, the concentration of formiminoglutamic acid (FIGLU) is increased in urine.

1048. Niacin deficiency causes:

A. Dementia
B. Diarrhea
C. Dermatitis
D. All of the above

Niacin is also known as nicotinic acid / niacinamide / nicotinamide / pellagra preventing factor. Pellagra is a wasting disease due to deficiency of nicotinic acid, characterized by **dementia**, **diarrhea**, **dermatitis**, glossitis and stomatitis.

- **Remember 3 Ds of pellagra, i.e. dementia, diarrhea, dermatitis.**

1049. Normal TIBC is.......... microgram/dL:

A. 50-100 **B.** 150-250
C. 100-150 **D.** 300-350

1050. Iron is transported by:

A. Ferritin **B.** Apotransferrin
C. Transferrin **D.** Apoferritin *(KERALA 1996)*

Despite the fact that iron is the *second* most abundant metal in the earth's crust, iron deficiency is the world's *most common* cause of anemia. When it comes to life, iron is more precious than gold. The body hoards the element so effectively that over millions of years of evolution, humans have developed no physiological means of iron excretion and iron absorption is the sole mechanism by which iron stores are physiologically manipulated. The majority of iron (80%) is located within the red blood cells, myoglobin of muscle cells, and iron-containing enzymes. In the body, iron is stored as **ferritin** (a protein-iron complex) or hemosiderin. There are small amounts of ferritin found in blood circulation which is a good indicator of tissue ferritin stores. In the plasma, **iron is transported by transferrin** (a glycoprotein synthesized by the liver). Normally, about 1/3 of the transferrin is saturated by iron. Transferrin transfers iron to cells which utilize it for hemoglobin synthesis. Iron is absorbed from the gut (duodenum and to a lesser extent, the stomach, ileum, and colon) via two pathways. Iron that is derived from hemoglobin, myoglobin, and animal proteins is subjected to gastric acids which release it from the *apo*proteins and leave the heme. Heme is absorbed by the mucosal cells and degraded to release iron. Nonheme iron is absorbed utilizing three proteins.

PROTEIN	ACTIONS
Luminal mucins	Bind iron at acid pH of stomach, keeping it soluble
Integrin-like molecule	In duodenum mucosal cells, iron is bound and transported across the cell membrane
Mobilferrin	Cytosolic protein accepts iron within the cell and delivers it to ferritin or transferrin

The principal measurements of iron supply used in clinical diagnosis are the **serum iron (SI)**, the **transferrin iron-binding capacity (TIBC)**, and the serum ferritin level. The serum iron is a measure of the amount of iron bound to transferrin, while the TIBC is a measure of the total binding capacity of transferrin. *The normal serum iron should be between 50 and 150 μg/dL*; the **normal TIBC between 300 and 360 μg/dL.** It is also important to calculate the percent saturation of transferrin (**% saturation = SI ÷ TIBC**). A normal individual has a% saturation of between 30 and 50%. Iron-deficiency states are associated with saturation levels below 20%, while clinically dangerous iron *overload* occurs if the saturation exceeds 50 to 60%. **Ferritin** found in the circulation is in equilibrium with tissue ferritins. The serum measurement correlates with the level of total-body **iron stores**. The adult male has a serum ferritin level of 50 to 150 μg/L, while most adult women demonstrate levels between 15 and 50 μg/L. Once iron stores are depleted, the serum ferritin level declines to levels below 15 μg/L.

1051. In a patient with internuclear ophthalmoplegia, the lesion is *most likely* to be at the level of the:

A. Median longitudinal fasciculus **B.** Third nerve nucleus
C. Reticular activating system **D.** Lateral lemniscus *(AIIMS May 2002)*

Internuclear ophthalmoplegia results from damage to the **medial longitudinal fasciculus** (ascending from the abducens nucleus in the pons to the oculomotor nucleus in the midbrain-hence the term "internuclear").

1052. A patient has history of recurrent hemoptysis, truncal obesity and cushingoid habitus and has increased ACTH *not* suppressible by dexamethasone suppression test. Which of the following is *most likely* to be the diagnosis:

A. Adrenal adenoma
B. Pituitary tumor
C. Ectopic ACTH secreting tumor
D. Iatrogenic Cushing's syndrome *(AIIMS May 2002)*

Failure of dexamethasone administration to suppress cortisol production is seen in patients with adrenal hyperplasia secondary to an ACTH-secreting pituitary *macro*adenoma or an **ACTH-producing tumor of nonendocrine origin** and in those with adrenal neoplasms.

1053. *True* regarding adult polycystic kidney disease I and II respectively is:

A. Chromosome 16 and 5 **B.** Chromosome 16 and 4
C. Chromosome 11 and 5 **D.** Chromosome 21 and 18 *(PGI May 2001)*

Autosomal dominant polycystic kidney disease (ADPKD) has a prevalence of 1:300 to 1:1000 and accounts for about 10 percent of end stage renal disease (ESRD) in the USA. 3 forms of ADPKD have been identified. ADPKD-1 accounts for 90% of cases, and the gene has been localized to the short arm of chromosome 16. The gene for ADPKD-2 has been mapped to the short arm of chromosome 4. A third form has been documented but has not been mapped to a gene at this point.

1054. Anosmia is seen in:

A. Kallmann's syndrome **B.** Down syndrome
C. Turner syndrome **D.** Patau syndrome *(PGI May 2001)*

Congenital anosmias are *rare* but important. **Kallmann's syndrome** is a neuronal migration defect for which the X-linked gene (KAL) has been cloned and is characterized by congenital anosmia and hypogonadotropic hypogonadism.

1055. Kartagener's syndrome is associated with:

A. Bronchiectasis **B.** Situs inversus
C. Sinusitis **D.** All *(PGI May 2001)*

1056. In Kartagener's syndrome all are seen *except*:

A. Cystic fibrosis **B.** Dextrocardia
C. Sinusitis **D.** Absence of cilia

Just about 50% of patients with primary ciliary dyskinesia fall into the subgroup of *Kartagener's syndrome*, in which **situs inversus** accompanies **bronchiectasis** and **sinusitis**.

1057. Ultrastructural abnormalities reported in immotile cilia syndrome are:

A. Dynein deficiency **B.** Absence of radial spokes
C. Absence of central microtubule **D.** All of the above

Also known as immotile cilia syndrome, the **Kartagener's syndrome** consists of bronchiectasis, sinusitis and situs inversus. The basic defect is in ciliary motility due to structural abnormality of cilia (**absent** or irregular **dynein** arms, **absence of radial spokes** and **absence of central microtubule**).

1058. Which of the following is seen in ITP:

A. Thrombocytosis **B.** Increased prothrombin time
C. Increased bleeding time **D.** Increased clotting time *(AI 2002)*

Idiopathic thrombocytopenic purpura is an autoimmune disorder. It is of 3 types:

- Acute ITP
- Chronic ITP
- Relapsing ITP

In 70% of cases there is a history of rubella, rubeola or viral respiratory infection about 2 weeks prior to the onset of purpura. The disease begins with development of petechiae, ecchymosis and easy bruising. These are features of reduced platelet count. In pediatric age group boys and girls are equally affected unlike in adults where women are 5 times more commonly affected. Severe manifestations include hematuria, GI bleeding and epistaxis. Thrombocytopenia is the only abnormality found in CBC. **Bleeding time is prolonged**. Bone marrow examination reveals normal or increased number of megakaryocytes. Steroids are the drug of choice and prednisolone should be given in a dose of 2 mg/kg/day for 2 weeks and then tapered in another 2 weeks. Splenectomy should be done if the child continues to bleed despite treatment with steroids and IV IgG.

1059. Treatment of acute gout includes all *except*:

A. NSAID
B. Colchicine
C. Allopurinol
D. All of the above

- NSAIDs are the treatment of choice.
- Give indomethacin 50 mg qid or Naproxen 250 mg 8 hourly for 10 days.
- Colchicine 1mg stat followed by 0.5 mg two hourly is highly effective but may cause vomiting or diarrhea.

- Allopurinol is a xanthine oxidase inhibitor, which is used for long-term prophylaxis. Xanthine oxidase is an enzyme, which converts xanthine and hypoxanthine to uric acid, thus it lowers uric acid production. Dose is 300-900 mg OD. Colchincine—0.5 mg BD should be given in the beginning of treatment as **allopurinol may precipitate acute gout.**

1060. Postural tremors are seen in all *except*:

A. Benign essential familial tremor
B. Heavy metal poisoning
C. Lithium toxicity
D. Spinocerebellar degeneration

Causes of Tremor

Rest tremor	Postural tremor	Intention tremor
• Idiopathic Parkinson's disease • Postencephalitic parkinsonism • Drug induced parkinsonism	• Thyrotoxicosis • Benign essential familial tremor • Severe cerebellar lesion • Heavy metal poisoning • Lithium • Antidepressants • Sympathomimetics • Anxiety • Wilson's disease • Neurosyphilis • Alcohol	• Multiple sclerosis • Spinocerebellar degeneration • Vascular disease • Tumor

- Asterixis is also known as liver flap or flapping tremor. "It is a nonrhythmic, asymmetric lapse in voluntary sustained posture of the extremities, head, and trunk". It is not specific for hepatic encephalopathy and can occur in any type of metabolic encephalopathy.

1061. Which of the following is *not* a feature of hypothyroidism:

A. Myxedema
B. Carpal tunnel syndrome
C. Menorrhagia
D. Increased appetite

Features of Hypothyroidism

General	Dermatological	Neuromuscular	Cardiorespiratory
• Tiredness • Goiter • Somnolence • Weight gain • Cold intolerance • Hoarseness	• Dry and flaky skin • Alopecia • Purplish lips • Malar flush • Carotenemia • Vitiligo • Erythema ab igne (garny tartan) • Myxedema	• Myotonia • Cerebellar ataxia • Depression • Psychosis • Deafness • Carpal tunnel syndrome • Delayed relaxation of tendon reflex • Muscle stiffness and pains	• Bradycardia • Hypertension • Angina • Heart failure • Xanthelasma • Pleural effusion • Pericardial effusion
Reproductive	**Gastrointestinal**	**Hematological**	
• Menorrhagia • Infertility • Galactorrhea • Impotence	• Constipation • Ileus • Ascites	• Macrocytosis • Anemia	

1062. Pulsus paradoxus is *not* seen in:

A. Cardiac tamponade
B. Chronic obstructive airways disease
C. Chronic constrictive pericarditis
D. Intermittent positive pressure ventilation

Causes of Paradoxical Pulse

- Cardiac tamponade
- Constrictive pericarditis
- Chronic obstructive airways disease
- Restrictive cardiomyopathies
- Hypovolemic shock
- Severe bronchial asthma

1063. Chronicity is *least* common in:

A. Poststreptococcal glomerulonephritis
B. Membranous glomerulonephritis
C. Minimal change glomerulonephritis
D. Focal glomerulonephritis

Despite massive proteinurea renal functions remain normal in minimal change disease. 90% of children with MCD give rapid response to oral corticosteroids, although relapses may occur. Long-term prognosis is 'excellent' and even in steroid dependent patients disease usually resolves on puberty.

1064. Wermer's syndrome (multiple endocrine neoplasia type I) is characterized by all of the following *except*:

A. Tumors of anterior pituitary
B. Tumors of parathyroid
C. Pancreatic adenomas
D. Pheochromocytoma

Multiple endocrine neoplasia type-1 or Wermer's syndrome consists of:

1. Neoplasm of **p**arathyroid
2. Neoplasm of **p**ituitary
3. Neoplasm of **p**ancreatic islet cells.

- *This syndrome is inherited as an **autosomal dominant trait**.*

1065. Treatment of choice in *Taenia saginata* and *Taenia solium* infestation is:

A. Metronidazole
B. Niclosamide
C. Praziquantel
D. Albendazole

A single dose of praziquantel (5 to 10 mg/kg) is the drug of choice for *Taenia saginata* and *Taenia solium* infestation.

1066. Which of the following is *not* a feature of mumps:

A. Caused by paramyxovirus
B. Aseptic meningitis
C. Orchitis
D. Incubation period is less than 2 weeks

Mumps is an acute, systemic, communicable viral infection characterized by swelling (which is generally bilateral, although the onset on the two sides may *not* be synchronous) of one or both parotid glands. Mumps is caused by a **paramyxovirus**. Features of mumps are as under:

- Parotitis
- **Orchitis** and oophoritis
- Pancreatitis
- Submaxillary mumps
- **Aseptic meningitis**
- Juvenile diabetes
- Sublingual mumps
- Encephalitis
- Deafness

- The incubation period of mumps ranges from 14 to 18 days.

1067. *Most common* complication of mumps in adults is:

A. Otitis media
B. Orchitis
C. Myocarditis
D. Encephalitis

Apart from parotitis, **orchitis** is the most common complication of mumps in adults and is seen in about 20% of cases.

1068. Which is *true* regarding von Willebrand's disease:

A. Prolonged bleeding time
B. *Rare* inherited bleeding disorder
C. Autosomal recessive disease
D. All of the above

von Willebrand's disease is an autosomal dominant disease characterized by **prolonged bleeding time** and deficiency of factor VIII. It is the most common inherited bleeding disorder having an incidence of 1 in 800 to 1000 individuals.

1069. Carbamazepine is the *drug of choice* in:

A. Absence attacks
B. Complex partial seizures
C. Myoclonus
D. Infantile spasm

A Guideline for the Management of Focal Onset Seizure

First line drugs	Alternative drugs
• Carbamazepine • Phenytoin • Valproic acid	• Lamotrigine • Gabapentin • Phenobarbital • Primidone

Focal onset seizures consist of simple partial seizure, complex partial seizure and tonic clonic seizure with *secondary* generalization.

1070. When carbamazepine is administered one should avoid:

A. Sulphamethoxazole
B. Amoxycillin
C. Ceftriaxone
D. Erythromycin

Carbamazepine should not be used with erythromycin because erythromycin inhibits metabolism of carbamazepine.

1071. Which of the following is a highly emetic drug:

A. Cisplatin
B. Methotrexate
C. Vincristine
D. 5 fluorouracil

Cisplatin is a platinum coordination complex. It is a highly **emetic drug**. The most important toxicity is renal impairment, which is dependent of total dose administered. Maintaining good hydration can reduce this. Tinnitus, deafness, neuropathy and hyperuricemia are other problems. Shock like state sometimes occurs during IV infusion. *Other* drugs causing nausea and vomiting are as under:

- Digitalis
- Estrogens
- Ferrous sulfate
- Levo dopa
- Opiates
- Potassium chloride
- Tetracycline
- Theophylline

1072. Which of the following is seen in infectious mononucleosis:

A. Lymphocytosis
B. Thrombocytopenia
C. Increased serum transaminase
D. All of the above

Infectious mononucleosis: The TLC is usually elevated after the 5th day of disease and may be 10,000 to 20,000 per μ liter. **Lymphocytosis** is usually present, with > 10% atypical lymphocytes. Neutropenia and **thrombocytopenia** are common during the 1st month of disease. Liver function is abnormal in more than 90% of cases. **Serum levels of aminotransferases and alkaline phosphatase are mildly elevated**; the serum concentration of bilirubin is elevated in about 40% of patients.

1073. Pernicious anemia is due to:

A. Iron deficiency
B. Atrophic gastritis
C. Low folic acid
D. None

In pernicious anemia, the **gastric glands that contain parietal cells are destroyed**. Besides HCl, parietal cells also secrete intrinsic factor therefore type A **atrophic gastritis** also results in malabsorption of (*extrinsic factor*) vitamin B_{12}.

1074. Which of the following drug causes acute pancreatitis:

A. Valproic acid
B. Furosemide
C. 6-mercaptopurine
D. All of the above

Drugs Causing Acute Pancreatitis

Association is definite	Association is probable
• Azathioprine	• Acetaminophen
• Sulfonamides	• Nitrofurantoin
• Thiazide diuretics	• Methyldopa
• Furosemide	• Erythromycin
• Estrogens	• Salicylates
• Tetracycline	• Metronidazole
• Valproic acid	• NSAIDs
• Pentamidine	• ACE inhibitors
• Dideoxyinosine	
• 6-mercaptopurine	

1075. *Staphylococcus aureus* commonly inhabits:

A. Nasopharynx
B. Throat
C. Ear
D. Skin

The mucous membrane of the **anterior nasopharynx** is the principal site of carriage of *Staphylococcus aureus* in human beings. Other sites include the axillae, the vagina, and the perineum and occasionally the GI tract.

1076. Daily requirement of vitamin K in adult male is:

A. 20 to 50 microgram
B. 10 to 20 microgram
C. 45 to 80 microgram
D. More than 150 microgram

Daily Vitamin K Requirement

Category	Weight in Kg	Vitamin K, µg
Infants	6	5
	9	10
Children	13	15
	20	20
	28	30
Males	45	**45**
	66	**65**
	72	**70**
	79	**80**
	77	**80**
Females	46	45
	55	55
	58	60
	63	65
	65	65

1077. Antidote of choice in methyl alcohol poisoning is:

A. Atropine
B. PAM
C. Neostigmine
D. Ethanol

- Gastrointestinal decontamination is indicated soon after ingestion of methanol. Gastric lavage should be done by Ryle's tube insertion.
- Supportive measures must include volume replacement, respiratory care.
- Seizures should be treated by anticonvulsants.
- Acidosis should be corrected with sodium bicarbonate.
- **Ethanol therapy** is indicated in patients who are symptomatic.

1078. Thyroid dysfunction is caused by:

A. Amiodarone
B. Lithium
C. Phenytoin
D. All of the above

Drugs Causing Thyroid Dysfunction

- Acetazolamide
- Amiodarone
- Bromsulfophthalein
- Chlorpropamide
- Clofibrate
- Colestipol and nicotinic acid
- Dimercaprol
- Gold salts
- Iodides
- Lithium
- Oral contraceptives
- Phenindione
- Phenothiazines
- Phenylbutazone
- Phenytoin
- Sulfonamides
- Tolbutamide

1079. Fungal meningitis is caused by:

A. *Cryptococcus*
B. *Actinomycetes*
C. *Sporotrichosis*
D. All of the above

The fungus *Cryptococcus neoformans* causes cryptococcosis. It commonly leads to **meningoencephalitis**. This form of the infection is usually fatal without appropriate therapy. Clinical features include headache, nausea, staggering gait, dementia, irritability, confusion, and blurred vision. Both fever and nuchal rigidity are often mild or lacking thus making the diagnosis difficult. Papilledema is present in 33% of cases. Cranial nerve palsies, typically asymmetric, occur in about 25% of cases. With progression of the infection, deepening coma and signs of brainstem compression appear. Treatment schedule is as under:

- Patients with AIDS and cryptococcosis are treated initially with intravenous amphotericin B and later with fluconazole.
- In patients without AIDS, cryptococcosis should be treated with amphotericin B alone or in combination with flucytosine.

1080. In a patient of fever, nausea and mild pain in right hypochondrium, the most *probable* diagnosis is:

A. Viral hepatitis
B. Acute cholecystitis
C. Gastritis
D. Pleurisy

Acute cholecystitis begins with an attack of biliary colic. The pain is more generalized in the right upper abdomen. Peritoneal signs of inflammation such as increased pain with jarring or on deep respiration may be present. The patient has anorexia and nausea. Vomiting is more common and may produce symptoms and signs of vascular and extracellular volume depletion. Jaundice is rare early in the course of acute cholecystitis but may occur when edematous inflammatory changes involve the bile ducts and surrounding lymph nodes. A low-grade fever is present and shaking chills or rigors are common.

1081. *Treatment of choice* for typhoid carriers:

A. Chloramphenicol
B. Ciprofloxacin
C. Cholecystectomy
D. Ampicillin

A quinolone (**ciprofloxacin**) is a good choice for the treatment of long-term carriers of *Salmonella typhi*.

1082. Hypomagnesemia is caused by which of the following:

A. Alcoholism
B. Hyperthyroidism
C. Both
D. None

Principal Causes of Hypomagnesemia

- Ethanol
- Primary hyperaldosteronism
- Diabetes mellitus
- Hyperthyroidism
- Hyperparathyroidism
- Hypoparathyroidism

1083. Which is *false* regarding Eaton-Lambert syndrome:

A. Guanidine gives relief
B. Neostigmine also effective
C. Ptosis
D. Associated with oat cell carcinoma

Lambert-Eaton myasthenic syndrome (LEMS) occurs in association with either a malignancy or with autoimmune disease. It is characterized by:

- Weakness
- Myalgias
- Fatigability
- Ptosis
- Dysautonomic features
- The disorder afflicts men > women
- In most cases the tumor is small cell carcinoma of lung
- Guanidine hydrochloride and 3, 4-diaminopyridine are beneficial in either autoimmune or paraneoplastic LEMS. Plasma exchange and immunosuppression are also effective.

1084. *True* about Ludwig's angina is:

A. Caused by *Anaerobic streptococci*
B. A severe form of cellulitis
C. Originates from an infected mandibular molar
D. All of the above

Anaerobic streptococci, or *peptostreptococci*, are part of the normal flora of the oral cavity, bowel, and vagina. They are involved, usually along with other organisms, in brain abscess, sinusitis, dental abscess, and other odontogenic infections (*Ludwig's angina*, abscesses of the retropharyngeal or lateral pharyngeal space). **Ludwig's angina** is a severe form of cellulitis, which originates from an infected mandibular molar, involves the submandibular space, and extends throughout the floor of the mouth. This results in elevation of the tongue, dysphagia, and dyspnea. Glottal edema may occur, requiring emergency tracheotomy.

1085. The treatment of eosinophilic myositis is:

A. Steroids
B. Aspirin
C. Persantine
D. Hydralazine

Eosinophilic myositis is a *rare* disease which represents 1 feature of the spectrum of hypereosinophilic syndrome. Some patients respond to glucocorticoids, methotrexate, or leukapheresis.

1086. Which is the diagnostic test in pancreatic insufficiency:

A. Schilling test
B. Serum lipase
C. Serum amylase
D. Fecal fat estimation

The **Schilling test** is used in the diagnosis of patients with suspected pernicious anemia, but it can also be used as *a diagnostic test for pancreatic insufficiency*. In this test intrinsic factor (Co^{57}) cobalamin and Hog R protein (Co^{58}) cobalamin are given together. Because proteases are necessary to cleave R protein, the ratio of labeled cobalamin excreted in urine is an index of exocrine dysfunction. It is a time-consuming and expensive test.

1087. HLA linkage is seen in:
- **A.** IDDM
- **B.** NIDDM
- **C.** Secondary diabetes due to pancreatic disease
- **D.** Diabetes due to insulin antagonist

HLA Association of Endocrine Disorders

Disorder	HLA
• **IDDM**	BfF1,DR2, DR3,DR4
• **Hyperthyroidism**	B8, DR3
• **Adrenal insufficiency**	Dw3
• **Subacute thyroiditis**	B35
• **Hashimoto's thyroiditis**	DR5
• **Congenital adrenal hyperplasia**	B47

1088. Trace element *not* needed is:
- **A.** Chromium
- **B.** Molybdenum
- **C.** Magnesium
- **D.** Cesium

Element	Deficiency leads to
Mn	Bleeding disorder (due to increased prothrombin time)
Mo	Esophageal cancer
Cr	Impairment of glucose tolerance

1089. Risk of development of atherosclerosis is *inversely* proportional to:
- **A.** LDL levels
- **B.** VLDL levels
- **C.** Chylomicron level
- **D.** HDL levels

1090. Which of the following *decreases* the risk of atherosclerosis:
- **A.** LDL
- **B.** VLDL
- **C.** HDL
- **D.** Hypertriglyceridemia

There is an *inverse* relationship between the level of HDL cholesterol and the risk of coronary events. Factors affecting risk of atherosclerosis are summarized below:

Increasing risk of atherosclerosis	Decreasing risk of atherosclerosis
• LDL • VLDL • Hypertriglyceridemia	• HDL

1091. Sinus bradycardia is seen in:
- **A.** Typhoid fever
- **B.** Hypothyroid state
- **C.** Athletes
- **D.** All of the above

The normal sinus rate under basal conditions in adults is 60 to 100 beats per minute. **Sinus bradycardia** is defined as sinus rate less than 60 beats per minute, and sinus *tachycardia* when it is more than 100 beats per minute.

Important causes of sinus bradycardia

• Trained athletes	• Typhoid fever
• Normal elderly patients	• Hypothermia
• Hypothyroidism	• Advanced liver disease
• Brucellosis	• Vasovagal syncope
• Severe hypoxia	• Hypercapnia
• Acidosis	• Acute hypertension

1092. Hallucination of obnoxious smell occurs in lesion of ....lobe:

A. Frontal **B.** Parietal
C. Temporal **D.** Occipital

Olfactory hallucinations are seen when there is involvement of the uncus of the temporal lobe. Pituitary adenomas, craniopharyngiomas, suprasellar meningiomas, and aneurysms of the anterior part of the circle of Willis extending forward and damaging olfactory structures may result in olfactory hallucinations.

1093. The *highest* frequency wave in EEG is .... wave:

A. Alpha **B.** Beta
C. Gamma **D.** Theta

Frequencies of Various EEG Waves

EEG wave	Frequency
• **Delta**	< 4 Hertz
• **Theta**	4 to 7 Hertz
• **Alpha**	8 to 13 Hertz
• **Beta**	> 13 Hertz

Mnemonic: β is **b**est.

1094. External cardiac massage is usually done in the:

A. Lower 1/3 of sternum **B.** Xiphisternum
C. Middle of sternum **D.** Manubrium

Basic life support is also known as CPR. It consists of the following 3 important steps, which constitute the ABC of life:

- **A**irway, ensures that airway is clear and patient is in proper position.
- **B**reathing, if spontaneous breathing is not there, positive pressure ventilation should be started using an Ambu® bag with the help of a mask or *preferably* an endotracheal tube.
- **C**irculation is established by chest compression at the lower 1/3rd of sternum at a rate of 100/minute also known as external cardiac massage.

1095. Features of rheumatic carditis are all *except*:

A. Aschoff bodies **B.** Lymphatic infiltration
C. Myocardial fibrosis **D.** Intramyocardial microemboli

Aschoff bodies consist of foci of fibrinoid necrosis surrounded by **lymphocytes** and macrophages with occasional plasma cells. These bodies are pathognomic of rheumatic fever and are finally replaced by **fibrous scar**.

1096. Goldblatt hypertension is seen in:

A. Renovascular disease **B.** Drug induced
C. Adrenal medullar tumor **D.** Children

Sir Harry Goldblatt was a US physician. He experimentally deprived blood supply of a part of a dog's kidney that resulted in **hypertension** in that dog. This condition may also occur in humans as a result of vascular disease.

1097. Air embolism is diagnosed by:

A. Loud P2 **B.** Continuous murmur
C. Mill-wheel sound **D.** Crescendodecrescendo murmur

If air enters the vein in any quantity it will cause a hissing sound in the wound and go to the right heart and lung causing an air lock obstruction in pulmonary artery. A loud precordial murmur the so-called "**mill-wheel murmur**" is present. It has been suggested that this term should be replaced by "**squelching gum boot murmur**".

- *Squelch* is the sound of liquid, mud, slush, etc. moving under pressure or suction, as in wet shoes.

1098. Hepatic granulomas are caused by:

A. Sarcoidosis
B. Sulfonamides
C. Schistosomiasis
D. All of the above

Causes of Hepatic Granulomas

INFECTIONS	SYSTEMIC DISEASES	DRUGS
• Tuberculosis	• Sarcoidosis	• Sulfonamides
• *Mycobacterium avium intracellulare*	• Hodgkin's lymphoma	• Isoniazid
• Brucellosis	• Non-Hodgkin's lymphoma	• Allopurinol
• Leprosy	• Primary biliary cirrhosis	
• Epstein-Barr virus	• Berylliosis	
• Cytomegalovirus	• Crohn's disease	
• Chickenpox	• Wegener's granulomatosis	
• Schistosomiasis	• Granulomatous hepatitis	
• Q fever	• Idiopathic	
• Syphilis		

1099. Progressive dementia *without* focal motor signs is seen in:

A. Motor neuron disease
B. Alzheimer's disease
C. Parkinson's disease
D. Huntington's chorea

Alzheimer's disease is the *most common* cause of *pre*senile dementia. It generally begins after 45 years of age with memory loss and decline in intellect. Symptoms of focal cerebral disease may be prominent mainly aphasia and loss of topographical memory due to lesion of parietal lobe. Stooped posture is common **but focal *motor* signs such as hemiplegia do not occur**.

1100. Tubercular nephritis is characterized by:

A. Pus cells without organism in the acidic urine
B. Pus cell with organism in the acidic urine
C. Pus cell without organism in the alkaline urine
D. Pus cell with organism in the alkaline urine

Sterile pyuria indicates infection with unusual bacterial agents such as *C. trachomatis*, *U. urealyticum*, and *Mycobacterium tuberculosis* or with a fungus. It is also seen in noninfectious urologic conditions such as stones, anatomic abnormality, nephrocalcinosis, vesicoureteral reflux, interstitial nephritis and polycystic disease. Urinalysis gives abnormal results in 90% of cases, revealing pyuria and hematuria. **The demonstration of culture-negative pyuria in acidic urine should raise the suspicion of tuberculosis.** An IVP is helpful in diagnosis. Culture of 3 morning urine specimens yields a definitive diagnosis in *majority* of cases.

1101. Which of the following combination is *not* synergistic:

A. Penicillin and streptomycin in endocarditis
B. Amphotericin B and flucytosine in cryptococcal meningitis
C. Penicillin and tetracycline in pneumococcal meningitis
D. Sulphamethoxazole and trimethoprim in UTI

Synergistic activity—Against some bacteria, 2 antibacterial agents are more active than 1. Synergistic activity is defined as *"a lowering of the minimal inhibitory concentration of each of 2 drugs tested in combination against a specific bacterium"*. The combination of trimethoprim and sulphamethoxazole has synergistic activity against many gram-negative bacteria. Most other antimicrobial combinations show indifferent activity (i.e. the combination is no better than the more active of the two agents alone), and **some combinations (e.g. penicillin plus tetracycline against pneumococci) may be antagonistic (i.e. the combination is worse than either drug alone).** The reason for this is that penicillin acts only on *rapidly dividing* bacteria by inhibiting their cell wall formation leading to lysis of bacteria by osmotic pressure. As tetracycline is a bacteriostatic drug, it stops bacterial division, thus nullifying the action of penicillin.

1102. Which of the following is *not* a feature of Bartter's syndrome:

A. Hypertension
B. Hypokalemia
C. Polyuria
D. Autosomal recessive inheritance

Features of Juxtaglomerular Hyperplasia (Bartter's Syndrome)

- Hypokalemia
- Normal to low blood pressure
- Autosomal recessive
- Failure to thrive
- Renal potassium wasting
- Metabolic alkalosis
- Weakness
- Polyuria

1103. Pericarditis in rheumatoid arthritis is:

A. Serous
B. Fibrinous
C. Serofibrinous
D. Adhesive

Clinically apparent heart disease attributed to the rheumatoid process is a *rare* possibility. But evidence of **serofibrinous pericarditis is found at autopsy in 50% of the cases**. Glucose level in pericardial fluid is low and is often associated with the occurrence of pleural effusion. Chronic constrictive pericarditis also may occur rarely.

1104. Leonine facies is seen in which disease:

A. Leprosy
B. Syphilis
C. Jaws
D. Trypanosomiasis

Advanced *un*treated and polar lepromatous **leprosy** may result in development of so called **leonine facies**. It consists of partial collapse of nose, nasal congestion and loss of eyebrows (madarosis).

1105. Chloroma is associated with:

A. Dehydration
B. Myelogenous leukemia
C. Melanoma
D. Wilms' tumor

In **AML** any extramedullary site may be infiltrated by the leukemic cells. Tumor like accumulations within soft tissue or bone is known as **chloromas** (due to their green color). They are more common with M_1 and M_2 variety. *Chloro = green (e.g. chlorophyll).*

1106. Black urine is seen in:

A. Porphyria
B. Rifampicin
C. Pyridium
D. Alkaptonuria

• **Yellow or orange urine**	Jaundice, sulfasalazine, rifampicin, thiamine
• **Red urine**	Porphyria, hemoglobinuria, myoglobinuria, pyridium
• **Dark brown or black urine**	Ochronosis (Alkaptonuria), melanoma

1107. The treatment of geographic tongue is:

A. Scrapping
B. Vitamin B_1
C. Vitamin B_{12}
D. Nothing

Geographic tongue (benign migratory glossitis or wandering rash) is an asymptomatic inflammatory condition of the tongue caused by rapid loss and regrowth of filiform papillae, leading to appearance of denuded red patches "wandering" across the surface of the tongue. **No treatment is required.**

1108. Angular oral fissures are treated with:

A. Riboflavin
B. Pyridoxine
C. Cyanocobalamin
D. Vitamin C

Features of Riboflavin Deficiency

• Sore throat	• Angular stomatitis	• Normochromic, normocytic anemia
• Edema of the oral mucous membranes	• Glossitis	• Hyperemia of the oral mucous membranes
• Cheilosis	• Seborrheic dermatitis	

1109. Temperature regulation is mostly controlled by:
- **A.** Pons
- **B.** Medulla
- **C.** Thalamus
- **D.** Hypothalamus

• **Reflex responses activated by warmth**	Anterior hypothalamus
• **Reflex responses activated by cold**	Posterior hypothalamus

1110. Progressive dysphagia is seen in:
- **A.** Carcinoma esophagus
- **B.** Globus hystericus
- **C.** Presbycusis
- **D.** Achalasia

Progressive dysphagia and weight loss of short duration are the early symptoms in a large number of patients of **carcinoma esophagus**. Dysphagia may be associated with pain on swallowing, pain radiating to the chest or back, regurgitation or vomiting, and aspiration pneumonia.

1111. Hutchinson's pupil is:
- **A.** Seen in syphilis
- **B.** Unilateral constricted pupil
- **C.** Irregular pupil
- **D.** Argyll Robertson pupil

Hutchinson's pupil is a condition in which 1 pupil is dilated while the other is not. The pupil on the side of the lesion is dilated and the other is contracted. This condition occurs due to compression of the 3rd cranial nerve for example in meningitis.

1112. Echolalia is a disorder of:
- **A.** Speech
- **B.** Mood
- **C.** Perception
- **D.** Personality

Echolalia is a disorder of speech in which the patient 'parrots' the fragments of heard conversations.

1113. Factor deficiency in Christmas disease is:
- **A.** II
- **B.** VII
- **C.** VIII
- **D.** IX

1114. Christmas disease is treated by:
- **A.** FF plasma
- **B.** FF blood
- **C.** Antibiotics
- **D.** Steroids

Factor IX deficiency is also known as hemophilia B or **Christmas disease**. It occurs in 1 in 1 lakh male babies. **Fresh frozen plasma** or a plasma fraction enriched in the prothrombin complex proteins is used to control bleeding.

1115. Sweaty feet syndrome is associated with:
- **A.** G6PD deficiency
- **B.** Isovaleric acidemia
- **C.** Branched chain ketonuria
- **D.** Phenylalanine deficiency

Isovaleric acidemia is an inherited (autosomal recessive) metabolic disease affecting leucine metabolism due to deficiency of Isovaleryl CoA dehydrogenase. Isovaleric acid accumulates in the blood during periods of increased amino acid metabolism producing a characteristic **sweaty feet odor**. Death may occur.

1116. Dementia is seen in:

A. Alzheimer's disease
B. Creutzfeldt-Jakob disease
C. Huntington's disease
D. All

Some Causes of Dementia

- Alzheimer's disease
- Huntington's disease
- Familial Creutzfeldt-Jakob disease
- Fatal familial insomnia
- Gerstmann-Straussler-Scheinker disease

1117. Recurrent painful orogenital ulcerations with arthritis are seen in:

A. Gonorrhea
B. Reiter's disease
C. Syphilis
D. Behçet's syndrome

Behçet's syndrome is a multisystem, chronic, recurrent disease marked by ulceration of the mouth and genitalia and by iritis, uveitis, arthritis, and thrombophlebitis. Recurrent painful orogenital ulceration is the most important feature of this syndrome.

1118. Volume of air taken into the lungs in normal respiration is known as:

A. Vital capacity
B. Timed vital capacity
C. Tidal volume
D. Inspiratory reserve volume

Various Lung Volumes

• **Tidal volume**	The amount of air which moves into the lung with each inspiration (or which comes out with each expiration)
• **Inspiratory reserve volume**	The excess air above the tidal volume which can be inspired with maximum inspiratory effort.
• **Expiratory reserve volume**	It is the volume of air that can be expelled by an active expiratory effort after passive expiration
• **Residual volume**	It is the volume of air that is left in lung after maximum expiratory effort.
• **Vital capacity**	The maximum amount of air that can be expired after a maximum inspiratory effort.
• **FEV 1**	Fraction of vital capacity expired in one second.

1119. The drug *not* used in donovanosis is:

A. Sulphonamide
B. Tetracycline
C. Penicillin
D. Streptomycin

Disease	**Organism**	**Drugs**
Donovanosis (granuloma inguinale)	*Calymmatobacterium granulomatis*	Tetracycline, erythromycin, quinolones, gentamicin, chloramphenicol, azithromycin, ceftriaxone, trimethoprim-sulfamethoxazole

*Streptomycin, once commonly used for this condition, is not widely used nowadays.

1120. Drug *not* used in herpes infection:

A. Acyclovir
B. Vinblastine
C. Vidarabine
D. Idoxuridine

Drugs Useful in HSV Infection

Mucocutaneous infections	HSV eye infections	HSV encephalitis
• Acyclovir • Famciclovir • Valacyclovir	• Idoxuridine • Trifluorothymidine • Vidarabine • Cidofovir	• IV Acyclovir

1121. The features of Weber's syndrome include:

A. 7th cranial nerve palsy **B.** 8th cranial nerve palsy
C. 3rd cranial nerve palsy **D.** Paraplegia

1122. Ipsilateral 3rd nerve palsy with contralateral hemiplegia with *tremors* is known as:

A. Millard-Gubler syndrome **B.** Benedict's syndrome
C. Weber's syndrome **D.** Foville's syndrome

Syndrome	Lesion	Features
• **Weber's syndrome**	Midbrain	Ipsilateral 3rd nerve palsy with contralateral hemiplegia
• **Benedict's syndrome**	Midbrain	Ipsilateral 3rd nerve palsy with contralateral hemiplegia with *tremors*.
• **Medial medullary syndrome**	Medulla	Contralateral hemiplegia and loss of sense of position and vibration with ipsilateral flaccid tongue weakness
• **Millard-Gubler syndrome**	Pons	Ipsilateral 6th,7th nerve palsy with crossed hemiplegia
• **Foville's syndrome**	Pons	MGS + Gaze palsy

1123. AIDS is caused by ....virus:

A. CMV **B.** EBV
C. Human T cell virus type I **D.** HTLV-III

In 1983, human immunodeficiency virus (HIV) was 1st isolated from a patient with lymphadenopathy, and by 1984 it was established to be the causative agent of AIDS. The virus belongs to the lentivirus subfamily of family retroviridae was previously called lymphadenopathy associated virus (LAV) or human T lymphotropic virus (HTLV-III).

1124. Which of the following is *not* predisposed to by contraceptive therapy:

A. Carcinoma breast **B.** Hepatic adenomas
C. Thromboembolism **D.** Budd-Chiari syndrome

Complications of Contraceptive Therapy

- Thromboembolism
- Hepatic adenoma
- Budd-Chiari syndrome
- Hepatocellular carcinoma

1125. *Most common* presenting feature of bladder carcinoma is:

A. Painless profuse intermittent hematuria
B. Dysuria
C. Clot colic
D. Sterile acid pyuria

Hematuria is the 1st sign of bladder cancer in 80 to 90% of patients, followed by urinary frequency or irritative symptoms.

1126. Which of the following disease increase the risk of active tuberculosis:

A. Sarcoidosis
B. Leprosy
C. Silicosis
D. Rheumatoid arthritis

Conditions Known to Increase the Risk of 'Active' Tuberculosis among Persons Infected with Tubercle Bacilli

- Silicosis
- Hemophilia
- Insulin-dependent diabetes mellitus
- Jejunoileal bypass surgery
- Gastrectomy
- Lymphoma
- Chronic renal failure
- Immunosuppressive treatment
- Malignant neoplasms
- Leukemia
- Hemodialysis

1127. The normal respiratory quotient of fat is:

A. 0.5
B. 0.9
C. 0.7
D. 1.0

Respiratory quotient may be defined as the ratio of volume of CO_2 produced to the volume of O_2 consumed per unit time. It is also known as respiratory exchange ratio. RQ of carbohydrate is 1 and that of fat is 0.7.

1128. HLA associated with hemochromatosis:

A. B 27
B. A
C. DW 5
D. B 14

HLA Association of Hematological Diseases

Disease	HLA
• **Idiopathic hemochromatosis**	A3 , B14
• **Pernicious anemia**	DR 5
• **Hodgkin's disease**	DP3,DP4

1129. Bence Jones proteins are excreted in the urine in:

A. Multiple myeloma
B. Waldenstrom's macroglobulinemia
C. Both
D. None

Bence Jones protein is a protein that occurs in the urine of patients with multiple myeloma and occasionally in patients with other diseases of the reticuloendothelial system. When urine samples are heated to 50°C to 60°C, a precipitate is formed. It dissolves when the urine is boiled and reappears when the urine cools. It may be found in the following conditions:

- Multiple myeloma
- Heavy chain diseases
- Waldenstrom's macroglobulinemia
- Primary amyloidosis

1130. Parasites causing lung injury include:

A. Strongyloides
B. Paragonimus
C. Both
D. None

Paragonimus: Adult flukes reside mainly in the lungs, but ectopic localization is relatively common.
Strongyloidiasis: First of all filariform larvae in soil contaminated with fecal matter penetrate the skin or mucous membranes. The larvae travel through the bloodstream to the lungs, where they break into the alveolar spaces, ascend the bronchial tree, are swallowed, and reach the small intestine.

1131. Mad as a hatter refers to.............poisoning:

A. Arsenic
B. Cadmium
C. Mercury
D. Selenium

Acute inhalation of **mercury** vapor can cause neurologic toxicity which is manifested by tremors, emotional liability, headaches, and polyneuropathy. Chronic exposure to metallic mercury produces a characteristic intention tremor, a group of findings including excitability, memory loss, insomnia, timidity, and delirium that was first described in workers with occupational exposure in the felt-hat industry-therefore the name **"mad as a hatter".**

☺ Hatter is a person who designs, makes, trims, or sells women's hats. Hatters became disoriented, or "mad," from nerve-destroying mercury salts used to treat felt fabric hence the term "mad as a hatter".

1132. Clonidine is indicated in all *except*:

A. Morphine withdrawal **B.** Migraine
C. Hypertension **D.** Cardiac arrhythmias

Indications of Clonidine

- Hypertension
- Dysmenorrhea
- Menopausal flushing
- Opioid (narcotic) abstinence syndrome
- Nicotine dependence
- Gilles de la Tourette's syndrome
- Migraine prophylaxis

1133. ABO hemolytic disease of newborn occurs when the blood group of mother is:

A. A **B.** B
C. AB **D.** O

ABO incompatibility occurs in type A or B newborns of **type O mothers** because they (mother) produce anti-A and anti-B antibodies of IgG type which cross the placenta and destroy fetal RBCs. Type A and B mother produce anti-A and anti-B antibodies of IgM class which does not cross placenta and do not produce ABO incompatibility.

1134. Heel pad thickness is useful in:

A. Hyperthyroidism **B.** Acromegaly
C. PEM **D.** Hypogonadism

Soft tissue X-rays of patients of **acromegaly** demonstrate increased thickness of the heel pad (> 18 mm in women and > 21 mm in men).

1135. Acromegaly is characterized by all *except*:

A. Diabetes
B. Enlarged nasal sinuses
C. Muscular hypertrophy
D. Increased heel pad thickness

Growth hormone excess results in **acromegaly**, which is a chronic, debilitating disease associated with **bony and soft tissue overgrowth**. Soft tissue X-rays of these patients demonstrate **increased thickness of the heel pad** (>18 mm in women and >21 mm in men). Patients with associated **diabetes** mellitus have increased mortality.

1136. Diabetes insipidus is treated with:

A. Thiazides **B.** Desmopressin
C. Both **D.** None

Desmopressin has a prolonged antidiuretic activity and is completely devoid of pressor effects of vasopressin. When given *intranasally* in dose of 10 and 20 μ grams it exerts an antidiuretic action for 10 to 24 hours. **Desmopressin is the drug of choice in the treatment of patients with diabetes insipidus.** The only way to treat patients with nephrogenic diabetes insipidus is by solute restriction and the administration of **thiazides**.

1137. Testosterone is secreted by:

A. Leydig cells
B. Germ cells
C. Sertoli cells
D. Adrenal medulla

Testosterone is secreted by Leydig cells.

1138. *Raised* platelet count may be found in:

A. Postoperative period
B. Acute hemorrhage
C. Splenectomized patients
D. All of the above

Platelets are acute-phase reactants, and patients with systemic inflammation, tumors, **bleeding**, **postoperative stress**, **splenectomy** and mild iron deficiency have an increased platelet count. It is a benign condition called secondary or reactive thrombocytosis.

1139. Visceral larva migrans is caused by:

A. *Toxocara canis*
B. *Ancylostoma braziliensis*
C. Strongyloidiasis
D. Filariasis

Visceral larva migrans is a syndrome caused by nematodes in human hosts that are normally parasitic for nonhuman host species. In humans, the nematode larvae do not typically develop into adult worms but instead migrate through host tissues and produce eosinophilic inflammation. The **most common form of visceral larva migrans is toxocariasis** due to larvae of the *Toxocara canis* or, less commonly, the *Toxocara cati*.

1140. Drug induced neutrophilia is *not* seen with:

A. Glucocorticoids
B. Lithium
C. NSAIDs
D. Alpha methyl dopa

Some Causes of Neutrophilia

- Glucocorticoids
- NSAIDs
- Lithium
- Bacterial infection
- Fungal infection
- Viral infection

1141. Clot solubility in 5M urea is a test of:

A. Factor 13
B. Factor 12
C. Platelet function
D. Plasmin inhibitor

5 M urea test is a test for **factor XIII-dependent fibrin cross-linking**. It should be done when the PT and PTT are *both* normal but there is a strong history of bleeding.

1142. Patients with lymphedema are prone to recurrent cellulitis with:

A. *Staphylococcus aureus*
B. *Streptococcus pyogenes*
C. *Escherichia coli*
D. *Proteus mirabilis*

Streptococci are responsible for recurrent cellulitis among patients with chronic lymphedema resulting from elephantiasis, lymph node dissection, or Milroy's disease. Recurrent staphylococcal cutaneous infections are more common among individuals who have eosinophilia and elevated serum levels of IgE **(Job's syndrome)** and among nasal carriers of staphylococci.

1143. *Non*oliguric renal failure is commonly seen in:

A. Snake bite
B. Hypovolemic shock
C. Aminoglycoside toxicity
D. Myeloma

Aminoglycosides are responsible for nonoliguric renal failure. Streptomycin is *least* toxic while other commonly used aminoglycosides are more commonly implicated.

1144. Acute myeloblastic leukemia (AML) is characterized by:
- **A.** Auer rods in blast cells
- **B.** Philadelphia chromosome
- **C.** High leukocyte alkaline phosphatase
- **D.** Peak incidence in childhood

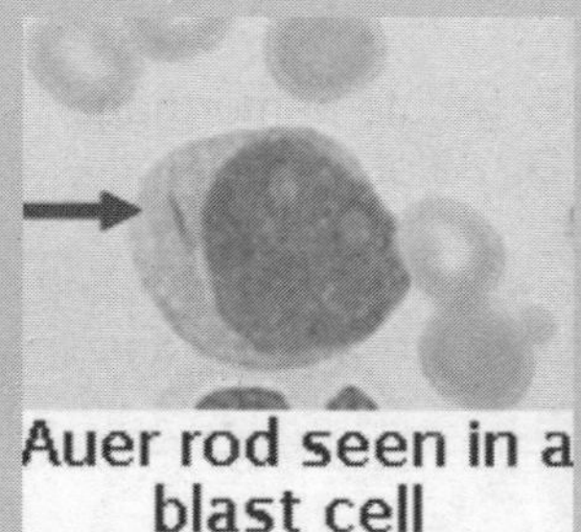
Auer rod seen in a blast cell

The diagnosis of AML is established by the presence of at least 30% myeloblasts in blood and/or bone marrow. Myeloblasts have nuclear chromatin that is uniformly fine or lacelike in appearance and large nucleoli (2 to 5 / cell). Specific cytoplasmic granules, **Auer rods**, or the nuclear folding and cleft formation are characteristic of AML.

1145. Digitalis given to atrial flutter often produces:
- **A.** Atrial fibrillation
- **B.** Atrial tachycardia
- **C.** Atrial asystole
- **D.** Atrial bigeminy

A characteristic pharmacological property of **digitalis** is that it reduces conduction of impulse at AV node and promotes conduction in atrial and ventricular conduction systems. Thus the result of using digitalis in a patient of atrial flutter is that it converts it into **atrial fibrillation**.

1146. A patient with spontaneous pneumothorax involving more than 50% of hemithorax is best treated with:
- **A.** Needle aspiration
- **B.** Closed drainage by tube in underwater seal
- **C.** Let spontaneous remission occurs
- **D.** Open thoracotomy

Development of spontaneous pneumothorax involving more than 50% of hemithorax is a medical emergency and warrants immediate closed drainage by tube in underwater seal.

1147. In a patient with liver cirrhosis factors pointing towards an alcoholic etiology include:
- **A.** Peripheral neuropathy
- **B.** Splenomegaly
- **C.** Hepatitis B surface antigen
- **D.** Macronodular cirrhosis

Alcoholic cirrhosis, also known as Laennec's cirrhosis, is the most common type of cirrhosis encountered in the western countries .It is characterized by diffuse fine scarring; fairly uniform loss of liver cells, and small regenerative nodules, and therefore it is sometimes referred to as **micronodular cirrhosis**. Some times alcoholic cirrhosis may progress to macronodular cirrhosis. Chronic intake of high doses of alcohol causes **peripheral neuropathy in 5 to 15% of alcoholics**, which is due to thiamine deficiency.

1148. Xylose absorption tests are good screening test for:
- **A.** Fat absorption
- **B.** Pernicious anemia
- **C.** Carbohydrate absorption
- **D.** Amino acid absorption

D-Xylose absorption is a good screening test for carbohydrate malabsorption. In this test 25 g of oral D-xylose is given. 5 hour urinary excretion should be more than 4.5 gm with peak blood level more than 30 mg/dL.

1149. The contraindications of amantadine include all *except*:

A. Heart failure
B. Severe renal disease
C. History of convulsion
D. Pregnancy

Contraindications of Amantadine

- Hypersensitivity
- Seizure disorder
- Congestive heart failure
- Renal failure
- Peptic ulcer
- Psychosis

1150. Which of the following is *not* an adverse effect of phenytoin:

A. Gum hyperplasia
B. Osteomalacia
C. Gynecomastia
D. Megaloblastic anemia

Side Effects of Phenytoin

Neurologic	Systemic
• CNS depression • Ataxia • Confusion • In coordination	• Lymphadenopathy • Osteomalacia • Skin rash • Facial coarsening • Hirsutism • Gum hyperplasia • Arrhythmia • Circulatory collapse • Hypotension • Insomnia • Megaloblastic anemia

1151. Myasthenia gravis is characterized by all of the following *except*:

A. Proximal muscle involvement
B. Fatigue with exertion
C. Spontaneous regression sometimes
D. Absent deep reflexes

The limb weakness in myasthenia gravis is often *proximal* and asymmetric. Although there is muscle weakness, **deep tendon reflexes are often preserved.**

1152. Myasthenia gravis is usually associated with:

A. Hyperparathyroidism
B. Thymoma
C. Thyroid adenoma
D. *Salmonella* infection

Myasthenia gravis is associated with tumors or hyperplasia of the thymus gland in about 15% cases.

1153. Myasthenia gravis is associated with:

A. Thymoma
B. Ca lung
C. Red cell aplasia
D. Glucagonoma

Diseases Associated with Myasthenia Gravis

- Thymoma
- Hyperplasia
- Skin disorders
- Thyroiditis
- Graves' disease
- Rheumatoid arthritis
- Lupus erythematosus

1154. Aggravation of myasthenia is a feature of all of the following drugs *except*:

A. Gentamicin
B. Neomycin
C. Edrophonium
D. Succinylcholine

Drugs Aggravating Myasthenia Gravis

- Aminoglycosides
- D-Penicillamine
- Polymyxins
- Succinylcholine

1155. Lipofuscin, the golden yellow pigment is seen in heart muscle:

A. Hypertrophy
B. Atrophy
C. Hyperplasia
D. Infarction

Lipofuscin is an insoluble lipid pigments found in cardiac and smooth muscle cells. It is also called aging pigment. This is seen in cells undergoing **atrophy**. Its presence is not injurious to the cell.

1156. Mode of action of streptokinase:

A. Antiplatelet action
B. Anticoagulant
C. Vasodilator
D. Fibrinolytic

Streptokinase combines with circulating plasminogen to form plasmin which converts insoluble fibrin to soluble fibrin fragments (fibrinolysis).

1157. Hyperglycemia is caused by all *except*:

A. Fluconazole
B. Furosemide
C. Glucocorticoids
D. Phenytoin

Drugs Causing Hyperglycemia

- Glucocorticoids
- Growth hormone
- Niacin
- Oral contraceptives
- Phenytoin
- Pentamidine
- Thiazides
- Asparaginase
- Chlorthalidone
- Diazoxide
- Encainide
- Ethacrynic acid
- Furosemide

1158. Pulsating tinnitus is seen in:

A. Glomus jugulare tumor
B. Glioma of frontal lobe
C. Tuberculoma in occipital lobe
D. Lithium toxicity

The differential diagnosis of **pulsatile tinnitus** includes vascular tumors such as **glomus jugulare tumors**, aneurysms, and stenotic lesions.

1159. Grey baby syndrome is caused by:

A. Tetracycline
B. Cotrimoxazole
C. Chloramphenicol
D. Amoxycillin

Grey baby syndrome is caused by chloramphenicol if it is given to newborns in high doses (>100mg/kg/day). It is due to inability of newborn to metabolize and excrete chloramphenicol leading to its accumulation.

1160. Klüver-Bucy syndrome is characterized by:

A. Rage reactions
B. Loss of recognition of people
C. Loss of fear
D. All of the above

Klüver-Bucy syndrome is a behavioral syndrome which usually follows bilateral temporal lobe removal. It is characterized by **loss of recognition of people, loss of fear, rage reactions,** hyper sexuality, memory deficit, and overreaction to certain stimuli.

1161. Angiotensinogen is synthesized in the:

A. Liver
B. Lungs
C. Kidneys
D. Adrenals

Angiotensinogen is an α_2 globulin which is synthesized in **liver.**

1162. Deletion of chromosome 22 occurs in 90% of:

A. Meningioma
B. Retinoblastoma
C. Neuroblastoma
D. Wilms' tumor

Solid tumors	Chromosomal region affected
• Wilms' tumor	11p13
• Germ cell tumors, testis	12p
• Retinoblastoma	13q14
• Meningioma	22q
• Neuroblastoma	1p31 to 3p36

1163. The antihypertensive which causes gingival hyperplasia is:

A. Metoprolol
B. Hydralazine
C. Nifedipine
D. Sodium nitroprusside

Gingival hyperplasia is an uncommon side effect of amlodipine. Other calcium channel blocking agents, such as diltiazem, felodipine, verapamil, and, most commonly, **nifedipine can also cause gingival hyperplasia.**

1164. Deficiency of which vitamin is associated with hyposmia:

A. Vitamin A
B. Vitamin B_6
C. Vitamin D
D. Vitamin B_{12}

The epithelial degeneration due to vitamin A deficiency causes anosmia.

1165. Deficiency of which metal is associated with hyposmia:

A. Zinc
B. Iron
C. Chromium
D. Magnesium

Profound **zinc** deficiency can results in losses and distortion of the sense of smell.

1166. Malabsorption of amino acids is seen in:

A. Homocystinuria
B. Alkaptonuria
C. Phenylketonuria
D. Cystinuria

Cystinuria is the *most common* inborn error of amino acid transport. **It is characterized by impaired tubular reabsorption and excessive urinary excretion of the amino acids cystine, ornithine, lysine and arginine.** A similar transport defect is also present in the intestinal mucosa.

Mnemonic: **cola**

1167. Calcium channel blocker with *maximum* peripheral actions:

A. Verapamil
B. Diltiazem
C. Nifedipine
D. Lisinopril

Relative Peripheral Actions of CCBs

Diltiazem	+
Verapamil	++
Nifedipine	+++

1168. Intestinal parasitic disease in immunocompromised patient is:

A. Strongyloides **B.** Ascaris
C. Trichuris **D.** Hookworm

In immunocompromised hosts, large numbers of strongyloides larvae can disseminate widely and this can be fatal.

1169. Dysgeusia is seen with the use of:

A. Cotrimoxazole **B.** Clotrimazole
C. Ciprofloxacin **D.** Captopril

Total hypogeusia	Decreased sensitivity to all tastants.
Partial hypogeusia	Decreased sensitivity to some tastants.
Dysgeusia	Distortion in the perception of a tastant, i.e. the perception of the wrong quality when a tastant is presented or the perception of a taste when there has been no tastant ingested.
Side effects of captopril	
• Diarrhea • Fatigue	• Dysgeusia • Nausea

1170. Treatment of traveler's diarrhea (watery diarrhea, no blood in stool or fever, 1-2 unformed stools per day with distressing enteric symptoms) is:

A. Sulfamethoxazole **B.** Loperamide
C. Metronidazole **D.** Chloramphenicol and streptomycin

In traveler's diarrhea having watery diarrhea without blood in stool + distressing abdominal pain/fever + > 2 unformed stools per day, treatment is **antibacterial drug + loperamide**.

1171. There is no correlation between X-ray appearance and clinical state of the patient in ....pneumonia:

A. *Mycoplasma* **B.** Pneumococcal
C. Friedlander's **D.** Staphylococcal

Clinical, radiologic, and laboratory findings in *Mycoplasma pneumoniae* infections are not specific and do not serve as a basis for an accurate diagnosis.

1172. Hepatic enzyme inducers are all *except*:

A. Phenobarbitone **B.** Phenytoin
C. Valproic acid **D.** Carbamazepine

Some Hepatic Enzyme Inducers

• Barbiturates	• Chloral hydrate	• Ethanol
• Phenytoin	• Rifampicin	• Tobacco
• Carbamazepine	• Griseofulvin	• Phenylbutazone

1173. Mechanism of action of quinidine is:

A. Potassium channel blocker **B.** Sodium channel blocker
C. Calcium channel blocker **D.** Chloride channel blocker

Mechanism of action of quinidine is by **decreasing the number of Na^+ channels** and preventing their reactivation.

1174. The following is *true* of tetralogy of Fallot *except*:

A. Increased lung vascularity
B. Clubbing
C. Cyanosis
D. Squatting

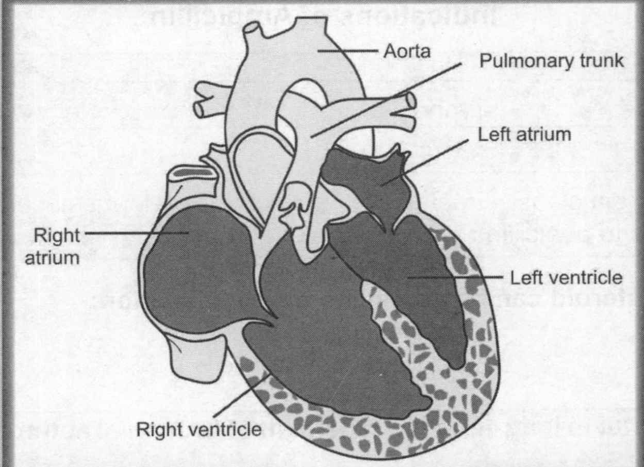

Tetralogy of Fallot is 1 of the most common forms of congenital heart disease. It is by far the most common condition with clinical cyanosis and **diminished vascularity on chest film**, especially in a patient with a right aortic arch and/or a skeletal anomaly. It is also the most common *cyanotic* condition seen in children and adults. The pathologic anatomy of the classic cyanotic tetralogy of Fallot consists of 4 morphologic abnormalities viz. a large **ventricular septal defect** located in the left ventricular outflow tract, usually involving the anterior septum immediately adjacent to the right and posterior aortic cusps; **obstruction or atresia of the right ventricular infundibulum**; **an aorta arising from both ventricles above the large subaortic VSD** in the so-called dextroposed position; and **right ventricular hypertrophy**. Cyanosis is one of the most obvious manifestations of TOF but it may not be present at birth. In the first year of life the cyanosis is most prominent on the mucus membranes of the lips and mouth and in the finger and toe nails. **Clubbing** of fingers and toes becomes apparent by the age of 1-2 years. Dyspnea occurs on excretion and *typically* the child assumes a **squatting** posture for the relief of dyspnea.

1175. Pickwickian syndrome consists of:

A. Decreased pulmonary function
B. Polycythemia
C. Obesity
D. All of the above

Pickwickian syndrome consists of obesity, decreased pulmonary function, and polycythemia.

1176. Mode of action of vigabatrin is:

A. GABA agonist
B. GABA antagonist
C. NMDA antagonist
D. Carbonic anhydrase inhibitor

Vigabatrin is an inhibitor of GABA transaminase which leads to **increased concentration of GABA** which is an inhibitory neurotransmitter.

1177. All predispose to ARDS *except*:

A. Fat embolism
B. Hypertransfusion
C. Septicemia
D. Status asthmaticus

Conditions Predisposing to ARDS

- Airway contusion
- Indirect lung injury
- Sepsis syndrome
- Severe non-thoracic trauma
- Hypertransfusion
- Cardiopulmonary bypass
- Direct injury to alveolar epithelium
- Aspiration
- Diffuse infection
- Near-drowning
- Toxic inhalation
- Fat embolism

1178. Ampicillin is used in all *except*:

A. UTI
B. LRTI
C. Typhoid
D. Infectious mononucleosis

Indications of Ampicillin

• UTI	• RTI	• Meningitis
• Gonorrhea	• Typhoid	• Bacillary dysentery
• Cholecystitis	• SABE	• Septicemia

Most patients of infectious mononucleosis 'treated' with ampicillin develop a macular rash; this rash is not predictive of future adverse reactions to penicillins.

1179. Which of the following steroid can be administered by inhalation:

A. Hydrocortisone
B. Dexamethasone
C. Prednisolone
D. Beclomethasone

Inhaled steroids are very useful in long-term management of bronchial asthma. Steroids that can be given by inhalation are:

- Beclomethasone
- Budesonide
- Fluticasone

1180. Side effect of steroid inhalation is:

A. Cushing syndrome
B. Sedation
C. Oropharyngeal candidiasis
D. None

Frequent Side Effects of Steroid Inhalation

- Oropharyngeal candidiasis
- Upper respiratory infections
- Insomnia
- Pain in nasal sinuses
- Nasal discharge
- Dysphonia

1181. Prognosis is related to incubation period in:

A. Cholera
B. Diphtheria
C. Rabies
D. Tetanus

In rabies rates of infection and mortality are dependent on incubation period. It is highest from bites on the face, intermediate from bites on the hands and arms, and lowest from bites on the legs.

1182. Drug of choice in chloramphenicol *resistant* typhoid fever is:

A. Ampicillin
B. Septran®
C. Ceftazidime
D. Ciprofloxacin

The drug of choice for multidrug resistant (MDR) typhoid is **ciprofloxacin**. *However* in children the drug of choice is **ceftriaxone**.

1183. Hereditary hypoparathyroidism is characterized by:

A. Nephrocalcinosis
B. Candidiasis
C. Bilateral cataract
D. Subcutaneous calcification

Characteristic skin manifestations of hereditary hypoparathyroidism are alopecia and **candidiasis**.

1184. Ipratropium bromide is an:

A. Sympatholytic
B. Antiemetic
C. Anticholinergic
D. Antipsychotic

Ipratropium bromide is an **anticholinergic drug** used in bronchial asthma as a bronchodilator inhaler.

1185. Simvastatin acts by:

A. Dissolution of plasma cholesterol
B. Inhibition of HMG Co A reductase
C. Decrease bile salt production
D. Inhibition of LDL secretion

Conversion of HMG-CoA to mevalonate is an early and rate limiting step in the formation of endogenous cholesterol. **Simvastatin acts by selectively and competitively inhibiting HMG-CoA reductase.**

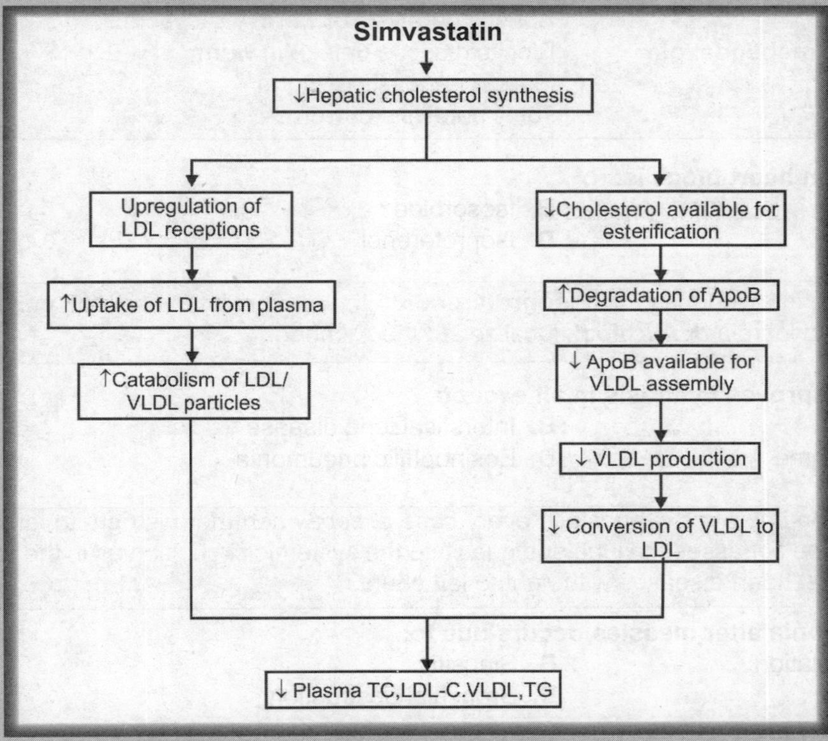

1186. Melphalan is the *drug of choice* of:

A. Nephroblastoma
B. Multiple myeloma
C. Craniopharyngioma
D. Retinoblastoma

Melphalan is the drug of choice of **m**ultiple myeloma. It is an alkylating agent which causes cross-linking or abnormal base pairing of DNA strands.

1187. Hypersensitive cholestatic jaundice is caused by:

A. Rifampicin
B. Chlorpromazine
C. Halothane
D. Phenobarbitone

Hypersensitivity Reactions of Chlorpromazine

- Cholestatic jaundice
- Photosensitivity
- Agranulocytosis

1188. The *drug of choice* in guinea worm infestation is:

A. Niridazole
B. Albendazole
C. Levamisole
D. Mebendazole

Niridazole inhibits glucose uptake by parasites and is the drug of choice in guinea worm infestation (25 mg/kg/day). It is not available in India and metronidazole can be used which produces similar results.

1189. Antihelmintic drug which acts by flaccid paralysis of worms:

A. Albendazole
B. Piperazine
C. Levamisole
D. Pyrantel pamoate

Mode of Action of Common Antihelmintic Drugs

• **Pyrantel pamoate**	Spastic paralysis of worm
• **Albendazole and mebendazole**	Blocks glucose uptake in worm
• **Piperazine**	Flaccid paralysis of worm
• **Levamisole**	Tonic paralysis of worm

1190. *Drug of choice* in heart block is:

A. Nifedipine
B. Isosorbide
C. Steroids
D. Isoproterenol

Atropine (0.5 to 2.0 mg intravenously) and **isoproterenol** (1 to 4 μg/min intravenously) increase the heart rate in patients with sinus bradycardia or **AV block** localized to the AV node.

1191. 100% oxygen improves cyanosis in all *except*:

A. TOF
B. Interstitial lung disease
C. Bronchial asthma
D. Eosinophilic pneumonia

100% oxygen inhalation improves cyanosis in every case *except* when there is right to left shunting of blood so that deoxygenated blood bypasses the lung and goes into the systemic circulation as in the case seen in TOF and various other congenital heart diseases with right to left shunt.

1192. Bronchopneumonia after measles occurs due to:

A. Immunomodulation
B. Sinusitis
C. Aspiration
D. Bronchial obstruction

The complications of measles are divided into 3 groups, and are due to immunomodulation:

- Respiratory tract
- Central nervous system
- Gastrointestinal tract.

1193. Cells seen in M-5 type of leukemia:

A. Lymphocytes
B. Neutrophils
C. Eosinophils
D. Monocytes

The French-American-British Classification of AML

M0	Minimally differentiated leukemia
M1	Myeloblastic leukemia without maturation
M2	Myeloblastic leukemia with maturation
M3	Hypergranular promyelocytic leukemia
M4	Myelomonocytic leukemia
M5	Monocytic leukemia
M6	Erythroleukemia
M7	Megakaryoblastic leukemia

1194. Diuretic used in hypokalemic state is:

A. Frusemide **B.** Thiazide
C. Spironolactone **D.** Bumetanide

Potassium Sparing Diuretics

Spironolactone	Aldosterone antagonist
Triamterene	Acts on membrane of distal tube to inhibit sodium absorption
Amiloride	Acts on membrane of distal tube to inhibit sodium absorption

1195. Neutropenia can be the feature of all *except*:

A. ALL **B.** Felty's syndrome
C. AIDS **D.** Typhoid fever

Some Causes of Neutropenia

Decreased production	
• Tuberculosis	• Measles
• Typhoid fever	• Infectious mononucleosis
• Tularemia	• Viral hepatitis
• Brucellosis	• AIDS
• Malaria	• Tumor invasion, myelofibrosis
• Leishmaniasis	• Vitamin B_{12} and folic acid deficiency
• Cyclic neutropenia	• Chédiak-Higashi syndrome
• Aplastic anemia	• Infantile genetic disorders
• Drug induced	• Idiopathic
Transient neutropenia	
• Overwhelming bacterial infection (acute endotoxemia)	
• Hemodialysis	
• Cardiopulmonary bypass	
Peripheral destruction of neutrophils	
• Antineutrophil antibodies and/or splenic or lung (alveolar macrophage) trapping	
• Felty's syndrome, rheumatoid arthritis, lupus erythematosus	
• Drugs as haptens such as aminopyrine, α-methyl dopa, phenylbutazone, mercurial diuretics, some phenothiazines	
• Wegener's granulomatosis	

1196. Antibiotic which is safe in renal failure:

A. Kanamycin **B.** Penicillin
C. Gentamicin **D.** Minocycline

While using **minocycline** caution is *not* required in renal impairment. No dosage reduction should be done in renal impairment. It should be taken with food or milk.

1197. Russell bodies are found in:

A. Plasma cell tumor
B. Gonadal tumor
C. Parkinson's disease
D. Ovarian tumor

Plasma cells which are actively producing immunoglobins some times become 'overloaded' with their synthetic products, producing large homogenous eosinophilic inclusions known as **Russell bodies**. They are found in **multiple myeloma**.

1198. Nickel exposure is associated with which cancer:

A. Larynx
B. Kidney
C. Lung
D. Pharynx

Nickel exposure is associated with an increased risk of cancer of the lung.

1199. Eclampsia differs from pre-eclampsia by the presence of:

A. Pregnancy
B. Convulsions
C. Albuminuria
D. Hypertension

• **Pregnancy induced hypertension**	Hypertension without proteinuria
• **Preeclampsia**	Hypertension with proteinuria
• **Eclampsia**	Pre-eclampsia with *seizure* activity

1200. All are seen in 3rd nerve palsy *except*:

A. Mydriasis
B. Ptosis
C. Outward deviation of eye
D. Miosis

The 3rd cranial nerve innervates the medial, inferior, and superior recti, inferior oblique, levator palpebrae superioris, and the iris sphincter.
Total paralysis of the oculomotor nerve lesion causes **ptosis**, a dilated pupil (**mydriasis**), and leaves the **eye "down and out"** because of the unopposed action of the lateral rectus and superior oblique.

1201. Which test is used in the diagnosis of anthrax:

A. Casoni's test
B. Ascoli's test
C. Atoloni's test
D. Frei's test

Ascoli's reaction [Alberto Ascoli]: It is a precipitation test for **anthrax** and is used for detection of anthrax bacilli in animal hides and meat. It is also called Ascoli's test.

1202. Test used in the diagnosis of infectious mononucleosis:

A. Paul-Bunnell test
B. Ascoti's test
C. Atoloni's test
D. Frei's test

Paul-Bunnell test is a test for heterophil antibodies in the serum of patients thought to have **infectious mononucleosis.**

1203. Steroids are used along with anti-tuberculous therapy in the following:

A. TB meningitis
B. Ureteric obstruction in genitourinary TB
C. TB of the eye
D. Pericardial effusion
E. All of the above

Steroid should be used along with appropriate ATT in the conditions where the anatomical integrity of the organ involved in tuberculosis is very important such as in **CNS tuberculosis, genitourinary tuberculosis, tubercular pericardial effusion** and **tuberculosis of eye**. Steroids prevent fibrosis and scarring that occurs during healing of a tubercular lesion induced by ATT, thus minimizing the complications.

1204. Salt losing nephropathy is a feature of:

A. Amyloid kidney
B. Interstitial nephritis
C. Lupus nephritis
D. Post-streptococcal glomerulonephritis *(AIIMS 1995)*

Interstitial nephritis: Nephritis associated with pathological changes in the renal interstitial tissue that may be primary or due to a toxic agent such as a drug or chemical is known as interstitial nephritis. The final outcome is the destruction of the nephrons and severe reduction of renal function. **Salt-losing syndrome** is a condition of greatly increased sodium loss from the body as a result of renal disease, adrenocortical insufficiency, or gastrointestinal disease.

1205. Romana's sign is seen in infestation with:

A. *Toxoplasma*
B. *Trypanosoma cruzi*
C. *Loa loa*
D. *Wuchereria*

Romana's sign is pathognomic of acute Chagas' disease. It consists of unilateral painless edema of the palpebrae and periocular tissues. The acute symptoms resolve spontaneously in all patients, who then enter the asymptomatic or indeterminate phase of chronic ***Trypanosoma cruzi*** infection.

1206. Fenfluramine is used to treat:

A. Gout
B. Radiation sickness
C. Dressler's syndrome
D. Obesity

Fenfluramine is an appetite suppressant used in the treatment of exogenous obesity.

1207. Fanconi's syndrome is inherited as:

A. X-linked trait
B. Autosomal recessive
C. Autosomal dominant
D. All of the above

Idiopathic Fanconi syndrome may be inherited as an autosomal dominant, autosomal recessive or X-linked trait. Sporadic cases are also seen.

1208. The following are interstitial lung diseases *except*:

A. Pulmonary alveolar proteinosis
B. Idiopathic pulmonary fibrosis
C. Bronchial asthma
D. Pneumoconiosis

Bronchial asthma is a **hyperreactive *airway* disease** associated with chronic inflammation of the bronchial mucosa. **Some causes of interstitial lung diseases are given below:**

- **Sarcoidosis**
- Langerhans cell granulomatosis (eosinophilic granuloma)
- Granulomatous vasculitides
- **Idiopathic pulmonary fibrosis**
- Collagen vascular diseases
- Systemic lupus erythematosus
- **Pulmonary alveolar proteinosis**

1209. The amount of factor VIII required to raise the plasma factor VIII concentration by 100% is:

A. 45 units/kg
B. 85 units/kg
C. 125 units/kg
D. 105 units/kg

1unit is defined as the amount of factor VIII present in 1ml of plasma of normal subjects. As the plasma volume is 45 ml/kg, 45 units/kg of factor VIII will be required to increase the level from 0 to 100%.

1210. Allergic bronchopulmonary aspergillosis is seen in:

A. Asthma
B. Carcinoma bronchus
C. Tuberculous cavity
D. Bronchiectasis

Some cases of **bronchiectasis** are due to exposure to a toxic substance that starts a severe inflammatory response, such as inhalation of a toxic gas like ammonia or aspiration of acidic gastric contents. An immune response in the airway can also trigger inflammation, destructive changes, and bronchial dilatation. This mechanism is responsible for bronchiectasis with **allergic bronchopulmonary aspergillosis (ABPA)**, which is due to an immune response to *Aspergillus* organisms that are present in the airway.

1211. Pleurisy is common in which of the following connective tissue disease:

A. SLE
B. Systemic sclerosis
C. Polyarteritis nodosa
D. Mixed connective tissue disease

Pleurisy and pleural effusions are common features of SLE. Lupus pneumonitis causes fever, breathlessness, and cough. X-rays show fleeting infiltrates or areas of plate-like atelectasis or both. This syndrome responds to glucocorticoids.

1212. All are features of hypereosinophilic syndrome *except*:
- **A.** Blood eosinophilia
- **B.** Bone marrow eosinophilia
- **C.** Associated with parasites
- **D.** Tissue eosinophilia

The idiopathic **hypereosinophilic syndrome** consists of a heterogeneous group of disorders with the common feature of
1. Persistent **blood eosinophilia** of unknown origin.
2. Associated organ system dysfunction, involving the CVS, CNS, renal, pulmonary, GI tract, and dermis.
3. The **bone marrow is involved in 100% cases**.
4. **Eosinophils are found in the affected tissues** and cause tissue damage by local deposition of toxic eosinophil proteins such as eosinophil cationic protein and eosinophil major basic protein.

1213. Pleural effusion with low glucose content is characteristic:
- **A.** Rheumatic arthritis
- **B.** Rheumatoid arthritis
- **C.** Mesothelioma
- **D.** Malignant effusions

1214. Raised glucose in pleural effusion is *not* seen in:
- **A.** Filarial effusion
- **B.** Nephrotic syndrome
- **C.** Rheumatoid arthritis
- **D.** Tuberculosis

(AIIMS 1991)

Pleuropulmonary manifestations of **rheumatoid arthritis** are commonly present in men. They include pleural disease, interstitial fibrosis, pleuropulmonary nodules, pneumonitis, and arteritis. **The pleural fluid contains very low levels of glucose in the absence of infection.**

1215. Which one of the following is an immunostimulant:
- **A.** Miconazole
- **B.** Levamisole
- **C.** Ketoconazole
- **D.** Albendazole

Levamisole acts as an immunorestorative agent in the presence of immunosuppression resulting from recent surgery and chemotherapy but *does not* stimulate the immune response to above normal levels. This may be related to T-cell activation and proliferation, augmentation of monocyte and macrophage activity (including phagocytosis and chemotaxis), and an increase in neutrophil mobility, adherence, and chemotaxis.

1216. Busulfan causes:
- **A.** Hemorrhagic cystitis
- **B.** Neurotoxicity
- **C.** Pulmonary fibrosis
- **D.** Alopecia

Some Drugs Causing Pulmonary Fibrosis

- Acyclovir
- Amiodarone
- Busulfan
- Gold
- Azathioprine
- Bleomycin
- Chlorambucil
- Cyclophosphamide

1217. Amantadine an anti-flu drug is useful in:
- **A.** Acromegaly
- **B.** Interstitial lung disease
- **C.** Parkinsonism
- **D.** Toxoplasmosis

Amantadine, either alone or combined with an anticholinergic agent, is useful for mild **Parkinsonism**. It acts by enhancing the release of endogenous dopamine.

1218. Myocardial isoenzyme of CK which is specific for myocardial infarction is:

A. CK-BB
B. CK-MB
C. CK-MM
D. All of the above

The **MB isoenzyme of CK has the big advantage total over CK** that it is *not* present in *significant* concentrations in extracardiac tissue and therefore is **more specific for MI**.

1219. What is morbilli:

A. Rubella
B. Smallpox
C. Monkey pox
D. Measles

Measles virus belongs to the genus **Morbillivirus** and the family Paramyxoviridae.

1220. Opportunistic lung infection in AIDS is due to:

A. *Pneumocystis carinii*
B. *Klebsiella*
C. *Mycoplasma*
D. Mucormycosis

Pneumocystis carinii Pneumonia is More Common in Following Group

- Premature infants
- Patients receiving immunosuppressive therapy such as glucocorticoids or anticancer drugs
- Malnourished children
- Organ transplantation
- Children with primary immunodeficiency diseases
- People with AIDS

1221. Hyperpathia is observed in...........:

A. Pontine hemorrhage
B. Pyramidal tact lesions
C. Thalamic syndrome
D. Sarcoidosis

Hyperpathia is a broad term which consists of:

- **Hyperesthesia** means exaggerated perception of sensations in response to mild stimuli (light touch or stroking of the skin).
- **Allodynia** describes the situation in which an ordinarily non-painful stimulus, once perceived, is experienced as painful, even excruciating.
- **Hyperalgesia** denotes an exaggerated response to a noxious stimulus.

Atheromatous occlusion of the penetrating branches of **th**alamic and thalamogeniculate arteries produce hyperpathia.

1222. Todd's paralysis is seen in:

A. Head injury
B. Strokes
C. Epilepsy
D. Subarachnoid hemorrhage

Patients of **partial seizure** may display a localized paresis for minutes to many hours in the involved region following the seizure which is known as **Todd's paralysis**.

1223. Gaze nystagmus is seen in:

A. Miners
B. Infants
C. Myasthenia gravis
D. Spinal cord lesions

Causes of Gaze-evoked Nystagmus

- Sedatives
- Anticonvulsants
- Alcohol
- Muscle paresis
- Myasthenia gravis
- Demyelinating disease
- Cerebellopontine angle
- Brainstem and cerebellar lesions

1224. In pericardial effusion all are seen *except*:

A. Raised JVP
B. Hepatomegaly
C. Pedal edema
D. Loud heart sounds

Pericardial effusion is associated with pain, ECG changes characteristic of pericarditis and an enlargement of the cardiac shadow. **Heart sounds tend to become faint** the so called 'distant' heart sounds as they appear to come from a distance.

1225. Which of the following is *not* used to treat acute pulmonary edema:

A. IV fluids
B. IV furosemide
C. IV morphine
D. Oxygen

Acute pulmonary edema is due to marked elevation of pulmonary capillary pressure which leads to alveolar edema, associated with extreme shortness of breath, rales over the lung fields, and the transudation and expectoration of blood-tinged fluid. Acute pulmonary edema may be fatal if not treated properly.

Management of Acute Pulmonary Edema

- **Morphine** is administered intravenously 2-5 mg IV.
- 100% **oxygen** should be administered, preferably under positive pressure.
- The patient should be maintained in the sitting position which reduces venous return.
- Intravenous loop diuretics, such as **furosemide** (40 to 100 mg) IV stat.
- Intravenous sodium nitroprusside at 20 to 30 μg/min in patients whose systolic arterial pressure is >100 mmHg.
- Inotropic support should be provided by dopamine.
- 1.0 mg digoxin IV should be given.
- Aminophylline (theophylline ethylenediamine), 240 to 480 mg IV, is effective in reducing bronchoconstriction.
- Rotating tourniquets should be applied to the extremities if the above measures fail.

1226. The *most common* neutrophil defect is:

A. Myeloperoxidase deficiency
B. Chédiak-Higashi syndrome
C. CD 3b deficiency
D. Job's syndrome

The **most common neutrophil defect is myeloperoxidase deficiency**. It is inherited as an autosomal recessive trait affecting 1 in 2000 persons.

1227. Transmural myocardial infarction in ECG is characterized by:

A. ST segment elevation
B. Pathological Q waves
C. Prolonged QRS
D. T waves inversion

Transmural infarction is present if the ECG demonstrates Q waves or loss of R waves; nontransmural infarction may be present if the ECG shows only transient ST-segment and T-wave changes.

1228. The following are contraindications of heart transplantation *except*:

A. Age *less than* 55 years
B. Pulmonary hypertension
C. IDDM
D. Pulmonary embolism

Contraindications of Cardiac Transplantation

- Infection
- Recent pulmonary infarction
- IDDM
- Pulmonary hypertension
- Circulating cytotoxic antibodies
- Peptic ulcer disease
- Malignancy
- COPD
- Alcoholism
- Peripheral or cerebrovascular disease

1229. The normal AV ratio in fundoscopy is:

A. 3:4
B. 1:2
C. 3:2
D. 1:3

The normal AV ratio in fundoscopy is 3:4.

1230. Dancing carotids (a sign in aortic regurgitation) is also known as:

A. Hill's sign
B. Quincke's sign
C. Corrigan's sign
D. Traube's sign

Some Physical Signs of Aortic Regurgitation

• **Corrigan's sign**	Visible arterial pulsations in neck, so called 'dancing' carotids.
• **de Musset's sign**	Nodding of head with heart beat.
• **Duroziez's sign**	Femoral artery is compressed and auscultated proximal to the compression. A diastolic murmur is audible.

1231. In ataxia-telangiectasia which is seen:

A. IgG absent
B. IgM present
C. IgA structure abnormality
D. IgA low

Features of Ataxia-Telangiectasia

- Autosomal recessive
- Cerebellar ataxia
- Oculocutaneous telangiectasia
- Immunodeficiency
- Defect at q22-23 on chromosome 11
- Thymus is hypoplastic
- Peripheral T cells are reduced
- Low serum IgE and IgA

1232. Liver biopsy is done by using..........needle:

A. Vim Silverman
B. Abrams
C. Kocher
D. Menghini

Liver biopsy is a common procedure of considerable diagnostic importance. The **Menghini** or trucut needles are best for this procedure.

1233. The half-life of chloroquine is:

A. 6 hours
B. 7 days
C. 12 days
D. 24 hours

Average half-life of chloroquine varies from **3-10 days or more** .The terminal elimination half-life is 1 to 2 months.

1234. Leukemoid reaction is seen in:

A. Acute infection
B. Hodgkin's disease
C. None
D. Both

Neutrophilia may result from any one of the following:

- Increased neutrophil production
- Marrow release
- Defective margination

The most important acute cause of neutrophilia is infection.

Neutrophilia from **acute infection** is due to both increased production and increased marrow release. **"Persistent neutrophilia of 30,000 to 50,000 cells/μL or > is known as leukemoid reaction"**. In a leukemoid reaction, the circulating neutrophils are mature. **Leukemoid reaction is common in patients of Hodgkin's disease.**

1235. In a patient with brain abscess which investigation is *contraindicated:*

A. CT scan **B.** Lumbar puncture
C. EEG **D.** Angiogram

Lumbar puncture is contraindicated in following conditions:
- Raised ICT which may be due to any SOL such as brain abscess, tumor
- Spontaneous subarachnoid hemorrhage
- Bleeding disorders
- Skin sepsis
- Spinal deformity

1236. The pathogenesis of cholera is by:

A. Stimulating the small intestine to secrete large amount of fluid
B. Ulceration of the mucosa of the intestine
C. Inhibition of absorption of fluids
D. None of the above

- **Cholera** is a toxin-mediated disease.
- The characteristic watery diarrhea is due to the action of cholera toxin (CTX), which is a potent protein enterotoxin released by the organism in the small intestine.
- This result is the intracellular accumulation of high levels of cyclic AMP.
- This cyclic AMP inhibits the absorptive sodium transport system in villus cells and **activates the excretory chloride transport system in crypt cells**, and this lead to the accumulation of sodium chloride in the intestinal lumen.
- **Because water moves passively to maintain osmolality, isotonic fluid accumulates in the lumen.**
- When the volume of that fluid exceeds the capacity of the rest of the gut to resorb it, watery diarrhea starts.

1237. Central necrosis of liver is seen in:

A. CCF **B.** Yellow fever
C. Phosphorus poisoning **D.** Carbon tetrachloride toxicity

- Many drugs and chemical toxic reactions such as **C**hloroform and **C**arbon tetrachloride poisoning cause mainly **C**entrilobular necrosis.
- Midzonal necrosis is seen in yellow fever.
- **Peripheral necrosis** in **Phosphorus poisoning**.

1238. Carcinoembryonic antigen is seen in:

A. Colorectal carcinoma **B.** Alcoholic cirrhosis
C. Emphysema **D.** Diabetes mellitus

Conditions Associated with Raised Carcinoembryonic Antigen

Adenocarcinomas of	Non-neoplastic Conditions
• Colon	• Pancreatitis
• Pancreas	• Hepatitis
• Lung	• Smoking
• Breast	• Inflammatory bowel disease
• Ovary	

1239. The normal fecal fat excretion is:

A. < 6 gm/day
B. 8 gm/day
C. 10 gm/day
D. 15 gm/day

Normal fecal fat excretion is less than 6 g for 24 hour.

1240. Enzyme appearing early in myocardial infraction:

A. CPK
B. LDH
C. SGOT
D. SGPT

Enzyme	Starts to rise	Peak	Return to normal
CK	4-6 hours	12 hours	48-72 hours
LDH	12 hours	2-3 days	After a week

1241. Recurrent chest pain and syncope is commonly seen in:

A. Aortic stenosis
B. Aortic regurgitation
C. Mitral valve prolapse
D. Mitral stenosis

The three cardinal symptoms of aortic stenosis are:
- Exertional dyspnea
- Angina pectoris
- Syncope

1242. Maximum specificity in VDRL test is seen in case of:

A. Primary syphilis
B. Tertiary syphilis
C. Secondary syphilis
D. GPI

Sensitivity of Different Tests in Different Stages

Test	Primary	Secondary	Latent	Tertiary
• **VDRL**	78%	100%	95%	70%
• **FTA-ABS**	85%	100%	100%	95%
• **MHA-TP**	75%	100%	100%	93%

1243. Niclosamide is *not* effective for treatment of:

A. *Tinea saginata*
B. Hymenolepiasis
C. *Tinea solium*
D. *Echinococcus granulosus*

Indications of Niclosamide

- Diphyllobothriasis
- Taeniasis
- Hymenolepiasis
- Dipylidiasis

1244. A person cannot identify familiar object when placed in the palm when he is blindfolded this condition is called:

A. Aphakia
B. Aphonia
C. Aphasia
D. Astereognosis

Stereognosis is defined as the ability of an individual to identify common objects by palpation, recognizing their shape, texture, and size. Individual who are unable to identify common objects in one hand but can do so in the other are said to have **astereognosis** of the abnormal hand.

1245. Obesity predisposes to all *except*:

A. Hypoventilation
B. Hyperventilation
C. Hypertension
D. Diabetes mellitus

Conditions Associated with Obesity

- High blood pressure
- Prostate cancer
- Obstructive sleep apnea (hypoventilation)
- Diabetes mellitus
- Colonorectal cancer
- Osteoarthritis
- Gallbladder disease
- Acanthosis nigricans

1246. The treatment of *choice* in symptomatic sinus node dysfunction is:

A. Diltiazem
B. Propranolol
C. Permanent pacemaker
D. Verapamil

Permanent pacemaker is the only satisfactory treatment for patients with symptomatic sinus node dysfunction.

1247. S_4 is caused by:

A. Atrial contraction
B. Mitral valve bellowing
C. Turbulent blood flow
D. Papillary muscle action

4th heart sound (S_4) is caused by an effective atrial contraction.

1248. The most sensitive and reliable indicator of rejection following renal transplant is:

A. Blood urea
B. Urinary hydroxyproline
C. Creatinine clearance
D. T4/T8 ratio

Rejection usually present only with a rise in **serum creatinine**, with or without oliguria.

1249. *Most common* arrhythmia encountered in digitalis toxicity:

A. Complete heart block
B. Bigeminus rhythm
C. Sick sinus syndrome
D. Atrial fibrillation

Although various cardiac arrhythmia are produced by digitalis, pulsus bigeminus is most common of them. Other arrhythmias are ventricular extrasystole, ventricular tachycardia or VF.

1250. The outstanding symptom of acute pancreatitis is:

A. Abdominal bloating
B. Jaundice
C. Agonizing upper abdominal pain
D. Constipation

The main symptom of acute pancreatitis is severe abdominal pain.

1251. Mitral valve prolapse is characterized by:

A. Diastolic click
B. Chest pain
C. Soft S1
D. Right ventricular atrophy

Many patients of MVP have chest pain that is substernal, sustained, not related to exertion.

1252. Characteristic signs of vitamin A deficiency include:

A. Dryness of the conjunctiva
B. Keratomalacia
C. Bitot's spot
D. All of the above

Classification of Vitamin A Deficiency

Classification	Primary signs
X 1A	Conjunctival xerosis
X 1B	Bitot's spots
X 2	Corneal xerosis
X 3A	Corneal ulceration
X 3B	Keratomalacia
	Secondary signs
X N	Night blindness
X F	Fundal changes
X S	Corneal scarring

Treatment guidelines: According to the WHO guideline 2 lakh IU of vitamin A should be given orally on presentation and on the following day. A third dose is recommended on 28th day. Half dose is given if the child is *less than* 12 months and 1/4th if *less than* 6 months. For IM route half of the oral dose is recommended. 1 ampoule of injection Aquasol® contains 1 lakh IU of vitamin A.

1253. Which vitamin deficiency occurs in intestinal malabsorption:

A. Vitamin A
B. Vitamin B_1
C. Vitamin B_{12}
D. Vitamin C

Some Causes of Vitamin A Deficiency

- Sprue (intestinal malabsorption)
- Proteinuria (increased excretion)
- Intestinal bypass surgery ((intestinal malabsorption)
- Total parenteral nutrition

1254. Peripheral stigmata of Laënnec's cirrhosis include all *except*:

A. Clubbing
B. Testicular atrophy
C. Purpura
D. None of the above

Clinical Features of Cirrhosis

- Hepatomegaly
- Spider telangiectasia
- Loss of libido
- Testicular atrophy
- Breast atrophy
- Menorrhagia
- Fetor hepaticus
- Fever
- Jaundice
- Palmar erythema
- Hair loss
- Impotence
- Menstrual irregularity
- Epistaxis
- Splenomegaly
- Clubbing
- Ascites
- Cyanosis
- Gynecomastia
- Amenorrhea
- Purpura
- Collateral vessels
- Hepatic encephalopathy
- Pigmentation

*Cirrhosis of the liver associated with chronic excessive alcohol ingestion is known as Laënnec's cirrhosis.

1255. Which of the following is *not* associated with tetany:

A. Chvostek's sign
B. Erb's sign
C. Coles' sign
D. Trousseau's sign

Features of Hypocalcemia

• Paresthesias	• Anxiety	• Laryngospasm
• Carpal spasm	• Seizures	• Chvostek's sign
• Pedal spasm	• Bronchospasm	• Trousseau's sign
• Erb's sign	• Long QT interval	• Irritability

* Neonatal hypocalcemia is defined as total serum calcium less than 7 mg/dl and ionized calcium less than 4 mg/dl. Hypomagnesemia and alkalosis lower the threshold for tetany whereas hypokalemia and acidosis raise the threshold for tetany.

1256. Adrenal 'reserve' is best tested by means of infusion with:

A. Glucocorticoids **B.** Hypothyroidism
C. Metyrapone **D.** ACTH

The functional reserve of the adrenal gland is tested by administration of ACTH. If the reserves are adequate the cortisol levels increase in adrenal venous blood.

1257. Plucked chicken skin appearance is pathognomic of:

A. Pseudoxanthoma elasticum
B. Homocystinuria
C. Marfan's syndrome
D. Any of the above

Plucked chicken skin is characteristic of **pseudoxanthoma elasticum** in which there is an abnormal deposition of calcium on the elastic fibers of the skin, eye, and blood vessels.

1258. Idoxuridine is the *drug of choice* in:

A. Chickenpox **B.** Adenovirus infection
C. Herpes virus infection **D.** Rubella

Idoxuridine is a thymidine analogue which is effective only against DNA viruses. Only clinical indication is **herpes simplex infection**.

1259. Pink frothy expectoration is seen in:

A. Pulmonary edema
B. Pulmonary tuberculosis
C. Bronchogenic carcinoma
D. Mucormycosis

Pulmonary edema manifests with bilateral wet rales. The patient is anxious and excessive sweating is present. The **sputum is pink, frothy and blood-tinged**.

1260. Fungal infection commonly seen in diabetics is:

A. Actinomycosis **B.** Mucormycosis
C. Aspergillosis **D.** Coccidioidomycosis

Rhinocerebral mucormycosis is an otherwise *rare* fungal infection that may develop during or after an episode of diabetic ketoacidosis.

1261. Hypothermia is characterized by all *except:*

A. Common in old age
B. External rewarming treatment of choice
C. Give warm dialysate
D. Steroids has no role

Hypothermia is defined as "a core body temperature of 35°C or below." It is of three types:
- Mild (35 to 32° C)
- Moderate (< 32 to 28° C)
- Severe (< 28°C)

Risk factors

- Extremes of age (especially the **elderly**)
- **Ethanol use**
- Poverty
- Neuroleptic medications
- Homelessness
- Malnutrition
- Mental illness
- Hypothyroidism

Rewarming can be active or passive, internal or external. **The most efficient rewarming technique is extracorporeal blood warming which is done by hemodialysis or cardiopulmonary bypass**.

1262. The characteristic ECG change in hypothermia is:
A. T wave inversion
B. PR prolonged
C. J wave
D. ST segment depressed

The characteristic ECG changes in hypothermia is the Osborn or **J wave** which is a positive deflection at the junction of the QRS complex and the ST segment.

1263. Chickenpox rash:
A. Appears in the second day of the illness
B. Appears on the trunk first
C. Maximum density on trunk
D. Lesions at all stages of development seen
E. All of the above are correct

Incubation period of chickenpox is 14-21 days. It mainly affects children less than 10 years of age and is highly infectious.1st sign of disease is rash and **appears on trunk** on the **second day** of illness. Then the rash spreads to involve face and finally the limbs. **Maximum density of rash is seen over trunk**. Spots appear in crops and **all stages of lesions are seen at a given time.** Drug of choice is acyclovir given in a dose of 20 mg/kg/dose qid for 7 days.

1264. Features of megaloblastic anemia include:
A. Poikilocytosis
B. Paresthesia
C. Macrocytosis with anisocytosis
D. Hyper segmentation of neutrophils
E. All of the above

Important Features of Megaloblastic Anemia

- Macrocytosis
- Anisocytosis
- Poikilocytosis
- Neutrophils show hypersegmentation of the nucleus
- Romberg sign may be positive
- Ataxia
- Weakness
- Paresthesias
- Numbness
- Positive Babinski signs

1265. Which one of the following is AIDS defining illness:
A. *Mycobacterium tuberculosis* meningitis
B. *Cryptococcus neoformans* meningitis
C. Cytomegalovirus meningitis
D. *Histoplasma capsulatum* meningitis

Cryptococcus neoformans is the major cause of meningitis in patients with AIDS. It is the initial AIDS-defining condition in 2% of patients.

1266. Cutting of the pituitary stalk decreases all of the following hormones *except*:
A. ACTH **B.** GH
C. Prolactin **D.** FSH

Interruption of the **pituitary stalk** leads to reduction in the release of GH, LH, FSH, TSH, and ACTH from the anterior pituitary. *However*, the level of **prolactin rises after cutting the stalk**, indicating that the normal hypothalamic influence on prolactin secretion is *inhibitory*.

Anterior lobe of the pituitary	Posterior lobe of the pituitary
• Growth hormone	• Vasopressin
• Prolactin	• Oxytocin
• Luteinizing hormone	
• Follicle-stimulating hormone	
• Thyroid-stimulating hormone	
• Adrenocorticotropin	

1267. A middle aged patient was brought to the hospital in stuporous conditions with loss of power in all four limbs. Waxy flexibility of muscle tone in the limbs was detected. The *most likely* diagnosis is:
A. Hysterical stupor **B.** Organic stupor
C. Catatonic stupor **D.** Depressive stupor

Catatonia is a hypomobile syndrome found in patients of major psychosis. The patients are awake with eyes open but make no voluntary or responsive movements. They blink spontaneously and do not appear distressed. They may demonstrate "**waxy flexibility**," in which limbs maintain their posture when lifted by the doctor. Upon recovery, these patients have some memory of events that occurred during their **catatonic stupor**.

1268. Which one of the following drugs causes hyperprolactinemia:
A. Domperidone **B.** Metoclopramide
C. Cisapride **D.** lansoprazole

Drugs Causing Hyperprolactinemia

Dopamine receptor antagonists	Dopamine-depleting agents
• Phenothiazines	• Methyldopa
• Butyrophenones	• Reserpine
• Thioxanthenes	• Hormones
• Metoclopramide	• Estrogens
• Sulpiride	• Antiandrogens
• Respiradone	• Opiates
	• Verapamil

1269. An Indian adult who has never traveled abroad comes with a history of high fever, headache, jaundice, marked oliguria and shock with TLC of 16,000/cumm.The *most likely* diagnosis is:
A. Viral hepatitis **B.** Leptospirosis (Weil's disease)
C. Yellow fever **D.** Hemolytic uremic syndrome

Severe leptospirosis (Weil's syndrome) is characterized by:
- **Jaundice**
- Renal dysfunction
- Hemorrhagic diathesis
- Hepatomegaly
- Tenderness in the right upper quadrant
- Splenomegaly
- Renal failure
- Hypovolemia
- Acute tubular necrosis with **oliguria** or anuria.
- **Leukocytosis**

1270. Causes of hypersensitivity pneumonitis are all *except*:

A. Silicosis
B. Bird fancier's lung
C. Farmer's lung
D. Coffee worker's lung

Types of Hypersensitivity Pneumonitis

- Bagassosis
- **Bird fancier's**, or handler's lung
- Cephalosporium HP
- Cheese washer's lung
- Chemical worker's lung
- **Coffee worker's lung**
- Compost lung
- Detergent worker's disease
- Familial HP
- **Farmer's lung**
- Fish meal worker's lung
- Furrier's lung
- Mushroom worker's lung
- Hot tub lung
- Humidifier or air-conditioner lung
- Japanese summer house HP
- Laboratory worker's HP
- Lycoperdonosis
- Paulis HP
- Pituitary snuff taker's lung
- Potato riddler's lung
- Sauna taker's lung
- Sequoiosis
- Streptomyces albus HP
- Suberosis
- Tap water lung
- Miller's lung
- Thatched roof disease
- Tobacco worker's disease
- Winegrower's lung
- Wood trimmer's disease
- Woodman's disease
- Woodworker's lung
- Malt worker's lung
- Maple bark disease

1271. Cisapride is contraindicated in all *except*:

A. Severe GI hemorrhage
B. GI obstruction
C. Pregnancy
D. Severe anemia

Contraindications of Cisapride

- Gastrointestinal hemorrhage
- Mechanical obstruction
- Pregnancy

1272. The causes of pericarditis include all *except*:

A. Uremia
B. Hypertension
C. Rheumatic fever
D. Tuberculosis

Causes of Pericarditis

Infectious	Immunological	Miscellaneous
• Viruses • Pyogenic bacteria • Mycobacterial tuberculosis • Fungus • Other parasites	• Rheumatic fever • SLE • Scleroderma • Dressler's syndrome • Drug hypersensitivity	• Radiation • Neoplasm • Trauma • Cardiac surgery • Uremia • Myocardial infraction

1273. Cerebral edema is characteristically seen in poisoning by:

A. Methanol
B. Lead
C. CO
D. All of the above

Cerebral edema can be caused by any *metabolic* encephalopathy such as that caused by enteric fever, hepatic encephalopathy and certain poisonous substances such as methanol, lead, carbon monoxide, etc.

1274. Cavernous breathing is seen in:

A. Pleural effusion
B. Consolidation
C. Carcinoma lung
D. Cavity lung

When a bronchus communicates directly with a large abnormal air space either in the **lung (cavity)** or pleural space (pneumothorax) it gives rise to hallow resonating breath sound which is known as **cavernous or amphoric breathing**.

1275. The principal cause of chyluria is:

A. Lymphosarcoma
B. Hypercholesterolemia
C. Hyperlipidemia
D. Filariasis

The presence of 'chyle' in the urine is known as chyluria. It gives a milky appearance to the urine. **Filariasis is the most common cause of chyluria** which occurs in 1-2% of cases; 10 to 20 years after initial infestation. It presents as **painless passage of milky white urine**; particularly after a fatty meal. Occasionally the chyle may clot leading to renal colic. On standing, a clot forms in the urine which does not dissolve on shaking with equal amount of ether. Chyluria may also be caused by ascariasis, malaria, tuberculosis and tumor and differential diagnosis includes gross pyuria, phosphaturia and caseous material from tuberculosis. Intravenous urography and / or lymphangiography will often demonstrate a *lymphourinary fistula*. *Treatment* consists of a low fat and high protein diet, increased fluid intake to prevent clot colic and finally laparotomy and ligation of the dilated lymphatics.

1276. Third heart sound when heard is:

A. Always pathological
B. Indicative of aortic stenosis
C. Suggestive of poor ventricular function
D. Suggestive of mitral stenosis

The 3rd Heart Sound (S_3)

- It is a low-pitched sound that is produced in the ventricle 0.15 seconds after A_2.
- **It is normal in children** and in patients with **high cardiac output**.
- **If present in patients over 40 years old, an S_3 indicates impairment of ventricular function** or AV valve regurgitation or any other conditions that increase the rate or volume of ventricular filling.

1277. Nitroblue tetrazolium test (NBT) is a test of:

A. Humoral immunity
B. Phagocytosis
C. Complement pathway
D. Cellular immunity

Nitroblue tetrazolium test is a test of the capability of leukocytes to change nitroblue tetrazolium from a colorless state to deep blue color. Failure to produce this reaction shows that the leukocytes do not have the capability of reacting in a normal manner to the ingestion of the particular bacteria **(phagocytosis)** used in the test.

1278. The critical narrowing of coronary vessels to cause angina is:

A. >50%
B. >70%
C. >80%
D. >60%

Critical narrowing of the coronary artery is said to be present when the lumen is reduced to less than 70% of the normal.

1279. Serum angiotensin converting enzyme levels are raised in:

A. Cat scratch fever
B. Miliary TB
C. Brucellosis
D. Sarcoidosis

Abnormalities of Blood in Sarcoidosis

- Lymphocytopenia
- Raised ESR
- Eosinophilia
- Hyperglobulinemia
- Elevated level of angiotensin-converting enzyme

1280. *Drug of choice* in carotid sinus syncope is:

A. Ephedrine **B.** Adrenaline
C. Reserpine **D.** Propranolol

The pharmacological treatment of **carotid sinus syncope** involves use of atropine or the **ephedrine** group of drugs.

1281. Alpha coma is characterized by the following *except*:

A. EEG shows waves of 8-12 hertz **B.** Prognosis good
C. Diffuse cortical damage **D.** None of the above

A pattern of "**alpha coma**" consists of, invariant 8 to 12 Hz activity resembling the normal alpha rhythm of waking but not responsive to environmental stimuli. α coma results from high pontine or **diffuse cortical damage** and is a **poor prognostic sign**.

1282. Dohle bodies are inclusions seen in:

A. Eosinophil **B.** Monocyte
C. Neutrophil **D.** Basophil

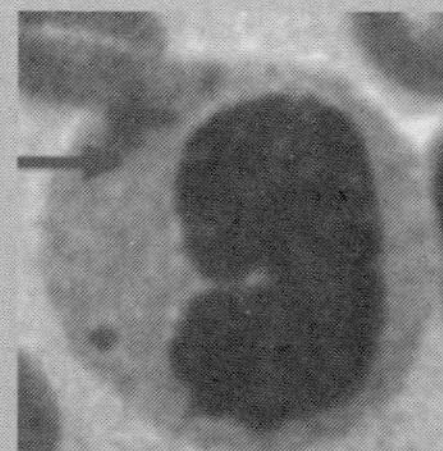

Dohle bodies are blue-staining non-granular areas seen in the periphery of the cytoplasm of **neutrophils** in severe infections and other toxic states. They are aggregates of rough endoplasmic reticulum.

1283. Spur cell anemia is a feature of:

A. Liver disease **B.** Myelofibrosis
C. Acute blood loss **D.** Renal failure

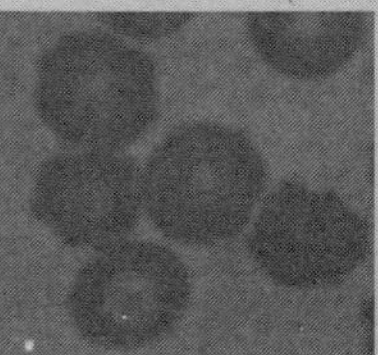

Spur cell are distorted RBCs having several irregularly distributed thorn like projections. They are also called **acanthocytes**. Hemolytic anemia with spur cells occur in some patients with severe **hepatocellular disease** usually advanced alcoholic cirrhosis.

1284. Keshan disease is due to deficiency of:

A. Selenium
B. Cobalt
C. B_{12}
D. Zinc

Selenium is a component of glutathione peroxidase enzyme and it plays an important role in the control of oxygen metabolism. It is required for the growth of cells in tissue culture. It is curative and preventive of **Keshan disease**, which is a syndrome consisting of multifocal myocardial necrosis and reduced serum Se. This disorder is found in China, where the soil is deficient in Se.

1285. All of the following are *true* of MVP *except*:

A. More common in females
B. Ejection click heard best on lying down
C. Sudden death is rare
D. Associated with arrhythmias

Mitral valve prolapse is more common in females. Arrhythmias, most commonly ventricular premature contractions and paroxysmal supraventricular and ventricular tachycardia frequently occur leading to palpitations, light-headedness, and syncope. **Sudden death may occur *rarely***. The click and murmur of MVP occur earlier with standing.

1286. Parkinsonism may occur because of chronic exposure to:

A. Chromium
B. Molybdenum
C. Manganese
D. Nickel

Causes of Secondary Parkinsonism

- Manganese dust
- Carbon monoxide poisoning
- Carbon disulfide
- Post encephalitic syndrome

1287. Photodermatitis and corneal microdeposits are side effects of:

A. Verapamil
B. Flecainide
C. Amiodarone
D. Procainamide

Amiodarone is a long acting antiarrhythmic drug. It's most prominent action is prolongation of APD and ERP at AV node conducting tissue, ventricular fibers. Its common side effects are as under:

- Bradycardia
- Photosensitization
- Corneal microdeposits
- AV block
- Skin pigmentation
- Hypothyroidism

1288. Rhabdomyoma of the heart is seen in association with:

A. Friedreich's ataxia
B. Noonan's syndrome
C. Turner's syndrome
D. Tuberous sclerosis

Rhabdomyomas are hamartomatous growths. They are multiple in about 90% of patients and are often associated with **tuberous sclerosis**, adenoma sebaceum, and benign kidney tumors in about 30% of patients.

1289. All of the following are endocrine manifestation of renal cell carcinoma *except*:

A. Erythrocytosis
B. Hypercalcemia
C. Stauffers' syndrome
D. Peptic ulcer

Some Endocrine Manifestations of Renal Cell Carcinoma

- Erythrocytosis
- Nonmetastatic hepatic dysfunction (Stauffers' syndrome)
- Hypercalcemia
- Acquired dysfibrinogenemia

1290. The normal cardiac index is:

A. 2-3
B. 4-5
C. More than 5
D. 2.6-3.6

The cardiac output per minute per square meter of body surface is known as **cardiac index**. The average cardiac index is 3.2 liter.

1291. General paralysis of insane (GPI) usually follows primary infection after:

A. 1 year
B. 5 years
C. 3 years
D. 10 years or more

GPI usually occurs 20 years after the primary infection of syphilis.

1292. The total daily loss of iron amounts to about:

A. 0.1 mg
B. 0.5 mg
C. 10 mg
D. 1 mg

The daily iron loss in adult males is 1 mg/day and in females 2 mg/day. Other factors that are required for erythropoiesis are folate, cyanocobalamin, thyroxin, vitamin C and E, androgens, copper and manganese.

1293. Dementia is not a feature of:

A. Hyperparathyroidism
B. Hyperthyroidism
C. Hypothyroidism
D. Cushing's disease

Endocrine Causes of Dementia

- Endocrine and other organ failure
- Hypothyroidism
- Adrenal insufficiency and Cushing's syndrome
- Hypo- and hyperparathyroidism

1294. Which is *not* an ionotropic agent:

A. Dopamine
B. Amrinone
C. Dobutamine
D. Amiodarone

Amiodarone is an antiarrhythmic drug, used in ventricular arrhythmias such as VT and VF.

1295. AIDS was first diagnosed in patients suffering from:

A. *Cryptococcus neoformans* meningitis
B. *Pneumocystis carinii* pneumonia (PCP)
C. Tuberculosis
D. Kaposi sarcoma

The acquired immune deficiency syndrome (AIDS) was first recognized in the USA in 1981, in a patient suffering from *Pneumocystis carinii* pneumonia.

1296. HELLP includes all *except*:

A. Thrombocytopenia
B. Hemolytic anemia
C. Eosinophilia
D. Hepatic dysfunctions

Hematologic Manifestations of Pre-eclampsia

H	**H**emolysis
EL	**E**levated **L**iver function tests
LP	**L**ow **P**latelets

1297. Hormones secreted by small cell carcinoma lungs all *except*:

A. Vasopressin
B. GHRH
C. ACTH
D. GIP

Hormones Produced by Small Cell Lung Cancer

- Growth hormone
- Adrenocorticotropic hormone
- Arginine vasopressin
- Growth hormone-releasing hormone
- Corticotropin-releasing hormone
- Atrial natriuretic peptide

1298. The cardiac anomaly seen in Osler-Rendu-Weber syndrome:

A. High output cardiac failure
B. Pulmonary stenosis
C. VSD
D. Dilated cardiomyopathy

The major CVS anomaly of **Osler-Rendu-Weber syndrome** is AV fistula which leads to **high output cardiac failure**. The arteriovenous fistula may be found in liver, lung or mucus membranes. Compression of a large arteriovenous fistula causes reflex slowing of the heart rate (**Nicoladoni-Branham sign**).

1299. Visual cortex is supplied by:

A. Anterior and middle cerebral artery
B. Middle cerebral artery
C. Posterior and middle cerebral artery
D. Posterior cerebral artery

The visual cortex is supplied by posterior and middle cerebral artery.

1300. 'Punch drunk' state is associated with:

A. Boxing
B. Parkinsonism
C. Alcoholism
D. Chorea

Recurrent head trauma in professional boxers can lead to dementia, also called the **"punch drunk" syndrome** or dementia pugilistica.

1301. *Drug of choice* for cytomegalovirus:

A. Acyclovir
B. Ganciclovir
C. Amantadine
D. Idoxuridine

Ganciclovir is the drug of choice for cytomegalovirus infection.

1302. Granulomatous hepatitis is caused by:

A. Amiodarone
B. Allopurinol
C. Halothane
D. None

When the cause of granulomatous infiltration of liver is not found, diagnosis of granulomatous hepatitis should be considered. It is an uncommon disorder of unknown etiology which responds to corticosteroids. Hepatic granulomas have occasionally been observed in patients taking **amiodarone.**

1303. Hamman's crunch is seen in:

A. Caries tooth
B. Mediastinal emphysema
C. Fracture mandible
D. Niemann Pick disease

Hamman's sign is a sign of **mediastinal emphysema.** A crunching or clicking noise with the heartbeat is heard in auscultation.

1304. Wilms' tumor is characterized by wh'ch chromosomal aberration:

A. 11 p-
B. 13 p-
C. 13q-
D. 11 q-

Tumor Suppressor Genes Associated with Familial Cancer Syndromes

• Wilms' tumor	11p13
• Hereditary multiple exostoses	11p11-13
• Li-Fraumeni syndrome	17q13
• Neurofibromatosis type I	17q11.2
• Neurofibromatosis type II	22q12
• Tuberous sclerosis	16p13.3
• von Hippel-Lindau	3p25-26
• Basal cell nevus	9q22.3
• Familial ovarian cancer	17q21
• Familial breast cancer	13q12-13
• Familial melanoma	9p21
• Familial polyposis coli	5q21
• Familial retinoblastoma	13q24

1305. One of the following statements about tetanus is *true*:

A. Caused by *Clostridium tetani* **B.** Central spores
C. Aerobic infection **D.** Cannot be prevented

Tetanus is characterized by increased muscle tone and spasms, due to tetanospasmin, which is a powerful protein toxin elaborated by ***Clostridium tetani***. Tetanus occurs in several clinical forms, including generalized, neonatal, and localized form.

1306. Lev's disease is:

A. Sclerodegeneration of the conducting system
B. Calcification and sclerosis of the fibrous cardiac skeleton
C. Seen as a result of surgical trauma to the conducting system
D. Congenital disorder of the conducting system

- In **Lev's disease**, there is **calcification** and **sclerosis** of the fibrous cardiac skeleton.
- Lenegre's disease is a primary sclerodegenerative disease within the conducting system itself with no involvement of the myocardium or the fibrous skeleton of the heart.

1307. The exanthem of Rocky Mountain spotted fever (RMSF) usually appears 1st on the:

A. Face **B.** Extremities
C. Abdominal wall **D.** Neck

Rash appears in 15% of patients on the 1st day of disease and in 50% during the first 3 days. It appears first on **wrists and ankles** and then spread to involve **extremities** and the trunk.

1308. Keratoderma blenorrhagica is pathognomic of:

A. Behçet's disease **B.** Lyme's disease
C. Glucagonoma **D.** Reiter's syndrome

Keratoderma blenorrhagica consists of hyperkeratotic scaling lesions on the palms, soles, and nails. They occasionally occur in other areas also. This condition is pathognomic of **Reiter's syndrome.**

1309. Alveolar hypoventilation is observed in:

A. Guillain-Barré syndrome **B.** Bronchiectasis
C. Status asthmaticus **D.** Chronic bronchitis

The alveolar hypoventilation may occur in a condition in which there is phrenic nerve palsy such as in poliomyelitis, **Guillain-Barré syndrome,** etc.

1310. Malignant hypertension is diagnosed when:

A. Associated malignancy is present
B. Papilledema associated with elevated BP
C. Diastolic BP 120 mm Hg
D. All of the above

Malignant hypertension is said to be present when **severe hypertension is associated with papilledema** and retinal hemorrhage and retinal exudates.

1311. The sick cell syndrome is characterized by:

A. Hyponatremia
B. Hypokalemia
C. Hypernatremia
D. Hyperkalemia

In **"sick-cell" syndrome** there is **hyponatremia** due to a subnormal setting of the hypothalamic osmoreceptors. It is usually associated with a chronic, debilitating disease.

1312. Dysdiadochokinesia is a sign of:

A. Hysteria
B. Epilepsy
C. Tabes dorsalis
D. Cerebellar ataxia

Clinical Signs of Cerebellar Ataxia

- Dysmetria
- Dysdiadochokinesia
- Drunken gait
- Intention tremor
- Abnormal rebound
- Nystagmus

1313. Characteristic histological appearance of cells in Niemann-Pick disease is:

A. Multinuclear
B. Foam cells
C. Eosinophilic
D. Crystals in cytoplasm

In Niemann-Pick disease the lipid laden phagocytic **foam cells** are found in spleen, liver, bone marrow, tonsil, GI tract and lungs.

1314. Vitamin B_6 deficiency is caused by all *except*:

A. Penicillamine
B. Isoniazid
C. Cyclosporine
D. Cycloserine

Drugs Causing Pyridoxine Deficiency

- Penicillamine
- Cycloserine
- Isoniazid
- Carbonyl reagents

1315. Fever is caused by :

A. Leukotrienes
B. Histamine
C. Interleukin
D. Prostaglandins

Fever is a natural response of the body that helps in fighting off foreign substances, such as microorganisms, toxins, etc. Body temperature is set by the thermoregulatory center, located in an area in the brain called **hypothalamus**. Body temperature is not constant all day, but actually is lowest at 6 AM and highest around 4-6 PM. Substances that cause fever are known as "**pyrogens**." There are **two types of pyrogens; exogenous and endogenous**. Those that originate outside the body, such as bacterial toxins, are called "exogenous" pyrogens. Pyrogens formed by the body's own cells in response to an outside stimulus (such as a bacterial toxin) are called "endogenous" pyrogens. There are several "endogenous" pyrogens. These are made up of small groups of amino acids, the building blocks of proteins. These natural pyrogens have other functions in addition to inducing fever; they have been named "**cytokines**". When cytokines are injected into humans, fever and chills develop within an hour. **Interferon**, **tumor necrosis factor**, and various **interleukins** are the major fever producing cytokines. The production of fever is a very complex process; somehow, these cytokines cause the thermoregulatory center in the hypothalamus to reset the normal temperature level. The body's initial response is to conserve heat by vasoconstriction, a process in which blood vessels narrow and prevent heat loss from the skin and elsewhere. This alone will raise temperature by two to three degrees. Certain behavioral activities also occur, such as adding more clothes, seeking a warmer environment, etc. If the hypothalamus requires more heat, then shivering occurs.

1316. Primary atypical pneumonia is caused by:

A. *Mycoplasma* **B.** *Mycobacterium kansasii*
C. *Pneumocystis carinii* **D.** Photochromogens

Organisms Causing Atypical Pneumonia

- *M. pneumoniae* (Primary)
- Oral anaerobes
- *Coxiella burnetii*
- *Coccidioides immitis*
- *L. pneumophila*
- *P. carinii*
- *Francisella tularensis*
- *C. pneumoniae*
- *C. psittaci*
- *H. capsulatum*

1317. Calcitonin is secreted from:

A. C cells of thyroid **B.** Oxyphil cells of parathyroid
C. Chief cells of parathyroid **D.** Acinar cells of thyroid

Calcitonin is secreted by **C cells or clear cells** of thyroid. So this hormone is also known as thyrocalcitonin.

1318. Which of the following drugs may precipitate gout:

A. Streptomycin **B.** Pyrazinamide
C. Rifampicin **D.** Isoniazid

Drugs Precipitating Gout

- Salicylates
- Diuretics
- Alcohol
- Levo dopa
- *Ethambutol*
- *Pyrazinamide*
- Nicotinic acid
- Cyclosporine

1319. The formation of 25 hydroxy cholecalciferol takes place in the:

A. Liver **B.** Kidneys
C. Intestines **D.** Pancreas

In the **liver**, **vitamin D is converted to 25 hydroxy cholecalciferol** by hepatic mitochondrial and/or microsomal enzymes.

1320. Water hammer pulse is seen in:

A. AR
B. Pregnancy
C. Anemia
D. All of the above

Water hammer pulse is characteristic of hyperdynamic circulation and is seen in conditions like aortic regurgitation, severe anemia, pregnancy and mitral regurgitation.

1321. Atherosclerosis in the coronary circulation *most commonly* affects:
A. Left anterior descending artery **B.** Left circumflex
C. Right coronary **D.** All of the above

In the coronary circulation, the proximal **left anterior descending coronary artery** is the vessel *most commonly* affected by atherosclerosis.

1322. Dressing apraxia is seen in lesion of which lobe:
A. Dominant temporal **B.** Nondominant temporal
C. Dominant parietal **D.** Nondominant parietal

Dressing apraxia is caused by lesion of bilateral (or right sided) dorsal parietal lobe.

1323. Palmomental reflex is present in lesions of:
A. Parietal lobe **B.** Frontal lobe
C. Occipital lobe **D.** Temporal lobe

Palmomental response is contraction of the chin *ipsilateral* to a scratch stimulus diagonally applied to the palm. It is seen in **frontal lobe lesion**.

1324. Frequency of rest tremor in Parkinson's disease is:
A. 2/sec **B.** 4-6/sec
C. 8/sec **D.** 14/sec

The resting tremor of Parkinson disease has a frequency of **4-6 hertz.**

1325. *Des*ferrioxamine is used in treatment of poisoning with:
A. Iron **B.** Gold
C. Lead **D.** Copper

Ferrioxamine is a long chain iron containing complex. It is obtained from *Actinomycetes*. If iron is removed from this complex it is converted into *des*ferrioxamine, which has a very high affinity for iron. **1 gram of *des*ferrioxamine binds to 85 mg of elemental iron**. It binds with iron forming a stable nontoxic complex which is excreted in urine. It is indicated in acute iron poisoning and transfusion associated iron overload as seen in patients of thalassemia. Dose is 0.5-1 gm/day IM in chronic iron overload.

1326. Stokes Adam syndrome is associated with:
A. Auricular fibrillation
B. Supraventricular tachycardia
C. Atrial flutter
D. Complete heart block

Complete heart block or 3rd degree heart block is said to be present when atrial contraction is normal *but* no impulse is conducted to the ventricle. Ventricles beat with their own rhythm due to escape mechanism. **If it is associated with fainting it is known as Stokes Adam syndrome.**

1327. How long can blood be stored with CPDA:
A. 12 days **B.** 21 days
C. 35 days **D.** 48 days

CPD blood has a **shelf life of 3 weeks** (CPD*A*-1 to 5 weeks).There is considerable reduction in platelets within 24 hours and functional usefulness is lost after this time.

1328. Negri bodies are *most often* found in:

A. Midbrain
B. Basal ganglia
C. Frontal cortex
D. Hippocampus

In rabies there is intense cerebral edema associated with wide spread degeneration of neurons. **Negri bodies** are cytoplasmic, round or oval or bullet shaped, multiple, eosinophilic inclusions found in neurons, ***most commonly*** **in hippocampus** and Purkinje's cells.

1329. Skin pigmentation in 'bronze' diabetes is due to:

A. Hemosiderin
B. Melanin
C. Acaroids
D. Lipofuscin

In hemochromatosis there is deposition of **hemosiderin** in various organs, particularly in liver and pancreas. Skin pigmentation is found in 85% of cases and diabetes mellitus in 80% (**bronze diabetes**).

1330. *Most common* presentation of *unilateral* renal artery stenosis is:

A. Uremia
B. Hypertension
C. Peripheral edema
D. Polycythemia

Stenosis of the renal artery accounts for 2 to 5% of hypertension. ***Most common*** **presentation of unilateral renal artery stenosis is hypertension.**

1331. Vitamin K is required for:

A. Over dosage of Dindevan (phenindione)
B. Hemophilia
C. Over dosage of heparin
D. Christmas disease

Administering vitamin K_1 IV (1 to 40 mg) is the *only* specific treatment of **phenindione poisoning.**

1332. *Not* a feature of hereditary spherocytosis:

A. Normal or decreased MCV
B. Increased RBC surface area/volume
C. Autosomal dominant
D. Increased mean corpuscular hemoglobin *(AIIMS 1991)*

Hereditary spherocytosis has an autosomal dominant inheritance pattern. It is characterized by spherical red cells due to a molecular defect in 1 of the proteins in the cytoskeleton of the red cell membrane, leading to a loss of membrane and hence decreased ratio of surface area to volume and consequently spherocytosis. **RBC surface area is reduced** and because for a given volume, sphere has got the minimal possible surface area the RBCs tends to acquire this shape to compensate for the deficit in RBC surface membrane.

1333. Congenital 17 hydroxylase deficiency leads to:

A. Hypertension
B. Virilism
C. Hermaphroditism
D. Hyperkalemia

17 α hydroxylase enzyme is required to convert progesterone into 17 hydroxyprogesterone. Deficiency of this enzyme leads to impairment in production of 17 hydroxyprogesterone so progesterone is now converted into desoxycorticosterone .This is manifested clinically by primary amenorrhea, sexual infantilism, and hypertension. **Hypertension is due to increased production of desoxycorticosterone (DOC).**

1334. Overdoes of LSD is *most likely* to be associated with:

A. Deafness
B. Bradycardia
C. Pupillary dilatation
D. Blindness

Effects of LSD Overdose

Within minutes	Half an hour
• Tachycardia • Hypertension • Pupillary dilation • Tremor • Hyperpyrexia	• Mood changes • Visual illusions • Synesthesias • Extreme liability of mood

1335. What percent of gouty individuals have nephrolithiasis:
A. 5%
B. 30-35%
C. 40%
D. 50-60%

40% of patients of gout have nephrolithiasis.

1336. Mode of action of actinomycin D is to prevent:
A. RNA synthesis
B. DNA elongation
C. DNA synthesis
D. None of the above

Although **dactinomycin** is an antibiotic, it is not used as an antimicrobial agent. Its antineoplastic action is due to binding to DNA by intercalation between base pairs and **inhibition of** DNA-dependent **RNA synthesis**.

1337. Treatment of Vincent's angina is:
A. Penicillin
B. Penicillin + metronidazole
C. Amphotericin B
D. Metronidazole

Vincent's angina is also known as acute necrotizing ulcerative gingivitis or trench mouth. Clinical features are halitosis and ulcerations of the interdental papillae. Oral anaerobic bacteria are the etiological agent of this condition. **Oral penicillin + metronidazole** or with clindamycin *alone* is the drug of choice.

1338. Meralgia paresthetica involves:
A. Axillary nerve
B. Median nerve
C. Sural nerve
D. Lateral cutaneous nerve of thigh

Meralgia paresthetica is a condition in which there is pain and hyperesthesia on the outer surface of thigh. It is due to involvement of **lateral femoral cutaneous branch** involving segment L_2 and L_3.

1339. In which of the following condition, tissue *and* blood eosinophilia is seen:
A. Bacillary dysentery
B. Entamoeba histolytic infection
C. *Trichinella* infestation
D. Giardiasis
(DELHI 1991)

Tissue and blood eosinophilia is seen in *Trichinella* infestation due to larval migration and muscle invasion.

1340. The enzyme avidin inactivates.............in the egg:
A. Riboflavin
B. Thiamine
C. Pyridoxine
D. Biotin

Avidin is a protein which is isolated from *raw* egg white. It is an inhibitor of **biotin**, thereby causing a deficiency in biotin.

1341. 'P' wave in the ECG disappears in:
A. Atrial tachycardia
B. Atrial flutter
C. Mitral valve prolapse
D. Atrial fibrillation

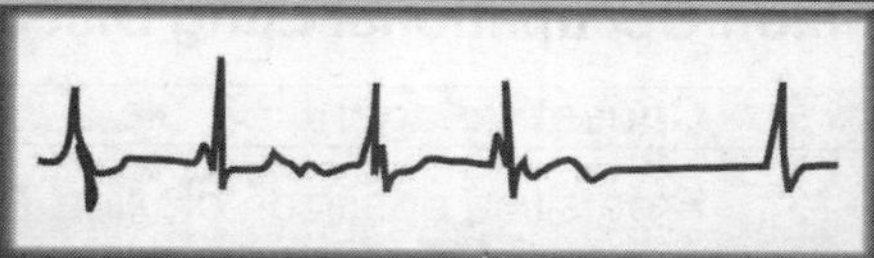

Atrial fibrillation is characterized by unorganized atrial activity **without distinct P waves** on the surface ECG.

1342. Treatment of choice in ventricular fibrillation is:
A. Electrical cardioversion
B. Carotid massage
C. IV lignocaine
D. IV nifedipine

Electrical cardioversion and defibrillation is the most effective methods for terminating arrhythmias.

1343. Ebstein's anomaly is associated with:
A. Tricuspid regurgitation
B. Cardiomyopathy
C. Coarctation of aorta
D. Right ventricular hypertrophy

In **Ebstein's anomaly** there is downward displacement of the tricuspid valve into the right ventricle which leads to tricuspid regurgitation.

1344. Sustained heaving cardiac impulse indicates:
A. Mitral regurgitation
B. Aortic regurgitation
C. Mitral stenosis
D. Aortic stenosis

When the left ventricle contracts and pushes through the blood through a **stenosed aortic valve**, it leads to characteristic **heaving** apex beat.

1345. pH of the gastric juice is:
A. 1.0
B. 2.5-3
C. 0.5-2.5
D. 3-3.5

The pH of gastric juice is about 1, while the pH of pancreatic juice is 8.

1346. Drug of choice in herpes simplex encephalitis is:
A. Interferon
B. Amantadine
C. Vidarabine
D. Acyclovir

Acyclovir is the drug of choice of herpes simplex encephalitis (IV10 mg/kg 8 hourly for 10 days).

1347. Bancroftian filariasis is transmitted by:
A. *Culex*
B. *Aedes*
C. *Mansonia*
D. Tick

Natural vectors for *W. bancrofti* are ***Culex fatigans*** mosquitoes in urban areas and anopheline or aedean mosquitoes in rural areas.

1348. Drug of choice to treat metabolic acidosis in cardiac arrest is:
A. Ringer lactate
B. Normal saline
C. $NaHCO_3$
D. Isolyte P

Drug of choice to treat metabolic acidosis in cardiac arrest is **$NaHCO_3$** (1 mEq/kg).

1349. Cotton dust is associated with:
A. Byssinosis
B. Bagassosis
C. Asbestosis
D. Silicosis

Common Occupational Lung Diseases

Disease	Causative agent
• Silicosis	Free silica or silicon dioxide
• Anthracosis	Coal
• Byssinosis	Cotton fiber dust
• Bagassosis	Sugar cane dust
• Asbestosis	Asbestos
• Farmer's lung	Moldy hay or grain dust

1350. Extrapyramidal symptoms are best treated with:

A. Haloperidol
B. Procyclidine
C. Trihexyphenidyl
D. Metoclopramide

Extrapyramidal symptoms are best treated with **trihexyphenidyl**, 2 mg 12 hourly, or *benztropine* mesylate, 1 to 2 mg 12 hourly.

1351. Juvenile Huntington's disease is marked by:

A. Chorea
B. Tremors
C. Athetosis
D. Tics

Huntington's disease is a familial, autosomal dominant, degenerative brain disease. It has an incidence of 10/100,000. The 2 important clinical features are:

- **Chorea**
- Behavioral disturbance

If the onset occurs before the age of 20, it is called juvenile Huntington's disease.

1352. Paroxysmal hypotension is seen in:

A. Infectious mononucleosis
B. Leukemia
C. Lymphoma
D. Carcinoid syndrome

Manifestations of the carcinoid syndrome:

- Cutaneous flushing
- Diarrhea
- Valvular heart disease
- Telangiectasias
- Wheezing
- Paroxysmal hypotension.

1353. Drug of choice for treating *Schistosoma hematobium* is:

A. Pyrantel pamoate
B. Metronidazole
C. Praziquantel
D. None of the above

The drug of choice for *Schistosoma hematobium* infection is **praziquantel**.

1354. Lardaceous spleen is seen in:

A. Alcoholic hepatitis
B. Malaria
C. Chronic active hepatitis
D. Diffuse amyloidosis

Amyloidosis of spleen may be asymptomatic or may produce moderate to massive splenomegaly. One of the 2 patterns of deposition may be seen.

- **Sago spleen**: Deposition is mainly limited to splenic follicles producing tapioca like granules.
- **Lardaceous spleen**: Here the follicles are spared and the amyloid deposits in the walls of splenic sinuses and connective tissue framework of red pulp given a large map like areas of amyloidosis.

1355. Synkinesia is seen in:

A. Trigeminal neuralgia **B.** Bell's palsy
C. Migraine **D.** All of the above

Faulty regeneration of the 7th nerve fibers during recovery of **Bell's palsy** sometimes results in very troublesome phenomena.

- If fibers that were previously connected with the orbicularis oculi muscle regenerate to innervate the orbicularis oris, closure of the lids will cause a retraction of the mouth.
- If fibers that were previously connected with the face regenerate to innervate the lacrimal gland, faulty tearing ("**crocodile tears**") may occur along with any activity of the facial muscles, such as eating.
- Another *rare* facial **synkinesia** is in which eyelids are closed when the patient opens the jaw.

1356. Milk alkali syndrome consists of all of the following *except*:

A. Azotemia **B.** Alkalosis
C. Hypercalcemia **D.** Hypercalciuria

The **milk-alkali syndrome** is caused due to an excessive intake of calcium and *absorbable* antacids such as milk or calcium carbonate. Features include:

- Hypercalcemia
- Alkalosis
- Renal failure

1357. Monckeberg's sclerosis involves:

A. Externa **B.** Media
C. Intima **D.** All the layers

There are 3 morphological types of arteriosclerosis:

- Atherosclerosis—Fibrofatty plaques formation in intima.
- Monckeberg's *medial* calcific sclerosis—Calcification of media of muscular arteries.
- Arteriolosclerosis—Proliferation or thickening of walls of small arteries and arterioles.

1358. Postural hypotension and failure of ejaculation is *most commonly* seen in treatment with:

A. Guanethidine **B.** Propranolol
C. Minoxidil **D.** Na^+ nitroprusside

Side Effects of Guanethidine

- Headache
- Peripheral edema (most common)
- Bradycardia
- Orthostatic hypotension
- Drooping eyelids
- Nocturia
- Loss of hair on scalp
- Angina
- Pulmonary edema
- Weakness
- Dryness of mouth
- Skin rash
- Muscle pain
- Diarrhea
- Difficulty in ejaculating
- Blurred vision
- Tremors
- Nausea or vomiting

1359. Rheumatic activity involves mostly.................valves:

A. Aortic and tricuspid **B.** Mitral and tricuspid
C. Aortic and pulmonary **D.** Mitral and aortic

In rheumatic carditis murmur of mitral regurgitation and/or aortic regurgitation due to valvulitis is *always* present and in their absence carditis should *not* be diagnosed.

1360. Somatostatin inhibits secretion of all *except*:

A. Prolactin **B.** Insulin
C. Glucagon **D.** Growth hormone

Hormones Inhibited by Somatostatin

• Gastrin	• VIP
• GIP	• Secretin
• Motilin	• Insulin
• Glucagon	• Pancreatic polypeptide
• Growth hormone	

1361. Clinical features of CRF appear when renal function is reduced to:

A. 20% of normal
B. 30% of normal
C. 50% of normal
D. 70% of normal

• **Diminished renal reserve**	GFR < 50% of normal
• **Renal insufficiency**	GFR < 20-50% of normal
• **Chronic renal failure**	GFR < 25% of normal
• **End stage renal disease**	GFR < 05% of normal

1362. In chronic renal failure all are seen *except:*

A. Hyperphosphatemia
B. Hypomagnesemia
C. Hyponatremia
D. Metabolic acidosis

Fluid and Electrolyte Disturbances in Uremia

- Volume expansion and contraction
- Hypernatremia and hyponatremia
- Hyperkalemia and hypokalemia
- Metabolic acidosis
- Hyperphosphatemia
- Hypocalcemia

1363. Following are CNS complications of AIDS:

A. Dementia
B. CNS lymphoma
C. Aseptic meningitis
D. All of the above

Neurologic Problems in HIV-infected Patients

• Toxoplasmosis	• Mycobacterium tuberculosis
• Cryptococcosis	• Syphilis
• Cytomegalovirus	• CNS lymphoma
• Progressive multifocal leukoencephalopathy	• Aseptic meningitis
• HTLV-I	• AIDS dementia complex

1364. Which is *false* about adrenal adenoma:

A. Half are malignant
B. Presents as abdominal mass
C. Should be excised
D. Causes Cushing's syndrome

About 20 to 25% of patients with **Cushing's syndrome** have an adrenal neoplasm. They are usually unilateral, and **50% are malignant**. When an adenoma or carcinoma is found to be present, adrenal exploration should be done and the tumor excised.

1365. Which of the following is *not* a differential diagnosis to botulism:

A. Polio
B. Stroke
C. Guillain-Barré syndrome
D. Tick palsy

Differential Diagnosis of Botulism

- Myasthenia gravis
- Guillain-Barré syndrome
- Lambert-Eaton syndrome
- Poliomyelitis
- Tick paralysis
- Diphtheria
- Mushroom poisoning
- Drugs
- Hypermagnesemia

1366. Which of the following is a 17-ketosteroid:

A. Progesterone
B. Pregnenolone
C. 17-hydroxypregnenolone
D. All

Adrenal steroids contain either 19 or 21 carbon atoms in their molecules. C_{19} steroids have a ketone group at C_{17} and are called 17-ketosteroids. The C_{19} steroids have predominantly androgenic activity. Progesterone, pregnenolone, 17-hydroxypregnenolone, etc. are 17 ketosteroids.

1367. One of the following is *not* a chromosomal breakage syndrome:

A. Bloom's syndrome
B. Xeroderma pigmentosa
C. Friedreich's ataxia
D. Fanconi anemia

Chromosomal Instability Syndromes

- Bloom syndrome
- Fanconi anemia
- ICF syndrome
- Nijmegen breakage syndrome
- Seckel syndrome
- Xeroderma pigmentosa

1368. M spike on serum electrophoresis is seen in:

A. α chain disease
B. Lymphoblastic leukemia
C. Waldenstrom's macroglobulinemia
D. AIDS

In plasma cell disorders such as multiple myeloma, **Waldenstrom's macroglobulinemia**, primary amyloidosis, and the heavy chain diseases when electrophoresis is done there is a sharp spike a region called an **M component** (M stands for monoclonal).

1369. All can cause acute tubular necrosis *except*:

A. Cyclosporine
B. Hypovolemia
C. Ceftriaxone
D. Aminoglycosides

Causes of Acute Tubular Necrosis

Ischemia	Toxins
• HYPOVOLEMIA	• RADIOCONTRAST
• LOW CARDIAC OUTPUT	• CYCLOSPORINE
• RENAL VASOCONSTRICTION	• AMINOGLYCOSIDES
• SYSTEMIC VASODILATATION	• CISPLATIN
• ABRUPTIO PLACENTAE	• ETHYLENE GLYCOL
• POSTPARTUM HEMORRHAGE	• ACETAMINOPHEN
	• ILLEGAL ABORTIFACIENTS
	• URIC ACID
	• RHABDOMYOLYSIS
	• HEMOLYSIS
	• PLASMA CELL DYSCRASIA
	• OXALATE

1370. *Most common* presentation of primary biliary cirrhosis:

A. Pruritus
B. Jaundice
C. Abdominal mass
D. Pain

In **primary biliary cirrhosis** the *earliest* symptom is **pruritus**, which may be generalized or limited initially to the palms and soles.

1371. 'Hung up' knee jerk is seen in:

A. Chorea
B. Hypothyroidism
C. Cerebral palsy
D. Athetosis

In **hypothyroidism** relaxation phase of the deep tendon reflexes is characteristically prolonged and is known as **hung-up reflex**.

1372. All of the following reduce gastric acid secretion *except*:

A. Cimetidine
B. Ranitidine
C. Pirenzepine
D. Carbenoxolone

Carbenoxolone sodium has no effect on volume or pH of gastric acid and acts by augmentation of mucus production which remains adherent to gastric mucosa and 'protecting' it from the acid.

1373. Continuous murmur is seen in:

A. PDA
B. Small (restrictive) ASD with MS
C. AV malformation
D. All of the above

Causes of Continuous Murmur

- Proximal coronary artery stenosis
- Mammary soufflé
- Pulmonary artery branch stenosis
- Bronchial collateral circulation
- Small ASD with MS
- Intercostal AV fistula
- PDA
- Coronary AV fistula
- Ruptured aneurysm of sinus of Valsalva
- ASD
- Cervical venous hum
- Anomalous left coronary artery

1374. Risus sardonicus is associated with:

A. Bell's palsy
B. Rabies
C. Poliomyelitis
D. Tetanus

In tetanus sustained contraction of the facial muscles results in a grimace or sneer (**risus sardonicus**), and contraction of the back muscles produces an arched back (opisthotonos).

1375. As an emetic, morphine acts at:

A. Dorsal medullary centre
B. Chemo trigger zone
C. Peripherally
D. Hypothalamus

The morphine *directly* stimulates chemotrigger zone (CTZ) producing nausea and vomiting.

1376. Which of the following is *true* of psoriatic arthritis:

A. Involves distal joints of hand and foot
B. Pencil in cup deformity
C. Sacroiliitis
D. All of the above

The term **psoriatic arthritis** may be used for all cases in which psoriasis and inflammatory polyarthritis are present and rheumatoid factor is absent from the serum. The classic radiologic features of psoriatic arthritis include a destructive arthritis involving the DIP joints of the hands and/or feet, bony ankylosis of interphalangeal joints, destruction of interphalangeal joints, bony proliferation, resorption of the terminal tufts, diffuse "sausage" swelling of the digits, and absence of osteoporosis. Erosions in psoriatic arthritis generally involve the "bare areas" (those areas within the joint capsule where the articular cartilage is thin or absent). In some patients, erosion of the subchondral bone is seen either exclusively or together with erosion in the bare areas. When subchondral erosion is extensive, the joint space may appear to be wider than usual and, in some cases; extensive bone resorption produces a "**pencil and cup**" deformity. Radiographs of the back show the typical findings of ankylosing spondylitis and **bilateral sacroiliitis**.

1377. Membranous glomerulonephritis can be caused by:

A. Penicillamine
B. Captopril
C. Gold
D. All of the above

Drugs Causing Membranous Nephropathy

- Penicillamine
- Mercury
- Trimethadione
- Gold
- Captopril
- Chlormethiazole

1378. Immunoglobulin administration is indicated in:

A. Rabies
B. Gas gangrene
C. Poliomyelitis
D. Typhoid

Indications of Immunoglobulin Administration

- Viral hepatitis A and B
- Mumps
- Chickenpox
- Leukemia
- Measles
- Poliomyelitis
- Premature infants
- Immunocompromised states

1379. First generation cephalosporins are *not* effective against:

A. *Pseudomonas*
B. *Proteus*
C. *Streptococci*
D. *Staphylococci*

The **1st generation cephalosporins** are **effective against** penicillinase producing, methicillin-susceptible staphylococci and streptococci. They have potent activity against many strains of *E. coli*, *Klebsiella pneumoniae*, and *Proteus mirabilis* and are among the drugs of choice in empirical therapy for community acquired urinary tract infections. They are **not effective against** *B. fragilis*, enterococci, methicillin-resistant staphylococci, *Pseudomonas*, *Acinetobacter*, *Enterobacter*, indole-positive *Proteus*, and *Serratia* and poor activity against *H. influenzae*.

1380. *Initial* site of cryptococcal infection is:

A. Meninges
B. Bone
C. Lungs
D. Skin

Cryptococcal infection is acquired by inhalation of fungus into the lungs. Pulmonary infection usually resolves spontaneously and is mostly asymptomatic. Silent hematogenous spread to the brain may occur leading to formation of clusters of cryptococci in the perivascular areas of gray matter, in the basal ganglia, and, to a lesser extent, in other areas of the CNS. The inflammatory response around these foci is usually of low grade.

1381. Which of the following is *false* about Tamm-Horsfall mucoprotein:

A. Normal urinary constituent
B. Tubular in origin
C. Abnormal urinary constituent
D. Seen in multiple myeloma

Tamm-Horsfall mucoprotein is a normal mucoprotein in the urine. It does not come from plasma but is **produced by the ascending limb of the loop of Henle**. When this protein is concentrated *at low pH*, it forms gel. These conditions may be met when the urine is exposed to myoglobin, hemoglobin, albumin, Bence-Jones protein, and contrast media. It is seen in **multiple myeloma** during immunofluorescent microscopy.

1382. Systolic murmur conducted from apex to axilla occurs in:

A. Mitral regurgitation **B.** Tricuspid regurgitation
C. Ventricular septal defect **D.** Mitral valve prolapse

The pansystolic murmur of **mitral regurgitation** and is best heard in the mitral area. It radiates to the axilla and also to the back when anterior leaflet of the mitral valve is abnormal.

1383. Quick reduction of blood pressure is done in:

A. Cerebral infarct **B.** Hypertensive encephalopathy
C. Myocardial infarction **D.** Any patient with hypertension

Malignant hypertension is a medical emergency and should be treated immediately. It should be distinguished from severe hypertension, because very aggressive therapy in malignant hypertension could result in a potentially hazardous reduction in myocardial and cerebral perfusion. **The initial aims of therapy are**

- **Correction of medical complications**
- **Reduction of diastolic pressure by 1/3rd, but not below 95 mmHg.**

1384. Nephrotic syndrome can be caused by all *except*:

A. Malaria **B.** Syphilis
C. Hepatitis **D.** *Mycoplasma*

1385. Systemic diseases which cause nephrotic syndrome are all *except*:

A. Systemic lupus erythematosus **B.** Amyloidosis
C. Diabetes mellitus **D.** Atherosclerosis

Important Causes of Nephrotic Syndrome

Primary glomerular diseases	Systemic diseases	Other causes
• Membranous glomerulonephritis	• Diabetes mellitus	• Dermatitis herpetiformis
• Lipoid nephrosis	• Amyloidosis	• Myasthenia gravis
• Focal segmental glomerulonephritis	• SLE	• Bullous pemphigoid
• Membranoproliferative glomerulonephritis	• Malaria	• Primary biliary cirrhosis
• IgA nephropathy	• Syphilis	• Sjögren's syndrome
	• Hepatitis B	• Hashimoto's disease
	• AIDS	• Crohn's disease
	• Gold	• α_1 antitrypsin deficiency
	• Penicillamine	• Fanconi's syndrome
	• Street heroin	• Weber-Christian disease
	• Carcinomas and melanomas	• Guillain-Barré syndrome
	• Bee sting allergy	• Sickle cell disease
	• Hereditary nephritis	• Sarcoidosis

1386. Bence Jones proteins in the urine are characteristic of:

A. Multiple myeloma **B.** Acute glomerulonephritis
C. Nephrotic syndrome **D.** Chromic glomerulonephritis

Bence Jones protein, named after Sir Henry Bence Jones, a British Physician, is a protein that occurs in the urine of patients with **multiple myeloma** and sometimes in patients with other diseases of the reticuloendothelial system. When urine samples are heated to 50° to 60°C, a precipitate forms.

1387. Chronic lymphatic leukemia occurs usually in the ....decade of life:

A. 1st **B.** 4th
C. 7th **D.** 3rd

The most common chronic leukemia/lymphoma is B cell chronic lymphatic leukemia, which often presents with asymptomatic lymphocytosis in patients with a **median age of 60**.

1388. Incubation period of mumps is:

A. 2-8 days **B.** 7 days
C. 10 days **D.** 18 days

The incubation period of mumps is **14-18 days**, with extremes of 7 and 23 days.

1389. Down syndrome is due to:

A. Trisomy 21 **B.** Trisomy 18
C. Trisomy 13 **D.** Trisomy 8

1390. Edward's syndrome is:

A. Trisomy 21 **B.** Trisomy 18
C. Trisomy 13 **D.** 5 P

1391. Patau syndrome is due to:

A. Trisomy 21 **B.** Trisomy 18
C. Trisomy 13 **D.** 5 P

Trisomy	**Trisomy 13**	**Trisomy 18**	**Trisomy 21**
Syndrome	**Patau's Syndrome**	**Edwards syndrome**	**Down syndrome**
Birth weight	NBW	IUGR	NBW
Skin	Scalp defects		
CNS	Holoprosencephaly Neural tube defect	Microcephaly ,muscular hypertonia	Muscular hypotonia
Face	Micro ophthalmia, cleft lip, cleft palate	Micrognathia	Up slanting eyes, flat face, prominent tongue, small ear
Cardiac anomalies	VSD/PDA/ASD Dextrocardia	VSD/ASD/PDA	AV canal defect/VSD/PDA
Abdomen	Polycystic kidney	Omphalocele	
Extremities		Camptodactyly (Permanent flexion of the fingers or toes), overlapping of fingers	Brachydactyly, Simians crease, clinodactyly of 5th finger (Hypoplasia of the middle phalanx), wide space between 1st and 2nd toe

1392. Vitamin D resistant rickets is inherited as:

A. Autosomal dominant
B. Autosomal recessive
C. X-linked recessive
D. X-linked dominant

X-linked hypophosphatemia is also known as *phosphate diabetes* or ***vitamin D-resistant rickets***. It is an **X-linked dominant** disorder characterized by rickets in an otherwise well-nourished, healthy-appearing child. When the child begins to walk and bear weight, lower limb deformities appear and become progressively worse.

1393. Alpha fetoproteins levels of greater than..........is suggestive of primary hepatomas:

A. 100 μg% **B.** 25 μg%
C. 400 μg% **D.** 500 μg%

Alpha fetoproteins (AFP) levels > **500** μg/L are found in about 80% of patients with hepatocellular carcinoma.

1394. Syphilis causes all *except*:

A. Linear calcification of aorta
B. Aortic regurgitation
C. Coronary ostial stenosis
D. None of the above

Common Features of Cardiovascular Syphilis

- Uncomplicated aortitis
- Coronary ostial stenosis
- Aortic regurgitation
- Calcification of the ascending aorta
- Saccular aneurysm

1395. The following does *not* occur with asbestosis:

A. Methemoglobinemia
B. Pulmonary fibrosis
C. Pleural mesothelioma
D. Pleural calcification

Health Hazards Associated with Asbestosis

- Pulmonary fibrosis
- Mesothelioma
- Calcification along the parietal pleura

1396. Cirrhosis of liver with portal hypertension occurs in all *except*:

A. Cystic fibrosis
B. $\alpha_1$antitrypsin deficiency
C. Wilson's disease
D. Congenital hepatic fibrosis

Causes of Cirrhosis or/and Liver Disease

INFECTIOUS DISEASES	INHERITED	DRUGS	OTHER
• Brucellosis • *Echinococcus* • Schistosomiasis • Toxoplasmosis • Viral hepatitis (Hepatitis B, C, D, E, G) • Cytomegalovirus	• $\alpha_1$antitrypsin deficiency • Fanconi's syndrome • Galactosemia • Gaucher's disease • Glycogen storage disease • Hemochromatosis • Hereditary fructose intolerance • Hereditary tyrosinemia • Wilson's disease	• Arsenicals • Isoniazid • Methotrexate • Methyldopa • Oral contraceptives • Oxyphenisatin • Perhexilene • Pyrrolidizine	• Chronic inflammatory bowel disease • Cystic fibrosis • Diabetes mellitus • Graft-versus-host disease • Jejunoileal bypass • Sarcoidosis

1397. Cardiac manifestations of Graves' disease would include all of the following *except*:

A. Wide pulse pressure **B.** Atrial fibrillation
C. Pleuropericardial scratch **D.** Aortic insufficiency

Important Features of Graves' Disease

- Nervousness
- Emotional changes
- Tremor
- Amenorrhea
- Systolic murmurs
- Insomnia
- Frequent bowel movements
- Perspiration
- *Wide pulse pressure*
- Cardiac enlargement
- Heat intolerance
- Weight loss
- Proximal muscle weakness
- *Atrial arrhythmias*
- *Means-Lerman scratch*

1398. All of the following conditions produce restrictive cardiomyopathy *except*:

A. Hypothyroidism
B. Amyloidosis
C. Hypereosinophilic syndrome
D. Endomyocardial fibrosis

Causes of Restrictive Cardiomyopathy

- Amyloidosis
- Hemochromatosis
- Eosinophilia
- Glycogen deposition
- Sarcoidosis
- Neoplastic infiltration
- Endomyocardial fibrosis
- Fabry's disease
- Myocardial fibrosis

1399. Japanese encephalitis is caused by:

A. Human retrovirus
B. Enteroviruses
C. Flaviviruses
D. Cytomegalovirus

Japanese encephalitis virus is found throughout Asia. It is very common in eastern parts of Uttar Pradesh. Epidemics usually occur in rainy seasons leading to high mortality especially in children. This **flavivirus** is particularly common in areas where irrigated rice fields attract the natural avian vertebrate hosts and provide abundant breeding sites for mosquitoes such as *Culex tritaeniorhyncus*, which transmit the virus to humans.

1400. Hurler's syndrome is associated with:

A. Dwarfism
B. Corneal clouding
C. Hepatosplenomegaly
D. All of the above

Important Features of Hurler's Syndrome (MPS 1H)

- Autosomal recessive inheritance
- Enzyme deficient is α–L-iduronidase
- Abnormal accumulation of heparan and dermatan sulphate
- Onset at the age of 6-8 months
- Dwarfism
- Corneal clouding
- Hepatosplenomegaly
- Valvular lesions
- Coronary artery lesions
- Skeletal deformities
- Joint stiffness
- Mental retardation

1401. Nerve involved in intracranial aneurysm is:

A. 1st
B. 2nd
C. 3rd
D. 10th

An expanding aneurysm may cause 3rd cranial nerve palsy.

1402. Which is *not* a feature of sarcoidosis:

A. Cardiomyopathy
B. Malabsorption
C. Hypercalcemia
D. Paratracheal lymph nodes

Features of Sarcoidosis

Pulmonary manifestations	Extrapulmonary manifestations
• Bilateral hilar enlargement due to paratracheal nodes • Pulmonary opacities • Pulmonary fibrosis • Cor pulmonale • Pleural effusion • "**Egg shell**" calcification of hilar nodes • Atelectasis	• **Skin**—erythema nodosum, cutaneous sarcoids, lupus pernio. • **Bones**—arthritis and arthralgia • **CNS**—cerebral, meningeal, cranial or peripheral nerve involvement • Hepatosplenomegaly • Nephrocalcinosis • **CVS**—myocarditis, cardiomyopathy and arrhythmias • Parotid gland enlargement • Conjunctivitis, uveitis, iridocyclitis • Disorder of calcium metabolism with hypercalciuria, with / without hypercalcemia

1403. Bullous lesion occurs in:
A. Diabetes mellitus
B. Hemochromatosis
C. Uremia
D. Porphyria

Cutaneous photosensitivity is the major clinical feature of **porphyrias** in which fluid-filled vesicles and **bullae develop** on sun-exposed areas of the body.

1404. Papillary necrosis is *most commonly* seen in:
A. Diabetes mellitus
B. Acute pyelonephritis
C. Sickle cell anemia
D. Analgesic nephropathy

Analgesic nephropathy is characterized by **papillary necrosis** and tubulointerstitial inflammation.

1405. All secondaries produce a *hot spot* on bone scan *except*:
A. Myeloma
B. Lymphoma
C. Small cell lung carcinoma
D. Renal cell carcinoma

The boney lesions of **multiple myeloma** are **lytic** in nature and are rarely associated with osteoblastic new bone formation; therefore, they produce **cold spots** on bone scan.

1406. All of the following are chromosomal anomalies *except*:
A. Down syndrome
B. Hypoplastic left heart syndrome (HLHS)
C. Edward's syndrome
D. Turner's syndrome

• **Turner's syndrome**	X O
• **Down syndrome**	Trisomy 21
• **Edward's syndrome**	Trisomy 18

1407. The part of RNA which *does not* code for proteins is:
A. Exon
B. Codon
C. Introns
D. Meson

• **Intron**	***Non*coding** space between the discrete coding regions (exons) of the DNA of the gene.
• **Exon**	Coding region of the DNA of genes
• **Codon**	Sequence of three bases in a strand of DNA or mRNA that is the genetic code for a specific amino acid
• **Meson**	Particle of mass intermediate between that of the electron and that of the proton. Mesons of more than one variety and of positive, neutral, and negative charges occur

1408. Pseudodementia is a feature of:

A. Endogenous depression **B.** Severe depression
C. Alzheimer's disease **D.** Multiple strokes

Psychiatric diseases can simulate dementia. **Severely depressed** individuals sometimes appear demented. This phenomenon is called **pseudodementia**.

1409. Enzyme marker of malignant hyperthermia is:

A. Serum CPK **B.** SGOT
C. LDH **D.** SGPT

Malignant hyperthermia is diagnosed in susceptible persons by elevated **creatine phosphokinase** levels and histochemical studies on muscle biopsy, and by a history of exposure to halothane.

1410. The most effective treatment of atrial flutter is:

A. IV lignocaine **B.** Quinidine
C. Low dose phenytoin **D.** DC shock

The most effective treatment of **atrial flutter** is direct-current **cardioversion**.

1411. Initial dose of heparin in deep vein thrombosis is:

A. 10,000 U/day **B.** 1 lakh U/day
C. 50.000 U/day **D.** 2 lakh U/day

Heparin should be administered IV as an initial bolus of 7500 to 10,000 IU, followed by a continuous infusion of 1000 to 1500 IU/hour.

1412. Ocular muscle *most commonly* involved in thyrotoxic myopathy is:

A. Superior oblique **B.** Inferior rectus
C. Inferior oblique **D.** Superior rectus

In thyrotoxicosis the weakness of the extraocular muscles, particularly elevators (**inferior oblique**), results in diplopia.

1413. Hematuria, RBC casts and proteinuria are suggestive of:

A. Nephrotic syndrome **B.** Acute nephritis
C. Renal cell carcinoma **D.** Chronic renal failure

Gross or microscopic hematuria, RBC casts, and proteinuria are necessary for the diagnosis of acute glomerulonephritis.

1414. Birefringent crystals in urine are seen with:

A. Phosphaturia **B.** Cystinuria
C. Uricosuria **D.** Struvite stones

Uric acid stones are radiolucent. Uric acid dihydrate forms teardrop-shaped crystals which are strongly birefringent.

1415. Function of the thalamus is:

A. Arousal **B.** Relay centre
C. Pain perception **D.** Pain location

Thalamus acts as a **relay centre** for the impulses ascending via lateral spinothalamic tract, ventral spinothalamic tract and medial lemniscus. These impulses are transmitted to postcentral gyrus via thalamic radiation.

1416. In tuberculosis in an AIDS patient the chest X-ray looks like:

A. Miliary shadow **B.** Consolidation
C. Cavity **D.** Collapse

Tuberculosis is an important problem in patients with HIV infection. The chest X-ray in patients with disseminated disease shows **miliary shadow**, pleural effusions, and hilar and/or mediastinal adenopathy.

1417. Ectopic ACTH syndrome is seen *most commonly* with:
A. Renal cell carcinoma
B. Bronchogenic carcinoma
C. Lymphoma
D. Pituitary adenoma

Most of the cases of ectopic ACTH syndrome are due to bronchogenic carcinoma of small cell (oat cell) type.

1418. Cyclosporine A inhibits:
A. B cells
B. CD_4
C. T cells
D. CD_8

Cyclosporine inhibits T lymphocyte proliferation. It is nephrotoxic and hepatotoxic and other side effects are anorexia, lethargy, hirsutism, gum hyperplasia and seizures.

1419. The following are the toxicity of cyclosporine *except*:
A. Nephrotoxicity
B. Tremor
C. Hirsutism
D. Hypokalemia

Common Side Effects of Cyclosporine

• Anaphylaxis	• Hemolytic-uremic syndrome	• Gingival hyperplasia
• Hyperkalemia	• Hypertension	• Nephrotoxicity
• Tremor	• Hirsutism	• Trembling

1420. Constrictive pericarditis is *not* caused by:
A. Tuberculosis
B. Rheumatic arthritis
C. Pyogenic infection
D. None of the above

Causes of Chronic Constrictive Pericarditis

• Tuberculosis (most common)	• Histoplasmosis	• Acute viral pericarditis
• Bacterial infections	• Neoplastic disease	• Rheumatoid arthritis
• SLE	• CRF	• Chronic dialysis

1421. All are *true* about idiopathic hypertrophic aortic stenosis *except*:
A. Autosomal dominant with complete penetrance
B. Sudden death
C. May have associated MR
D. Verapamil may ameliorate symptoms

Idiopathic hypertrophic aortic stenosis is genetically heterogeneous that is it may be AD or AR or X-linked. It usually leads to MR due to hypertrophic obstructive cardiomyopathy. Sudden death may be the first manifestation of this disease. Verapamil and diltiazem may ameliorate symptoms.

1422. Causes of atrial fibrillation include:
A. Thyrotoxicosis
B. Cardiomyopathy
C. Chronic lung disease
D. All of the above

Causes of Atrial Fibrillation

• Rheumatic heart disease	• Chronic lung disease	• Thyrotoxicosis
• Nonrheumatic mitral valve disease	• Atrial septal defect	• Miscellaneous cardiac abnormalities

1423. Hormone producing carcinoma bronchus manifests:
- **A.** Hormonal changes earlier than other changes
- **B.** Hormonal changes after other changes
- **C.** Simultaneously
- **D.** During remission

Paraneoplastic syndromes are common in patients of lung cancer and may be the 1st sign of this condition.

1424. Treatment of hypertensive emergency is:
- **A.** Nitroprusside
- **B.** Propranolol
- **C.** Guanethidine
- **D.** Frusemide

Malignant hypertension is a medical emergency and requires immediate treatment. Nitroprusside is the drug of choice of this condition given in a dose of 0.25 to 8.0 μg/kg per minute.

1425. All are the features of sickle cell anemia *except*:
- **A.** Leukopenia
- **B.** Pulmonary hypertension
- **C.** Heart failure
- **D.** Acute chest syndrome

1426. *Not* a feature of sickle cell anemia:
- **A.** Fish vertebrae
- **B.** Enlarged heart
- **C.** Leukopenia
- **D.** Pulmonary hypertension *(UP 1997)*

Common Features of Sickle Cell Anemia

- Chronic anemia
- Leg ulcers
- Priapism
- *Salmonella* osteomyelitis
- Pulmonary infarction
- Acute chest syndrome
- Pulmonary hypertension
- Stroke
- Heart failure
- Retinal detachment
- Blindness
- Aseptic necrosis of the femoral head
- Hematuria
- Renal papillary necrosis
- Splenic infarction
- Fish mouth vertebra

1427. Selective protein loss occurs in:
- **A.** Tropical sprue
- **B.** Celiac disease
- **C.** Intestinal lymphangiectasia
- **D.** Whipple's disease

The primary laboratory finding in intestinal lymphangiectasia is hypoproteinemia with decreased serum levels of albumin, immunoglobulins IgG, IgA, and IgM, transferrin, and ceruloplasmin.

1428. Cause of *secondary* hyperparathyroidism is:
- **A.** Cardiac failure
- **B.** Werner syndrome
- **C.** Solitary adenoma
- **D.** CRF

Secondary hyperparathyroidism occurs in:
- Renal failure
- Osteomalacia (vitamin D deficiency)
- Pseudohypoparathyroidism

1429. All are ECG manifestations in Wolf Parkinson white syndrome *except*:

A. Narrow QRS
B. Low PR interval
C. Normal QT interval
D. Initial slur

Normally the atria and ventricle are connected electrically by bundle of His. Some people *however* have an extra-conducting tissue which forms a direct connection between atrium and ventricle. This is usually situated in the left side of heart. A wave of depolarization which should have reached the ventricle through the bundle of His via AV node is short circuited via this tract leading to ventricular pre-excitation. This **shortens the PR interval** and gives a **slurred upstroke in QRS complex** known as delta wave.

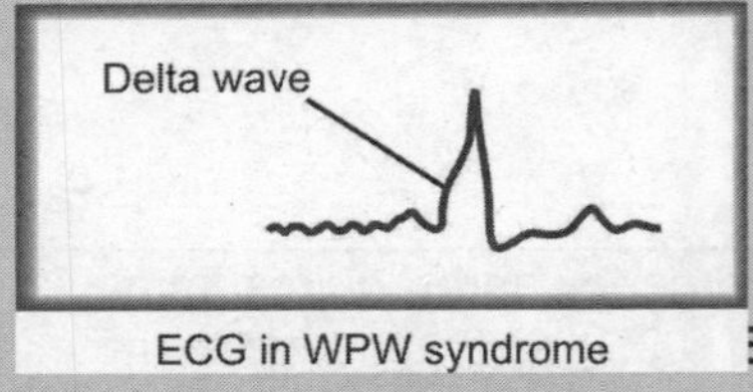

ECG in WPW syndrome

1430. Microscopic appearance of *Pneumocystis carinii* shows:

A. Interstitial pneumonia
B. Eosinophilic infiltrate of interstitium
C. Fibrosis of alveoli
D. Pulmonary hemorrhage

Malnourished infants with *Pneumocystis carinii* pneumonia show an intense plasma cell infiltrate (**Syn. interstitial plasma cell pneumonia**).

1431. Neurofibrillary tangles and plaques are seen in the brain in:

A. Picks disease
B. Huntington's chorea
C. Alzheimer's disease
D. Parkinsonism

The *most important* microscopic findings in **Alzheimer's disease** are neuritic "senile" plaques and neurofibrillary tangles (NFTs).

1432. Ebstein's anomaly is caused by:

A. Carbamazepine
B. Imipramine
C. Lithium
D. Amphetamin

The use of lithium is associated with an increased incidence of neonatal goiter and congenital cardiovascular malformations, especially Ebstein's anomaly.

1433. Meconium ileus is a manifestation of:

A. Hirschsprung's disease
B. Fibrocystic disease of pancreas
C. Achalasia cardia
D. Celiac disease

Meconium ileus is a manifestation of fibrocystic disease of pancreas (cystic fibrosis).

1434. Pheochromocytoma is associated with:

A. Vitiligo
B. Ash leaf amelanotic macules
C. Acanthosis nigricans
D. Café au lait spots

Pheochromocytoma is often associated with neurofibromatosis and if one finds **café au lait spots**, vertebral abnormalities, or kyphoscoliosis in a patient with hypertension pheochromocytoma should be suspected.

1435. In nontropical sprue there is deficiency of all *except*:

A. Iron
B. B_{12}
C. Folic acid
D. Vitamin A

Reduced Serum Level of the following is Seen in Non-tropical Sprue

• Serum calcium	• Serum magnesium
• Serum albumin	• Serum zinc
• Serum cholesterol	• Serum iron
• Serum carotenes	• Serum vitamin A
• Vitamin B_{12}	• Carbohydrate absorption

1436. Patients with sickle cell anemia are prone to infections with:

A. *Staphylococcus aureus* **B.** *Pneumococcus*
C. *Haemophilus influenza* **D.** *Gonococcus*

Patients with sickle cell anemia are prone to infections with pneumococcal and meningococcal organisms.

1437. In an AIDS patient presenting with fever, cough a diagnosis of *Pneumocystis carinii* pneumonia is best established by:

A. Transtracheal biopsy
B. Bronchoalveolar lavage
C. Staining of intranuclear inclusion and silver staining
D. Aspiration and culture

Fiberoptic bronchoscopy with bronchoalveolar lavage (BAL) is sensitive and it remains the mainstay of *Pneumocystis carinii* diagnosis.

1438. Pseudocoma results from infarction or hemorrhage in:

A. Pons **B.** Medulla
C. Hypothalamus **D.** Mid brain

In **locked-in state** or **pseudocoma** patients are awake but deefferented, i.e. has no means of producing speech or limb, face, or pharyngeal movements. Infarction or hemorrhage of the **ventral pons** is the cause.

1439. α Interferon 3-5 million units thrice in a week for 3-6 months is useful in the treatment of:

A. Wilson's disease **B.** Chronic hepatitis B
C. Chronic autoimmune hepatitis **D.** Antitrypsin deficiency

In chronic hepatitis B interferon α should be given for 4 months by subcutaneous injections.

- Daily dose is 5 million units
- Three times a week at a dose of 10 million units

1440. Cirrhosis of liver in adult population is commonly due to all of the following *except*:

A. Hepatitis A **B.** Hepatitis C
C. Hepatitis B **D.** Hepatitis E

Hepatitis A is a self-limiting disease and does not progress to chronic liver disease.

1441. Cerebellar ataxia is a *rare* complication of:

A. Chickenpox **B.** Mumps
C. Measles **D.** Glandular fever

Measles can sometimes leads to **subacute sclerosing pan encephalitis (SSPE)** which is a prolonged, chronic, rare form of measles encephalitis. It manifests as progressive intellectual deterioration, seizures, myoclonus, **ataxia**, and visual disturbances.

1442. Generalized edema can be produced by deficiency of:

A. Vitamin A **B.** Vitamin D
C. Folic acid **D.** Thiamine

The two major manifestations of thiamine deficiency are:
- Wet beriberi –generalized edema
- Dry beriberi and the Wernicke-Korsakoff syndrome

1443. Weil's syndrome usually present as:
A. Aseptic meningitis **B.** Lobar pneumonia
C. Diarrhea and vomiting **D.** Jaundice

Severe leptospirosis with profound jaundice (Weil's syndrome) develops in 5 to 10% of infected individuals.

1444. External cardiac massage is given at least at the rate of:
A. 40/minute **B.** 60 /minute
C. 80/minute **D.** 120/minute

4 Major Steps in Cardiopulmonary Resuscitation

- Make certain the victim has an open airway.
- Start respiratory resuscitation immediately.
- Feel for the carotid pulse in the groove alongside the thyroid cartilage.
- If pulse is absent, begin cardiac massage. Use **80-100 compressions a minute** with one lung inflation after each group of five chest compressions.

1445. *True* about coarctation of aorta is:
A. Most common site is distal to origin of subclavian artery
B. BP *always* comes down after repair
C. Increased incidence in Down syndrome
D. Notching of *superior* border of rib is seen

In **coarctation of aorta** narrowing or constriction of the lumen of the aorta can occur anywhere along its length but the most common site is **distal to the origin of the left subclavian artery** near the insertion of the ligamentum arteriosum.

1446. Lymphocytic choriomeningitis is caused by:
A. Arenavirus **B.** Coronavirus
C. Reovirus **D.** Parvovirus

Lymphocytic choriomeningitis is an acute viral disease of the CNS manifested by flu-like symptoms (fever, malaise, headache) sometimes followed by acute septic meningitis. It is caused by LCM virus (**Arenavirus**).

1447. Regarding Dandy Walker syndrome, all are seen, *except*:
A. Hydrocephalus **B.** Posterior fossa cyst
C. Arachnoid cyst **D.** Cerebellar vermis deficiency

Features of Dandy Walker Syndrome

- Absence or severe hypoplasia of the vermis of cerebellum
- Cystic distention of roof of 4th ventricle
- Bulging of 4th ventricle in posterior fossa
- Hydrocephalus

1448. Bilateral anterior uveitis, skin depigmentation is seen in:
A. Vogt-Koyanagi-Harada syndrome **B.** Alport's disease
C. Fabry's disease **D.** Weinberg disease

A history of aseptic meningitis, nontraumatic uveitis, tinnitus, hearing loss, and/or dysacousis points to the diagnosis of the **Vogt-Koyanagi-Harada syndrome**. The face and scalp are the most common locations of pigment loss.

1449. Xanthelasma is:

A. Premalignant
B. Deposit around eyelids
C. More common in females
D. Deposit over trunk

Xanthelasma or xanthoma is a raised, yellow plaque, commonly found in the upper and lower lids near the inner canthus and often symmetrical in the 2 lids and on both sides.

1450. An overdose of morphine is treated with:

A. IV naloxone
B. IV nalorphine
C. IV methadone
D. IV steroids

Naloxone is a competitive antagonist of all types of opioid receptors. Given intravenously (0.4-0.8 mg) in rapidly antagonizes all actions of morphine.

1451. Vinyl chloride has been implicated in:

A. Angiosarcoma of liver
B. Hepatomas
C. Angiofibroma of nose
D. Bladder cancer

Angiosarcoma of liver consists of vascular spaces lined by malignant endothelial cells. Etiologic factors of angiosarcoma of liver are thorium dioxide, polyvinyl chloride, arsenic, and androgenic anabolic steroids.

1452. Casal necklace is seen in:

A. Beriberi
B. Pityriasis rosea
C. Scabies
D. Pellagra

Casal necklace is seen in **pellagra**. There are bilaterally symmetrical lesions on the neck which consist of erythema and progress to vesiculation and crusting.

1453. Ormond's disease is:

A. Retroperitoneal fibrosis
B. Retroperitoneal carcinomatosis
C. Intra-abdominal desmoid
D. Reactive mesenteric adenitis

Retroperitoneal fibrosis is also known as **Ormond's disease**. It may cause physical compression of the ureters, and even the vena cava and aorta. It is usually associated with methysergide therapy.

1454. Sensory neuropathy is *not* seen in:

A. Diabetes
B. Lead poisoning
C. Beriberi
D. Alcoholism

Common Features of Lead Poisoning

- **ABDOMINAL PAIN**
- **FATIGUE**
- **HEADACHE**
- **ANEMIA**
- **JOINT PAIN**
- **PERIPHERAL MOTOR NEUROPATHY**

1455. Onion skin spleen is seen in:

A. SLE
B. Thalassemia
C. ITP
D. Scleroderma

The morphological hallmark of **SLE** induced angiopathy is acute necrotizing vasculitis of small arteries and arterioles. When it occurs in spleen the central penicilliary arteries are involved leading to concentric periarterial fibrosis in the spleen producing the characteristic **Onion skin appearance**.

1456. Metastatic tumor causing spinal cord compression are all *except*:

- **A.** Carcinoma prostate
- **B.** Meningioma
- **C.** Carcinoma lung
- **D.** Carcinoma breast

Common Metastatic Tumor Causing Spinal Cord Compression

• Carcinoma breast	• Carcinoma lung	• Carcinoma prostate
• Plasma cell dyscrasia	• Lymphoma	• Kidney

1457. Hypochromic microcytic anemia is seen in all *except*:

- **A.** Hypothyroidism
- **B.** Thalassemia
- **C.** Sideroblastic anemia
- **D.** Iron deficiency anemia *(AIIMS 1991)*

Anemia develops in 1/3rd to half of the patients with hypothyroidism. The anemia is usually mild or moderate with a hemoglobin level of 8-12 gm/dL. The MCV is usually in the normal range and **microcytosis and hypochromia occurs only when it is associated with iron deficiency**.

1458. *False* regarding chronic iron deficiency anemia is:

- **A.** Increased bone marrow macrophage iron ingestion
- **B.** Decreased transferrin iron binding capacity
- **C.** Decreased ferritin
- **D.** Decreased serum iron level *(AIIMS 1991)*

Iron deficiency anemia is recognized from the combination of abnormal iron supply studies and microcytic, hypochromic RBC morphology. The serum iron falls to very low levels (<30 μg/dL), while **the transferrin iron binding capacity increases**, resulting in a percent saturation of < 10%. The ferritin level is always < 15 μg/L.

1459. Magnetic gait is seen in:

- **A.** Hepatic encephalopathy
- **B.** Parkinsonism
- **C.** Hemiparesis
- **D.** Normal pressure hydrocephalus *(KERALA 1999)*

Normal pressure hydrocephalus (NPH) is a disorder usually involving the elderly that presents primarily with difficulty in walking. The difficulty has been described as a "**magnetic gait**," one in which the patient feels that his or her feet are stuck to the floor as if there were magnets on the soles of their shoes. A person with NPH usually has problems initiating their gait - *typically* having to take many tiny steps in order to get going and/or if trying to stop. If severe, the patient may be completely unable to walk and be confined to a wheelchair. The second common feature of NPH is **impaired bladder control**. Early on, the most common complaint is urgency-having to rush to the bathroom as soon as the urge is felt. Later in the disease, urinary incontinence may develop. **Declining short-term memory** is the third feature of NPH. The degree of forgetfulness is above that normally attributed to aging. If advanced, the patient can become quite demented which may make the diagnosis difficult to distinguish from Alzheimer's disease.

1460. In children *not* a common presentation of AIDS:

- **A.** *Pneumocystis carinii* pneumonia
- **B.** Lymphocytic interstitial pneumonitis
- **C.** Kaposi sarcoma
- **D.** Failure to thrive *(AIIMS 1993)*

Many children with HIV infection do not gain weight or grow normally (**failure to thrive**). HIV-infected children frequently are slow to reach important milestones in motor skills and mental development such as crawling, walking and speaking. As the disease progresses, many children develop neurologic problems such as difficulty in walking, poor school performance, seizures, and other symptoms of HIV encephalopathy. *Like adults with HIV infection*, children with HIV develop life-threatening **opportunistic infections**, although the incidence of various opportunistic infections differs in adults and children. For example, toxoplasmosis is seen less frequently in HIV-infected children than in HIV-infected adults, while serious bacterial infections occur more commonly in children than in adults. Also, as children with HIV become sicker, they may suffer from chronic diarrhea due to opportunistic pathogens. *Pneumocystis carinii* pneumonia (PCP) is the leading cause of death in HIV-infected children with AIDS. PCP, as well as cytomegalovirus (CMV) disease, usually are primary infections in children, whereas in adults these diseases result from the reactivation of latent infections. A lung disease called **lymphocytic interstitial pneumonitis** (LIP), rarely seen in adults, also occurs frequently in HIV-infected children. Children with HIV suffer the usual childhood bacterial infections — only more frequently and more severely than uninfected children. These bacterial infections can cause seizures, fever, pneumonia, recurrent colds, diarrhea, dehydration and other problems that often result in extended hospital stays and nutritional problems. HIV-infected children frequently have severe candidiasis, a yeast infection that can cause unrelenting diaper rash and infections in the mouth and throat that make eating difficult. **Kaposi's sarcoma occurs mainly in gay and bisexual men with HIV disease; it is infrequent in HIV-infected women, children, and injection drug users.**

1461. Dapsone is *not* used in:

A. Alcoholic liver disease
B. Actinomycotic mycetoma
C. Dermatitis herpetiformis
D. Leprosy *(AIIMS 1993)*

Common Indications of Dapsone

- Leprosy
- Dermatitis herpetiformis
- Actinomycotic mycetoma
- Cicatricial pemphigoid
- Subcorneal pustular dermatosis
- Granuloma annulare
- Pemphigoid
- Systemic lupus erythematosus
- Prophylaxis of malaria
- Pneumocystis carinii

1462. Hemiballism is caused by lesions of:

A. Caudate nucleus
B. Contra lateral subthalamic nuclei
C. Putamen
D. Substantia nigra

Hemiballism or **hemichorea are wide, flinging or throwing movements of 1 arm and leg. These movements are irregular in timing and force, like those of chorea. Hemiballism is usually seen in elderly patients due to a stroke. Lesions of contralateral subthalamic nucleus (corpus luysi) due to vascular insult or neoplastic infiltration results in acute hemiballism.**

- **Balismos means jumping.**
- **Fling means to throw, especially with force or violence; hurl; cast.**

1463. Diagnostic features of allergic bronchopulmonary aspergillosis (ABPA) include all of the following *except*:

A. Changing pulmonary infiltrates
B. Peripheral eosinophilia
C. Serum precipitins against *Aspergillus fumigatus*
D. Occurrence in patients with old cavitary lesions *(AI 2003)*

Diagnostic Features of Allergic Bronchopulmonary Aspergillosis

Major diagnostic criteria	Other diagnostic features
• Bronchial asthma • Pulmonary infiltrates • Peripheral eosinophilia (more than 1000/micro liter) • Immediate wheal-and-flare response to *Aspergillus fumigatus* • Serum precipitins to *Aspergillus fumigatus* • Elevated serum IgE • Central bronchiectasis	• History of brownish plugs in sputum • Culture of *Aspergillus fumigatus* from sputum • Elevated IgE (and IgG) class antibodies specific for *Aspergillus fumigatus*

Ref: *Harrison's Principles of Internal Medicine; 14th edition*

1464. Which of the following is the *best* indicator of iron deficiency?

A. Serum iron levels **B.** Serum ferritin levels
C. TIBC **D.** Serum transferrin levels *(UP 2001)*

The Principles measurements of iron supply used in clinical diagnosis are the serum iron (SI), the transferrin iron-binding capacity (TIBC), and the serum ferritin level. The level of **serum ferritin**, an iron storage protein, provides a **relatively accurate** estimate of body iron stores in the absence of inflammatory disease. Once iron stores are depleted, the serum ferritin level declines to levels below 15 microgram/liter.

Ref: *Harrison's Principles of Internal Medicine; 14th edition and Nelson Textbook of Pediatrics; 16th edition; page 1470*

1465. A patient with recent onset primary 'generalized' epilepsy develops drug reaction and skin rash due to phenytoin sodium. The *most appropriate* course of action is:

A. Shift to clonazepam **B.** Restart phenytoin sodium after 2 weeks
C. Shift to sodium valproate **D.** Shift to ethosuximide *(AIIMS 11 May 2003)*

Antiepileptic drugs of choice

Focal onset seizure	Generalized tonic-clonic	Absence	Myoclonic	Atonic
• Carbamazepine • Phenytoin • Valproic acid	• Valproic acid • Carbamazepine • Phenytoin	• Ethosuximide • Valproic acid	• Valproic acid	• Valproic acid

Ref: *Harrison's Principles of Internal Medicine; 14th edition*

1466. Which of the following is *true* about pericarditis?

A. Pain increases on leaning forward
B. Pain decreases in supine position
C. Pain increases in inspiration
D. Pain increases on eating *(JIPMER 2002)*

The **pain of pericarditis** is severe. It is typically retrosternal and left precordial, referred to the back and the trapezius ridge. Often the pain is pleuritic as a result of accompanying pleural inflammation, i.e. sharp and **aggravated by inspiration**, coughing, and changes in body position.

Ref: *Harrison's Principles of Internal Medicine; 15th edition; page 1365*

1467. Hemorrhagic pericarditis occurs in all of the following conditions *except*:

A. Transmural myocardial infarction **B.** Dissecting aneurysm of aorta
C. Metastatic disease of pericardium **D.** *Constrictive* pericarditis *(AIIMS 11 May 2003)*

Hemorrhagic pericarditis refers to an exudate made up of blood mixed with a fibrinous or suppurative effusion. It is most commonly caused by tuberculosis or by malignant neoplastic involvement of the pericardial space, most often due to spread of lung and breast carcinomas, melanocarcinomas, lymphomas and leukemias. It can also occur in bacterial infections or in patients with bleeding disorders. It often follows cardiac surgery. The clinical significance is that of a **suppurative pericarditis**.

Ref: *Robbins Pathologic Basis of Disease; 4th edition; page 650*

1468. Chylous ascites is caused by all of the following *except*:

A. Colloid carcinoma of stomach **B.** Tuberculosis
C. Trauma **D.** Nephrotic syndrome *(AIIMS Nov 2002)*

Chylous ascites is most often the result of lymphatic obstruction from trauma, tumor, tuberculosis, filariasis, or congenital abnormalities. It also may be seen in the nephrotic syndrome.

Ref: *Harrison's Principles of Internal Medicine*

1469. In a patient with cirrhosis the causative organism for spontaneous bacterial peritonitis is:

A. *Escherichia coli* **B.** Staphylococci
C. Streptococcus **D.** Pseudomonas *(BHU June 2002)*

Patients with ascites and cirrhosis may develop acute bacterial peritonitis without an obvious primary source of infection. Patients with very advanced liver disease are particularly susceptible to **spontaneous bacterial peritonitis** (SBP).[1] The microbiology of SBP is also distinctive; while enteric Gram negative bacilli such as *Escherichia coli* are most commonly encountered, Gram – positive organisms such as streptococci, enterococci or even pneumococci are sometimes found.

[1] Ref: *Harrison's Principles of Internal Medicine; 15th edition; volume 1; page 829*

1470. Sleep apnea is defined as a temporary pause in breathing during sleep lasting for at least:

A. 40 seconds **B.** 30 seconds
C. 20 seconds **D.** 10 seconds *(AIIMS 11 May 2003)*

Sleep apnea may be defined as 'an intermittent cessation of airflow at the nose and mouth during sleep'. *By convention*, **apneas of at least 10 second duration have been considered important**, although in most patients they are 20 to 30 second in duration and may be as long as 2 to 3 minutes. **Sleep apnea syndrome** is the *clinical disorder* that arises from recurrent sleep apneas. Sleep apneas can be central or obstructive in type. In **central sleep apnea (CSA)** the neural derive to all the respiratory muscles is transiently abolished while in **obstructive sleep apnea (OSA)** airflow stops despite continuing respiratory drive because of occlusion of the oropharyngeal airway.

Ref: *Harrison's Principles of Internal Medicine; 15th edition; volume 2; page 1520*

1471. *Most common* cause of papillary necrosis is:

A. Diabetes mellitus **B.** Hemolytic uremic syndrome
C. Analgesic nephropathy **D.** Hypertension *(BHU June 2002)*

A distinct clinicopathologic syndrome has been described in heavy users of analgesic mixtures containing phenacetin in combination with aspirin, acetaminophen, or caffeine. **Analgesic nephropathy** is characterized by papillary necrosis and tubulointerstitial inflammation.

1472. *Most common* presentation of neurocysticercosis is:

A. Seizures
B. Focal neurological deficits
C. Dementia
D. Radiculopathy *(AI 2003)*

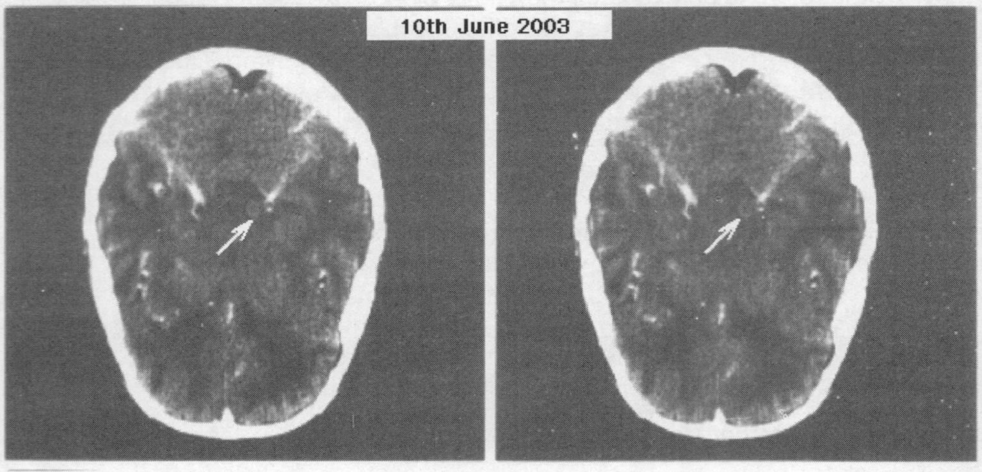

CT-scan of a patient named Ashish Mishra; 9-year-old male child; demonstrating RING ENHANCING LESION with perifocal white matter edema due to neurocysticercosis. Patient presented with simple partial seizure
(Courtesy: Dr. Sharad Chandra MBBS, DCH, MIAP; Consultant Pediatrician; Fatima Hospital, Mahanagar, Lucknow)

Neurocysticercosis generally occurs in a previously healthy and normal child. **Seizures are the *most common* mode of presentation (90%);** partial seizure being *more frequent* than generalized. It may also mimic cerebral tumor and present by features of raised intracranial tension (15%). It may also be detected accidentally in plain X-ray skull or CT-scan where calcification may be seen. Neurocysticercosis is of the following types depending upon the site of the cyst. Of these, the parenchymal variety is *most common* and found in 95% of cases. It consists of single or few-isolated lesion in parenchyma of brain.

- Parenchymal
- Racemose
- Meningoencephalitic
- Disseminated
- Intra-ventricular

1473. A 55-year-old man who has been on bed rest for the past 10 days complains of breathlessness and chest pain. The chest X-ray is normal. The next investigation should be:
A. Lung ventilation-perfusion scan **B.** Pulmonary arteriography
C. Pulmonary venous angiography **D.** Echocardiography *(AI 2003)*

Lung scanning is the Principles imaging test for the diagnosis of pulmonary thromboembolism. Small particulate aggregates of albumin labeled with a gamma-emitting radionuclide are injected IV and are trapped in the pulmonary capillary bed. Selective pulmonary angiography is the *most specific* examination available for establishing the definitive diagnosis of PTE and can detect emboli as small as 1 to 2 mm.

1474. The *most common* cause of tricuspid regurgitation is secondary to:
A. Rheumatic heart disease **B.** Dilatation of right ventricle
C. Coronary artery disease **D.** Endocarditis due to intravenous drug abuse *(AI 2003)*

Most commonly, **tricuspid regurgitation** is 'functional' and **secondary to marked dilatation of the right ventricle** and the tricuspid annulus.

1475. Absence seizures are characterized on EEG by:
A. 3Hz spike and wave **B.** 1-2Hz spike and wave
C. Generalized poly spikes **D.** Hypsarrhythmia *(AI 2003)*

The *electrophysiologic hallmark* of **typical absence seizures** is a generalized, symmetric, **3 Hz spike-and-wave discharge** that begins and ends suddenly on a normal EEG background.

1476. Normal anion gap metabolic acidosis is caused by:
A. Cholera **B.** Starvation
C. Ethylene glycol poisoning **D.** Lactic acidosis *(AI 2003)*

1477. Normal anion gap is seen in:
A. Starvation acidosis **B.** Renal tubular acidosis
C. Salicylate poisoning **D.** Diabetic ketoacidosis *(BHU June 2002)*

1478. Normal anion gap acidosis is seen in:
A. Chronic renal failure **B.** Diarrhea
C. Diabetic ketoacidosis **D.** Methanol poisoning *(MANIPAL 2002)*

Anion gap represents *unmeasured* anions in plasma and is calculated as = $[Na^+] - ([Cl^-] + [HCO_3^-])$. The **normal anion gap is 10 to 12 mmol/L**. The unmeasured anions include anionic proteins, phosphate, sulfate, and organic anions.

Causes of High-Anion-Gap Metabolic Acidosis

Lactic acidosis	Toxins	Renal failure
• Diabetic ketoacidosis • Alcoholic ketoacidosis • Starvation ketoacidosis	• Ethylene glycol • Methanol • Salicylates	• Acute • Chronic

1479. All of the following cause high-anion-gap metabolic acidosis *except*:
A. Lactic acidosis **B.** Salicylate poisoning
C. Ethylene glycol poisoning **D.** Ureterosigmoidostomy *(AIIMS Nov 2002)*

1480. Metabolic abnormality of ureterosigmoidostomy is:
A. Hypochloremic alkalosis **B.** Hypochloremic acidosis
C. Hyperchloremic alkalosis **D.** Hyperchloremic acidosis *(UP 2003)*

Ureterosigmoidostomy is a method of urinary diversion and was first used by Henri Chaput in 1894. The procedure was subsequently modified by Coffey and Grey Turner. In this procedure the ureters are cut obliquely and pulled into the gut by a stitch. The typical biochemical changes are **hyperchloremic acidosis** with potassium depletion and are seen in *every* patient. These changes are due to a combination of reabsorption of urea and chloride and progressively diminishing renal function due to chronic pyelonephritis.

1481. *Best* method to diagnose bronchiectasis is:
A. X-ray **B.** Bronchography
C. MRI **D.** HRCT *(KARNATAKA 2001)*

Chest radiograph is important in the evaluation of suspected **bronchiectasis** but the findings are often nonspecific. Bronchography can provide excellent visualization of bronchiectatic airways but this technique has now been replaced by computerized tomography which also provides an excellent view of dilated airways, as seen in cross sectional images. With the advent of high resolution CT-scanning (**HRCT**), in which the images are 1 mm thick, the sensitivity for detecting bronchiectasis has improved event further.

Ref: *Harrison's Principles of Internal Medicine*; 15th edition; page 1486

1482. In the diagnosis of pheochromocytoma, 1 of the following radionuclide scans is useful:
A. MIBG scan **B.** MIDA scan
C. DTPA scan **D.** DMSA scan *(KARNATAKA 2001)*

Surgical removal of **pheochromocytoma** is facilitated if the location of the tumor or tumors can be established preoperatively. CT or MRI of the adrenals is usually successful in identifying intra-adrenal lesions. An additional localization technique involves a radionuclide scintiscan after administration of the radiopharmaceutical (^{131}I) meta-iodobenzylguanidine (**MIBG**). This agent is concentrated by the amine uptake process and produces an external scintigraphic image at the site of the tumor.

1483. 'H' shaped vertebra seen in:

A. Phenylketonuria **B.** Sickle cell anemia
C. Hemangioma **D.** Osteoporosis *(KARNATAKA 2001)*

In 1966 Reynolds described "**H**" or "step-off" **vertebra** in patients with **sickle cell disease**. He considered this feature to be characteristic of sickle cell hemoglobinopathy and extremely rare in other hematologic disorders.

1484. The morphology of RBC in disseminated intravascular coagulation is:

A. Microcytes **B.** Macrocytes
C. Schistocytes **D.** Eliptocyte *(KARNATAKA 2001)*

The laboratory manifestations of **disseminated intravascular coagulation** include thrombocytopenia and the presence of **schistocytes** or fragmented RBCs that arise from cell trapping and damage within fibrin thrombi; prolonged prothrombin time and partial thromboplastin time and thrombin time and a reduced fibrinogen level from depletion of coagulation proteins; and elevated fibrin degradation products (FDP) from intense secondary fibrinolysis. The D-dimer immunoassay, which specifically measures cross-linked fibrin derivatives, is a more specific FDP assay.

1485. Progressive multifocal leukoencephalopathy (PML) is characterized by all of the following *except*:

A. Caused by JC virus **B.** Late manifestation of AIDS
C. Cognitive impairment *common* **D.** Brainstem can be involved *(KARNATAKA 2001)*

Progressive multifocal leukoencephalopathy (PML) is a progressive disorder characterized by multifocal areas of demyelination, which vary greatly in size and are scattered **throughout the central nervous system**. There are characteristic cytologic alterations in both astrocytes and oligodendrocytes. Oligodendrocytes have enlarged, densely staining nuclei that contain viral inclusions formed by crystalline arrays of **JC virus** particles. Patients often present with **visual deficits (45%)**, *typically* a homonymous hemianopia, and mental impairment (38%) (dementia, confusion, personality change). Motor weakness may not be present early but eventually occurs in 75% of cases. Almost all patients (>95%) have an underlying immunosuppressive disorder. **More than 60% of currently diagnosed PML cases occur in patients with AIDS**.

1486. Wimberger's ring is present in:

A. Rickets **B.** Scurvy
C. Secondary syphilis **D.** Tuberculosis *(KARNATAKA 2001)*

In **scurvy** there often are characteristic signs such as **Wimberger's ring**, the white line of Frankel, the Truemmerfeld zone, and subperiosteal hemorrhage, which aid in distinguishing this condition.

1487. All of the following are advantages of using isoniazid in antitubercular treatment *except*:

A. It reduces load of TB bacilli
B. It kills intracellular TB bacilli
C. It acts on dormant bacilli
D. It has preventable side effects like peripheral neuropathy *(MANIPAL 2002)*

Isoniazid (INH) is a synthetic, bactericidal antitubercular agent that is active against many mycobacteria, primarily those that are actively dividing. INH ranks among the most powerful drug in the treatment of tuberculosis and it can easily penetrate the cell membrane (thus active against intracellular as well as extracellular bacilli). **Its action is *most marked* on rapidly multiplying bacilli and is less active against slow multipliers.** It gets widely distributed in the body including CSF. Its ease of administration, freedom from toxicity and low cost makes it an ideal component of any antitubercular regime. Patients may experience GI irritation, peripheral neuropathy, and hyperglycemia and liver damage. The addition of pyridoxine helps to prevent the occurrence of peripheral neuropathy.

1488. The *only* drug available for treatment of nephrogenic diabetes insipidus is:

A. Chlorpropamide **B.** Thiazide
C. Desmopressin **D.** Furosemide *(MANIPAL 2002)*

Treatment of **nephrogenic diabetes insipidus** is aimed at maintaining adequate hydration. In the infant, low-solute feedings and high water intake are generally adequate. Addition of a **thiazide** diuretic reduces urine flow by inhibiting sodium reabsorption in the distal convoluted tubule. Administration of vasopressin and its analogues has no role in the management of this disorder.

1489. Narcolepsy is:

A. Narcotic induced epilepsy **B.** Narcotic induced depression
C. Attacks of sleep and paralysis **D.** Narcotic withdrawal reaction *(MANIPAL 2002)*

1490. Narcolepsy is characterized by all of the following *except*:

A. Sleep paralysis **B.** Cataplexy
C. Hallucination **D.** Snoring *(AIIMS Nov 2002)*

The *most common* symptoms of **narcolepsy** are excessive daytime sleepiness with involuntary daytime sleep episodes, disturbed nocturnal sleep, and cataplexy (sudden weakness or loss of muscle tone without loss of consciousness that is elicited by emotion). Some patients also experience muscular paralysis and/or hallucinations at sleep onset or upon awakening. Nearly all narcoleptics are positive for the human leukocyte antigen DR15.

1491. Regarding Barrett's esophagus, which of the following statements is *incorrect*:

A. Is due to chronic gastroesophageal reflux
B. Is lined by columnar epithelium
C. Is associated with elevated lower esophageal sphincter pressure
D. Is associated with increased incidence of adenocarcinoma of esophagus *(KARNATAKA 2001)*

Barrett's esophagus or **columnar lined lower esophagus** is a 'metaplastic' change in the mucus lining of the esophagus in response to chronic gastroesophageal reflux. It is still not known that why some people with gastroesophageal reflux disease (GERD) develop esophagitis while the others develop Barrett's esophagus without significant esophagitis. In Barrett's esophagus, the junction between squamous esophageal mucosa and gastric mucosa moves 'proximally'. If a peptic stricture occurs in Barrett's esophagus it always occurs at the new squamo-columnar junction. When the intestinal metaplasia occurs there is an increased risk of adenocarcinoma of the esophagus in the order of 25 times that of the general population.

1492. The *normal* PR interval is in seconds:

A. 0.05-0.08 **B.** 0.12-0.16
C. 0.8-1.6 **D.** 1.2-2.3 *(MANIPAL 2002)*

The PR interval (**normally 120 to 200 millisecond**) measures the time between atrial and ventricular depolarization, which includes the physiologic 'delay', imposed by stimulation of cells in the AV junction area. The QRS interval (normally 100 ms or less) reflects the duration of ventricular depolarization. The QT interval includes both ventricular depolarization and repolarization times and varies inversely with the heart rate.

Interval	Average	Range
• **PR interval**	0.18	0.12 - 0.20
• **QRS duration**	0.08	0.08 - 0.10
• **QT interval**	0.40	0.40 - 0.43
• **ST interval (QT – QRS)**	0.32	....

1493. Cardiac output is decreased by:

A. Increased sympathetic activity **B.** Tachycardia
C. Increased preload **D.** Decreased venous return *(MANIPAL 2002)*

The amount of blood pumped out of each ventricle per beat (**stroke volume**) is about 80 ml in a resting man of average size in the supine position. The output of the heart per unit time is the **cardiac output**. In a resting supine man it averages about 5.5 liter per minute (80 ml x 69 beats per minute). The output per minute per square meter of body surface area (**cardiac index**) is 3.2 liter. *Variations in cardiac output can be produced by changes in the heart rate or stroke-volume*. The heart rate is primarily controlled by the cardiac innervation (sympathetic stimulation increasing the heart rate and parasympathetic stimulation decreasing it).

Effect of various conditions on cardiac output

No change	Increase	Decrease
• Sleep • Moderate changes in environmental temperature	• Anxiety and excitement (50–100%) • Eating (30%) • Exercise (up to 70%) • High environmental temperature • Pregnancy • Epinephrine • Histamine	• Sitting or standing from lying position (20-30%) • Rapid arrhythmias • Heart disease

The body typically regulates its own heart rate, with tachycardia being the first symptom of congestive cardiac failure. Various chronotropic drugs (e.g. isoproterenol) can be used to increase the heart rate and thereby increase the cardiac output. Cardiac output may also be increased by increasing the stroke volume. The cardiac index increases with left ventricular end-diastolic pressure (LVEDP) up to a point, after which there is a decline in the cardiac index. One may manipulate the preload (or LVEDP) with either fluid boluses or diuretics in an effort to maximize cardiac output on a given Frank-Starling curve. If judicious fluid management does not sufficiently increase cardiac output, the heart failure must be treated with drugs that increase cardiac contractility such as digoxin, dopamine, and dobutamine, or decrease the resistance (after load) against which the heart is pumping. Afterload reducers are vasodilators and include nitroprusside, hydralazine, and captopril.

1494. The *most common* cause of pseudohermaphroditism is:
- **A.** Ovarian dysgenesis
- **B.** Ovarian tumor
- **C.** Congenital adrenal hyperplasia
- **D.** PCOD *(MANIPAL 2002)*

Congenital adrenal hyperplasia due to classic 21-hydroxylase deficiency is the *most common* cause of ambiguous genitalia in the newborn.

1495. All of the following are true about congenital heart disease *except*:
- **A.** ASD is associated with fixed split in 2nd sound
- **B.** Transposition of great vessels is associated with boot shaped heart
- **C.** Down syndrome is associated with endocardial cushion defect
- **D.** VSD is the *most common* type in children *(SGPGI 2003)*

1496. Tetralogy of Fallot constitutes all of the following *except*:
- **A.** VSD
- **B.** Hypertrophy of the right ventricle
- **C.** Hypoplasia of aorta
- **D.** Pulmonary stenosis *(SGPGI 2003)*

1497. All of the following are seen in tetralogy of Fallot *except*:
- **A.** VSD
- **B.** Overriding aorta
- **C.** Pulmonary stenosis
- **D.** Left ventricular hypertrophy *(MANIPAL 2002)*

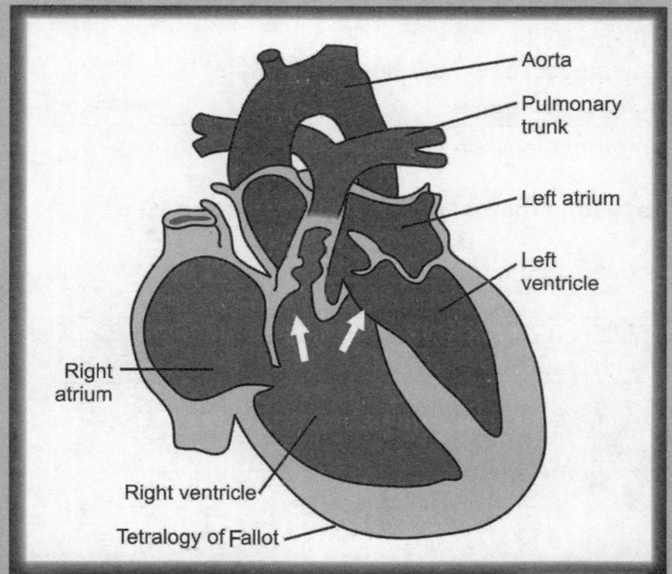

Tetralogy of Fallot is 1 of the *most common* forms of congenital heart disease. It is by far the *most common* condition with clinical cyanosis and diminished vascularity on chest film, especially in a patient with a right aortic arch and/or a skeletal anomaly. **It is also the *most common* cyanotic condition seen in children and adults.** The pathologic anatomy of the classic cyanotic tetralogy of Fallot consists of 4 morphologic abnormalities viz. a large ventricular septal defect (VSD) located in the left ventricular outflow tract, usually involving the anterior septum immediately adjacent to the right and posterior aortic cusps; obstruction or atresia of the right ventricular infundibulum; an aorta arising from both ventricles above the large subaortic VSD in the so-called dextroposed position; and right ventricular hypertrophy. Cyanosis is 1 of the most obvious manifestations of TOF but it may not be present at birth. In the 1st year of life the cyanosis is most prominent on the mucus membranes of the lips and mouth and in the finger and toe nails. Clubbing of fingers and toes becomes apparent by the age of 1 – 2 years. Dyspnea occurs on exertion and *typically* the child assumes a squatting posture for the relief of dyspnea. There is usually polycythemia and the CXR reveals a '**boot shaped heart**' with poorly developed lung musculature. The diagnosis should be confirmed by echocardiography and cardiac catheterization. Indications for operation include severe cyanosis, dyspnea or exertion and syncopal attacks. The choice of operation depends upon the anatomical considerations and age and general condition of the patient. There are 2 approaches to the operative treatment of tetralogy of Fallot. In **palliative procedures** systemic blood is diverted into the pulmonary circulation to improve oxygenation. Palliative procedures include right subclavian to pulmonary artery anastomosis (*Blalock-Taussig*) or a modification in which an interposition graft is used or an aortic-pulmonary artery anastomosis done (Pott's procedure). **Total correction** is done via a median sternotomy. Repair is often undertaken in the third year of life and ideally before the child reaches school age.

1498. In *most* patients with multiple sclerosis, CSF proteins are:

A. Increased **B.** Decreased
C. Normal **D.** Absent *(MANIPAL 2002)*

CSF abnormalities consist of mononuclear cell pleocytosis, an elevation in the level of total immunoglobulins, and the presence of oligoclonal immunoglobulins. CSF cell counts are generally < 20/μL in **multiple sclerosis**, and counts above 50/μL are unusual but may occur at the onset of disease. Pleocytosis of more than 75 cells/μL or a finding of polymorphonuclear leukocytes in CSF makes the diagnosis of multiple sclerosis unlikely. In about 80% of patients, CSF IgG is increased with a **normal total protein level**, due to the selective production of IgG within the CNS. Occasional MS patients exhibit mild elevations in the total CSF protein content.

1499. Which of the following is the *treatment of choice* for cryptococcal meningitis?

A. Fluconazole **B.** Itraconazole
C. Flucytosine **D.** Amphotericin B *(AIIMS Nov 2002)*

- Patients with AIDS and cryptococcosis are treated initially with intravenous amphotericin B (with or without flucytosine) and later with fluconazole.
- In patients without AIDS, cryptococcosis may be treated with amphotericin B alone or in combination with flucytosine.

Ref: *Harrison's Principles of Internal Medicine; 14th edition*

1500. A male child of 15 years, with a mental age of 9 years has an IQ of:

A. 50 **B.** 60
C. 70 **D.** 80 *(AI 2003)*

Intelligence Quotient (IQ) is obtained *by dividing the mental age by chronological age and multiplying by 100.* Higher the IQ, more brilliant the child. 80% of people have an IQ of or near 100.

$$IQ = \frac{\text{Mental age}}{\text{Chronological age}} \times 100$$

$$= \frac{9}{15} \times 100$$

$$= 60$$

WHO Category	IQ
• Mild mental retardation	50-70
• Moderate mental retardation	35-49
• Severe mental retardation	20-34
• Profound mental retardation	Under 20

1501. During cardiopulmonary resuscitation intravenous calcium gluconate is indicated under all of the following circumstances *except*:

A. After 1 minute of arrest *routinely* **B.** Hypocalcemia
C. Calcium channel blocker toxicity **D.** Electromechanical dissociation *(AI 2003)*

In the past calcium was recommended in treatment of electromechanical dissociation and asystole but there is no evidence of its efficacy and there is evidence for harmful effects as calcium is implicated in the cytoplasmic calcium accumulation in the final common pathway of cell death. This results from calcium entering cells following ischemia and during reperfusion of ischemic organs. Administration of calcium in resuscitation of asystolic patient is not recommended. Calcium is indicated for treatment of hypocalcemia, hyperkalemia, hypermagnesemia, and calcium channel blocker overdose.

1502. Diagnosis of rotavirus diarrhea is confirmed by:

A. Stool culture
B. Antigen detection in blood by ELISA
C. Antigen detection in stool by ELISA
D. Antibody detection in blood by ELISA *(AI 2000)*

1503. The *most specific* investigation for rotavirus infection is:

A. Stool antigen
B. Serum ELISA
C. Microscopy
D. Stool culture *(AIIMS May 2002)*

A variety of specific commercial **immunoassays** are available to detect **rotavirus antigen** in **fecal specimens**. DNA probe diagnosis also appears to be sensitive and specific.

Ref: *Harrison's Principles of Internal Medicine*

1504. The ECG changes seen in hyperkalemia are all of the following *except*:

A. Flat P waves
B. Peaked P waves
C. Tall T waves
D. Progressive widening of QRS *(BHU June 2002)*

Hyperkalemia produces a sequence of changes in ECG usually beginning with narrowing and peaking (tenting) of the T waves. Further elevation of extracellular potassium ions leads to AV conduction disturbances, diminution in P-wave amplitude, and widening of the QRS interval. Severe hyperkalemia causes cardiac arrest with a slow sinusoidal type of mechanism ("sine-wave" pattern) followed by asystole.

1505. Polymyositis involves all of the following muscles *except*:

A. Brachialis
B. Ocular muscles
C. Vastus medialis
D. Shoulder girdle *(BHU June 2002)*

In **primary idiopathic polymyositis** there may be weakness of the muscles of the trunk, the pectoral and pelvic girdles, the upper arms and thighs, the neck, and the pharynx. **Ocular muscles are almost never affected** except in a rare association with myasthenia gravis.

Ref: *Harrison's Principles of Internal Medicine*

1506. The *drug of choice* in the treatment of PSVT is:

A. Amiodarone
B. Adenosine
C. Procainamide
D. Propranolol *(BHU June 2002)*

Verapamil (2.5 to 10 mg intravenously) or **adenosine** (6 to 12 mg intravenously) is the agent of choice in paroxysmal supra-ventricular tachycardia.

1507. The patent ductus arteriosus connects aorta and:

A. Pulmonary trunk
B. Left pulmonary artery
C. Subclavian artery
D. Descending aorta *(BHU June 2002)*

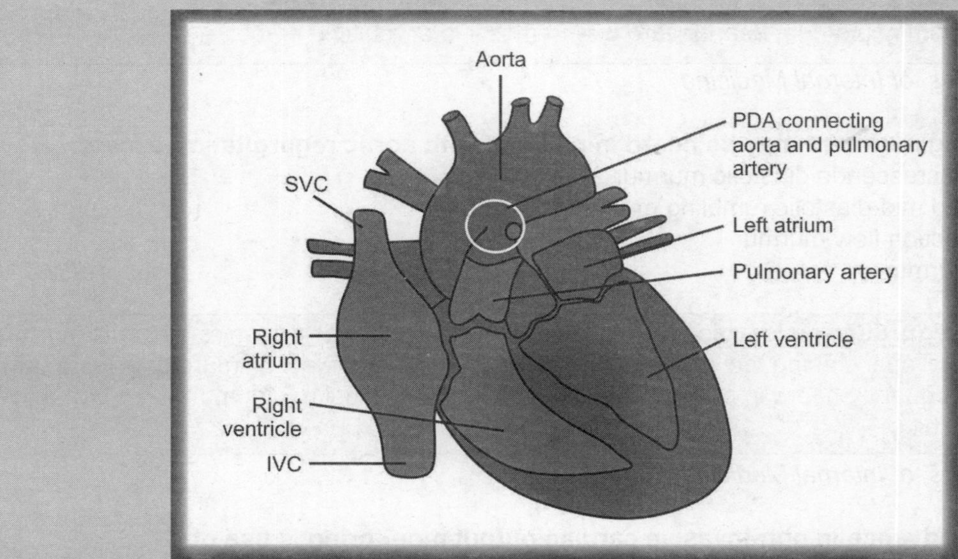

The ductus arteriosus is a vessel leading from the **bifurcation of the pulmonary artery to the aorta** just distal to the left subclavian artery. Normally, the vascular channel is open in the fetus but closes immediately after birth.

1508. Neurological complications of meningitis include all of the following *except*:

A. Seizures
B. Increases intracranial pressure
C. Cerebral hematoma
D. Subdural effusions *(AIIMS Nov 2002)*

Acute bacterial meningitis (ABM) is one of the most potentially serious infections in infants and older children and is associated with a high rate of acute complications and risk of chronic morbidity. ABM should be included in the differential diagnosis of altered mental status such as lethargy or irritability, or evidence of other neurological dysfunctions in febrile infants. During the first 2 months of life, the bacteria that cause meningitis reflect the maternal flora or environment of the infant (group B *Streptococcus*, Gram-negative enteric bacilli, and *Listeria monocytogenes*). ABM in children between 2 months to 12 years of age is usually due to *Streptococcus pneumoniae*, *Neisseria meningitides*, or *Haemophilus influenzae* type b. **Increased intracranial pressure** is due to cell death (cytotoxic cerebral edema), cytokine-induced increased capillary vascular permeability (vasogenic cerebral edema) and increased hydrostatic pressure (interstitial cerebral edema) after obstructed reabsorption of CSF in the arachnoid villus or obstruction to the flow of fluid to the ventricles. **Seizures** (focal or generalized) due to cerebritis, infarction or electrolyte disturbances occur in 20-30% of patients with meningitis. Collection of fluid in the subdural space (**subdural effusion**) develops in 10-30% of patients with meningitis and is especially common in infants. In the presence of increased ICP or a depressed level of consciousness, symptomatic subdural effusion should be treated by aspiration through the open fontanel.

Reference and further reading: *Nelson Textbook of Pediatrics; 16th edition; page 751 – 757*

1509. Following cranial nerve is *most commonly* involved in patients with sarcoidosis:

A. II Cranial nerve　**B.** III Cranial nerve
C. VII Cranial nerve　**D.** IX Cranial nerve *(AIIMS Nov 2002)*

All components of the nervous system can be involved in **sarcoidosis**. Neurologic findings are observed in about 5% of patients. **Seventh nerve involvement** with unilateral facial paralysis is *most common*.

Ref: *Harrison's Principles of Internal Medicine*

1510. The *most common* cause of acute cor pulmonale is:

A. Pneumonia
B. Pulmonary thromboembolism
C. Chronic obstructive pulmonary disease
D. Primary spontaneous pneumothorax *(AIIMS Nov 2002)*

Cor pulmonale is enlargement of the right ventricle secondary to diseases of the lung, thorax, or pulmonary circulation. In the USA about 50,000 people die each year from pulmonary emboli (acute cor pulmonale). Probably half die within the 1st hour from acute right heart failure due to massive or multiple emboli.

Ref: *Harrison's Principles of Internal Medicine*

1511. All of the following murmurs may be heard in patients with aortic regurgitation *except*:

A. High-pitched decrescendo diastolic murmur
B. Soft, low pitched mid-diastolic rumbling murmur
C. Mid-systolic ejection flow murmur
D. Pan-systolic murmur *(AIIMS Nov 2002)*

The murmur of **aortic regurgitation** is typically a high-pitched, blowing, decrescendo diastolic murmur, heard best in the third intercostal space along the left sternal border. A mid-systolic ejection murmur is frequently audible in AR. A third murmur frequently heard in patients with severe AR is the Austin Flint murmur, a soft, low-pitched, rumbling mid-diastolic bruit.

Ref: *Harrison's Principles of Internal Medicine*

1512. The most recent advance in non-invasive cardiac output monitoring is use of:

A. PA catheter　**B.** Thermodilution technique
C. Echocardiography　**D.** Electrical impedance cardiograph technology *(AIIMS Nov 2002)*

Impedance cardiography (ICG) is a non-invasive monitoring technique, which is especially known for noninvasive measurement of cardiac output. It measures the impedance changes of the thorax caused from the pumping heart to monitor cardiac parameters. Common ECG shows the electrical activity of the heart but by ICG one can see the heart 'beating'.

1513. ASD is seen in all *except*:

A. Turner's syndrome
B. Ellis–van Creveld syndrome
C. Down syndrome
D. Holt-Oram syndrome *(PGI May 2001)*

Atrial septal defects can occur in any portion of the atrial septum. Rarely there may be near absence of atrial septum creating a functional single atrium. Isolated secundum ASDs account for about 7% of congenital heart defects. The majority of cases of ASD are 'sporadic', however, autosomal dominant inheritance does occur as a part of **Holt-Oram syndrome** (hypoplastic or absent radii, first degree heart block, and ASD). Ostium primum defects occur commonly in patients with **Down syndrome**. Common atrium (absence of the entire septum) is the usual lesion in the **Ellis-van Creveld syndrome**, in which it is associated with polydactylism and ectodermal abnormalities.

1514. Selective media for TB bacilli is:

A. NNN media
B. Dorset media
C. Lowenstein-Jensen media
D. Nutrient agar *(PGI May 2001)*

Definitive diagnosis of tuberculosis is dependent on the isolation and identification of *Mycobacterium tuberculosis* from a diagnostic specimen (e.g. sputum specimen obtained from a patient with a productive cough). Specimens may be inoculated onto egg- or agar-based medium (e.g., **Lowenstein-Jensen** or Middlebrook 7H10) and incubated at 37°C under 5% CO_2. Because most species of mycobacteria, including *Mycobacterium tuberculosis*, are slow growing, 4 to 8 weeks may be required before growth is detected.

1515. Drug of choice in anaphylaxis:

A. Epinephrine
B. Chlorpheniramine
C. Wait and watch
D. Nebulised salbutamol *(UP 2003)*

1516. A 70-year-old man was administered penicillin intravenously. Within 5 minutes, he developed generalized urticaria, swelling of lips, hypotension and bronchospasm. The *first choice* of treatment is to administer:

A. Chlorpheniramine injection
B. Epinephrine injection
C. High-dose hydrocortisone tablet
D. Nebulised salbutamol *(AIIMS Nov 2002)*

The life-threatening **anaphylactic response** of a sensitized person appears within minutes after administration of specific antigen and is manifested by respiratory distress often followed by vascular collapse or by shock without antecedent respiratory difficulty. Early recognition of an anaphylactic reaction is mandatory, since death occurs within minutes to hours after the 1st symptoms. Symptoms such as pruritus and urticaria can be controlled by administration of 0.2 to 0.5 mL of 1:1000 **epinephrine** subcutaneously, with repeated doses as required at 20-minutes intervals for a severe reaction.

1517. A 30-year-old man presented with nausea, fever and jaundice of 5-days duration. The biochemical tests revealed a bilirubin of 6.7 mg/dl (conjugated 5.0 mg/dl) with SGOT/SGPT (AST/ALT) of 123/900 IU/ml. The serological tests showed presence of HBsAg, IgM anti-HBc and HBeAg. The *most likely* diagnosis is:

A. Chronic hepatitis B infection with high infectivity
B. Acute hepatitis B infection with high infectivity
C. Chronic hepatitis B infection with low infectivity
D. Acute hepatitis B infection with low infectivity *(AIIMS Nov 2002)*

A diagnosis of hepatitis B infection can usually be made by detection of HBsAg in serum. Another serologic marker that may be of value in patients with hepatitis B is HBeAg. Its Principles clinical usefulness is as an indicator of relative infectivity.

1518. The *drug of choice* for chemoprophylaxis in contacts of a patient of pneumonic plague is:

A. Penicillin
B. Rifampicin
C. Erythromycin
D. Tetracycline *(AIIMS Nov 2002)*

Short-term antibiotic prophylaxis is recommended for persons known to have had face-to-face or other direct contact with a patient with suspected or confirmed pneumonic plague.

Drugs	Daily doses	Interval in hours
• **Tetracycline**		
Adults	1-2 g	6 or 12
Children ≥ 9 year	25-50 mg/kg	6 or 12
• **Doxycycline**		
Adults	100-200 mg	12 or 24
Children ≥9 year	2-4 mg/kg	12 or 24
• **Septran®**		
Adults	1.6-3.2 g	12
Children ≥2 month	40 mg/kg	12

1519. All of the following statements regarding the ECG in acute pericarditis are *true except*:

A. T-wave inversions develop before ST elevations return to baseline
B. Global ST segment elevation is seen in early pericarditis
C. Sinus tachycardia is a common finding
D. PR segment depression is present in majority of patients *(AI 2003)*

Acute pericarditis is the *most common* pathologic process involving the pericardium. There is **widespread elevation of the ST segments**, involving 2 or 3 standard limb leads and V2 to V6, with reciprocal depressions only in aVR and sometimes V1. Usually there are no significant changes in QRS complexes, except for some reduction in voltage in patients with large pericardial effusions. After several days, **the ST segments return to normal, and only then do the T waves become inverted.**

Ref: *Harrison's Principles of Internal Medicine*

1520. Troponin T is preferable to CPK-MB in the diagnosis of acute MI in all of the following situations *except*:

A. Bedside diagnosis of MI
B. Postoperatively after CABG
C. Re-infarction after 4 days
D. Small Infarcts *(AI 2003)*

Cardiac-specific troponin T (cTnT) and **cardiac-specific troponin I** (cTnI) have different amino acid sequences than the skeletal muscle forms of these proteins. As cTnT and cTnI are not normally detectable in the blood of healthy individuals but may increase after myocardial infarction to levels over 20 times higher than the cut off value (usually set only slightly above the noise level of the assay), measurement of cTnT or cTnI is of considerable diagnostic utility. Levels of cTnI may remain elevated for 7 to 10 days after myocardial infarction, and cTnT levels may remain elevated for up to 10 to 14 days. In view of the prolonged elevation of cardiac-specific troponins (>1 week), episodes of recurrent ischemic discomfort and **suspected recurrent myocardial infarction are more readily diagnosed with a serum cardiac marker that remains elevated in the blood more briefly, such as CKMB or myoglobin.**

Ref: *Harrison's Principles of Internal Medicine*

1521. A 60-year-old man is diagnosed to be suffering from Legionnaire's disease after he returns home from attending a convention. He could have acquired it:

A. From a person suffering from the infection while traveling in the aeroplane
B. From a chronic carrier in the convention center
C. From inhalation of the aerosol in the air-conditioned room at convention center
D. By sharing an infected towel with a fellow delegate at the convention *(AI 2003)*

Legionella pneumophilia colonizes water tanks kept at less than 60°C such as in **hotel air-conditioning** and hot water systems. It causes outbreaks of **Legionnaire's disease**. There are flue like symptoms (fever, malaise, myalgia), which precede a dry cough and dyspnea. Extrapulmonary features include anorexia, diarrhea and vomiting, hepatitis, renal failure, confusion, and coma. Chest X-ray demonstrates bibasal consolidation. Lymphopenia, hyponatremia and deranged liver function test may be present. Urine analysis may show hematuria. Diagnosis is established by Legionella serology and treatment consists of high dose of erythromycin. There is 10% mortality.

Ref: *Oxford Handbook of Clinical Medicine; 5th edition; page 160*

1522. The following are true regarding Lyme disease, *except*:

A. It is transmitted by ixodes tick
B. Erythema chronicum migrans may be a clinical feature
C. *Borrelia recurrentis* is the etiological agent
D. Rodents act as natural hosts *(AI 2003)*

Lyme disease is a **tick borne infection caused by *Borrelia burgdorferi***. It was originally described in Lyme, but is now widespread. The tick (*Ixodes dammini*) is so small and the initial bite so mild that the patient may not recall having been bitten. It presents with erythema chronicum migrans with or without malaise; cognitive impairment; lymphadenopathy; arthralgia (later on erosive arthropathy); Myocarditis; heart block; meningitis; ataxia; amnesia; cranial nerve palsies; neuropathy; lymphocytic meningoradiculitis (Bannwarth's syndrome). Diagnosis is clinical ± serology.

Ref: *Oxford Handbook of Clinical Medicine; 5th edition; page 602*

1523. A 30-year-old HIV positive patient presents with fever, dyspnea and non-productive cough. Patient is cyanosed. His chest X-ray reveals bilateral, symmetrical interstitial infiltrates. The *most likely* diagnosis is:

A. Tuberculosis **B.** Cryptococcosis
C. *Pneumocystis carinii* pneumonia **D.** Toxoplasmosis *(AI 2003)*

Pneumocystis carinii is an opportunistic pathogen whose natural habitat is the lung. The organism is an important cause of pneumonia in the compromised host. The frequency of pneumocystosis among patients infected with human immunodeficiency virus (HIV) far exceeds that among other immunocompromised hosts. Impaired cellular immunity is the major host factor that predisposes to pneumocystosis, although defects in B cell function also play a role. Patients with *Pneumocystis carinii* pneumonia develop dyspnea, fever, and non-productive cough. Physical findings include tachypnea, tachycardia, and cyanosis, but lung auscultation reveals few abnormalities. The classic findings on chest radiography consist of bilateral diffuse infiltrates beginning in the perihilar regions, but a variety of atypical manifestations (nodular densities, cavitary lesions) have also been reported. Patients who receive aerosolized pentamidine have an increased frequency of upper-lobe infiltrates and pneumothorax.

1524. *True* regarding methemoglobinemia is:

A. Oxygen saturation is normal **B.** Amyl nitrite is used in the treatment of symptomatic cases
C. Hemoglobin is in the ferrous form **D.** Levels greater than 5% are almost always fatal *(SGPGI 2003)*

Iron of both oxygenated and deoxygenated hemoglobin is normally in the ferrous (Fe^{++}) state, which is essential for its oxygen transporting function. Oxygenation of hemoglobin iron to **ferric (Fe^{+++}) state** yields **methemoglobin**, which is nonfunctional and colors the blood brown (in sufficient concentration it causes cyanosis). Accumulation of large amounts of the brown, reversibly oxidized methemoglobin in red cells can occur for 3 reasons: (A) a dominantly inherited abnormality in hemoglobin, 1 of the hemoglobins M, in which the structural lesion prevents the reduction of methemoglobin to hemoglobin; (B) a recessively inherited deficiency in the enzyme methemoglobin reductase; and (C) exposure to hemoglobin-oxidizing chemicals or drugs such as nitrites, xylocaine, or benzene derivatives. Methemoglobinemia induced by drugs or chemicals is spontaneously reversible when the agent is withdrawn. However, high levels of the pigment amounting to **more than 30 to 40% of the total pigment can be life threatening** and are best **treated by the infusion of methylene blue**, 1 to 2 mg per kg body weight.

1525. Reye's syndrome is caused by:

A. Ibuprofen **B.** Mefenamic acid
C. Salicylates **D.** Naproxen *(SGPGI 2003)*

Fatty liver with encephalopathy or **Reye's syndrome** is an acute illness encountered exclusively in children below 15 years of age. It is characterized clinically by vomiting and signs of progressive central nervous system damage, signs of hepatic injury, and hypoglycemia. There is mitochondrial dysfunction with decreased activity of hepatic mitochondrial enzymes. Its cause is unknown, although viruses and drugs, particularly **salicylates**, have been implicated. The onset of disease follows a URTI, especially influenza or chickenpox and within 1 to 3 days, persistent vomiting occurs, together with stupor, which progresses rapidly to generalized convulsions and coma. The liver is enlarged, but jaundice is characteristically absent or minimal. Elevations in serum aminotransferases and prothrombin time, hypoglycemia, metabolic acidosis, and elevated serum ammonia levels are the major laboratory findings. The mortality rate in Reye's syndrome is approximately 50%. Treatment consists of infusions of glucose and fresh frozen plasma, as well as IV mannitol to reduce the cerebral edema. Chronic liver disease has not been reported.

1526. All of the following are X-linked transmissions *except*:

A. Down syndrome
B. Duchenne muscle dystrophy
C. Hemophilia
D. G-6-PD deficiency *(SGPGI 2003)*

1527. All of the following autosomal recessive *except*:

A. Congenital adrenal hyperplasia
B. Cystic fibrosis
C. Hemophilia
D. Wilson's disease *(SGPGI 2003)*

Common X-linked *recessive* diseases

- Christmas disease
- Glucose-6-phosphate dehydrogenase deficiency
- Hunter's syndrome
- Nephrogenic diabetes insipidus
- Duchenne muscular dystrophy (DMD)
- Hemophilia
- Lesch-Nyhan syndrome

*There are few X-linked *dominant* disorders but a 'notable' example is 1 form of vitamin D resistant rickets.

1528. Turner's syndrome karyotype is:

A. 45, XXY
B. 45 XO
C. 45, XX
D. 45, XY *(MANIPAL 2002)*

1529. A 19-year-old female with short stature wide spread nipples and primary amenorrhea *most likely* has a karyotype of:

A. 47, XX +18
B. 46, XXY
C. 47, XXY
D. 45 X *(AI 2003)*

Primary amenorrhea, sexual infantilism, short stature, multiple congenital anomalies, and bilateral streak gonads in phenotypic women characterize **Turner syndrome**. About 50% of the patients have a **45, X karyotype**, about 25% have mosaicism with no structural abnormality (46, XX/45, X), and the remainders have a structurally abnormal X chromosome with or without mosaicism. Lymphedema of the hands and feet, webbing of the neck, low hairline, redundant skin folds on the back of the neck, a shield like chest with widely spaced nipples, and growth retardation are suggestive of this condition in infancy.

1530. Which endocrine disorder is associated with epiphyseal dysgenesis?

A. Hypothyroidism
B. Cushing's syndrome
C. Addison's disease
D. Hypoparathyroidism *(AI 2003)*

Hypothyroidism is present in about 1 in every 5000 neonates and manifests itself as persistence of physiologic jaundice, a hoarse cry, constipation, somnolence, and feeding problems. Physical characteristics of the cretin include short stature; coarse features with a protruding tongue, broad, flat nose, and widely set eyes; sparse hair; dry skin; a protuberant abdomen with an umbilical hernia; impaired mental development; retarded bone age; **epiphyseal dysgenesis**; and delayed dentition.

1531. Normal value in blood analysis is:

A. PaO_2 of arterial blood 105
B. PaO_2 of arterial blood 110
C. SaO_2 of 90
D. SaO_2 of blood 97 *(SGPGI 2003)*

Normal values in blood gas analysis		
Arterial O_2 tension	PaO_2	95 ± 5 mmHg
Arterial CO_2 tension	$PaCO_2$	40 ± 2 mmHg
Arterial O_2 saturation	SaO_2	97 ± 2%
Arterial blood pH	pH	7.40 ± 0.02
Arterial bicarbonate	HCO_3^-	24 ± 2 mEq/L

1532. In a diabetic it was found that he was suffering from orbital mucormycosis. The treatment to be given to him would include:

A. Amphotericin B **B.** Itraconazole
C. Fluconazole **D.** Ketoconazole *(SGPGI 2003)*

Extensive debridement of craniofacial lesions appears to be very important. Orbital exenteration may be required. Intravenous **amphotericin B** is clearly of value in **craniofacial mucormycosis** and should be employed in the other forms of mucormycosis as well. Regulation of diabetes mellitus and a decrease in the dose of immunosuppressive drugs facilitate the treatment of mucormycosis.

Ref: *Harrison's Principles of Internal Medicine*

1533. Which of the following is an *acquired* stem cell defect as a cause of anemia:

A. G-6-PD deficiency
B. Pure red cell aplasia
C. Paroxysmal nocturnal hemoglobinuria
D. Shwachman syndrome *(SGPGI 2003)*

Paroxysmal nocturnal hemoglobinuria (PNH) is distinctive among hemolytic disorders because it is an **intracorpuscular defect acquired at the stem cell level**.

1534. *First* abnormality of Alport's syndrome is:

A. Microscopic hematuria **B.** Proteinuria
C. Sensorineural deafness **D.** Lenticonus *(UP 2003)*

The diagnosis of classic **Alport's syndrome** is based on X-linked inheritance of hematuria, sensorineural deafness, and lenticonus. The mean age for onset of renal disease is 6 years but it has been noted as early as 1st few months of life. **Hematuria is the *most common* manifestation**; initially it is microscopic but episodes of gross hematuria do occur, sometimes in relation to exercise and respiratory tract infection.

1535. MEN II syndrome is associated with all of the following *except*:

A. Pheochromocytoma **B.** Pituitary adenoma
C. Medullary carcinoma thyroid **D.** Parathyroid hyperplasia *(SGPGI 2003)*

MEN type 2A is the combination of **medullary thyroid carcinoma**, **hyperparathyroidism**, and **pheochromocytoma**. Three subtypes of MEN 2A are *familial* medullary thyroid carcinoma (FMTC), MEN 2A with cutaneous lichen amyloidosis, and MEN 2A with Hirschsprung disease. **MEN type 2B** is the combination of medullary thyroid carcinoma, pheochromocytoma, mucosal neuromas, intestinal ganglioneuromatosis, and marfanoid-like features.

1536. *True* about Sydenham's chorea is all of the following *except*:

A. Usually occurs 6 months after rheumatic fever
B. Occurs in 1/3rd of cases of rheumatic fever
C. The jerks are exaggerated on movement
D. ASLO titer and other markers are not specific *(SGPGI 2003)*

Sydenham's chorea occurs in less than 10% of patients with rheumatic fever. The latent period between the onset of the initiating streptococcal infection and the onset of Sydenham's chorea may be as long as several months. There is no definitive laboratory test for establishing a diagnosis of Sydenham's chorea, and the diagnosis is one of exclusion.

1537. *Most common* cause of sporadic encephalitis is:

A. Japanese B virus
B. Herpes simplex virus
C. Human immunodeficiency virus
D. Rubeola virus *(AI 2003)*

Approximately 2,000 cases of encephalitis are reported to the Centers for Disease Control in Atlanta, GA each year. The viruses causing primary encephalitis can be epidemic or sporadic. The poliovirus is an epidemic cause. Arthropod-borne viral encephalitis is responsible for most epidemic viral encephalitis. The viruses live in animal hosts and mosquitoes that transmit the disease. The **most common form of non-epidemic or sporadic encephalitis is caused by the herpes simplex virus, type 1** (HSV-1) and has a high rate of death. Mumps is another example of a sporadic cause.

1538. All of the following are associated with SLE *except*:

A. Thrombocytopenia **B.** Leukopenia
C. Lymphocytosis **D.** Anemia *(SGPGI 2003)*

Hematologic abnormalities of SLE include **anemia** (usually normochromic normocytic but occasionally hemolytic), **leukopenia**, lymphopenia, and **thrombocytopenia**. The Westergren erythrocyte sedimentation rate correlates with disease activity in some patients.

Ref: *Harrison's Principles of Internal Medicine; 14th edition*

1539. All of the following parameters indicate prerenal azotemia *except*:

A. Urine sodium is less than 20 **B.** Urine to serum creatinine ratio is >20
C. FeNa is >1 **D.** Serum BUN to creatinine ratio is <20 *(SGPGI 2003)*

In children with hypovolemia the need for volume replacement is critical. It may be impossible to distinguish whether oliguria is due to hypoperfusion or impending acute tubular necrosis (ATN). Urine examination may prove helpful in this regard; in patients with **hypovolemia**, the urine is concentrated (osmolality > 500 mOsm/kg); Na^+ less than 20 mEq/L; and **fractional excretion of sodium is usually less than 1%.** By contrast, in patients with ATN, the urine is dilute (osmolality < 350 mOsm/kg); Na^+ more than 40 mEq/L; and fractional excretion of sodium is usually more than 1%. If hypovolemia is present the intravascular compartment should be expanded by administration of IV isotonic saline (20 ml/kg) over 30 minutes.

$$\text{Fractional excretion of sodium (\%)} = \frac{\text{Urinary Na x plasma Cr}}{\text{Plasma Na x urinary Cr}} \times 100$$

1540. All of the following changes are seen in hemolytic anemia *except*:

A. Increased reticulocyte count **B.** Increased hemoglobinuria
C. Increased haptoglobin **D.** Iron deficiency *(SGPGI 2003)*

Haptoglobin is an alpha globulin, which is present in high concentration (~1.0 g/L) in the plasma. It binds specifically and tightly to the protein (globin) in hemoglobin and the hemoglobin-haptoglobin complex is cleared within minutes by the mononuclear phagocyte system. Thus **patients with significant hemolysis, either intravascular or extravascular, have low or absent levels of serum haptoglobin.** Laboratory evaluation of hemolysis can be done as under:

Test	Extravascular	Intravascular
• **Routine blood film**	Polychromatophilia	Polychromatophilia
• **Reticulocyte count**	Raised	Raised
• **Bone marrow examination**	Erythroid hyperplasia	Erythroid hyperplasia
• **Plasma bilirubin**	Raised unconjugated	Raised unconjugated
• **Plasma haptoglobin**	Low, absent	Absent
• **Plasma hemoglobin**	Normal or raised	High
• **Lactate dehydrogenase**	Raised (variable)	High (variable)
• **Urine bilirubin**	0	0
• **Urine hemosiderin**	0	+
• **Urine hemoglobin**	0	+ In severe cases

1541. The primary defect, which leads to sickle cell anemia, is:

A. An abnormality in porphyrin part of hemoglobin
B. Replacement of glutamate by valine in β-chain of HbA
C. A nonsense mutation in the β-chain of HbA
D. Substitution of valine by glutamate in the α-chain of HbA *(AI 2003)*

Hereditary disorders of hemoglobin may be classified into 2 broad groups viz. the **hemoglobinopathies** and the **thalassemias**. The hemoglobinopathies are characterized by production of **structurally defective hemoglobin** due to abnormalities in the formation of the globin moiety of the molecule, whereas thalassemias are characterized by a **reduced rate of production of normal hemoglobin** due to absent or decreased synthesis of 1 or more types of globin polypeptide chains. **Hemoglobin S found in sickle cell anemia** is characterized by the *substitution of a valine for glutamic acid* as the 6th amino acid in the beta-globin chain, resulting from a DNA substitution of thymine for adenine.

1542. de Quervain's thyroiditis is characterized by all *except*:

A. Tender enlargement of thyroid **B.** Increased ESR
C. Increased RAIU **D.** Fever *(MANIPAL 2001)*

Subacute thyroiditis is also known as granulomatous, giant cell, or **de Quervain's thyroiditis**. It is a disease of viral origin. Symptoms of thyroiditis usually start after an episode of upper respiratory infection and include asthenia, fever, malaise, and symptoms referable to stretching of the thyroid capsule, mainly pain over the thyroid or pain referred to the lower jaw, ear, or occiput. These symptoms may exist in a suppressed state for weeks before the diagnosis is suspected. **Two laboratory findings are characteristic of this disease: a high erythrocyte sedimentation rate and a depressed radioactive iodine uptake.** The disease is usually self-limiting and acute cases should be managed with oral prednisolone for 7 days and then it is gradually tapered off over the next month.

1543. Metabolic acidosis occurs in all *except:*

A. Diarrhea **B.** Renal tubular acidosis
C. Pyloric stenosis **D.** CRF *(MANIPAL 2001)*

Causes of Metabolic Acidosis

Increased anion gap (> 16mEq per L)	Normal anion gap (8–16 mEq per L)
• Chronic renal insufficiency • Diabetic ketoacidosis • Hyperalimentation • Inherited aminoacidurias • Lactic acidosis • Starvation • Poisoning (methyl alcohol, ethylene glycol, salicylates)	• Renal tubular acidosis • Diarrhea • Alkali ingestion

Ref: *Nelson Textbook of Pediatrics; 16th edition; page 208*

1544. Recent studies show that relapses of *P. vivax* is due to:

A. Exoerythrocytic stage
B. Erythrocytic stage
C. Liver hypnozoites
D. Vivax stage in peripheral smears *(MANIPAL 2001)*

In *Plasmodium vivax* and *Plasmodium ovale* infections, a proportion of the intrahepatic forms do not divide immediately but remain dormant for months to years before reproduction begins. These dormant forms, or **hypnozoites**, are the cause of the relapses that characterize infection with these 2 species.

1545. Erysipelas is caused by:

A. Viruses **B.** *Staphylococcus aureus*
C. Pseudomonas **D.** *Streptococcus* *(MANIPAL 2001)*

Erysipelas is caused by *Streptococcus pyogenes*. The characteristic features are well-defined indurated margins, particularly along the nasolabial fold; rapid progression; and intense pain. Flaccid bullae may develop during the 2nd or 3rd day of illness, but extension to deeper soft tissues is rare. Treatment with penicillin is effective.

1546. Broca's area is situated at:

A. Inferior frontal gyrus **B.** Superior frontal gyrus
C. Inferior temporal gyrus **D.** Superior temporal gyrus *(MANIPAL 2001)*

Broca's area is the area of the left hemisphere of the brain at the posterior end of the **inferior frontal gyrus**. It contains the motor speech area and controls movements of tongue, lips, and vocal cords. Loss of speech may follow hemorrhage into this area.

1547. Mesna is used to treat:

A. Nausea and vomiting **B.** Neuritis
C. Hemorrhagic cystitis **D.** Drug fever *(MANIPAL 2001)*

1548. Sodium-2-mercapto ethane sulfonate (mesna) is used as a protective agent in:

A. Radiotherapy **B.** Cancer chemotherapy
C. Lithotripsy **D.** Hepatic encephalopathy *(AIIMS 11 May 2003)*

Mesna is indicated to reduce the incidence of ifosfamide-induced or (cyclophosphamide-induced) hemorrhagic cystitis.

1549. *True* about acute intermittent porphyria (AIP) are all *except:*

A. Dark urine **B.** Acute abdominal pain
C. Skin manifestation **D.** Neuropsychiatric features *(MANIPAL 2001)*

Acute intermittent porphyria (AIP) or Swedish porphyria, pyrroloporphyria, or intermittent acute porphyria, is an autosomal dominant disorder resulting from a partial PBGD (**porphobilinogen deaminase**) deficiency. The deficient enzyme activity is found in all tissues including RBCs in the majority of patients (85%). *However*, a subset of patients (15%) shows deficient enzyme activity only in non-erythroid cells. The majority of individuals with PBGD deficiency remain biochemically and clinically normal and clinical expression of the disease is usually linked to environmental or acquired factors (nutritional status, drugs, steroids, other chemicals and so on). The cardinal feature of the disease is a neurological dysfunction that may affect the peripheral, central or autonomic nervous system. AIP is the *most common* genetic porphyria. Abdominal pain, which may be generalized or localized, is the *most common* symptom and often the initial sign of an attack. Other GIT features may include nausea, vomiting, constipation or diarrhea, abdominal distention, and ileus. Urinary retention, incontinence, and dysuria are observed. The urine develops a port-wine color in severe cases due to a high content of porphobilin. Tachycardia and hypertension and less frequently fever, sweating, restlessness and tremors are observed. Neuropathy is a common feature of AIP and muscle weakness often begins proximally in the legs but may involve arms or distal extremities. Motor neuropathy involving cranial nerves lead to bulbar paralysis, respiratory deficiency and death. Mental symptoms such as anxiety, insomnia, depression, disorientation, hallucinations, and paranoia can occur in acute attacks. Seizures can be due to neurologic effects or to hyponatremia.

1550. Resistance against anti-TB drug primarily starts from:

A. INH **B.** Rifampicin
C. PZM **D.** Streptomycin *(MANIPAL 2001)*

Strains of *Mycobacterium tuberculosis* resistant to individual drugs arise by spontaneous point mutations in the mycobacterial genome, that occurs at low but predictable rates. As there is no cross-resistance among the commonly used drugs, the possibility that a strain will be resistant to 2 drugs is very low. The development of drug-resistance is invariably the result of 'monotherapy' (failure to prescribe at least 2 drugs to which tubercle bacilli are susceptible or of the patient to take properly prescribed therapy). Drug resistant tuberculosis may be either primary or acquired. **In North America and Europe primary resistance is very uncommon and isoniazid resistance is *most common*.** Drug resistant tuberculosis can be prevented by adherence to the Principles of sound therapy, i.e. the inclusion of at least 2 bactericidal drugs to which the organisms is susceptible and the verification that the patient completes the prescribed course. Although the 6 months regimen (HRZE 2 + HR 4) is highly effective for patients with initial isoniazid resistant disease, it is sensible to extend treatment to 9 months and to give ethambutol throughout; alternately rifampin, pyrazinamide and ethambutol may be given for 6 months.[1] The treatment *regimen of choice* for virtually all forms of tuberculosis in both adults and children consists of a 2-month initial phase of isoniazid, rifampin and pyrazinamide followed by a 4-month continuation phase of isoniazid and rifampin. Except for patients who seem unlikely on epidemiological grounds to be initially infected with a drug-resistant strain, ethambutol (or streptomycin) should be included in the regimen for first 2 months or until the result of drug susceptibility testing become available.

[1] Ref: *Harrison's Principles of Internal Medicine; 15th edition; volume 1; page 1031*

1551. Cause of candidiasis all *except*:

A. OC pills **B.** DM
C. Hypertension **D.** Pregnancy *(MANIPAL 2001)*

Candida vaginitis or moniliasis is caused by *Candida albicans. Candida albicans* is present in vagina in about 20% of women without causing any symptom. Infection is more likely in patients of **diabetes**; during **pregnancy**; and patients taking broad-spectrum antibiotics, corticosteroid therapy or **oral pills**. It is commonly associated with HIV infection and in thyroid, and parathyroid diseases. Patients present with vaginal discharge with intense vulvovaginal pruritus. Discharge is thick, curdy white and in flakes, often adherent to the vaginal wall. Vulva may be red and swollen. Diagnosis is confirmed by direct smear of the discharge or the flakes or by culture in Nickerson's or Sabouraud's media. Local fungicidal preparations containing Nystatin or imidazole in the form of vaginal cream or pessary are prescribed. 1 pessary is to be introduced high in vagina at bed time for consecutive 2 weeks. Single dose oral therapy with fluconazole or itraconazole is also effective.

1552. Organism causing dental caries:

A. *Streptococcus mutans* **B.** *Streptococcus sanguis*
C. *Staphylococcus aureus* **D.** *Bacteroides* *(JIPMER 2002)*

Dental caries is a destructive disease of the hard tissues of the teeth due to infection with *Streptococcus mutans* and other bacteria.

Ref: *Harrison's Principles of Internal Medicine*

1553. Streptococci cause toxic shock syndrome due to:

A. Streptolysin - S **B.** Pyrogenic exotoxin
C. M protein **D.** Streptolysin – O *(AIIMS 1998, AI 2001)*

Exactly why certain patients develop streptococcal toxic shock syndrome is not known; however, early studies of the streptococcal strains isolated from these patients demonstrated a strong association with the production of **pyrogenic exotoxin A**. In more recent case series, particularly from Europe, the syndrome has also been associated with strains producing either exotoxin B or exotoxin C.

Ref: *Harrison's Principles of Internal Medicine*

1554. Which of the following is *false* regarding Wiskott-Aldrich syndrome?

A. Increased IgE **B.** Decreased IgM
C. Increased IgA **D.** Decreased CD4 / CD8 ratio *(AIIMS 1993, 1997)*

Wiskott-Aldrich syndrome is an X-linked genetic disease characterized by eczema, thrombocytopenia, and repeated infections. Serum concentrations of IgM are usually decreased, while IgA and IgG are normal and IgE is frequently increased.[1]

Further reading: *Nelson Textbook of Pediatrics; 16th edition; page 604* and [1] *Harrison's Principles of Internal Medicine*

1555. All of the following are associated with increased bone age *except*:

A. Congenital adrenal hyperplasia **B.** Gonadal tumors
C. Turner syndrome **D.** Polyostotic dysplasia *(KERALA 1998)*

An essential investigative method for evaluating 'short-stature' is bone-age measurement. It is done by X-rays of wrist and elbow; bone age is computed from appearance of epiphyseal centers and fusion of epiphysis with metaphysis. A child with delayed bone age has a better chance for future height gain than those with appropriate or advanced bone age. **Children with familial genetic short stature have a bone age appropriate for chronological age, whereas those with an endocrine cause such as growth hormone deficiency and hypothyroidism have delayed bone age.**

- In **congenital adrenal hyperplasia** the excessive androgen levels result in accelerated growth, so that **bone age exceeds chronological age**. Since epiphyseal closure is hastened by excessive androgens, growth stops, but truncal development continues, the characteristic appearance being a short child with a well-developed trunk.

1556. A 62-year-old man with carcinoma of lung presented to emergency department with respiratory distress. His EKG showed electrical alternans. The *most likely* diagnosis is:

A. Pneumothorax **B.** Pleural effusion
C. Cardiac tamponade **D.** Constrictive pericarditis *(AIIMS 11 May 2003)*

Echocardiography is the *most effective* diagnostic laboratory technique available for pericardial effusion, since it is sensitive, specific, simple, noninvasive, and may be performed at the bedside. In patients with large effusions the heart may swing freely within the pericardial sac; when severe, the extent of this motion alternates and may be associated with electrical alternans. **Electrical alternans** (a beat-to-beat alternation in 1 or more components of the EKG signal) is a common type of nonlinear cardiovascular response to a variety of perturbations. For example, total electrical alternans (P-QRS-T) with sinus tachycardia is a relatively specific sign of pericardial effusion, often with **cardiac tamponade**.

Ref: *Harrison's Principles of Internal Medicine*

1557. Atrial fibrillation may occur in all of the following conditions *except*:

A. Mitral stenosis **B.** Hypothyroidism
C. Dilated cardiomyopathy **D.** Mitral regurgitation *(AIIMS 11 May 2003)*

Some Causes of Atrial Fibrillation

- Emotional stress
- Acute hypoxia
- Following surgery
- Hypercapnia
- Following exercise
- Metabolic or hemodynamic derangements
- Acute alcoholic intoxication
- Rheumatic heart disease
- Non-rheumatic mitral valve disease
- Hypertensive cardiovascular disease
- Chronic lung disease
- Atrial septal defect
- Thyrotoxicosis
- Tachycardia phase of the tachycardia-bradycardia syndrome
- Miscellaneous cardiac abnormalities

Ref: *Harrison's Principles of Internal Medicine*

1558. The occurrence of hyperthyroidism following administration of supplemental iodine to subjects with endemic iodine deficiency goiter is known as:

A. Jodbasedow effect
B. Wolff-Chaikoff effect
C. Thyrotoxicosis factitia
D. de Quervain's thyroiditis *(AI 2004)*

In both endemic and sporadic nontoxic multinodular goiter, administration of iodides may lead to the development of thyrotoxicosis (jodbasedow)

1559. Which of the following imaging modalities is 'most sensitive' for evaluation of extra-adrenal pheochromocytoma:

A. Ultrasound **B.** CT
C. MRI **D.** MIBG scan *(AIIMS 11 May 2003)*

MIBG scanning may be particularly valuable in locating an ectopic pheochromocytoma when CT-scan shows normal adrenals.[1]

Pheochromocytomas produce, store, and secrete catecholamines. They are usually derived from the adrenal medulla but may also develop from chromaffin cells in or about sympathetic ganglia (extra-adrenal pheochromocytomas or paragangliomas). CT or MRI scan of adrenal is usually successful in identifying intra-adrenal lesions. **Extra-adrenal tumors within the chest can frequently be identified by CXR or CT-scan. MRI is useful in identifying extra-adrenal tumors in the abdomen.** If these studies are unsuccessful in locating the tumor, abdominal aortography may identify extra-adrenal pheochromocytomas in the abdomen, since a large aberrant artery often supplies these lesions. An additional localization technique involves a radionucleotide scan after administration of the radiopharmaceutical (MIBG). This agent is concentrated by the amine uptake process and produces an external scintigraphic image at the site of the tumor. MIBG scanning may be useful in characterizing lesions discovered by CT, as well as in localizing extra-renal pheochromocytomas. Percutaneous fine needle aspiration is contraindicated.[2]

[1] Ref: *Bailey and Love's Short Practice of Surgery; 23rd edition; page 747*
[2] Ref: *Harrison's Principles of Internal Medicine; 15th edition; page 2108*

1560. All are correct about potassium balance *except*:
- **A.** Most of the potassium is intracellular
- **B.** Three quarter of the total body potassium is found in skeletal muscle
- **C.** Intracellular potassium is released into extracellular space in response to severe injury or surgical stress
- **D.** Acidosis leads to movement of potassium from extracellular to intracellular fluid compartment

(AIIMS 11 May 2003)

Potassium is the major intracellular cation. The normal plasma potassium concentration is 3.5 to 5.0 mmol per liter, whereas its concentration inside the cells is about 150 mmol per liter. Insulin increases sodium-potassium-ATPase activity leading to potassium ion shift into muscle and liver cells. Beta-2-adrenergic agonists promote whereas alpha-adrenergic agonists impair potassium ion uptake by cells. **Organic acidoses are not usually associated with pH-related potassium ion shift, since anions such as lactate and beta-hydroxybutyrate can be readily taken up by the cells. The converse, movement of potassium ions into the cells, may be seen with metabolic alkalosis.** Tissue destruction or breakdown results in 'release' of intracellular potassium ions.

Ref: *Harrison's Principles of Internal Medicine; 15th edition; page 278*

1561. Which of the following is *not* a usual feature of right middle cerebral artery territory infarct:
- **A.** Aphasia
- **B.** Hemiparesis
- **C.** Facial weakness
- **D.** Dysarthria

(AIIMS 11 May 2003)

- The symptoms and signs of an ischemic stroke vary depending on the location of the occlusion and the extent of the spared collateral flow. Symptoms and signs of carotid system disease *most commonly* affect the distribution of the **middle cerebral artery**, and the patient may exhibit a contralateral hemiparesis, hemisensory deficit, and hemianopia. **If the 'dominant-hemisphere' is involved, there is usually some degree of aphasia.**[1]
- Human language functions depend more on 1 cerebral hemisphere than on the other. This hemisphere is concerned with categorization and symbolization and has often been called the **dominant hemisphere**. The other hemisphere is not less developed or 'non-dominant'; instead it is 'specialized' in the area of spatiotemporal relations and is concerned with recognition of faces, identification of objects by their form and the recognition of musical themes. That is why, the concept of 'cerebral dominance' has been replaced by a concept of 'complementary specialization' of the hemispheres; 1 for language functions and sequential analytic processes (**categorical hemisphere**) and 1 for visuospatial relations (**representational hemisphere**). In right-handed individuals (who constitute 91% of human population) the left hemisphere is the dominant or categorical hemisphere; in about 30% of left-handed individuals, the right hemisphere is the categorical hemisphere. *However*, in the remaining 70% of left-handers, the left hemisphere is the categorical hemisphere.[2]

[1] Ref: *Harrison's Principles of Internal Medicine*
[2] Ref: *Review of Medical Physiology by W.F. Ganong; 13th edition; page 224*

1562. Dystrophin-gene mutation leads to:

A. Myasthenia gravis
B. Motor neuron disease
C. Poliomyelitis
D. Duchenne muscular dystrophy

(AIIMS 11 May 2003)

Duchenne dystrophy is caused by a mutation of the gene responsible for producing dystrophin. The **dystrophin-gene**, estimated at 2000 kb in size, is one of the largest identified human genes. It is localized to the short arm of the X chromosome at Xp21. At present, mutations of the gene can be identified (in approximately 2/3rd of Duchenne patients) using a battery of cDNA probes.

Ref: *Harrison's Principles of Internal Medicine*

1563. Hypocalcemia is characterized by all *except*:

A. Numbness and tingling of circumoral region
B. Hyperactive tendon reflexes and positive Chvostek's sign
C. Shortening of Q - T interval in ECG
D. Carpopedal spasm

(AIIMS 11 May 2003)

A decrease in the concentration of Ca^{++} in plasma results in increased neuromuscular irritability and tetany. It is characterized by peripheral and perioral paresthesias, carpal spasm, pedal spasm, anxiety, seizures, bronchospasm, laryngospasm, Chvostek's, Trousseau's, and Erb's signs, and **'lengthening' of the QT interval of the ECG**.

Ref: *Harrison's Principles of Internal Medicine*

1564. The level of alpha-fetoprotein is raised in all of the following *except*:

A. Cirrhosis of liver
B. Hepatocellular carcinoma
C. Yolk-sac tumor
D. Dysgerminoma

(AIIMS 11 May 2003)

Conditions associated with raised alpha-fetoprotein

Neoplastic conditions	Non-neoplastic conditions
• Hepatocellular carcinoma • Gonadal germ cell tumor	• Cirrhosis • Hepatitis

- In men germ cell tumors are divided into non-seminoma and seminoma subtypes. Non-seminomatous germ cell tumors comprise 4 histological subtypes, viz. embryonal carcinoma, teratoma, choriocarcinoma, and endodermal sinus (yolk-sac) tumor. Seminoma represents 50% of all germ cell tumors.
- Fewer than 5% of all ovarian tumors are germ cell in origin. They include teratomas, dysgerminoma, endodermal sinus tumor, and embryonal carcinoma.
- Many GCTs produce tumor markers that can be measured in the blood and then used to monitor response to treatment and for follow-up care. Endodermal sinus tumors secrete alpha-fetoprotein and choriocarcinoma, and dysgerminomas occasionally secrete beta human chorionic gonadotropin (βHCG). Dysgerminoma may secrete lactate dehydrogenase and placental alkaline phosphatase.

(http://www.emedicine.com/med/topic3306.htm)
Ref: *Harrison's Principles of Internal Medicine; 15th edition; page 494, 617*

1565. Which of the following conditions is associated with Coombs' positive hemolytic anemia:

A. Thrombotic thrombocytopenia purpura
B. Progressive systemic sclerosis
C. Systemic lupus erythematosus
D. Polyarteritis nodosa

(AIIMS 11 May 2003)

Anemia of chronic disease occurs in most patients when **lupus** is active. Hemolysis occurs in a small proportion of those with **positive Coombs' tests**; it is usually responsive to high-dose glucocorticoids; resistant cases may respond to splenectomy.

Ref: *Harrison's Principles of Internal Medicine*

1566. The severity of mitral stenosis is clinically best decided by:

A. Length of diastolic murmur
B. Intensity of diastolic murmur
C. Loudness of first heart sound
D. Split of second heart sound

(AIIMS 11 May 2003)

Since the opening snap occurs when the left ventricular pressure falls below the left atrial pressure, the time interval between A_2 closure and opening snap varies inversely with the severity of the MS. The intensities of the opening snap and S_1 correlate with the mobility of the anterior mitral leaflet. The opening snap is followed by a low-pitched, rumbling, **diastolic murmur**, heard best at the apex with the patient in the left lateral recumbent position. **In general, the duration of this murmur correlates with the severity of the mitral stenosis.**

Ref: *Harrison's Principles of Internal Medicine*

1567. The risk of developing infective endocarditis is *least* in a patient with:

A. Small ventricular septal defect
B. Severe aortic regurgitation
C. Severe mitral regurgitation
D. Large atrial septal defect

(AIIMS 11 May 2003)

Patients of **congenital heart disease** (CHD) having a high velocity of blood ejected through a 'hole' or stenotic orifice are more susceptible to endocarditis. Therefore children with VSD, left sided valvular disease and systemic pulmonary arterial communication (including palliative shunts) are at the 'highest' risk. **PDA, VSD, TOF, TGA, AS, and palliative shunts are the 'most frequent' structural lesions associated with endocarditis.** In older children congenital bicuspid aortic valves and mitral valve prolapse (MVP) pose additional risks for endocarditis. Surgical 'repair' of CHD may reduce but does not eliminate the risk of endocarditis except the repair of a simple ASD or PDA. **Endocarditis is 'unusual' in sites with a small pressure gradient, as in atrial septal defects.**[1]

[1] Ref: *Harrison's Principles of Internal Medicine*

1568. Kenny Packs were used in the treatment of:

A. Poliomyelitis
B. Muscular dystrophy
C. Polyneuropathies
D. Nerve injury

(AIIMS 11 May 2003)

As a nurse in the outback in Australia, Sister Kenny found that there was no treatment for "infantile paralysis." And, she was told to treat the symptoms present. That's exactly what she did, and the child recovered. What worked for her were pieces of wool (torn from blankets) that were soaked in hot water and rung out so they wouldn't burn the skin. Properly done, they provided relief for the affected muscles. Next, she attempted to retrain the muscles. This was the beginning of the famous Kenny Method to treat polio. However, Sr. Kenny's unorthodox methods were not embraced by the medical doctors (either in Australia or England).

Ref: www.geocities.com/arojann.geo/sisterkenny.html

1569. In a patient with polyuria and polydipsia with passage of dilutes urine is suffering from abnormality involving:

A. Aldosterone
B. ADH
C. Insulin
D. Growth hormone

(MANIPAL 2002)

Diabetes insipidus (DI) is a disease characterized by excessive thirst and passage of large amount of urine. DI may result from either a lack of arginine-vasopressin (AVP; antidiuretic hormone) or failure of the AVP-sensitive renal epithelial cells of the collecting duct to respond normally to the hormone. On this basis DI can be subdivided into central diabetes insipidus (CDI) and nephrogenic diabetes insipidus (NDI). Although polyuria and polydipsia are the 'hallmarks' of DI the family members may not recognize these symptoms immediately. The urine is pale or colorless with a specific gravity between 1.001 and 1.010. Other renal function studies are normal.

1570. The immunological response giving protection to Hepatitis A for long periods:

A. IgM
B. IgG
C. IgA
D. IgD

(MANIPAL 2002)

Antibodies to hepatitis A virus can be detected during acute phase when SGPT activity is elevated and fecal HAV shedding is still occurring. This early antibody response is predominantly of the IgM class and persists for several months, rarely for 6 to 12 months. During convalescence, anti-HAV of the IgG class becomes the predominant antibody. **Following acute hepatitis A infection, anti-HAV of the IgG class remains detectable indefinitely, and patients with serum anti-HAV are immune to reinfection.** Indeed, neutralizing antibody activity parallels the appearance of anti-HAV, and the IgG anti-HAV present in immune globulin accounts for the protection it affords against HAV infection.

Ref: *Harrison's Principles of Internal Medicine*

1571. Loss of speech with inability to read, understand in a patient is referred to as:

A. Dyslexia **B.** Aphasia
C. Disconnection syndrome **D.** Apraxia *(MANIPAL 2002)*

Dyslexia is an imprecise term concerning a condition in which an individual with normal vision is unable to interpret written language. These individuals can see and recognize letters but are unable to spell and write words. They have no difficulty in recognizing the meaning of objects and pictures.

1572. The blocking antibodies in pernicious anemia are:

A. Directed against parietal cells
B. Prevents binding of IF and B_{12}
C. Prevents absorption of IF and B_{12} complex
D. Are directed against enterocytes in ileum *(MANIPAL 2002)*

The *most common* cause of cobalamin deficiency in temperate climates is **pernicious anemia**, in which intrinsic factor secretion ceases due to atrophy of the gastric mucosa. Patients with pernicious anemia also have abnormal circulating antibodies related to their disease: **90% have anti-parietal cell antibody**, while 60% have anti-intrinsic factor antibody.

Ref: *Harrison's Principles of Internal Medicine*

1573. Hypertrophic pulmonary osteoarthropathy is seen *more commonly* with which of the following lung carcinomas:

A. Squamous cell carcinoma **B.** Adenocarcinoma
C. Epidermoid carcinoma **D.** Oat cell carcinoma *(MANIPAL 2002)*

Skeletal-connective tissue syndromes seen in patients of lung cancer include clubbing in 30% of cases (usually non-small cell carcinomas) and **hypertrophic pulmonary osteoarthropathy in 1 to 10% of cases (usually adenocarcinomas)** with periostitis and clubbing giving pain, tenderness, and swelling over the affected bones and a positive bone scan.

Ref: *Harrison's Principles of Internal Medicine*

1574. "Pathergy" test is specific for:

A. Caplan's syndrome **B.** Sjögren's syndrome
C. Behçet's syndrome **D.** Felty's syndrome *(KARNATAKA 2001)*

Nonspecific skin inflammatory reactivity to any scratches or intradermal saline injection (**pathergy test**) is a common and specific manifestation of **Behçet's syndrome**.

Ref: *Harrison's Principles of Internal Medicine*

1575. "Onychodystrophy" is found in:

A. Rheumatic arthritis **B.** Rheumatoid arthritis
C. Psoriatic arthritis **D.** Reiter's arthritis *(KARNATAKA 2001)*

Most patients of **psoriatic arthritis** have **onychodystrophy** (onycholysis, ridging and pitting of nails), the course of which does not parallel that of the synovitis.

Ref: *Harrison's Principles of Internal Medicine*

1576. All the following are characteristic of "right ventricular infarction" *except*:

A. Jugular venous distension
B. Basal crepitation of lung
C. Tender palpable liver
D. Volume expansion is the treatment *(KARNATAKA 2001)*

Clinically significant right ventricular infarction causes signs of severe right ventricular failure (**jugular venous distention**, Kussmaul's sign, **hepatomegaly**) with or without hypotension. Treatment consists of **volume expansion** to maintain adequate right ventricular preload and efforts to improve left ventricular performance with attendant reduction in pulmonary capillary wedge and pulmonary arterial pressures.

Ref: *Harrison's Principles of Internal Medicine*

1577. A young female presents with history of dyspnea on exertion. On examination, she has a wide, fixed split of S_2 with ejection systolic murmur (III/IV) in left second intercostal space. Her EKG shows left axis deviation. The *most probable* diagnosis is:

A. Total anomalous pulmonary venous drainage
B. Tricuspid atresia
C. Ostium primum atrial septal defect
D. Ventricular septal defect with pulmonary artery hypertension *(AIIMS 11 May 2003)*

Atrioventricular septal defects (ostium primum and AV canal or endocardial cushion defects): The ostium primum defect is situated in the lower portion of the atrial septum and overlies the mitral and tricuspid valves. In most instances there is also a cleft in the anterior leaflet of the mitral valve. AV septal defect (AV canal defect or endocardial cushion defect) consists of contagious atrial and ventricular septal defects with markedly abnormal AV valves. In complete form of AV septal defect there is a single AV valve, common to both ventricles. The lesion is common among children with Down syndrome and may occasionally occur with pulmonary stenosis. The basic abnormality in ostium primum defect is the combination of a left to right shunt across the atrial defect with mitral (or occasional tricuspid) insufficiency. The shunt is usually moderate to large. The physiology of this lesion is similar to an ostium secundum ASD. In AV septal defect the left to right shunt is at both atrial and ventricular levels. Many children with ostium primum defect are asymptomatic and the condition is discovered during a routine physical examination. The auscultatory features include normal or accentuated first heart sound; **wide, fixed-splitting of second heart sound**; **a pulmonary systolic ejection murmur**; and a low pitched mid diastolic rumbling murmur. ECG in complete septal defect is 'distinctive'. In patients with an ostium primum defect, the right ventricular conduction defect is characteristically accompanied by **left axis deviation** and by superior orientation and counterclockwise rotation of the QRS loop in the frontal plane. Varying degrees of right ventricular and right atrial hypertrophy may occur with each type of defect, depending on the height of the pulmonary artery pressure.

1578. Which of the following is *not* seen in cerebral malaria?

A. Heavy parasitemia
B. ARDS
C. Thrombocytopenia
D. Hyperglycemia *(AIIMS 1997)*

Cerebral malaria manifests as diffuse symmetric encephalopathy; focal neurologic signs are unusual. Adults with severe *falciparum* malaria may develop non-cardiogenic pulmonary edema even after several days of antimalarial therapy. The pathogenesis of this variant of the **adult respiratory distress syndrome** is unclear. Mortality is over 80%. Slight coagulation abnormalities are common in falciparum malaria, and **mild thrombocytopenia** is usual. An important and common complication of severe malaria, **hypoglycemia** is associated with a poor prognosis and is particularly problematic in children and pregnant women.

Ref: *Harrison's Principles of Internal Medicine*

1579. *Most common* primary immunodeficiency is:

A. AIDS
B. Wiskott-Aldrich syndrome
C. Isolated IgA immunodeficiency
D. Common variable immunodeficiency *(AI 1994)*

The primary immunodeficiencies are relatively common. The **most frequent, isolated IgA deficiency** occurs in approximately 1 in 600 individuals in North America.

Ref: *Harrison's Principles of Internal Medicine*

1580. Subdural effusion is a complication of which of the following parasite?

A. *Pseudomonas*
B. *Haemophilus influenzae*
C. *Staphylococcus aureus*
D. *Streptococcus pneumonia* *(AI 2000)*

Collection of fluid in the subdural space develops in 10 to 30% of children with meningitis and is asymptomatic in 85 to 90% of cases. Subdural effusions are especially common in infants. Symptomatic subdural effusion may result in a bulging fontanel, diastasis or sutures, enlarging head circumference, vomiting, seizures, and fever. CT or MRI-scanning confirms the presence of subdural effusion. Symptomatic subdural effusion should be treated by aspiration through the open fontanel. The most serious manifestation of infection with *Haemophilus influenzae* type-b is meningitis.[1] **Subdural effusion**, the *most common* complication, is suspected when, despite 2 or 3 days of appropriate antibiotic therapy, the infant has seizures, hemiparesis, or continued obtundation.[2]

Ref: [1] *Nelson Textbook of Pediatrics; 16th edition; page 755-756*
[2] *Harrison's Principles of Internal Medicine*

1581. Congenital long QT syndrome can lead to:

A. Complete heart block
B. Polymorphic ventricular tachycardia
C. Acute myocardial infarction
D. Recurrent supraventricular tachycardia *(AIIMS 11 May 2003)*

A malignant form of ventricular arrhythmia called *torsades de pointes* (**polymorphic ventricular tachycardia associated with long QT intervals**) occurs in patients with long QT-syndrome and is a cause of syncope and sudden death. About 50% cases of long QT-syndrome are familial.

Ref: *Nelson Textbook of Pediatrics; 16th edition; page 1421*

1582. *Most common* organism causing septicemia in splenectomized patient is:

A. *Haemophilus influenzae*
B. Pneumococci
C. *Pseudomonas aeruginosa*
D. *Staphylococcus aureus* *(AI 2000)*

Encapsulated bacteria such as *Streptococcus pneumoniae* (more than 60% of cases), *Haemophilus influenzae* and *Neisseria meningitidis* are the *most common* organisms associated with post-splenectomy sepsis.

Ref: *Nelson Textbook of Pediatrics; 16th edition; page 1527*

1583. Phlegmasia cerulea dolens in deep vein thrombosis denotes:

A. Black leg
B. Red leg
C. Blue leg
D. White leg *(BHU June 2002)*

Deep thrombosis of the iliac, femoral, or popliteal veins is suggested by unilateral leg swelling, warmth, and erythema. In some patients, deoxygenated hemoglobin in stagnant veins imparts a cyanotic hue to the limb, a condition called **phlegmasia cerulea dolens**.

Ref: *Harrison's Principles of Internal Medicine*

1584. All of the following are implicated in the causation of hepatocellular carcinoma *except*:

A. Alcoholic cirrhosis
B. Hepatitis C
C. Hepatitis B
D. Hepatitis A

(BHU June 2002)

The main reason for the high incidence of **hepatocellular carcinoma** in parts of Asia and Africa is the frequency of chronic infection with hepatitis B virus and hepatitis C virus. These chronic infections frequently lead to cirrhosis, which itself is an important risk factor for hepatocellular carcinoma.

Ref: *Harrison's Principles of Internal Medicine; 14th edition*

1585. All of the following are useful *intravenous* therapy for hypertensive emergencies *except*:

A. Fenoldopam
B. Urapidil
C. Enalapril
D. Nifedipine

(AI 2003)

Malignant hypertension is a medical emergency requiring immediate therapy. Drugs useful for treatment of malignant hypertension can be divided into 2 groups on the basis of the time they take in onset of action. Those in the first group act within a few minutes but are unsatisfactory for long-term management. [1]

Immediate onset drugs	Delayed onset drugs [2]
• Nitroprusside (continuous IV) • Nitroglycerine (continuous IV) • Diazoxide (IV bolus) • Fenoldopam (continuous IV) • Esmolol (continuous IV)	• Enalaprilat (IV) • Hydralazine (IV, IM) • Labetalol (IV) • Nicardipine (IV)

In **hypertension emergency** patients with cerebrovascular disease nitroprusside, enalaprilate, labetalol, urapidil are recommended. In patients with acute coronary syndrome esmolol, metoprolol, beta-blockers of course, nitroglycerin, labetalol are the drugs of choice. In acute LV failure enalaprilate, furosemide, nitroprusside, nitroglycerin are the drugs that could be recommended but in patients with aortic dissection we should reduce the pulsation of the arteries so nitroprusside and esmolol could be the drugs of choice. [3]

[1] Ref: *Harrison's Principles of Internal Medicine; 15th edition; page 1429*
[2] Ref: *Harrison's Principles of Internal Medicine; 15th edition; page 1424*
[3] http://www.eshonline.org/education/esh2002/transcriptions/farsang.htm

1586. Father-to-son inheritance is *never* seen in case of:

A. Autosomal dominant inheritance
B. Autosomal recessive inheritance
C. X-linked recessive inheritance
D. Multifactorial inheritance

(AIIMS 11 May 2003)

An important aspect of all X-linked inheritance is the **absence of male-to-male (i.e., father-to-son) transmission of the trait**.

Ref: *Harrison's Principles of Internal Medicine; 14th edition*

1587. A young man with tuberculosis presents with massive recurrent hemoptysis. For angiographic treatment which vascular structure should be evaluated first:

A. Pulmonary artery
B. Bronchial artery
C. Pulmonary vein
D. Superior vena cava

(AIIMS Nov 2002, 11 May 2003)

The **bronchial arteries** are the part of **high-pressure** systemic circulation and originate either from the aorta or from the intercostal arteries and are the source of bleeding in bronchitis or bronchiectasis or with endobronchial tumors. Embolotherapy involves an angiographic procedure in which a vessel proximal to the bleeding site is cannulated, and a material (gel foam) is injected to occlude the bleeding vessel.

Ref: *Harrison's Principles of Internal Medicine; 15th edition; page 205 and 207*

1588. The syndromic management of urethral discharge includes treatment of:

A. *Neisseria gonorrhoeae* and herpes genitalis
B. *Chlamydia trachomatis* and herpes genitalis
C. *Neisseria gonorrhoeae* and *Chlamydia trachomatis*
D. Syphilis and chancroid *(AI 2003)*

Chlamydia trachomatis, *Neisseria gonorrhoeae* and sometimes herpes simplex virus causes symptomatic urethritis (**urethral syndrome** in women).

Ref: *Harrison's Principles of Internal Medicine; 15th edition; page 841*

1589. A 60-year-old hypertensive patient on angiotensin II receptor antagonists (losartan) is posted for hernia repair surgery. The antihypertensive drug should be:

A. Continued till the day of operation
B. Discontinued 24 hrs preoperatively
C. Discontinued one week preoperatively
D. Administered in an increased dosage on the day of operation *(AIIMS 11 May 2003)*

Recent evidence suggests that withdrawal of antihypertensive therapy (**losartan**) prior to surgery may be **undesirable**. However, the anesthesiologist must be aware of such therapy.

Ref: *1998 United States Pharmacopeial Convention*

1590. Which of the following is *not* an oncologic emergency:

A. Spinal cord compression
B. Superior vena caval syndrome
C. Tumor lysis syndrome
D. Carcinoma cervix Stage III 'B' with pyometria *(AIIMS 11 May 2003)*

Common oncologic emergencies

Structural-obstructive	Metabolic	Treatment related
• Superior vena cava syndrome • Pericardial effusion/tamponade • Intestinal obstruction • Urinary obstruction • Malignant biliary obstruction • Spinal cord compression • Increased intracranial pressure • Neoplastic meningitis • Seizures • Intracerebral leukocytostasis • Hemoptysis • Airway obstruction	• Hypercalcemia • SIADH • Lactic acidosis • Hypoglycemia • Adrenal insufficiency	• Tumor lysis syndrome • Human antibody infusion reactions • Neutropenia and infection • Pulmonary infiltrates • Typhlitis • Hemorrhagic cystitis

Ref: *Harrison's Principles of Internal Medicine; 15th edition; page 646-650*

1591. Which of the following markers in the blood is the *most reliable* indicator of recent hepatitis B infection:

A. HBsAg
B. IgG anti-HBs
C. IgM anti-HBc
D. IgM anti-HBe *(AIIMS 11 May 2003)*

In patients with hepatitis-B surface antigenemia of unknown duration, testing for IgM anti-HBc may be useful to distinguish between acute or **recent infection** (**IgM anti-HBc-positive**) and chronic HBV infection (IgM anti-HBc-negative and IgG anti-HBc-positive).

Ref: *Harrison's Principles of Internal Medicine; 15th edition; page 1731*

1592. Development of testes is dependant upon which of the following:

A. X chromosome
B. Y chromosome
C. XY chromosomes
D. XX chromosomes *(MANIPAL 2002)*

Development of the testis requires a Y-chromosome, but the short arm of the Y-chromosome is critical for sex determination; a testis-determining factor at this site has been identified and the gene for it has been cloned and designated *SRY*.

Ref: *Nelson Textbook of Pediatrics; 17th international edition; page 1922*

1593. Hypocalcemia is characterized by all of the following features *except*:

A. Numbness and tingling of circumoral region
B. Hyperactive tendon reflexes
C. Shortening of Q-T interval in ECG
D. Carpopedal spasm *(AI 2003)*

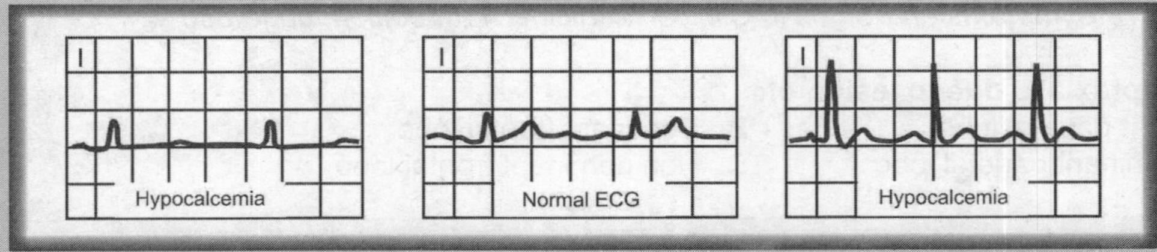

Neuromuscular and neurologic manifestations of chronic hypocalcemia include muscle spasms, carpopedal spasm, facial grimacing, and, in extreme cases, laryngeal spasm and seizures. **The QT interval on the ECG is prolonged**, in contrast to its shortening with hypercalcemia.

Ref: *Harrison's Principles of Internal Medicine; 14th edition*

1594. All of the following are 'poor' prognostic factors for acute myeloid leukemia, *except*:

A. Age more than 60 years
B. Leukocyte counts more than 1,000,000/micro liter
C. Secondary leukemia
D. Presence of t (8;21) *(AI 2003)*

The *most important* prognostic factor in acute myeloid leukemia is attainment of CR, which is defined after examination of both blood and bone marrow and should last for at least 4 weeks or more. Age at diagnosis remains the *most important* pretreatment risk factor, with more than 60 years being associated with a poorer prognosis. Chromosomal findings at diagnosis are an independent prognostic factor. **Patients with t (8; 21), inv (16), or t (15; 17) have extremely good prognosis.**

Ref: *Harrison's Principles of Internal Medicine; 15th edition; page 708*

1595. All of the following are the electrocardiographic features of severe hyperkalemia *except*:

A. Peaked T waves
B. Presence of U waves
C. Sine wave pattern
D. Loss of P waves *(AI 2003)*

- **Hyperkalemia** produces a sequence of changes in ECG starting with narrowing and peaking of the T-waves (**tented T-waves**). Further elevation of extracellular potassium ion concentration leads to atrioventricular conduction disturbances, **diminution in P-wave amplitude**, and widening of the QRS interval. Severe hyperkalemia finally causes cardiac arrest with a slow sinusoidal type of mechanism ("**sine-wave**" pattern) followed by asystole.
- An abnormal increase in U-wave amplitude is *most commonly* due to drugs (quinidine, procainamide, disopyramide) or hypokalemia.

Ref: *Harrison's Principles of Internal Medicine; 14th edition*

1596. A laborer involved with repair-work of sewers was admitted with fever, jaundice and renal failure. The most appropriate test to diagnose the infection in this patient is:

A. Weil-Felix test
B. Paul-Bunnell test
C. Microscopic agglutination test
D. Microimmunofluorescence test *(AI 2003)*

Certain occupational groups are especially at high risk of contracting **leptospirosis**. This group includes veterinarians, agricultural workers, **sewage workers**, slaughterhouse employees, and workers in the fishing industry. Weil's syndrome, the most severe form of leptospirosis, is characterized by jaundice, renal dysfunction, hemorrhagic diathesis, and high mortality. A definite diagnosis of leptospirosis is based either on isolation of the organism from the patient or on seroconversion or a rise in antibody titer in the **microscopic agglutination test** (MAT).

Ref: *Harrison's Principles of Internal Medicine; 14th edition*

1597. Following are the features of corticospinal involvement *except*:

A. Cogwheel rigidity
B. Spasticity
C. Planter extensor response
D. Exaggerated deep tendon reflexes *(AI 2003)*

Rigidity is a feature of **Parkinson disease** and may be of two types; **cogwheel rigidity** in which the resistance to movement diminishes in jerky steps and this is probably due to a combination of tremor and rigidity. In cases without tremor rigidity is of the **lead-pipe variety**.

Ref: *Chamberlain's Symptoms and Signs in Clinical Medicine; 11th edition; page 388*

1598. Dressing apraxia is due to lesion of:

A. Dominant parietal lobe
B. Dominant frontal lobe
C. Non-dominant parietal lobe
D. Non dominant frontal lobe *(AIIMS 1998)*

Apraxia may be defined as *the inability to perform a particular movement, although the patient is aware of what he/she wishes to do and has no paralysis preventing him/her from doing it*. **Dressing apraxia** is a feature of bilateral (or **right sided**) dorsal **parietal lobe lesions**. The patient with dressing apraxia is unable to align the body axis with the axis of the garment and can be seen struggling as he or she holds a coat from its bottom or extends his or her arm into a fold of the garment rather than into its sleeve.

Ref: *Chamberlain's Symptoms and Signs in Clinical Medicine; 11th edition; page 420 and Harrison's Principles of Internal Medicine; 14th edition*

1599. A lesion of ventrolateral part of spinal cord will lead to loss (below the level of lesion) of:

A. Pain sensation on the ipsilateral side
B. Proprioception on the contralateral side
C. Pain sensation on the contralateral side
D. Proprioception on the ipsilateral side *(AI 2003)*

A **peripheral nerve** consists of the axons of 3 different types of neurons viz. primary sensory afferents, motor neurons and sympathetic postganglionic neurons. Primary afferent neurons are classified by their diameter, degree of myelination and conduction velocity. The largest diameter fibers known as A-beta respond maximally to light touch and/or moving stimuli and are present primarily in the nerves that innervate the skin. In normal people, the activity of these neurons does not produce pain. Two other classes of primary afferents are the small-diameter myelinated A-delta fibers and unmyelinated C-fibers. Some tissues like cornea are innervated by A-delta and C afferents. A-delta and C-fibers respond maximally only to intense painful stimuli and produce the subjective experience of pain after electrical stimulation and are known as **primary afferent nociceptors**. The axons of primary afferent nociceptors enter the spinal cord via the dorsal root. They terminate in the dorsal horn of the spinal gray matter. The terminals of primary afferent axons 'contact' spinal neurons, which transmit the pain signal to brain sites involved in pain perception. Majority of spinal neurons contacted by primary afferent nociceptors send their axons to the contralateral thalamus. **These axons form the contralateral spinothalamic tract, which lies in the anterolateral white matter of the spinal cord**, the lateral edge of the medulla, and the lateral pons and midbrain.

Further reading: *Harrison's Principles of Internal Medicine; 15th edition; page 55*

1600. All of the following are *true* regarding cerebellar lesion *except*:
A. Hypotonia B. Dysdiadochokinesia
C. *Resting* tremors D. Ataxia (MANIPAL 2002)

1601. Past pointing, intention tremor, slurred speech, and 'drunken' gait are seen in the lesions of?
A. Pons B. Medulla
C. Cerebellum D. Caudate nucleus (JHARKHAND 2003)

1602. All of the following are seen in cerebellar lesions *except*:
A. Ataxia B. Dysarthria
C. *Spontaneous* tremors D. Hypotonia (SGPGI 2003)

The signs of **unilateral cerebellar disease** are on the same side of body as the lesion. The signs are as under:
- **Loss of muscle tone:** Hypotonia is obvious only in 'acute' cerebellar lesions. There is undue flaccidness of the limbs that can be moved through unusually large range of movements;
- **Muscular in-coordination** can be seen in the **ataxic (drunken) gait**, which is so often present. The patient tends to fall on the affected side. Ataxia of arms can be demonstrated by asking the patient to make a fist and then to pronate and supinate the forearm rapidly. On the side of the lesion this cannot be properly accomplished (dysdiadochokinesia). **Intention tremor** is another example of muscle in-coordination. When the patient attempts to touch the nose with the finger, the arm and hand become increasingly 'shaky' until the nose is reached (dysmetria).
- The *most common* ocular disturbance is **nystagmus**, usually lateral but sometimes rotatory.
- **Speech defects** generally take the form of 'staccato' speech.

Ref: *Chamberlain's Symptoms and Signs in Clinical Medicine; 11th edition; page 415*

1603. Which of the following is *not* a usual feature of 'right' middle cerebral artery territory infarct:
A. Aphasia
B. Hemiparesis
C. Facial weakness
D. Dysarthria (AIIMS Nov 2002)

1604. Lesion in left inferior frontal gyrus leads to:
A. Compromised language output
B. Difficulty in articulation
C. Inability to comprehended written language
D. Inability to comprehended hearing (UP 2000, AIIMS 1997)

Motor aphasia may be defined as a condition in which the *sensory appreciation of words is normal and the articulatory apparatus is unharmed, yet the patient is unable to speak words, which have a meaning both to him and to the listener.* **Motor aphasia is commonly associated with a right hemiplegia from left middle cerebral artery thrombosis which also affects the area of the left inferior frontal gyrus known as Broca's area (area 44).**

Ref: *Chamberlain's Symptoms and Signs in Clinical Medicine; 11th edition; page 340-341*

1605. Inhibition of 5-lipoxygenase is useful in:
A. Cardiac failure B. Bronchial asthma
C. Hepatic failure D. Arthritis (AIIMS Nov 2002)

Zileuton is a leukotriene antagonist **anti-asthmatic agent**. Zileuton is indicated in patients with chronic asthma to improve asthma symptoms, forced expiratory volume in 1 second (FEV_1), morning and evening peak expiratory flow rates, and to decrease the use of an inhaled $beta_2$-agonist. **Zileuton is an inhibitor of 5-lipoxygenase**, the enzyme that catalyzes the formation of leukotrienes from arachidonic acid.

Ref: *1998 United States Pharmacopeial Convention*

1606. A 56-year-old man has painful rashes over his right upper eyelid and forehead for the last 48 hours. He underwent chemotherapy for non-Hodgkin's lymphoma one year ago. His temperature is 98ºF, blood pressure is 138/76 mmHg and pulse rate is 80 per minute. Examination shows no other abnormalities. Which of the following is the *most likely* diagnosis:

A. Impetigo
B. Herpes zoster
C. Pyoderma gangrenosum
D. Erysipelas

(AIIMS Nov 2002)

Patients with Hodgkin's disease and **non-Hodgkin's lymphoma** are at greatest risk for progressive herpes zoster and cutaneous dissemination develops in about 40% of these patients. Herpes zoster is characterized by a unilateral vesicular eruption within a dermatome, often associated with severe pain.

Ref: *Harrison's Principles of Internal Medicine; 14th edition*

1607. A 25-year-old female presented with mild pallor and moderate hepatosplenomegaly. Her hemoglobin was 9.2 gram per liter and fetal hemoglobin level was 65%. She has not received any blood transfusion till date. She is *most likely* to be suffering from:

A. Thalassemia major
B. Thalassemia intermedia
C. Hereditary persistent fetal hemoglobin homozygous state
D. Hemoglobin D, homozygous state

(AIIMS Nov 2002)

Hereditary persistence of fetal hemoglobin may be considered as a subset of beta-thalassemia in which few beta chains are synthesized, but the thalassemic features are mild or absent, and fetal hemoglobin represents much of the circulating hemoglobin.

Ref: *Harrison's Principles of Internal Medicine; 14th edition*

1608. A 41-year-old patient presented with chronic diarrhea for 3 months. A D-xylose absorption test was ordered to look for:

A. Carbohydrate malabsorption due to mucosal disease
B. Carbohydrate malabsorption due to chronic pancreatitis
C. Fat malabsorption due to mucosal disease
D. Fat malabsorption due to chronic pancreatitis

(AIIMS Nov 2002)

Xylose absorption test is the *most commonly* employed test of carbohydrate absorption. In this test the patient ingests 25 gram D-xylose. Abnormal D-xylose absorption is found most frequently in diseases affecting the **mucosa** of the proximal small intestine, such as celiac sprue and tropical sprue.

Ref: *Harrison's Principles of Internal Medicine; 14th edition*

1609. Which of the following statements is *true* regarding drugs used in parkinsonism?

A. Amantadine causes ankle edema
B. Levodopa is particularly effective in reducing tremor
C. Amantadine is more effective than levodopa
D. Antimuscarinics are effective in drug induced parkinsonism

(AIIMS Nov 2002)

- **Levodopa**, the metabolic precursor of dopamine, provides symptomatic benefit in most patients with parkinsonism and is often particularly helpful in relieving bradykinesia.
- **Amantadine** may cause congestive heart failure and **peripheral edema**; presumed to be due to redistribution of fluid, not a gain of body water.

Ref: *Harrison's Principles of Internal Medicine; 15th edition; page 2401*

1610. All of the following are used in the treatment of parkinsonism *except*:

A. Bromocriptine
B. Riluzole
C. Ropinirole
D. Pramipexole

(BHU June 2002)

Dopamine agonists that were initially available were **bromocriptine** and pregolide, which are ergot derivatives. **Pramipexole** and **ropinirole** are new dopamine agonists. [1]
Riluzole is indicated in the treatment of amyotrophic lateral sclerosis. Riluzole presynaptically inhibits glutamate release in the central nervous system and postsynaptically interferes with the effects of excitatory amino acids. Another pharmacological property of riluzole that may be related to its effect is inactivation of voltage-dependent sodium channels.

Ref: *Harrison's Principles of Internal Medicine; 15th edition; page 2400-2403* [1]

1611. Which of the following is the *most common* tumor associated with type-I neurofibromatosis:

A. Optic nerve glioma
B. Meningioma
C. Acoustic neuroma
D. Low grade astrocytoma *(AIIMS 11 May 2003)*

The majority of tumors in Neurofibromatosis type-I or von Recklinghausen's disease are benign (neurofibromas). Malignant transformation of tumors is rare but is responsible for the severity of NF1. The distribution of malignant tumors is very different from that of the general population: **50% of the tumors are central nervous system tumors** (ependymoma, astrocytoma, medulloblastoma, meningioma, glioma), **33% of which are optic gliomas**. The risk of pheochromocytoma or neurofibrosarcoma is significantly elevated, for NF1 patients and those of leukemia and multiple cancers are also increased.

Frequencies of tumors in NF1 patients in Great Britain (*Narod et al., 1991*)

NF1-associated cancers	**Observed cases**
Leukemias	7
Acute lymphoid	4
Chronic myeloid	3
Lymphomas	3
Hodgkin's	2
Non-Hodgkin's	1
Central nervous system tumors	**60**
Ependymoma	1
Optic gliomas	**34**
Astrocytoma	13
Medulloblastoma	3
Meningioma	3
Other glioma	6
Sympathetic nervous system tumor	2
Neuroblastoma	1
Pheochromocytoma	1
Soft-tissue sarcoma	18
Rhabdomyosarcoma	5
Neurofibrosarcoma	12
Other fibrosarcoma	1
Total	**90**

http://www.orpha.net/data/patho/GB/uk-NF1.html

1612. A patient undergoing surgery suddenly develops hypotension. The monitor shows that the end-tidal CO_2 has decreased abruptly by 15 mmHg. What is the probable diagnosis:

A. Hypothermia
B. Pulmonary embolism
C. Massive fluid deficit
D. Myocardial depression due to anesthetic agents *(AIIMS 11 May 2003)*

End-tidal carbon dioxide is *most commonly* used as a noninvasive substitute for $PaCO_2$ (tension of carbon dioxide in arterial blood) in evaluating the adequacy of ventilation during laparoscopic surgery because the gradient between $PaCO_2$ and P_ECO_2 (tension cf CO_2 in expired air) in healthy patients under general anesthesia is between 2 mmHg and 9 mmHg. However, for patients with compromised cardiopulmonary function, the gradient between $PaCO_2$ and P_ECO_2 may become large and unpredictable so direct estimation of $PaCO_2$ by arterial blood gas analysis may be necessary to detect hypercarbia. **A P_ECO_2 monitor is also valuable for early detection of venous gas embolism.** Patients with massive pulmonary thromboembolism present with systemic arterial hypotension and usually have anatomically widespread thromboembolism.

Ref: http://www.emro.who.int/Publications/EMHJ/0401/30.htm

1613. The *most common* cause of death in a patient with primary amyloidosis is:

A. Renal failure
B. Cardiac involvement
C. Bleeding diathesis
D. Respiratory failure

(AIIMS 11 May 2003)

The kidney is the *most commonly* targeted organ in primary amyloidosis, manifesting as proteinuria or nephrotic syndrome in 75% of cases. **The *most common* causes of death in patients with systemic amyloidosis are extra-renal amyloid deposits in the heart, or liver**. Cardiac death in AL patients is caused by progressive cardiomyopathy with resultant heart failure, or sudden death from ventricular arrhythmia.

Ref: http://www.wvsma.com/amyloidosis.htm

1614. The *most common* infectious agent associated with chronic pyelonephritis is:

A. *Proteus vulgaris*
B. *Klebsiella pneumoniae*
C. *Staphylococcus aureus*
D. *Escherichia coli*

(AIIMS 11 May 2003)

Chronic pyelonephritis is renal injury induced by recurrent or persistent renal infection. It occurs almost exclusively in patients with major anatomic anomalies, including urinary tract obstruction, struvite calculi, renal dysplasia, or, most commonly, vesicoureteral reflux (VUR) in young children. **The pathogens are generally the same as those causing acute pyelonephritis. Possible pathogens include**

- *Escherichia coli* (>80% of cases)
- Proteus spp.
- Klebsiella spp.
- Enterococcus spp.
- Coagulase negative Staphylococcus spp.
- *Staphylococcus aureus*
- Streptococcus spp.

Ref: http://www.bsac.org.uk/pyxis/UTI/Acute%20pyelonephritis/Acute%20pyelonephritisF.htm

1615. IV bicarbonate is given in:

A. Metabolic alkalosis
B. Metabolic acidosis
C. Head injury
D. Uncompensated respiratory acidosis

(MANIPAL 2002)

Intravenous **$NaHCO_3$**, which was formerly used in large quantities in management of cardiac arrest, is no longer considered routinely necessary and may be dangerous in large quantities. However, the patient who is having persistent **metabolic acidosis**, after successful defibrillation and intubation should be given 1 mEq/kg of $NaHCO_3$ initially and an additional 50% of the dose repeated every 15 minutes.

Ref: *Harrison's Principles of Internal Medicine; 15th edition; page 232*

1616. *Chlamydia* is *best* treated by:

A. Tetracycline
B. Ampicillin
C. Gentamicin
D. Cephalexin

(MANIPAL 2002)

One-week course with doxycycline or tetracycline should be given for uncomplicated genital infections, but a 2-week course of therapy is recommended for complicated chlamydial infections.

Further reading: *Harrison's Principles of Internal Medicine; 15th edition; page 1081*

1617. A 23-year-old woman has experience episode of myalgias, pleural effusion, pericarditis and arthralgias without joint deformity over course of several years. The best laboratory-screening test to diagnose her disease would be:

A. CD4 Lymphocyte count **B.** Erythrocyte sedimentation rate
C. Antinuclear antibody **D.** Assay for thyroid hormones *(AI 2003)*

Systemic lupus erythematosus is a disease of unknown cause in which tissues and cells are damaged by pathogenic autoantibodies and immune complexes. **Ninety percent of patients are women**. Almost all patients experience **arthralgias** and **myalgias**; most develop intermittent arthritis. **Pericarditis** is the *most frequent* manifestation of *cardiac* lupus; effusions can occur and occasionally lead to tamponade; constrictive pericarditis is rare. Pleurisy and pleural effusions are common manifestations of SLE. **Antinuclear antibodies are the best screening test for SLE.**

Ref: *Harrison's Principles of Internal Medicine; 14th edition*

1618. A postoperative cardiac surgical patient developed sudden hypotension, raised central venous pressure, pulses paradoxus at the 4th postoperative hour. The *most probable* diagnosis is:

A. Excessive mediastinal bleeding **B.** Ventricular dysfunction
C. Congestive cardiac failure **D.** Cardiac tamponade *(AI 2003)*

Paradoxical pulse is an important clue to the presence of **cardiac tamponade** consists of a greater than normal (10 mmHg) inspiratory decline in systolic arterial pressure.

Ref: *Harrison's Principles of Internal Medicine; 14th edition*

1619. The diffusion capacity of lung (DL_{co}) is decreased in all of the following conditions *except*:

A. Interstitial lung disease
B. Goodpasture's syndrome
C. Emphysema
D. Primary pulmonary hypertension *(AI 2003)*

Between 50 and 70% of patients of Anti-GBM disease have pulmonary hemorrhage; the clinical complex of anti-GBM nephritis and lung hemorrhage is known as **Goodpasture's syndrome**. Patients with lung involvement frequently have microcytic, hypochromic, iron-deficiency anemia due to alveolar hemorrhage, and abnormal bilateral hilar and basilar interstitial shadowing on CXR that may be difficult to distinguish from pulmonary edema or infection. The **diffusion capacity for carbon dioxide** is a useful method to distinguish among the latter diagnoses, being **increased in patients with lung hemorrhage due to uptake of carbon monoxide by alveolar blood**, and reduced in patients with infection or pulmonary edema.

Ref: *Harrison's Principles of Internal Medicine; 14th edition*

1620. Prolactin secretion is inhibited by:

A. Growth hormone **B.** Somatostatin
C. Dopamine **D.** TSH *(MANIPAL 2002)*

1621. Prolactin secretion will be *inhibited* by:

A. Haloperidol **B.** GABA
C. Neurophysin **D.** Dopamine *(AIIMS Nov 2002)*

The **major hypothalamic inhibitory factor for prolactin is dopamine**, but peptide inhibitory factors such as endothelin and calcitonin may have a role.

Ref: *Harrison's Principles of Internal Medicine; 14th edition*

1622. Epidemics of poliomyelitis are *most commonly* caused by?

A. Type I **B.** Type II
C. Type III **D.** Type II and III *(CUPGME 2003)*

Poliovirus strains have been classified into 3 types, viz. type 1, 2 and 3 on the basis of neutralization tests. **Type-1 is the *most common* and causes 'most' epidemics.** Type-2 usually causes endemic infections. Type-3 strains have caused epidemics. The immunity produced is type specific.

Ref: *Textbook of Microbiology by R. Ananthanarayan and C. K. J. Paniker; 6th edition; page 454*

1623. Which of the following is associated with primary hemochromatosis?

A. HLA DW5 **B.** HLA-A3
C. HLA DW6 **D.** HLA DW7 *(CUPGME 2003)*

About **70% of individuals with hemochromatosis are HLA-A3**, but only 28% of the general population are HLA-A3. Also present in many patients of idiopathic **hemochromatosis** are B-7, B-14, or Bw-35 because they are closely linked to HLA-A3.

Ref: *Robbins Pathologic Basis of Disease; 4th edition; page 950*

1624. A 6-year-old child is brought with history of hemophilia, and swollen and painful right knee joint. Factor VIII serum level is 10%. Which of the following is the preferred treatment?

A. Cryoprecipitate **B.** Factor VIII concentrate
C. Fresh frozen plasma **D.** Desmopressin acetate *(CUPGME 2003)*

Each unit of factor VIII infused, defined as the amount present in 1 mL normal plasma, will raise the plasma level of the recipient by 2 percent per kilogram of body weight. An uncomplicated episode of soft tissue bleeding or **an early hemarthrosis can be treated with 1 infusion of sufficient factor VIII concentrate to raise the factor VIII level to 15 or 20%.**

Ref: *Harrison's Principles of Internal Medicine; 14th edition*

1625. *Most common* cause of acute cor pulmonale is?

A. Pulmonary thromboembolism **B.** Lung disease
C. Aortic stenosis **D.** Pulmonary stenosis *(CUPGME 2003)*

Cor pulmonale (pulmonary heart disease) constitutes right ventricular enlargement secondary to pulmonary hypertension caused by disorders that affect either the function or the structure of the lungs. Based on the suddenness of development of the pulmonary hypertension, 2 forms of cor pulmonale may develop. **Acute cor pulmonale** refers to the right ventricular dilatation that follows **massive pulmonary thromboembolism. Chronic cor pulmonale** means right ventricular hypertrophy secondary to prolonged 'pressure' overload whether related to narrowing or obstructions of major arteries or compression of septal arteries.

Ref: *Robbins Pathologic Basis of Disease; 4th edition; page 617*

1626. Which of the following is the best indicator of chronic renal failure?

A. Red cell casts **B.** Hyaline casts
C. Granular casts **D.** Broad casts *(CUPGME 2003)*

Broad casts arise in the dilated tubules of enlarged nephrons that have undergone compensatory hypertrophy in response to reduced renal mass (i.e., **chronic renal failure**).

Ref: *Harrison's Principles of Internal Medicine; 14th edition*

1627. HLA B-27 is associated with all *except*:

A. Sjögren's syndrome **B.** Juvenile rheumatoid arthritis
C. Psoriatic arthritis **D.** Ankylosing spondylitis *(CUPGME 2003)*

Studies have demonstrated that **HLA-B8, -DR3, and -DRw52** are prevalent in primary **Sjögren's syndrome** patients as compared with the normal control population.

Ref: *Harrison's Principles of Internal Medicine; 14th edition*

1628. Albendazole is effective against infection with all of the following *except*:

A. Ascariasis
B. Neurocysticercosis
C. *Echinococcus granulosus*
D. Schistosomiasis

(KARNATAKA 2001)

Although a number of drugs are available for the treatment of *Schistosoma mansoni* infection, praziquantel and oxamniquine are the drugs of choice.

Treatment of Schistosomiasis

Species	*Drug*
Schistosoma haematobium	Praziquantel, Metrifonate
Schistosoma mansoni	
• Americas and Caribbean	Oxamniquine, Praziquantel
• Africa and Middle East	Oxamniquine Praziquantel
Schistosoma japonicum or *Schistosoma mekongi*	Praziquantel

Ref: *Harrison's Principles of Internal Medicine; 14th edition*

1629. CD10 is a marker in:

A. ALL
B. AML
C. CML
D. CLL

(BHU June 2002)

Antigens and receptors on the surface of normal hemopoietic cells at various stages of differentiation may also be present on the leukemic **blast cells** of the same lineage. It is therefore possible to classify acute leukemia not only by morphological criteria, but also in terms of **cell surface markers**. This is particularly useful in the lymphoblastic leukemias. The surface markers used for classification of acute lymphoblastic leukemia are as under:

- Immunoglobulin bond to the cell surface membrane (SIg) is a B-lymphoid cell marker;
- Sheep erythrocyte rosette formation (E) is a T-lymphoid cell surface marker equating with T-11 surface antigen;
- Surface and internal antigens detected by the use of specific antibodies include the common acute lymphoblastic leukemia antigen (CALLA or CD10), T and B-lymphoid cell surface antigens, cytoplasmic μ chains;
- Estimation of deoxynucleotidyl transferase (TdT) by immunofluorescence after reaction with monoclonal anti-TdT is useful in diagnosis of ALL in which the levels are high (in contrast to most cases of AML).

Ref: *de Gruchy's Clinical Hematology in Medical Practice; 5th edition; page 246 – 247 and Robbins Pathologic Basis of Disease; 4th edition; page 725*

1630. Takayasu's arteritis *most common*ly involves:

A. Abdominal aorta
B. Subclavian artery
C. Renal artery
D. Common carotid artery

(BHU June 2002)

Takayasu's arteritis involves medium- and large-sized arteries, with a strong predilection for the aortic arch and its branches; the pulmonary artery also may be involved.

Artery	*Involvement (%)*
• Subclavian	93
• Common carotid	58
• Abdominal aorta	47
• Renal	38
• Aortic arch or root	35
• Vertebral	35
• Coeliac axis	18
• Superior mesenteric	18
• Iliac	17
• Pulmonary	10-40
• Coronary	<10

Ref: *Harrison's Principles of Internal Medicine; 14th edition*

1631. Which one of the following conditions may lead to exudative pleural effusion?

A. Cirrhosis B. Nephrotic syndrome
C. Congestive heart failure D. Bronchogenic carcinoma *(AI 2003)*

A **pleural effusion** is fluid in the pleural space and effusions can be divided by their protein concentration into **transudates** (less than 30 gm per liter) and **exudates** (more than 30 gm per liter).

- **Transudates** may be due to increased venous pressure (cardiac failure, constructive pericarditis, fluid overload) or hypoproteinemia (cirrhosis, nephrotic syndrome, malabsorption). It also occurs in hypothyroidism and Meigs' syndrome (right pleural effusion and ovarian fibromas).
- **Exudates** are mostly due to increased leakiness of pleural capillaries due to infection, inflammation or malignancy. Common causes are pneumonia, tuberculosis, pulmonary infarction, rheumatoid arthritis, systemic lupus erythematous, bronchogenic carcinoma, malignant metastases, lymphoma, mesothelioma, and lymphangitis carcinomatosis.

Ref: *Oxford Handbook of Clinical Medicine; 5th edition; page 182*

1632. A high amylase level in pleural fluid suggests a diagnosis of:

A. Tuberculosis B. Malignancy
C. Rheumatoid arthritis D. Pulmonary infarction *(AIIMS 11 May 2003)*

1633. All of the following are causes of decreased glucose in pleural effusion *except*:

A. Squamous cell carcinoma B. Rheumatoid arthritis
C. Empyema D. Cirrhosis *(SGPGI 2003)*

1634. Decreased pleural fluid glucose is seen in all of the following *except*:

A. Empyema B. Cirrhosis
C. Rheumatoid arthritis D. Malignancy *(SGPGI 2003)*

A **glucose concentration** of < 60 mg/dL in an exudative pleural effusion indicates TB, malignancy, para-pneumonic effusion, or rheumatoid disease. In most rheumatoid pleural effusions, glucose is < 30 mg/dL. Very **high amylase levels** occur in pleural effusions associated with acute pancreatitis, chronic pancreaticopleural fistulas, and esophageal rupture. In about 10% of malignant pleural effusions, amylase is slightly to moderately elevated.

Ref: http://www.merck.com/pubs/mmanual/section6/chapter80/80c.htm

1635. All of the following are *true* statements regarding acid base balance *except*:

A. Diarrhea is associated with normal anion gap
B. Respiratory acidosis is associated with increased $PaCO_2$
C. Lactic acidosis can produce an increase in anion gap
D. Hyperkalemia is associated with metabolic *alkalosis* *(SGPGI 2003)*

Metabolic acidosis leads to **hyperkalemia** as a result of cellular shifts in which H^+ is exchanged for K^+ or Na^+.

Ref: *Harrison's Principles of Internal Medicine; 14th edition*

1636. Which test is performed to detect *reversible* myocardial ischemia:

A. Coronary angiography B. MUGA scan
C. Thallium scan D. Resting echocardiography *(AIIMS 11 May 2003)*

The most widely used test in the diagnosis of ischemic heart disease involves recording the 12-lead electrocardiogram before, during, and after exercise on a treadmill or using a bicycle ergometer. The information gained from an exercise test can be enhanced by stress myocardial perfusion imaging after the intravenous administration of a radioisotope such as **thallium 201** or technetium 99m sestamibi during exercise.

Ref: *Harrison's Principles of Internal Medicine; 14th edition*

1637. The relevance of fibrin degradation products is in:

A. Hemolytic uremic syndrome B. von Willebrand's disease
C. TTP D. DIC *(SGPGI 2003)*

The **laboratory features of DIC** include thrombocytopenia and the presence of schistocytes or fragmented RBCs that arise from cell trapping and damage within fibrin thrombi; prolonged prothrombin time and partial thromboplastin time and thrombin time and a reduced fibrinogen level from depletion of coagulation proteins; and raised **fibrin degradation products** (FDP) from intense secondary fibrinolysis.

Ref: *Harrison's Principles of Internal Medicine; 14th edition*

1638. Familial amyloidotic polyneuropathy is due to amyloidosis of nerves caused by deposition of:

A. Amyloid associated protein
B. Mutant calcitonin
C. Mutant transthyretin
D. Normal transthyretin *(AIIMS Nov 2002)*

No definitive treatment exists for **familial amyloidotic polyneuropathy** (FAP), an autosomal dominant disease associated with a **mutant form of the protein transthyretin** (prealbumin). Symptoms usually begin in middle life with peripheral neuropathy, autonomic dysfunction, cardiomyopathy, vitreous opacities, and occasionally renal failure. Death results from cardiomyopathy, malnutrition, or complications of autonomic neuropathy about 10 years after the onset of disease. Treatment of FAP has been limited to supportive measures including cardiac pacemakers, dialysis, parenteral nutrition, and physical therapy. In 1990, investigators in Sweden proposed liver transplantation as a treatment to remove the major source of mutant transthyretin production. Since then, several patients with FAP in Sweden. Spain, and now the USA have received liver transplants.

Ref: http://www.acponline.org/journals/annals/15jan94/liver.htm

1639. The *severity* of mitral regurgitation is decided by all of the following clinical findings *except*:

A. Presence of mid-diastolic murmur across the mitral valve
B. Wide *split* of second heart sound
C. Presence of left ventricular S_3 gallop
D. Intensity of systolic murmur across mitral valve *(AIIMS 11 May 2003)*

The **physical signs of mitral regurgitation** depend on its severity. When the condition is 'mild', signs of cardiac failure are not present, precordium is quite, and auscultation reveals a high-pitched holosystolic murmur at the apex, which radiates to the axilla. With 'severe' regurgitation signs of CHF may be present. The heart is enlarged, with a heaving apical left ventricular impulse and often an apical systolic thrill. The second heart sound may be accentuated if pulmonary hypertension is present. In patients with severe MR, the aortic valve may close prematurely, resulting in wide splitting of the second heart sound. The third heart sound is generally prominent. A holosystolic murmur is heard at the apex, which radiates to the axilla. A short mid-diastolic 'rumbling' murmur caused by increased blood flow across the mitral valve is also present.

Ref: *Nelson Textbook of Pediatrics; 17th edition*

1640. All of the following type of lymphoma are *commonly* seen in the orbit *except*:

A. Non-Hodgkin's lymphoma, mixed lymphocytic and histiocytic
B. Non-Hodgkin's lymphoma, lymphocytic poorly differentiated
C. Burkitt's lymphoma
D. Hodgkin's lymphoma *(AIIMS 11 May 2003)*

Various types of reticular tumors (lymphoma, lymphosarcoma, reticulo-sarcoma, and Hodgkin's disease) and chloroma are hemopoietic tumors that may occur in orbit.[1]

Burkitt's lymphoma is a childhood tumor that has 2 major clinical presentations.

- The endemic (African) form generally presents as a jaw or abdominal tumor that spreads to extranodal sites, especially to the bone marrow and meninges.
- The nonendemic (American) form has an abdominal presentation with massive disease; ascites; and skin, bone, and peripheral node involvement. Like the African form, it also spreads to the bone marrow and CNS (although less often).[2]

Ref: *Parsons' Diseases of the Eye; 18th edition; page 385*[1] and *Harrison's Principles of Internal Medicine; 14th edition*[2]

1641. The nephrotic syndrome with *best* prognosis is seen in which of the following nephropathies:

A. Minimal change disease **B.** Focal segmental disease
C. Membranoproliferative **D.** Mesangioproliferative *(SGPGI 2003)*

Renal biopsy is not required in the majority of children with nephrotic syndrome as most cases are due to **minimal change disease** and respond to 'empiric' treatment with glucocorticoids.

1642. All of the following familial syndromes are associated with the development of pheochromocytoma *except*:

A. Sturge-Weber syndrome **B.** von Recklinghausen's neurofibromatosis
C. MEN Type II b **D.** Prader-Willi syndrome *(AIIMS Nov 2002)*

About 80-90% of pheochromocytomas occur sporadically, and most often these are solitary tumors. The remaining **10-20% are associated with 4, possibly more, familial syndromes:**

- One hereditary pattern is **simple familial predisposition to pheochromocytomas** transmitted as autosomal dominant trait;
- Second familial syndrome is **MEN type 2a**, also known as Sipple's syndrome;
- A third familial subgroup is **MEN type 2b** (or sometimes MEN type 3); and
- The fourth familial syndrome is the association of pheochromocytoma with **von Recklinghausen's neurofibromatosis and other neurocutaneous phakomatosis syndromes.**

Phakomatosis are familial, slowly progressive neurocutaneous disorders, which form the 'borderland' between malformations and neoplasms. They include neurofibromatosis, von Hippel-Lindau's disease, Sturge-Weber syndrome and tuberous sclerosis.

Ref: *Robbins Pathologic Basis of Disease; 4th edition; page 1263 and 1441*

1643. Congenital transmission is seen in all of the following *except*:

A. Cryptococcus **B.** Herpes
C. Toxoplasmosis **D.** Cytomegalovirus *(BHU June 2002)*

- Of the 70% of **neonatal herpes simplex virus infections** caused by HSV-2, almost all result from contact with infected genital secretions at the time of delivery. *However*, **congenitally** infected infants have been reported.
- **Congenital toxoplasmosis** is an infection of newborns that results from the transplacental passage of parasites from an infected mother to the fetus.
- **Congenital cytomegalovirus** infection can result from either primary or reactivation infection of the mother. However, clinical disease in the fetus or newborn is almost exclusively related to primary maternal infection.

Ref: *Harrison's Principles of Internal Medicine; 14th edition*

1644. All of the following heart sounds occur shortly after S_2 *except*:

A. Opening snap **B.** Pericardial knock
C. Ejection click **D.** Tumor plop *(AI 2003)*

Ejection click is a sharp sound, which **occur immediately after the first heart sound (S_1)**. It occurs with the sudden opening of the appropriate semilunar valve in conditions where this opening is delayed (e.g. in aortic valve stenosis, hypertension, pulmonary valve stenosis), or where the opening of the valve is abnormally rapid. As is the case of the opening snap of the mitral valve, the ejection click is an indication of the 'mobility' of the appropriate semilunar valve.

Ref: *Chamberlain's Symptoms and Signs in Clinical Medicine; 11th edition; page 232*

1645. A patient with a mid-diastolic murmur with loud S_1 and S_2 at the apex is *most likely* suffering from:

A. Mitral incompetence
B. Mitral stenosis
C. Aortic regurgitation
D. Pulmonary regurgitation *(SGPGI 2003)*

In **mitral stenosis** the first heart sound (S_1) is generally accentuated and snapping. In patients with pulmonary hypertension, the pulmonary component of the second heart sound (P_2) is often accentuated, and the 2 components of the second heart sound are closely split. The opening snap is followed by a low-pitched, rumbling, diastolic murmur, heard best at the apex.

Ref: *Harrison's Principles of Internal Medicine; 14th edition*

1646. In a patient presenting with episodic jaundice and 'conjugated' hyperbilirubinemia had 'normal' liver biopsy. The *most likely* diagnosis is:

A. Crigler-Najjar syndrome
B. Rotor's syndrome
C. Dubin-Johnson syndrome
D. Gilbert's syndrome

(SGPGI 2003)

Rotor's syndrome is much less common than Dubin-Johnson syndrome. **It presents with asymptomatic conjugated hyperbilirubinemia with no pigmentation in liver**.

Ref: *Robbins Pathologic Basis of Disease; 4th edition; page 921*

1647. *True* regarding multiple respiratory papillomatosis is all of the following *except*:

A. Causative organism is HPV
B. Usually seen in children
C. *Mainstay* of treatment is steroids
D. Tracheostomy is avoided as it causes seeding further below

(SGPGI 2003)

Recurrent respiratory papillomatosis (RRP): Papillomas are the *most common* respiratory tract neoplasms in children. They are simple warty benign tumors caused by human papilloma virus (HPV). The most commonly associated types of HPV are 6 and 11 and half of the children are below 5 years of age. These benign squamous lesions can produce chronic hoarseness in the infant. The *most common* site is larynx, specifically at the vocal cords but in 31% of cases these lesions occur in other areas of respiratory tract, viz. nose, pharynx, trachea, bronchi and lungs. With the increase in grown on vocal cords, hoarseness increases and communication becomes difficult. Respiratory distress may develop in severe cases. Symptoms often occur first during sleep. Progressive respiratory distress during sleep, exertion, daily activity, and finally at rest requires surgical intervention. **Endoscopic surgical removal is the treatment of choice**. Most surgeons in North America prefer excision with CO_2 laser. Other types of medical management include injection of cidofovir.

Ref: *Nelson Textbook of Pediatrics; 17th edition; page 1413 – 1414*

1648. A patient with CRF is having normocytic anemia. Which of the following drugs is *most likely* to correct it:

A. Iron
B. Folic acid
C. Erythropoietin
D. Vitamin B_{12}

(JHARKHAND 2003)

Normochromic-normocytic anemia occurs regularly in **chronic renal failure**. Erythropoiesis is depressed in chronic renal failure, due to the effects of retained toxins on bone marrow, to diminished biosynthesis of erythropoietin by the diseased kidney or to the presence of erythropoietin inhibitors. The administration of erythropoietin results in a dramatic increase in hematocrit and hemoglobin concentration, suggesting that a reduced level of serum erythropoietin is the most important of these factors. **Administration of recombinant human erythropoietin is the treatment of choice for anemia in patients with advanced renal insufficiency**, both before and after initiation of dialysis. The starting dose is approximately 25 to 50 units per kilogram body weight three times per week, either subcutaneously or intravenously.

Ref: *Harrison's Principles of Internal Medicine; 14th edition*

1649. All of the following are associated with increased pigmentation *except*:

A. Hypopituitarism
B. Addison's disease
C. Hemochromatosis
D. Biliary cirrhosis

(SGPGI 2003)

Systemic diseases causing hyperpigmentation

Localized	*Diffuse*
• Seborrheic keratoses (sign of Leser-Trelat) • Acanthosis nigricans (endocrine disorders, paraneoplastic) • Lentigines (Peutz-Jeghers, LEOPARD syndromes, xeroderma pigmentosum) • Nevi [Carney complex (LAMB and NAME syndromes)] • Cafe au lait spots (neurofibromatosis, Albright's syndrome) • Urticaria pigmentosa • Incontinentia pigmenti • Dyskeratosis congenita	• **Addison's disease** • Nelson's syndrome • Ectopic ACTH syndrome • Porphyria cutanea tarda • **Hemochromatosis** • Vitamin B_{12}, folate deficiency • Pellagra • Malabsorption, Whipple's disease • Melanosis secondary to metastatic melanoma • **Biliary cirrhosis** • Scleroderma • POEMS syndrome • Eosinophilia-myalgia syndrome • Drugs and metals

Ref: *Harrison's Principles of Internal Medicine; 14th edition*

1650. All of the following are *true* statements regarding diabetic ketoacidosis *except*:

A. The fluid deficit to be corrected within 6 hours
B. Usually associated with > 2-3 liters of fluid deficit
C. In *most cases* the blood sugar level is above 300 mg%
D. Potassium deficit may be present to the cells in spite of hyperkalemia *(SGPGI 2003)*

Therapy of ketoacidosis also requires IV fluids. The **usual fluid deficit is 3 to 5 liter**, and both salt solutions and free water are needed. Between 1 and 2 liter of isotonic saline or Ringer's lactate should be given rapidly IV on arrival, with additional amounts determined by urine output and clinical assessment of the fluid state. Potassium replacement is always necessary, but the time of administration will vary. The **initial potassium level is often high despite a total-body deficit** because of the severe acidosis. **Hyperglycemia may occur but is usually mild and rarely, if ever, exceeds 300 mg/dL.**

Ref: *Harrison's Principles of Internal Medicine; 14th edition*

1651. *True* regarding primary hypothyroidism is:

A. Delayed relaxation of ankle jerks **B.** T_3 is best for replacement
C. TSH levels are decreased **D.** None of the above *(SGPGI 2003)*

The relaxation phase of the deep tendon reflexes in hypothyroidism is characteristically **prolonged**, the so-called **hung-up reflex**.

Ref: *Harrison's Principles of Internal Medicine; 14th edition*

1652. The *best* drug in treatment of motion sickness, among the following is:

A. Domperidone **B.** Metoclopramide
C. Ondansetron **D.** Promethazine *(SGPGI 2003)*

Antihistamines such as dimenhydrinate, meclizine, and **promethazine hydrochloride** are effective for the control of nausea and vomiting due to **motion sickness**.

Ref: *Harrison's Principles of Internal Medicine; 14th edition*

1653. Lyme disease caused by:

A. *Leptospira* **B.** *Borrelia*
C. *Treponema* **D.** *Bordetella* *(PGI May 2001)*

Borrelia burgdorferi is the causative agent of the Lyme disease.

Ref: *Harrison's Principles of Internal Medicine; 14th edition*

1654. A patient presents with respiratory symptoms i.e. cough, hemoptysis and glomerulonephritis. His c-ANCA level in serum is raised. The *most likely* diagnosis is:

A. Goodpasture's syndrome
B. Classic polyarteritis nodosa
C. Wegener's granulomatosis
D. Kawasaki syndrome *(AIIMS Nov 2002)*

Wegener's granulomatosis is characterized by granulomatous vasculitis of the upper and lower respiratory tracts together with glomerulonephritis. A high percentage of these patients develop ANCA; c-ANCA is the predominant ANCA in this disease. A *typical* patient presents with severe upper respiratory tract findings such as paranasal sinus pain and drainage and purulent or bloody nasal discharge with or without nasal mucosal ulceration. Renal disease generally dominates the clinical picture and, if left untreated, accounts directly or indirectly for most of the mortality in this disease.

Ref: *Harrison's Principles of Internal Medicine; 14th edition*

1655. The pathogenesis of hypochromic anemia in lead poisoning is due to:

A. Inhibition of enzymes involved in heme biosynthesis
B. Binding of lead to transferrin, inhibiting transport of iron
C. Binding of lead to cell membrane of erythroid precursors
D. Binding of lead to ferritin inhibiting their breakdown into hemosiderin *(AIIMS Nov 2002)*

The **pathogenesis of anemia in lead poisoning** is not fully known but it appears that the main factor is an interference with bone marrow hemopoiesis. There is also some hemolytic element, probably due to direct RBC membrane damage. There is evidence of **inhibition of enzymes involved in heme synthesis.** Globin synthesis is also impaired.

Ref: *de Gruchy's Clinical Hematology in Medical Practice; 5th edition; page 210*

1656. Dystrophic calcification is seen in:

A. Rickets
B. Hyperparathyroidism
C. Atheromatous plaque
D. Vitamin A intoxication *(AIIMS Nov 2002)*

Dystrophic calcification is encountered in areas of necrosis, whether they are of coagulative, caseous, or liquefactive variety, and also in the foci of enzymatic necrosis of fat. **Calcification is almost inevitable in the atheromas of advanced atherosclerosis.** It also commonly develops in aging and damaged heart valves.

Ref: *Robbins Pathologic Basis of Disease; 4th edition; page 35*

1657. Following is true regarding opening snap:

A. It is a high-pitched diastolic sound
B. It is due to opening of stenosed aortic valve
C. It indicated pulmonary arterial hypertension
D. It precedes the aortic component of second heart sound *(AIIMS Nov 2002)*

The **opening snap** has considerable importance in clinical evaluation of mitral stenosis. It is associated with the sudden movement of the valve as it opens in **early diastole** and is of a relatively sharp character. Its intensity depends upon the mobility of the mitral valve and the severity of the stenosis.

Ref: *Chamberlain's Symptoms and Signs in Clinical Medicine; 11th edition; page 231*

1658. In type II respiratory failure, there is:

A. Low PaO_2 and low $PaCO_2$
B. Low PaO_2 and high $PaCO_2$
C. Normal PaO_2 and high $PaCO_2$
D. Low PaO_2 and normal $PaCO_2$ *(AIIMS Nov 2002)*

Types of respiratory failure

Type	PaO_2	$PaCO_2$	$PA\text{-}aO_2$
I	Low	Normal or low	High
II	Low	High	Normal
III	Low	High	High

Type I, or oxygenation failure, may be caused by any disorder that produces ventilation-perfusion imbalance, shunt, or diffusion impairment. It may, therefore, be caused by any disorder that affects the airways, parenchyma, or blood vessels of the lung. Examples include ARDS, COPD, asthma, pulmonary edema, pneumonia, PE, and interstitial fibrosis

Type II, or ventilation failure, occurs when a primary fall in minute ventilation causes alveolar ventilation to be insufficient to maintain the $PaCO_2$ in the normal range. The **increase in $PaCO_2$ is accompanied by a fall in the PaO_2** as predicted by the alveolar gas equation, and therefore, the $PA\text{-}aO_2$ does not increase. Ventilation failure can be caused by any disorder that decreases central respiratory drive, interferes with the transmission of signals from the CNS to the respiratory muscles, or causes respiratory muscle weakness. Examples include drug intoxication, amyotrophic lateral sclerosis, Guillain-Barre syndrome multiple sclerosis, myasthenia gravis, muscular dystrophy, and polymyositis

Type III, or combined oxygenation-ventilation failure, occurs when minute ventilation cannot be increased sufficiently to maintain a normal $PaCO_2$ in the presence of marked V/Q imbalance. In theory, any disorder causing Type I failure can also cause Type III failure. In fact, however, only a few of these disorders commonly result in CO_2 retention. These are ARDS, asthma, and COPD

1659. Which of the following imaging modality is *most sensitive* to detect 'early' renal tuberculosis:

A. IV urography
B. Ultrasound
C. Computed tomography
D. MRI

(AIIMS Nov 2002)

In the **very earliest stages of renal tuberculosis** the normally clear-cut outline of a renal papilla may be rendered indistinct by the presence of ulceration in **intravenous urography**.

Ref: *Bailey and Love's Short Practice of Surgery; 23rd edition; page 1195*

1660. Microangiopathic hemolytic anemia is seen in all *except*:

A. HUS
B. ITP
C. Malignant hypertension
D. Prosthetic valves

(PGI May 2001)

The **microangiopathic hemolytic anemias** are 'mechanical' hemolytic anemias in which RBC fragmentation is due to contact between RBCs and the abnormal intima of partially thrombosed, narrowed, or necrotic small blood vessels.

Causes of mechanical hemolytic anemias

- Hemolytic uremic syndrome (HUS)
- Disseminated intravascular coagulation
- Malignant hypertension
- SLE
- Polyarteritis nodosa
- Acute glomerulonephritis
- Hemangiomas
- March hemoglobinuria
- Thrombotic thrombocytopenic purpura
- Disseminated carcinoma
- Eclampsia
- Scleroderma
- Wegener's granulomatosis
- Renal transplant rejection
- Cardiac hemolytic anemia

Hemolytic anemia is an occasional complication of open-heart surgical procedures, particularly those involving the use of valve prostheses (mainly aortic but also mitral) and the use of Teflon grafts for the repair of ostium primum ASD and other defects. Hemolysis is due to direct mechanical trauma to the RBCs, consequent on the development of turbulent blood flow in the vicinity of the prosthesis or Teflon graft. The condition is known as *cardiac hemolytic anemia*.

Ref: *de Gruchy's Clinical Hematology in Medical Practice; 5th edition; page 206 – 207*

1661. 'c' wave in JVP corresponds to:

A. Atrial systole
B. Ventricular systole
C. Atrial diastole
D. Ventricular diastole
(PGI May 2001)

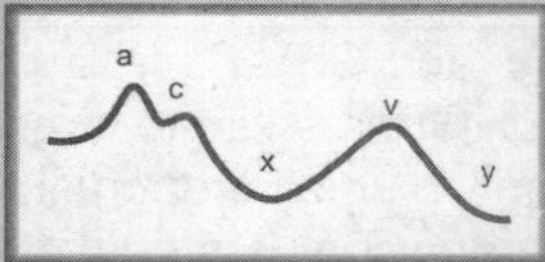

The pulsation observed in the jugular veins reflects the pressure changes in the right atrium. When the atrium contracts and the pressure in the atrium rises to force blood into the right ventricle, this rise in atrial pressure can be seen in the jugular veins as the 'a' wave. When the atrium relaxes and the ventricular systole begins, the intra-ventricular pressure rises above that in the atrium resulting in closure of the tricuspid valve. As the valve cusps 'balloon' into the atrial cavity, there is a temporary halt in the falling intra-atrial pressure and a transient rise, shown as the 'c' wave.

Ref: *Chamberlain's Symptoms and Signs in Clinical Medicine; 11th edition; page 222 – 223*

1662. *False* about pyloric stenosis:

A. Hypokalemia
B. Hyponatremia
C. Metabolic acidosis
D. Hypochloremia
(PGI May 2001)

The typical infant of **hypertrophic pyloric stenosis** is a 7-week-old; first-born male child who presents with non-bilious vomiting which increasingly becomes 'projectile' over several days or weeks. Ultimately the infant does not hold down even water and become severely dehydrated showing **metabolic alkalosis and severe depletion of potassium ion and chloride ion**. The potassium deficit may not be apparent until the late stages because the serum potassium ion concentration is maintained even after severe losses. The serum pH is high and urine pH is also high initially but it eventually drops as severe potassium ion deficit leaves only hydrogen ions for exchange with sodium ion in the distal tubule of kidney (**paradoxical aciduria**). The diagnosis can be made by palpation of the typical olive in the right upper quadrant and occasionally vigorous peristaltic waves can be seen passing from left to right across the epigastrium. Ultrasonography will diagnose the condition in 95% of cases. Correction of electrolyte abnormalities and metabolic alkalosis is essential before the operation and for severe depletion a solution containing normal saline with potassium (2-4 mEq/kg in 24 hours) is required. After the fluid 'resuscitation', a *Fredet Ramstedt's pyloromyotomy* is performed.

1663. Which of the following symbol represent adopted individuals:

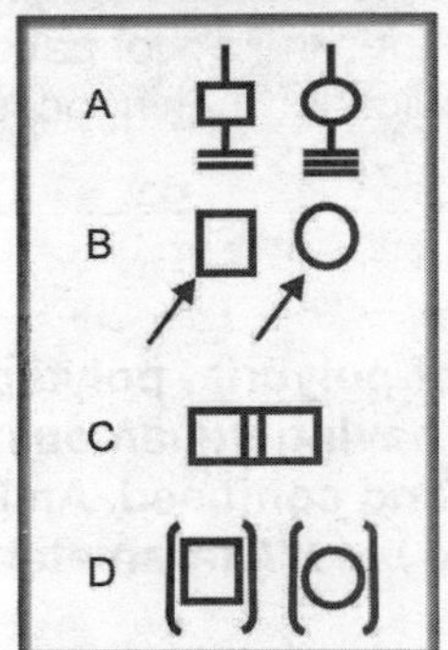

(AI 2003)

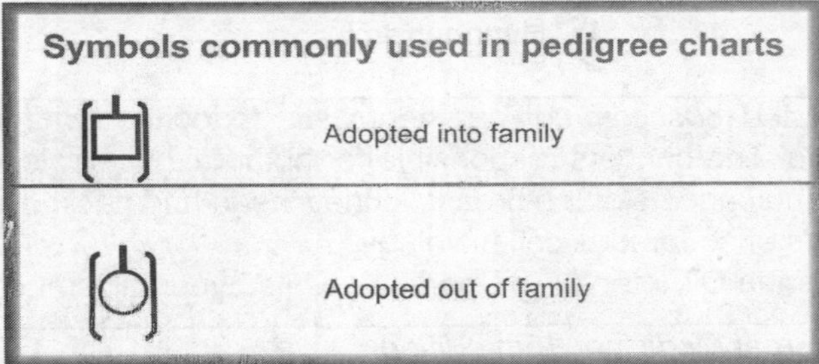

Reference and further reading: *Nelson Textbook of Pediatrics; 17th edition; page 377*

1664. Choose the *false* statement regarding hepatitis G virus:

A. Also called GB virus **B.** Blood borne RNA virus
C. Mostly infected with C virus **D.** Responds to Lamivudine (*KARNATAKA 2001*)

Hepatitis-G virus (HGV), which includes HGV, and GBV-C virus was identified by polymerase chain reaction of the plasma of a patient with chronic hepatitis. HGV is a single stranded RNA virus, which shares a 27% homology with hepatitis-C virus. HGV accounts for only a small proportion of cases of non-A-E hepatitis and most HGV infections are not associated with hepatic inflammation. It is not yet clear whether HGV is a pathogen or not. No conclusive evidence shows that HGV causes fulminant or chronic disease and currently there is no method to prevent infection with HGV.

Reference and further reading: *Nelson Textbook of Pediatrics; 17th edition; page 1331*

1665. A 35-year-old non-smoker presents with 2 episodes of mild hemoptysis. There is no history of fever or any constitutional symptoms. A plain X-ray of chest is found to be normal. Which one of the following should be the next step in the diagnostic evaluation of this patient?

A. Bronchography
B. High-resolution computed tomography
C. Contrast-enhanced computed tomography
D. Fiber-optic bronchoscopy (*AIIMS Nov 2003*)

Fiber-optic bronchoscopy is particularly helpful for localizing the site of bleeding and for visualization endobronchial lesions.

Ref: *Harrison's Principles of Internal Medicine; 15th edition; page 206*

1666. A 15-year-old boy presents to you with history of fever, altered sensorium and purpuric rash for two days. On examination, the patient is found stuporous. He has a BP of 90/60 mmHg and extensive palpable purpura over the legs. Which of the following would be the most appropriate initial choice of antibiotic?

A. Vancomycin **B.** Penicillin G
C. Ciprofloxacin **D.** Gentamicin (*AIIMS Nov 2003*)

N. meningitidis typically causes an acute infective illness, and more than 90% of the patients who become ill have meningococcemia and/or meningitis. Between 30 and 40% of patients with meningococcal disease have meningococcemia without clinical signs of meningitis. The *most striking* feature is rash, which develops in 75% of patients and may be maculopapular, petechial, or ecchymotic. Penicillin G remains the drug of choice for meningococcal disease.

Ref: *Harrison's Principles of Internal Medicine; 14th edition;*

1667. A 55-year-old man, a chronic smoker is brought to emergency with history of polyuria, polydipsia, nausea and altered sensorium for last two days. He had been diagnosed as having squamous cell carcinoma of lung two months prior to this. On examination, he was lethargic and confused. An ECG was normal except for a narrowed QT interval. Which one of the following is the *most likely* metabolic abnormality?

A. Hypernatremia **B.** Hypercalcemia
C. Hypokalemia **D.** Hyponatremia (*AIIMS Nov 2003*)

Hypercalcemia of malignancy, the *most common* paraneoplastic endocrine syndrome, is responsible for approximately 40% of all hypercalcemia. The cancers responsible for humoral hypercalcemia of malignancy in patients are non-small cell lung cancer and cancers of the breast, kidney, head and neck, and bladder. HHM is particularly common in patients with cancers of squamous cell histology.
Hypocalcemia typically prolongs the QT interval (ST portion), while hypercalcemia shortens it

Ref: *Harrison's Principles of Internal Medicine; 15th edition;*

1668. Tumor lysis syndrome is associated with all of the following laboratory features, *except*:

A. Hyperkalemia **B.** Hypercalcemia
C. Hyperuricemia **D.** Hyperphosphatemia *(AIIMS Nov 2003)*

Tumor lysis syndrome is characterized by various combinations of hyperuricemia, **hyperkalemia, hyperphosphatemia**, lactic acidosis, and **hypocalcemia** and is caused by the mass destruction of a large number of rapidly proliferating neoplastic cells. Frequently, ARF develops as a result of tumor lysis syndrome. It is most frequently associated with the treatment of Burkitt's lymphoma, acute lymphoblastic leukemia, and other high-grade lymphomas, but it also may be seen with chronic leukemias and, rarely, with solid tumors.

1669. All of the following drugs are useful in the treatment of a patient with *acute* bronchial asthma *except*:

A. Ipratropium **B.** Salbutamol
C. Montelukast **D.** Hydrocortisone *(AIIMS Nov 2003)*

Montelukast sodium is a selective and orally active leukotriene receptor antagonist that inhibits the cysteinyl leukotriene CysL T_1 receptor. Montelukast is indicated for the prophylaxis and chronic treatment of asthma in patients' ages 2 years and older. **Montelukast should not be used as rescue medication to treat acute asthma episodes.** Patients should be advised to have appropriate rescue medication available. Use of montelukast may not eliminate the need for inhaled (ICS) or systemic corticosteroids. Safety and effectiveness of montelukast in patients younger than 2 years of age have not been established.

2 to 5 years of age	6 to 14 years of age	15 years of age and older
One 4-mg cherry chewable tablet daily in the evening	One 5-mg cherry chewable tablet daily in the evening	One 10-mg tablet daily in the evening

1670. A normal anion gap metabolic acidosis occurs in patients with:

A. Diarrhea **B.** Diabetic ketoacidosis
C. Methyl alcohol poisoning **D.** Acute renal failure *(AIIMS Nov 2003)*

There are 4 principal causes of a high anion gap acidosis: (1) lactic acidosis, (2) ketoacidosis, (3) ingested toxins and (4) acute and chronic renal failure.

1671. A 41-year-old male patient presented with recurrent episodes of bloody diarrhea for 5 years. Despite regular treatment with adequate doses of sulfasalazine, he has had several exacerbations of his disease and required several weeks of steroids for the control of flares. What should be the next line of treatment for him:

A. Methotrexate **B.** Azathioprine
C. Cyclosporine **D.** Cyclophosphamide *(AIIMS Nov 2003)*

Azathioprine also may have a limited role as a "steroid-sparing agent" in the patient with chronic ulcerative colitis who must be maintained on glucocorticoids to control disease activity.

1672. A 55-year-old male patient was diagnosed to have chronic hepatitis C. He responded to treatment with interferon, however, after one year of follow up he showed a relapse of disease. Which of the following would be the next most appropriate choice?

A. Ribavirin and interferon
B. Lamivudine and interferon
C. Nevirapine and lamivudine
D. Indinavir and ribavirin *(AIIMS Nov 2003)*

The most effective way to increase the efficacy of interferon therapy of chronic hepatitis C is to add ribavirin, an oral guanoside neucleoside.

Ref: *Harrison's Principles of Internal Medicine; 15th edition; page 1748*

1673. In malignant hyperthermia the increased heat production is due to:
- **A.** Increased muscle metabolism by excess of calcium ions
- **B.** Thermic effect of blood
- **C.** Increased sympathetic discharge
- **D.** Mitochondrial thermogenesis

(AIIMS Nov 2003)

Malignant hyperthermia is an inherited disease of skeletal-muscle sarcoplasmic reticulum which causes a rapid increase in intracellular Ca^{++} levels in response to halothane and other inhalational anesthetics or to scoline. Elevated temperature, increased muscle metabolism, rigidity, rhabdomyolysis, acidosis, and cardiovascular instability develop rapidly. Cessation of anesthesia and administration of *dantrolene sodium* are the immediately indicated methods.

1674. Which of the following management procedures of acute upper gastrointestinal bleed should possible be avoided:
- **A.** Intravenous vasopressin
- **B.** Intravenous beta-blockers
- **C.** Endoscopic sclerotherapy
- **D.** Balloon tamponade

(AIIMS Nov 2003)

Vasopressin has been the most extensively used drug for initial control of variceal bleeding. Nitroglycerine may be as effective. However the initial treatment of esophageal varices in most centers is endoscopy sclerotherapy using 5% ethanolamine oleate. If the rate of blood loss prohibits endoscopic evaluation a Sengstaken-Blakemore tube may be inserted to provide temporary hemostasis.

Ref: *Bailey & Love's Short Practice of Surgery; 23rd edition; page 940*

1675. Early diagnosis of acute hepatitis B infection is made by:
- **A.** Presence of HBeAg in serum
- **B.** Presence of IgM anti-HBc in serum
- **C.** Presence of HBsAg in serum
- **D.** Presence of IgG anti-HBc in serum

(AIIMS Nov 2003)

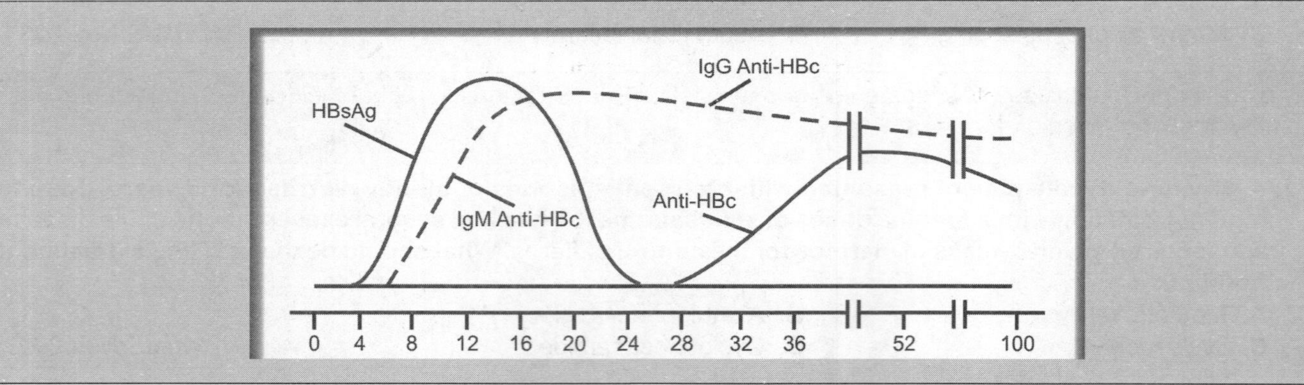

1676. Duchenne muscular dystrophy is a disease of:
- **A.** Neuromuscular junction
- **B.** Sarcolemmal proteins
- **C.** Disuse atrophy due to muscle weakness
- **D.** Muscle contractile proteins

(AI 2004)

Duchenne dystrophy is caused by a mutation of the gene responsible for producing dystrophin which is a 427-kDa protein localized to the inner surface of the sarcolemma of the muscle fiber.

1677. Which of the following is the drug of first choice for non-gonococcal urethritis?
- **A.** Ceftriaxone
- **B.** Doxycycline
- **C.** Ciprofloxacin
- **D.** Minocycline

(AI 2004)

Before the introduction of azithromycin, chlamydial infections could not be eradicated by single-dose or short-term antimicrobial treatment. A week of treatment with doxycycline or tetracycline should be given for uncomplicated genital infections.

1678. Ataxia telangiectasia is characterized by all of the following *except*:

A. Chronic sinopulmonary disease **B.** Decreased level of alfa fetoprotein
C. Chromosomal breakage **D.** IgA deficiency *(AI 2004)*

Ataxia-telangiectasia is an autosomal recessive genetic disorder characterized by cerebellar ataxia, oculocutaneous telangiectasia, and immunodeficiency. The AT gene belongs to a conserved family of genes that monitor DNA repair and coordinate DNA synthesis with cell division. Immunodeficiency may be clinically manifest by recurrent and chronic *sinopulmonary infection* leading to bronchiectasis, although not all patients have overt immunodeficiency. Although B lymphocyte development is normal, most patients are *deficient in serum IgE and IgA*, and a smaller number have reduced serum levels of IgG, particularly of the IgG2, IgG4 subclasses. IgM and IgD are usually normal.

1679. Hemoglobin A 1c level in blood explains:

A. Chronic pancreatitis **B.** Hepato-renal syndrome
C. Long term status of blood sugar **D.** Acute rise of sugar *(AI 2004)*

It is also standard practice to measure hemoglobin A1c levels quarterly in all patients of diabetes mellitus. Hemoglobin A1c is an electrophoretically fast-moving hemoglobin component that is present in normal persons and increases in amount in the presence of hyperglycemia.

1680. The *first* investigation of choice in a patient with suspected subarachnoid hemorrhage should be:

A. CSF examination
B. Magnetic Resonance Imaging (MRI)
C. Contrast-enhanced computed tomography
D. Non-contrast computed tomography *(AI 2004)*

The hallmark of aneurysmal rupture is blood in the CSF and more than 95% of patients have enough blood to be seen on a high quality **non-contrast CT-scan** obtained within 72 hours.

Ref: *Harrison's Principles of Internal Medicine; 15th edition; page 2389*

1681. Elevated serum ferritin, serum iron and percent transferrin saturation are *most consistent* with the diagnosis of:

A. Iron deficiency anemia **B.** Anemia of chronic disease
C. Hemochromatosis **D.** Lead poisoning *(AI 2004)*

Determination	**Normal**	**Symptomatic Hemochromatosis**
Plasma iron, micromol/L (microg/dL)	9-27 (50-150)	32-54 (180-300)
Total iron-binding capacity, μmol/L (microg/dL)	45-66 (250-370)	36-54 (200-300)
Transferrin saturation, percent	22-46	50-100
Serum ferritin, microg/L	10-200	900-6000
Urinary iron, mg/24 h	0-2	9-23
Liver iron, microg/g dry wt	300-1400	6000-18,000
Hepatic iron index $\frac{\text{(microg/g dry wt)}}{\text{56 x age}}$	<1.0	>2

1682. Estimation of the following hormones is useful while investigating a case of gynecomastia *except*:

A. Testosterone **B.** Prolactin
C. Luteinizing hormone **D.** Estradiol *(AI 2004)*

Endocrine evaluation of **gynecomastia includes measurement of serum androstenedione or 24-h urinary 17-ketosteroids (usually elevated in feminizing adrenal states), measurement of plasma estradiol and hCG, and measurement of plasma luteinizing hormone (LH) and testosterone.**

1683. Estimation of the following hormones is useful while investigating a case of gynecomastia, *except*:

A. Testosterone **B.** Prolactin
C. Luteinizing hormone **D.** Estradiol *(AI 2004)*

Endocrine evaluation of **gynecomastia** includes measurement of serum androstenedione or 24-h urinary 17-ketosteroids (usually elevated in feminizing adrenal states), measurement of plasma **estradiol** and hCG, and measurement of plasma **luteinizing hormone** (LH) and **testosterone.**

1684. Which of the following is the *treatment of choice* for Kawasaki disease?

A. Cyclosporine
B. Dapsone
C. IV immunoglobulin
D. Methotrexate *(AIIMS May 2005)*

Kawasaki disease is an acute, febrile, multisystem disease of children. Although the disease is generally benign and self-limited, it is associated with coronary artery aneurysms in about 1/4th of cases, with an overall case fatality rate of 0.5 to 2.8 %. **High-dose intravenous gamma globulin** (2 g/kg as a single infusion over 10 hour) together with aspirin (100 mg/kg per day for 14 days followed by 3 to 5 mg/kg per day for several weeks) has been shown to be effective in reducing the prevalence of coronary artery abnormalities when administered early in the course of the disease.

Ref: *Harrison's Principles of Internal Medicine; 14th edition*

1685. Which one of the following is *not* a feature of multiple myeloma?

A. Hypercalcemia **B.** Anemia
C. Hyperviscosity **D.** Elevated alkaline phosphatase *(AIIMS May 2005)*

Multiple myeloma is a malignant proliferation of plasma cells derived from a single clone. The tumor, its products, and the host response to it result in a number of organ dysfunctions and symptoms of bone pain or fracture, renal failure, susceptibility to infection, **anemia**, **hypercalcemia**, and occasionally clotting abnormalities, neurologic symptoms, and vascular manifestations of **hyperviscosity**.

Serum alkaline phosphatase is usually normal even with extensive bone involvement because of the absence of osteoblastic activity.

Ref: *Harrison's Principles of Internal Medicine; 14th edition*

1686. Which one of the following diseases is an autosomal dominant disorder?

A. Hemochromatosis
B. Phenylketonuria
C. Maturity-onset diabetes of the young
D. Glucose-6-phosphate dehydrogenase deficiency *(AIIMS May 2005)*

Evidence suggest that the transmission of **maturity-onset diabetes of the young (MODY)** occurs as an **autosomal dominant trait**.

Ref: *Harrison's Principles of Internal Medicine; 14th edition*

1687. Which of the following lymphomas is associated with HTLV-I virus infection?

A. Burkitt's lymphoma
B. B-cell lymphoma
C. Adult T-cell leukemia and lymphoma
D. Hodgkin's disease *(AIIMS May 2005)*

HTLV-I is the causative agent of the **adult T-cell leukemia/lymphoma** endemic to the Caribbean and southern Japan.

Ref: *Harrison's Principles of Internal Medicine; 14th edition*

1688. D-dimer is the *most sensitive* diagnostic test for:

A. Pulmonary embolism
B. Acute pulmonary edema
C. Cardiac tamponade
D. Acute myocardial infarction *(AIIMS May 2005)*

The quantitative ***plasma* D-*dimer enzyme-linked immunosorbent assay*** level is elevated (>500 ng/ml) in more than 90% of patients with **pulmonary thromboembolism**, reflecting plasmin's breakdown of fibrin and indicating endogenous thrombolysis.

Ref: *Harrison's Principles of Internal Medicine; 14th edition*

1689. The *most appropriate* drug for the treatment of bulimia nervosa is:

A. Amitriptyline **B.** Lithium
C. Fluoxetine **D.** Sertraline *(AIIMS May 2005)*

It is generally accepted that antidepressants are helpful in **bulimia nervosa** but not anorexia nervosa. The serotonin uptake inhibitor **fluoxetine** has an advantage over other antidepressants. If used, a dose of 60 mg daily is suggested in adults instead of the usual dosages recommended for depression.

Ref: *Harrison's Principles of Internal Medicine; 14th edition*

1690. Carcinoid syndrome produces valvular disease primarily involving:

A. Pulmonary valves **B.** Tricuspid valves
C. Mitral valve **D.** Aortic valve *(AIIMS May 2005)*

Manifestations of the **carcinoid syndrome** include the triad of cutaneous flushing, diarrhea, and valvular heart disease and, sometimes, telangiectasias, wheezing, and paroxysmal hypotension. Endocardial fibrosis can cause valvular heart disease, **usually affecting the proximal side of the tricuspid and pulmonary valves** and leading to tricuspid insufficiency, pulmonary stenosis, and secondary right-sided heart failure.

Ref: *Harrison's Principles of Internal Medicine; 14th edition*

1691. All of the following conditions are observed in marasmus, *except*:

A. Hepatomegaly **B.** Muscle wasting
C. Low insulin levels **D.** Extreme weakness *(AIIMS May 2005)*

Marasmus is manifested by stunted growth, loss of adipose tissue, generalized wasting of protein mass, and no edema and is thought to be due to the combined effects of protein and energy malnutrition.

Features	Marasmus	Kwashiorkor
• **Muscle wasting**	Present	Hidden by edema and fat
• **Fat wasting**	Severe	Fat is retained
• **Edema**	None	Present
• **Weight for height**	Very low	Low
• **Mental changes**	Quite and apathetic	Irritable
• **Appetite**	Good	Poor
• **Skin changes**	None	Diffused pigmentation
• **Hair changes**	Rare	Sparse, easily pluckable
• **Diarrhea**	Common	Common
• **Fatty liver and hepatomegaly**	Never	Sometimes

1692. Bart's hydrops fetalis is lethal because:

A. Hb Bart's cannot bind oxygen
B. The excess α-chain form insoluble precipitates
C. Hb Bart's cannot release oxygen to fetal tissues
D. Microcytic red cells become trapped in the placenta *(AI 2005)*

Hemoglobin-Bart's hydrops fetalis is the *most severe* manifestation of alpha thalassemia gene. It is common in south east Asia, but rare in other part of the World. Affected infants are homozygous for α° determinant (- -/- -), with both parents having heterozygous α° thalassemia. There is almost total suppression of α-chain synthesis with a gross excess of γ chains. The γ-chain tetramer, Hb-Bart's, has a high oxygen affinity, and tissue hypoxia results.

Ref: *de Gruchy 's Clinical Hematology in Medical Practice; 5th edition; page 165*

1693. Which of the following is a cause of reversible dementia?

A. Subacute combined degeneration
B. Picks disease
C. Creutzfeldt-Jakob disease
D. Alzheimer's disease *(AI 2005)*

1694. Vitamin B_{12} deficiency can give rise to all of the following, *except*:

A. Myelopathy **B.** Optic atrophy
C. Peripheral neuropathy **D.** Myopathy *(AI 2005)*

Subacute combined degeneration of the spinal cord *is a progressive disorder that is due to vitamin B_{12} deficiency and produces weakness, clumsiness, tingling, and other abnormal sensations.* This disorder affects about 1 of 10,000 people, usually those who are older than 40. It is **due to a deficiency of vitamin B_{12}**, which typically also causes pernicious anemia. Usually, the deficiency is not related to diet but to the body's inability to absorb vitamin B_{12} from the intestine. **In this disorder, the columns of sensory nerve fibers in the spinal cord degenerate. The brain, nerves of the eyes, and peripheral nerves are sometimes damaged.** The disorder begins with a general feeling of weakness. Tingling, a pins-and-needles sensation, and numbness are felt in both hands and feet. These sensations tend to be constant and to gradually worsen. People who have this disorder may not be able to feel vibrations and may lose the sense of where their limbs are. The limbs feel stiff, movements become clumsy, and walking may become difficult. Reflexes may be decreased, increased, or absent. Vision may be reduced. People who have this disorder may become irritable, apathetic, drowsy, suspicious, and confused. Their emotions may change rapidly and unpredictably. ***Rarely, dementia develops***. The diagnosis is made based on blood tests to measure levels of vitamin B_{12} and its metabolites. Recovery is more likely if the disorder is treated early. When treated within a few weeks after symptoms appear, most people recover completely. If treatment is delayed, the progression of symptoms may be slowed or stopped, but recovery of lost function is unlikely. Injections of vitamin B_{12} should be given immediately and must be continued indefinitely to prevent symptoms from recurring. Sometimes, large doses of vitamin B_{12} taken by mouth are equally effective.

Ref: *http://www.merck.com/mmhe/sec06/ch093/ch093j.html*

1695. Which one of the following is used in therapy of toxoplasmosis:

A. Artesunate **B.** Thiacetazone
C. Ciprofloxacin **D.** Pyrimethamine *(AI 2005)*

Immunologically competent adults and older children who have only lymphadenopathy do not require specific therapy unless they have persistent and severe symptoms. Patients with ocular **toxoplasmosis** should be treated for one month with **pyrimethamine** plus either sulfadiazine or clindamycin.

Ref: *Harrison's Principles of Internal Medicine; 14th edition*

1696. Which of the following drugs is useful in prophylaxis of migraine?

A. Propranolol **B.** Sumatriptan
C. Domperidone **D.** Ergotamine *(AI 2005)*

Drugs effective for the prophylaxis of migraine
• Amitriptyline • Propranolol • Nadolol • Atenolol • Timolol • Metoprolol • Papaverine • Cyproheptadine • Verapamil • Phenelzine • Valproic acid • Methysergide

1697. Antipsychotic drug-induced parkinsonism is treated by:

A. Anticholinergics **B.** Levodopa
C. Selegiline **D.** Amantadine *(AI 2005)*

Parkinsonism is a frequent complication of treatment with dopamine-depleting agents such as reserpine or antipsychotic dopamine antagonists such as the phenothiazines or butyrophenones. Discontinuing the antipsychotic drug when possible, substituting an antipsychotic with greater anticholinergic potency, or **adding an anticholinergic drug** such as trihexyphenidyl best manages drug-induced parkinsonism.

Ref: *Harrison's Principles of Internal Medicine; 14th edition*

1698. Which of the following infestation leads to malabsorption?

A. *Giardia lamblia* **B.** *Ascaris lumbricoides*
C. *Necator americanus* **D.** *Ancylostoma duodenale* *(AI 2005)*

Giardia lamblia is a cosmopolitan protozoal parasite that inhibits the small intestines of humans and other mammals. The development of lactose intolerance and **significant malabsorption** in some infected adults and children are clinical signs of the loss of brush border enzyme activities.

Ref: *Harrison's Principles of Internal Medicine; 14th edition*

1699. All of the following can cause osteoporosis, *except*:

A. Hyperparathyroidism **B.** Steroid use
C. Fluorosis **D.** Thyrotoxicosis *(AI 2005)*

Cause of osteoporosis
• Hypogonadism • Rheumatoid arthritis • Hyperadrenocorticism • Malnutrition • *Chronic glucocorticoid administration* • Alcoholism • *Hyperparathyroidism* • Epilepsy • *Thyrotoxicosis* • Primary biliary cirrhosis • Malabsorption • Chronic obstructive pulmonary disease • Scurvy • Menkes' syndrome • Calcium deficiency

- Osteogenesis imperfecta
- Immobilization
- Homocystinuria due to cystathionine synthase deficiency
- Chronic heparin administration
- Ehlers-Danlos syndrome
- Systemic mastocytosis
- Marfan's syndrome
- Adult hypophosphatasia
- Other metabolic bone diseases

1700. Hypercalcemia associated with malignancy is *most often* mediated by:

A. Parathyroid hormone (PTH)
B. Parathyroid hormone related protein (PTHrP)
C. Interleukin-6 (IL-6)
D. Calcitonin
(AI 2005)

Hypercalcemia of malignancy, the *most common* paraneoplastic endocrine syndrome, is responsible for approximately 40 percent of all hypercalcemia. **Parathyroid hormone related peptide (PTHrP) causes nearly all cases of humoral hypercalcemia of malignancy**.

Ref: *Harrison's Principles of Internal Medicine; 14th edition*

1701. All of the following are the causes of 'relative' polycythemia, *except*:

A. Dehydration
B. Dengue hemorrhagic fever
C. Gaisbock syndrome
D. High altitude
(AI 2005)

The term polycythemia means an increase above normal in the number of RBCs in the circulating blood. It is important to distinguish between *absolute polycythemia* (an increase in the total red cell mass) and *relative, polycythemia,* which occurs when, through loss of blood plasma, the concentration of the red cells in the circulating blood, becomes greater than normal.

In **Gaisbock syndrome** or *stress erythrocytosis* the total red blood cell mass is normal, and the plasma volume is below normal. Thus they have a moderately elevated hematocrit, usually 50 to 60 percent, and **relative polycythemia**.

Ref: *Harrison's Principles of Internal Medicine; 14th edition*

1702. 5'-nucleotidase activity is increased by:

A. Bone diseases
B. Prostate cancer
C. Chronic renal failure
D. Cholestatic disorders
(AI 2005)

The enzyme 5′-nucleotidase catalyzes the hydrolysis of phosphate from the 5′ position of the pentose component of the nucleotide. **Elevated levels of 5′-nucleotidase are generally associated with hepatobiliary disease.** The principal value of the 5′-nucleotidase measurement is to confirm the hepatic origin of an elevated alkaline phosphatase level in children or pregnant women or in those settings where coincident bone disease may be present.

Ref: *Harrison's Principles of Internal Medicine; 14th edition*

1703. Normal CSF glucose level in a normoglycemic adult is:

A. 20-40 mg/dl
B. 40-70 mg/dl
C. 70-90 mg/dl
D. 90-110 mg/dl
(AI 2005)

Normal CSF values in adults	
• Protein	20-50 mg per dl
• Sugar	40-70 mg per dl
• Total leukocyte count	Less than 5 per ml
• Differential leukocyte count	$L_{60-70}\,M_{30-50}\,P_0$

Ref: *Harrison's Principles of Internal Medicine; 14th edition*

1704. All of the following may cause ST segment elevation on ECG, *except*:

A. Early repolarization variant
B. Constrictive pericarditis
C. Ventricular aneurysm
D. Prinzmetal's angina *(AI 2005)*

In chronic **constrictive pericarditis** the electrocardiogram frequently displays low voltage of the QRS complex and **diffuse flattening or inversion of the T waves**. P mitrale may be present in patients with sinus rhythm; atrial fibrillation is present in about one-third of patients.

Ref: *Harrison's Principles of Internal Medicine; 14th edition*

1705. The *most sensitive* test for the diagnosis of myasthenia gravis is:

A. Elevated serum Ach-receptor binding antibodies
B. Repetitive nerve stimulation test
C. Positive edrophonium test
D. Measurement of jitter by single fiber electromyography *(AI 2005)*

Single Fiber EMG (SFEMG) is the *most sensitive* clinical test of neuromuscular transmission and shows increased jitter in some muscles in almost all patients with myasthenia gravis. Jitter is greatest in weak muscles but may be abnormal even in muscles with normal strength. Patients with mild or purely ocular muscle weakness may have increased jitter only in facial muscles. Increased jitter is a nonspecific sign of abnormal neuromuscular transmission and can be seen in other motor unit diseases. Normal jitter in a weak muscle excludes abnormal neuromuscular transmission as the cause of weakness.

Comparison of Diagnostic Techniques: *Intravenous edrophonium chloride* is often diagnostic in patients with ptosis or ophthalmoparesis, but is less useful when other muscles are weak. Elevated serum concentrations of *AChR binding antibodies* virtually assures the diagnosis of myasthenia gravis, but normal concentrations do not exclude the diagnosis. Repetitive nerve stimulation confirms impaired neuromuscular transmission but is not specific to myasthenia gravis and is frequently normal in patients with mild or purely ocular disease. **The measurement of jitter by SFEMG is the most sensitive clinical test of neuromuscular transmission and is abnormal in almost all patients with myasthenia gravis.** A normal test in a weak muscle excludes the diagnosis of myasthenia gravis, but an abnormal test can occur when other motor unit disorders cause defects in neuromuscular transmission.

Ref: *http://www.myasthenia.org/information/summary.html*

1706. *Not* a neurologic channelopathy:

A. Hypokalemic periodic paralysis
B. Episodic ataxias
C. Familial hemiplegic migraine
D. Huntington's disease *(AIIMS May 2004)*

1707. All of the following are neurological channelopathies, *except*:

A. Hypokalemic periodic paralysis
B. Episodic ataxia type 1
C. Familial hemiplegic migraine
D. Spinocerebellar ataxia 1 *(AI 2005)*

Ion channels are membrane-bound proteins that perform key functions in virtually all human cells. Such channels are critically important for the normal function of the excitable tissues of the nervous system, such as muscle and brain. Until relatively recently it was believed that dysfunction of ion channels in the nervous system would be incompatible with life. However, an increasing number of diseases associated with dysfunctional ion channels are now recognized. Such **neurological channelopathies** are frequently genetically determined but may also arise through autoimmune mechanisms.

Ref: *http://www.pmj.bmjjournals.com/cgi/content/full/81/951/20*

Classification of inherited neurological channelopathies according to type of channel affected		
	Muscle	**Central nervous system**
Voltage gated channels	*Hypokalemic periodic paralysis* Hyperkalemia periodic paralysis Andersen's syndrome Myotonia congenita Paramyotonia congenita Malignant hyperthermia	*Episodic ataxia type 1* Episodic ataxia type 2 *Familial hemiplegic migraine* Several inherited epilepsy syndromes
Ligand gated channels	Congenital myasthenia gravis	Hyperexplexia Autosomal dominant nocturnal frontal lobe epilepsy

Classification of neurological channelopathies according to channel				
Channel	**Muscle**	**Gene**	**CNS**	**Gene**
Sodium channel	Hypokalemic periodic paralysis	SCN4A	Generalized epilepsy with febrile seizures plus syndrome (GEFS+), severe myoclonic epilepsy of infancy	SCN1A SCN1B SCN2A
	Hyperkalemic periodic paralysis	SCN4A		
	Paramyotonia congenita	SCN4A		
	Potassium aggravated myotonia	SCN4A		
Chloride channel	Myotonia congenita: Thomsen's, Becker's	CLCN1		
Calcium channel	Hypokalemic periodic paralysis	CACNA1S	Episodic ataxia type 2	CACNA1A
	Malignant hyperthermia	CACNA1S CACNL2A	Familial hemiplegic migraine	
Potassium channel	Andersen's syndrome	KCNJ2	Episodic ataxia type 1	KCNA1
	Hypokalemic periodic paralysis	KCNE3	Benign familial neonatal convulsions	KCNQ2 KCNQ3
	Hyperkalemic periodic paralysis	KCNE3		
Ryanodine receptor	Malignant hyperthermia	RYR1	Ryanodine receptor	
Glycine receptor		Hyperexplexia	GLRA1	
Acetylcholine receptor			Autosomal dominant frontal lobe epilepsy	CHRNB2 CHRNA4

1708. All of the following are calcium channelopathies, *except:*

A. Episodic ataxia type 1
B. Spinocerebellar ataxia type 6
C. Familial hemiplegic migraine
D. Hypokalemic periodic paralysis

(AIIMS May 2005)

Channel	**Muscle**	**Gene**	**CNS**	**Gene**
Calcium channel	Hypokalemic periodic paralysis	CACNA1S	Episodic ataxia type 2	CACNA1A
	Malignant hyperthermia	CACNA1S CACNL2A	Familial hemiplegic migraine	

1709. At what value of one-hour glucose challenge test will you recommend a standard glucose tolerance test?

A. 120 mg/dl **B.** 140 mg/dl
C. 150 mg/dl **D.** 160 mg/dl *(AIIMS May 2005)*

National Diabetes Data Group of the National Institutes of Health (revised the criteria for the diagnosis of diabetes 1979):

1. Fasting (overnight): Venous plasma glucose concentration ≥7.8 mmol/L (140 mg/dl) on at least 2 separate occasions.
2. Following ingestion of 75 gram of glucose: Venous plasma glucose concentration ≥11.1 mmol/l (200 mg/dl) at 2 hour and on at least 1 other occasion during the 2-hour test; i.e. 2 values ≥11.1 mmol/L (200 mg/dl) must be obtained for diagnosis.

Ref: *Harrison's Principles of Internal Medicine; 14th edition*

1710. A 50-year-old man, an alcoholic and a smoker presents with a 3-hour history of severe retrosternal chest pain and increasing shortness of breath. He started having this pain while eating, which was constant and radiated to the back and interscapular region. He was a known hypertensive. On examination, he was cold and clammy with a heart rate of 130/min, and a BP of 80/40 mm Hg. JVP was normal. All peripheral pulses were present and equal. Breath sounds were decreased at the left lung base and chest X-ray showed left pleural effusion. Which one of the following is the *most likely* diagnosis?

A. Acute aortic dissection **B.** Acute myocardial infarction
C. Rupture of the esophagus **D.** Acute pulmonary embolism *(AI 2005)*

Acute aortic dissection presents with the sudden onset of pain, which is often described as very severe and tearing and is associated with diaphoresis. The pain may be localized to the front or back of the chest, often the interscapular region, and typically migrates with propagation of the dissection. In dissections involving the ascending aorta, the chest X-ray often reveals a widened superior mediastinum. A pleural effusion (usually left-sided) also may be present.

Ref: *Harrison's Principles of Internal Medicine; 14th edition*

1711. A 30-years-old male patient presents with complaints of weakness in right upper and both lower limbs for last 4 months. He developed digital infarcts involving 2nd and 3rd fingers in right side and 5th finger in left side. On examinations, BP was 160/140 mm Hg, all peripheral pulses were palpable and there was asymmetrical neuropathy. Investigations showed Hb-12 gm, TLC-12000 Cu mm, Platelets-4,30,000, ESR-49 mm. Urine examination showed proteinuria and RBC 10-15 per HPF with no casts. Which of the following is the *most likely* diagnosis?

A. Polyarteritis nodosa **B.** Systemic lupus erythematosus
C. Wegener's granulomatosis **D.** Mixed cryoglobulinemia *(AI 2005)*

Classic polyarteritis nodosa (PAN) is a multi-system, necrotizing vasculitis of small and medium-sized muscular arteries in which involvement of the renal and visceral arteries is characteristic. Nonspecific signs and symptoms are the hallmarks of classic PAN. Fever, weight loss, and malaise are present in over one-half of cases. Patients usually present with vague symptoms such as weakness, malaise, headache, abdominal pain, and myalgias.

Organ System	*% Incidence*	*Clinical Manifestations*
Renal	60	Renal failure, hypertension
Musculoskeletal	64	Arthritis, arthralgia, myalgia
Peripheral nervous system	51	Peripheral neuropathy, mononeuritis multiplex
Gastrointestinal tract	44	Abdominal pain, nausea and vomiting, bleeding, bowel infarction and perforation, cholecystitis, hepatic infarction, pancreatic infarction
Skin	43	Rash, purpura, nodules, cutaneous infarcts, livedo reticularis, Raynaud's phenomenon

Cardiac	36	Congestive heart failure, myocardial infarction, pericarditis
Genitourinary	25	Testicular, ovarian, or epididymal pain
Central nervous system	23	Cerebral vascular accident, altered mental status, seizure

Renal involvement *most commonly* manifests as ischemic changes in the glomeruli, whereas in microscopic polyangiitis glomerulonephritis is the predominant renal lesion. Hypertension may be related to both the renal polyarteritis and the glomerulitis and may dominate the clinical picture. An elevated erythrocyte sedimentation rate (ESR) is almost always present.

Ref: *Harrison's Principles of Internal Medicine; 14th edition*

1712. All of the following conditions are known to cause diabetes insipidus, *except*:

A. Multiple sclerosis **B.** Head injury
C. Histiocytosis **D.** Viral encephalitis *(AI 2005)*

Any lesion, which damages the neurohypophyseal unit, may result in **diabetes insipidus** (DI). Tumors of this region particularly craniopharyngiomas and optic gliomas are common cause of DI. 25 to 50% patients of **histiocytosis** have diabetes insipidus due to histocytic infiltration of hypothalamus and pituitary. **Encephalitis**, sarcoidosis, tuberculosis, actinomycosis and leukemia are occasional cause. **Head injury**, especially basal skull fractures may produce DI immediately or after a delay of several months. Operative procedures near the pituitary or hypothalamus may result in transient or permanent DI. In a minority of instances it is hereditary. Diabetes insipidus also occurs as a part of a rare syndrome in which it is associated with diabetes mellitus, optic atrophy, and sensorineural deafness (Wolfram's syndrome). Diabetes insipidus is increasingly recognized in newborns. It has been reported following birth asphyxia, intraventricular hemorrhage (IVH), intravascular coagulopathy, *Listeria monocytogenes* sepsis, and group B beta hemolytic streptococcal meningitis.

Ref: *Nelson's Textbook of Pediatrics; 12th edition; page 1438*

1713. Increased susceptibility to breast cancer is likely to be associated with a mutation in the following gene:

A. p53 **B.** BRCA-1
C. Retinoblastoma (Rb) **D.** H-Ras *(AIIMS Nov 2004)*

Another putative tumor suppressor gene, **BRCA-1**, has been identified at the chromosomal locus 17q21. **Women who inherit a mutated allele of this gene from either parent have an about 85 to 90 % lifetime chance of developing breast cancer**, as well as about a 33 % chance of developing ovarian cancer.

Ref: *Harrison's Principles of Internal Medicine; 14th edition*

1714. The *most common* pathogens responsible for nosocomial pneumonias in the ICU are:

A. Gram-positive organisms **B.** Gram-negative organisms
C. Mycoplasma **D.** Virus infections *(AI 2005)*

Legionellae are responsible for 10 to 50 % of nosocomial pneumonias when a hospital's water system is colonized with the organisms. Legionnaires' disease was first recognized in 1976, when an outbreak of pneumonia took place at a hotel in Philadelphia. Investigators from the CDC identified the causative aerobic **gram-negative bacterium** in lung specimens obtained from the victims at autopsy and named this organism *Legionella pneumophila*.

Ref: *Harrison's Principles of Internal Medicine; 14th edition*

1715. Ropinirole is *most useful* for treatment of:

A. Parkinson's disease **B.** Wilson's disease
C. Hoffman's syndrome **D.** Carpal tunnel syndrome *(AIIMS Nov 2004)*

Ropinirole is used to treat the **symptoms of Parkinson's disease**, including tremors, stiffness, and slowness of movement.

Ref: *http://www.ropinirole.com/*

1716. In which of the following arthritis erosions are *not* seen?

A. Rheumatoid arthritis
B. Systemic lupus erythematosus (SLE)
C. Psoriasis
D. Gout

(AIIMS May 2005)

Almost all patients of **SLE** experience arthralgias and myalgias; most develop intermittent arthritis. **Erosions are rare**; subcutaneous nodules occur.

Ref: *Harrison's Principles of Internal Medicine; 14th edition*

1717. Flapping tremors are seen in the following conditions, *except*:

A. Uremic encephalopathy
B. Parkinsonism
C. Hepatic encephalopathy
D. Carbon dioxide narcosis

(AIIMS May 2005)

Asterixis (flapping tremor), which may superficially resemble a tremor, is an intermittent inhibition of muscle contraction that occurs with **metabolic encephalopathy**.

Ref: *Harrison's Principles of Internal Medicine; 14th edition*

1718. All of the following are *true* regarding tetralogy of Fallot, *except*:

A. Ejection systolic murmur in second intercostals space
B. Single second heart sound
C. Predominantly left to right shunt
D. Normal jugular venous pressure

(AIIMS May 2005)

In **T of F** when the obstruction is severe, the pulmonary blood flow is reduced markedly, and a large volume of desaturated systemic venous blood is shunted from **right to left** across the ventricular septal defect.

Ref: *Harrison's Principles of Internal Medicine; 14th edition*

1719. Which one of the following is *not* a feature of irritable bowel syndrome:

A. Abdominal pain
B. Constipation
C. Rectal bleeding
D. Bloating

(AIIMS May 2005)

Symptoms not compatible with IBS

- Visible or occult blood in stool
- Weight loss
- Fever

Ref: *Harrison's Principles of Internal Medicine; 14th edition*

1720. In which of the following conditions of malabsorption, an intestinal biopsy is diagnostic?

A. Celiac disease
B. Tropical sprue
C. Whipple's disease
D. Lactose intolerance

(AIIMS May 2005)

Whipple's disease is a rare disorder characterized clinically by arthralgia, abdominal pain, and diarrhea, progressive weight loss, dilated lacteals in the bowel wall, and impaired intestinal absorption. The diagnosis is established by demonstrating the presence in the mucosa of macrophages containing large cytoplasmic granules that stain brilliant magenta with the periodic acid—Schiff (PAS) reagent.

Ref: *Harrison's Principles of Internal Medicine; 14th edition*

1721. Hemolytic anemia may be characterized by all of the following, *except*:

A. Hyperbilirubinemia
B. Reticulocytosis
C. Hemoglobinuria
D. Increased plasma haptoglobin level

(AIIMS May 2005)

Patients with significant hemolysis, either intravascular or extravascular, have low or absent levels of serum haptoglobin.

Ref: *Harrison's Principles of Internal Medicine; 14th edition*

1722. Recurrent facial/oropharyngeal/laryngeal edema in a patient having low C_4, normal C_3 and normal factor B. The pathogenesis is *most likely* due to:

A. Immune complex disease
B. C 1 esterase inhibitor deficiency
C. Hereditary deficiency of Qi
D. Classical pathway activation by IgM

(AIIMS May 2005)

Reduced levels of **C1 esterase inhibitor (alpha$_2$-neuraminoglycoprotein)** are associated with **hereditary angioneurotic edema** (giant urticaria). The protein is an inhibitor of esterase activity of the complement component C1.

Ref: *Nelson's Textbook of Pediatrics; 12th edition; page 472*

1723. There is mutation of gene coding for the ryanodine receptors in malignant hyperthermia. Which of the following statements *best* explains the increased heat production in malignant hyperthermia?

A. Increased muscle metabolism by excess of calcium ions
B. Thermic effect of food
C. Increased sympathetic discharge
D. Mitochondrial thermogenesis

(AIIMS May 2005)

Malignant hyperthermia is an inherited disorder of skeletal-muscle sarcoplasmic reticulum that causes a rapid increase in intracellular calcium levels in response to halothane and other inhalational anesthetics or to succinylcholine.

Ref: *Harrison's Principles of Internal Medicine; 14th edition*

1724. All of the following conditions are observed in gout, *except:*

A. Uric acid nephrolithiasis
B. Deficiency of enzyme xanthine oxidase
C. Increase in serum urate concentration
D. Renal disease involving interstitial tissues

(AIIMS May 2005)

Allopurinol, a substrate and competitive inhibitor of *xanthine oxidase*, is the most widely used antihyperuricemic agent and is used in treatment of gout.

Ref: *Harrison's Principles of Internal Medicine; 14th edition*

1725. Which of the following statement is *false* regarding Wilson's disease?

A. It is an autosomal recessive disorder
B. Serum ceruloplasmin level is less than 20 mg/dl
C. Urinary copper excretion is less than 100 microgram per day
D. Zinc acetate is effective as maintenance therapy

(AIIMS May 2004)

The **diagnosis of Wilson's disease** is confirmed by the demonstration of either:

- A serum ceruloplasmin level less than 200 mg/L *and* Kayser-Fleischer rings or
- A serum ceruloplasmin level less than 200 mg/L *and* a concentration of copper in liver biopsy greater than 250 microgram/g dry weight.
- Most symptomatic *patients excrete more than 100 microgram copper per day in urine* and have histologic abnormalities on liver biopsy.

Ref: *Harrison's Principles of Internal Medicine; 14th edition*

1726. *False* regarding Creutzfeldt-Jakob disease:

A. It is a neurodegenerative disease
B. It is caused by infectious proteins
C. Myoclonus is rarely seen
D. Brain biopsy is specific for diagnosis

(AIIMS May 2004)

Creutzfeldt-Jakob disease *typically* presents as a rapidly progressive dementia with prominent associated myoclonus.

Ref: *Harrison's Principles of Internal Medicine; 14th edition*

1727. Which of the following is *not* a feature of juvenile myoclonic epilepsy?

A. Myoclonus on awakening
B. Generalized tonic-clonic seizures
C. Automatism
D. Absence seizure

(AIIMS May 2004)

Juvenile myoclonic epilepsy is a **generalized seizure disorder** of unknown cause that starts in early adolescence and is usually characterized by bilateral myoclonic jerks that may be single or repetitive. The **myoclonic seizures are *most frequent* in the morning after awakening** and can be produced by sleep deprivation. Consciousness is maintained unless the myoclonus is especially severe. Many patients also experience generalized tonic-clonic seizures, and up to 33% have absence seizures.

Ref: *Harrison's Principles of Internal Medicine; 14th edition*

1728. A 20-year-old female presents with history of dyspnea on exertion. On examination she has wide fixed split of S_2 with ejection systolic murmur (III/VI) in left second intercostals space. Her EKG shows left axis deviation. The *most probable* diagnosis is:

A. Total anomalous pulmonary venous connection
B. Tricuspid atresia
C. Ostium primum atrial septal defect
D. Tetralogy of Fallot

(AIIMS May 2004)

Atrial septal defect is a common cardiac anomaly in adults that occurs more frequently in females. The *second heart sound is widely split and is relatively fixed* in relation to respiration. A middiastolic rumbling murmur, loudest at the fourth intercostal space and along the left sternal border. In patients with an **ostium primum defect**, the right ventricular conduction defect is characteristically accompanied by *left axis deviation* and by superior orientation and counterclockwise rotation of the QRS loop in the frontal plane.

Ref: *Harrison's Principles of Internal Medicine; 14th edition*

1729. The *only* thrombolytic agent approved for the treatment of acute ischemic stroke is:

A. Tissue plasminogen activator
B. Streptokinase
C. Urokinase
D. Pro-urokinase

(AIIMS May 2004)

It seems clear that thrombolysis works in ischemic cerebrovascular disease. Thrombolysis should only be administered using the strict protocol of the National Institute of Neurological Disorders and stroke recombinant tissue plasminogen activator study, with adequate protection of patients by full disclosure of the possible risks.

Ref: *Harrison's Principles of Internal Medicine; 14th edition*

1730. The *most common* cause of sporadic viral encephalitis is:

A. Japanese B encephalitis
B. Herpes simplex encephalitis
C. HIV encephalitis
D. Rubeola encephalitis

(AIIMS May 2004)

Herpes simplex virus is the most commonly identified cause of acute, sporadic viral encephalitis in the USA.

Ref: *Harrison's Principles of Internal Medicine; 14th edition*

1731. A 27-year-old man is noted to have blood pressure of 170/100 mm Hg. He has prominent aortic ejection click and murmurs heard over the ribs on both sides anteriorly and over the back posteriorly. In addition, the pulses in the lower extremities are feeble and he complains of mild claudication with exertion. The *most likely* diagnosis is:

A. ASD
B. Aortic stenosis
C. Coarctation of aorta
D. Cardiomyopathy

(AIIMS Nov 2004)

Narrowing or constriction of the lumen of the aorta may occur anywhere along its length but is *most common* after the origin of the left subclavian artery near the insertion of the *ligamentum arteriosum*. Coarctation occurs in about 7% of patients with CHD, male female ratio is 2:1, and is *most frequent* in patients with gonadal dysgenesis.

Reference and further reading: *Harrison's Principles of Internal Medicine; 15th edition*

1732. A 62-year-old diabetic female patient presented with history of progressive right sided weakness of one-month duration. The patient was also having speech difficulty. Fundus examination showed papilledema. Two months ago, she also had a fall in her bathroom and struck her head against a wall. The most likely clinical diagnosis is:

A. Alzheimer's disease
B. Left parietal glioma
C. Left MCA territory stroke
D. Left chronic subdural hematoma *(AIIMS Nov 2004)*

Chronic subdural hematomas are *most common* in infants and adults over 60-years of age. They present with progressive neurological deficits more than 2 weeks after the trauma. These collections can be removed by drilling burr holes and washing them out with warm saline.

Ref: *Bailey & Love's Short Practice of Surgery; 23rd edition; page 551*

1733. All of the following can cause hypercalcemia, *except*:

A. Prolonged immobilization
B. Tumor lysis syndrome
C. Sarcoidosis
D. Multiple melanoma *(AIIMS Nov 2004)*

Tumor lysis syndrome is characterized by various combinations of hyperuricemia, hyperkalemia, hyperphosphatemia, lactic acidosis, and hypocalcemia and is caused by the mass destruction of a large number of rapidly proliferating neoplastic cells.

Ref: *Harrison's Principles of Internal Medicine; 14th edition*

1734. Humoral immunodeficiency is suspected in a patient and he is under investigation. Which of the following infections would *not* be consistent with the diagnosis?

A. Giardiasis
B. *Pneumocystis carinii* pneumonia
C. Recurrent sinusitis
D. Recurrent subcutaneous abscesses *(AIIMS Nov 2004)*

Abnormalities of cell-mediated immunity predispose to disseminated virus infections, such as herpes simplex, varicella zoster and cytomegalovirus. In addition, patients so affected almost invariably develop mucocutaneous candidiasis and frequently acquire systemic fungal infections. **Pneumonia caused by *Pneumocystis carinii* is also common**.

Ref: *Harrison's Principles of Internal Medicine; 14th edition*

1735. In a patient with *Listeria* meningitis who is allergic to penicillin, the *antimicrobial of choice* is:

A. Vancomycin
B. Gentamicin
C. Trimethoprim-sulfamethoxazole
D. Ceftriaxone *(AIIMS Nov 2004)*

Penicillin-allergic patients of *Listeria monocytogenes* may be treated with trimethoprim-sulfamethoxazole.

Ref: *Harrison's Principles of Internal Medicine; 14th edition*

1736. Migratory thrombophlebitis is associated with the following malignancies, *except*:

A. Lung cancer
B. Prostate cancer
C. Pancreas cancer
D. Gastrointestinal cancer *(AIIMS Nov 2004)*

Unusual clinical features associated with **gastric adenocarcinomas** include migratory thrombophlebitis, microangiopathic hemolytic anemia, and acanthosis nigricans.

Other initial manifestations of **carcinoma pancreas** include venous thrombosis and migratory thrombophlebitis, gastrointestinal hemorrhage resulting from varices due to compression of the portal venous system by tumor, and splenomegaly caused by cancerous encasement of the splenic vein.

Ref: *Harrison's Principles of Internal Medicine; 14th edition*

Many endocrine syndromes are associated with small cell **lung cancer** (SCLC) because of the secretion of neuroendocrine hormones. These include Cushing syndrome (which involves adrenocorticotropic hormone [ACTH]), syndrome of inappropriate antidiuretic hormone (ADH) secretion, hyperparathyroidism, carcinoid syndrome, gynecomastia (which involves gonadotropins), hyperpigmentation (which involves melanocyte-stimulating hormone), hypoglycemia (which involves an insulin-like substance), and hypocalcemia (which involves calcitonin). Other features include the following: anemia, thrombocytopenia, **migratory thrombophlebitis**, leukocytosis, thrombocytosis and glomerulonephritis.

Ref: *http://www.emedicine.com/radio/topic405.html*

1737. Which of the following is the *most common* extra-renal involvement in autosomal dominant polycystic kidney disease?

A. Mitral valve prolapse
B. Hepatic cysts
C. Splenic cyst
D. Colonic diverticulosis

(AIIMS Nov 2004)

Extrarenal manifestations of autosomal dominant **polycystic kidney** disease are frequent and underscore the systemic nature of the defect. **Hepatic cysts occur in 50 to 70% of patients.**

Ref: *Harrison's Principles of Internal Medicine; 14th edition*

1738. Which of the following is generally *not* seen in ITP?

A. More common in females
B. Petechiae, ecchymosis and bleeding
C. Palpable splenomegaly
D. Increased megakaryocytes in bone marrow

(AIIMS Nov 2004)

Acute idiopathic thrombocytopenic purpura is the *most common* of all thrombocytopenic purpura of childhood and is associated with petechiae, mucocutaneous bleeding and occasionally hemorrhages into tissues. There is profound deficiency of circulating platelets. **The liver, spleen and lymph nodes are not enlarged.**

Ref: *Nelson's Textbook of Pediatrics; 12th edition; page 1249*

1739. Which of the following arbovirus diseases has *not* been reported in India?

A. Japanese encephalitis
B. Yellow fever
C. Chikungunya fever
D. KFD

(AIIMS Nov 2004)

Yellow fever is a zoonotic disease caused by an arbovirus. **There is no evidence that yellow fever has ever been present in Asia.**

Ref: *Park's Textbook of Preventive and Social Medicine; 17th edition; page 216*

ANSWERS

1 D 2 B 3 B 4 A 5 C 6 B 7 D 8 D 9 C 10 A
11 B 12 C 13 D 14 B 15 B 16 C 17 B 18 A 19 C 20 B
21 B 22 A 23 C 24 D 25 C 26 C 27 C 28 D 29 D 30 A
31 C 32 D 33 B 34 B 35 A 36 A 37 A 38 A 39 D 40 D
41 A 42 D 43 C 44 D 45 B 46 A 47 B 48 C 49 C 50 A
51 C 52 D 53 D 54 D 55 C 56 D 57 C 58 C 59 C 60 D
61 D 62 A 63 D 64 D 65 B 66 B 67 D 68 B 69 C 70 A
71 A 72 B 73 A 74 A 75 C 76 C 77 B 78 D 79 B 80 B
81 B 82 B 83 A 84 C 85 B 86 B 87 D 88 A 89 B 90 B
91 D 92 B 93 D 94 C 95 C 96 D 97 D 98 B 99 C 100 C
101 D 102 C 103 B 104 B 105 D 106 D 107 B 108 D 109 A 110 B
111 C 112 B 113 C 114 A 115 A 116 A 117 A 118 C 119 A 120 D
121 D 122 B 123 D 124 C 125 D 126 A 127 C 128 C 129 C 130 C
131 C 132 C 133 D 134 C 135 C 136 C 137 D 138 B 139 A 140 A
141 B 142 B 143 D 144 C 145 C 146 C 147 D 148 C 149 D 150 B
151 C 152 B 153 B 154 C 155 A 156 C 157 A 158 C 159 C 160 B
161 C 162 A 163 B 164 C 165 C 166 D 167 A 168 A 169 C 170 A
171 D 172 C 173 C 174 C 175 D 176 B 177 D 178 B 179 C 180 C
181 D 182 A 183 D 184 C 185 C 186 C 187 D 188 A 189 D 190 D
191 D 192 B 193 A 194 A 195 C 196 A 197 D 198 C 199 C 200 B
201 C 202 A 203 B 204 C 205 D 206 A 207 D 208 D 209 C 210 B
211 A 212 C 213 D 214 D 215 A 216 C 217 A 218 C 219 A 220 C
221 B 222 B 223 A 224 D 225 B 226 A 227 A 228 A 229 D 230 A
231 D 232 D 233 C 234 D 235 C 236 B 237 B 238 A 239 B 240 A
241 D 242 A 243 C 244 B 245 B 246 C 247 C 248 C 249 D 250 A
251 A 252 C 253 C 254 C 255 D 256 D 257 D 258 B 259 D 260 B
261 D 262 A 263 B 264 C 265 B 266 D 267 B 268 A 269 B 270 B
271 A 272 A 273 C 274 A 275 B 276 D 277 D 278 C 279 C 280 B
281 A 282 C 283 D 284 A 285 B 286 A 287 A 288 C 289 A 290 A
291 C 292 C 293 A 294 B 295 D 296 B 297 D 298 D 299 B 300 D
301 D 302 A 303 C 304 D 305 C 306 D 307 A 308 D 309 D 310 A
311 D 312 A 313 D 314 A 315 B 316 C 317 B 318 A 319 A 320 A
321 C 322 C 323 D 324 C 325 B 326 C 327 C 328 B 329 D 330 A
331 B 332 B 333 C 334 C 335 C 336 D 337 B 338 B 339 A 340 C
341 C 342 A 343 D 344 C 345 B 346 B 347 C 348 A 349 C 350 C
351 A 352 B 353 C 354 D 355 A 356 D 357 B 358 B 359 B 360 A
361 B 362 A 363 A 364 D 365 B 366 A 367 A 368 C 369 C 370 C
371 C 372 A 373 D 374 B 375 C 376 A 377 D 378 B 379 B 380 C
381 A 382 B 383 A 384 B 385 D 386 A 387 C 388 B 389 A 390 B
391 A 392 C 393 B 394 C 395 C 396 B 397 B 398 C 399 C 400 C
401 B 402 B 403 C 404 D 405 A 406 B 407 A 408 D 409 A 410 D
411 C 412 C 413 B 414 B 415 B 416 C 417 C 418 A 419 B 420 C
421 C 422 B 423 D 424 A 425 A 426 C 427 B 428 A 429 A 430 B
431 B 432 D 433 C 434 C 435 C 436 C 437 D 438 A 439 B 440 A
441 C 442 A 443 B 444 C 445 C 446 D 447 B 448 C 449 B 450 C
451 D 452 B 453 A 454 C 455 C 456 C 457 A 458 A 459 C 460 D

461 C	462 C	463 B	464 B	465 C	466 B	467 D	468 A	469 C	470 D
471 C	472 B	473 D	474 A	475 B	476 C	477 A	478 D	479 D	480 B
481 B	482 D	483 D	484 C	485 C	486 A	487 D	488 C	489 A	490 C
491 B	492 B	493 B	494 C	495 D	496 B	497 B	498 A	499 D	500 A
501 A	502 B	503 D	504 A	505 B	506 B	507 C	508 C	509 C	510 B
511 B	512 A	513 D	514 C	515 D	516 C	517 C	518 C	519 A	520 C
521 A	522 A	523 B	524 B	525 D	526 B	527 C	528 B	529 C	530 C
531 C	532 C	533 B	534 A	535 A	536 A	537 B	538 A	539 D	540 B
541 A	542 A	543 D	544 C	545 A	546 D	547 C	548 C	549 B	550 A
551 A	552 C	553 B	554 B	555 A	556 A	557 D	558 C	559 D	560 B
561 B	562 D	563 D	564 B	565 A	566 C	567 A	568 D	569 A	570 B
571 A	572 A	573 A	574 A	575 B	576 D	577 D	578 A	579 D	580 A
581 C	582 A	583 A	584 D	585 A	586 C	587 C	588 C	589 C	590 A
591 B	592 C	593 C	594 B	595 D	596 D	597 B	598 C	599 D	600 A
601 D	602 D	603 B	604 D	605 C	606 A	607 C	608 D	609 C	610 A
611 C	612 D	613 D	614 D	615 A	616 B	617 A	618 B	619 A	620 A
621 B	622 C	623 D	624 A	625 B	626 A	627 B	628 C	629 A	630 C
631 B	632 C	633 A	634 A	635 C	636 D	637 A	638 B	639 D	640 C
641 D	642 D	643 A	644 B	645 B	646 C	647 A	648 B	649 A	650 C
651 C	652 C	653 B	654 D	655 C	656 A	657 C	658 D	659 D	660 A
661 C	662 C	663 A	664 A	665 A	666 B	667 A	668 C	669 D	670 D
671 A	672 D	673 B	674 A	675 A	676 C	677 A	678 D	679 C	680 C
681 D	682 C	683 D	684 D	685 D	686 D	687 B	688 C	689 C	690 B
691 D	692 C	693 A	694 A	695 C	696 D	697 B	698 B	699 A	700 D
701 A	702 B	703 D	704 A	705 C	706 A	707 A	708 D	709 D	710 C
711 C	712 A	713 C	714 D	715 C	716 D	717 B	718 A	719 C	720 B
721 B	722 B	723 C	724 A	725 B	726 C	727 C	728 A	729 D	730 C
731 B	732 B	733 B	734 C	735 B	736 C	737 B	738 A	739 B	740 C
741 B	742 B	743 D	744 D	745 B	746 C	747 B	748 B	749 C	750 A
751 D	752 B	753 A	754 C	755 B	756 C	757 D	758 B	759 C	760 A
761 C	762 D	763 C	764 B	765 B	766 B	767 B	768 D	769 D	770 D
771 B	772 A	773 A	774 C	775 D	776 A	777 D	778 B	779 B	780 D
781 A	782 A	783 A	784 D	785 B	786 C	787 C	788 B	789 D	790 D
791 C	792 C	793 A	794 A	795 C	796 D	797 D	798 D	799 B	800 C
801 A	802 A	803 D	804 C	805 A	806 A	807 A	808 D	809 A	810 A
811 C	812 B	813 B	814 C	815 A	816 A	817 D	818 A	819 D	820 D
821 B	822 D	823 C	824 C	825 D	826 C	827 C	828 A	829 A	830 D
831 A	832 A	833 B	834 C	835 A	836 B	837 A	838 C	839 D	840 B
841 C	842 B	843 A	844 B	845 D	846 C	847 C	848 B	849 D	850 C
851 A	852 D	853 B	854 D	855 B	856 A	857 A	858 B	859 A	860 C
861 B	862 A	863 B	864 A	865 B	866 A	867 C	868 A	869 C	870 D
871 D	872 B	873 D	874 B	875 C	876 C	877 B	878 A	879 C	880 A
881 B	882 D	883 C	884 A	885 A	886 C	887 B	888 C	889 B	890 C
891 B	892 C	893 B	894 B	895 A	896 B	897 D	898 D	899 A	900 A
901 C	902 C	903 A	904 C	905 A	906 D	907 D	908 C	909 A	910 C
911 D	912 C	913 A	914 C	915 B	916 B	917 C	918 A	919 A	920 D
921 A	922 C	923 A	924 B	925 D	926 B	927 D	928 B	929 D	930 A

931 D 932 B 933 C 934 B 935 C 936 B 937 D 938 A 939 A 940 C
941 B 942 C 943 D 944 B 945 C 946 B 947 B 948 D 949 C 950 C
951 C 952 D 953 A 954 A 955 B 956 B 957 B 958 A 959 A 960 A
961 D 962 D 963 C 964 D 965 B 966 D 967 D 968 A 969 B 970 B
971 C 972 A 973 C 974 B 975 C 976 A 977 B 978 B 979 D 980 D
981 B 982 B 983 A 984 C 985 C 986 A 987 B 988 A 989 A 990 B
991 B 992 C 993 A 994 B 995 C 996 C 997 D 998 A 999 D 1000 C
1001 C 1002 D 1003 B 1004 C 1005 A 1006 A 1007 B 1008 B 1009 A 1010 A
1011 B 1012 D 1013 C 1014 A 1015 D 1016 A 1017 D 1018 A 1019 A 1020 A
1021 C 1022 D 1023 A 1024 A 1025 B 1026 D 1027 B 1028 B 1029 B 1030 B
1031 D 1032 D 1033 B 1034 B 1035 A 1036 C 1037 C 1038 B 1039 D 1040 C
1041 C 1042 C 1043 A 1044 D 1045 A 1046 D 1047 C 1048 D 1049 D 1050 C
1051 A 1052 C 1053 B 1054 A 1055 D 1056 A 1057 D 1058 C 1059 C 1060 D
1061 D 1062 D 1063 C 1064 D 1065 C 1066 D 1067 B 1068 A 1069 B 1070 D
1071A 1072 D 1073 B 1074 D 1075 A 1076 C 1077 D 1078 D 1079 A 1080 B
1081 B 1082 C 1083 B 1084 D 1085 A 1086 A 1087 A 1088 D 1089 D 1090 C
1091 D 1092 C 1093 B 1094 A 1095 D 1096 A 1097 C 1098 D 1099 B 1100 A
1101 C 1102 A 1103 C 1104 A 1105 B 1106 D 1107 D 1108 A 1109 D 1110 A
1111 B 1112 A 1113 D 1114 A 1115 B 1116 D 1117 D 1118 C 1119 C 1120 B
1121 C 1122 B 1123 D 1124 A 1125 A 1126 C 1127 C 1128 D 1129 C 1130 C
1131 C 1132 D 1133 D 1134 B 1135 B 1136 C 1137 A 1138 D 1139 A 1140 D
1141 A 1142 B 1143 C 1144 A 1145 A 1146 B 1147 D 1148 C 1149 D 1150 C
1151 D 1152 B 1153 A 1154 C 1155 B 1156 D 1157 A 1158 A 1159 C 1160 D
1161 A 1162 A 1163 C 1164 A 1165 A 1166 D 1167 C 1168 A 1169 D 1170 B
1171 A 1172 C 1173 B 1174 A 1175 D 1176 A 1177 D 1178 D 1179 D 1180 C
1181 C 1182 D 1183 B 1184 C 1185 B 1186 B 1187 B 1188 A 1189 B 1190 D
1191 A 1192 A 1193 D 1194 C 1195 A 1196 D 1197 A 1198 C 1199 B 1200 D
1201 B 1202 A 1203 E 1204 B 1205 B 1206 D 1207 D 1208 C 1209 A 1210 D
1211 A 1212 C 1213 B 1214 C 1215 B 1216 C 1217 C 1218 B 1219 D 1220 A
1221 C 1222 C 1223 C 1224 D 1225 A 1226 A 1227 B 1228 A 1229 A 1230 C
1231 D 1232 D 1233 B 1234 D 1235 B 1236 A 1237 D 1238 A 1239 A 1240 A
1241 A 1242 C 1243 D 1244 D 1245 B 1246 C 1247 A 1248 C 1249 B 1250 C
1251 B 1252 D 1253 A 1254 D 1255 C 1256 D 1257 A 1258 C 1259 A 1260 B
1261 B 1262 C 1263 E 1264 E 1265 B 1266 C 1267 C 1268 B 1269 B 1270 A
1271 D 1272 B 1273 D 1274 D 1275 D 1276 C 1277 B 1278 B 1279 D 1280 A
1281 B 1282 C 1283 A 1284 A 1285 B 1286 C 1287 C 1288 D 1289 D 1290 D
1291 D 1292 D 1293 B 1294 D 1295 B 1296 C 1297 D 1298 A 1299 C 1300 A
1301 B 1302 A 1303 B 1304 A 1305 A 1306 B 1307 B 1308 D 1309 A 1310 B
1311 A 1312 D 1313 B 1314 C 1315 C 1316 A 1317 A 1318 B 1319 A 1320 D
1321 A 1322 D 1323 B 1324 B 1325 A 1326 D 1327 B 1328 D 1329 A 1330 B
1331 A 1332 B 1333 A 1334 C 1335 C 1336 A 1337 B 1338 D 1339 C 1340 D
1341 D 1342 A 1343 A 1344 D 1345 A 1346 D 1347 A 1348 C 1349 A 1350 C
1351 A 1352 D 1353 C 1354 D 1355 B 1356 D 1357 B 1358 A 1359 D 1360 A
1361 A 1362 B 1363 D 1364 B 1365 B 1366 D 1367 C 1368 C 1369 C 1370 A
1371 B 1372 D 1373 D 1374 D 1375 B 1376 D 1377 D 1378 C 1379 A 1380 C
1381 C 1382 A 1383 B 1384 D 1385 D 1386 A 1387 C 1388 D 1389 A 1390 B
1391 C 1392 D 1393 D 1394 D 1395 A 1396 D 1397 D 1398 A 1399 C 1400 D

1401 C 1402 B 1403 D 1404 D 1405 A 1406 B 1407 C 1408 B 1409 A 1410 D
1411 A 1412 C 1413 B 1414 C 1415 B 1416 A 1417 B 1418 C 1419 D 1420 D
1421 A 1422 D 1423 A 1424 A 1425 A 1426 C 1427 C 1428 D 1429 A 1430 A
1431 C 1432 C 1433 B 1434 D 1435 C 1436 B 1437 B 1438 A 1439 B 1440 A
1441 C 1442 D 1443 D 1444 C 1445 A 1446 A 1447 C 1448 A 1449 B 1450 A
1451 A 1452 D 1453 A 1454 B 1455 A 1456 B 1457 A 1458 B 1459 D 1460 C
1461 A 1462 B 1463 D 1464 B 1465 C 1466 C 1467 D 1468 A 1469 A 1470 D
1471 C 1472 A 1473 A 1474 B 1475 A 1476 A 1477 B 1478 B 1479 D 1480 D
1481 D 1482 A 1483 B 1484 C 1485 C 1486 B 1487 C 1488 B 4189 C 1490 D
1491 C 1492 B 1493 D 1494 C 1495 B 1496 C 1497 D 1498 C 1499 D 1500 B
1501 A 1502 C 1503 A 1504 B 1505 B 1506 B 1507 A 1508 C 1509 C 1510 B
1511 D 1512 D 1513 A 1514 C 1515 A 1516 B 1517 B 1518 D 1519 A 1520 C
1521 C 1522 C 1523 C 1524 A 1525 C 1526 A 1527 C 1528 B 1529 D 1530 A
1531 D 1532 A 1533 C 1534 A 1535 B 1536 B 1537 B 1538 C 1539 C 1540 C
1541 B 1542 C 1543 C 1544 C 1545 D 1546 A 1547 C 1548 B 1549 C 1550 A
1551 C 1552 A 1553 B 1554 D 1555 C 1556 C 1557 B 1558 A 1559 D 1560 D
1561 A 1562 D 1563 C 1564 D 1565 C 1566 A 1567 D 1568 A 1569 B 1570 B
1571 A 1572 A 1573 B 1574 C 1575 C 1576 B 1577 C 1578 D 1579 C 1580 B
1581 B 1582 B 1583 C 1584 D 1585 D 1586 C 1587 B 1588 C 1589 A 1590 D
1591 C 1592 B 1593 C 1594 D 1595 B 1596 C 1597 A 1598 C 1599 C 1600 C
1601 C 1602 C 1603 A 1604 A 1605 B 1606 B 1607 C 1608 A 1609 A 1610 B
1611 A 1612 B 1613 B 1614 D 1615 B 1616 A 1617 C 1618 D 1619 B 1620 C
1621 D 1622 A 1623 B 1624 B 1625 A 1626 D 1627 A 1628 D 1629 A 1630 B
1631 D 1632 B 1633 D 1634 B 1635 D 1636 C 1637 D 1638 C 1639 D 1640 C
1641 A 1642 D 1643 A 1644 C 1645 B 1646 B 1647 C 1648 C 1649 A 1650 C
1651 A 1652 D 1653 B 1654 C 1655 A 1656 C 1657 A 1658 B 1659 A 1660 B
1661 B 1662 C 1663 D 1664 D 1665 D 1666 B 1667 B 1668 B 1669 C 1670 A
1671 B 1672 A 1673 A 1674 B 1675 C 1676 B 1677 B 1678 B 1679 C 1680 D
1681 C 1682 B 1683 B 1684 C 1685 D 1686 C 1687 C 1688 A 1689 C 1690 B
1691 A 1692 C 1693 A 1694 D 1695 D 1696 A 1697 A 1698 A 1699 C 1700 B
1701 D 1702 D 1703 B 1704 B 1705 D 1706 D 1707 D 1708 B 1709 B 1710 A
1711 A 1712 A 1713 B 1714 B 1715 A 1716 B 1717 B 1718 C 1719 C 1720 C
1721 D 1722 B 1723 A 1724 B 1725 C 1726 C 1727 C 1728 C 1729 A 1730 B
1731 C 1732 D 1733 B 1734 B 1735 C 1736 B 1737 B 1738 C 1739 B

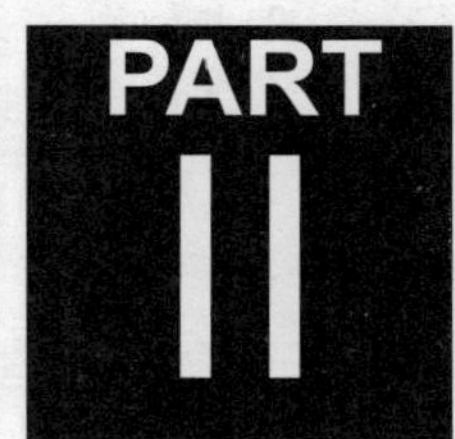

Pediatrics

Pediatrics

1. **A 2-year-old child whose weight is 6.7 kg was brought to the hospital with a history of diarrhea and vomiting for 2 days. On examination, the skin when pinched up took almost 3 seconds to return to normal. *Most likely* diagnosis is:**
   A. No dehydration
   B. Some dehydration
   C. Severe dehydration
   D. Only skin pinching is not reliable in making a diagnosis *(AI 2002)*

Acute Diarrheal Disease

- Diarrhea is defined as passage of three or more loose watery stools in 24 hours.
- A loose stool is one which takes the shape of container.
- Dysentery is defined as diarrhea with visible blood in stool.
- Persistent diarrhea is defined as continuation of an acute episode for 14 or more days.
- A child with diarrhea should be assessed for dehydration, blood in stool, malnutrition and any serious systemic infection.

Clinical Classification of Dehydration

	ADD with no dehydration	ADD with some dehydration	ADD with severe dehydration	
General Condition	Well and alert	Restless, irritable	Lethargic, unconscious, floppy	
Eyes	Normal	Sunken	Very sunken, dry	
Tears	Present	Absent	Absent	
Mouth and Tongue	Moist	Dry	Very dry	
Thirst	Not thirsty	Thirsty, drinks eagerly	Unable to drink	
Skin Pinch	Goes back quickly	Goes back slowly	Goes back very slowly	
Management	Continue feeding and give extra home available fluids	Give ORS 75 ml/kg in four hours	100 ml/kg of Ringer lactate should be given IV	
Ingredients	**Bicarbonate ORS**	**Citrate ORS**	Children >10 kg	Children <10 kg
Glucose	111 mmol/L	111 mmol/L		
Sodium ions	90 mmol/L	90 mmol/L	30 ml/kg is given in half hour	30 ml/kg is given in one hour
Chloride ions	80 mmol/L	80 mmol/L		
Bicarbonate ions	30 mmol/L	Nil	70 ml/kg is given in two and a half hours	70 ml/kg is given in five hours
Potassium ions	20 mmol/L	20 mmol/L		
Citrate	Nil	10 mmol/L		

***Two or more of the above mentioned signs should be present, along with a red sign, to assign a category.**

2. **In which of the following conditions, transient rash is seen:**
   A. Chickenpox
   B. Exanthem subitum
   C. Scarlet fever
   D. Eczema herpeticum *(UP 1997)*

3. A half-year-old infant develops high grade fever which subsided after three days following which there was appearance of a generalized rash which also subsided after 48 hours without any residual pigmentation. Most probable diagnosis is:

A. Rubella
B. Measles
C. Roseola infantum
D. Fifth disease

(AI 2002)

ROSEOLA INFANTUM is also known as **Exanthem subitum**. In 90% of cases it is caused by human herpes virus 6. Onset of illness is sudden with high grade fever and bulging anterior fontanelle. Seizures are seen in 5-35% of cases. Child looks relatively well despite high grade fever. Fever falls by 3-4th day and *as the temperature returns to normal a macular or maculopapular rash appears over the body.* This rash starts from the truck and then spread to arms and neck and sometimes involves face and neck also. **Rash fades within 3 days**. There is no residual pigmentation.

4. Which of the following is the *drug of choice* in status epilepticus in children:

A. Carbamazepine | **B.** Diazepam
C. Phenobarbitone | **D.** Phenytoin

(UP 1993)

Treatment Protocol of Status Epilepticus

1.	Give **IV diazepam** in a dose of 0.3 mg/kg (or 1 mg/year dose); may be repeated if seizure does not stop within 5 minutes.
2.	Give loading dose of Epsolin (phenytoin) (20 mg/kg) IV; not more than 1mg/kg/minute.
3.	If seizure is not controlled, gives inj. Gardinal (phenobarbitone) 20 mg/kg IV; not more than 1 mg/kg/minute.
4.	Start diazepam infusion in a dose of 0.01 mg/kg/minute and dose may be increased up to 0.03 mg/kg/minute. Maintain a seizure free period of 12 hours, then taper off.
5.	General anesthesia with thiopentone 4 mg/kg is the last option.

5. In India which of the following is *not* an important cause of *post-neonatal* mortality:

A. Tetanus
B. Diarrhea
C. Malnutrition
D. Respiratory infection

(AI 2002)

Causes of Infant Mortality in India

Neonatal mortality	Post-neonatal mortality
• Low birth weight	• Acute diarrheal disease
• Birth injury	• Acute respiratory infection
• Congenital abnormalities	• Other infectious diseases
• Hemolytic disease of newborn (HDN)	• Malnutrition
• Diarrheal disease	• Congenital abnormalities
• Acute respiratory infection	• Accidents
• Tetanus neonatorum	

6. Renal biopsy was done of a child less than 6 years of age having *nephrotic syndrome*, which is responsive to steroids. Under light microscopy what will be seen:

A. Nothing
B. Loss of foot process
C. Tubule atrophy
D. Crescents

(AIIMS 2001)

Nephrotic syndrome is characterized by heavy proteinuria leading to hypoproteinemia, edema and hyperlipidemia. Causes of nephrotic syndrome in children are as under:	
Idiopathic (90 %)	**Glomerulonephritis associated (10 %)**
• Minimal change disease (85%)	• Membranous
• Focal sclerosis (10%)	• Membrano-proliferative
• Mesingio-proliferative (5%)	
In minimal change disease the **glomeruli appear normal under light microscope**. More than 95% of these patients respond very well to steroids.	

7. All of the following causes of neonatal convulsion have bad prognosis *except*:
- **A.** Brain tumor
- **B.** Intraventricular hemorrhage
- **C.** Late hypocalcemia
- **D.** Meningitis

(AI 1991, SGPGI 1996)

8. *Best* prognosis in neonatal seizures is due to which of the following causes:
- **A.** Hypomagnesemia
- **B.** Hyponatremia
- **C.** Hypocalcemia
- **D.** Hypoglycemia

(SGPGI 2002)

Prognosis in Neonatal Seizure

Cause of seizure	Normal outcome
Late hypocalcemia	100%
Early hypocalcemia	50%
Subarachnoid hemorrhage	90%
Hypoglycemia	35-70%
Neonatal encephalopathy	30-50%
Intraventricular hemorrhage	10%
Meningitis	10-65%
Neural dysgenesis	0%
Idiopathic	75%

9. Acute febrile convulsion in children is treated with:
- **A.** Ethosuximide
- **B.** Diazepam
- **C.** Phenobarbitone
- **D.** Phenytoin

(AIIMS 1996)

10. Which of the following is *true* regarding febrile convulsions:
- **A.** It is a benign condition
- **B.** If first episode is not treated then recurrence occurs
- **C.** Phenobarbitone is given for 2 years
- **D.** Focal neurological deficit

(UP 1996)

11. Which of the following is *not* a clinical feature of simple febrile seizure:
- **A.** Convulsions are always generalized
- **B.** In treatment aspirin should be avoided
- **C.** Seizure does not last for > 15 minutes
- **D.** Convulsions are related with degree of elevation of temperature

(UP 1993)

12. All are *false* regarding simple febrile convulsions *except*:
- **A.** No spontaneous remission
- **B.** Follow high fever
- **C.** Recurrent in nature
- **D.** Occurs at 6 years onwards

(AIIMS 1997)

13. A three-year-old child presented with fever and a history of recurrent seizures in past. Which of the following steps should be taken to prevent recurrence of seizures:
A. Paracetamol 6 hourly
B. Phenobarbitone
C. Paracetamol 6 hourly and diazepam 12 hourly
D. Continue diazepam infusion *(AIIMS 2001)*

"FEBRILE SEIZURE MAY BE DEFINED AS BRIEF, SELF LIMITING, GENERALIZED AND TONIC CLONIC EVENT ASSOCIATED WITH FEVER AND NOT ASSOCIATED WITH ANY UNDERLYING NEUROLOGICAL DISEASE." They generally occur between 6 months to 5 years of age. The typical case is a child who has a generalized, tonic-clonic seizure during a febrile illness such as otitis media, respiratory infection, or gastroenteritis. *The seizure is more likely to occur during the* ***rising phase*** *of the temperature curve rather than well into the course of the illness.* A **simple febrile seizure** is a single, isolated event, brief, and symmetric in appearance. **Complex febrile seizures** have repeated seizure activity, last more than 15 minutes, or have focal features. No long-term prophylaxis is required. EEG is not of much use because inter-ictal EEG is often normal. **Seizures may be controlled by treating the fever with hydrotherapy and paracetamol along with IV or PR diazepam-0.3 mg/kg. Short-term prophylaxis with oral Diazepam (0.3 mg/kg/dose bid) should be given for three days.** As it is a BENIGN CONDITION, long-term anticonvulsant prophylaxis is not required. Phenobarbitone or sodium valproate may be used for long-term prophylaxis which is only ***rarely*** required.

14. Child doubles the height at the age of .... years:
A. 5½ **B.** 4½
C. 3½ **D.** 2 *(UP 1993)*

Length of a newborn child is approximately 50 cm and at one year it is 75 cm. Thereafter the height can be calculated by multiplying the age in year by 6 and then adding 77 to it (Height in cm = age in years x 6 + 77).

15. Which of the following causes furuncle:
A. *Pseudomonas* **B.** *Escherichia coli*
C. *Streptococcus* **D.** *Staphylococcus* *(UP 1995)*

Staphylococcus aureus is the most common etiologic agent of skin and soft tissue infections including furuncles. A furuncle is often known as a boil. It is a deep-seated necrotic infection of a hair follicle commonly found on buttocks, face, or neck. Furuncles are very painful and tender, and are often associated with fever and constitutional symptoms.

16. Carbamazepine is the *drug of choice* in which of the following conditions:
A. Absence attacks **B.** Partial complex seizure
C. Infantile spasm **D.** Post-anoxic myoclonus *(AI 1991, SGPGI 1999)*

17. *Drug of choice* in temporal lobe epilepsy is:
A. Ethosuximide **B.** Phenytoin
C. Carbamazepine **D.** Phenobarbitone *(UP 1999)*

Mesial temporal lobe epilepsy is the most common syndrome associated with complex-partial seizures. Drug of choice for **complex-partial seizure** is carbamazepine (10-20 mg/kg/day in 3 divided doses).

18. In petit mal (absence) epilepsy the *drug of choice* is:
A. Phenobarbitone **B.** Phenytoin
C. Valproic acid **D.** Ethosuximide *(UP 1995, 1997)*

19. Drug *not* used in absence seizure is:
A. Ethosuximide
B. Valproate
C. Phenytoin
D. Clonazepam *(AI 1994)*

Drug of Choice in Various Seizures

Focal-onset Seizures*	Generalized Tonic-clonic	Absence	Myoclonic	Atonic
		First line drugs		
Carbamazepine	Valproic acid	Ethosuximide	Valproic acid	Valproic acid
Phenytoin	Carbamazepine	Valproic acid		
Valproic acid	Phenytoin			
		Alternative drugs		
Lamotrigine	Phenobarbital	Acetazolamide	Clonazepam	Clonazepam
Gabapentin	Primidone	Clonazepam	Acetazolamide	
Phenobarbital		Phenobarbital		
Primidone				

*Simple-partial, complex-partial, and secondarily generalized tonic-clonic seizures.

20. Coarctation of aorta is common in:
- **A.** Noonan's syndrome
- **B.** Down syndrome
- **C.** Klinefelter syndrome
- **D.** Turner syndrome *(AI 1995)*

In **Turner syndrome** coarctation of aorta (20-50%) is the most frequent cardiovascular lesion, but hypertension of unknown etiology and other congenital heart defects may also occur.

21. Tonic neck reflex disappears at .... weeks:
- **A.** 36 **B.** 32
- **C.** 24 **D.** 18 *(UP 1995)*

22. Moro's reflex disappears by.......... month:
- **A.** 7 **B.** 3
- **C.** 5 **D.** 8 *(UP 1994)*

Neonatal Reflexes

REFLEX	APPEARS AT	NO LONGER OBTAINABLE
Moro's	Birth	3 months
Stepping	Birth	6 weeks
Placing	Birth	6 weeks
Rooting and sucking	Birth	4 months awake 7 months asleep
Palmar grasp	Birth	6 months
Plantar grasp	Birth	10 months
Adductor spread of knee jerk	Birth	7 months
Tonic neck	2 months	6 months
Neck righting	4-6 months	24 months
Landau	3 months	24 months
Parachute	9 months	Persists

23. Danger in epiglottitis is:

A. Defect in drinking
B. Defect in speech
C. Respiratory obstruction
D. Aspiration

(UP 1995)

Acute epiglottitis is a rapidly progressive cellulitis of the epiglottis that MAY CAUSE COMPLETE AIRWAY OBSTRUCTION and is therefore a life-threatening condition. Epiglottitis is most common among children between 2 and 4 years. All patients must be given antibiotics active against ***Haemophilus influenzae***, the organism that is responsible for nearly all pediatric cases. Children should be treated with intravenous cefuroxime, ceftriaxone or ampicillin/sulbactam combination.

24. Which of the following is *true* regarding Dawn phenomenon:

A. Early morning hyperglycemia
B. Early morning hypoglycemia
C. Hypoglycemia is followed by hyperglycemia
D. Insulin dose is decreased in treatment

(UP 1995)

The Somogyi effect	The Dawn phenomenon
It may be defined as rebound **hyperglycemia** which occurs, after an episode of hypoglycemia, due to release of counter regulatory hormones.	It is early morning rise in plasma glucose (**hyperglycemia**) due to increased insulin requirement.

25. In which of the following conditions, *iceberg phenomenon* is seen:

A. Filaria
B. Malaria
C. PEM
D. None of the above

(UP 1994)

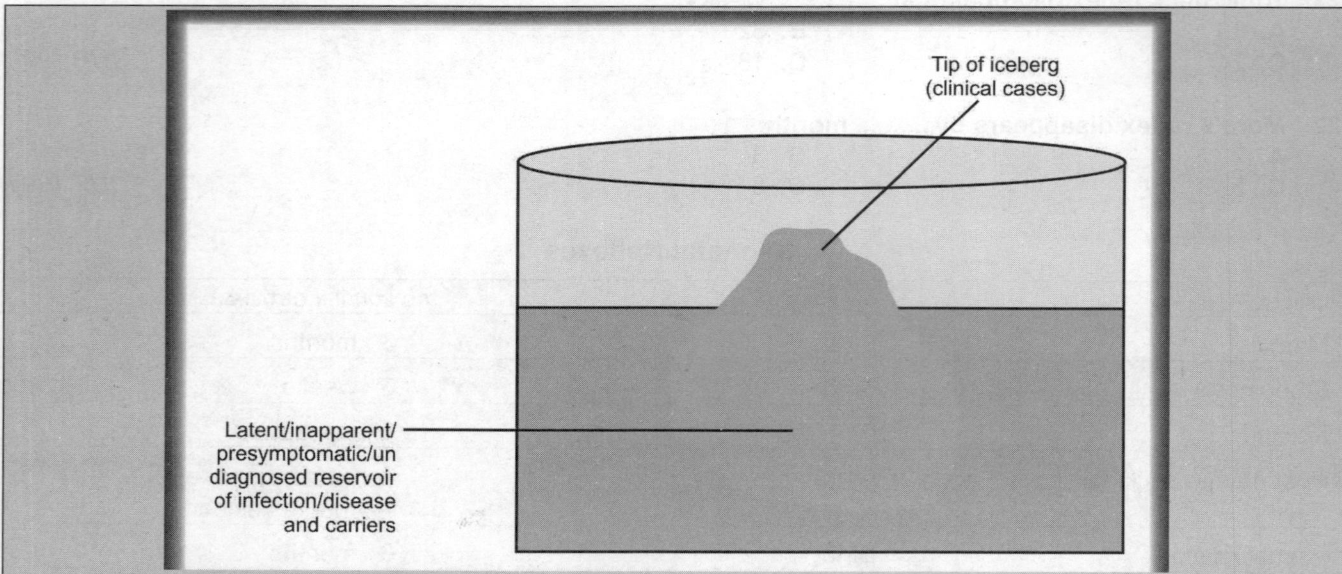

Disease in a community is just like an iceberg. The floating tip of the iceberg represents clinical cases, while the vast submerged portion represents the hidden mass of disease. This phenomenon is commonly seen in the following diseases:

- Anemia
- Protein-energy malnutrition (PEM)
- Mental illness
- Diabetes
- Hypertension

26. Osteomalacia is due to deficiency of:
- **A.** Vitamin A
- **B.** Vitamin D
- **C.** Vitamin B
- **D.** Vitamin C

(UP 1994)

Rickets may be defined as a disorder involving softening and weakening of the bones of children, primarily caused by lack of vitamin D and/or lack of calcium or phosphate which leads to decreased calcification of growing bones. **Rickets** is a condition caused by the lack of vitamin D, calcium, and phosphorus. Term ***osteomalacia*** is usually used for this disorder in the adult, in whom the epiphyseal growth plates are closed. Rickets is seen most often in infancy and childhood. It is marked by abnormal bone growth. Symptoms include soft bones causing defects, as bowlegs and knock-knees, swellings on the ends and sides of the bones, muscle pain, a swollen skull, chest defects, a curved spine, swollen liver and spleen, heavy sweating, and general tenderness of the body when touched. Prevention and treatment are a diet rich in calcium, phosphorus, and vitamin D and enough exposure to sunlight. Kinds of rickets include adult rickets, celiac rickets, renal rickets, and vitamin D resistant rickets.

27. Which of the following is the primary aim of neonatal resuscitation:
- **A.** To induce spontaneous cry
- **B.** To retain color
- **C.** To maintain breathing
- **D.** To restore heart rate

(UP 1994)

Establishment of spontaneous breathing after birth is the most crucial event for the survival of newborn baby and is the primary aim of neonatal resuscitation. A guideline for neonatal resuscitation is given below.

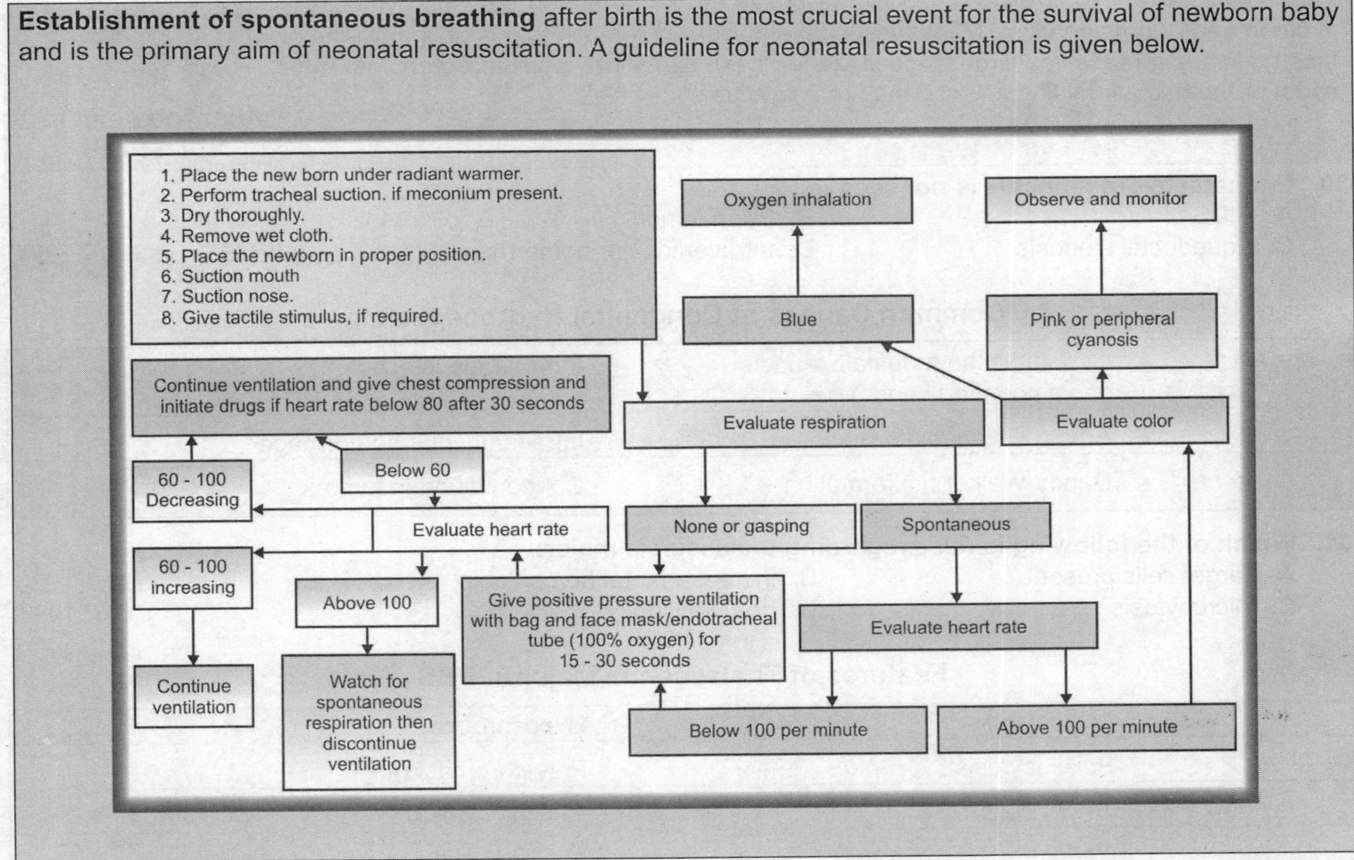

28. *Not* a feature of Friedreich's ataxia:
- **A.** Posterior column involvement
- **B.** Corticospinal tracts involvement
- **C.** Spinocerebellar tracts involvement
- **D.** None of the above

(UP 1994)

Friedreich's ataxia is the most common form of inherited ataxia. The primary site of involvement is the spinal cord and the peripheral nerves. Atrophy of the cerebellum and cerebral gyri can occur. Sclerosis and degeneration are seen mainly in the spinocerebellar tracts, lateral corticospinal tracts, and posterior columns. Degeneration of the glossopharyngeal, vagus, hypoglossal, and deep cerebellar nuclei may occur. The cerebral cortex is histologically almost normal except for loss of Betz cells in the precentral gyri. Peripheral nerves are extensively involved and they demonstrate a loss of large myelinated fibers. Features of Friedreich's Ataxia are as under:	
• Staggering gait	• Dysarthria
• Frequent falling	• Nystagmus
• Titubation	• Dysmetria
• Muscle weakness	• Absent deep tendon reflexes
• Extensor plantar responses	• Cardiomegaly

29. Which of the following is *true* regarding AML:
A. Prognosis is good
B. Peak incidence in childhood
C. Auer rods present
D. Philadelphia chromosomes
(UP 1994, PGI 1998)

The diagnosis of AML is established by the presence of at least 30 percent myeloblasts in blood and/or bone marrow. Myeloblasts have nuclear chromatin that is uniformly fine or lacelike in appearance and large nucleoli (2 to 5 / cell). Specific cytoplasmic granules, **Auer rods**, or the nuclear folding and clefting are characteristic of AML.

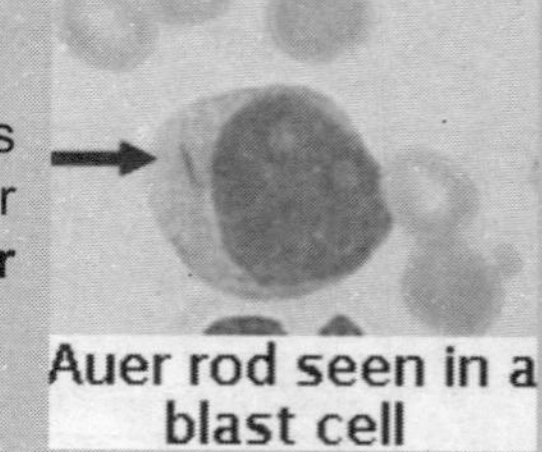
Auer rod seen in a blast cell

30. Neonatal hydrocephalus is *not* seen in:
A. AIDS
B. Brain tumor
C. Aqueductal stenosis
D. Intraventricular hemorrhage
(JIPMER 1993, UP 1994)

Common Causes of Congenital Hydrocephalus

• Congenital aqueductal stenosis (most common cause)	• Intrauterine infection
• Arnold-Chiari malformation	• Intraventricular hemorrhage
• Dandy-Walker malformation	• Congenital brain tumors

31. Which of the following is *false* regarding thalassemia major:
A. Target cells present
B. Increased fetal hemoglobin
C. Microcytosis
D. Iron deficiency
(UP 1994)

Features of Thalassemia Major in PBS

• Microcytosis	• Hypochromia
• Poikilocytosis	• Poly-chromasia
• Target cells	• Reticulocytosis
• Reduced osmotic fragility	• Iron overload
• Increased fetal hemoglobin	• Elevated unconjugated serum bilirubin

32. Deficiency of which of the following leads to pellagra:
A. Pyridoxine
B. Nicotinamide
C. Riboflavin
D. Thiamine
(UP 1994)

Pellagra is a chronic wasting disease typically associated with dermatitis, dementia, and diarrhea caused by deficiency of *Niacin* (nicotinic acid).

33. Fetal hemoglobin is increased in which of the following:
- **A.** Hereditary spherocytosis
- **B.** Pure red cell aplasia
- **C.** Polycythemia vera
- **D.** Juvenile CML

(AIIMS 1997)

34. *Not* a feature of juvenile CML:
- **A.** Lymphadenopathy
- **B.** Philadelphia chromosome positive
- **C.** Fetal hemoglobin is increased
- **D.** Thrombocytopenia

(AI 1994, KERALA 1999)

35. Which of the following is *true* regarding juvenile CML:
- **A.** Philadelphia chromosome
- **B.** High fetal hemoglobin content
- **C.** Low acid phosphatase
- **D.** Massive splenomegaly

(UP 1996)

Differentiating Features of Adult and Juvenile CML

Features	Adult type	Juvenile type
Age	10-12 years	1-2 years
Philadelphia chromosome	Always present	Never present
Fetal hemoglobin values	3-7%	30-70%
Splenomegaly	Massive	Mild to moderate
Lymphadenopathy	Occasional	Frequent
Skin rash	Not present	Frequently present on face
WBC count	Over 1,00,000	Less than 1,00,000
Thrombocytopenia	Uncommon	Common
Blast cells in GBP	Rare	Common
Complete remission	Frequent	Rare
Alkaline phosphatase in neutrophils	Decreased	Decreased

36. Which of the following is *false* regarding tricuspid atresia:
- **A.** Severe cyanosis
- **B.** Left ventricular hypertrophy
- **C.** Left axis deviation
- **D.** Right axis deviation

(AI 1992, UP 1997))

37. In which of the following conditions left axis deviation with left ventricular hypertrophy is seen:
- **A.** VSD
- **B.** Coarctation of aorta
- **C.** Tricuspid atresia
- **D.** TOF

(UP 1996, AI 2001)

In TRICUSPID ATRESIA there is complete absence of tricuspid valve. Therefore there is no direct communication between right atrium and right ventricle. More than 90% of patients have an associated VSD. An atrial level communication is essential for blood to exit the right atrium; therefore there is an obligatory right to left shunt at this level. The clinical picture consists of severe **cyanosis** due to obligatory admixture of systemic and pulmonary venous blood in the left ventricle. The ECG characteristically shows right atrial enlargement, **left axis deviation, and left ventricular hypertrophy**.

38. Which of the following is the characteristic feature of acute rheumatic fever:
- **A.** Hemoptysis
- **B.** Tender nodule
- **C.** Pan-systolic murmur
- **D.** Erythema marginatum

(UP 1994)

39. Which of the following is *not* a major criterion of rheumatic fever:
- **A.** Chorea
- **B.** Subcutaneous nodules
- **C.** Streptococcal antibodies
- **D.** Polyarthritis

(UP 1997)

40. Which of the following is an *essential* criterion in rheumatic fever:
- **A.** Chorea
- **B.** Arthralgia
- **C.** Erythema marginatum
- **D.** Acute streptococcal infection

(UP 1996)

The Jones Criteria for Rheumatic Fever

Major Criteria	Minor Criteria	
Carditis	**Clinical**	**Laboratory**
Migratory polyarthritis	Fever	Elevated ESR
Sydenham's chorea	Arthralgia	Elevated CRP
Subcutaneous nodules		Prolonged PR interval
Erythema marginatum		

PLUS (ESSENTIAL CRITERIA)

Supporting evidence of a recent group A streptococcal infection which includes any one of the following:
- Positive throat culture for *Streptococcus*
- Rapid antigen detection test
- Elevated or increasing streptococcal antibody test (**ASO titer** > 200 Todd's unit in adults or > 300 Todd's unit children).

*Diagnosis of rheumatic fever is highly probable if two major or one major and two minor criteria are present along with the evidence of previous *Streptococcus* infection.

41. Rib notching is seen in:
- **A.** Tricuspid regurgitation
- **B.** ASD
- **C.** VSD
- **D.** Coarctation of aorta

(UP 1996)

Causes of Inferior Rib Notching

Aortic	Coarctation, occlusion
Subclavian	Takayasu disease, Blalock-Tausig operation (unilateral)
Reduced pulmonary blood flow	Pulmonary atresia and stenosis, TOF, truncus type IV
Venous	SVC,IVC obstruction
Shunts	Pulmonary or intercostal AV fistula, intercostal pulmonary fistula
Other causes	Hyperparathyroidism, neurogenic tumor, idiopathic.

42. Shakir's tape is used for measurement of:
- **A.** Height
- **B.** Length of infant
- **C.** Mid arm circumference
- **D.** Head circumference

(DELHI 1996)

43. At Shakir's tape the red zone indicates .... cm:
- **A.** 14.5
- **B.** 13.5
- **C.** 11.5
- **D.** Less than 12.5

(UP 1995)

Measurement of mid arm-circumference (MAC) is an age independent criteria for assessment of nutritional status of a child between 1 and 5 years. The mid-arm circumference is relatively constant **(16.5 to 17.5 cm)** between 1 and 5 years. Any child having MAC value below 12.5 should be considered to be malnourished. It can be measured by **Shakir's tape** which is fiber glass tape.

Color of Shakir's tape	Measurement	Nutritional status
• Red color	Less than 12.5 cm	Wasted
• Yellow color	12.5 to 13.5 cm	Borderline
• Green color	More than 13.5 cm	Normal

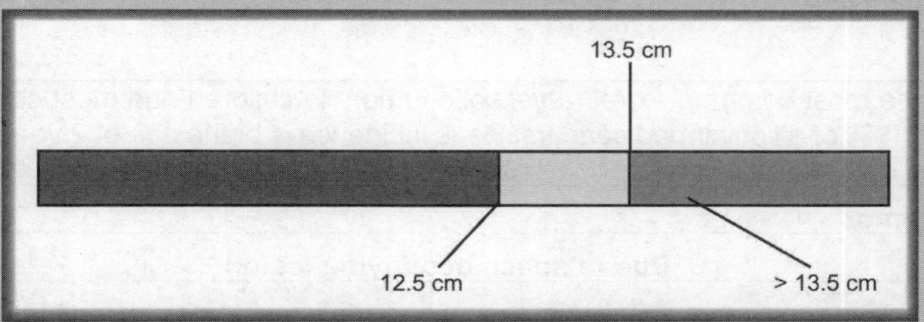

44. Toxic shock syndrome may occur due to:
A. Hepatitis B vaccine
B. Measles vaccine
C. DPT vaccine
D. BCG vaccine *(UP 1998)*

Toxic shock syndrome (TSS) may occur when the MEASLES VACCINE being used is contaminated or the vial is being used for more than one session in same day or on the next day. The vaccine should not be used 4 hours after opening the vial. TSS presents as severe diarrhea, vomiting and high grade fever within few hours of measles vaccination. Case fatality rate is high and child may die within 48 hours.

45. Which of the following is the *absolute contraindication* for DPT vaccine:
A. Cerebral palsy
B. Progressive neurological disease
C. ADD
D. Febrile convulsion *(UP 1998)*

Absolute Contraindication for DPT Vaccine

- An acute febrile illness
- Progressive neurological disease
- Uncontrolled cry, seizure or severe reaction following first dose.

46. Croup is *not* associated with:
A. Polio virus **B.** Adenovirus
C. Influenza virus **D.** RSV *(UP 1998)*

Croup (Croop): It is an acute viral disease of childhood, marked by a resonant barking cough, suffocative and difficult breathing, and laryngeal spasm. Difficulty in breathing is due to acute sub-glottic edema. Because of severe respiratory distress, the child is hypoxic. Viral agents account for nearly all cases of croup except that associated with diphtheria and acute epiglottis. The PARAINFLUENZA VIRUSES account for approximately two-third of all cases. Other viral causes of croup are as under:

- RSV
- Influenza virus
- Adenovirus
- Measles virus

47. Which of the following is *false* regarding neuroblastoma:
- **A.** Hepatomegaly
- **B.** Hypertension
- **C.** *Cafe au lait spots*
- **D.** Opsomyoclonus

(UP 1996)

48. Which of the following is *false* regarding neuroblastoma:
- **A.** Hepatomegaly
- **B.** Abdominal swelling
- **C.** Massive splenomegaly
- **D.** Proptosis

(UP 1996)

Neuroblastomas are the most common *extracranial* solid tumors in children and most common solid tumor in infancy. They constitute 10% of all childhood cancers. Peak incidence is at the age of 2 years. Clinical features may be classified as under:

• **Due to primary tumor**		
	Due to space occupying lesion	
Swelling	Pain	Breathlessness
Ascites	Constipation	Urinary retention
	Neurological features	
Horner's syndrome	Paraplegia	Quadriplegia
• **Due to metastasis**		
Bone pains	Proptosis	Hepatomegaly
Fever	Failure to thrive	Subcutaneous nodules
• **Paraneoplastic syndrome**		
Opsomyoclonus	Cerebellar ataxia	Secretory diarrhea
Flushing	Hypertension	Excessive sweating

49. A child present with change in color of hair, blue eyes and mental retardation. He is suffering from:
- **A.** Cystinuria
- **B.** PKU
- **C.** Malonyl urea
- **D.** Hemocystinuria

(UP 1997)

50. Which of the following *inborn error of metabolism* is associated with mental retardation:
- **A.** PKU
- **B.** Duchenne's syndrome
- **C.** Down syndrome
- **D.** McArdle syndrome

(AI 1992)

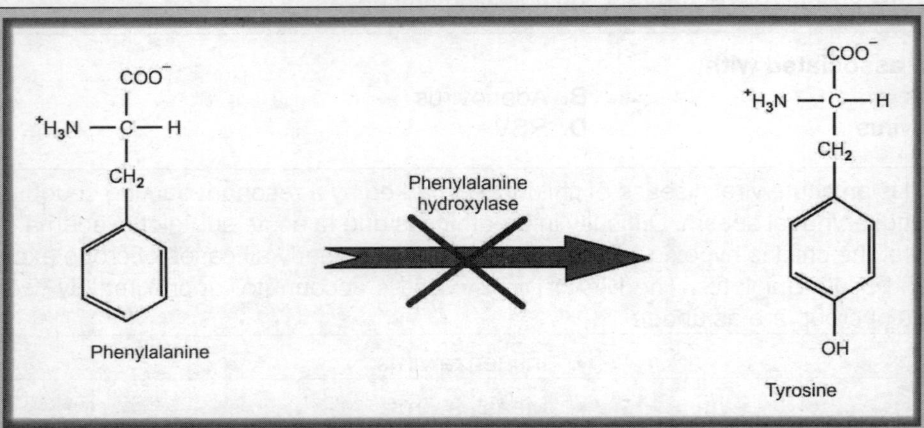

Phenylalanine hydroxylase

Phenylalanine

Tyrosine

PHENYLKETONURIA (PKU) is a genetic condition in which the body is unable to use one of the constituents of a normal diet—an amino acid, called phenylalanine (PHE) due to DEFICIENCY OF ENZYME PHENYLALANINE HYDROXYLASE. PHE is found in all protein foods such as meat, eggs, fish, milk and cheese and to a lesser extent in cereals, vegetables and fruits. In PKU, PHE cannot be converted to TYR, and so PHE accumulates in the blood. TYR deficiency *per se* does not occur because the diet provides sufficient TYR. Newborns with this disease are asymptomatic but ultimately present with LIGHT COLORED HAIR, BLUE EYES, ECZEMA AND MENTAL RETARDATION. Seizure and behavioral problems are also seen. Urine and sweat of these children have characteristic ***mousy odor*** due to phenyl acetic acid in urine and sweat. Blood for screening should be obtained after 72 hours of life and after giving protein feeds to reduce the possibility of false negative result.

Diagnostic criteria are as under:

1. Plasma phenylalanine level more than 20 mg/dL.
2. Normal plasma tyrosine level.
3. Increased urinary levels of metabolites of phenylalanine, i.e. phenyl pyruvic acid and hydroxy phenyl acetic acid.
4. Normal plasma concentration of cofactor tetrahydrobiopterin (BH_4)

51. Which of the following is *false* regarding Gilbert's syndrome:

A. Unconjugated hyperbilirubinemia
B. Normal liver biopsy
C. Normal LFT
D. Mild conjugated hyperbilirubinemia *(UP 1997)*

Syndrome	Inheritance	Enzyme deficient	Bilirubin
Crigler-Najjar-1	AR	Absent glucuronyl transferase	Unconjugated > 20 mg/dL
Crigler-Najjar-2	AD	Decreased glucuronyl transferase	Unconjugated < 20 mg/dL
Gilbert's syndrome	AD	Decreased glucuronyl transferase with decreased hepatic uptake	Unconjugated < 6 mg/dL
Dubin-Johnson syndrome	AR	Impaired biliary secretion **(dark grey discoloration of liver)**	Conjugated < 5 mg/dL
Rotor syndrome	AR	Decreased hepatic uptake, storage and secretion	Conjugated < 5 mg/dL

52. Rectal polyps usually present with which of the following:

A. Bleeding
B. Perforation
C. Obstruction
D. Malignant changes *(UP 1993)*

53. In children *most common* cause of bleeding per rectum is:

A. Hirschsprung's disease
B. Foreign body
C. Intussusception
D. Rectal polyp *(UP 1997)*

Causes of Bleeding Per Rectum

Neonates	Infants	Children
Anal fissure	Anal fissure	Rectal polyps
Necrotizing enterocolitis (NEC)	Intussusception	Vascular malformations
Volvulus neonatorum	Meckel's diverticulum	Tumors of GIT
	Polyps in intestine	

54. Which of the following is the *most common* cause of community acquired neonatal meningitis:

A. *Klebsiella pneumoniae*
B. *Neisseria*
C. *Entamoeba coli*
D. *Pseudomonas* *(SGPGI 2002)*

Common Etiological Agents of Acute Bacterial Meningitis

Up to 4 weeks	4-12 weeks	>12 weeks
Escherichia coli	*Haemophilus influenzae*	*Haemophilus influenzae*
Klebsiella pneumoniae	*Streptococcus pneumoniae*	*Streptococcus pneumoniae*
Listeria monocytogenes	Group B *Streptococcus*	*Neisseria meningitidis*
Enterococcus spp.	*Listeria monocytogenes*	
Salmonella spp.		

55. Organism which commonly causes meningitis in 6 month to 2 years of age is:

A. *Staphylococcus*
B. *Neisseria*
C. *Haemophilus influenzae*
D. *Streptococcus* *(AI 1993, 1996, 1998, 2001, AIIMS 1999)*

Organisms Causing Acute Bacterial Meningitis in Children (1 month to 15 years)

Haemophilus influenzae	40-60%
Neisseria meningitidis	25-40%
Streptococcus pneumoniae	10-20%
Streptococci	2-4%
Gram-negative bacilli	1-2%
Staphylococci	1-2%
Listeria species	1-2%

56. An eight-year-old girl presented with *low* grade fever, vomiting, headache and convulsions. Her CSF finding revealed protein 105 mg%, sugar 40 mg%, chloride 52 mg% with *predominant lymphocytes*. The diagnosis is:

A. Traumatic meningitis
B. Viral meningitis
C. Acute bacterial meningitis
D. Tubercular meningitis *(UP 2000)*

	Appearance	Pressure	Cells	Protein	Sugar
Normal	Watery	100-180 mm of CSF	0-5 all lymphocytes	20-40 mg%	40-80 mg%
Acute bacterial meningitis	Turbid	Raised	100-5000 neutrophil predominant	100-400 mg%	Low Organism may be seen
Tubercular meningitis	Clear or cloudy	Raised	10-500 Lymphocyte predominant	80-400 mg% or more	Low Organism may be seen
Viral encephalitis	Clear	Normal	20-2000 Lymphocyte predominant	150 mg%	Normal C/S sterile

*Low chloride is seen in tubercular meningitis due to chloride loss as a result of protracted vomiting and is not specific for TBM.

57. *Most common* cause of neonatal death in India is:

A. Birth injury
B. Malabsorption
C. Prematurity
D. Congenital malformation *(UP 1993)*

Causes of Neonatal Mortality in India

Causes	0-28 days
• **Prematurity** (including LBW)	**254**
• Birth injury/asphyxia	233
• Neonatal sepsis	208
• Multiple pregnancy (twins/triplets)	40
• Respiratory distress syndrome	44
• Neonatal pneumonia	37
• Congenital malformation	33
• Neonatal tetanus	18
• Postnatal aspiration	15
• Diarrhea and dysentery	11
• Sudden death	2
• Others (undetermined)	105
Total	**1000**

Prematurity including low birth weight was the *most important* cause of neonatal deaths. Other important causes of neonatal deaths were birth injury/asphyxia and neonatal sepsis. Deaths due to prematurity, congenital malformation, respiratory distress syndrome, neonatal pneumonia, postnatal aspiration were more common during first seven days of life. Deaths due to birth injury/asphyxia, neonatal sepsis, neonatal tetanus and sudden deaths were more common during 8-28 days of life. Deaths due to diarrhea, dysentery and sudden death were recorded only in the late neonatal period.

* *Indian Pediatrics 2001; 38: 1022-1025*

58. Which of the following is *not* caused by thiamine deficiency in children:

A. Infantile tremor syndrome
B. Wernicke's encephalopathy
C. Korsakoff's psychosis
D. Congestive heart failure *(UP 1993)*

In India, the **infantile tremor syndrome** was described in 1950's. This syndrome was first thought to be due to B_{12} deficiency by Jadhav *et al* based on 6 cases with megaloblastic anemia and improvement with B_{12}. These finding were reproduced by Garewal *et al* who found megaloblastic anemia in 20 and low B_{12} levels (below 100 pg/ml) in 88% of cases. However, several others failed to find megaloblastic anemia and failed to get improvement with B_{12}. **This may imply that B_{12} deficiency is a cause in a subset of these cases.**

59. Bull neck in diphtheria occurs due to:

A. Cellulitis
B. Lymphadenopathy
C. Retropharyngeal abscess
D. Laryngeal edema *(AIIMS 1992, AI 1996)*

60. Diphtheric neuropathy occurs in .... week of infection:

A. 4th
B. 3rd
C. 2nd
D. 1st *(UP 2001)*

Diphtheria is an acute infectious disease caused by *Corynebacterium diphtheriae*. Incubation period is 2-5 days. Tonsillar and pharyngeal diphtheria is the most common clinical type which presents with low grade fever, sore throat and difficulty in swallowing. Within 1 to 2 days a white membrane appears on tonsil, **cervical lymph nodes may be enlarged accompanied by severe edema** (BULL NECK APPEARANCE). Myocarditis and neuropathy are important complications. Generalized polyneuritis usually occurs 3-6 weeks after the illness.

61. Which of the following is a common cause of bronchiolitis:

A. Mycoplasma
B. Parainfluenza virus
C. Adenovirus
D. RSV

(UP 1997)

Acute bronchiolitis is caused by respiratory syncytial virus in 50-60% of cases. Other viruses responsible for acute bronchiolitis are parainfluenza virus 1, parainfluenza virus 2, adenovirus, influenza virus and rhinovirus. Rarely *Mycoplasma* and *Chlamydia* may also cause this disease.

Clinical Syndromes Produced by Respiratory Syncytial Virus

Most frequent	Occasional	Infrequent
Pneumonia and bronchiolitis in young children	Common cold in adults	Pneumonia in elderly and immunosuppressed patients

62. Blast cells of acute lymphocytic leukemia in childhood have:

A. Excessive mitochondria
B. Antibodies on WBC
C. CALLA +ve
D. Surface antigen

(AI 1993, UP 1996)

The blast cells of ALL may or may not react to **C**ommon **A**cute **L**ymphocytic **L**eukemia **A**ntigen (**CALLA**). They are classified as CALLA +ve or CALLA –ve.

63. Cirrhosis is *not* seen in:

A. Cystinuria
B. Alpha$_1$-antitrypsin deficiency
C. Wilson disease
D. Galactosemia

(UP 1996)

Causes of Liver Cirrhosis

Infections	Inherited and metabolic	Drug and chemicals	Miscellaneous
Brucellosis	Glycogen storage disease	Oral contraceptives (Budd-Chiari)	Diabetes mellitus
Echinococcus	Hemochromatosis	Oxyphenisatin	Graft-versus-host disease
Schistosomiasis	Hereditary fructose intolerance	Perhexilene maleate	Jejuno-ileal bypass
Toxoplasmosis	Hereditary tyrosinemia	Pyrrolidizine alkaloids (veno-occlusive disease)	Sarcoidosis
Viral hepatitis B, C, D, E, G; CMV	Wilson's disease	Arsenicals	Chronic inflammatory bowel disease
	Alpha$_1$-antitrypsin deficiency	Isoniazid	Cystic fibrosis
	Fanconi's syndrome	Methotrexate	Alcoholism
	Galactosemia	Methyldopa	
	Gaucher's disease		

64. Thiamine deficiency causes:

A. Glossitis
B. Cheilosis
C. Angular stomatitis
D. Beriberi disease

(UP 1997)

The two major manifestations of thiamine deficiency are CVS (wet beriberi) and nervous systems (dry beriberi and the Wernicke-Korsakoff syndrome).

65. Mayer-Rokitansky-Kuster-Hauser syndrome is due to:
A. 45 XO
B. 47 XXY
C. 46 XX
D. Trisomy 18 *(UP 1999)*

Women with Mayer-Rokitansky-Kuster-Hauser syndrome have a 46-XX karyotype, female secondary sex characteristics, and normal ovarian function, including cyclic ovulation, but have absence or hypoplasia of the vagina.

66. Glucose-6-phosphate dehydrogenase deficiency is:
A. AR **B.** AD
C. X-linked **D.** Y-linked *(AI 1991)*

67. Which of the following is *not* an X-linked disorder:
A. Ocular albinism
B. Hemophilia A
C. Congenital adrenal hyperplasia
D. Testicular feminization *(UP 1999)*

X-linked Disorders

• Ocular albinism	• Color blindness
• Testicular feminization	• Hemophilia A
• Chronic granulomatous disease	• Glucose-6-phosphate dehydrogenase deficiency
• Hypophosphatemic rickets	• Duchenne/Becker muscular dystrophy
• Fragile-X syndrome	• Fabry's disease

68. Which of the following drug *does not* cause hemolytic anemia in G6PD deficiency:
A. Nitrofurantoin **B.** Dapsone
C. INH **D.** Primaquine *(AI 1992, UP 1998)*

Drug Causing Hemolytic Anemia in G-6-PD Deficiency

• Aminosalicylic acid	• Phenacetin
• Antimalarials, e.g. primaquine	• Probenecid
• Aspirin	• Procainamide
• Chloramphenicol	• Quinidine
• Co-trimoxazole	• Sulfonamides
• Dapsone	• Vitamin C
• Nalidixic acid	• Vitamin K
• Nitrofurantoin	

69. In a child with bronchial asthma, steroid should be given:
A. Orally
B. Subcutaneously
C. Aerosol
D. Intravenously *(UP 1999)*

Global Initiative for Asthma Guidelines for Asthma Management

GRADE	LONG-TERM MANAGEMENT	QUICK RELIEF
Step 1	No daily medication needed	Short acting bronchodilator-SOS Inhaled salbutamol preferred.
Step 2 Use spacer or nebulizer for infants below 2 years. Cromal—5 inhaler Flohale—50 inhaler Flohale—125 inhaler Flohale—100 rotacap Flohale—250 rotacap Budecort inhaler—100 / 200 mcg Beclate inhaler/rotacap 100/200 mcg. Daily medication required	Sodium cromoglycate (Cromal) 1-5 mg/dose t.d.s. or low dose inhaled **steroids as aerosol** 1. Beclomethasone 200-400 microgram/day. 2. Budesonide 100-400 microgram/ day. 3. Fluticasone 50-100 microgram/ day. 4. Theophylline SR (20 mg/kg/day) 1. Oxygen by mask @ 5 liter/	minute to achieve oxygen saturation of > 90%. 2. Salbutamol 0.15 mg/kg/dose. (Minimum 2.5 mg)—Asthalin respirator solution 5 mg/ml every 20 minutes for 3 doses, diluted in normal saline with oxygen @ 6 liter/minute. 3. Hydrocortisone 10 mg/kg (IV) followed by oral wysolone 2 mg/ kg/ day. **Step 3**
Flohale—50 inhaler Flohale—125 inhaler Flohale—100 rotacap Flohale—250 rotacap Budecort inhaler—100 / 200 mcg Beclate inhaler /rotacap 100/200 mcg. Daily therapy required.	Medium dose inhaled steroids. 1. Beclomethasone 400-800 microgram/day. 2. Budesonide 400-600 microgram/ day. 3. Fluticasone 100-200 microgram/ day. 4. Theophylline SR (20 mg/kg/ day) or long acting beta agonist (salmeteral)—salmeter/serobid inhaler 25 mcg dose 1-2 puffs b.d. not recommended for children below 4 years. 1. Oxygen by mask @ 5 liter/	minute to achieve Oxygen saturation of > 90%. 2. Salbutamol 0.15 mg/kg/dose. (Minimum 2.5 mg)—Asthalin respirator solution 5 mg/ml every 20 minutes for 3 doses, diluted in normal saline with oxygen @ 6 liter/minute. 3. Hydrocortisone 10 mg/kg (IV) followed by oral wysolone 2 mg/ kg/day. **Step 4**
Flohale—50 inhaler Flohale—125 inhaler Flohale—100 rotacap Flohale—250 rotacap Budecort inhaler—100/200 mcg Beclate inhaler/rotacap 100/200 mcg Daily therapy required.	High dose inhaled steroids. 1. Beclomethasone 800-1000 microgram/day. 2. Budesonide > 600 microgram/day. 3.Fluticasone 200-400 microgram/ day (along with oral steroid if needed) 4. Theophylline SR (20 mg/kg/ day) or long acting beta agonist (salmeteral)—salmeter/serobid inhaler 25 mcg dose 1-2 puffs b.d. not recommended for children below 4 years. 1. Oxygen by mask @ 5 liter/	minute to achieve Oxygen saturation of > 90%. 2. Salbutamol 0.15 mg/kg/dose. (Minimum 2.5 mg)—Asthalin respirator solution 5 mg/ml every 20 minutes for 3 doses, diluted in normal saline with oxygen @ 6 liter/minute. 3. Hydrocortisone 10 mg/kg (IV) followed by oral wysolone 2 mg/ kg/ day.

70. The chest X-ray film of a newborn with respiratory distress showing multiple air containing lesions in left hemithorax and mediastinal shift indicates:

A. Congenital lung cysts
B. Pneumatoceles
C. Neonatal emphysema
D. Diaphragmatic hernia

(AIIMS 1991. AI 2001)

71. A newlyborn child with respiratory distress and Apgar score of 3 in one minute is resuscitated with IPPR. On examination he has cyanosis, apex beat shifted to right side and scaphoid abdomen. The diagnosis is:

A. TOF
B. Dextrocardia
C. Diaphragmatic hernia
D. Pneumothorax

(UP 1998)

The large diaphragmatic hernias that compromise lung growth are **posterolateral** in position and are caused by defective closure of the pleuroperitoneal canal. The remnant of this canal in the normally developed diaphragm is the **foramen of Bochdalek. Infants with congenital diaphragmatic hernias are severely distressed at birth with cyanosis and shifting of apex beat**, and because the **abdomen** contains fewer contents than normal, it appears **scaphoid**. Radiographically, the abdominal contents, which may include stomach, bowel, spleen, and liver, can be identified within the thorax. **About 85% of congenital hernias are left-sided.** The ipsilateral lung is more severely hypoplastic, but because of mediastinal shift a lesser degree of contralateral hypoplasia is also present.

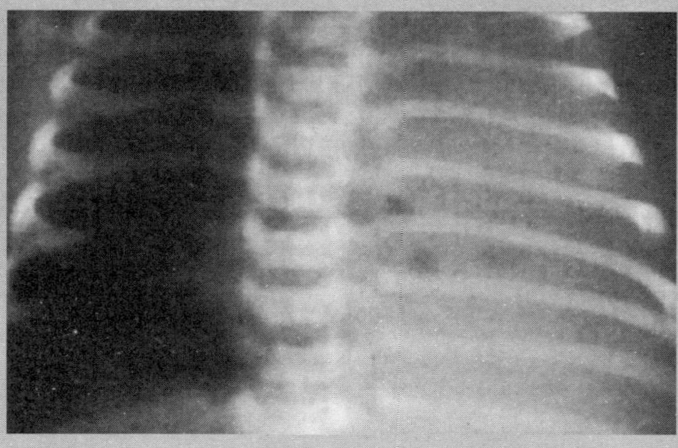

72. In Down syndrome, defect is:

A. Trisomy 18
B. Trisomy 21
C. Trisomy 13
D. 45 XO

(UP 1999)

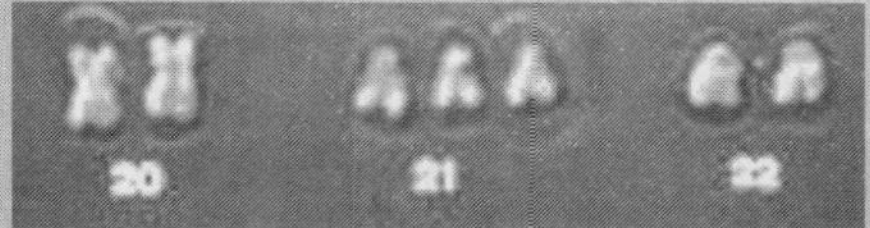

Down syndrome results when the child inherits all or part of an extracopy of chromosome 21. The most common chromosomal abnormality that produces Down syndrome is **Trisomy 21,** a defect in which an extra, third copy of chromosome 21 is present in every cell in the body.

73. Which of the following is the *most common* renal lesion in children and young adults:

A. Hemolytic-uremic syndrome
B. Minimal change nephrotic syndrome (MCNS)
C. MPGN
D. Interstitial nephritis

(UP 2001)

Idiopathic (90 %)	Glomerulonephritis associated (10 %)
• Minimal change disease (85%) • Focal sclerosis (10%) • Mesingio-proliferative (5%)	• Membranous • Membrano-proliferative

74. Best treatment for a neonate born to hepatitis B infected mother is:

A. Immunoglobulin (HBIG) and hepatitis B vaccine
B. Hepatitis B vaccine
C. Immunoglobulin
D. Isolation

(AI 1999)

75. A newborn of HBsAg positive mother should be vaccinated at:

A. One year **B.** 6 months
C. 1 month **D.** Birth *(UP 1998)*

Newborn of HBsAg +ve mother should be managed with hepatitis B active and passive immunization. The **first immunization and HBIG** (0.5ml) should be given **within first 12 hours of life** and the vaccine should be repeated at the age of 1 and 6 months.

76. *False* regarding childhood polycystic kidney is:

A. It can be diagnosed by USG
B. It presents with hypertension and renal insufficiency
C. Abdominal mass present
D. It is autosomal dominant *(UP 2001)*

Autosomal recessive polycystic kidney disease is a rare genetic disease with an incidence between 1:10,000 and 1:40,000. Its gene has been localized to chromosome 6. Most of cases are diagnosed in infancy, presenting as bilateral **abdominal masses**. Death in the neonatal period is most commonly due to pulmonary hypoplasia. **Hypertension and impaired urinary concentrating ability** are common features. **Ultrasound** is the most common technique used to diagnose autosomal recessive polycystic kidney disease.

77. Which of the following is *false* regarding Gaucher's disease in children:

A. Spleen is always markedly enlarged
B. X-linked recessive trait
C. Neuropsychological defects in the child
D. Deficiency of glucosylceramide β-glucosidase *(UP 1999)*

Gaucher's disease consists of 3 clinically distinct genetic diseases involving the storage of glucosylceramide (glucocerebroside). Inheritance pattern is **autosomal recessive**. **Splenomegaly** is the initial finding in most patients with weight of spleen being more than 3 kg. Liver is usually enlarged. Patients with infantile Gaucher's disease have severe involvement of CNS leading to decreased brain size, neuronal degeneration and active neuronophagia. There is loss of neurons in spinal cord as well. All clinical problems are due to storage of glucosylceramide because of **deficiency of β-glucosidase**. Onset of **infantile Gaucher's disease (type II)** usually occurs within the first few months of life with the following symptoms:

• Hepatosplenomegaly	• Developmental retardation
• Strabismus	• Difficulty in swallowing
• Laryngeal spasm	• Opisthotonos
• Pseudobulbar palsy	• Recurrent aspiration and chronic bronchopneumonia

The juvenile form of **Gaucher's disease (type III)** presents with dementia, behavioral changes, seizures, extrapyramidal and cerebellar signs. Pathological fractures are a major problem in some patients.

Diagnosis of Gaucher's disease is based on clinical picture alongwith identification of Gaucher's cells in bone marrow. Serum acid phosphatase levels are greatly elevated. However, the best diagnostic method is measurement of **GLUCOSYLCERAMIDE β GLUCOSIDASE** activity in leukocytes.

78. A child can climb steps with alternate limb at:

A. 4 years of age **B.** 3 years of age
C. 2 years of age **D.** 1 year of age *(AIIMS 1993)*

79. Which of the following is used to assess the motor function of a 4-year-old child:

A. Ascends with alternate step from staircase with holding the railing
B. Skips smoothly
C. Stands on single leg for 15 seconds
D. Hopes *(AIIMS 1998, UP 2000)*

Motor Development Pattern from One Year Onwards

• 12 months	Walks with one hand held or walks holding the furniture
• 15 months	Walks alone and crawls upstairs
• 18 months	Runs stiffly and sits on small chairs, walks upstairs with support of one hand and explores drawers and dustbins
• 24 months	Runs well, walks up and down stairs with one step at a time, climbs on furniture and opens doors
• 30 months	Jumps
• 36 months	**Goes upstairs alternating feet**, rides tricycle and stand momentarily on one foot
• 48 months	**Hops** on one foot, climbs, use scissors to cut pictures and throws ball overhand
• 60 months	Skips

80. Ossification centre which develops before birth is:

A. Lower end of femur
B. Lower part of tibia
C. Talus
D. Coracoid

(UP 1997)

Ossification centre of distal end of femur and proximal end of tibia are present at birth.

81. Which of the following is *true* regarding microcephaly:

A. It is a metabolic disease
B. It is a familial disorder
C. Autosomal recessive disease
D. Result of mild encephalitis

(KARNATAKA 2000)

82. Which of the following maternal disorders may lead to microcephaly:

A. Rubella
B. SLE
C. Hurler syndrome
D. Hepatitis A

(UP 1993, AIIMS 1994)

Causes of Microcephaly

Intrauterine infections	Perinatal and postnatal disorders	Developmental disorders
Congenital rubella	Birth asphyxia (HIE)	Hereditary microcephaly (RECESSIVE)
CMV infection	Severe malnutrition in early infancy	Autosomal trisomy syndromes **mainly trisomy 21**
Congenital syphilis	Neonatal herpes viral infection	Maternal PKU
Congenital toxoplasmosis		Fetal alcohol syndrome
		Fetal exposure to ionizing radiation
		Seckel dwarfism
		Cornelia de Lange syndrome
		Rubinstein Taybi syndrome
		Smith Lemii Opitz syndrome

83. Breastfeeding should be started earliest by .... hours:

A. More than 24
B. More than 48
C. 2-4
D. More than 72

(UP 1994)

Breastfeeding should be started within ½ to 1 hour of birth.

84. Fatty liver *does not* occur in:

A. Alcoholic liver disease
B. Diabetes mellitus
C. Marasmus
D. kwashiorkor

(AIIMS 1991, UP 1996)

Features	Marasmus	Kwashiorkor
Muscle wasting	Present	Hidden by edema and fat
Fat wasting	Severe	Fat is retained
Edema	None	Present
Weight for height	Very low	Low
Mental changes	Quite and apathetic	Irritable
Appetite	Good	Poor
Skin changes	None	Diffused pigmentation
Hair changes	Rare	Sparse, easily pluck able
Diarrhea	Common	Common
Fatty liver and hepatomegaly	**Never**	**Sometimes**

* Other causes of fatty liver include alcoholism, diabetes mellitus, obesity, hepatotoxins and certain chronic illnesses.

85. A child presents with increased oral secretion and chocking. He has:

A. Cyanotic heart disease
B. Pyloric stenosis
C. Tracheoesophageal fistula
D. Achalasia cardia

(AIIMS 1991, AI 2001)

TYPES OF TRACHEOESOPHAGEAL FISTULA	INCIDENCE
• Lower segment communicates with trachea and upper end blind	85%
• Both end blind	12%
• Upper end communicates with trachea	2%
• Both ends communicate with trachea	1%

Clinical features are that the newborn regurgitates 1st and every feed. Saliva pours continuously from his/her mouth. This is pathognomic of esophageal atresia and *does not* occur in any other condition.

86. Hair on end appearance on skull X-ray and greatly expanded diploë is seen in:

A. Meningioma
B. Multiple myeloma
C. Congenital hemolytic anemia
D. Paget's disease

(AIIMS 1991, 1997)

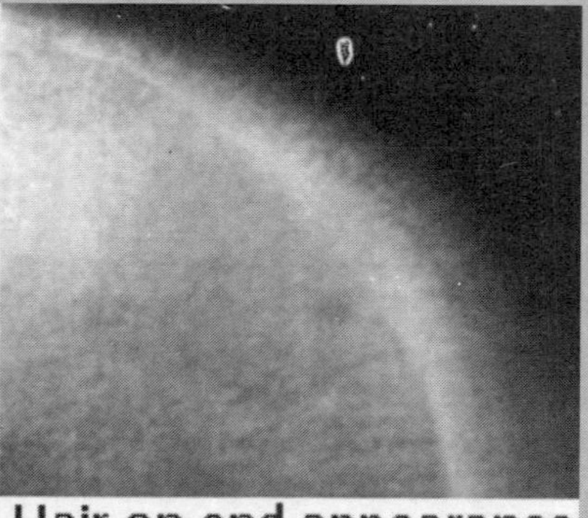

Hair on end appearance

In **congenital hemolytic anemia** such as thalassemia major (Cooley's anemia) the vault is greatly thickened and has the typical "**hair-on-end**" appearance. CT scan demonstrates the thickening with very little inner or outer table bone due to the greatly expanded erythropoietic diploë.

87. Which of the following is *not* treated by steroids:

A. MPGN | B. Membranous glomerulonephritis
C. Focal segmental glomerulonephritis | D. Lupus glomerulonephritis *(AIIMS 1991)*

The general outcome of all types of **Membranoproliferative glomerulonephritis** is poor. **No definite therapy exists.** Although complete recovery has been sometimes reported, most patient progress to end stage renal disease (ESRD).

88. In children, Cushing syndrome is *best* diagnosed by:

A. Steroid assay | B. Dexamethasone suppression test
C. CT scan | D. ACTH level *(AIIMS 1991)*

Cortisol levels in the blood are measured to diagnose **Cushing syndrome.** They are normally elevated at 8 am and decrease to less than 50% at 8 pm except in children less than 3 years of age in whom diurnal rhythm has not been established. In patients of Cushing syndrome this diurnal rhythm is lost and **cortisol levels at 8 pm are elevated.**

89. In hypothyroidism which of the following appears first:

A. Decreased BMR | B. Decreased T3
C. Increased TSH | D. Delayed ankle jerk *(AI 1991)*

90. Congenital hypothyroidism is diagnosed *earliest* by which of the following:

A. Decreased T3 level in blood
B. Increased TSH level in blood
C. Increased radioactive iodine uptake
D. Protein bound iodine estimation in blood *(AIIMS 1991)*

Causes and Incidence of Congenital Hypothyroidism

Cause	Incidence
• Thyroid dysgenesis	1 in 4000 (most common cause)
• TBG deficiency	1 in 5000
• Thyroid hormone synthesis defects	1 in 30,000
• Hypothalamic pituitary hypothyroidism	1 in 50,000
• Hypothyroxinemia	1 in 1,00,000

Newborn screening for congenital hypothyroidism is routinely done in developed countries and a spot T4 measurement is the method of choice. **TSH estimation** is done in cases with low T4 value to confirm the diagnosis.

91. *Not* a causative agent of lung abscess:

A. *Entamoeba histolytica* | B. *Pneumococcus*
C. *Staphylococcus* | D. *Klebsiella* *(AI 1991)*

Common Causes of Lung Abscess in Children

- Bacteroides
- *Fusobacterium*
- Anaerobic *streptococci*
- *Staphylococcus aureus*
- *Klebsiella*
- *Entamoeba histolytica*
- Nocardia
- Actinomyces
- *Mycobacterium*

92. Long-standing unconjugated hyperbilirubinemia of newborn is *not* caused by:
A. Crigler-Najjar syndrome **B.** Cretinism
C. Septicemia **D.** Breast milk jaundice *(AIIMS 1991)*

93. Which of the following conditions is *not* associated with prolonged *unconjugated* hyperbilirubinemia in a newborn:
A. Breast milk jaundice **B.** Hypothyroidism
C. Septicemia **D.** Crigler-Najjar syndrome *(UP 1993)*

Causes of Persistent Neonatal Jaundice

Unconjugated hyperbilirubinemia	Conjugated hyperbilirubinemia
• Breast milk jaundice	• Neonatal hepatitis
• Hypothyroidism	• Extrahepatic biliary atresia
• Crigler Najjar syndrome	• Inborn errors of metabolism
• Intestinal obstruction or stasis	• Total parenteral nutrition
• ABO or Rh incompatibility	

Neonatal jaundice which may be physiological or pathological usually disappears by 2 weeks of age. If it persists beyond this age it is known as **persistent neonatal jaundice**.

94. Wilms' tumor is *not* associated with:
A. Beckwith syndrome **B.** Aniridia
C. Polycystic kidney **D.** Hemihypertrophy *(AI 1991, 1994, AIIMS 1997)*

95. *False* regarding Wilms' tumor is:
A. Derived from renal blastema **B.** Always associated with hematuria
C. Fever may be present **D.** Abdominal mass present *(AI 1991)*

Wilms' tumor or nephroblastoma is a childhood tumor derived from **renal blastema** made up of mixture of primitive renal epithelial and stromal elements along with heterologous tissues. In children Wilms' tumor accounts for almost all the renal neoplasms and it is diagnosed at a median age of 3 years. It is associated with congenital anomalies in 13% of patients. The most common associations are genitourinary abnormalities (5-7%), **hemihypertrophy** (3%) and **sporadic aniridia** (2%). Less frequently associated abnormalities are:

Syndrome of pseudohermaphroditism and nephropathy	
Beckwith-Wiedemann syndrome	Macroglossia, gigantism and umbilical hernia
Klippel-Trenaunay syndrome	Hemangiomas and lower extremity hypertrophy
Translocation involving B and C group chromosomes	

Tumor is bilateral in 5-13% of cases and metastasizes most frequently to the lungs (80%). Most frequent clinical sign is an **abdominal mass** (95%). Mass is smooth and firm and rarely crosses the midline. 50% of children have additional symptoms such as abdominal pain, vomiting or **fever**. Hypertension is seen in 30-60% of cases due to increased renin level caused by renal ischemia. Polycythemia, Cushing syndrome and symptomatic hypoglycemia may occur due to paraneoplastic syndromes.

96. Koplik's spots are pathognomic of:
A. Chickenpox **B.** Typhoid
C. Rubeola **D.** Rubella *(AI 1992)*

97. Which of the following is *false* regarding measles:
A. Koplik's spots
B. Incubation period 20-22 days
C. Sequence of appearance of rash is characteristic
D. Caused by paramyxovirus *(UP 1999)*

Measles or rubeola is an acute highly infectious disease of children caused by a specific **RNA paramyxovirus.** Incubation period is commonly 10 days from exposure to onset of fever and 14 days from exposure to appearance of rash. Prodromal stage begins 10 days after the exposure and lasts until 14th day. It is characterized by fever, sneezing, and nasal discharge, and cough, redness of eyes, lacrimation and photophobia. A day or two before appearance of rash, **Koplik's spots appear in the buccal mucosa opposite the first and second upper molar. These are pathognomic of measles.** Eruptive phase is characterized by a typical red macular and maculopapular rash which starts from behind the ears and spreads rapidly in a few hours to the face and neck. Thereafter it extends down the body and reaches lower extremities in 3 days. It may remain discrete but it often becomes confluent.

98. *Not* a feature of Wilson's disease in children:

A. Hemolytic anemia
B. Chronic active hepatitis
C. Fanconi syndrome
D. Sensory changes

(AIIMS 1991)

Wilson's disease is an inherited disorder of copper metabolism leading to impairment of the normal excretion of hepatic copper. This results in toxic accumulations of the metal in liver, brain, and other organs. Wilson's disease should be considered in any patient under the age of 40 with:

• UNEXPLAINED DISORDER OF THE CNS	• CHRONIC ACTIVE HEPATITIS
• UNEXPLAINED PERSISTENT ELEVATIONS OF SGPT	• HEMOLYTIC ANEMIA IN THE PRESENCE OF HEPATITIS
• UNEXPLAINED CIRRHOSIS	• FAMILY HISTORY OF WILSON'S DISEASE

***Sensory changes, except headache, never occur**. Hematuria, proteinuria, Fanconi syndrome and renal tubular acidosis may rarely be seen due to copper accumulation in kidney.

99. *Not* included in apgar score in neonates:

A. Color
B. Muscle tone
C. Respiratory rate
D. Heart rate

(AIIMS 1997, AI 2001)

100. Calculate the apgar score of a newborn with heart rate 110, good cry, blue extremities, active movement and grimace:

A. 9
B. 8
C. 6
D. 4

(AIIMS 1991)

Apgar score	**0**	**1**	**2**
Heart rate	Nil	Less than 100	More than 100
Color	**Blue**	**Pink** but extremities **blue**	**Pink**
Tone	Limp	Flexion of extremities	Active movement
Response to catheter in nostril	No response	Grimace	Cough or sneeze
Respiratory effort	Absent	Slow irregular	Good crying

*It is a quantitative rating test with a maximum score of 10 used to measure the vital signs of a newborn a minute or so after birth: a score greater than 7 signifies good health and less than 3 indicates need of urgent resuscitation.

• Heart rate 110	2
• Good cry	2
• Blue extremities	1
• Active movement	2
• Grimace	1
Total score	8

101. Isolation period of mumps is until:

A. Headache subsides
B. Swelling subsides
C. Pain subsides
D. Fever subsides

(KERALA 1994)

102. Which of the following is *false* regarding mumps:

A. Swelling persists for 3-7 days
B. Incubation period is of 2-3 weeks
C. Unilateral swelling is common
D. Painful parotid swelling

(AI 1992)

103. In children which of the following is the *most common* complication of mumps:

A. Aseptic meningitis
B. Otitis media
C. Myocarditis
D. Orchitis

(AIIMS 1991, 1994)

The virus is present in nasopharynx for a period extending from 2 days before the onset of symptoms to the 2 days after the onset of symptoms AND ISOLATION IS RECOMMENDED UNTIL SWELLING SUBSIDES. Incubation period of mumps is 2-3 weeks, usually 18 days. It is characterized by pain and swelling in either one or both the parotid glands. Swelling slowly subsides within 3-7 days. Parotitis is generally BILATERAL, although the onset on the two sides may not be synchronous and at times only one side is affected. THE MOST COMMON COMPLICATION OF MUMPS IN CHILDREN IS ASEPTIC MENINGITIS. It may develop before, during, after, or in the absence of parotitis. Symptoms are stiff neck, headache, and drowsiness. Pleocytosis of the cerebrospinal fluid, with up to 1000 cells/microliter, develop in up to half of the cases, but clinical signs of meningeal irritation are seen in only 5 - 25 % of patients.

104. Cardiac anomaly *commonly* seen in congenital rubella is:

A. TOF
B. ASD
C. PDA
D. VSD

(AIIMS 1992, AI 1993, 1996)

105. All are associated with congenital rubella *except*:

A. Pulmonary stenosis
B. Patent ductus arteriosus
C. ASD
D. VSD

(AIIMS 1991)

Common Features of Congenital Rubella Syndrome

Cardiac features	Extracardiac features
Patent ductus arteriosus (most common)	Cataracts
Pulmonary stenosis and/or arterial stenosis	Deafness
Atrial septal defect	Microcephaly

106. In which of the following diseases *Saber-shaped tibia* is seen:

A. Renal osteodystrophy
B. Gonorrhoea
C. Rickets
D. Congenital syphilis

(AIIMS 1991)

Saber-shaped tibia is the deformity of the tibia caused by gummatous periostitis due to **syphilis,** in which it curves outward.

Saber means a heavy cavalry sword with a slightly curved blade.

107. Which of the following is *not* beneficial in the management of acute attack of bronchial asthma in children:

A. IV hydrocortisone
B. Sodium cromoglycate nebulisation
C. High concentration of oxygen
D. Salbutamol nebulisation

(AI 1991, UP 1993)

Management of Severe Acute Asthma

1. Oxygen by mask @ 5 liter / minute to achieve oxygen saturation of > 90%.
2. **Nebulised Salbutamol** 0.15 mg / kg / dose. (minimum 2.5 mg)—Asthalin respirator solution 5 mg / ml every 20 minutes for 3 doses, diluted in normal saline with oxygen @ 6 liter / minute.
3. Hydrocortisone 10 mg / kg (IV) followed by oral wysolone 2 mg / kg / day.

*Sodium cromoglycate is used for long-term management of asthma and is of no use during an acute attack.

108. Pneumatoceles are commonly associated with:

A. Viral pneumonia
B. *Klebsiella* pneumonia
C. Staphylococcal pneumonia
D. Pneumococcal pneumonia *(AIIMS 1991, AI 1996, 1998)*

Empyema, pyopneumothorax and pneumatocele formation are common complication of *Staphylococcal pneumonia.* However *Staphylococcus, Klebsiella, Haemophilus influenzae* and pneumococcal pneumonia may also be associated with pneumatocele formation.

109. Which of the following is the *most common* cause of empyema in children *less than* 2 years of age:

A. *Pseudomonas*
B. *Staphylococcus*
C. *Escherichia coli*
D. Pneumococcus *(AIIMS 1991, AIIMS 1993)*

Empyema or purulent pleurisy is an accumulation of pus in pleural cavity. Most common cause is *pneumonia* caused by *Staphylococcus aureus.* Less frequently pneumococci or *Haemophilus influenzae* may also cause empyema.

110. Which of the following shows the *most* specific finding in pediatric age with nutritional/malabsorption state:

A. Malnutrition
B. Giardiasis
C. Abetalipoproteinemia
D. Tropical sprue *(UP 2000)*

Abetalipoproteinemia /Acanthocytosis/Bassen-Kornzweig syndrome is a rare, autosomal recessive disorder in which the microsomal triglyceride transfer protein is absent because of mutations in the MTP gene. Patients have total cholesterol levels <50 mg/dL and virtually no VLDL, IDL, LDL, or chylomicrons. Because dietary fat as well as vitamins A and E are transported from the intestine in chylomicrons, these patients have malabsorption of fat and fat-soluble vitamins. Vitamin E deficiency results in neurologic problems. If vitamin replacement is adequate patients can lead normal life. **Lipid droplets can be seen in intestinal mucosal cells obtained by peroral biopsy which is pathognomic for this disease.**

111. *Most common* cause of convulsion in a newborn on *first day* of life is:

A. Head injury
B. Anoxia
C. Hypoglycemia
D. Hypocalcemia *(AI 1992)*

Causes of Seizure on First Day of Life

• Birth asphyxia (**most common**)	• Intraventricular hemorrhage
• Narcotic withdrawal	• Pyridoxine dependency
• Hypoglycemia	• Hypocalcemia
• Accidental injection of lignocaine	• Inborn errors of metabolism such as PKU, maple serum urine disease, homocystinuria

112. *Not* a feature of necrotizing enterocolitis:

A. Abdominal distention
B. Blood in stool
C. Bilious vomiting
D. Increased bowel sound *(AI 1992)*

Feature of Necrotizing Enterocolitis

THE SYSTEMIC SIGNS	THE ABDOMINAL SIGNS
• Respiratory distress	• Abdominal distention
• Apnea	• Vomiting
• Bradycardia	• Paralytic ileus
• Lethargy	• Erythema of abdominal wall
• Temperature instability	• Bloody stools
• Poor feeding	• Abdominal mass
• Shock	• Ascites
• Bleeding	• Abdominal tenderness

113. Which of the following is *not* seen in congenital rubella syndrome:

A. PDA **B.** Deafness
C. Aortic stenosis **D.** Mental retardation *(AI 2002)*

Maternal infection with rubella in *early* pregnancy can lead to fetal infection. CONGENITAL RUBELLA SYNDROME (CRS) consists of triad of cataracts, sensorineural deafness and congenital heart disease. *Most common* cardiac defects are patent ductus arteriosus and pulmonary stenosis. Psychomotor retardation is seen in 62% of cases. Other abnormalities include:

TRANSIENT	PERMANENT	DEVELOPMENTAL
LOW BIRTH WEIGHT	DEAFNESS	MENTAL RETARDATION
THROMBOCYTOPENIA	PULMONARY STENOSIS	DIABETES MELLITUS
HEPATOSPLENOMEGALY	PATENT DUCTUS ARTERIOSUS	BEHAVIORAL DISORDERS
JAUNDICE	GLAUCOMA	
PNEUMONIA	CATARACT	

The most important factor in the pathogenicity of rubella virus for the fetus is gestational age at the time of infection. Maternal infection during the 1st trimester causes fetal infection in nearly half of the cases, while the maternal infection early in the 2nd trimester leads to fetal infection in 1/3rd of cases. Fetal malformations are more common after maternal infection in the 1st trimester and are more severe and they involve more organ systems.

114. Pincer grasp develops by........ months:

A. 5-7 **B.** 9-12
C. 8-9 **D.** 12-24 *(UP 1999)*

Pincer finger thumb grasp develops around the age of 9 months. It is used to pick up small objects.

115. Cyanosis with plethora is *not* seen in:

A. Transposition of great vessels
B. Total anomalous pulmonary damage
C. Ebstein anomaly
D. TOF *(AIIMS 1991)*

Tetralogy of Fallot is the most common cyanotic congenital heart disease. There is diminished pulmonary vascularity in chest X-ray due to pulmonary stenosis.

116. In children suprasellar calcification suggests:

A. Meningioma
B. Neuroblastoma
C. Craniopharyngioma
D. Glioma *(AI 1992, AIIMS 1996, AI 1997)*

Suprasellar calcification in a flocculent, granular, or curvilinear pattern is present on skull x-rays in most children and in some adults with CRANIOPHARYNGIOMA.
Craniopharyngiomas are benign, slow growing neoplasms which represent 6% of intracranial neoplasms in children, and 3% of intracranial neoplasms in general. **The classic CT findings are sellar or suprasellar mass with calcification**, cyst formation, and enhancement. CT detects calcification in 80% of pediatric cases and 40% of adults.

117. *Not* a characteristic feature of infantile pyloric stenosis:
A. More common in male child **B.** Vomiting at birth
C. Visible peristalsis **D.** Presence of lump *(AIIMS 1991)*

Hypertrophic pyloric stenosis is the *most common* cause of upper GI obstruction of the young infant. It is **more common in males** and **develops usually between the 3rd and 6th weeks of life**. The clinical features of non-bilious projectile vomiting, **visible gastric peristaltic waves**, and a **palpable pyloric mass** are diagnostic. The radiological findings are confirmatory and consist of gastric dilatation with a deficiency of small-bowel gas. Ultrasound examination is the diagnostic investigation of choice for hypertrophic pyloric stenosis. Ramstedt's operation is the treatment of choice.

118. Which of the following is the *treatment of choice* in infantile myoclonus:
A. Clonazepam **B.** Phenytoin
C. Phenobarbitone **D.** ACTH *(AI 1992)*

Infantile myoclonic seizure is also known as infantile spasm or lightning major or jack knife epilepsy. They occur below 2 years of age and involve more than one group of muscles. Most common type constitutes a sudden dropping of head and flexion of arms. EEG shows random high voltage slow waves and spikes (hypsarrhythmia). Therapeutic trial with **ACTH**, corticosteroids, or pyridoxine is indicated.

119. *Most common* cause of ambiguous genitalia in children is:
A. Mixed gonadal dysgenesis
B. 21-hydroxylase deficiency
C. Klinefelter syndrome
D. Testicular feminization *(AI 1992)*

Congenital adrenal hyperplasia due to **21-hydroxylase deficiency** is the most common cause of ambiguous genitalia in the newborn.

120. *False* regarding systemic juvenile rheumatoid arthritis is:
A. Rheumatoid factor positive **B.** Leukocytosis
C. Hepatosplenomegaly **D.** Fever *(AI 1998, 2000)*

121. Which of the following types of juvenile rheumatoid arthritis is associated with iridocyclitis:
A. Rheumatoid factor +ve **B.** Systemic
C. Pauciarticular **D.** Polyarticular *(AI 1991)*

JRA	Systemic	Polyarticular RF -ve	Polyarticular RF +ve	Pauciarticular Type I	Pauciarticular Type II
Percentage	20%	25%	10%	30%	15%
Sacroiliitis	No	No	Rare	No	Common
Iridocyclitis	No	Rare	No	50% chronic	20% acute
Rheumatoid factor	Negative	Negative	100%	Negative	Negative
ANA	Negative	25%	75%	60%	Negative
Boys/girls	60% boys	90% girls	80% girls	80% girls	90% boys

122. Which of the following is the *most common* complication of amebic liver abscess in children:

A. Secondary infection
B. Rupture into peritoneal cavity
C. Recurrence
D. Rupture into right lung

(AI 1991)

Most common complication of amebic liver abscess in children is **rupture into peritoneum.**

123. In kwashiorkor the diagnosis is based on which of the following:

A. Edema and mental changes
B. Edema and skin changes
C. Bitot's spots and hepatomegaly
D. Weight loss and mental changes

(AI 1991)

Diagnostic Criteria of Kwashiorkor

Essential criteria	Nonessential criteria
Growth retardation	Hair changes, skin changes, mineral and vitamin deficiency
Muscle wasting with retention of subcutaneous fat	Hepatomegaly, clubbing and non specific ECG changes
Psychomotor changes such as **mental** apathy and lack of interest in surroundings	Diarrhea, vomiting, anorexia
Hypoalbuminemic pitting **edema** with serum albumin less than 2.5 gm/dL	Superadded infections such as tuberculosis, bronchopneumonia, pyoderma etc

124. *False* negative tuberculin reaction *does not* occur in children in which of the following condition:

A. Atypical mycobacteria
B. 4-6 weeks following measles
C. Patient on corticosteroid therapy
D. Very severely malnourished child

(UP 1993)

A positive tuberculin test (induration of 10 mm or more) indicates the presence of tuberculous infection or disease. *However*, a negative tuberculin test does not exclude tuberculosis because it is negative in children with tuberculosis, who are immunocompromised due to severe PEM, drugs such as corticosteroids or post-measles state. Tuberculin test cross-reacts with atypical mycobacteria.

125. In children which of the following is *not* used in treatment of asthma:

A. Sedatives
B. Salbutamol
C. Adrenaline
D. Steroids

(AI 1992, AIIMS 1997)

Management of Acute Asthma

1. Adrenaline (1 in 10,000)—0.1 ml/kg subcutaneous stat. Up to 3 doses can be used at 20 minutes interval.
2. Nebulised salbutamol is a better alternative of adrenaline.
3. Injection hydrocortisone 10 mg/kg/dose.
4. Oxygen inhalation.

*Sedatives are contraindicated

126. A newborn exclusive fed with goat's milk will develop which of the following diseases as compared to being fed with breast milk:

A. Megaloblastic anemia
B. Microcytic anemia
C. Rickets
D. Scurvy

(SGPGI 2002)

Cows and human milk are relatively poor sources of folic acid but contain enough foliate to prevent nutritional deficiency. However **goat's milk is a poor source of foliate and may cause megaloblastic anemia.**

127. Cerebrospinal fluid examination of a one day old term male baby reveals a cell count of 10RBCs/HPF, sugar 45 mg/dL and protein 40 mg/dL. *Most likely* diagnosis is:

A. Hypoglycemia **B.** Intracranial bleed
C. Meningitis **D.** None of the above *(KARNATAKA 2000)*

Normally the CSF contains no RBC and at the most 5 leukocytes/cubic mm *except* in newborns in which up to 500 RBCs and up to 15 leukocytes/cubic mm, including granulocytes, are insignificant. Normal protein and sugar contents of CSF are given below in the table.

Appearance	Pressure	Cells	Protein	Sugar
Watery	100-180 mm of CSF	0-5 all lymphocytes	20-40 mg%	40-80 mg%

128. In which of the following ossification centre appears *first*:

A. Upper end of tibia **B.** Femur
C. Talus **D.** Ossicles *(UP 1995)*

Malleus	With exception of its anterior process, it is ossified from a single endochondral ossification centre which appears near the neck of bone in 4th month of fetal life.
Incus	4th month of fetal life
Stapes	4th month of fetal life
Talus	6th month of fetal life
Femur	Begins in the middle of the shaft in the 7th month of fetal life
Upper end of tibia	At birth

129. Which of the following is a *live* attenuated vaccine:

A. ATS **B.** Salk
C. BCG **D.** DPT *(KARNATAKA 2000)*

Disease	Vaccine
Anthrax	Inactivated a virulent bacteria
Tuberculosis (BCG)	**Living bacteria** (attenuated *Mycobacterium bovis*)
Hepatitis A	Killed virus antigen
Cholera	Inactivated bacteria
Meningococcal A, C, Y, W135	Bacterial polysaccharide of 4 serotypes
Plague	Inactivated bacteria
Rabies (human diploid)	Inactivated virus
Yellow fever	**Live attenuated vaccine**
Japanese encephalitis	Inactivated virus
Typhoid	
Phenol and heat-killed Ty_{21a} Vi	Killed whole bacteria Live mutant bacteria Vi capsular polysaccharide
Polio	Salk polio vaccine contains all 3 types of poliovirus inactivated by formalin Sabin OPV is **live** vaccine

130. Which of the following is *true* regarding neonatal herpes:

A. Spontaneous recovery occurs **B.** Caused by HSV II
C. Hepatosplenomegaly is diagnostic **D.** All are correct *(PGI 2000)*

There are two types of Herpes simplex viruses, type 1 and 2. HSV-2 is the predominant cause of neonatal disease (80%).

131. A child has pedal edema ++, facial edema. His blood pressure is 190/110. He has gross hematuria but ascites is absent. He is suffering from:

A. CRF | **B.** Renal vein thrombosis
C. Nephrotic syndrome | **D.** Acute glomerulonephritis *(PGI 2000)*

Acute nephritic syndrome presents as sudden onset, hematuria which may be microscopic or macroscopic, oliguria and edema. Majority of cases in pediatric population are due to post-streptococcal glomerulonephritis. This condition follows a throat or skin infection with nephritogenic group A β streptococcal infection. Common strains for pharyngitis are type 12 and 25 while type 49 is associated with pyoderma. 10-21 days after such episode the child, generally between 3 and 12 years of age presents with hematuria, edema, hypertension and oliguria. Proteinuria is often in the range of 2+ or 3+. Facial edema usually precedes hematuria. Pleural effusion or ascites may occur. Treatment consists of salt and fluid restriction and protein restriction to about 0.6 gm/kg/day. A course of procaine penicillin 50000 IU/kg/day IM OD for 10 days should be given to eradicate the streptococci. Diuretics are used to control edema while nifedipine or atenolol or enalapril is used to control hypertension.

132. For a 2-year-old child calories as supplied in ICDS diet are:

A. 1000 Kcal | **B.** 500-600 Kcal
C. 300-400 Kcal | **D.** 200 Kcal *(SGPGI 2002)*

Under Integrated Child Development Services program (ICDS) 300-400 Kcal are to be provided per day. Children are also administered 200000 IU of vitamin A at 6 months.

133. *False* regarding sacral myelomeningocele is:

A. Lax anal sphincter is seen | **B.** Bladder incontinence
C. Hydrocephalus | **D.** Spasticity is a feature of lower limb *(AI 1995)*

134. *False* regarding myelomeningocele in children is:

A. Absent hydrocephalus | **B.** Fecal and urinary incontinence
C. Areflexic paraparesis | **D.** Neural tube defect *(UP 2001)*

NEURAL TUBE DEFECTS or dysraphism constitute a group of congenital abnormalities of CNS due to failure of neural tube to close spontaneously. **Myelomeningocele constitutes the most severe form of dysraphism.** Folic acid deficiency is believed to play a role in its etiology. There is a sac like cystic midline swelling present on the back which is covered by a thin membrane. It may be located anywhere along the neural axis but 3/4th of them are present in lumbosacral region. There is variable degree of **LOWER MOTOR NEURON PARALYSIS OF LOWER EXTREMITIES** along with sensory loss in perineal area and lower limbs. **FECAL AND URINARY INCONTINENCE** may occur due to neurogenic bladder and bowel. **HYDROCEPHALUS**, CTEV and congenital dislocation of hip (CDH) may be associated with this condition.

135. Zinc deficiency causes:

A. Hypogonadism | **B.** Impaired glucose tolerance
C. Cardiomyopathy | **D.** Tetany *(AI 1996)*

Common Feature of Zinc Deficiency

• Growth retardation	• Diarrhea
• Alopecia	• Immunologic dysfunction
• Dermatitis	• Failure to thrive
• Psychological disturbances	• **Gonadal atrophy**
• Impaired spermatogenesis	• Congenital malformations

136. A 2-year-old child presented with respiratory distress. On examination there is wheezing. *Most likely* diagnosis is:
A. RSV infection
B. Severe pneumonia
C. Adenovirus
D. Rhinovirus
(AIIMS 2000)

137. In bronchiolitis, the treatment of choice is:
A. Zidovudine
B. Vidarabine
C. Amantidine
D. Ribavirin
(AI 1996)

Bronchiolitis is defined as ***first*** *episode of* ***expiratory wheezing*** *which is of* ***acute onset*** *in a* ***child less than 2 years*** *of age who has features of viral respiratory illness such as coryza, otitis media* ***or*** *fever with or without respiratory distress, pneumonia or atopy.* **RSV is the etiological agent in about 60% of cases** although other viruses such as parainfluenza 1 and 2, adenovirus, rhinovirus may also cause this disease. The child is tachypneic with respiratory rate between 60 to 80 per minute. Cyanoses may or may not be present. Management consists of humidified oxygen, bronchodilators and other supportive measures. **Ribavirin,** a synthetic nucleoside analogue that inhibits a wide range of RNA and DNA viruses, reduces the severity of disease and shortens the hospital stay if given early in the course of disease. Ribavirin inhalation solution should be administered using the Viratek SPAG Model SPAG-2 only. This is done by attaching an infant oxygen hood to the SPAG-2 aerosol generator.

138. *Not* a complication of chickenpox:
A. Enteritis
B. Pneumonia
C. Encephalitis
D. Reye syndrome
(AI 1993)

139. Which of the following is the *most common* complication of chickenpox:
A. Diarrhea
B. Encephalitis
C. Secondary bacterial infection
D. Pneumonia
(PGI 2000)

Most common complication of chickenpox is secondary bacterial infection of skin lesions while the most common CNS complication is postinfectious encephalitis. In about 10% of cases, Reye syndrome is associated with chickenpox. Other complications of chickenpox are as under:

• Varicella pneumonia	• Purpura fulminans
• Thrombocytopenia	• Myocarditis
• Pericarditis	• Endocarditis
• Hepatitis	• Glomerulonephritis
• Arthritis	• Acute myositis
• Keratitis	• Vesicular conjunctivitis
• GB syndrome	• Transverse myelitis
• 7th nerve palsy	• Optic neuritis
• Hypothalamic syndrome	• Ataxia, nystagmus, tremors

140. Which of the following is *true* regarding Klinefelter syndrome:
A. Breast adenoma
B. Subnormal intelligence
C. Pituitary adenoma
D. Short stature
(AI 1996, 1998)

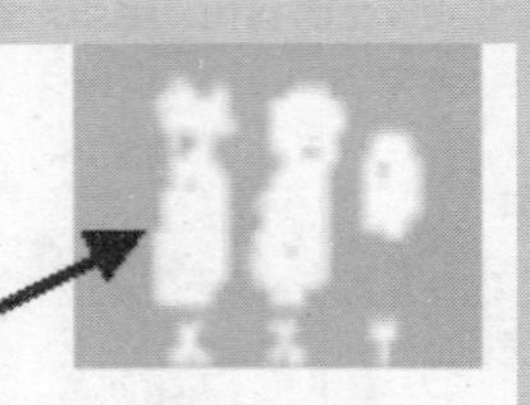

KLINEFELTER SYNDROME has an incidence of 1 in 500 males. It occurs when a male inherits an extra X-chromosome (**47 XXY**) that interferes with the development of male characteristics. American endocrinologist Harry F. Klinefelter first described this disorder in 1942. Features of this syndrome are as under:

• HISTOLOGIC EVIDENCE OF IMPAIRED SPERMIOGENESIS	• SMALL TESTES
• AZOOSPERMIA	• GYNECOMASTIA
• DECREASED FACIAL HAIR	• DECREASED PUBIC HAIR
• DECREASED PENILE SIZE	• DECREASED LIBIDO OR POTENCY
• DECREASED TESTOSTERONE (PLASMA)	• INCREASED GONADOTROPINS (URINE AND PLASMA)
• MILD MENTAL DEFICIENCY	• The risk of breast cancer is 20 times that of normal men, but only about a fifth that in women.

141. In which of the following syndromes nuchal fold thickness is increased:
A. Paul Bunnel syndrome **B.** Cri du chat syndrome
C. Turner syndrome **D.** Down syndrome *(SGPGI 1999, AI 1999, UP 2000)*

Prenatal diagnosis of Down syndrome:
Ultrasound (11-20 weeks) nuchal fold >4 mm, double bubble in abdomen, short femur, clinodactytly and macroglossia.

142. Which of the following is the characteristic feature of fragile X syndrome:
A. Large testis **B.** Large nose
C. Large eyes **D.** Long face *(UP 2000)*

Fragile X syndrome: It is a condition caused by an X-linked mutation associated with a fragile site near the tip of the long arm of the X chromosome. Most males and 30% of females with this syndrome are mentally retarded. This syndrome is the **most common inherited cause of mental retardation**. **Males develop greatly enlarged testicles (macro-orchidism)** usually after puberty, but this change has been reported as early as 5 months of age along with large head and ears.

143. *Not* seen in neonatal septicemia:
A. Band-neutrophils **B.** Increased ESR
C. Increased CRP **D.** Leukocytosis *(AI 1996)*

For diagnosis of neonatal sepsis the following 5 criteria are used (Philip criteria):	
TLC < 5000	Band-neutrophil ratio 0.2 or more
Positive C reactive protein	Elevated haptoglobin
ESR 15 mm or more in 1st hour	
If all the **five** are normal then the *probability* is that infection is absent (99% accuracy). If 3 of the 5 tests are abnormal then *probability* of infection is 90%.	

144. IUGR is *not* caused by:
A. CRF **B.** Diabetes
C. Smoking **D.** Alcohol *(AIIMS 1991)*

Common Causes of IUGR

Fetal factors	Placental factors	Maternal factors
Chromosomal disorders Such as autosomal trisomies	Decreased placental weight or cellularity or both	Toxemia
Chronic fetal infections such as CMV inclusion disease, congenital rubella, syphilis	Decrease in surface area	Hypertensive or renal disease or both
Familial dysautonomia	Villous placentitis (bacterial, viral or parasitic)	Hypoxemia (high altitude, cyanotic cardiac or pulmonary disease)
Radiation injury	Chorioangioma Hydatidiform mole	Sickle cell anemia
Multiple gestation	Placental separation	Narcotics, cigarettes
Pancreatic aplasia	Twin transfusion syndrome	Alcohol
	Localized transfer lesion	Antimetabolites

145. Phenytoin is *not* used for which of the following conditions:
A. Focal cortical epilepsy
B. Psychomotor epilepsy
C. Petit mal epilepsy
D. Grand mal epilepsy
(UP 1995)

Indication of Phenytoin

• Grand mal epilepsy	• Trigeminal neuralgia
• Status epilepticus	• Cardiac arrhythmias (digitalis induced)
• Partial (focal) seizure	

146. In vitamin A deficiency X3A means:
A. Corneal scar
B. Corneal ulcer
C. Corneal xerosis
D. Conjuctival xerosis
(UP 1995)

Classification of Vitamin A Deficiency

Classification	Primary Signs
X 1A	Conjuctival xerosis
X 1B	Bitot's spots
X 2	Corneal xerosis
X 3A	Corneal ulceration
X 3B	Keratomalasia
	Secondary signs
X N	Night blindness
X F	Fundal changes
X S	Corneal scarring

TREATMENT GUIDELINES—According to the WHO guideline 2 lakhs I.U. of vitamin-A should be given orally on presentation and on the following day. A third dose is recommended on 28th day. Half dose is given if the child is less than 12 months and 1/4th if less than 6 months. For IM route half of the oral dose is recommended.

147. Diarrhea in children is *most commonly* caused by:
A. *Pneumococcus*
B. Rotavirus
C. *Escherichia coli*
D. Vibrio cholerae
(AI 1995)

Rotaviruses belong to the family Reoviridae. Each virion consists of a 100 nm triple-shelled icosahedral capsid surrounding a genome composed of 11 segments of double-stranded RNA. **Rotaviruses are the most important cause of acute diarrheal disease with severe dehydration in infants and young children and account for up to 50 percent of all cases** of diarrhea requiring hospitalization and intravenous fluid therapy. Rotavirus infects and kills the mature villus tip cells of the small intestine. The mature epithelial cells are replaced by immature absorptive cells that cannot absorb carbohydrates or other nutrients *efficiently*. Therefore rotavirus infection leads to osmotic diarrhea due to nutrient malabsorption. By the age of 3 years, almost every individual has been infected by rotaviruses at least once.

148. Neonatal jaundice at birth or before 24 hours is commonly due to:

A. Physiological
B. Biliary atresia
C. Congenital hyperbilirubinemia
D. Erythroblastosis *(AI 1995)*

Jaundice occurring before age 24 hours is generally considered "pathologic" and requires further evaluation. Although some healthy infants appear slightly jaundiced by 24 hours, the presence of jaundice before 24 hours requires (at least) a serum bilirubin measurement. If indicated, further evaluation for possible hemolytic disease or other diseases should be done. Phototherapy and/or exchange transfusion may be indicated for rapidly rising TSB levels in the first 24 hours of life. **Jaundice within 24 hour of life is due to erythroblastosis fetalis until proved otherwise.**

149. Defective hepatic conjugation is *not* seen in:

A. Novobiocin therapy
B. Crigler Najjar syndrome
C. Gilbert's syndrome
D. Neonatal jaundice *(AI 1996)*

Novobiocin and some cholecystographic dyes interfere in bilirubin uptake.

150. *False* regarding childhood ITP is:

A. Splenectomy for chronic case
B. Decreased bone marrow megakaryocytes
C. Preceding viral infection
D. Prolonged bleeding time *(AIIMS 1992)*

Idiopathic thrombocytopenic purpura is an autoimmune disorder. It is of 3 types:

1. Acute ITP
2. Chronic ITP
3. Relapsing ITP

In 70% of cases there is a history of rubella, rubeola or viral respiratory infection about 2 weeks before the onset of purpura. The disease begins with development of petechiae, ecchymosis and easy bruising. These are features of reduced platelet count. In pediatric age group boys and girls are equally affected unlike in adults where women are 5 times more commonly affected. Severe manifestations include hematuria, GI bleeding and epistaxis. Thrombocytopenia is the only abnormality found in CBC. Bleeding time is prolonged. **Bone marrow examination reveals normal or increased number of megakaryocytes.** Steroids are the drug of choice and prednisolone should be given in a dose of 2mg/kg/day for 2 weeks and then tapered in another 2 weeks. Splenectomy should be done if the child continues to bleed despite treatment with steroids and IV IgG.

151. Microcytic, hypochromic anemia is *not* seen in:

A. Beta thalassemia
B. CRF
C. Iron deficiency anemia
D. Lead poisoning *(AI 1991)*

Anemia of renal disease is typically a normocytic, normochromic anemia with a low reticulocyte production index.

DIFFERENTIAL DIAGNOSIS BASED ON GBP FOR MICROCYTIC ANEMIA	
Iron deficiency	Microcytic hypochromic
Thalassemia	Microcytic hypochromic with target cells
Sideroblastic anemia	Variable

Lead poisoning can produce anemia with impaired hemoglobin formation and ringed sideroblasts (SIDEROBLASTIC ANEMIA). Chronic or repeated malarial infections cause hypergammaglobulinemia and normochromic, normocytic anemia.

152. Unconjugated hyperbilirubinemia is *not* seen in:

A. Hemolytic anemia
B. Hypothyroidism
C. Dubin Johnson syndrome
D. Gilbert's syndrome *(AI 1998)*

Syndrome		Enzyme deficient	Bilirubin
Crigler-Najjar-1	AR	Absent glucuronyl transferase	Unconjugated > 20 mg/dL
Crigler-Najjar-2	AD	Decreased glucuronyl transferase	Unconjugated < 20 mg/dL
Gilbert's Syndrome	AD	Decreased glucuronyl transferase with decreased hepatic uptake	Unconjugated < 6 mg/dL
Dubin Johnson syndrome	AR	Impaired biliary secretion **(dark grey discoloration of liver)**	**Conjugated < 5 mg/dL**
Rotor syndrome	AR	Decreased hepatic uptake, storage and secretion	Conjugated < 5 mg/dL

153. *Not* found in TOF:

A. Severity of cyanosis is directly related to severity of pulmonary stenosis
B. Ventricular septal defect
C. Left ventricular hypertrophy
D. Pulmonary stenosis *(UP 1999)*

The four components of the tetralogy of Fallot are:

- **Ventricular septal defect**
- **Obstruction to right ventricular outflow**
- **Aortic override of the ventricular septal defect**
- **Right ventricular hypertrophy**

Severity of cyanosis is directly related to severity of pulmonary stenosis because as the severity of pulmonary stenosis increases there is increased shunting of deoxygenated blood through the VSD.

154. *False* regarding polio is:

A. Fasciculation seen
B. Normal sensorium
C. Autonomic involvement
D. 70% of cases have muscle paralysis *(AIIMS 1994)*

Poliomyelitis is an infection of human alimentary tract but the virus may infect the CNS leading to paralysis in 1% of cases.

155. In rheumatic fever *most common* valvular lesion is:

A. Aortic regurgitation
B. Aortic stenosis
C. Mitral regurgitation
D. Mitral stenosis *(AIIMS 1994)*

156. *False* regarding rheumatic heart disease in India:

A. Most common MR
B. Aortic valve is most commonly involved
C. Progresses rapidly
D. Starts in young age *(AIIMS 1994)*

Mitral regurgitation is the most common valvular involvement in children with rheumatic heart disease. AR is less common than MR. Other lesions are MS and TR.

157. *True* regarding AIDS in children is:

A. Presents with lymphadenopathy
B. Pneumonitis often important
C. Kaposi sarcoma rarely occurs
D. All are correct

(AIIMS 1994)

Failure to thrive, hepatosplenomegaly, unexplained persistent fever, parotitis, persistent oral thrush, recurrent gastroenteritis, otitis media and lymphadenopathy are common presentation of childhood AIDS. Neoplasms are relatively uncommon in pediatric HIV patients. While lymphocytic interstitial pneumonia (LIP) is relatively common clinical presentation of pediatric AIDS.

158. In which of the following disorders deficiency of glucuronyl transferase is seen:

A. Intrahepatic cholestasis
B. Rotor syndrome
C. Dubin Johnson syndrome
D. Crigler-Najjar syndrome

(PGI 1997)

159. Unconjugated hyperbilirubinemia is *not* seen in:

A. Crigler-Najjar syndrome
B. G6PD deficiency
C. Rotor syndrome
D. Thalassemia

(AIIMS 1994)

Syndrome	Inheritance	Enzyme deficient	Bilirubin
Crigler-Najjar-1	AR	Absent glucuronyl transferase	Unconjugated > 20 mg/dL
Crigler-Najjar-2	AD	Decreased glucuronyl transferase	Unconjugated < 20 mg/dL
Gilbert's syndrome	AD	Decreased glucuronyl transferase with decreased hepatic uptake	Unconjugated < 6 mg/dL
Dubin Johnson syndrome	AR	Impaired biliary secretion **(dark grey discoloration of liver)**	Conjugated < 5 mg/dL
Rotor syndrome	AR	Decreased hepatic uptake, storage and secretion	**Conjugated** < 5 mg/dL

160. *Most common* chromosomal anomaly is:

A. Fragile X syndrome
B. Trisomy 21
C. Trisomy 18
D. Trisomy 13

(AIIMS 1994)

Down syndrome is the most common chromosomal disorder occurring with a frequency of 1: 700 newborns.

161. Mycoplasma pneumonia is treated with:

A. Oral penicillin
B. Erythromycin
C. Co-trimoxazole
D. Rifampicin

(AIIMS 1994, AI 1996)

Oral erythromycin (250 to 500 mg every 6 hr for adults, 20 to 50 mg/kg daily in 3 or 4 doses for children) is the drug of choice for mycoplasmal respiratory infections.

162. *Not* a major criterion of rheumatic fever:

A. Arthritis
B. Subcutaneous nodule
C. Carditis
D. Increased ASO titre

(AIIMS 1994)

The Jones Criteria for Rheumatic Fever

Major criteria	Minor criteria	
Carditis	**Clinical**	**Laboratory**
Migratory polyarthritis	Fever	Elevated ESR
Sydenham's chorea	Arthralgia	Elevated CRP
Subcutaneous nodules		Prolonged PR interval
Erythema marginatum		
PLUS (ESSENTIAL CRITERIA)		
Supporting evidence of a recent group A streptococcal infection which includes any one of the following: • Positive throat culture for *Streptococcus* • Rapid antigen detection test • Elevated or increasing streptococcal antibody test (**ASO titer** > 200 Todd's unit in adults or > 300 Todd's unit children).		

*Diagnosis of rheumatic fever is highly probable if two major or one major and two minor criteria are present along with the evidence of previous *Streptococcus* infection.

163. In children *most common* cause of subdural effusion is:

A. *Meningococcus*
B. *Streptococcus*
C. *Haemophilus influenzae*
D. *Staphylococcus* *(AIIMS 1993)*

Subdural effusion can occur after any acute bacterial meningitis but it is most commonly associated with *Haemophilus influenzae* meningitis.

164. A child on 10th day of birth was found to have 10% decrease in weight after exclusive breastfeeding. It was passing golden yellow soft stools. *Anxious* parents report to the pediatrician. The *most appropriate* advice is:

A. Start the child on high protein diet **B.** More frequent breastfeeding
C. Reassurance **D.** Investigate for lactic acidosis *(AIIMS May 2002)*

- The **normal newborn baby losses up to 10% of its weight during the first week of life**, but regains it in the next few days. It doubles its birth weight by 4 months, triples it by 1 year and increases it 4 times by 2 years.
- The baby may pass meconium *in utero* or soon after birth, but all healthy newborn babies *must* evacuate within 24 hours of birth. During the first 2-3 days the baby passes black, tarry 'meconium' stools which are followed by greenish (transitional) stools for the next 1 or 2 days. **The normal breastfed baby usually passes 4-8 semisolid sticky golden yellow stools every day.** Some babies may pass stools after *each* feed due to the **'exaggerated' gastrocolic reflex**. The stools are often very small (at times like droppings of the birds) with normal consistency. The babies continue to gain weight.

165. Mediastinal widening is seen in:

A. Prolymphatic leukemia **B.** T cell ALL
C. CML with blast crisis **D.** Histocytic lymphoma *(AIIMS 1993, AI 1995)*

A mediastinal mass which reflects involvement of thymus is frequently seen with T cell ALL.

166. Obstructive hydrocephalus in children is *most commonly* caused by:

A. Aqueductal stenosis
B. Arnold-Chiari malformation
C. Meningitis
D. Dandy Walker syndrome *(JIPMER 1993, AIIMS 1993)*

The most common cause of *obstructive* hydrocephalus is congenital aqueductal stenosis. Other causes are as under:

Obstructive hydrocephalus	Communicating hydrocephalus
Aqueductal stenosis (congenital or acquired)	Arnold-Chiari malformation
Midline brain tumors	Post-infectious (meningitis, toxoplasmosis, CMV infection)
Vein of Galen malformation	Secondary to subarachnoid hemorrhage
Posterior fossa subdural hematoma	Secondary to excessive production of CSF (papilloma of choroid plexus)
Dandy Walker syndrome	Diseases of connective tissue (Hurler syndrome, achondroplasia)
	Vitamin A intoxication

167. Which of the following is the *most common* cause of portal hypertension in children:

A. Postnecrotic
B. Veno-occlusive disease
C. Budd-Chiari syndrome
D. Extrahepatic compression *(AI 1998)*

The most common cause of portal hypertension in children is extrahepatic portal venous obstruction (50-70%).

168. Which of the following is the *most common* organism causing neonatal septicemia in USA:

A. *Escherichia coli*
B. *Streptococcus viridans*
C. *Staphylococcus aureus*
D. Group B streptococci *(AIIMS 1993)*

Neonatal sepsis is a clinical syndrome characterized by systemic signs of infection and accompanied by bacteremia in the 1st month of life. If the disease occurs with in the first week it is known as **early onset sepsis** and if it occurs from 8-28 days it is known as **late onset sepsis**. Mortality is 15 - 50% in early onset sepsis and 10 -15% in late onset sepsis. Microbiological etiology of neonatal sepsis varies in different parts of the world and often changes over the years. Group B streptococci (GBS) are the most common cause of neonatal sepsis and meningitis in USA. *However in India *Klebsiella pneumoniae* (30%), *Staphylococcus aureus* (13%) and *Escherichia coli* (12.2%) are the main organisms responsible for neonatal sepsis.

FREQUENCY OF CLINICAL SIGNS IN NEONATAL SEPTICEMIA AND MENINGITIS

Clinical sign	Septicemia (%)	Meningitis (%)
• Hyperthermia	51	61
• Hypothermia	15	0
• Respiratory distress	33	47
• Apnea	22	7
• Cyanosis	24	0
• Icterus	35	28
• Hepatomegaly	33	32
• Refusal to feed	28	49
• Vomiting	25	0
• Abdominal distention	17	0
• Diarrhea	11	17
• Seizures	0	40
• Bulging fontanelle	0	28
• Neck rigidity	0	15

* Neonatal morbidity and mortality. Report of the National Neonatal Perinatal Database. *Indian Pediatr 1999;* **36:** 167-169.

169. The height of children in 2-10 years increases:

A. 10 cm/year
B. 6 cm/year
C. 2 cm/year
D. 4 cm/year

(AI 1997)

Growth Velocity in Children

Age	Height
At birth	50 cm
6 months	62 cm (+12)
1 year	75 cm (+25)
2 years	85 cm
2-5 years	Increases @ 6-8 cm/year
5 years and above	Increases @ 5 cm/year

170. *Not* a feature of Down's syndrome:

A. Hypertonicity
B. Mental retardation
C. Simian crease
D. Brushfield spots

(AI 1994)

Down's syndrome or mongolism: Patients have mild to moderate MENTAL RETARDATION and **hypotonia**. There is an extrachromosome usually at number 21 .The characteristic features are as under:

- Sloping forehead, small ear canals, gray or very light yellow spots at the periphery of the iris (BRUSHFIELD SPOTS), short broad hands with a single palmar crease (SIMIAN CREASE), and a flat nose or absent bridge, low-set ears, and dwarfed physique.
- Brachycephaly with flat occiput, small head, flat rounded face, upward slant of the eyes, small nose with depressed nasal bridge, inner epicanthic folds, protruding tongue and small misshapen ears form the characteristic mongoloid facies. The hands are short, the fingers are short and the fifth finger is short and incurved (clinodactyly).

171. Correct sequence of development in puberty in girls is:

A. Menarche, pubarche, thelarche
B. Thelarche, menarche, pubarche
C. Pubarche, thelarche, menarche
D. Thelarche, pubarche, menarche

(AI 2000)

172. In girls the first sign of puberty is:

A. Clitorache
B. Ditroanche
C. Menarche
D. Thelarche

(PGI 1999)

In girls, puberty usually begins with breast development (THELARCHE) but occasionally with the appearance of pubic hair (PUBARCHE). MENARCHE usually occurs about two years after breast development begins.

173. Which of the following is the *earliest* sign of puberty in males:

A. Change in voice
B. Moustaches
C. Pubarche
D. Testicular enlargement

(UP 1994)

Puberty marks the transition of a child into an adult. In boys, TESTICULAR ENLARGEMENT (more than 3 ml) marks the onset of puberty and is followed by the appearance of pubic hair and development of external genitalia.

174. Bronze baby syndrome occurs due to:

A. Phototherapy
B. Wilson's disease
C. Hemochromatosis
D. Aortic regurgitation

(PGI 1998)

The bronze baby syndrome refers to a dark, grayish brown discoloration of the skin sometimes seen in infants undergoing PHOTOTHERAPY. This discoloration may last for several months.

175. In which of the following leukemias, *chloroma* is seen:

A. CML B. AML
C. ALL D. CLL *(PGI 1999)*

In AML any extramedullary site may be infiltrated by the leukemic cells. Tumor like accumulations within soft tissue or bone is known as CHLOROMAS (due to their green color). They are more common with M1 and M 2 variety. Chloro = green (e.g. chlorophyll).

176. *False* regarding transient tachypnea of newborn (TTN) is:

A. Reticulogranular pattern are seen B. Fluid in intralobar fissure
C. Mild pleural effusion D. Prominent perihilar streaking *(PGI 1998)*

TRANSIENT TACHYPNEA OF NEWBORN is also known as Wet Lung disease or RDS type II. It is a common, mild, self-limiting disorder affecting near term or term infants and is characterized by tachypnea with mild retraction and mild cyanosis. The infant usually develops tachypnea (RR > 80 /min) within 2-6 hours. Symptoms typically persist for 12-24 hours in mild TTN and may persist for more than 72 hours in severe TTN. It is very difficult to distinguish TTN from HMD *except* by sudden recovery and absence of reticulogranular pattern in X ray. **Radiological findings are as under:**

1. Prominent perihilar streaking
2. Mild to moderate cardiomegaly
3. Coarse fluffy densities which represent liquid filled alveoli
4. Increased lung volume due to air trapping associated with bronchiolar collapse
5. **Fluid may be seen in minor fissure, pleural space** or both. **Widening of interlobar fissure** and prominence of right lung minor fissure are occasional finding.

177. *Not* a characteristic feature of petit mal seizures:

A. 3 Hz spike and wave pattern in EEG
B. Onset after the age of 14 years
C. Absence of motor activity during seizures
D. Short duration of seizure *(SGPGI 1996)*

Absence seizures (Petit mal): Absence seizures are characterized by sudden, **brief** lapses of consciousness **without loss of postural control.** The seizure typically lasts for only seconds, consciousness returns as suddenly as it was lost, and there is no post-ictal confusion. **Absence seizures almost always begin in childhood (ages 4 to 8)** or early adolescence and are the main seizure type in 15 to 20 % of children with epilepsy. The electrophysiologic hallmark of typical absence seizures is a generalized, symmetric, **3 Hz spike-and-wave discharge** that begins and ends suddenly on a normal EEG background.

178. Infant triples weight at the age of.......... months:

A. 5 B. 11
C. 18 D. 24 *(AIIMS 1996)*

The child doubles its birth weight by 4 months, triples it by 1 year and increases it 4 times by two years.

179. *Not* seen in systemic juvenile rheumatoid arthritis:

A. Iridocyclitis
B. High fever
C. Rheumatoid rashes
D. Hepatosplenomegaly *(AIIMS 2001)*

180. Characteristic feature of Still disease is:

A. Maculopapular rash
B. Renal involvement
C. Neutropenia
D. Rheumatoid factor +ve *(AIIMS 1996)*

Clinical features of Still disease (systemic JRA)	Percent
• High intermittent fever	100%
• Arthritis/ Arthralgia/ myalgia during febrile period	100%
• Rheumatoid rash	95%
• Chronic arthritis	90%
• Hepatosplenomegaly and / or lymphadenopathy	85%
• Leukocytosis	85%
• Pleuritis and / or pericarditis	60%
• Severe anemia	40%
• Abdominal pain	20%
• Rheumatoid factor	Absent
• Antinuclear antibody	Absent
• Iridocyclitis	Absent

181. Which of the following is *true* regarding porencephaly:

A. Neural tube defects
B. Vascular lesion due to degenerative vessel disease and head injury
C. Dandy-Walker syndrome
D. Fetal alcohol syndrome *(AI 1999)*

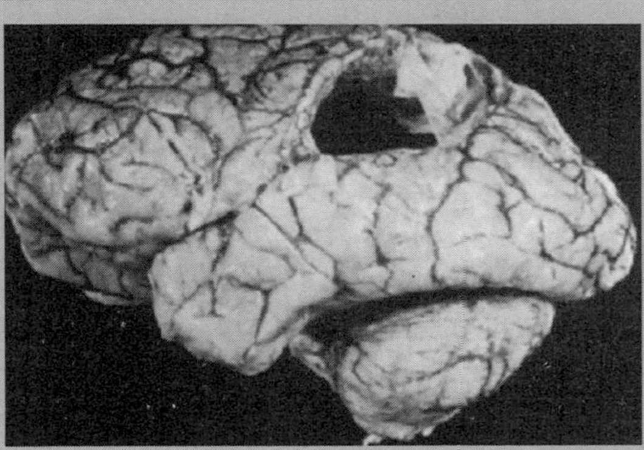

PORENCEPHALY: Neuroimaging of mentally retarded infants or those with sensory motor abnormalities (epilepsy, spasticity, and paresis) may reveal a single focal loss of brain substance filled with CSF. Aside from this defect, the brain is surprisingly normal. The porencephalic area communicates with the ventricle, the subarachnoid space, or both. **Vascular insufficiency may account for brain loss and the development of an abnormal cortex.**

182. A child presented with *diarrhea* followed by development of *rashes* and *petechiae*. *Most likely* diagnosis is:

A. *Giardia* **B.** *Shigella*
C. *Campylobacter* **D.** *Vibrio* *(SGPGI 2002)*

If the infection is due to *Shigella dysenteriae* type I hemolysis, anemia and hemolytic syndrome are common symptoms. They manifest as rash and petechiae.

183. A child has anti-mongoloid slant, pulmonary stenosis, short stature and undescended testis. This child has:

A. Down syndrome **B.** Turner syndrome
C. Noonan's syndrome **D.** Klinefelter syndrome *(AI 1997)*

Features of Noonan's syndrome are as under:

• XY Turner phenotype	• Webbing of the neck
• Pectus carinatum or pectus excavatum	• Cubitum valgum
• **Pulmonary valvular stenosis** or ASD	• Hypertelorism
• Epicanthus	• **Antimongoloid palpebral slant**
• Ptosis	• Micrognathia
• Clinodactyly	• Hernia
• Vertebral anomalies	• Low set ears
• **Cryptorchidism**	• Small testis
• Mental retardation	• Short stature

184. Secondary lactose intolerance is seen with which of the following:

A. Yersinia enterocolitis
B. Entamoeba
C. Shigella infection
D. Rotavirus diarrhoea *(AIIMS 1991)*

Rotaviruses are nonenveloped, icosahedral, with double capsid. Their electron microscope appearance shows a 60-80 nm wheel with radiating spokes (Latin, rota = wheel). The rotavirus genome contains double stranded (ds) RNA in 11 segments that can be separated by polyacrylamide gel electrophoresis (PAGE). Affected host cells are mature enterocytes lining the middle and upper end of the intestinal villi. Histopathology of infected intestines shows villous atrophy and blunting, due to the death of mature enterocytes and infiltration of lamina propria with mononuclear cells. Subsequently there is repopulation of the villous tips with immature secretory cells (crypt hyperplasia). Cell dysfunction and death results in a net secretion of intsetinal fluid, hence the watery diarrhea. Activation or enteric nervous sytem may also play a role. Repopulation with immature secretory cells may contribute to the secondary lactose intolerance that is sometimes seen.

185. ***False* regarding thumb sucking is:**

A. Must be treated vigorously in the first year of life
B. It is a sign of insecurity
C. It is a source of pleasure
D. Can lead to malocclusion *(JIPMER 1991)*

Thumb sucking is normal in early infancy. It is a source of pleasure in children and is a sign of insecurity. It can lead to malocclusion of teeth if it persists beyond 5 years. *Best policy* is to ignore thumb sucking and concentrate on positive aspects of child's behavior. **No treatment is required below 5 years of age.**

186. A two-year-old HIV positive boy presents with history of croup, fever, cough, diffuse wheezing, and crypts all over. Examination reveals hyperinflated chest. His management should be started with:

A. Ganciclovir
B. Erythromycin
C. Co-trimoxazole
D. Nebulised ribavirin *(AIIMS 2001)*

***Pneumocystis carinii* pneumonia** (PCP) is the most common and lethal opportunistic infection in HIV positive pediatric population. Trimethoprim-sulfamethoxazole (cotrimoxazole) is the drug of choice for all forms of pneumocystosis. Trimethoprim-sulfamethoxazole is administered orally or intravenously at a dosage of 15 to 20 mg of TMP/kg per day and 75 to 100 mg of SMZ/kg per day in 3 or 4 divided doses. Trimethoprim-sulfamethoxazole is well tolerated by non-AIDS patients, but > 50% of AIDS patients experience serious adverse reactions, including fever, rash, neutropenia, thrombocytopenia, hepatitis, and hyperkalemia.

187. Which of the following congenital diseases is characterized by reduced production of RBCs:

A. Sickle cell anemia **B.** Diamond Blackfan syndrome
C. Polycythemia vera **D.** Paroxysmal nocturnal hemoglobinuria *(AIIMS 2001)*

The selective absence of erythroid progenitors in an *otherwise normal marrow* is known as pure red cell aplasia (PRCA). Hereditary PRCA is known as **Diamond-Blackfan syndrome** and in this condition anemia is detected within the 1st year of life. In Diamond-Blackfan syndrome other physical anomalies are present in about 30 % of cases.

188. Thalassemia is because of:

A. Deficiency of spectrin **B.** Defect in spleen
C. Defect in hemoglobin synthesis **D.** All of the above *(PGI 1997)*

189. *True* about β thalassemia is:

A. Decreased α chain, decreased β chain
B. Increased β chain, increased α chain
C. Decreased β chain, increased α chain
D. Increased β chain, decreased α chain *(AIIMS 2001)*

The fundamental abnormality in thalassemia is impaired production of either the alpha or beta hemoglobin chain. Hemoglobin synthesis requires the coordinated production of heme and globin. Heme is the prosthetic group that mediates reversible binding of oxygen by hemoglobin. Globin is the protein that surrounds and protects the heme molecule. Heme is synthesized in a complex series of steps involving enzymes in the mitochondrion and in the cytosol of the cell. Two distinct globin chains (each with its individual heme molecule) combine to form hemoglobin. One of the chains is designated **alpha**. The second chain is called "**non-alpha**". With the *exception* of the very first weeks of embryogenesis, one of the globin chains is always alpha. The fetus has a distinct non-alpha chain called gamma. After birth, a different non-alpha globin chain, called beta, pairs with the alpha chain. **The combination of two alpha chains and two non-alpha chains produces a complete hemoglobin molecule (a total of four chains per molecule).** The combination of two alpha chains and two gamma chains form "fetal" hemoglobin, termed "hemoglobin F". With the exception of the first 10 to 12 weeks after conception, fetal hemoglobin is the primary hemoglobin in the developing fetus. The combination of two alpha chains and two beta chains form "adult" hemoglobin, also called "hemoglobin A". Although hemoglobin A is called "adult", it becomes the predominant hemoglobin within 12 to 16 weeks of birth. **The genes that encode the alpha globin chains are on chromosome 16. Those that encode the non-alpha globin chains are on chromosome 11.** The genes in the beta globin locus are arranged sequentially from 5' to 3' beginning with episolon. The beta globin locus ends with the adult beta globin gene. The sequence of the genes is: epsilon, gamma, delta, and beta. **There are two copies of the gamma gene on each chromosome 11. The others are present in single copies.** Therefore, each cell has two beta globin genes, one on each of the two chromosomes 11 in the cell. These two beta globin genes express their globulin protein in a quantity that precisely matches that of the four alpha globulin genes.

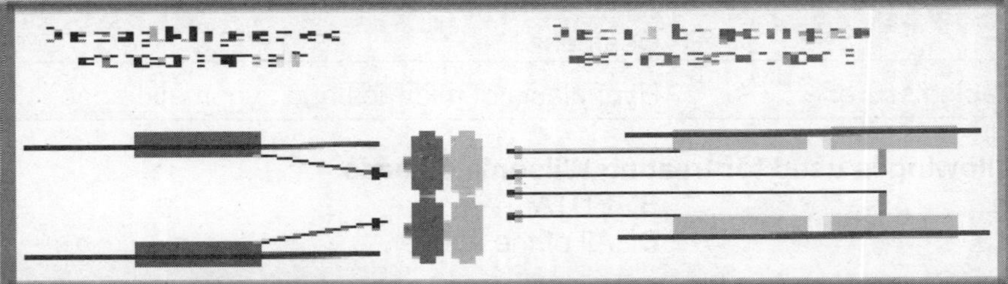

Embryonic hemoglobins	Fetal hemoglobin	Adult hemoglobins
Gower 1- zeta(2), epsilon(2) Gower 2- alpha(2), epsilon (2) Portland- zeta(2), gamma (2)	Hemoglobin F- alpha(2), gamma(2)	Hemoglobin A- alpha(2), beta(2) Hemoglobin A2- alpha(2), delta(2)

Unlike the **deletions** that constitute most of the alpha thalassemia syndromes, beta thalassemias are caused by **mutations** on chromosome 11 that affect all aspects of beta globin production: transcription, translation, and the stability of the beta globin product. **Excessive alpha chains** precipitate in red cell membrane and damage it leading to hemolytic anemia.

190. Wilms' tumor *commonly* metastasis to which of the following organ:
A. Liver B. Brain
C. Lymph node D. Lung *(AIIMS 1994)*

Hematogenous spread occurs (10-12%) in Wilms' tumor and *most commonly* involves lungs and liver and rarely to brain and bones.

191. A 5-year-old child of normal intelligence presents with features of hypotonia. There were fasciculation in his tongue and he keeps his body in a frog like position. *Most likely* diagnosis is:
A. Limb girdle atrophy B. Spinal muscular atrophy
C. GB syndrome D. Down syndrome *(AIIMS 2000)*

192. Infantile spinal muscular atrophy is a group of disorders which affect:
A. Motor neurons B. Pyramidal tracts
C. Peripheral nerves D. Neuromuscular junctions *(PGI 1998)*

Infantile spinal muscular atrophy or ***Werdnig Hoffmann disease*** is a recessive trait. The primary pathological change in this disease is atrophy of anterior horn cell (motor neuron) in the spinal cord and of motor nuclei in brainstem with secondary atrophy of motor nerve roots and of muscles. Onset of symptoms occurs before the age of two years and early manifestations are **weakness and hypotonia** of proximal and distal limbs, intercostal muscles and bulbar muscles. Legs adopt a typical **'frog leg' position**. As the diaphragm is *not* involved, diaphragmatic function in the presence of weakness of intercostal muscles results in characteristic paradoxical breathing. Extraocular muscles are not involved and tendon reflexes are almost always absent. **Mental development is normal**. Death results due to respiratory failure and aspiration pneumonia. Differential diagnoses include all diseases leading to floppy baby. Diagnosis is basically clinical and electromyography shows evidence of denervation of muscle, i.e. fibrillation potentials and **fasciculations**.

193. *Not* a feature of Treacher-Collins syndrome:
A. Deafness B. Colobomas of lower eyelid
C. Hypoplasia of zygomatic bone D. Mongoloid slant of palpable fissure *(KERALA 1999)*

Mandibulofacial dysostosis is also known as **Franceschetti-Klein syndrome** or **Treacher-Collins syndrome**. Important features are as under:

Micrognathia	Colobomas of lower eyelid
Sunken cheek bones	Blind fistulas between the angles of mouth and ears
Deformed pinnas	Atypical hair growth extending towards cheek
Receding chin	Large mouth
Facial clefts	Deafness
Anti-mongoloid palpable fissure	Hypoplasia of mid face and zygomatic bone

194. Which of the following is used for treating Wilson's disease:
A. Penicillamine B. EDTA
C. BAL D. All of the above *(KERALA 1999)*

Penicillamine is the drug of choice of Wilson's disease. Penicillamine is administered orally in an initial dose of 1 g daily in single or divided doses along with 25 mg/d of pyridoxine once daily.

195. Which of the following is the marker for neural tube defect:
A. Acetyl phosphatidyl esterase
B. Acetyl cystine
C. Acetyl glucorinidase
D. Acetyl cholinesterase *(AIIMS 1999)*

196. Increased levels of acetyl cholinesterase in amniotic fluid indicate which of the following:

A. Edward syndrome
B. Down syndrome
C. Esophageal atresia
D. Open neural tube defects *(AI 1999, UP 2000)*

Amniotic fluid should be examined for a number of compounds such as alpha-fetoprotein (AFP), acetyl cholinesterase (AChE), bilirubin and pulmonary surfactant. **Increased level of APF along with presence of acetyl cholinesterase (AChE) signifies presence of neural tube defect (NTD) with 98% accuracy.** AFP levels are also elevated in anencephaly, abdominal wall defects, intestinal atresia and congenital nephrosis.

197. The age of onset of JRA is before:

A. 16 years **B.** 13 years
C. 8 years **D.** 12 years *(KERALA 1999)*

American Rheumatism Association has defined JRA as **"ARTHRITIS OF ONE OR MORE JOINTS WITH ONSET BELOW THE AGE OF 16 YEARS AND WHICH PERSISTS FOR AT LEAST 6 WEEKS WITH EXCLUSION OF OTHER SPECIFIC DISEASES"**.	
• Age of onset	Less than 16 years
• Duration of disease	More than 6 weeks
• Presence of arthritis	**Swelling or effusion or 2 of the following:** 1. Painful joint or limited joint movement 2. Tenderness 3. Warmth
• Subtypes **after 6 months of disease**	Systemic JRA with arthritis, fever and rash. Polyarticular JRA i.e. >4 joints are involved Pauciarticular JRA i.e. <5 joints are involved
• Other	Other forms of juvenile arthritis should be excluded

198. Inborn error of metabolism associated with mental retardation is:

A. Scheie syndrome **B.** Homocystinuria
C. Pentosuria **D.** Alkaptonuria *(AI 2001)*

Homocystinuria is the second most common inborn error of metabolism and it occurs due to deficiency of cystathionine β synthetase. It is an autosomal recessive disorder. Deficiency of cystathionine β synthetase leads to increased concentration of homocytine and its precursor methionine in blood and other body fluids. Untreated patients are asymptomatic in infancy but subsequently develop **MENTAL RETARDATION**, skeletal disorders, thromboembolism and numerous ocular complications. Ectopia lentis is the most notable ophthalmic finding while other ocular findings are microcystic peripheral retinal degeneration, glaucoma, secondary papillary block, rental detachment, myopia, cataract, strabismus, optic atrophy, iris atrophy, uveitis, keratitis, and spherophakia. **Homocystinuria is one of the few metabolic disorders that can be treated.** Pyridoxine (vitamin B6) combined with dietary restriction of methionine results in benefit in 40% of cases.

199. Trans-placental transmission is *not* seen in:

A. Toxoplasma **B.** Rubella
C. Mump **D.** Syphilis *(TN 1990)*

Maternal Diseases Associated with Specific Syndromes in Newborns

Syphilis	**R**ubella
Toxoplasmosis	**C**MV
AIDS	**H**erpes virus infection

- **STARCH** *complex*

200. Fetal lung maturity is assessed by:

A. USG
B. Bilirubin contents of amniotic fluid
C. Amniocentesis
D. L/S ratio

(KERALA 1994)

- The pulmonary immaturity of the fetal lungs can be assessed by determination of **LECITHIN/SPHINGOMYELIN RATIO** in the amniotic fluid.
- L/S ratio of 2 or more indicates adequate lung maturity, while a ratio of less than 1.5 is associated with HMD.
- Amniotic fluid 'shake test' is a simple bedside test for assessment of lung maturity. Estimation of phosphotidyl glycerol is a more specific indicator of lung maturity (especially in diabetic mothers), and its absence is always associated with development of HMD.

201. Central cyanosis with *systolic murmur* at birth is seen in which of the following conditions:

A. Endocardial cushion defect
B. TGA
C. Ventricular septal defect
D. PDA

(AIIMS 2001)

In **transposition of great arteries** (TGA) the aorta arises from right ventricle and pulmonary artery from left ventricle. 50% of patients have an associated VSD (leading to *ejection systolic murmur*). In patients with an intact interventricular septum a communication is *must* either as PDA or as patent foramen ovale. The **newborn is clinically cyanosed within few hours of life** due to mixing of oxygenated and deoxygenated blood. Initial management consists of:

1. Make certain that there is adequate mixing between 2 parallel circuits.
2. Maximization of mixed venous oxygen saturation.

If the patient does not respond to the above measures foramen ovale should be enlarged by balloon atrial septostomy (**Rashkind procedure**). In this procedure a deflated balloon is inserted into a vein, passed through the foramen ovale, and then inflated and pulled vigorously through the atrial septum to enlarge the opening and improve oxygenation of the blood. Definitive management consists of surgical correction with an **arterial switch operation** in early neonatal period.

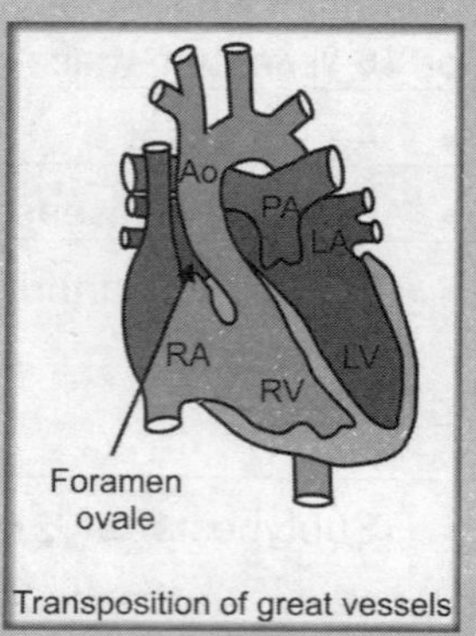

Transposition of great vessels

202. *Not* seen in nephrotic syndrome:

A. Hypercholesterolemia
B. Massive proteinuria
C. Hypoalbuminemia
D. Hematuria

(TN 1995)

203. *Not* seen in a child with nephrotic syndrome:

A. Reduced serum calcium
B. Uremia
C. Hyperlipidemia
D. Hypoproteinemia

(JIPMER 1990)

Nephrotic syndrome is characterized by heavy proteinurea (>40 mg/m²/hour), **hypoproteinemia**, edema and **hyperlipidemia**. More than 90% of children with nephrotic syndrome have some form of idiopathic nephrotic syndrome of which 85% show minimal change disease as renal pathology while the incidence of focal sclerosis is 10% and that of mesangial proliferation is 5%. In remaining 10% of cases nephrotic syndrome is due to some form of glomerulonephritis of which membranous and membranoproliferative are more common. The basic pathological abnormality in nephrotic syndrome is heavy proteinurea due to increased glomerular capillary wall permeability. The protein loss generally exceeds 2 gm/day and is composed mainly of albumin. Thus it may be said that hypoproteinemia is essentially hypoalbuminemia. Edema appears when the serum albumin level falls below 2.5 gm/dL due to decrease in plasma oncotic pressure. Almost all serum lipids (cholesterol and triglyceride) and lipoprotein levels are elevated. Laboratory findings are as under:

• Proteinuria	3+ or 4+ (>2 gm/24 hours)
• Serum cholesterol	Elevated
• Serum triglyceride	Elevated
• Serum albumin	<2 gm/dL
• Total serum calcium	Reduced
• C3 level	Normal
• Renal function	Generally normal but may be reduced

If the age of child is between 1 and 8 years it is most likely that he is having minimal change disease and oral steroid therapy should be started as prednisolone 2 mg/kg/day (maximum 60 mg/kg/day) in 3 divided doses without further investigation. Renal biopsy is indicated if the age of child is <1 years or >8 years. A combination of furosemide (1-2 mg/kg/day) and spironolactone is useful in reducing edema. Average time required for response of prednisolone is about 2 weeks and response is defined as the point at which the urine becomes free of protein. If the child continues to have proteinuria of 2+ or more after one month prednisolone therapy then the nephrotic syndrome is termed as *steroid resistant* and is an indication of renal biopsy. Five days after the urine becomes free of protein (-ve, trace or 1+) the total dose of prednisolone is given as a single dose with breakfast on alternate day for 3-6 months. After such a period prednisolone is discontinued abruptly.

A relapse is defined as recurrence of edema and not merely proteinuria which resolves spontaneously. Repeated relapse and severe corticosteroid toxicity are indication of cyclophosphamide therapy (3 mg/kg/day OD) along with alternate day prednisolone for 3 months. TLC must be monitored during cyclophosphamide therapy and it should be withheld if TLC falls below 5000.

204. Which of the following is the *most common* malignancy in children:

A. Neuroblastoma **B.** Wilms' tumor
C. Lymphoma and leukemia **D.** Retinoblastoma *(AI 1999)*

Acute leukemia and lymphomas (Hodgkin's and Non Hodgkin's) account for 60% of cases of childhood malignancies. Remaining 40% comprise of solid tumors of which Wilms' tumor is most common. Other solid tumors commonly seen in pediatric age group are neuroblastoma, Ewing's sarcoma, osteosarcoma, soft tissue sarcoma, and retinoblastoma and brain tumors.

205. Which of the following is *true* regarding brain tumor in children:

A. Hemiparesis is present
B. Usually causes papilledema
C. Usually infratentorial
D. Most common tumor in children is Wilms' tumor *(AI 2000)*

Intracranial tumors are the second most common neoplasms in children and are only exceeded by leukemia. Two-third of all intracranial tumors of children between 2-12 years are infratentorial.

206. Which of the following is the *first* constant symptom of brain tumor in children:

A. Personality disturbances **B.** Headache
C. Vomiting **D.** Increased head size *(UP 2001)*

In infratentorial tumors early features of raised intracranial pressure include **ENLARGEMENT OF HEAD**, vomiting, headache and visual symptoms.

207. Which of the following intracranial tumors in children has *poor* prognosis:

A. Hemangioma **B.** Medulloblastoma
C. Glioma **D.** Glioma multiforme *(AI 1994)*

Medulloblastoma is the second most common posterior fossa tumor in children. It is most prevalent in pre school children. Tumor is rapidly progressive and is capable of local spread via CSF. It carries poor prognosis.

208. *Most common* infratentorial tumor in children is:

A. Ependymoma **B.** Medulloblastoma
C. Glioma of midline of cerebellum **D.** Astrocytoma *(AI 1994)*

209. In children *most common* posterior fossa tumor is:

A. Meningioma **B.** Astrocytoma
C. Glioblastoma multiforme **D.** Medulloblastoma *(AIIMS 1995, AI 1997)*

Cerebellar **ASTROCYTOMAS** are the most common posterior fossa tumor of childhood (12% of all brain tumors) and have best prognosis.

210. ***Most common*** **childhood tumor is:**

A. Lymphangioma
B. Meningioma
C. Ependymoma
D. Glioma
(AI 1996)

In 80% of brain tumors of children the basic cell is glial and the tumor is known as glioma.

211. Which of the following is *not* a tumor of first decade of life:

A. Ameloblastoma
B. Rhabdomyosarcoma
C. Neuroblastoma
D. Retinoblastoma
(AIIMS 1992)

Ameloblastoma presents at an age of 11 years upwards, but most patients present in 4th or 5th decade of life.

212. ***Not*** **a feature of neonatal necrotizing enterocolitis:**

A. Pneumoperitoneum
B. Metabolic acidosis
C. Increased bowel sound
D. Abdominal distention
(AI 1998)

Necrotizing enterocolitis (NEC) is the most common serious surgical disorder among infants in neonatal intensive care unit. NEC is an acute intestinal necrosis syndrome of unknown etiology. Prematurity is the single greatest risk factor for NEC. Clinical features can be divided into systemic and abdominal signs:

SYSTEMIC SIGNS	ABDOMINAL SIGNS
• Respiratory distress	• **Abdominal distention**
• Apnea	• Vomiting
• Bradycardia	• **Paralytic ileus**
• Lethargy	• Erythema of abdominal wall
• Temperature instability	• Bloody stools
• Poor feeding	• Abdominal mass
• Shock	• Ascites
• Bleeding	• Abdominal tenderness

X-ray abdomen may show bowel wall edema and ***pneumatosis cystoides intestinalis*** which is diagnostic of NEC. Portal and hepatic venous air, pneumobilia and pneumoperitoneum may be present. Thrombocytopenia, persistent metabolic acidosis and severe refractory hyponatremia are the most common triad of laboratory findings seen in NEC.

213. Combination of retinitis pigmentosa and icthyosis is seen in:

A. Down syndrome
B. Turner syndrome
C. Refsum's disease
D. Mohr's syndrome
(JIPMER 2002)

Refsum's disease (RD) is a neurocutaneous syndrome which is characterized *biochemically* by the accumulation of phytanic acid in plasma and tissues. Patients with RD are unable to degrade phytanic acid because of a deficient activity of phytanoyl-CoA hydroxylase (PhyH), a peroxisomal enzyme catalyzing the first step of phytanic acid alpha-oxidation. Refsum first described this disease in the year 1946. Peripheral polyneuropathy, cerebellar ataxia, **retinitis pigmentosa**, and **ichthyosis** are the major clinical components. The symptoms evolve slowly and insidiously from childhood through adolescence and early adulthood.

214. A mother while kissing her baby found that the baby's skin is salty. Baby is suffering from:

A. Niemann-Pick disease
B. Cystic fibrosis
C. Thalassemia
D. Fanconi syndrome
(TN 1990)

215. ***False*** **regarding cystic fibrosis is:**

A. Increased sweat Na^+ concentration
B. Dry mouth
C. Steatorrhea
D. Sterility
(UP 1996)

Cystic fibrosis is an autosomal recessive disease resulting from mutations in a gene located on chromosome 7. Sweat glands are unable to reabsorb chloride, leading to increased sweat chloride concentration. The airway epithelia are unable to secrete chloride into the lumen combined with active sodium absorption. The resultant dehydration of luminal mucus layer, defective mucociliary action and accumulation of thick viscous secretions lead to recurrent lower respiratory tract infections and obstructive pulmonary diseases.

• Chronic airway infection	• Exocrine pancreatic insufficiency
• Bronchiectasis	• Intestinal dysfunction
• Bronchiolectasis	• Abnormal sweat gland function
• Urogenital dysfunction	• Steatorrhea or malabsorption due to lack of pancreatic enzyme
• Males are usually infertile due to failure of development of vas and epididymis	• Females usually develop secondary amenorrhea

216. Which of the following *do not* regress:
- **A.** Salmon patch
- **B.** Strawberry angioma
- **C.** Port wine stain
- **D.** Lymphangiomyomatosis circumscripta

(AIIMS 2001)

Lesion	Appearance	Regression	Treatment
Salmon patch	At birth	One year	None
Port wine stain (Naevus flammeus)	At birth	**Does not occur**	Excision and grafting
Venous angioma (cavernous angioma)	At birth	Does not occur	Sclerotherapy or therapeutic embolisation
Strawberry angioma	1-3 weeks	7-8 years	Not required
Arterial angioma (plexiform angioma)	At birth	Never	surgery

***Salmon patch and Strawberry angioma Show Spontaneous regression.**

217. In bed wetting the *drug of choice* is:
- **A.** Trazodone
- **B.** Tranylcypromine
- **C.** Imipramine
- **D.** Selegiline

(AIIMS 1999)

218. *Most common* cause of nocturnal enuresis in children is:
- **A.** NIDDM
- **B.** Spina bifida
- **C.** UTI
- **D.** Psychological stress

(UPSC 1996)

The word enuresis is derived from the Greek word "ENOUREIN" which means to void urine. Bladder control is normally achieved between 1-5 years and a majority of children are dry during day by 3 years and at night by 5 years. Nocturnal enuresis (bed wetting) means involuntary voiding at night with day time control. It is a very common condition and has a prevalence of about 15% in children above 5 years. Boys are three times more commonly affected. **Emotional stress** precipitates bed wetting in a previously normal child. It has been observed that these children are heavy sleepers and have lower nocturnal ADH level. Psychological and behavioral problems are common in such children. A urine culture should be done and diabetes mellitus, diabetes insipidus and other renal disorder should be ruled out. **Imipramine 50 mg HS OD is useful.** Vasopressin nasal spray is also effective but the benefits are temporary.

219. *Most common* renal lesion in children is:
- **A.** Diffuse glomerulonephritis
- **B.** Focal glomerulonephritis
- **C.** Membranoproliferative glomerulonephritis
- **D.** Lipoid nephrosis *(TN 1995)*

Minimal change disease is also known as nil disease, lipoid nephrosis, or foot process disease. It is the most common cause of glomerulonephritis in children.

220. Which of the following is *true* regarding erysipelas:
- **A.** Anaerobic infection
- **B.** Subcutaneous inflammation due to *Streptococcus*
- **C.** Lymphangitis due to *Streptococcus*
- **D.** Lymphangitis due to *Staphylococcus* *(JIPMER 1990)*

Erysipelas is a form of **streptococcal cellulitis**. The symptoms include fever, chills, nausea, vomiting, painful and warm skin, and hot, red lesions on the face and head .The skin often has a peau d'orange texture. Superficial bullae may form, usually 2 or 3 days after onset. Erysipelas shows predilection for certain characteristic locations. They are the malar area of the face, often with extension over the bridge of the nose to the contralateral malar region and the lower extremities.

221. In a newborn, Harlequins skin change is due to:
- **A.** Polycythemia
- **B.** Septicemia
- **C.** Autonomic dysfunction
- **D.** Icthyosis *(JIPMER 1993)*

HARLEQUIN SIGN is a benign transient color change seen in newborn babies in which one half of the body blanches while the other half becomes redder, with a clear line of demarcation. This sign is commonly seen in low birth weight infants. It may be **due to an imbalance in the autonomic vascular regulatory mechanism**. Color change is transient lasting only a few minutes and occasionally affects a portion of trunk or face. Pattern is reversed by changing the infant's position. Multiple episodes can occur but are not indicative of permanent autonomic imbalance.

222. *False* regarding breath holding spells is:
- **A.** Attacks of cyanosis can occur
- **B.** Child may lose consciousness
- **C.** Antiepileptic treatment is necessary
- **D.** Occurs between 6 months to 5 years of age *(AIIMS 1997)*

223. *False* regarding breath holding spells in children is:
- **A.** It must be immediately attended to prevent hypoxia and onset of seizure
- **B.** Parents are advised to ignore and not to reinforce these attacks
- **C.** It does not contribute to increased risk of seizure disorder
- **D.** It is fairly common in the first two years of life *(KARNATAKA 1994)*

Breadth holding is not uncommon during the 1st years of life. It is a *method* used by infants and toddlers in an attempt to control their environment and their caregivers. Whereas some children hold their breath until they lose consciousness, sometimes leading to a seizure, ***there is no increased risk of their later developing a seizure disorder***. ***Parents are best advised to ignore the behavior and leave the room in response***. Without sufficient reinforcement the behavior soon disappears.

224. In X-ray batwing appearance is due to:
- **A.** Pulmonary embolism
- **B.** Mitral stenosis
- **C.** Cardiogenic pulmonary edema
- **D.** Bronchial asthma *(KERALA 1994)*

Advanced cardiogenic pulmonary edema gives a central **batwing appearance** on chest X-ray.

225. *Not* a constituent of ORS:

A. Glucose without salt
B. Glucose with salt
C. Na^+
D. K^+ *(KERALA 1994)*

WHO formula of ORS		
Sodium chloride	3.5 gm	
Sodium bicarbonate	2.5 gm	
Potassium chloride	1.5 gm	
Glucose	20.0 gm	
Home made ORS		
Ingredients	**Weight in grams**	**Household measure**
Common salt	3.5	3/4th teaspoon
Baking soda	2.5	½ teaspoon
Cane sugar	40	8 level teaspoons
Lemon	1 lemon	Supplies potassium

226. Dandy-Walker syndrome is because of obstruction of:

A. Arachnoid granulations
B. Foramen of Magendie and Luschka
C. Foramen of Munro
D. Foramen of Morgagni *(JIPMER 1992)*

227. *Not* a clinical feature of Dandy-Walker syndrome:

A. Arachnoid cyst
B. Agenesis of cerebellar vermis
C. Hydrocephalus
D. Posterior fossa cyst *(AIIMS 1998)*

Dandy-Walker syndrome is a congenital defect of midline cerebellar structures in which **hydrocephalus** is due to atresia of foramina of Luschka and Magendie. Other features are as under:

- Absence or severe hypoplasia of vermis of cerebellum
- Gross cystic distention of roof of fourth ventricle which bulges out posteriorly
- Agenesis of corpus callosum
- Anomalies of cell migration

228. Minimum level of bilirubin to start phototherapy in a 3-day-old full term baby with jaundice is:

A. 15 mg%
B. 18 mg%
C. 12 mg%
D. 9 mg% *(AIIMS 1999)*

229. Neonatal jaundice seen after 48 hours of birth with bilirubin <5 mg% is due to:

A. Physiological jaundice
B. Neonatal hepatitis
C. Hemolytic disease of newborn
D. ABO incompatibility *(KERALA 1994)*

Physiological Jaundice: About 60-70% of healthy newborn babies are likely to develop physiological jaundice. Physiological jaundice appears between 24 and 72 hrs of age, its maximum intensity is seen on the 4th and 5th day of life, and the peak serum **bilirubin level does not exceed 15 mg/dl.** This type of jaundice usually disappears before 14 days of life and does not need any specific therapy.

MANAGEMENT OF HYPERBILIRUBINEMA IN HEALTHY TERM NEWBORN—AAP GUIDELINES

Age in hrs	Consider phototherapy Total serum bilirubin in mg%	Phototherapy	Exchange transfusion If intensive phototherapy fails	Exchange transfusion and extensive phototherapy
< / = 24 hrs	observation	observation	observation	observation
25-48 hrs	> / = 12 mg%	> / = 15 mg%	> / = 20 mg%	> / = 25 mg%
49-72 hrs	> / = 15 mg%	> / = 18 mg%	> / = 25 mg%	> / = 30 mg%
> 72 hrs	> / = 17 mg%	> / = 20 mg%	> / = 25 mg%	> / = 30 mg%

TREATMENT OF JAUNDICED PREMATURE INFANTS

Weight	Phototherapy	Exchange transfusion
< 1000 gm	Start phototherapy within 24 hrs.	10-12 mg%
1000-1500 gm	7-9 mg%	12-15 mg%
1500-2000 gm	10-12 mg%	15-18 mg%
2000-2500 gm	13-15 mg%	18-20 mg%

230. One gram of hemoglobin librates how many milligram of bilirubin:

A. 55 **B.** 34
C. 10 **D.** 40 *(AIIMS 1997)*

One gram of hemoglobin produces **34 mg** of bilirubin.

231. Normal caloric requirement of a five-year-old child is:

A. 2000 calories
B. 1500 calories
C. 800 calories
D. 1000 calories *(PGI 1993)*

Age	Caloric requirement
• 1 year	1020
• 2-3 years	1320
• 4-5 years	1720
• 6-9 years	2130
• 10-12 years	2480
• 13-15 years	2580-3080

232. *Earliest* manifestation of rickets is:

A. Harrison's groove
B. Craniotabes
C. Pigeon chest
D. Rachitic rosary *(AIIMS 1997)*

Earliest sign of rickets is craniotabes which may be defined as an abnormal softening of the skull bones. Bones of the occipital region are more severely affected and may become thin like paper.

233. Which of the following is *true* regarding TOF:
- **A.** Spells associated with hypoxia and cyanosis
- **B.** Usually present after 7 years
- **C.** No supportive treatment is required
- **D.** Murmur intensify during spells

(UP 1995)

Tetralogy of Fallot is the most common cyanotic congenital heart disease. Paroxysmal dyspneic spells or anoxic blue spells are characterized by dyspnea, restlessness, increased cyanosis, gasping respiration and syncope. During the attack there is disappearance or reduction in intensity of systolic murmur.

234. In children hydrocephalus is commonly caused by:
- **A.** Brain tumors
- **B.** Postinflammatory obstruction
- **C.** Perinatal injury
- **D.** Congenital anomaly

(AI 1996, 1998)

235. *Not* a sign of hydrocephalus in a neonate:
- **A.** Depressed fontanelle
- **B.** Crack pot sign
- **C.** Sunset sign
- **D.** Enlarged head

(AIIMS 1997)

Hydrocephalus results from an increased volume of CSF either due to increased production or obstruction in its path. It may also result when there is impaired absorption. The ventricles become dilated and intracranial pressure is increased. Normal total volume of CSF is about 50 ml in an infant and 150 ml in an adult. Normal rate of production is 20 ml per hour. CSF is secreted by choroid plexus situated in lateral ventricles by ultrafiltration of plasma and energy dependent active secretion. It then circulates through fourth ventricle and reaches the basal cisterns via foramina of Luschka and Magendie and to the subarachnoid space at the base and cortex of brain. Normal pressure of CSF is 180 mm of water.

CAUSES OF HYDROCEPHALUS

Congenital	Acquired
• Aqueductal stenosis	• Postinflammatory (ABM, TBM) **Most common cause in children**
• Arnold-Chiari malformation	• Posterior fossa tumor
• Dandy-Walker syndrome	• Cortical atrophy (**hydrocephalus ex vacuo**)
• Intrauterine infections	
• Intracranial hemorrhage	
• Congenital tumors	

A large head or rapidly increasing head size is the single most important clinical feature. Sutures and fontanelle remain prominent are not closed and in fact the fontanelles are bulging. Macewan's or crack pot sign may be positive. Child may have impaired upward gaze (sun set sign), cranial nerve palsy and other features of upper motor neuron lesion. It is important to remember that all large heads are not hydrocephalus and the differential diagnosis includes

• Macrocephaly	• Megalencephaly
• Neurocutaneous syndromes	• Subdural effusions
• Achondroplasia	• Hemolytic anemias
• Familial large heads	

If the condition is suspected a CT scan or MRI should be done to make precise diagnosis. Surgical intervention in the form of ventriculoperitoneal shunt (VP shunt) is not required in every case. Medical management should be started if surgery is not indicated. Acetazolamide (Tab. Diamox 250 mg) in a dose 50 mg/kg/day in 3 or 4 divided doses is the drug of choice and it reduces CSF formation by up to 60%. Glycerol is an alternative of acetazolamide and the dose is 0.5-1 ml/kg/dose diluted in twice the volume of fruit juice or milk, 6 hourly.

236. In an AIDS patient, diarrheal syndrome can be due to:

A. *Cryptosporidium*
B. Adenovirus
C. Rotavirus
D. *Escherichia coli* *(AIIMS 1997)*

Cryptosporidium causes diarrheal disease in immunocompetent human hosts and more commonly among persons with AIDS or other forms of immunodeficiency. No drug effective against *Cryptosporidium* has been identified, although PAROMOMYCIN (500 to 750 mg qid) may be partially effective in some patients infected with AIDS.

237. In human milk the percentage of lactose is:

A. 4.5 gm%
B. 7.2 gm%
C. 8.0 gm%
D. 6.7 gm% *(AIIMS 1997)*

Constituents (gm %)	**Human milk**	**Cow's milk**
Water	88	88
Protein	0.9	3.3
Casein	0.4	2.7
Lactalbumin	0.4	0.4
Lactglobulin	0.2	0.2
Fat	3.8	3.8
% polyunsaturated	8	2
Lactose	**7**	**4.8**
Vitamin A (IU)	1898	1025
Thiamine (microgram)	160	440
Riboflavin (microgram)	360	1750
Niacin (microgram)	1470	940
Pyridoxine (microgram)	100	640
Pathothenate (mg)	2	3
Folacin (microgram)	52	55
B12 (microgram)	0.3	4
Vitamin C (mg)	43	11
Vitamin D (IU)	22	14
Vitamin E (mg)	2	0.4
Vitamin K (microgram)	15	60
Calcium (mg/100gm)	34	117

238. *True* regarding hemorrhagic disease of newborn:

A. Prolonged bleeding time
B. Defective platelet count
C. Prolonged thrombin time
D. Prolonged prothrombin time *(AIIMS 1997)*

239. Abnormal finding seen in classical hemorrhagic disease in children is:

- **A.** Fibrinogen activated partial thromboplastin time
- **B.** Activated partial thromboplastin time
- **C.** Thrombin time
- **D.** Platelet count

(AI 1999)

Hemorrhagic disease of the newborn (HDNB) was first identified over 100 years ago by Townsend. It presents as unexpected bleeding, often with gastrointestinal hemorrhage and ecchymosis, and, in many cases, intracranial hemorrhage. In 1961, the Committee on nutrition of the American Academy of Pediatrics (AAP) recommended that vitamin K_1 0.5 to 1.0 mg be administered intramuscularly to all newborns shortly after birth to prevent this problem. **Hemorrhagic disease of newborn (HDN)** occurs in 1 of every 400 neonates who are not given vitamin K prophylaxis. In a typical case a healthy newborn develops bleeding and bruising 48 hours after birth. **Platelet count is normal** while **prothrombin time** and **activated partial thromboplastin** time are **increased**. If active bleeding is present 10 ml/kg of fresh frozen plasma (FFP) and 1mg/kg of vitamin K should be given intravenously. *Vitamin K_1 should be given as a single intramuscular dose of 0.5 mg (birth-weight 1500 g or less) or 1.0 mg (birth weight greater than 1500 g) to all newborns within the first 6 h after birth following initial stabilization of the baby to prevent HDN.*

240. Kwashiorkor is *not* characterized by:

- **A.** Fatty infiltration of pancreas
- **B.** Fatty liver
- **C.** Patchy depigmented hair
- **D.** Edema

(AI 1999)

Kwashiorkor is characterized by pitting **edema**. The child is listless, lethargic, apathetic and miserable. Hairs are thin, dry, brittle and lusterless. They become straight and hypopigmented grayish white or reddish brown in color. During recovery growing part of hair are pigmented giving appearance of a flag (the flag sign).The skin lesions appear as large areas of erythema followed by hyperpigmentation. Skin becomes dry and hyperkeratotic. Alternate areas of hypo and hyperpigmentation give a resemblance to pavement (**pavement dermatosis**). Mosaic pattern may also be seen (mosaic dermatosis). **Liver is enlarged and fatty**.

241. Watson-Schwartz test is used to diagnose:

- **A.** Wilson's disease
- **B.** Hemochromatosis
- **C.** Acute intermittent porphyria
- **D.** All of the above

(AIIMS 1997)

Watson-Schwartz test is a test used in **acute porphyria** to differentiate porphobilinogen from urobilinogen.

242. In G6PD deficiency, hemolytic anemia *does not* occur with:

- **A.** Estrogen
- **B.** Nitrofurantoin
- **C.** Primaquine
- **D.** Salicylates

(AIIMS 1997)

Some Drugs Causing Hemolytic Anemia in G6PD Deficiency

- **Aminosalicylic acid**
- Antimalarials, e.g. **primaquine**
- Aspirin
- Chloramphenicol
- Co-trimoxazole
- Dapsone
- Nalidixic acid
- **Nitrofurantoin**
- Phenacetin
- Probenecid
- Procainamide
- Quinidine
- Sulfonamides
- Vitamin C
- Vitamin K

243. *False* regarding tricuspid atresia is:

A. Split S_2
B. Pulmonary oligemia
C. Patent foramen ovale
D. Left axis deviation

(AIIMS 1997)

In **tricuspid atresia** there is no outlet from the right atrium to the right ventricle and the entire systemic venous return goes to the left side of heart by means of a **patent foramen ovale** (PFO).

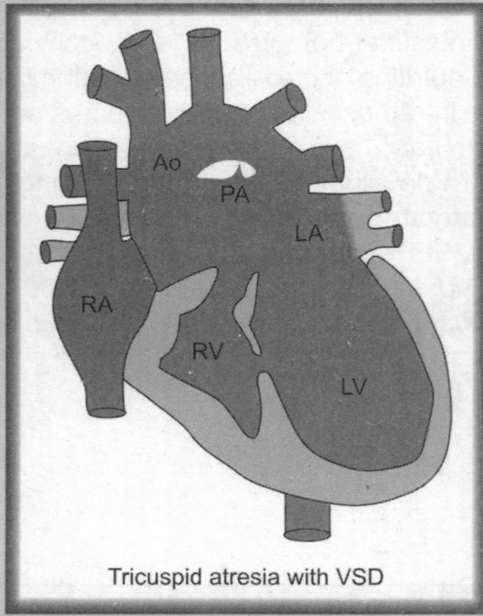

Tricuspid atresia with VSD

Pulmonary blood flow depends on the size of the VSD or PDA; the only means by which the pulmonary circulation is perfused. Cyanosis, polycythemia, easy fatigability, dyspnea on exertion and occasional hypoxic episodes develop as a result of compromised pulmonary blood flow. Clubbing and cyanosis are present and there is a heaving left ventricular apical impulse. Most of the patients have pan systolic murmurs audible along the left sternal border and the **2nd heart sound is single**. **CXR demonstrates pulmonary under-circulation** while **left axis deviation** and left ventricular hypertrophy are almost invariably evident on ECG. Symptomatic newborns require a shunt procedure to increase the pulmonary blood flow and the Blalock Taussig procedure is the preferred anastomosis. The Fontan operation is another approach to surgical management.

244. *Not* a feature of neonatal tetanus:

A. Mortality is 95%
B. Refusal to feed is common initial symptom
C. Usually occurs in first 8 days of life
D. It is caused by *Clostridium tetani*

(AIIMS 1997)

Tetanus is an acute disease caused by exotoxin of ***Clostridium tetani***. *Clostridium tetani* is gram-positive, anaerobic spore forming bacteria having terminal spores (**drum stick appearance**). *Clostridium tetani* are noninvasive and produce two types of toxins, namely tetanospasmin and tetanolysin. Tetanospasmin is neurotoxic and is responsible for clinical sign and symptoms of tetanus. Common cause is infection of umbilical stump after birth and the first symptom is usually seen on 8th day of life (**8th day disease**). First symptom is difficulty in sucking and excessive cry. Soon baby becomes stiff and spasms begin to appear. By this time difficulty in swallowing is obvious. Treatment consists of neutralizing the circulating toxins and removing the source of toxin, i.e. killing the bacteria. Human tetanus immunoglobulin (TIG) 3000 units should be given IM. **Penicillin is the drug of choice** and bactericidal to *Clostridium tetani*. Dose is 200000 IU/kg/day in four divided doses. Cleaning of umbilical cord is equally important. The child should be nursed in a quite, dark environment and diazepam 0.1 mg/kg should be given IV four hourly to control spasm. Neonatal tetanus is a severe disease having a mortality of 45-55%.

245. Chronic iridocyclitis is present in:

A. Pauciarticular rheumatoid factor +ve
B. Juvenile systemic Rh -ve arthritis
C. Polyarticular Rh factor + ve
D. Pauciarticular type I

(AIIMS 1997

Pauciarticular JRA		Polyarticular JRA	
Type I	**Type II**	**Rh factor +ve**	**Rh factor -ve**
Mainly in girls Chronic iridocyclitis	Mainly in boys Acute iridocyclitis	10% of total JRA ANA +ve in majority Severe arthritis	15-20% of total JRA Severe arthritis Iridocyclitis may occur

246. Prior to discharge of a patient of *Haemophilus influenzae* meningitis, which of the following essential investigations should be done:

A. Development screening test **B.** ECG
C. ABER **D.** EEG *(AIIMS 1997)*

Deafness is a common complication of *Haemophilus influenzae* meningitis. Vaccination of infants against type B ***Haemophilus influenzae*** meningitis prevents a major cause of acquired deafness. ABER should be done after recovery to detect hearing loss.

247. In acute poliomyelitis the *most common* cause of death is:

A. Intercostal muscle paralysis **B.** Respiratory failure
C. Cardiac arrest **D.** Convulsions *(AIIMS 1997)*

In acute bulbar poliomyelitis, function of respiratory centre is impaired and irregularities of rate and rhythm of breading leads to respiratory failure and sudden collapse.

248. Drug of choice in community acquired neonatal pneumonia is:

A. Metronidazole + Amikacin **B.** Ampicillin + Chloramphenicol
C. Cefotaxime + Amikacin **D.** Ampicillin + Gentamicin *(AIIMS 1997)*

Treatment of choice of community acquired neonatal pneumonia is intravenous **ampicillin and gentamicin** for 10 days.

249. Persistent Moro's reflex at 12 weeks indicates:

A. Normal child **B.** Brain damage
C. Irritable child **D.** Hungry child *(UP 1996)*

MORO REFLEX is also known as embrace reflex or startle reflex. It is a reflex seen in infants in response to stimuli, e.g. that produced by suddenly striking the surface on which the infant rests. To elicit this reflex the head is momentarily allowed to fall back and then is resupported by the examiner's hand. The child symmetrically abducts and extends the arms, flexes the thumbs. This movement is followed by flexion and adduction of upper extremities. **Persistence of Moro's reflex beyond 12 weeks indicates neurological damage.**

250. Asymmetric Moro's reflex is *not* seen in:

A. Hemiparesis
B. Fracture of clavicle
C. Sternomastoid tumor
D. Brachial plexus injury *(PGI 1997)*

Moro's reflex appears by 28-30 weeks but lacks complete adduction phase until 38 weeks of gestation. Moro's reflex is depressed or absent in infants with cerebral depression but it is exaggerated in cases of cerebral irritability. Incomplete response is obtained in preterm infants with gestational age < 35 weeks. **Asymmetric Moro's reflex is suggestive of brachial palsy, fracture of clavicle or humerus and hemiparesis.** Babies with kernicterus show a characteristic Moro's response in which extension of arms is not followed by flexion but there is downward rolling of eyeballs (setting sun sign), lid lag and peculiar grin.

251. Bacterial *endocarditis* is *most commonly* seen in:

A. AS **B.** ASD
C. VSD **D.** PDA *(UP 1994)*

252. Infective endocarditis is least *common* with:

A. Aortic regurgitation
B. Small ventricular septal defect
C. Atrial septal defect
D. Ventricular septal defect

(AI 1994, AIIMS 1998)

The **common congenital lesions involved in infective endocarditis are those with VSD** or aortic disease. Isolated VSD, VSD with AR, TOF, tricuspid atresia, aortic stenosis or bicuspid aortic valve in coarctation of aorta are the most common lesions associated with endocarditis.

253. All are *false* regarding typhoid in children *except*:

A. Urine culture positive in 4-6 days
B. Mild splenomegaly is usual
C. Meningitis is always seen
D. Leukocytosis is characteristic

(AI 1994)

Typhoid fever is an acute systemic febrile illness seen exclusively in humans. It is caused by *Salmonella typhi.* This disease is endemic in India and is transmitted by feco-oral route through contaminated water and food. Older children are more commonly infected although 10% of patients are below 5 years of age and 2% even below 2 years of age. Incubation period is 10-14 days. Disease starts with acute onset of fever which gradually rises over next 2-3 days. Fever is high and continuous and by the end of next week small **soft splenomegaly** appears along with clinical features of mild bronchitis. In 30% of cases liver involvement is pronounced with tenderness and jaundice. Right hypochondrial pain and tenderness indicates presence of acalculus cholecystitis. Every organ in the body may be involved and may manifest as pneumonia, myocarditis, osteomyelitis, meningitis, arthritis, etc. Intestinal hemorrhage and perforation may occur in 2nd or 3rd week of illness. Isolation of organism from blood culture in the 1st week and from stool and urine in subsequent weeks is the ideal diagnostic test. Leucopenia and eosinopenia in a typical clinical setting is highly suggestive of diagnosis. Chloramphenicol is the drug of choice and should be given 50-100 mg/kg/day 8 hourly for 2 weeks. It takes about one week to control the fever. Other effective parenteral antibiotics include high-dose ampicillin, cefotaxime, cefoperazone, and the 4-fluoroquinolones but none has been as rapidly acting or as effective as **ceftri-axone** (100 mg/kg/day for 5 days). Differential diagnosis includes infections associated with prolonged fever, such as the rickettsioses, brucellosis, tularemia, leptospirosis, miliary tuberculosis, viral hepatitis, infectious mononucleosis, cytomegalovirus infections, and malaria, as well as noninfectious causes of fever, such as lymphoma.

254. *False* regarding pseudotumor cerebri:

A. CT scan shows ring enhancing lesion
B. Ventricular system is of normal size or small
C. No focal neurological deficit
D. ICT is raised

(AIIMS 1997)

Pseudotumor cerebri: As the name itself indicates this condition produces clinical features that mimic those of brain tumor. Increased intracranial pressure is caused by diffuse cerebral edema. Common causes of pseudotumor cerebri are as under:

• Amiodarone	• Hypervitaminosis A
• Glucocorticoids	• Oral contraceptives
• Mineralocorticoid	• Tetracycline
• Hypoparathyroidism	• Galactosemia
• Idiopathic	• Obese adolescent girl

It is more common when glucocorticoids are being tapered off or after have been discontinued. **Clinical features are as under:**

• Headache	• Morning vomiting
• Papilledema	• 6th nerve palsy

It is important to note that the signs of focal neurological disease are absent and diagnosis should be suspected in a child with raised intracranial pressure in whom neither a mass lesion nor enlargement of ventricular system is found. **Lateral ventricles may be reduced in size** because of compression by edematous brain. CSF is normal. CT or MRI scan are required to rule out a focal mass lesion. If neuroradiologic studies are normal, the subarachnoid pressure should be measured by lumbar puncture to confirm that it is elevated. If it is elevated the diagnosis of pseudotumor cerebri (**idiopathic intracranial hypertension**) is made by exclusion. No treatment is required in mild cases. Repeated removal of CSF via lumber puncture helps patients with severe increase in intracranial pressure. Corticosteroids are very effective but relapse occurs when therapy is discontinued. Weight reduction is useful in obese children. Treatment with a carbonic anhydrase inhibitor such as acetazolamide lowers intracranial pressure by reducing the production of cerebrospinal fluid.

255. *False* regarding cartilage hair hypoplasia syndrome:

- **A.** T cell dysfunction
- **B.** Lymphocytosis
- **C.** Sparse hair
- **D.** Short limb dwarfism *(AIIMS 1997)*

Cartilage hair hypoplasia (CHH) is a unique form of bone dysplasia which results in short limb dwarfism, sparse hair which lacks a central pigmented core and neutropenia. Inheritance pattern is autosomal recessive. Only a small percentage of short limbed dwarfs show immune defects even though testing implies a virtual absence of T cell function.

256. *Not* a clinical feature of VSD:

- **A.** A loud pan systolic murmur is present at the right sternal border
- **B.** Infective endocarditis is also seen
- **C.** Congestive cardiac failure is common
- **D.** Second heart sound is split and variable with respiration *(AIIMS 1997)*

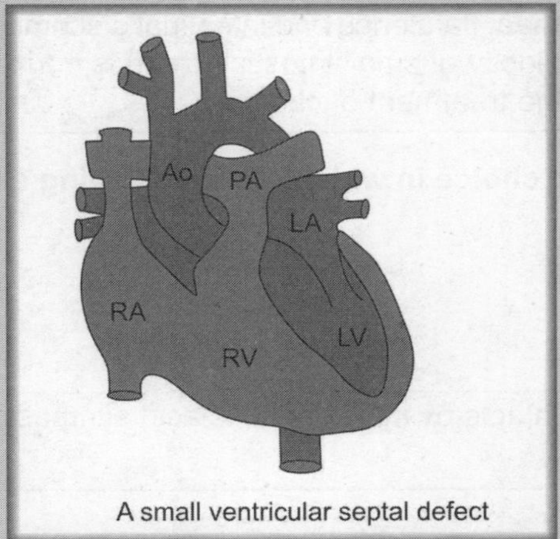

A small ventricular septal defect

Ventricular septal defect (VSD) is the *most common* congenital heart disease (CHD). The majority of defects are of membranous type in posteroinferior position. Characteristically, there is a loud, harsh, or blowing left parasternal pansystolic murmur, heard best over the lower **left** sternal border and frequently accompanied by a thrill. The second heart sound is narrowly split in large shunts. As the left to right shunt is limited in neonates, the systolic murmur may be inaudible during the first few days of life. In small defects, the child is asymptomatic and growth is normal while moderate to large defects present with repeated pulmonary infections, reduced exercise tolerance, failure to thrive (FTT) or pulmonary hypertension. **Congestive cardiac failure** may be precipitated in large defects. About 50% of small defects close spontaneously during the first year of life. **Infective endocarditis** occurs in less than 1% of cases.

257. In children lactase deficiency is characterized by:

- **A.** Low lactic acid level in blood
- **B.** High pH of stool
- **C.** Abdominal bloating, craps and diarrhea
- **D.** Dumping syndrome *(SGPGI 1996)*

258. An eight-year-old boy takes part in an icecream competition comes to the hospital with pain in abdominal distention and bloating. He also has previous similar episodes on eating icecream/milk products. Which of the following enzymes is deficient:

A. Maltase
B. Salivary amylase
C. Lactase
D. Sucrase *(AIIMS 1999)*

259. The characteristic feature of lactase deficiency in children is:

A. Low lactic level in blood
B. High pH of stool
C. Abdominal distention, cramps and diarrhea
D. Dumping syndrome *(UP 1993)*

260. Which of the following is affected by lactase deficiency:

A. Soya bean **B.** Meat
C. Cereals **D.** Milk ingestion *(UP 1998)*

261. Characteristic feature of lactase deficiency is:

A. Acidity of stool
B. Abnormal muscle cells
C. Abdominal pain, distention and diarrhea after meat ingestion
D. Decreased serum lactic acid *(AIIMS 1991)*

Congenital lactose intolerance presents with **severe diarrhea, abdominal pain and distention** soon after diet containing lactose (**milk**) is started. Symptoms disappear if milk is replaced by "**clear** liquid diet". Blood glucose concentration increases normally after oral administration of glucose or galactose but not after lactose. Lactose administration leads to explosive diarrhea, flatulence and intestinal discomfort. Lactic acid produces an **acid pH in stool** and maintains the diarrhea. In biopsy of small intestine there is normal morphology with markedly deficient lactase activity. A lactose free diet is the treatment of choice.

262. Erythromycin is *not* the drug of choice in which of the following childhood infections:

A. *Chlamydia trachomatis*
B. *Pneumocystis carinii*
C. *Bordetella pertussis*
D. *Mycoplasma pneumoniae* *(UP 1993)*

Trimethoprim-sulfamethoxazole, which acts by inhibiting folic acid synthesis, is the drug of choice for all forms of pneumocystosis.

263. Nadas' criteria are used for:

A. Malnutrition **B.** Dehydration
C. Mental retardation **D.** Presence of heart disease *(AIIMS 1997)*

Nadas' Criteria

Major	Minor
Systolic murmur of grade III or associated with thrill	Systolic murmur of < grade III
Diastolic murmur	Abnormal S2
Cyanosis	Abnormal ECG
CHF	Abnormal CXR
	Abnormal BP
One major and two minor criteria are essential for indicating the **presence of heart disease**.	

264. ***False*** **regarding hemolytic-uremic syndrome is:**

A. Viral prodrome
B. Burr cells are seen
C. ARF
D. Always fatal *(JIPMER 1991)*

265. An infant with a history of diarrhea 15 days back, presented with fever, purpuric rash, anemia and tachycardia. The diagnosis is:

A. Prerenal azotemia
B. Henoch-Schönlein purpura
C. Idiopathic thrombocytopenia
D. Hemolytic-uremic syndrome *(AIIMS 1998, UP 2000)*

Hemolytic-uremic syndrome is an acute disorder characterized by ARF with or without oligoanuria, microangiopathic hemolytic anemia and thrombocytopenia. These features develop about 2 weeks after an episode of gastroenteritis or less commonly an episode of URTI. Exact etiological agent is not known although *Coxsackievirus*, *Arboviruses*, *Echovirus*, *Shigella*, *Salmonella*, *Streptococcus pneumoniae*, Group A β hemolytic *Streptococcus* and *Mycoplasma* have been implicated. More than 50% of children have microangiopathy affecting the glomeruli and arterioles. There is widening of subendothelial space and in immunofluorescent studies the main finding is fibrin deposition with in capillary walls, lumen and in the mesangium. These changes are characteristic of hemolytic-uremic syndrome and are known as *thrombotic microangiopathy*. The platelets and RBCs are damaged when they pass through *altered* capillary and arteriolar network and are subsequently *trapped* in spleen. Hemolytic anemia is Coombs' *negative* and the RBCs are fragmented, irregular and anisocytotic. Burr cells and Helmet cells are also seen.

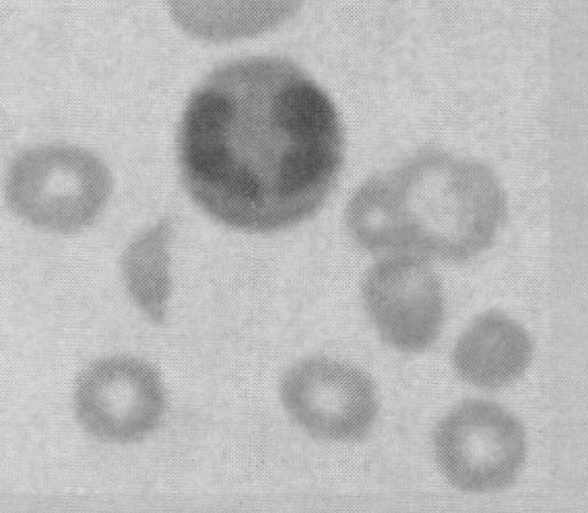

HELMET CELLS

BURR CELLS

Clinical features: Onset is acute with extreme pallor, purpura or bruising, irritability, lethargy and reduced urine output. Hypertension, edema, splenomegaly, mild jaundice, seizures and signs of congestive cardiac failure such as hepatomegaly, cardiomegaly, pulmonary edema, tachycardia, gallop rhythm and venous distention may develop. About 90% of patients now survive the acute phase.

Laboratory data: Hemoglobin level of 5-7 gm% is common associated with reticulocytosis and thrombocytopenia. TLC of 15 to 20000/cubic mm with predominance of polymorphs is a common finding. An unexplained significant hypokalemia is sometimes seen. This is a paradoxical finding in a patient of ARF and hemolytic anemia.

266. Microcytic hypochromic anemia is ***not*** **seen in:**

A. Fanconi anemia
B. Iron deficiency anemia
C. Thalassemia major
D. Lead poisoning *(AIIMS 1997)*

Fanconi anemia is the best recognized constitutional pancytopenia. Children with **Fanconi anemia** (autosomal recessive) and **dyskeratosis congentia** have **macrocytosis** as well as mild **poikilocytosis** and **anisocytosis** and their RBCs contain higher levels of hemoglobin F than are found in acquired aplasia.

267. ***Not*** **a clinical feature of scurvy in children:**

A. Retrobulbar hemorrhage
B. Intracerebral hemorrhage
C. Perifollicular hemorrhage
D. Hemorrhage into periosteum of long bones *(AIIMS 1997)*

Ascorbic acid (vitamin C) is a potent reducing substance which is essential for normal function of collagen. Adrenals and lenses are particularly rich in vitamin C. During vitamin C deficiency there is impaired formation of collagen and chondroitin sulfate. Although scurvy can occur at any age but it is extremely rare in neonatal period. Majority of cases occur between the age of 6 and 24 months. **Clinical features of child hood scurvy are as under:**	
• Irritability	• Tachypnea
• Digestive disturbances	• Loss of appetite
• Generalized tenderness	• Pseudo-paralysis (frog leg position)
• Edematous swelling of shaft of leg bones	• Subperiosteal hemorrhage
• Petechial hemorrhage in skin and mucus membrane	• Swollen joints
• Subdural hemorrhage	• Anemia
• Scorbutic rosary	• Purpura and ecchymoses
• Subarachnoid and intracerebral hemorrhages	• Retrobulbar hemorrhage

268. Delayed eruption of teeth is seen in:

A. Down syndrome　**B.** Hypopituitarism
C. Hypothyroidism　**D.** All of the above　*(AIIMS 1997)*

Conditions Associated with Delayed Eruption of Teeth

• Hypopituitarism	• Hypothyroidism
• Cleidocaranial dysostosis	• Down syndrome
• Progeria	• Albright osteodystrophy
• Incontinentia pigmenti	• Rickets
• Hunter syndrome	• Dubowitz syndrome
• Goltz syndrome	• de Lange syndrome
• Gardner syndrome	• Maroteaux Lamy syndrome

269. In a child with attack of *severe acute asthma*, the treatment of choice is:

A. IV hydrocortisone　**B.** SC Adrenaline
C. IV theophylline　**D.** Nebulised salbutamol　*(UP 1995)*

Management of Severe Acute Asthma

1. Oxygen by mask @ 5 liter / minute to achieve Oxygen saturation of > 90%.
2. **Nebulised Salbutamol** 0.15 mg / kg / dose. (Minimum 2.5 mg)—Asthalin respirator solution 5 mg / ml every 20 minutes for 3 doses, diluted in normal saline with Oxygen @ 6 liter / minute.
3. Hydrocortisone 10 mg / kg (IV) followed by oral wysolone 2 mg / kg / day.

*Sodium cromoglycate is used for long term management of asthma and is of no use during an acute attack.

270. *Not* a feature of Laurence-Moon-Biedl syndrome:

A. Retinitis pigmentosa
B. Polydactyly
C. Diabetes insipidus
D. Mental retardation　*(KERALA 1999)*

Laurence-Moon-Biedl syndrome consists of a combination of girdle-type obesity, sexual underdevelopment, **mental retardation**, retinal degeneration, **polydactyly,** and deformity of the skull. This condition is inherited as an autosomal recessive trait. Pleomorphic pigmentary retinal degeneration (**retinitis pigmentosa**), with progressive impairment of vision is also seen in this syndrome.

271. *False* regarding fetal alcohol syndrome is:

A. Growth retardation
B. Micrognathia
C. Brachycephaly
D. Altered palmer crease patterns *(AIIMS 1999)*

Some Features of Fetal Alcohol Syndrome

• Prenatal onset and persistence of growth deficiency for length, weight and head circumference	• Facial abnormalities including short palpebral fissures, epicanthic folds, maxillary hypoplasia, micrognathia and thin upper lip.
• Cardiac defects including primary septal defects	• Minor joint and limb abnormalities
• Altered palmer crease patterns	• Delayed mile stones and mental retardation

272. *Not* a feature of *D*own syndrome:

A. Respiratory tract infection
B. Pigmented birth marks
C. Hypotonia
D. Clinodactyly *(AIIMS 1991)*

273. *False* regarding Down syndrome is:

A. Duodenal atresia
B. Decreased femur length
C. Decreased humerus length
D. Decreased nuchal fold thickness *(AIIMS 1999)*

Some Features of Down Syndrome

Mongoloid face	**Ocular system**
Brachycephaly with flat occiput	Brushfield spots (gray or very light yellow spots at the periphery of the iris)
Small head, flat round face	Congenital cataract or cataract after 25 years
Mongoloid slant of eyes	Nystagmus, strabismus
Depressed nasal bridge	Blepharitis
Inner epicanthal folds	Keratoconus
Protruding tongue	Refractive error
Ears	**Endocrine**
Sensorineural/conductive deafness	Congenital hypothyroidism
Small, misshapen, low set ears	Girls fertile, boys sterile
Limbs	**Central nervous system**
Simian crease	Mental retardation
Short broad hands	**Hypotonia**
Clinodactyly (hypoplasia of middle phalanx of 5th finger)	Alzheimer's disease after 25-30 years
Gap between 1st and 2nd digits of toe	Reactive depression in adolescents
Short extremities	Autistic behavior
Cardiovascular system	**GIT**
Congenital heart disease (mainly septal defects) especially of the endocardial cushion	Atresia of gut (duodenal, esophageal and anal)
	Hirschsprung's disease

Genitalia	**Hematological system**
Small penis	Higher incidence of acute leukemia
Cryptorchidism	Congenital thrombocytopenia
Bulbous vulva	Neonatal jaundice
Immune system	**Orthopedic**
Frequent infections (ARI)	Joint laxity
Autoimmune diseases	Dislocation of patella and hip, atlanto-axial dislocation

Prenatal diagnosis of Down syndrome:
Ultrasound (11-20 weeks) nuchal fold >4 mm, double bubble in abdomen, short femur and humerus, clinodactytly and macroglossia.

274. Apt test is done for:

A. Neonatal tachypnea
B. Fetal hemoglobin
C. Neonatal asphyxia
D. Fetal maturation

(PGI 1998)

Apt test is a test done in infants to differentiate swallowed maternal blood in the stool from gastrointestinal bleeding from the infant. The blood could be swallowed during delivery or from a bleeding nipple fissure. To test:

1. A bloody stool or diaper is rinsed to obtain a pink supernatant.
2. The supernatant is centrifuged and the top fluid is removed.
3. To 5 parts of the removed solution, 1 part of 0.25 normal (1%) NaOH is added. Within **1 to 2 minute**, a color reaction takes place.

- A **yellow-brown color** indicates that the blood originated from the mother.
- A persistent **pink color** indicates that the blood is from the infant (fetal hemoglobin).

275. According to Indian Academy of Pediatrics, PEM grade III is:

A. 50-60%
B. 70-80%
C. 60-70%
D. 80-90%

(PGI 1998)

Grade of malnutrition (IAP)	% of expected weight
Grade I	71 % to 80 %
Grade II	61 % to 70 %
Grade III	51 % to 60 %
Grade IV	Less than 50 %

276. Spaulding sign is an indication of:

A. Dead fetus
B. Macerated fetus
C. Battered fetus
D. Putrefied fetus

(PGI 1999)

If a fetus dies *in utero* and *aseptic* autolysis starts, this process is known as maceration. The skull bones override each other. This can be demonstrated radiologically and is known as **Spaulding's sign.**

277. Which of the following is the *most common* cause of fecal soiling (*encopresis*) in a child:

A. Chronic constipation
B. Hirschsprung's disease
C. Gastroparesis
D. Gastrocolic reflex

(PGI 1999)

Fecal soiling or ***encopresis*** means passage of feces into inappropriate places at any age after which the bowel control should have been established. It is OFTEN ASSOCIATED WITH CHRONIC CONSTIPATION, fecal impaction and overflow incontinence. The condition may progress to *psychogenic* megacolon. It represents unconscious anger and defiance of the child.

278. Which of the following is *true* regarding coarctation of aorta:
- **A.** Right ventricular hypertrophy
- **B.** Upper rib notching due to erosion by dilated collateral vessels
- **C.** Most common distal to the origin of the left subclavian artery
- **D.** Most common presentation at 15-20 years of age

(AI 1999), (UP 2000)

279. *Not*ching of 4-9th ribs with double bulging is found in:
- **A.** Diaphragmatic hernia
- **B.** Coarctation of aorta
- **C.** Aortic dissection
- **D.** Aortic aneurysm

(AI 1998)

Coarctation of aorta: Constriction of aorta may occur at any point from transverse arch to iliac bifurcation but the most common site (98%) is **just below the origin of left subclavian artery** at the origin of ductus arteriosus (**juxtaductal coarctation**). This anomaly is twice more common in male. It is often associated with following conditions.

- Turner's syndrome (XO)
- Bicuspid aortic valve
- Parachute mitral valve
- Supravalvar mitral ring
- Subaortic stenosis
- Shone complex

When the left sided obstructive lesions occur together they are known as **Shone complex**. Classical signs of coarctation of aorta include a disparity in pulsation and blood pressure of arm and legs. Femoral, popliteal, posterior tibial and dorsalis pedes pulses are weak or may be absent (40% of cases) in contrast to the bounding pulses of arms and carotids. 90% children have systolic hypertension by the age of one year; the blood pressure being more than 95th percentile for age. Precordial impulse and heart sounds are usually normal. Notching of inferior border of ribs due to pressure erosion by enlarged collateral vessels is common by late childhood. **Rib notching is *not* seen in upper and lower 2 or 3 ribs.**

280. Pleomorphic rash is characteristic of:
- **A.** Erythema subitum
- **B.** Erythema infectiosum
- **C.** Chickenpox
- **D.** Smallpox

(DELHI 1996)

In **chickenpox** the skin lesions include maculopapules, vesicles, and scabs in various stages of evolution. **Rash is pleomorphic,** i.e. different stages of rash are seen at one given time, because rash appears in successive crops.

281. Which of the following is *true* regarding tuberculoma in childhood:
- **A.** No macrophages are seen
- **B.** Always associated with extracerebral tuberculosis
- **C.** Most common in brainstem
- **D.** Always associated with meningitis

(AI 1993)

282. In India *most common* cause of intracerebral calcification in children is:
- **A.** Toxoplasmosis
- **B.** AV malformation
- **C.** Tuberculoma
- **D.** Hyperparathyroidism

(JIPMER 1993)

Tuberculoma is the most common cause of childhood intracranial calcification in India. 50% of intracranial space occupying lesions in Indian children are due to tuberculoma. **Tuberculoma is always secondary to a primary tuberculous lesion else where in the body**. It may present with vomiting, headache, cerebellar ataxia, focal onset seizures and visual disturbances. Scanning of brain with CT scan or *preferably* MRI scan is the investigation of choice. Anti-tubercular chemotherapy should be started as soon as the diagnosis is made.

283. Which of the following should *not* be done if a women having tuberculosis delivers a baby:
- **A.** Disposal of sputum by burning
- **B.** Give ATT
- **C.** Stop breastfeeding
- **D.** Give baby BCG

(AI 2001)

Treatment protocol of baby born to mother with tuberculosis (diagnosed in the third trimester or during delivery)
- Breastfeeding must be continued
- BCG vaccine should be given at birth
- If chest X-ray is normal then 6 HR
- If chest X-ray is abnormal then 2 HRZ/7 HR
- Congenital tuberculosis: 2 HRZ/7 HR

Dosage of different antitubercular drugs	
Isoniazid (H)	5 mg/kg/day
Rifampicin (R)	10 mg/kg/day
Pyrazinamide (Z)	25 mg/kg/day
Streptomycin (S)	20 mg/kg/day
Ethambutol (E)	20 mg/kg/day
Prednisolone	1 mg/kg/day

284. Antibodies seen in a neonate after an intrauterine infection are:

A. IgD **B.** IgA
C. IgM **D.** IgG *(KERALA 1999)*

IgM is the earliest immunoglobulin to be synthesized by the fetus, beginning by about 20 weeks of intrauterine life. Because it is not transported across the placenta, **the presence of IgM in the fetus or newborn indicates intrauterine infection** and its detection is useful in the diagnosis of congenital syphilis, rubella and toxoplasmosis.

285. The correct dose of chloroquine in 4-6 years of age group is:

A. 600 mg **B.** 520 mg
C. 400 mg **D.** 150 mg *(UP 1993)*

The total dose of chloroquine to be given in a child is **25 mg/kg** of which 10mg/kg is given stat, then 5mg/kg after 6hrs and 5 mg/kg once daily for two days. As the approximate weight of a child of 4 years comes out to be [4 x 2] + 8 = 16kg the total dose of chloroquine will be 16 x 25 = **400 mg**.

286. Secondary hypertension in children is *most common*ly caused by:

A. Adrenal tumors **B.** Systemic vasculitis
C. Renal artery stenosis **D.** Renal disease *(PGI 1993)*

In children 75-90% cases of hypertension are due to underlying renal parenchymal disease primarily **acute glomerulonephritis**.

287. Which of the following fatty acids is necessary during 0-6 months of age:

A. Arachidonic acid **B.** Linolenic acid
C. Linoleic acid **D.** Palmitic acid *(JIPMER 1991)*

Human beings do not synthesize linoleic acid hence it must be supplied in diet. **Linoleic acid is the most essential fatty acid** because it serves as a basis of production of other essential fatty acids (linolenic acid and arachidonic acid).

288. A child has recurrent hypoglycemic attacks and hepatomegaly. He is *most likely* suffering from:

A. Neonatal hepatitis **B.** Neonatal diabetes
C. von Gierke disease **D.** Galactosemia *(DELHI 1993)*

Glycogen Storage Disease Type I or glucose-6-phosphatase deficiency or von Gierke disease: Children with GSD I are unable to release glucose from liver glycogen. If untreated, this results in prolonged periods of **hypoglycemia**. In early childhood they present with sweating, irritability, poor growth and muscle weakness. **Hepatomegaly** is seen due to excessive accumulation of glycogen that cannot be broken down normally. In addition to these problems, children with GSD I can develop frequent mouth ulcers and are at increased risk of infection. Treatment primarily consists of giving glucose drinks frequently during the day and, in most cases, continuously overnight through a nasogastric tube. As children get older, treatment with cornstarch, which releases glucose slowly into the gut, may be very effective. With such intensive treatment most children do well and their symptoms improve as they reach adulthood.

289. Preterm infant with PDA should be treated with:

A. Corticosteroids **B.** Indomethacin
C. Aspirin **D.** Prostaglandin E2 *(UP 1990)*

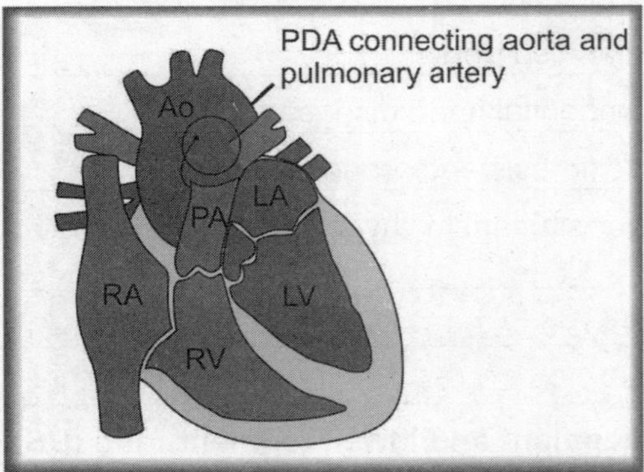

Dose of IV Indomethacin in Premature Infants with PDA

Age	Initial	Second and third
Less than 48 hrs	0.2 mg/kg	0.1 mg/kg
2-7 days	0.2 mg/kg	0.2 mg/kg
More than 7 days	0.2 mg/kg	0.25 mg/kg

- Ibuprofen therapy **(IV; first dose of 10 mg per kilogram, followed at 24-hour intervals by two doses of 5 mg per kilogram each or oral Ibuprofen 10 mg/kg—1st dose, 5 mg/kg—2 doses at 12 hourly intervals)** on the 3rd day of life is as efficacious as indomethacin for the treatment of patent ductus arteriosus in **preterm infants** with the respiratory distress syndrome and is significantly *less likely* to induce oliguria.

*Doses to be given at 12-18 hour interval

290. Which of the following is *not* an indication for antibiotics in diarrhea:

A. Organism with darting motility **B.** Septic focus
C. Severe dehydration **D.** Bloody diarrhea *(AI 1993)*

Unnecessary use of antibiotics in management of acute diarrheal disease will do more harm than good. Antibiotics should be considered when the cause of diarrhea has been clearly identified to be bacteria such as *Shigella* (bloody diarrhea), *Vibrio* (motile organism in hanging drop preparation) or if the patient has other focus of sepsis.

291. Upper and lower portion of body disproportion with growth retardation is characteristic of:

A. Congenital hypothyroidism **B.** Silver Russell syndrome
C. Turner syndrome **D.** Down syndrome *(AI 1993)*

Differential Diagnosis of Short Stature

1. Normal variants	
• Familial genetic short stature	• Constitutional growth delay
2. Disproportionate short stature	
• Skeletal dysplasias	• Untreated congenital hypothyroidism
• Rickets	
3. Proportionate short stature of prenatal onset	
• **IUGR** due to maternal toxemia, diabetes mellitus, intrauterine infections, alcohol, nicotine and drugs	
• **Dysmorphic syndromes** such as Silver Russell syndrome	
• **Chromosomal anomalies** such as Down syndrome, Turner syndrome	

4. Proportionate short stature of postnatal onset	
• **Malnutrition**	
• **Diseases of GI tract** such as celiac disease, chronic diarrhea	
• **Renal diseases** such as CRF, tubular disorders	
• **CVS disorders** such as cyanotic congenital heart disease, CHF	
• **Pulmonary diseases** such as cystic fibrosis and bronchial asthma	
• **Endocrine disorders** such as hypopituitarism, hypothyroidism, diabetes mellitus, Cushing's syndrome, hypogonadism	
• **Chronic infections** such as tuberculosis	
• **Psychosocial** short stature	
Normal upper segment and lower segment ratio (US: LS ratio)	
At birth	1.7
At 3 years	1.3
At 6 years	1.1
At 10 years	1.0

292. Epiphyseal dysgenesis is a *pathognomic* feature of which of the following conditions:

A. Hyperthyroidism **B.** Hypothyroidism
C. Hyperparathyroidism **D.** Hypoparathyroidism *(UP 1993)*

Hypothyroidism is present in about 1 in every 5000 neonates. It is manifested by persistence of physiologic jaundice, a hoarse cry, constipation, somnolence, and feeding problems. All neonates should be screened for hypothyroidism with measurements of the serum T4 or TSH because the clinical diagnosis is difficult and early treatment is crucial for normal intellectual development. Later in affected child, delay in reaching the normal milestones of development becomes evident, and the characteristics of the cretin appear. They include:

• SHORT STATURE	• BROAD AND FLAT NOSE	• DRY SKIN
• PROTRUDING TONGUE	• WIDELY SET EYES	• IMPAIRED MENTAL DEVELOPMENT
• MACROGLOSSIA	• SPARSE HAIR	• RETARDED BONE AGE
• EPIPHYSEAL DYSGENESIS	• DELAYED DENTITION	• PROTUBERANT ABDOMEN WITH AN UMBILICAL HERNIA

293. In tuberculous meningitis, the CSF finding includes:

A. Low sugar + high protein and lymphopenia
B. High sugar + high chloride
C. Low sugar + high protein and lymphocytosis
D. High sugar + low protein *(AI 1994)*

	Appearance	Pressure	Cells	Protein	Sugar
Normal	Watery	100-180 mm of CSF	0-5 all lymphocytes	20-40 mg%	40-80 mg%
Acute bacterial meningitis	Turbid	Raised	100-5000 Neutrophil predominant	100-400mg%	Low Organism may be seen
Tubercular meningitis	Clear or cloudy	Raised	10-500 Lymphocyte predominant	80-400 mg% or more	Low Organism may be seen
Viral encephalitis	Clear	Normal	20-2000 Lymphocyte predominant	150 mg%	Normal C/S sterile

294. L Asparaginase is particularly used in:

A. CLL **B.** ALL
C. CML **D.** AML *(AI 1995)*

Treatment Regimens for ALL

Remission induction phase (one month)
Prednisone : 40 mg/sq m/day Vincristine : 1.5 mg/ sq m /week IV for 4 weeks **L Asparaginase** : 200 IU /kg/day IV
CNS prophylaxis(beginning at 4 week)
Cobalt 60 cranial irradiation for 2.5 weeks total dose 1800 rads Intrathecal methotrexate : 12 mg/ sq m twice a week for 2.5 weeks maximum dose 15 mg
Continuation therapy for 30 months
6-mercaptopurine: 50 mg/sqmt / 24 hour PO Methotrexate : 20 mg/ sq m /wk intravenously

295. Hypokalemia in an infant is *not* due to:

A. Diarrhea **B.** Thiazide therapy
C. ARF **D.** β 2 agonists *(AI 1994)*

Daily maintenance requirement of potassium is 2 mEq/kg body weights. Some causes of hypokalemia in children are as under:		
Excessive renal loss		
• Tubular diseases (drugs, cystinosis)		
• Steroid (glucocorticoids, aldosterone)		
• Diuretics (Thiazide, Furosemide therapy)		
• Nonreabsorbable anions (penicillin, bicarbonate)		
Nonrenal loss		
• Vomiting	• Diarrhea	• Laxative abuse
Shift from extracellular to intracellular fluid		
• Insulin	• β 2 agonists	• Alkalosis
Limited intake		

* ARF causes hyperkalemia

296. Which of the following is a preventable cause of mental retardation in children:

A. Cerebral palsy **B.** Hypothyroidism
C. Down syndrome **D.** All of the above *(AI 1995, PGI 1998)*

Hypothyroidism is a preventable cause of mental retardation. Sodium-L-Thyroxine is the treatment of choice in hypothyroidism. The goal is to maintain T4 and TSH in normal range. It is available as 100μg tablet (Tab. Eltroxin) and the dosages are as under:

- **Newborns** 10-15 μg/ kg/day
- **Children** 4 μg/ kg/day
- **Adults** 2 μg/ kg/day

297. *False* regarding typhoid is:

A. Recurrence is common
B. Localizes in gallbladder
C. Chronic carrier state lasts for 3-4 months
D. Fecal carrier are more than urinary carrier *(AIIMS 1994)*

Carrier of typhoid may be temporary or chronic carriers. Persons who excrete the bacilli for more than a year after a clinical attack are known as chronic carriers. In these carriers the organism persists in gallbladder and biliary tract. A chronic carrier may excrete bacilli for several years (may be up to 50 years). Fecal carriers are more frequent than urinary carriers. Natural typhoid fever does not provide solid immunity and second attacks may occur.

298. In a 2-year-old child, seizure with chorioretinitis is suggestive of:

A. Hypoxia
B. Tay-Sachs disease
C. Congenital toxoplasmosis
D. Galactosemia *(AIIMS 1994, 1996)*

Congenital toxoplasmosis manifests as poor feeding, fever, maculopapular rash, lymphadenopathy, splenomegaly, hepatomegaly, jaundice, hydrocephalus, microcephaly, seizures. Cerebral calcification and chorioretinitis may be present at birth or may appear subsequently.

299. *False* regarding childhood malignancies:

A. AML is the most common type of leukemia
B. Neuroblastoma occurs in first 4 years of life
C. Lymphoma commonly presents with CNS symptoms
D. 66% of leukemia have splenomegaly *(AIIMS 1994)*

Acute leukemia is the **most common** form of childhood cancer and ALL accounts of 60% of leukemia cases in children.

300. Decreased serum alpha-fetoprotein level is seen in:

A. Exomphalos
B. Fetal death
C. Meningomyelocele
D. Down syndrome *(AIIMS 1992)*

Alpha-fetoprotein is an antigen present in the human fetus and in certain pathological conditions in the adult. The maternal serum level should be evaluated at 16 to 18 weeks of pregnancy to detect fetal abnormalities. It is increased in the following conditions:

• Anencephaly	• Meningomyelocele
• Encephalocele	• Omphalocele (Exomphalos)
• Meckel syndrome	• Congenital nephrosis
• Impending spontaneous abortion	• Fetal death
• Rh sensitization	• Presence of intestinal atresia
• **Decreased levels indicate an increased risk of having a baby with Down syndrome.**	

If an abnormal level of AFP is found, further tests such as ultrasound or amniocentesis should be done to establish the final diagnosis. Elevated serum levels are also found in adults with certain hepatic carcinomas or chemical injuries.

Omphalocele (Exomphalos) has an incidence of 1 in 6000. It occurs due to failure of all or part of midgut to return to coelom. When the sac remains unruptured, it is semitranslucent and consists of 3 layers; an outer layer of amniotic membrane, a middle layer of Wharton's jelly, and an inner layer of peritoneum. It is of two types; Exomphalos major and Exomphalos minor. Operation within first few hours of life is only hope of survival.

301. Congenital heart disease, which causes death in the first week of life, is:

A. Ventricular septal defect
B. Tetralogy of Fallot
C. Ebstein's anomaly
D. Hypoplastic left ventricle syndrome

In HYPOPLASTIC LEFT VENTRICLE SYNDROME the sign of heart failure are present within the 1st week of life and most patient die during the 1st month of life, usually the **1st week.**

302. In an infant congestive cardiac failure is diagnosed by:

A. Basal crypts **B.** Elevated JVP
C. Pedal edema **D.** Liver enlargement

In infants **CHF** is difficult to diagnose. The symptoms of congestive cardiac failure are as under:

- Poor feeding
- Poor weight gain
- Excessive sweating
- Irritability
- Weak cry
- Labored breathing
- Tachypnea and subcoastal retraction
- Flaring of alae nasi
- HEPATOMEGALY NEARLY ALWAYS OCCUR

303. In meningitis subdural effusion is *most commonly* due to:

A. Meningococcal **B.** Pneumococcal
C. *Haemophilus* **D.** Tuberculous

Meningitis is the most serious manifestation of **Haemophilus-b** infection. It mainly affects infants < 2 years of age. The most **common features** are:

- Fever
- Altered central nervous system function
- Neck rigidity may be present
- **Subdural effusion is the most common complication and it should be suspected when, the patient has seizures, hemiparesis or continued obtundation, despite 2-3 days of appropriate antibiotic therapy**
- The mortality from meningitis caused by *Haemophilus influenzae* b is about 5 %
- 6% of the survivors have **permanent sensorineural hearing loss**, and 1/4th have a significant handicap of some type such as partial hearing loss and delay in language development

304. The national schedule of immunization in a child begins at birth and end at:

A. 3rd year **B.** 4th year
C. 5th year **D.** 10th year

National Immunization Schedule

Age	Vaccine
• At birth	BCG+OPV
• 6 weeks	DPT + OPV
• 10 weeks	DPT + OPV
• 14 weeks	DPT + OPV
• 9 months	Measles
• 18 months	DPT + OPV
• 5 years	DT
• 10 years	TT
• 16 years	TT
• Pregnant women	TT (2 doses at 4 weeks interval)

305. First *permanent* tooth to erupt is:

A. First premolar
B. First molar
C. First incisor
D. Second premolar

Chronology of Human Dentition–Secondary or Permanent Teeth

Teeth	Maxillary	Mandibular
• First molar	6 – 7 years	6 – 7 years
• Central incisor	7 – 8 years	6 – 7 years
• Lateral incisor	8 – 9 years	7 – 8 years
• First premolar	10 – 11 years	10 – 12 years
• Second premolar	10 – 12 years	11 – 13 years
• Canine	11 – 12 years	9 – 11 years
• Second molar	12 – 13 years	12 – 13 years
• Third molar	17 – 22 years	17 – 22 years

306. The diagnosis of rheumatic fever is *best* confirmed by:
- **A.** ASO titer
- **B.** ECG changes
- **C.** Raised ESR
- **D.** Throat swab culture

307. Which of the following is *necessary* for diagnosis of rheumatic fever:
- **A.** Prior history of rheumatic fever
- **B.** Recent sore throat infection
- **C.** One major and two minor criteria
- **D.** Erythema marginatum *(AI 1993)*

308. A child presents with migratory polyarthritis, the investigation of choice to confirm the diagnosis is:
- **A.** ESR
- **B.** ASO titre
- **C.** Pharyngeal swab for culture and sensitivity
- **D.** ECG

The Jones Criteria for Rheumatic Fever

Major Criteria	Minor Criteria	
	Clinical	**Laboratory**
Carditis		
Migratory polyarthritis	Fever	Elevated ESR
Sydenham's chorea	Arthralgia	Elevated CRP
Subcutaneous nodules		Prolonged PR interval
Erythema marginatum		
PLUS (ESSENTIAL CRITERIA)		
Supporting evidence of a recent group A streptococcal infection which includes any one of the following:		
• Positive throat culture for *Streptococcus*		
• Rapid antigen detection test		
• Elevated or increasing streptococcal antibody test (**ASO titer** > 200 Todd's unit in adults or > 300 Todd's unit children).		

*Diagnosis of rheumatic fever is highly probable if ***two major*** or one ***major and two minor*** **criteria** are present along with the evidence of previous *Streptococcus* infection.

309. In congenital rubella *most commonly* occurring defect is:
- **A.** Blindness
- **B.** Mental retardation
- **C.** Deafness
- **D.** Microcephaly

310. Rubella maximally infects the fetus if the mother contacts the disease during........ weeks of pregnancy:

A. 5-6 B. 12-13
C. 20 D. 9-12

CONGENITAL RUBELLA: Maternal infection in early pregnancy can lead to fetal infection. The characteristic features of congenital rubella are as under:

- Cataract
- Heart disease
- Deafness

Other abnormalities include:

TRANSIENT	PERMANENT	DEVELOPMENTAL
• LOW BIRTH WEIGHT	• DEAFNESS	• MENTAL RETARDATION
• THROMBOCYTOPENIA	• PULMONARY STENOSIS	• DIABETES MELLITUS
• HEPATOSPLENOMEGALY	• PATENT DUCTUS ARTERIOSUS	• BEHAVIORAL DISORDERS
• JAUNDICE	• GLAUCOMA	
• PNEUMONIA	• CATARACT	

The most important factor in the pathogenicity of rubella virus for the fetus is gestational age at the time of infection. **Maternal infection during the 1st trimester causes fetal infection in nearly half of the cases**, while the maternal infection early in the 2nd trimester leads to fetal infection in 1/3rd of cases. Fetal malformations are more common after maternal infection in the 1st trimester and are more severe and they involve more organ systems.

311. IUGR can be caused by all *except*:

A. Captopril B. Caffeine
C. Atenolol D. Phenothiazine

- CAPTOPRIL can cause intrauterine growth retardation, fetal distress and hypotension, and cranial malformation
- CAFFEINE crosses the placenta and achieves blood and tissue concentrations in the fetus that are similar to maternal concentrations. Caffeine consumption by pregnant women may increase the risk of spontaneous abortion and IUGR.
- ATENOLOL and nadolol can also cause Intrauterine growth retardation

312. Feature of petit mal epilepsy in EEG is:

A. Spike and dome B. Continuous stunted spikes
C. Waves at the rate of 10/seconds D. Continuous tall spikes

PETIT MAL EPILEPSY: The hallmark of typical absence seizures is a generalized, symmetric, 3 Hz SPIKE-AND-WAVE DISCHARGE which begins and ends suddenly on a normal EEG background.

313. An 8-month-old child will *not* be able to do:

A. Pincer grasp B. Says mama baba
C. Stand without support D. Sitting stably

Pincer finger thumb grasp develop around the age of 9 months. It is used to pickup small objects.

314. Which of the following immunoglobulins is *most* affected in kwashiorkor:

A. IgM B. IgE
C. IgA D. IgD *(AI 1994)*

In addition to the impairment of physical growth and of cognitive and other physiologic functions, immune response changes occur early in the course of significant **malnutrition** in a child. These immune response changes correlate with poor outcomes and mimic the changes observed in children with acquired immune deficiency syndrome (AIDS). Loss of delayed hypersensitivity, fewer T lymphocytes, impaired lymphocyte response, impaired phagocytosis secondary to decreased complement and certain cytokines, and **decreased secretory immunoglobulin A (IgA)** are some changes that may occur.

315. The percentage of calories to be supplied by proteins is:

A. > 20%
B. 10-15 %
C. 15-20%
D. 5-10 %

Nutrients	Percentage of calories to be supplied
• Carbohydrate	45-55%
• Fat	35-45 %
• Protein	9-15 %

316. Early sign of rickets at 6 months of age is:

A. Craniotabes
B. Bent tibia
C. Double malleoli
D. Knock knees

Earliest sign of rickets is CRANIOTABES which may be defined as an abnormal softening of the skull bones. Those in the occipital region are more severely affected and may become almost paper thin.

317. *Most common* cause of bronchiolitis:

A. Respiratory syncytial virus
B. *Pneumococcus*
C. *Haemophilus*
D. Enterovirus

Respiratory syncytial virus infection may cause a wide range of respiratory diseases. In infants, 25-40% of infections result in lower respiratory tract involvement, and they include pneumonia, **bronchiolitis**, and tracheo-bronchitis. The disease begins frequently with rhinorrhea, low-grade fever, and mild systemic symptoms, along with cough and wheezing. Patients generally recover in 1 -2 weeks. In severe disease, tachypnea and dyspnea develop which eventually leads to frank hypoxia, cyanosis, and apnea. Diffuse wheezing, rhonchi, and rales are present. Chest X-ray shows hyperexpansion, peribronchial thickening and infiltrates. Disease is more severe in children born prematurely and in those with congenital cardiac disease, bronchopulmonary dysplasia, nephrotic syndrome, or immunosuppression.

318. Hyaline membrane in the lung is seen in:

A. Respiratory distress syndrome
B. Pneumococcal pneumonia
C. Acute viral hepatitis
D. Pulmonary edema

Hyaline membrane disease is also known as respiratory distress syndrome of the newborn.

319. Leukemoid reaction is seen in:

A. Acute infection
B. Erythroleukemia
C. Myelomatosis
D. Hemorrhage

Persistent neutrophilia of 30,000-50,000 cells/μL or greater is known as **leukemoid reaction**. It is a term used to distinguish this degree of neutrophilia from leukemia. In a leukemoid reaction, the circulating neutrophils are mature and not clonally derived. Leukemoid reaction is seen in ACUTE INFECTIONS.

320. The malignancies of childhood include:

A. AML
B. Wilms' tumor
C. ALL
D. All of the above

Occurrence of Malignant Neoplasms in Children under 15 Years of Age

	Rate (per million/Year)	
Neoplasm	**White**	**Black**
• Leukemia [ALL,AML,CML]	42.1	24.3
• CNS tumor	23.9	23.9
• Lymphoma	13.2	13.9
• Sympathetic nervous system	9.6	7.0
• Kidney tumor [Wilms' tumor]	7.8	7.8
• Bone tumor	5.6	4.8
• Soft tissue sarcoma	8.4	3.9
• Retinoblastoma	3.4	3.0
• Gonadal and germ cell tumor	2.2	2.6
• Liver tumor	1.9	0.4

321. In assessment of gestational age of a neonate the following are seen *except*:

A. Ocular **B.** Breast bud
C. Genitalia **D.** Scrotal skin *(JIPMER 2001)*

External Signs Used in Dubowitz Scoring to Assess Gestational Age of a Neonate

- Edema
- Skin color (infant not crying)
- Plantar creases
- Breast size
- Ear firmness
- Skin texture
- Lanugo (over back)
- Nipple formation
- Ear form
- Genitalia

322. The mechanism of diarrhea in giardiasis is prevention of absorption of fat by:

A. Mechanical coating of the walls of intestine
B. Production of exotoxins
C. Production of endotoxins
D. Secondary bacterial infection

Trophozoites of *Giardia* adhere to the epithelium and they do not cause invasive or locally destructive alterations at the site of attachment. The loss of brush border enzyme activities lead to development of lactose intolerance and significant malabsorption in a small number of infected adults and children. Generally the morphology of the bowel is unaltered but in chronically infected and symptomatic patients, the histopathological findings, including flattened villi and the clinical features resemble with those of tropical sprue and gluten-sensitive enteropathy. The pathogenesis of diarrhea in GIARDIASIS is not clearly known.

323. Bronchiolitis is treated with:

A. Humidified oxygen **B.** Steroids
C. Antibiotics **D.** All of the above

Bronchiolitis is caused by infection of respiratory syncytial virus. It is a member of the Paramyxoviridae family and genus Pneumovirus. Its replication leads to the fusion of neighboring cells into large multinucleated syncytia. Treatment of bronchiolitis is supportive and consists of:

- **HUMIDIFIED OXYGEN**
- Intravenous fluids
- Antipyretics
- Use of steroids should be avoided because it may increase the viral proliferation
- Antibiotics are of no use

324. *Most common* cause of meningitis in neonates is:

A. *Streptococcus*
B. *Haemophilus*
C. *Escherichia coli*
D. *Meningococcus*

Organism	Neonates
• Gram-negative bacilli **(mainly *Escherichia coli*)**	50-60 %
• Streptococci	20-40%
• *Listeria* species	2-10 %
• Staphylococci	5 %
• *S. pneumoniae*	0-5 %
• *H. influenzae*	0-3 %
• *N. meningitidis*	0-1 %

325. In children most *common complication* of measles is:

A. ASOM
B. Orchitis
C. Meningitis
D. Bronchopneumonia

The respiratory tract complications of measles manifest as laryngitis, croup, or bronchitis. **In young children, OTITIS MEDIA is the most common complication**. Pneumonia is the major reason for hospitalization in adults. The pneumonia is of generally of viral origin but secondary bacterial most commonly caused by streptococci, pneumococci, or staphylococci also occur. Primary giant cell (Hecht's) pneumonia is seen in immunocompromised and malnourished patients.

326. Post-measles bronchopneumonia is treated with:

A. Antibiotics and oxygen
B. No treatment is necessary
C. Steroid
D. Only oxygen

The pneumonia is generally of viral origin but secondary bacterial most commonly caused by streptococci, pneumococci, or staphylococci also occur. Therefore it is necessary to give ANTIBIOTICS that are active against gram-positive bacteria. Combination of clavulanic acid and amoxicillin (enhancin / augmentin) with an amino glycoside (amikacin / tobracin) is a good choice. Other supportive treatment such as intravenous fluids, antipyretics, OXYGEN and vitamin A should also be given.

327. Syphilis attack the fetus after the .... months:

A. 2nd
B. 7th
C. 4th
D. 3rd

Transmission of *T. pallidum* from a syphilitic woman to her fetus across the placenta can occur at any stage of pregnancy, **but the lesions of congenital** syphilis **generally develop after the 4TH MONTH OF GESTATION.** At this time the fetal immunologic competence begins to develop. This timing indicates that the pathogenesis of congenital syphilis depends on the immune response of the host rather than on a direct toxic effect of *T. pallidum*.

328. Child changes rattle from one hand to another at:

A. 1 year
B. 6 months
C. 3 months
D. 2 years

A child transfers object from hand to hand at the age of 28 weeks.

329. *Most common* complication of mumps in children is:

A. Orchitis
B. Aseptic meningitis
C. Myocarditis
D. Pancreatitis

Parotitis is generally BILATERAL, although the onset on the two sides may not be synchronous and at times only one side is affected. THE MOST COMMON COMPLICATION OF MUMPS IN CHILDREN IS ASEPTIC MENINGITIS. It **may develop before, during, after, or in the absence of parotitis.** Symptoms are stiff neck, headache, and drowsiness. Pleocytosis of the cerebrospinal fluid, with up to 1000 cells/μL, develop in up to half of the cases, but clinical signs of meningeal irritation are seen in only 5-25 % of patients.

330. Asperger's disorder is a:

A. Developmental delay
B. Neuromuscular disease
C. Degenerative disorder
D. Metabolic disorder

(JIPMER 2002)

In **Asperger's disorder**, affected individuals are characterized by **social isolation and eccentric behavior in childhood.** There are **impairments in two-sided social interaction and non-verbal communication.** Though grammatical, their speech is peculiar due to abnormalities of inflection and a repetitive pattern. Clumsiness is prominent both in their articulation and gross motor behavior. They usually have a circumscribed area of interest which usually leaves no space for more age appropriate, common interests. Some examples are cars, trains, French Literature, door knobs, hinges, meteorology, astronomy or history. The name "Asperger" comes from Hans Asperger, an Austrian physician who first described the syndrome in 1944.

331. Drug of choice initially in juvenile chronic arthritis is:

A. Salicylates
B. Prednisolone
C. Phenylbutazone
D. Indomethacin

A number of drugs are effective in suppressing the inflammatory process of juvenile rheumatoid arthritis, but aspirin is still the safest and most effecftive in a dose of 100 mg/kg/day.

332. Steroids are useful in:

A. Rapidly progressing glomerulonephritis
B. Membranous glomerulonephritis
C. Post-streptococcal glomerulonephritis
D. Minimal change glomerulonephritis

Minimal change glomerulonephritis IS HIGHLY STEROID-RESPONSIVE and has an excellent prognosis. Spontaneous remission occurs in 30-40% of childhood cases. About 90 % of children enter remission after 8 weeks of high-dose oral glucocorticoids. In a typical regimen, 60 mg of prednisone per m^2 of body surface area daily for 4 weeks, followed by 40 mg/m^2 on alternate days for an additional 4 weeks should be given to the patient.

333. Transient tachypnea of the newborn develops in:

A. Term baby by spontaneous vaginal delivery
B. Term baby by forceps
C. Preterm baby by cesarean section
D. Preterm with ventouse

(AIIMS May 2002)

Newborns at *higher risk* for development of transient tachypnea of the newborn (TTN) include those who are:

- Premature
- Delivered by **cesarean section**
- Born to mothers who smoked during pregnancy
- Born to mothers with diabetes
- Small for gestational age (SGA)

334. In childhood thyrotoxicosis, treatment of choice is:

A. Radioiodine
B. Lugol's iodine
C. Carbimazole
D. Surgery

(AIIMS 1992)

Although ^{131}I therapy may gain acceptance, the most common choice for therapy of thyrotoxicosis in children is between antithyroid drugs and subtotal thyroidectomy. Proponents of antithyroid drug therapy believe that there is a greater tendency for remission of thyrotoxicosis in children compared to adults and that antithyroid drug therapy avoids the psychic and physical problems caused by surgery in this age group. With drugs the need for surgery (or ^{131}I) can be delayed almost indefinitely until conditions become favorable. **Antithyroid drug therapy is the usual preferable initial therapy in children.**

335. Sitting height is equal to:

A. Head circumference
B. Upper segment
C. Chest circumference
D. Crown rump length

(DELHI 1996)

Crown rump length is the **sitting length** or distance from the top of the baby's head to its *rump* or buttock. This measurement is used more often than crown to heel length because the baby's legs are most often bent, making that dimension difficult.

336. Infantile diarrhea is *not* caused:

A. Adenovirus
B. Reovirus
C. Rotavirus
D. Caliciviruses

Acute infectious diarrheal disease is a leading cause of mortality in **infants** and young children in developing countries. **Two separate groups of viruses—the rotaviruses and the enteric caliciviruses, such as Norwalk virus—as well as a variety of bacterial pathogens are important etiologic agents of gastroenteritis.** The rotaviruse primarily affects young children. The Norwalk and related enteric caliciviruses affect adults and children both. Enteric **adenoviruses** are a minor cause of diarrheal illness in infants and children, accounting for only **10 %** of the cases. **Reovirus** is a **rare cause** of mild gastroenteritis in infants and children.

337. Blood and mucus in stools are *not* seen with:

A. *Shigella shigae*
B. *Escherichia coli*
C. *Entamoeba histolytica*
D. *Vibrio cholerae*

The stool in **cholera** has a typical appearance. Stools are in the form of non bilious, gray, slightly cloudy fluid with **flecks of mucus, no blood,** and have a sweet, inoffensive odor. It is called **"rice-water" stool** because it resemble to the water in which rice has been washed.

338. *Not* a cause nephrotic syndrome:

A. Membranous glomerulonephritis
B. Focal glomerulosclerosis
C. Post streptococcal glomerulonephritis
D. Minimal lesion glomerulonephritis

Causes of Nephrotic Syndrome in Children

1. Idiopathic (90 %)	2. Glomerulonephritis associated (10%)
• Minimal change disease (85%) • Focal sclerosis (10%) • Mesingioproliferative (5%)	• Membranous • Membranoproliferative

339. Poisoning with which of the following can cause unexplained ataxia in a child:

A. Salicylate
B. Lead
C. Mercury
D. Arsenic

Lead poisoning symptoms in childhood develop at blood **lead** levels > 3.9 μmol/L. The symptoms are abdominal pain and irritability followed by lethargy, anorexia, pallor due to anemia, **ataxia**, and slurred speech. Convulsions, coma, and death as a result of generalized cerebral edema and renal failure occur in the most severe cases. Subclinical lead poisoning (blood lead level >1.4 μmol/L) may cause mental retardation and selective deficits in language, cognitive function, balance, behavior, and school performance.

340. *Not* a characteristic feature of kwashiorkor:

A. Edema
B. Flag sign
C. Dermatitis
D. Alertness

Kwashiorkor is characterized by **pitting edema**. The child is listless, **lethargic**, apathetic and miserable. Hairs are thin, dry, brittle and lusterless. They become straight and hypopigmented grayish white or reddish brown in color. During recovery growing part of hair are pigmented giving appearance of a flag (the **flag sign**).The skin lesions appear as large areas of erythema followed by hyperpigmentation. Skin becomes dry, hyperkeratotic. Alternate areas of hypo and hyper pigmentation give a resemblance to pavement (**pavement dermatosis**). Mosaic pattern may also be seen (**Mosaic dermatosis**). Liver is enlarge and fatty.

341. In newborns, *most common* cause of pneumothorax is:

A. Resuscitation
B. Hyaline membrane disease
C. Pneumonia
D. Meconium aspiration

(UP 1998)

Air leaks occur when the alveoli become *over distended* and burst. **Pressure of the air delivered by mechanical ventilators is the *most common* cause of pneumothorax in newborns.** Meconium aspiration can also trap air and lead to over distention and air leaks. Some otherwise healthy babies can develop a "spontaneous" air leak that does not cause symptoms or distress.

342. The clinical sign in measles which appears last is:

A. Coryza
B. Fever
C. Rash
D. Koplik's spot

Measles: The clinical features are fever, general malaise, sneezing, nasal congestion, brassy cough, conjunctivitis, spots on the buccal mucosa (Koplik's spots), and a **maculopapular eruption** over the entire body. The characteristic erythematous, nonpruritic, maculopapular rash begins at the hairline and behind the ears, then spreads down the trunk and limbs including the palms and soles, and becomes confluent.

343. A child has mental age of 7 and chronological age of 7 years. His IQ is:

A. 100
B. 80
C. 120
D. 145

IQ = Mental age/chronological age x 100
= 7/7 x 100 = 100

344. *Not* a characteristic feature of thalassemia major:

A. Target cells
B. Splenomegaly
C. Hypochromic microcytic anemia
D. Decreased serum iron

Thalassemia major is also known as Cooley's anemia. It is characterized by fatigue, **splenomegaly**, and severe anemia, enlargement of the heart, slight jaundice, leg ulcers, and gallbladder stones. Increased bone marrow activity results in thickening of the cranial bones. The peripheral blood smear reveals severe abnormalities, marked anisocytosis with many small and colorless microcytic, **hypochromic red cells.** Abnormal forms, including **target cells**, stippled red cells and fragmented red cells are also present.

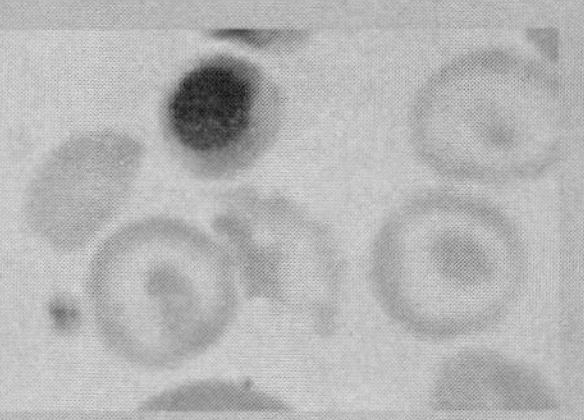

345. In the females, congenital adrenal hyperplasia causes which of the following conditions:

A. Infant hercules
B. Macrogenitosomia praecox
C. Female pseudohermaphroditism
D. None

Congenital adrenal hyperplasia is the most common adrenal disorder of infancy and childhood. It is due to any of several autosomal recessive mutations. Partial enzyme deficiencies may be expressed after adolescence, mainly in women with hirsutism and oligomenorrhea but there is minimal virilization. Late-onset adrenal hyperplasia accounts for 5-25% of cases of hirsutism and oligomenorrhea in women. Adrenal virilization in the female at birth is associated with FEMALE PSEUDOHERMAPHRODITISM. Virilization begins after the 5th month of intrauterine development. At birth there may be enlargement of the clitoris, partial or complete fusion of the labia, and occasionally a urogenital sinus in the female. If the labial fusion is nearly complete, the female infant has external genitalia resembling a penis with hypospadias.

346. *Most common* cause of aplastic anemia is:

A. Idiopathic
B. Petroleum products
C. Phenylbutazone
D. Chloramphenicol

Causes of Aplastic Anemia

Drugs	Chemicals	Hereditary	Other
Antimetabolites	Benzene	Shwachman syndrome	Non-A, non-B, non-C hepatitis
Chloramphenicol	Solvents	Dyskeratosis congenita	HIV virus
Phenylbutazone	Insecticides	Fanconi's anemia	Epstein-Barr virus
Sulfonamides			Radiation
Antimitotic agents			Paroxysmal nocturnal hemoglobinuria
Gold			Connective tissue disorders
			Graft-versus-host disease
			Pregnancy
			Idiopathic: 50-65% of cases

347. A mother is preparing to breastfeed her infant, it would be of value to her, if she knows:

A. Grasp reflex
B. Rooting reflex
C. Moro's reflex
D. Cough reflex

The turning of an infant's mouth toward the stimulus when the infant's cheek is stroked is known as ROOTING REFLEX. This reflex is present at birth .By the age 4 months it is gone when the infant is awake and by the age 7 months it is gone when the infant is asleep.

348. The essential feature in nephrotic syndrome is:

A. Proteinuria
B. Hyperlipidemia
C. Edema
D. Hypoalbuminemia

The **nephrotic syndrome** is characterized by a number of renal and extrarenal features. The most prominent of which are PROTEINURIA of >3.5 g per 1.73 m^2 per 24 hour, hypoalbuminemia, edema, hyperlipidemia, lipiduria, and hypercoagulability. The proteinuria, results from altered permeability of the glomerular filtration barrier for protein, namely the GBM and the podocytes and their slit diaphragms. The other components of the nephrotic syndrome and the metabolic complications are all secondary to urine protein loss.

349. *Not* a characteristic feature of Lowe's syndrome:

A. Defect in CNS and eye
B. Undescended testes
C. Mental deterioration
D. Hypophosphatemic rickets

Lowe's syndrome (Oculocerebrorenal dystrophy): It is transmitted as a sex-linked recessive. It is characterized by hypotonia, loss of reflexes, **mental deterioration, glaucoma, cataracts**, and renal tubular dysfunction. **Rickets**, osteopenica and pathologic facture develop due to metabolic acidosis and phosphate depletion.

350. *Most common* complication following meningococcal meningitis is:

A. Hydrocephalus
B. Arthritis
C. Subdural effusion
D. Waterhouse-Fredrickson syndrome

Fulminant meningococcemia, previously known as **Waterhouse-Frederickson syndrome**, occurs in 10-20% of patients with **meningococcal** disease. It is characterized by the development of shock, DIC, and multiple organ failure.

351. Oligohydramnios is associated with which of the following conditions:

A. Esophageal atresia
B. Renal agenesis
C. Anencephaly
D. All of the above

Fetal causes of **polyhydramnios** include *anencephaly*, presumably due to impaired swallowing on a neurologic basis, and gastrointestinal tract obstruction (*esophageal or duodenal atresia*). Maternal diabetes is also associated with a high incidence of polyhydramnios. Genitourinary tract anomalies that diminish fetal urine output, such as **bilateral renal agenesis** or **posterior urethral valves**, lead to oligohydramnios. Other causes of oligohydramnios include IUGR and ruptured membranes.

- **Oligohydramnios** is defined as *the volume of the amniotic fluid (AF) being less than 300 ml during the 3rd trimester of pregnancy.*

352. Flag sign is seen in which of the following diseases:

A. Kwashiorkor
B. Pellagra
C. Hypothyroidism
D. Marasmus

KWASHIORKOR is characterized by pitting edema. The child is listless, lethargic, apathetic and miserable. Hairs are thin, dry, brittle and lusterless. They become straight and hypopigmented grayish white or reddish brown in color. **During recovery growing part of hair are pigmented giving appearance of a flag (*the flag sign*).**The skin lesions appear as large areas of erythema followed by hyper pigmentation. Skin becomes dry, hyperkeratotic. Alternate areas of hypo and hyperpigmentation give a resemblance to pavement (*pavement dermatosis*).Mosaic pattern may also be seen (*Mosaic dermatosis*). Liver is enlarged and fatty.

353. The *etiological* agent for roseola infantum is:

A. Parvovirus
B. EBV
C. CMV
D. Human herpes virus 6 *(JIPMER 2002)*

Roseola infantum is also known as exanthem subitum. In 90% of cases it is caused by **human herpes virus 6** (HHV 6).

354. *Most common* cause of aseptic meningitis is:

A. Arbovirus
B. Enterovirus
C. Adenovirus
D. Herpes virus

Viruses Causing Aseptic Meningitis

Common	Less common	Rare
• **Enteroviruses (80% causes)** • Arboviruses • HIV • Herpes simplex virus –2	• Herpes simplex virus -1 • Lymphocytic choriomeningitis virus • Mumps virus	• Adenoviruses • CMV • Epstein-Barr virus • Influenza A, B • Measles parainfluenza • Rubella • Varicella-zoster virus

355. In an infant with galactosemia which of the following should be avoided:

A. Egg **B.** Rice
C. Milk **D.** Gluten

GALACTOSEMIA is treated by **removal of galactose-containing foods from the diet, especially milk**. Milk substitutes such as Nutramigen are given. Though soyabean preparations contain polysaccharide-bound galactose, they are well tolerated because the bound galactose is not readily liberated.

356. *False* regarding Reye's syndrome is:

A. Frequently complicates viral infection **B.** Deep jaundice is present
C. Prothrombin time is prolonged **D.** Disease may be precipitated by salicylates *(PGI 1996)*

REYE'S SYNDROME: The onset usually occurs after an URTI, especially influenza or chickenpox. Within 1 to 3 days, persistent vomiting starts, together with stupor, this progresses rapidly to generalized convulsions and coma. Hepatomegaly is present, but ***jaundice is characteristically absent or minimal***. **Elevations in** SGPT and **prothrombin time**, hypoglycemia, metabolic acidosis, and elevated serum ammonia levels are the chief laboratory findings. The cause is not known, although viral agents and drugs, mainly **salicylates**, have been blamed for this condition.

357. Brachycephaly occurs due to fusion of:

A. Coronal suture **B.** Lambdoid suture
C. Sagittal suture **D.** Parietal suture *(AIIMS 1997)*

When 1 or more sutures fuse *prematurely*, skull growth can be restricted perpendicular to the suture. If multiple sutures fuse while the brain is still increasing in size, intracranial pressure can increase.

- *Scaphocephaly* - Early fusion of the sagittal suture
- *Anterior plagiocephaly* - Early fusion of 1 coronal suture
- *Brachycephaly* - Early bilateral coronal suture fusion
- *Posterior plagiocephaly* - Early closure of 1 lambdoid suture
- *Trigonocephaly* - Early fusion of the metopic suture

In **brachycephaly**, there is **coronal synostosis bilaterally** (both sides), also involving sutures under the brain, in the upper face (behind the nose and eyes). These basal sutures are called frontoethmoidal and frontosphenoidal. This is relatively uncommon. When it occurs, there are often deformities in other parts of the body.

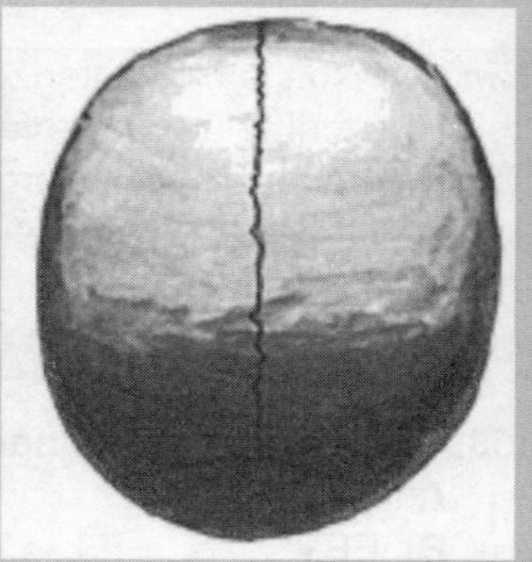

Brachycephaly

358. Autohemolysis test is positive in which of the following conditions:

A. Sickle cell disease **B.** Vitamin E deficiency
C. Hereditary spherocytosis **D.** β Thalassemia *(JIPMER 1995)*

The AUTOHEMOLYSIS TEST measures the amount of spontaneous hemolysis occurring after 48 hours of sterile incubation. In **hereditary spherocytosis**, about 10 to 50 % of the RBCs are lysed (versus fewer than 4 % of normal red blood cells).

359. Meconium is excreted by a newborn till:

A. 6 days
B. 3 days
C. 5 days
D. 2 days

The baby may pass meconium *in utero* or soon after birth, but **all healthy newborn babies *must* evacuate within 24 hours of birth**. **During the first 2-3 days the baby passes black, tarry (like tar) 'meconium' stools** which are followed by greenish (transitional) stools for the next 1 or 2 days. The normal breastfed baby usually passes 4-8 semisolid sticky golden yellow stools every day. Some babies may pass stools after *each* feed due to the 'exaggerated' gastrocolic reflex. The stools are often very small (at times like droppings of the birds) with normal consistency. The babies continue to gain weight.

- Tar means a thick, sticky, brown to black liquid with a pungent odor, obtained by the destructive distillation of wood, coal, peat, shale, etc.

360. A 2-year-old child has a weight of 6.4 kg and has vitamin A deficiency. The grade of malnutrition in this child is:

A. Second degree
B. Fourth degree
C. Third degree
D. First degree

Grade of malnutrition (IAP)	Percentage of expected weight
• Grade I	71 % to 80 %
• Grade II	61 % to 70 %
• Grade III	51 % to 60 %
• Grade IV	Less than 50 %

The expected weight of a 2-year-old child should be (2 × 2) + 8 = 12. Therefore the grade of malnutrition is of grade III according to IAP guidelines.

361. In kernicterus which is increased:

A. Conjugated bilirubin
B. Unconjugated bilirubin
C. None
D. Both

KERNICTERUS is a form of icterus neonatorum which occurs in infants during the 2nd–8th day of life. The basal ganglia and other areas of the brain and spinal cord are infiltrated with bilirubin.
In neonatal jaundice or type I or II Crigler-Najjar syndrome **extremely high concentrations (>20 mg/dL) of unconjugated bilirubin** can accumulate, and the resulting diffusion of bilirubin into the CNS can cause encephalopathy (**kernicterus**) and permanent impairment of nervous function.

362. Rotavirus immunity to children occurs above:

A. 5 years
B. 10 years
C. 3 years
D. 7 years

363. Diarrhea in infants is *most commonly* caused by which of the following viruses:

A. Rotavirus
B. Rhabdovirus
C. Myxovirus
D. Adenovirus

Rotavirus infection occurs worldwide and by the age of **3 years**, virtually every individual has been infected by rotaviruses at least once. **Rotaviruses are the single most important cause of severe dehydrating diarrhea in infants and young children** (under age 3).

364. *Not* caused by RSV:

A. Pneumonia in elderly
B. Cold in children
C. Coryza in adult
D. ARDS

RSV infection is the cause of wide range of respiratory diseases. In **infants**, 25-40% of infections result in lower respiratory tract involvement, and they include **pneumonia**, bronchiolitis, and tracheobronchitis. In **adults**, the most common symptoms of RSV infection are those of the **common cold**, with rhinorrhea, sore throat, and cough. RSV virus also causes lower respiratory tract disease with fever in adults, and **severe pneumonia in the elderly**.

365. Phenylketonuria is diagnosed by:

A. Guthrie test
B. Vanillylmandelic acid in urine
C. Gerhard's test
D. Ferric chloride test

The mental retardation in **classic phenylketonuria** can be prevented only if the dietary treatment is initiated before the child is 3 weeks of age. The diagnosis is difficult because the plasma phenylalanine concentrations are normal at birth in affected newborn but it rises rapidly after institution of protein (milk) feedings. Newborns in USA and European countries are routinely screened by using the **GUTHRIE BACTERIAL INHIBITION ASSAY** for determination of the concentration of phenylalanine in blood**.** Abnormal values are then confirmed with fluorometric or chromatographic assays.

366. *Most common* type of cerebral palsy is:

A. Spastic
B. Atonic
C. Extrapyramidal
D. None

Cerebral palsy is defined as *any nonprogressive central motor deficit dating to events in prenatal or perinatal periods.* **Spastic cerebral palsy is the most common type of cerebral palsy**. Other types are extrapyramidal cerebral palsy, atonic diplegia, and congenital cerebellar ataxia.

367. Sexual maturity rate (SMR) in girls does *not* include:

A. Breast development
B. Onset of menarche
C. Weight velocity
D. Pubic hair development

(JIPMER 2002)

The Stages of Development of Puberty in Girls

Sexual maturity rating	Average age (Years)	Features	What happens
1	8 2/3	Growth, breasts and pubic hair	Height spurt begins. Body fat at 15.7%. Breasts are **prepubertal**; no glandular tissue. No pubic hair.
2	11 1/4	Breasts	The **areola** (pigmented area around the nipple) enlarges and becomes darker. It raises to become a mound with a small amount of breast tissue underneath. This is called a **bud**.
2	11 3/4	Pubic hair and growth	A few long, downy, slightly darkened hairs appear along the **labia majora**. At the end of this stage, the body fat has increased to 18.9%.
3	11 2/3	Growth	**Peak height velocity** (maximum growth rate) is reached. Body fat is now 21.6%.
3	12	Breasts	Development of breast tissue past the edge of the areola.
3	12 1/3	Pubic hair	Moderate amount of more curly, pigmented, and coarser hair on the mons pubis (the raised, fatty area above the labia majora). Hair begins to spread more laterally. **Menarche** (first menstrual period) occurs in 20% of girls during this pubic hair stage
4	12 3/4	Pubic hair	Hair is close to adult pubic hair in curliness and coarseness. Area of pubis covered is smaller than adults, and there are no hairs on the middle surfaces of the thighs. Menarche occurs in 50% of girls.

4	13	Breasts	Continued development of breast tissue; in side view, areola and nipple protrude.
			26.7%.
5	14 1/2	Pubic hair and Body fat	Adult. It is normal for some long pigmented hairs to grow on the inner thighs. Body fat remains at 26.7%.
5	15 1/4	Breasts	Adult breasts.

*The average age listed here can vary widely; about 2 years either side of these listed ages will usually be considered normal.

368. Ghon's focus is:

A. Primary complex
B. Miliary TB
C. TB lymph nodes
D. Postprimary TB

Ghon's tubercle: A small, sharply defined shadow in X-ray of the lung seen in certain cases of **PULMONARY TUBERCULOSIS IN CHILDREN**. It is the primary lesion of tuberculosis in children. The tubercle bacilli in the lesion become encased in calcium and the only remaining sign of infection is a positive tuberculin skin test. The *Mycobacterium tuberculosis* organisms may remain viable and can cause endogenous and generalized reinfection with the tubercle bacillus.

369. All the following milestones are seen in a 16 weeks child *except*:

A. Kicks the ground on placing it on its feet
B. Brings objects to the mouth
C. Polysyllabic vowel sounds
D. Laughs loudly

(JIPMER 2002)

At 16 weeks

Prone	Lifts head and chest Head is approximately vertical axis Legs extended
Supine	Symmetrical posture predominates Hands in midline Reaches and **grasps objects and brings them to mouth**
Sitting	No head lag on pull to sitting position Head steady, held forward Enjoys sitting with full truncal support
Standing	When held erect, **pushes with feet**
Adaptive	Sees pellet but makes no move to it
Social	**Laughs out loud** May show displeasure if social contact is broken Excited at sight of food

*Polysyllabic vowel sounds are formed at 28 weeks.

370. *Not* a characteristic feature of cretinism:

A. Macroglossia
B. Dwarfism
C. Hyperpyrexia
D. Mental retardation

Some Features of Cretinism

• **Short stature**	• Broad and flat nose	• Dry skin
• Protruding tongue	• Widely set eyes	• **Impaired mental development**
• **Macroglossia**	• Sparse hair	• Retarded bone age
• Epiphyseal dysgenesis	• Delayed dentition	• Protuberant abdomen with an umbilical hernia

371. A child with IQ of 50 is graded as:

A. Moderately intelligent
B. Moderate mental retardation
C. Severe mental retardation
D. Mild mental retardation

Degree of retardation	IQ
• Border line	70-90
• Mild retardation	70-51
• **Moderate retardation**	**50–36**
• Severe retardation	35–21
• Profound retardation	0–20

372. *Earliest* change in raised intracranial tension in a child is:

A. Posterior clinoid erosion
B. Erosion of sella
C. Silver beaten appearance
D. Sutural separation

In infant and children SUTURAL DIASTASIS is the **first and most prominent feature of raised intracranial tension**, the younger the child more marked the sign. It may be the only sign of raised ICT in children. Sellar erosion may occur but is a late sign and indicates long-standing chronic raised ICT. In children less than 10 years if sellar erosion is present without sutural diastasis it is more likely to be due to local erosive lesion rather than raised ICT.

373. Which of the following is *true* regarding phocomelia:

A. It is a defect in long bones
B. Absence of brain
C. It is a defect in short bones
D. Reduplication of bones *(AI 1996, 1998)*

Phocomelia means a great reduction in size of proximal parts of the limbs. It is a congenital malformation in which the proximal portions of the extremities are poorly developed or absent. As a result the hands and feet are attached to the trunk directly or by means of a poorly formed bone. In some cases this occurs due to intake of thalidomide, a sleeping pill, during early pregnancy.

374. *Not* seen in myotonic dystrophy:

A. Cardiac defect
B. Cataract
C. Respiratory failure
D. Enlarged testes

Patients with MYOTONIC DYSTROPHY have **cardiac disturbances**. ECG abnormalities are common, including first-degree heart block and more extensive conduction system involvement. Mitral valve prolapse is also common. Complete heart block and sudden death may also occur. Congestive heart failure may result from cor pulmonale secondary to **respiratory failure**.

Other features of myotonic dystrophy are intellectual impairment, hypersomnia, posterior subcapsular **cataracts**, frontal baldness, **gonadal atrophy**, insulin resistance, and decreased esophageal and colonic motility.

375. *False* regarding Reye's syndrome:

A. Bilirubin of more than 3 mg%
B. Microfatty changes in liver without inflammatory changes
C. Increased prothrombin time
D. Cerebral edema

REYE'S SYNDROME **or fatty liver with encephalopathy** occurs exclusively in children less than 15 years of age. Its cause is unknown, although viral agents and drugs, especially **salicylates**, have been implicated. The clinical features are vomiting and signs of progressive central nervous system damage, signs of hepatic injury, and hypoglycemia. There is **extensive fatty vacuolization of the liver and renal tubules**. The major extrahepatic changes include fatty changes of the renal tubular cells, **cerebral edema**, and neuronal degeneration of the brain. The onset follows an upper respiratory tract infection, especially with influenza or chickenpox. Within 1 to 3 days, persistent vomiting occurs, together with stupor, which progresses rapidly to convulsions and coma.

Features of Reye's syndrome are as under:
- Despite hepatomegaly, jaundice is typically absent or minimal.
- Elevation of serum aminotransferases
- Increased prothrombin time
- Hypoglycemia
- Respiratory alkalosis
- Metabolic acidosis
- Elevated serum ammonia

376. Which of the following *does not* predispose to malignancy:

A. Down's syndrome
B. Cri du chat syndrome
C. Klinefelter syndrome
D. Turner's syndrome

Cri du chat syndrome: It is a hereditary congenital disorder due to a deletion of the short arm of chromosome 4 or 5 of the B group. It is so named because the infant's cry resembles the cry of a cat. It is characterized by mental retardation, microcephaly, dwarfism, epicanthal folds, and laryngeal defect.

377. *False* regarding Pierre Robin syndrome is:

A. Mandibular hypoplasia
B. Coloboma irides
C. Cleft palate
D. Respiratory distress *(JIPMER 1991)*

Features of Pierre Robin syndrome:
There is unusual smallness of the jaw, **mandibular hypoplasia** combined with **cleft palate**, downward displacement of the tongue and an absent gag reflex. **Micrognathia**, pseudomacroglossia, glossoptosis (dropping of the tongue downward out of normal position), high arched or cleft palate is present. **Obstruction of air passage** occurs during inspiration because the buccal cavity is small in size and the tongue, which is of normal size, may obstruct the airway.

378. *True* regarding nutritional rickets is:

A. Decreased cortical bone
B. Decreased calcification of mature bone
C. Decreased calcification of growing bone
D. Decreased production of steroid

Rickets may be defined as *a disorder involving softening and weakening of the bones of children, primarily caused by lack of vitamin D and/or lack of calcium or phosphate which leads to decreased calcification of growing bones*. It is seen most often in infancy and childhood. It is marked by abnormal bone growth. Symptoms include soft bones causing defects, as bowlegs and knock-knees, swellings on the ends and sides of the bones, muscle pain, a swollen skull, chest defects, a curved spine, swollen liver and spleen, heavy sweating, and general tenderness of the body when touched. Prevention and treatment are a diet rich in calcium, phosphorus, and vitamin D and enough exposure to sunlight. *Kinds of rickets include adult rickets, celiac rickets, renal rickets, and vitamin D resistant rickets.*

379. *True* regarding a 2-month-old child is:

A. Sustain head level with body when placed in ventral suspension
B. Hold head and chest off a flat surface with extended elbows
C. Lift head and chest off a flat surface with extended elbows
D. Show a positive parachute protective reflex *(SGPGI 1999)*

At 8 weeks
- Raises head slightly farther
- **Head sustained in plane of body on ventral suspension**
- Tonic neck posture predominates
- Head lags on pull to sitting position
- Follows moving object 180 degree
- Smiles on social contact
- Listens to voice and coos

380. Empyema in a child less than 2 years is *most commonly* caused by:

A. *Klebsiella* **B.** *Staphylococcus*
C. *Escherichia coli* **D.** *Pneumococcus*

EMPYEMA: Pus in a body cavity, especially in the pleural cavity. It is due to a primary infection in the lungs. The symptoms of acute state are chills, high fever, and sweating. The skin is gray and malar flushed, appetite is poor with marked malaise, and chest pain, cough, and emaciation. In the chronic state, weight loss, general malaise, and low-grade fever are seen. Common organisms associated with postpneumonia empyema in children are ***Staphylococcus aureus***, *Haemophilus influenzae, Streptococcus pneumoniae* and anaerobic bacteria.

381. *False* regarding Henoch-Schönlein purpura:

A. Nephritis **B.** Centrifugal rash
C. Thrombocytopenia **D.** Arthritis

HENOCH-SCHÖNLEIN PURPURA is the most common cause of NONTHROMBOCYTOPENIC PURPURA. It is a self-limited type of vasculitis which occurs in children and young adults. Patients have an acute inflammatory reaction in capillaries, mesangial tissues and small arterioles which leads to increased vascular permeability, exudation, and hemorrhage. Henoch-Schönlein purpura may be preceded by an upper respiratory tract infection or streptococcal pharyngitis or be associated with drug or food allergies. Patients develop a purpuric **rash** on the extensor surfaces of the arms, legs and on the buttocks. Patients also have polyarthralgias or **arthritis**, colicky abdominal pain, and hematuria from focal **glomerulonephritis**. Some patients may develop fatal acute renal failure, and 5-10% develops chronic nephritis.

382. *Not* a cause of floppy baby:

A. Prader Willi syndrome **B.** Little's disease
C. Werdnig-Hoffman syndrome **D.** Down syndrome *(JIPMER 1991)*

Differential Diagnosis of a "Floppy Infant"

Central nervous system disorders
• Kernicterus • Prader-Willi syndrome • Cerebral lipidosis • Chromosomal defects • Oculocerebrorenal syndrome (Lowe syndrome) • Congenital cerebellar ataxia • Atonic diplegia
Spinal cord diseases
• Spinal cord trauma • Werdnig-Hoffmann disease
Diseases of peripheral nerve
• Polyneuritis (GB Syndrome) • Familial dysautonomia • Congenital sensory neuropathy
Diseases of the neuromuscular junction
• Myasthenia gravis • Infantile botulism
Muscle diseases
• Mitochondrial myopathies • Nemaline myopathy • Central core disease • Glycogen storage disease of muscle and heart (Pompe disease) • Myotonic dystrophy • Congenital muscular dystrophy

383. *True* regarding diaphragmatic hernia is:

A. More common on right side **B.** Vomiting occurs early
C. Chest X-ray is not diagnostic **D.** Pulmonary hypoplasia is seen

DIAPHRAGMATIC HERNIA: The large diaphragmatic hernias that compromise lung growth are posterolateral in position and are caused by defective closure of the pleuroperitoneal canal. The remnant of this canal in the normally developed diaphragm is the **foramen of Bochdalek**. Typically, infants with congenital diaphragmatic hernias have severe respiratory distress at birth, and because the abdomen contains fewer contents than normal, it appears scaphoid. Radiographically, the abdominal contents, which may include stomach, bowel, spleen, and liver, can be identified within the thorax in plain X-ray chest. **About 85% of congenital hernias are left-sided.** The **ipsilateral lung is severely hypoplastic**, but because of mediastinal shift a lesser degree of contralateral hypoplasia is also present.

384. Which of the following is the *most common* age group affected by infantile colic:

A. 4-6 months **B.** 0-3 months
C. 6-9 months **D.** 9-12 months *(JIPMER 2002)*

Infantile colic is a common and *frustrating* condition affecting infants. It involves persistent and often violent crying for no *obvious* reason. There is also a considerable amount of flatulence present. *Typically*, it occurs within the 1st month postpartum and spontaneously self-resolves by the 3rd to 4th month.

385. In which of the following conditions, combination chemotherapy is *not* indicated:

A. Immunologically suppressed patients **B.** Primary complex
C. Acute epiglottitis **D.** Acute laryngotracheobronchitis *(JIPMER 1995)*

ACUTE LARYNGOTRACHEOBRONCHITIS or **croup** is an infection of the upper and lower respiratory tract that causes marked subglottic edema. Fever, hoarseness, a **"*seal's bark*" cough**, and inspiratory stridor are the usual clinical features. Most common etiological agent is parainfluenza virus, although it may also be caused by other viruses (e.g. influenza or respiratory syncytial virus) and by *Mycoplasma pneumoniae*. **As it is usually viral infection chemotherapeutic agents are of no use and antibiotics are not indicated to prevent suprainfection.** Use of steroid remains controversial and efficacy is not proved.

386. *Not* a usual feature of ascariasis:

A. Intussusception **B.** Loeffler's syndrome
C. Anemia **D.** Abdominal pain

Anemia is more common with hookworm infestations rather than ascariasis which presents with abdominal pain, intussusception and occasionally Loeffler's Syndrome.

387. In a term newborn, hypoglycemia occurs when the serum blood glucose level is *below*:

A. 30 mg/dl **B.** 40 mg/dl
C. 50 mg/dl **D.** 55 mg/dl *(MAHE 2001)*

On the basis of recent neurophysiologic, metabolic and statistical data, most pediatricians now attempt to maintain the neonatal glucose levels at or above 40 mg/dL.

388. In kernicterus, staining of brain is more intense in:

A. Corpus callosum **B.** Cerebral cortex
C. Basal ganglion **D.** Spinal cord

In the neonatal state and infancy, unconjugated bilirubin levels above 20 mg/dL may lead to **kernicterus** due to bilirubin deposition in the lipid-rich **basal ganglia**. Kernicterus is a pathological diagnosis and refers to *yellow staining of brain together with evidence of neuronal injury*. Grossly, bilirubin staining is most commonly seen in basal ganglia, various cranial nerve nuclei, other brainstem nuclei, cerebellar nuclei, hippocampus and anterior horn cells of spinal cord.

389. In cystic fibrosis *most common* organism is *Pseudomonas aeruginosa*. *Next most common organism* is:

A. *Staphylococcus aureus*
B. *Klebsiella*
C. *Pneumococci*
D. *Streptococcus pyogenes* (*JIPMER 1995*)

The patients of **cystic fibrosis** have a unique predisposition for chronic infection of airways by *Staphylococcus aureus* and *Pseudomonas aeruginosa*.

390. In pertussis antibiotic of choice is:

A. Penicillin
B. Ampicillin
C. Erythromycin
D. Gentamicin

Erythromycin is the drug of choice for **Pertussis**. It is given in a dose of 25-50 mg/kg/day in 3 divided doses for 2 weeks.

391. *True* about dietary treatment of galactosemia is:

A. Must be continued life long
B. Ensures normal intellectual development if started in the first week of life
C. Can be relaxed after puberty
D. Involves delayed weaning

The treatment of GALACTOSEMIA consists of the removal of galactose-containing foods from the diet, particularly milk. Milk substitutes such as Nutramigen should be used. The institution of a galactose-free diet leads to a marked improvement in all clinical features *except* for mental retardation. **Patients should be kept on galactose-free diets indefinitely** or at least until they have attained adequate physical and neurologic development.

392. A comatose child has garlic like odor to the breath. The *most probable* diagnosis is:

A. Lead poisoning
B. Flavism
C. Atropine poisoning
D. Arsenic poisoning

Acute ARSENIC POISONING results in increased permeability of small blood vessels and inflammation and necrosis of the intestinal mucosa. These changes manifest clinically as hemorrhagic gastroenteritis, fluid loss, and hypotension. Delayed cardiomyopathy associated with ECG abnormalities may develop. Symptoms are nausea, vomiting, diarrhea, abdominal pain, delirium, coma, and seizures. A **garlicky odor** detectable in the breath is characteristic. ATN and hemolysis may develop.

393. Croup syndrome is usually caused by:

A. Coxsackie B virus
B. Rhinovirus
C. Coxsackie A virus
D. Parainfluenza viruses

Croup (croop): It is an acute viral disease of childhood, marked by a **resonant barking cough,** suffocative and difficult breathing, and laryngeal spasm. Difficulty in breathing is due to acute subglottic edema. Because of severe respiratory distress, the child is hypoxic. Viral agents account for nearly all cases of croup *except* that associated with diphtheria and acute epiglottis. The **parainfluenza viruses** account for approximately 2/3rd of all cases.

394. Clinical manifestations of cystic fibrosis *do not* include:

A. Malabsorption
B. Cor pulmonale
C. Bronchiectasis
D. Hypertension

Clinical Manifestations of Cystic Fibrosis

- Meconium ileus
- Frequent respiratory tract infection
- **Bronchiectasis**
- Protein and fat malabsorption
- **Malabsorption** of fat-soluble vitamins
- Exocrine pancreatic insufficiency
- Intestinal dysfunction
- Urogenital dysfunction
- Foul-smelling stools
- **Cor pulmonale**

395. ***False*** **regarding childhood autism is:**

A. Isolated area of talent may be remarkable developed
B. Parental attitude and behavior do not attribute to it
C. Emergence of speech and social smile is often delayed
D. It represents a type of childhood neurotic disorder *(KARNATAKA 1994)*

AUTISM includes mental retardation, cerebral palsy, learning disability, communication disorder and attention deficit disorders. *Autism is not a disease*. It is one of the **developmental disorders** of the brain function. Its cause is not known in majority of cases but unlike other developmental disabilities, **prenatal and perinatal factors do *not* play a major role in its etiology**. Clinical features are **speech and language delay**, impairment of comprehension of language, fluent but unintelligible jargon, impairment of social interaction, hyperactivity, unusual interest in TV commercials, repetitive compulsive play activity, etc. Seizures are more common in autistic children than in general population. Some autistic children have **islands of brilliance.**

396. Cephalhematoma usually disappears within............. weeks:

A. 5-7 **B.** 2-12
C. 1-2 **D.** 3-5

CEPHALHEMATOMA: It is a mass composed of clotted blood, located between the periosteum and the skull of a newborn. The swelling is confined between suture lines and usually is unilateral. The cause is rupture of periosteal bridging veins due to pressure and friction during labor and delivery, resulting in the collection of clotted blood between the periosteum and the fetal skull. **The swelling reabsorbs slowly within 2-12 weeks of birth, depending on their size.**

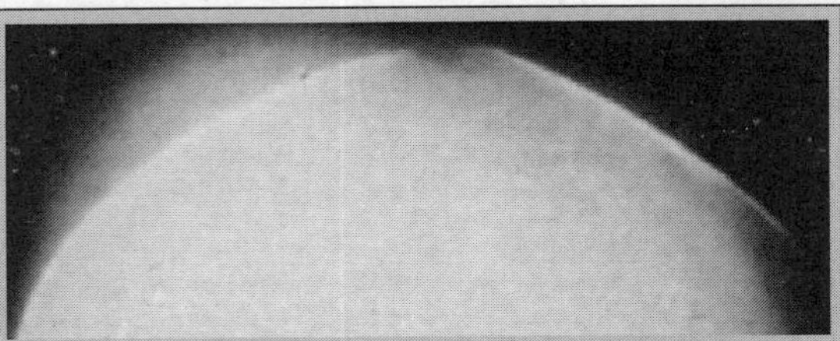

Rising Sun Appearance Typical of a Fresh Cephalhematoma

397. Scratch tests are best read within:

A. 4 hours **B.** 1 hour
C. 10 minutes **D.** 15-20 minutes

Scratch test: Placement of an appropriate dilution of a test material, suspected of being an allergen, in a lightly scratched area of the skin is known as scratch test. If the material is an allergen, **a wheal will develop within 15 minutes.**

398. Genotype in testicular feminization syndrome is:

A. 46 XY **B.** 45 XO
C. 47 XXY **D.** 46 XX *(MAHE 2001)*

Androgen insensitivity syndrome (testicular feminization syndrome):

- XY genotype/phenotypically females
- End organ insensitivity to androgen
- High circulating levels of androgens
- No ovarian or uterine tissue present, blind vagina
- Intra-abdominal testis present
- Increased incidence of gonadal neoplasms

399. Y chromosome is always present in which of the following conditions:

A. Gonadal dysgenesis **B.** True hermaphroditism
C. Klinefelter syndrome **D.** Turner syndrome *(SGPGI 1999)*

Disorder	Common chromosomal complement
• Klinefelter syndrome	47, XXY *or* 46, XY/47, XXY
• XX male	46, XX
• Gonadal dysgenesis (Turner syndrome)	45, X *or* 46, XX/45, X
• Mixed gonadal dysgenesis	46, XY/45, X *or* 46, XY
• True hermaphroditism	46, XX *or* 46, XY *or* mosaics

400. Cerebral palsy is defined as:

A. A nonprogressive neuromuscular disorder of cerebral origin
B. Progressive neuromuscular disorder of cerebral origin
C. Progressive neuromuscular disorder of cerebral origin
D. Nonprogressive neuromuscular disorder of peripheral origin

Cerebral palsy: It is defined as a group of **nonprogressing encephalopathies** often associated with changing motor impairment syndromes secondary to a lesion or anomaly of brain, arising in early stage of its development.

401. *True* regarding canals of Lambert in the alveolar spaces of lung:

A. Prevent atelectasis
B. Bronchoalveolar connections
C. None
D. Both

Canal of Lambert: It is one of the several **bronchoalveolar communications** in the lung. It is helpful in **preventing atelectasis**.

402. Normal reflex patterns at birth include:

A. Sucking and rooting reflex
B. Moro's reflex
C. Grasp reflex
D. All of the above

Neonatal Reflexes

Reflex	Appears at	No longer obtainable
• Moro's	Birth	3 months
• Stepping	Birth	6 weeks
• Placing	Birth	6 weeks
• Rooting and sucking	Birth	4 months awake 7 months asleep
• Palmar grasp	Birth	6 months
• Plantar grasp	Birth	10 months
• Adductor spread of knee jerk	Birth	7 months
• Tonic neck	2 months	6 months
• Neck righting	4-6 months	24 months
• Landau	3 months	24 months
• Parachute	9 months	Persists

403. Croup is *not* associated with:

A. Adenovirus
B. Enterovirus
C. Influenza virus
D. RSV

Viruses Causing Croup

- Parainfluenza virus (most common)
- Adenovirus
- RSV
- Influenza virus
- Measles virus

404. First clinical manifestation of abetalipoproteinemia is:

A. Convulsions
B. Tremors
C. Steatorrhea
D. Hypohydrosis

Abetalipoproteinemia is due to the absence of Apo B which results in defective chylomicron formation. Children with this disorder usually present with STEATORRHEA, acanthocytic red blood cells, ataxia, and retinitis pigmentosa.

405. *Not* a characteristic feature of Down's syndrome:

- **A.** Mental retardation
- **B.** Protruding tongue
- **C.** Simian crease
- **D.** Prominent occiput

Common Features of Down's Syndrome

• **General**	**Mental retardation** and hypotonia
• **Craniofacial**	Flat occiput; oblique palpebral fissure; epicanthic folds; Brushfield spots; **protruding tongue**; prominent and malformed ears; flat nasal bridge.
• **Thorax**	CHD especially endocardial cushion defect
• **Hands and feet**	**Simian's crease**; short broad hands; hypoplasia of middle pharynx of 5th figure; gap between 1st and 2nd toe
• **Other**	High arched palate; strabismus; broad and short neck; small teeth; intestinal atresia; imperforate anus

406. Calculate the percentage of burns on the head, neck and face in child of 1 year:

- **A.** 15 %
- **B.** 19 %
- **C.** 10%
- **D.** 13 %

Rule of nines is a formula for calculating the percentage of body surface areas and is particularly helpful in judging the portion of skin that has been burned. **In children**:

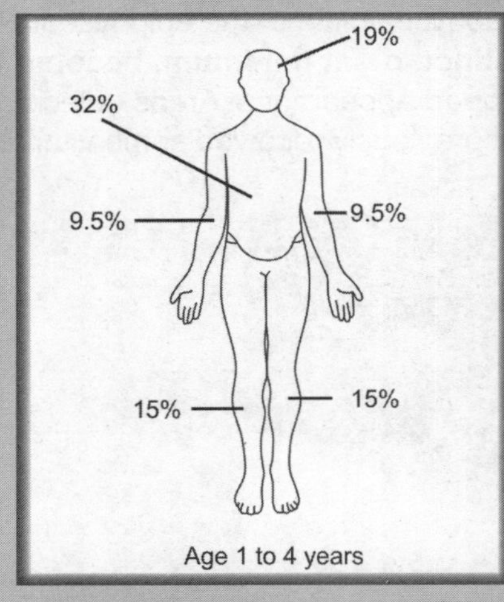

Age 1 to 4 years

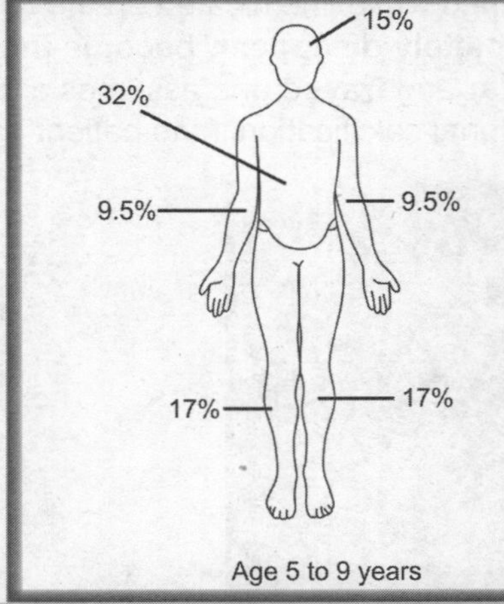

Age 5 to 9 years

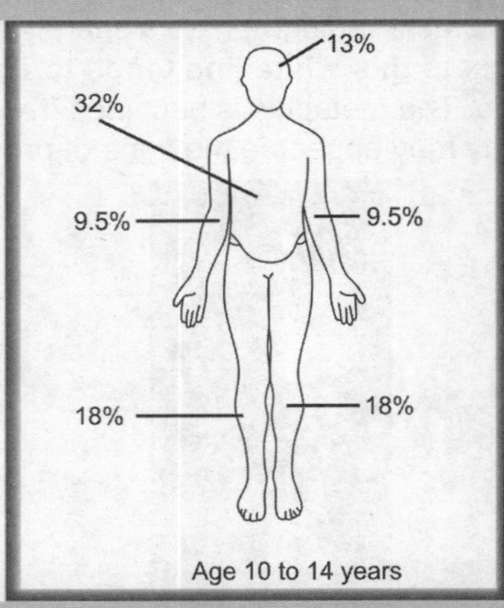

Age 10 to 14 years

407. The incubation period of hepatitis A is:

- **A.** 6 weeks to 6 months
- **B.** 2 days to 2 weeks
- **C.** 4 weeks
- **D.** 2 weeks to 2 months

Hepatitis A has an incubation period of about **4 weeks.**

408. Human colostrum in comparison with mature human milk contains more:

A. Protein
B. Fat
C. Water
D. Lactose

(KARNATAKA 1994)

Constituents (gm/100 gm)	Human milk	Human colostrum
• **Water**	88	87
• **Protein**	0.9	2.7
• **Fat**	3.8	2.9
• **Lactose**	7.0	5.3
• **Specific gravity**	1.030	1.040-1.060

409. Retrolental fibroplasia is because of:

A. Hyperoxia
B. Hypoxia
C. Hypocapnia
D. Increased CO_2

(PGI 1999)

Retrolental fibroplasia occurs in premature infants treated with oxygen at concentrations above ambient air levels. The increased arterial oxygen tensions that result may lead to severe arterial vasoconstriction with subsequent hypoxic damage to the immature retina. The exact level or duration of elevated arterial pO_2 that results in injury is not known, but arterial oxygen tension should be kept between 50-80 mmHg. **Immaturity and periods of relative retinal HYPEROXIA are considered to be major factors in the development of this disorder**.

410. *Not* a radiographic feature of rickets:

A. Increase in width of growth plate
B. Rickety rosary
C. Subperiosteal bleeding
D. Decrease in bone density

In rickets there is abnormal increased axial height of the cartilaginous portion of the epiphyseal plate and **irregular mineralization of the zone of provisional calcification**. The zone of provisional calcification is normally recognized on the radiograph as a sharply defined white line located on the metaphyseal side of the epiphyseal plate. **In rickets this white line tends to completely disappear, become indistinct, or, at minimum, become less dense.** The metaphysis becomes **irregular** and **frayed** and assumes a **cupped** appearance. Areas of increased density may appear in the zone of provisional calcification if the patient had previously received some vitamin D.

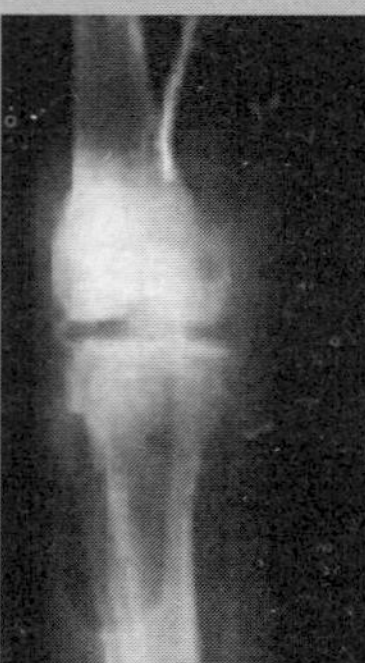

NORMAL KNEE

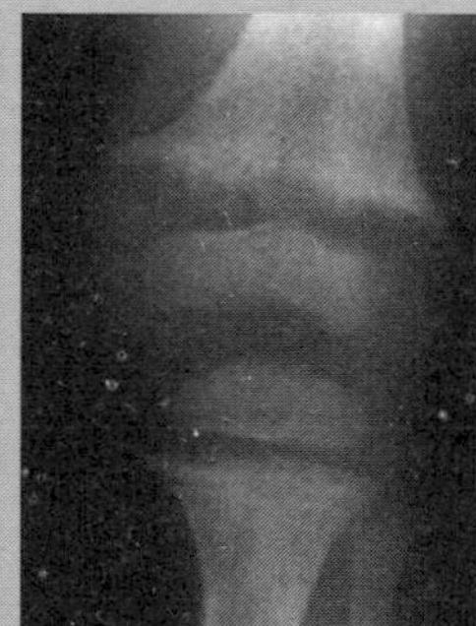

RICKETS

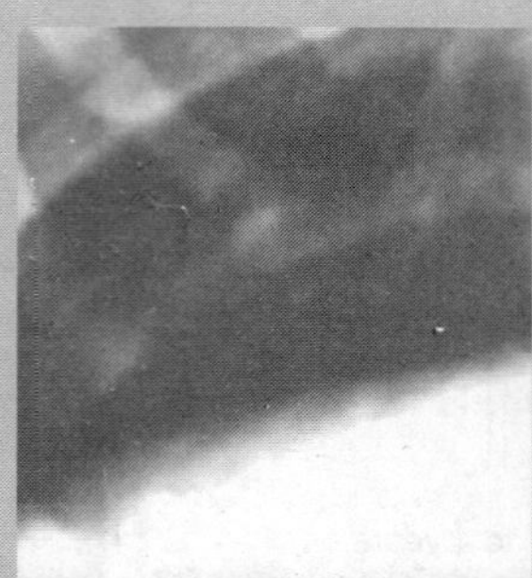

RACHITIC ROSARY

Aside from the changes described above, both the cortical and medullary structures of the **long and flat bones show a decrease in overall density.** The cortices appear thin and the trabeculae become indistinct and reduced in number. The **skull is markedly deformed** in very young infants, since the supine position results in flattening of the posterior part of the skull. Osteoid accumulation in the frontal and parietal bones results in the squared configuration commonly known as craniotabes. Later, in early childhood, enlarged and widened growth plates are noted and present as joint swellings. Swelling at the costochondral junction of the ribs is known as the rachitic **rosary** and can be palpated as well as viewed radiographically.

411. *Not* a recognized feature of Wilson's disease:
- **A.** Increased copper content of liver
- **B.** Increased ceruloplasmin
- **C.** Histopathological features of chronic active hepatitis
- **D.** Psychological disturbances

WILSON'S DISEASE is an inherited disorder of copper metabolism. There is impairment of the normal excretion of hepatic copper which results in **toxic accumulations of the Copper in liver**, brain, and other organs. In infants with Wilson's disease, the neonatal **deficiency of ceruloplasmin** and excess of hepatic copper persist indefinitely. **Psychiatric disturbances** are present in most patients with neurologic symptoms. Parenchymal liver disease is present in the form of **chronic active hepatitis** and cirrhosis.

412. Incubation period of pertussis is...........days:
- **A.** 3
- **B.** 7-10
- **C.** 28
- **D.** 15-28

The incubation period **of pertussis** ranges from 5 to 14 days but is usually **7-10 days**.

413. *Not* a complication of pertussis:
- **A.** Pneumonia
- **B.** Convulsions
- **C.** Cerebellar ataxia
- **D.** Subconjunctival hemorrhage

Complications of Pertussis

- *Pneumonia* (most frequent)
- Subcutaneous emphysema
- Otitis media
- *Convulsions*
- Epistaxis
- Rupture of diaphragm
- Rectal prolapse
- Inguinal hernia
- Ulcer of tongue
- Atelectasis
- Bronchiectasis
- Reactivation of tuberculosis
- Coma
- *Subconjunctival hemorrhage*
- Umbilical hernia
- Melena
- Dehydration
- Protein energy malnutrition

414. A 3-month-old girl weighs 4 kg and is suffering from loose motions. On examination, she is found to be suffering from moderate dehydration. The amount of ORS to be given to her in first four hours should be:
- **A.** 600 ml
- **B.** 300 ml
- **C.** 100 ml
- **D.** 500 ml

In cases of moderate dehydration the amount of ORS to be given in first four hours is 75 ml/kg.

415. *True* regarding transient tachypnea of newborn:
- **A.** It often leads to chronic lung disease
- **B.** In premature babies it is often fatal
- **C.** Onset of respiratory distress is immediately after birth and it rarely lasts beyond 72 hours
- **D.** It is the commonest respiratory disorder caused by absence of surfactant

Transient tachypnea of newborn is also known as wet lung disease or RDS type II. It is a common mild self-limiting disorder affecting near term or term infants and is characterized by tachypnea with mild retraction and mild cyanosis. The infant usually develops tachypnea (RR > 80 /min) within 2–6 hours. Symptoms typically persist for 12–24 hours in mild TTN and may persist for more than 72 hours in severe TTN.

416. In the case of CNS relapse ALL chemotherapy would consist of intrathecal:
- **A.** Methotrexate
- **B.** Prednisolone
- **C.** Adriamycin
- **D.** Methotrexate + cytosine arabinoside

Effective Treatment Regimens for ALL

Remission induction phase (one month)
Prednisone : 40 mg/sqmt/day Vincristine : 1.5 mg/sqmt/week IV for 4 weeks L Asparaginase : 200 IU /kg/day IV
CNS prophylaxis(beginning at 4 week)
Cobalt 60 cranial irradiation for 2.5 weeks total dose 1800 rads **Intrathecal methotrexate** : 12 mg/sqmt twice a week for 2.5 weeks maximum dose 15 mg
Continuation therapy for 30 months
6-mercaptopurine : 50 mg/sqmt / 24 hours PO Methotrexate : 20 mg/sqmt/wk intravenously

417. Drug of choice for neonatal convulsions:

A. Carbamazepine
B. Valproate
C. Phenobarbitone
D. Phenytoin

Drug of choice for neonatal convulsions is **phenobarbitone**; loading dose of 20 mg/kg is given slow diluted IV. It is followed by a maintenance dose of 5 mg/kg/day PO or IV.

418. In pulse polio program, target age group is:

A. Under 3 years
B. Under 10 years
C. Under 5 years
D. Under 1 year

Under pulse polio program the target age group is under 5 years.

419. 10-years-old child presented with 10 days continuous fever with soft, enlarged spleen. The diagnosis is:

A. Enteric fever
B. Hodgkin's disease
C. Meningitis
D. Malaria

Enteric fever presents with a step like daily increase in temperature (up to 40 to 41°C) associated with headache, malaise, and chills. **The cardinal of typhoid fever is prolonged, persistent fever** which may persist for 1-2 months in untreated patients. **Mild hepatomegaly and soft splenomegaly is detectable in the majority of patients of typhoid.**

420. Human colostrum has a relatively lower concentration of:

A. Sodium
B. Fat
C. Protein
D. IgA

COLOSTRUM: Breast fluid that may be secreted from the second trimester of pregnancy onward but that is most evident in the first 2 to 3 days after birth and before the onset of true lactation. This thin yellowish fluid contains a great number of proteins and calories in addition to immune globulins. Colostrum contains **several times as much protein as mature breast milk and more minerals but less carbohydrate and fat.**

421. Pseudopancreatic cyst in a child is commonly because of:

A. Drug induced pancreatitis
B. Choledochal cyst
C. Traumatic pancreatitis
D. Annular pancreatitis

Pancreatic pseudocyst is a sharply defined, encapsulated collection of pancreatic fluid enclosed by a wall of fibrous or granulation tissue, which arise as a consequence of **acute pancreatitis, pancreatic trauma, or chronic pancreatitis**.

422. Craniopharyngioma is *most commonly* located in:

A. Suprasellar **B.** Intraventricular
C. Intracerebral **D.** Infrasellar *(SGPGI 1999)*

Craniopharyngiomas occur almost exclusively in the region of the sella turcica, suprasellar cistern, or 3rd ventricle. Hydrocephalus may result from a tumor that obstructs the third ventricle. The epicenter of the tumor is *most commonly* the **suprasellar cistern**. Adamantinomatous-type tumors also can grow (entirely) within the sella, the third ventricle, or the sphenoid sinus or nasal cavity (although rarely).

423. *Not* a characteristic feature of fragile X syndrome:

A. Large testis **B.** Large nose
C. Large ear **D.** Large face *(AI 1999)*

Fragile X syndrome: It is a condition caused by an X-linked mutation associated with a fragile site near the tip of the long arm of the X chromosome. Most males and 30% of females with this syndrome are mentally retarded. This syndrome is the most common inherited cause of mental retardation. **Males also develop greatly enlarged testicles (macro-orchidism)** usually after puberty, but this change has been reported as early as 5 months of age **along with large head and ears.**

Fragile X Characteristics

- Long ears
- Prominent forehead
- Long face
- Prominent jaw
- Macrocephaly
- High arched palate
- Joint looseness
- Pes planus
- Soft skin
- Mitral valve prolapse
- Postnatal overgrowth
- Macro-orchidism after puberty
- Mental retardation
- Temper tantrum
- Hyperactivity
- Autism
- Extreme shyness

424. Hemolytic anemia in G6PD deficiency is *not* caused by:

A. Co-trimoxazole **B.** Nitrofurantoin
C. Rifampicin **D.** Nalidixic acid *(AIIMS 1995)*

Drugs Causing Hemolytic Anemia in G6PD Deficiency

- Aminosalicylic acid
- Antimalarials, e.g. primaquine
- Aspirin
- Chloramphenicol
- Co-trimoxazole
- Dapsone
- Nalidixic acid
- Nitrofurantoin
- Phenacetin
- Probenecid
- Procainamide
- Quinidine
- Sulfonamides
- Vitamin C
- Vitamin K

425. *Not* seen in kwashiorkor:

A. Edema
B. Fatty infiltration of liver
C. Depigmented areas in skin
D. Fatty infiltration of pancreas

Kwashiorkor is characterized by pitting edema. The child is listless, lethargic, apathetic and miserable. Hairs are thin, dry, brittle and lusterless. They become straight and hypopigmented grayish white or reddish brown in color. During recovery growing part of hair are pigmented giving appearance of a flag (the flag sign).The skin lesions appear as large areas of erythema followed by hyperpigmentation. Skin becomes dry, hyperkeratotic. Alternate areas of hypo and hyperpigmentation give a resemblance to pavement (pavement dermatosis).Mosaic pattern may also be seen (Mosaic dermatosis).**Liver is enlarged and fatty.**

426. In the treatment of severe malnutrition, calories required/kg body weight in phase III is:

A. 130
B. 300
C. 180
D. 125

Management of severe PEM consists of three phases:

1. **Initial phase** consists of 80 kcal/kg/day of energy along with 0.7 gm protein /kg/day according to the actual weight than the expected weight.
2. In **phase II** 100 kcal/kg/day of energy along with 1.0 gm protein /kg/day.
3. **Phase of high energy feeding** 150–180 kcal/kg/day of energy along with 2 gm protein /kg/day.

427. ***False*** **regarding primary complex in children:**

A. Effusion seen
B. Mediastinal lymphadenopathy
C. Connecting lymphatic channels
D. Ghon's focus in lung

Primary complex consists of:

- Ghon's focus in lung
- Mediastinal lymphadenopathy
- Connecting lymphatic channels

428. Tetanus is characterized by:

A. Incubation period is 2-3 day
B. Spasm of masseter occurs first
C. Accompanied by loss of consciousness
D. Can be cultured from wound

TETANUS is an acute infectious disease of the central nervous system caused by an exotoxin of the tetanus bacillus, *Clostridium tetani*. The toxin is produced anaerobically at the site of a wound. **The incubation period is usually 3 to 21 days**. The disease manifests by the onset of extremely painful muscular contractions that usually begin gradually but may appear suddenly. The contractions may be of brief duration or last some weeks. **First sign of tetanus is stiffness of the jaw**, esophageal muscles, and some of the muscles of the neck. This disease is usually fatal, with the patient expiring from asphyxia or exhaustion.
Masseter*: The muscle that closes the mouth and is the principal muscle in mastication.*

429. Death in diaphragmatic hernia is due to:

A. Hypoplastic lung
B. Cardiac malformation
C. Intestinal obstruction
D. Infections

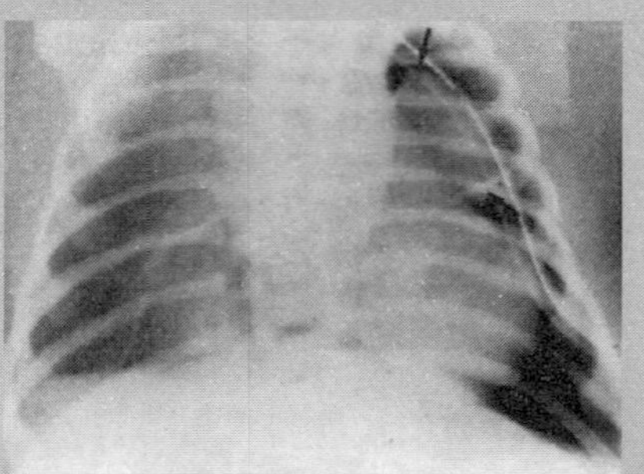

In **diaphragmatic hernia** death is usually due to **hypoxia** caused **by hypoplastic lung**

430. Neonatal sepsis and meningitis is ***most commonly*** **caused by:**

A. Group B *Streptococcus*
B. *Staphylococcus aureus*
C. *Streptococcus agalactiae*
D. *Enterococcus faecalis*

Group B *Streptococcus* is the most common cause of neonatal sepsis and meningitis in USA. Infection most commonly occur during the first few days of life (the early onset disease),mean age of onset being 20 hours and has got an incidence of 2-4 /1000 live births. A distinct form of disease occurs after the first week of life, mean age of onset being 24 days. This form of disease is known as late onset disease and has an incidence of 1-2 /1000 live births.

431. The goal of incubator care is to maintain the core temperature of infant at:

A. 36.6-37.5 °C **B.** 30.6-31.5 °C
C. 39.6-40.5 °C **D.** None

Human incubators, in use since 1880, have helped save the lives of babies born as much as 17 weeks prematurely. Incubators used in centers that specialize in care of infants born prematurely, called **neonatal intensive care units** [NICU], are equipped with electronic devices for monitoring the infants' temperature and the amount of oxygen in the infants' blood. The goal of incubator care is to maintain the core temperature of infant at 36.6-37.5 °C.

432. A 3-year-old can *not* do:

A. Climb upstairs **B.** Hobble 5 steps
C. Draw a circle **D.** Speak sentences *(AIIMS 1994)*

36 Months

Motor	**Goes up stairs alternating feet**; rides tricycle; stands momentarily on one foot
Adaptive	Tower of 9 cubes; imitates construction of bridge of 3 cubes; **copies a circle**; imitates a cross
Language	Knows age and sex; counts 3 objects correctly; repeats 3 numbers or **a sentence of 6 syllables**
Social	Plays simple games (in parallel with other children)helps in dressing (unbuttons clothing and puts on shoes); washes hands

433. *True* regarding about juvenile CML is:

A. Massive splenomegaly **B.** High HbF content
C. High alkaline phosphatase **D.** Philadelphia chromosome

Differentiating Features of Adult and Juvenile CML

Features	Adult type	Juvenile type
• **Age**	10-12 years	1-2 years
• **Philadelphia chromosome**	Always present	Never present
• **Fetal Hb values**	3-7%	30-70%
• **Splenomegaly**	Massive	Mild to moderate
• **Lymphadenopathy**	Occasional	Frequent
• **Skin rash**	Not present	Frequently present on face
• **WBC count**	Over 1,00,000	Less than 1,00,000
• **Thrombocytopenia**	Uncommon	Common
• **Blast cells in GBP**	Rare	Common
• **Complete remission**	Frequent	Rare
• **Alkaline phosphatase in neutrophils**	Decreased	Decreased

434. Phototherapy reduces unconjugated bilirubin to conjugated bilirubin by:

A. Structural isomerization **B.** Photo-oxidation
C. E-isomerization **D.** All of the above

When bilirubin absorbs light, 3 types of photochemical reactions occur:
1. **Photoisomerization** occurs in extravascular space of skin in which natural isomer of unconjugated bilirubin (4Z,15Z) is converted to less toxic polar isomer (4Z,15E) that diffuses into blood and is excreted with bile. This process is known as **E isomerization**.
2. **Structural isomerization** in which bilirubin is converted to lumirubin by intramolecular cyclization. This is the most important pathway for lowering of serum bilirubin levels.
3. **Photo-oxidation**

435. Which of the following is *false* regarding Turner syndrome:
A. Hypergonadotrophic hypogonadism
B. Horseshoe kidney
C. Coarctation of aorta
D. Breast development *(UP 1999)*

Turner syndrome is characterized by primary amenorrhea, sexual infantilism, short stature, multiple congenital anomalies, and bilateral streak gonads in phenotypic women. About 50% of the patients have a 45, X karyotype, about 25% have mosaicism with no structural abnormality (46, XX/45, X), and the remainder have a structurally abnormal X chromosome with or without mosaicism. The incidence is about 1 in 3000 newborn females. The external genitalia are unambiguously female but remain immature, and there is **no breast development** unless exogenous estrogen is given. The fallopian tubes and uterus are immature, and bilateral streak gonads are present in the broad ligaments.

Lymphedema of the hands and feet, webbing of the neck, low hairline, redundant skin folds on the back of the neck, a shield like chest with widely spaced nipples, and growth retardation are suggestive of this condition in infancy. Micrognathia, epicanthal folds, prominent low-set or deformed ears, a fishlike mouth, and ptosis are seen.

Short 4th metacarpals are seen in half of the cases, and 10-20 % have **coarctation of the aorta**. About half the patients have abnormal urograms, **horseshoe kidney** and malrotation being the most common anomalies. In adults, the average height rarely exceeds 150 cm. Associated conditions like renal malformations, pigmented nevi, hypoplastic nails, tendency to keloid formation, perceptive hearing loss, unexplained hypertension, glucose intolerance, and autoimmune thyroid disease may be present.

436. Emergency treatment of TGV:
A. Balloon septostomy
B. Digoxin
C. Oxygen
D. Ventilation

BALLOON ATRIAL SEPTOSTOMY OR RASHKIND PROCEDURE:
The surgical enlargement of an opening between the cardiac atria for palliative relief of congestive heart failure in newborns with certain heart defects [such as Transposition of Great vessels]. A deflated balloon is inserted into a vein, passed through the foramen ovale, and then inflated and pulled vigorously through the atrial septum to enlarge the opening and improve oxygenation of the blood.

437. Infantile myocarditis and pericarditis is *not* caused by:
A. Echovirus
B. Coxsackie A
C. Coxsackie B
D. Rotavirus

Causes of Viral Myocarditis in Children

- Coxsackievirus A
- Coxsackievirus B
- Echovirus
- Rubella
- Varicella
- Influenza

438. In infants which of the following drug is *contraindicated*:
A. Ciprofloxacin
B. Chloroquine
C. Theophylline
D. Barbiturate

Fluoroquinolones are not recommended for use in infants and children. They should not be used in children until absolutely necessary due to risk of cartilage toxicity to the growing cartilage associated with this group of drugs.

439. IUGR is defined as:

A. <7percentile of expected weight
B. <8 percentile of expected weight
C. <10 percentile of expected weight
D. <5 percentile of expected weight *(AI 1993)*

Fetuses weighing < 10th percentile for gestational age or less than two standard deviations below the mean for gestational age have been classified as IUGR.

440. Risk of kernicterus is *not* increased:

A. High level of serum albumin
B. Low level of serum albumin
C. Prematurity
D. Acidosis

Bilirubin enters the brain to cause kernicterus only in unbound form. Normally it is tightly bound to serum albumin (8.5 mg binds with 1 gm of albumin).This binding capacity is less in small and premature babies. Acidosis affects bilirubin solubility and its deposition into brain tissue.

441. Drug of choice in infantile myoclonic seizures is:

A. ACTH
B. Clonazepam
C. Phenytoin
D. Phenobarbitone

Drug of choice in infantile myoclonic seizure is **ACTH**.

442. A 5-year-old child has anemia of long duration. The investigation to be done is:

A. Peripheral smear
B. Estimation of hemoglobin %
C. RBC count
D. PCV

The most important investigations for anemia are:

- Complete blood count
- Reticulocyte count
- GENERAL BLOOD PICTURE

In patients with severe anemia and abnormalities in RBC morphology, a bone marrow aspirate and biopsy should be done.

443. Fetal hemoglobin equals adult hemoglobin at:

A. 2 months
B. Birth
C. 4 months
D. 6 months

Hemoglobin F contains gamma chain in place of beta chain found in adult hemoglobin. At birth it constitutes 70% of hemoglobin and thereafter its synthesis decreases rapidly and by the age of 6–12 months only a trace is present. In older children and adults its concentration is 2%.

444. Which of the following is caused by congenital 17 hydroxylase deficiency:

A. Hyperkalemia
B. Hermaphroditism
C. Hypertension
D. Virilism

(AIIMS 1992)

17-hydroxylase (17-OH) deficiency syndrome is a *rare* genetic disorder of steroid biosynthesis causing decreased production of glucocorticoids and sex steroids and increased synthesis of mineralocorticoid precursors. Reduced or absent levels of both gonadal and adrenal sex hormones result in sexual infantilism in 46, XX females and ambiguous genitalia in 46, XY males. **Excessive mineralocorticoid activity produces varying degrees of hypertension** and *hypo*kalemia. Patients usually are diagnosed with this condition during an evaluation of delayed puberty, absent secondary sexual characteristics or primary amenorrhea.

445. One-year-old child presenting with abdominal mass and calcification on X-rays is suggestive of:

A. Wilms' tumor
B. Neuroblastoma
C. Rhabdomyosarcoma
D. Teratoma

Neuroblastomas are the most common tumor of early childhood; most occur in children younger than five years. The adrenal medulla is the typical site for a neuroblastoma, but it may arise at other sites also. **The abdominal radiograph is useful in demonstrating the calcifications which is seen in about 50% of neuroblastomas.** Differential diagnosis is with Wilms' tumor.

446. Upper segment lower segment ratio at 3 years of age in a normal child is:

A. 1.7 **B.** 1.1
C. 1.3 **D.** 1.0 *(KARNATAKA 1996)*

Upper segment and lower segment ratio (US: LS ratio)	
• At birth	1.7
• At 3 years	1.3
• At 6 years	1.1
• At 10 years	1.0
Arm span	
• At birth	< length by 2.5 cm
• At 11 years and there after	Equals height

447. In ORS the function of glucose is to:

A. Increase Na^+ absorption by co-transport
B. Increase Na^+ K^+ pump activity
C. Increase osmolality of ORS
D. Give sweat taste to ORS *(PGI 1996)*

Oral rehydration is only possible if glucose is added to the salts because there is absorption of sodium ions along with glucose due to glucose facilitated sodium ion absorption (co-transport).

448. *Most common* cause of gastrointestinal hemorrhage in children is:

A. Mallory Weiss syndrome **B.** Portal hypertension
C. Peptic ulcer **D.** Erosive damage

Erosive damage to the mucosa of GI tract is the most common cause of GI hemorrhage in children.

449. All the following are features of cerebral palsy *except*:

A. Hypotonia **B.** Spasticity
C. Erb's palsy **D.** Quadriplegia *(JIPMER 2002)*

Cerebral palsy is a disorder of motor development. Cerebral palsy is a *static* encephalopathy which is characterized as a disorder of movement and posture associated with an abnormal pattern of persistent primitive reflexes and delayed evolution of postural reactions and consequent motor milestones. The classification is based on the predominant motor pattern. Two major categories are used in this scheme: **spastic (pyramidal)** and **extrapyramidal**. Approximately 65% of children with cerebral palsy have spastic cerebral palsy. The spastic group is further subdivided based on the pattern of body involvement.

Quadriplegia	It involves all 4 extremities and should be further described if there is asymmetry in the degree of involvement among the extremities.
Hemiplegia	It is restricted to 1 side of the body with the arm typically more severely involved than the leg.
Diplegia	It involves the lower extremities predominantly, although there can be minor fine motor abnormalities. This is the *most common* pattern in premature infants.
Triplegia	A single upper extremity spared. This likely represents hemiplegia superimposed on diplegia.
Monoplegia	In a lower extremity.

Extrapyramidal cerebral palsy, comprising 25% of cases, almost always represents a quadriplegic pattern of involvement. The subdivisions of this group are based on the type of movement disorder which predominates: rigidity, dystonia, choreoathetosis, and ataxia. Although not a movement disorder, hypotonic cerebral palsy is included in the extrapyramidal group. Rigidity is the most common of this group. The critical feature characterizing spasticity is **velocity dependent** increase of tone. The faster the attempt to passively move the joint, the greater the resistance. Gradual slow pressure produces movement more readily. There is also clasp knife effect: beyond a certain amount of stretch of the muscle, a sudden relaxation of the muscle allows movement more easily. The presence of a fixed contracture will interfere with the attempt to elicit these characteristics. Rigidity is characterized by consistent increased tone unrelated to speed of movement or joint position. The final 10% of cases are classified as mixed, displaying prominent spastic and extrapyramidal features.

450. *Not* seen in a child with nephrotic syndrome:

A. Hyperlipidemia
B. Increased alpha globulins
C. Uremia
D. Hypoproteinemia

In **nephrotic syndrome** the basic defect is heavy proteinuria. The protein loss generally exceeds 2 gm/day and consists mainly of albumin, leading to **hypoproteinemia**. Edema appears when serum albumin levels fall below 2.5 gm/dL. All **serum lipids and lipoproteins are increased** because the hypoproteinemia stimulates generalized protein synthesis in liver including lipoproteins. Decreased lipid catabolism is also responsible for it. **Renal function tests are normal**. Most common cause of nephrotic syndrome in children is idiopathic nephrotic syndrome (90%).

451. *Most common* cause of systemic hypertension in children is:

A. Congenital adrenal hyperplasia
B. Acute glomerulonephritis
C. Coarctation of aorta
D. Nephrotic syndrome

In children 75-90% cases of hypertension are due to underlying renal disease primarily **acute glomerulonephritis**.

452. *Not* a complication of chickenpox:

A. Pneumonia
B. Reye's syndrome
C. Enteritis
D. Meningitis

Complications of Chickenpox

• ACUTE CEREBELLAR ATAXIA	• MENINGEAL IRRITATION
• SECONDARY BACTERIAL SUPERINFECTION OF THE SKIN	• ASEPTIC MENINGITIS
• ENCEPHALITIS	• TRANSVERSE MYELITIS
• GUILLAIN-BARRE SYNDROME	• REYE'S SYNDROME
• VARICELLA PNEUMONIA	• INTERSTITIAL PNEUMONITIS

453. *Not* a recognized sign and symptom of raised ICT in a 9-month-old infant:

A. Papilledema
B. Diplopia
C. Increase in head size
D. Bulging fontanel

(SGPGI 1996)

Papilledema is not frequently seen in infants in whom the fontanels are open and the skull bones are not fused because these *openings* in the skull act as safety valve. Raised ICT manifests as an increase in head size, bulging fontanels, open sutures, protruding forehead and prominent scalp veins which appear thin and shiny in these children. The **sunset-sign** in which sclera is visible above the iris and cracked pot sign (**Macewan's sign**) may also be present.

454. A five-year-old child can remember how many digits:

A. 8
B. 4
C. 5
D. 10

At 5 years	
Motor	Skips
Adaptive	Draws triangle from copy; names heavier of 2 weights
Language	Names 4 colors; repeats sentence of 10 syllables; counts 10 pennies correctly
Social	Dresses and undresses; asks questions about meaning of words; domestic role playing

455. Triad of mental retardation, seizure and sebaceous adenoma is seen in:

A. Tuberous sclerosis
B. Hypothyroidism
C. Congenital syphilis
D. Toxoplasmosis

(AIIMS 1997)

Tuberous sclerosis is characterized by skin lesions, seizures, and mental retardation. The skin lesions include **adenoma sebaceum** (facial angiofibromas), ash leaf-shaped hypopigmented macules, shagreen patches (yellowish thickenings of the skin over the lumbosacral region of the back), and depigmented nevi. Rhabdomyomas of the myocardium and angiomyomas of the kidney, liver, adrenals, and pancreas may also occur. Neurologic features may include epilepsy, mental retardation, and hydrocephalus. On CT/MRI scan, the presence of subependymal nodules, which may be calcified, is characteristic. Treatment is symptomatic. Anticonvulsants for seizures, shunting for hydrocephalus are used.

456. Spasticity is *not* associated with:

A. LMN type paralysis
B. Quadriplegia
C. Clonus
D. Clasp knife rigidity

Motor unit consists of an upper motor neuron [UMN] and a lower motor neuron [LMN] and the muscle fibers supplied by it. Upper motor neuron originates in the cerebral cortex descends into corona radiata crosses the internal capsule then travels through the brain stem where it may terminate if it is that of a cranial nerve or may descend into the spinal cord. Here it synapses with the lower motor neuron which finally innervates the muscle fibers. Any lesion affecting the UMN is associated with spasticity of the muscles which it used to innervate. **Lesions associated with LMN injury result in flaccid paralysis.**

Clasp-knife phenomenon: Increased muscle resistance to passive movement of a joint followed by a sudden release of the muscle; commonly seen in patients with **spasticity**.

Clonus: Spasmodic alternation of muscular contractions between antagonistic muscle groups caused by a hyperactive stretch reflex from an upper motor neuron lesion. Sustained pressure or stretch of one of the muscles inhibits the reflex.

Spastic quadriplegia: Paralysis of all four extremities .There is usually associated mental defect. Pseudobulbar palsy is prominent and convulsions are common.

457. 98% of neonates void within:

A. 8 hours
B. 48 hours
C. 12 hours
D. 24 hours

17% of newborn void immediately after birth, 93% void by 24 hrs and 98% void by 48 hours. Rate of urine formation is 0.5–5.0 ml/kg/hour and the most common cause of delayed voiding is inadequate renal perfusion. However intrinsic renal anomalies or obstruction to the urinary tract may be the underlying cause.

458. Neonate with recurrent hypoglycemia attacks and hepatomegaly is likely to have:

A. von Gierke disease
B. Neonatal hepatitis
C. Galactosemia
D. Neonatal diabetes

Common Features of Galactosemia in Newborns

• Jaundice (unconjugated in 1st week) thereafter conjugated	• Hepatomegaly
• Bleeding	• Coagulopathy
• Lethargy	• Weight loss
• Feed intolerance	• Gram-negative septicemia
• Hypoglycemia	• Cataract
• Renal Fanconi syndrome	• Abnormal liver function test

459. Meningitis in preschool children is *most commonly* due to:

A. *Staphylococcus*
B. *Streptococcus*
C. *Pneumococcus*
D. *Haemophilus influenzae*

Organisms	Children (1 month -15 years)
• *H. influenzae*	40-60 %
• *N. meningitidis*	25-40 %
• *S. pneumoniae*	10-20 %
• Streptococci	2-4 %
• Gram-negative bacilli	1-2 %
• Staphylococci	1-2 %
• *Listeria* species	1-2 %

460 *False* regarding febrile convulsions:

A. Aspirin must be given during spike of fever
B. Temperature >38 degree centigrade
C. Occurs from six months to five years
D. Seizures occur early in disease *(JIPMER 1991)*

"Febrile convulsions are generalized, tonic-clonic, brief (< 15 minutes) and self-limiting events that occur in the presence of fever (more than 38 degree celsius) and in the absence underlying neurological disease". They generally occur between 6 months to 5 years of age. Most febrile seizures occur in the early phase of disease usually within 2–3 days. Seizures may be controlled by treating the fever with hydrotherapy and paracetamol, IV or PR diazepam-0.3 mg/kg. Phenobarbitone or sodium valproate may be used for long-term prophylaxis which is rarely required.

461. *Most common* site of childhood rhabdomyosarcoma is:

A. Trunk
B. Genitourinary system
C. Extremities
D. Head and neck *(AIIMS 2000)*

Rhabdomyosarcoma has a peak incidence at an age of 4 years. **Most frequent site is head and neck area** which accounts for 25% of cases. Next most frequent sites are extremities (20%) and genitourinary system (20%). Less common sites are trunk, orbit, intrathoracic area and retroperitoneum.

462. Normal calorie requirement for a 9-year-old child is:

A. 2000 calories **B.** 800 calories
C. 1700 calories **D.** 1000 calories

Age	Caloric requirement
• 1 year	1020
• 2–3 years	1320
• 4–5 years	1720
• 6–9 years	2130
• 10–12 years	2480
• 13–15 years	2580-3080

463. A 4-day-old healthy newborn has jaundice and serum bilirubin of 22 mg/dl, treatment of choice is:

A. Investigation of liver function
B. Phototherapy
C. Exchange transfusion
D. Observation

MANAGEMENT OF HYPERBILIRUBINEMIA IN HEALTHY TERM NEWBORN-AAP GUIDELINES				
Age in hrs	**Consider phototherapy Total serum bilirubin in mg%**	**Phototherapy**	**Exchange transfusion if intensive phototherapy fails**	**Exchange transfusion and extensive phototherapy**
< / = 24 hrs	observation	observation	observation	observation
20-48 hrs	> / = 12 mg%	> / = 15 mg%	> / = 20 mg%	> / = 25 mg%
49-72 hrs	> / = 15 mg%	> / = 18 mg%	> / = 25 mg%	> / = 30 mg%
> 72 hrs	> / = 17 mg%	> / = 20 mg%	> / = 25 mg%	> / = 30 mg%

TREATMENT OF JAUNDICED PREMATURE INFANTS		
Weight	**Phototherapy**	**Exchange transfusion**
< 1000 gm	Start phototherapy within 24 hrs	10-12 mg%
1000-1500 gm	7-9 mg%	12-15 mg%
1500-2000 gm	10-12 mg%	15-18 mg%
2000-2500	13-15 mg%	18-20 mg%

464. *True* regarding laryngeal papilloma is:

A. Seen in adults
B. Multiple
C. Cautery is treatment
D. Single

Papilloma is the most common laryngeal tumor of childhood but is rare in adults. When there are **multiple papillomas**, the tumor may implant in the distal tracheobronchial tree by aerogenous means. Distal spread of laryngeal papillomas occurs in about 2% of cases. An interval of about 10 years separates the discovery of the primary lesions and detection of implants in the distal airways.

465. Energy requirement of an infant is:

A. 50-60 Kcal/kg
B. 60-70 K Kcal/kg
C. 80-90 Kcal/kg
D. 110-120 Kcal/kg

Age (year)	Protein	Calories
• 0–0.5	2.2 gm/kg	115 kcal/kg
• 0.5–1	2 gm/kg	105 kcal/kg
• 1–3	23 gm	1300 kcal
• 4–6	30 gm	1700 kcal
• 7-10	34 gm	2400 kcal

466. The major toxicity of acetaminophen overdose involves:

A. Heart **B.** Acid base metabolism
C. Liver **D.** CNS

Early manifestations of poisoning with acetaminophen **(paracetamol)** are nausea, vomiting, diaphoresis, and pallor. CNS depression is absent. Within 24 to 48 hr, **hepatotoxicity** is manifested by right upper quadrant tenderness and mild hepatomegaly. Laboratory evidence of hepatic toxicity includes prolongation of the prothrombin time and elevation of serum bilirubin and SGPT/SGOT. Severe poisoning may cause hepatic failure.

467. Jaundice in newborn is physiological when:

A. Jaundice persists for more than 4 days in a term infant
B. Infant is visibly jaundiced in first 24 hr of birth
C. Total bilirubin concentration in serum increases by 1 mg/dl per day
D. Total bilirubin concentration in serum is above 15 mg/dl

1. Onset of jaundice in first 24 hours
2. Rise in serum bilirubin more than 0.5 mg/dl/hour
3. Signs of underlying illness in infant (vomiting, poor feeding, lethargy, apnea, tachypnea, temperature instability, weight loss)
4. Jaundice persisting after 8 days in term infant and 14 days in preterm infants
5. Any elevation of serum bilirubin that requires phototherapy.

AAP GUIDELINES TO START PHOTOTHERAPY

Age in hours	Total Serum Bilirubin Level [mg/dL]			
Actions	Consider Phototherapy	Phototherapy	Exchange Transfusion	Exchange Transfusion and Intensive Phototherapy
<=24	...	...	...	...
25-48	≥12	≥15	≥20	≥25
49-72	≥15	≥18	≥25	≥30
>72	≥17	≥20	≥25	≥30

468. Risk of neonatal chickenpox is the *maximum*, if maternal infection occurs:

A. Within 6 weeks of delivery
B. Within 4 days of delivery
C. During the first trimester
D. During the second trimester

The greatest risk of disease in newborn is when the maternal disease occurs within 4 days of delivery.

469. *Most common* cause of congenital hypothyroidism is:

A. Deficiency of deoximinase **B.** Defective release
C. Thyroid dysgenesis **D.** Pendre syndrome

Causes and Incidence of Congenital Hypothyroidism

Cause	Incidence
• Thyroid dysgenesis	1 in 4000
• TBG deficiency	1 in 5000
• Thyroid hormone synthesis defects	1 in 30,000
• Hypothalamic pituitary hypothyroidism	1 in 50,000
• Hypothyroxinemia	1 in 1,00,000

470. Retinoblastoma is bilateral in:

A. 100 % of cases
B. 1 % of cases
C. 50 % of cases
D. 30 % of cases

Retinoblastoma: It is a malignant glioma of the retina, usually unilateral, that occurs in young children and usually is hereditary. **In about 30 % of patients retinoblastoma is bilateral.** The initial diagnostic finding is usually a yellow or white light reflex seen at the pupil (**cat's eye reflex**).

471. A child can copy a circle first at:

A. One and half years
B. 4 years
C. 2 years of age
D. 3 years

	3 years
Motor	Goes up stairs alternating feet; rides tricycle; stands momentarily on one foot
Adaptive	Tower of 9 cubes; imitates construction of bridge of 3 cubes; **copies a circle**; imitates a cross
Language	Knows age and sex; counts 3 objects correctly; repeats 3 numbers or a sentence of 6 syllables
Social	Plays simple games (in parallel with other children) helps in dressing (unbuttons clothing and puts on shoes); washes hands

472. IUGR is caused by all *except*:

A. Diabetes
B. Chronic renal failure
C. Alcohol
D. Smoking

Etiology of Intrauterine Fetal Growth Retardation

Fetal factors	Placental factors	Maternal factors
Chromosomal disorders Such as autosomal trisomies	Decreased placental weight or cellularity or both	Narcotics, **alcohol**, **cigarettes**, antimetabolites
Chronic fetal infections such as CMV inclusion disease, congenital rubella, syphilis	Villous placentitis (bacterial, viral parasitic)	Hypoxemia (high altitude, cyanotic cardiac or pulmonary disease)
Familial dysautonomia	Tumor (chorioangioma, hydatidiform mole)	Hypertensive or **renal disease** or both
Radiation injury	Decrease in surface area	Sickle cell anemia
Multiple gestation	Placental separation	Toxemia
Pancreatic aplasia	Twin transfusion syndrome	
	Localized transfer lesion	

473. Acute coryza is *most common*ly caused by:

A. Rhinovirus
B. RSV
C. Influenza virus
D. Arenavirus

(AIIMS 1993)

Picornaviruses, especially rhinoviruses and certain echoviruses and coxsackieviruses, cause the common cold (acute coryza). **About 30 to 50% of all colds are caused by one of the > 100 serotypes of rhinoviruses.** At any one time only a few viruses are prevalent. Often a single virus is responsible during outbreaks in relatively closed populations, such as in a school or barrack. Adenoviruses most often lead to pharyngitis but may produce symptoms difficult to distinguish from other respiratory viruses.

474. Convulsions in a child with dehydration and vomiting can be due to:

A. Decreased serum magnesium
B. Decreased serum sodium
C. Decreased serum chloride
D. Decreased serum potassium

Reduction in serum sodium results from excessive loss due to dehydration and vomiting. As the serum sodium is reduced osmolarity of ECF is also reduced. As a result water enters the neurons causing cerebral edema which leads to convulsions.

475. Child born to diabetic mother can have all *except*:

A. Small left colon syndrome
B. Hypoglycemia
C. Hypocalcemia
D. Mental retardation

Specific Problems Frequently Observed in Infants of Diabetic Mothers

• Respiratory distress syndrome	• **Hypoglycemia**
• **Hypocalcemia**	• Polycythemia
• Jaundice	• Congenital anomalies
• Poor feeding	• Macrosomia
• Myocardial dysfunction	• Renal vein thrombosis
• Other thrombosis	• **Small left colon syndrome**

476. A neonate less than 7 days old presents with fever, features of meningitis, anorexia. CSF examination revealed increased protein decreased sugar and increased WBC. Most likely diagnosis is:

A. *Listeria monocytogenes*
B. *Shigella*
C. *Mycoplasma*
D. *Mycobacterium tuberculosis* (AIIMS 2000)

Common etiological agents of acute bacterial meningitis in neonates in India

- *Escherichia coli*
- *Klebsiella pneumoniae*
- *Listeria monocytogenes*
- *Enterococcus* spp.
- *Salmonella* spp.

Listeria monocytogenes is a gram-positive rod that grows on ordinary media in a temperature range of 4-42 °C. Greater success in isolation is achieved if the materials are stored in glucose broth at 4°C. Drug of choice for Listeria *monocytogenes* meningitis is ampicillin 300 mg/kg/day.

477. Infant born to mothers of advanced age has greater risk of:

A. Down's syndrome
B. Glycogenesis type II
C. Marfan's syndrome
D. Trisomy 18

Women at high risk of giving birth to a child with Down syndrome are

- Those over 40
- Those who have had a previous child with the syndrome
- Those who themselves have Down syndrome.

478. Neuroblastoma in children is characterized by all *except:*

A. Proptosis
B. Hypertension
C. Café au lait spots
D. Hepatomegaly

Neuroblastomas are the most common tumor of early childhood. It generally occurs in children < five years of age. The adrenal medulla is the typical site for a neuroblastoma. Neuroblastomas are often hormonally active, **producing catecholamines-hypertension-**or less active hormone precursors. Neuroblastomas tend to metastasize widely and early. Hepatic metastasis presents as **hepatomegaly**. Orbits are other frequent sites of metastasis leads to –**proptosis**, periorbital swelling/ecchymosis.

479. Bilateral cataract with direct van den Bergh's test positive in a 3-month old neonate who is exclusively breastfed is suffering from:

A. von Gierke disease
B. Toxoplasmosis
C. Galactosemia
D. Fructosemia

Direct van den Bergh's test is positive in conjugated jaundice.

Common Features of Galactosemia in Newborns	
• Jaundice (unconjugated in 1st week) thereafter conjugated	• Hepatomegaly
• Bleeding	• Coagulopathy
• Lethargy	• Weight loss
• Feed intolerance	• Gram-negative septicemia
• Hypoglycemia	• Cataract
• Renal Fanconi syndrome	• Abnormal liver function test

480. Drug of choice for an attack of familial periodic paralysis:

A. Adrenaline **B.** Potassium chloride
C. ACTH **D.** Calcium chloride

Familial periodic paralysis is also known as hypokalemic periodic paralysis. First attack usually occurs in late childhood. Large carbohydrate meal or rest after exertion may precipitate paralysis. The typical patient awakes paralysed in the morning after a day of heavy exercise followed by a heavy evening meal. During the attack the limbs are flaccid and reflexes are lost. Respiration may be affected and an attack may last for 24 hours. Potassium levels during the attack are low usually between 2-3 mEq/L. Therapy during the attack consist of oral **KCl 2-3 gm**, acetazolamide (Diamox) reduces the frequency of attack.

481. A 4 kg infant with severe dehydration (10%) needs the following amount of IV fluid in the first 24 hours:

A. 1200 ml **B.** 800 ml
C. 500 ml **D.** 100 ml

100 ml/kg of Ringer lactate should be given to correct the dehydration.30 % of it is given rapid IV and 70 % in 5 hours. Thereafter 100 ml/kg of isolyte P is given in 19 hr as a maintenance fluid requirement.

482. A 2-year-old child presented with cough, fever, and dyspnea. His *respiratory rate is 55/minute, chest in-drawing is present* but he has no cyanosis or convulsions. Most likely diagnosis is:

A. Very severe disease **B.** Severe pneumonia
C. Pneumonia **D.** Cough and cold *(AIIMS 2000)*

Clinical Classification of ARI

Clinical category	Diagnostic criteria	Treatment plan
Very severe pneumonia	Central cyanosis Unable to breastfeed or drink Convulsions Lethargy Unconsciousness Severe respiratory distress (e.g. head nodding)	Inpatient care IM or IV Chloramphenicol (100 mg/kg/day QID) or Ampicillin + Gentamicin Give oxygen
Severe pneumonia	**Lower chest Indrawing or Nasal flaring** and No signs of very severe pneumonia	Inpatient care IM or IV benzyl penicillin or ampicillin
Pneumonia	**Fast breathing** and No indicators of severe or very severe pneumonia	Home care Oral co-trimoxazole or amoxicillin or ampicillin or IM procaine penicillin
Cough and cold	No fast breathing and No indicators of severe or very severe pneumonia	Home care Home remedy for cough Paracetamol for fever

Fast breathing (tachypnea) is present if the respiratory rate is more than or equal to	
• In children less than 2 months	60/minute
• In children between 2 months and 12 months	50/ minute
• In children above12 months to 5 years	40/minute

483. All of the following cause splenomegaly *except*:

A. Malaria **B.** Kala azar
C. Tay-Sachs disease **D.** Typhoid

Common Causes of Splenomegaly

Bacterial Infection	Typhoid	Septicemia	Endocarditis	Abscess
Viral infection	EBV	CMV		
Protozoal	Malaria	Kala azar	Toxoplasma	
Hematological	Hemolytic anemias	Thalassemia	Osteopetrosis	Myelofibrosis
Neoplastic	Leukemia	Lymphoma	Hemangioma, hamartoma	Secondaries
Infiltration	Niemann-Pick disease	Gaucher's disease	Histiocytosis	
Congestive	Cirrhosis	Portal hypertension	CCF	
Cystic	Congenital	Acquired		
Other	SLE	Rheumatoid arthritis	Sarcoidosis	

484. Compared to oral digitalizing dose, parenteral dose of Digoxin should be:

A. 1/3 **B.** 1/4
C. 1/2 **D.** 2/3

Compared to oral digitalizing dose, parenteral dose of digoxin should be 2/3.

485. *Not* associated with a large fontanel:

A. Vitamin D deficiency rickets
B. Down's syndrome
C. Hypogonadism
D. Osteogenesis imperfecta

Disorders Associated with a Large Anterior Fontanel

• Achondroplasia	• Osteogenesis imperfecta
• Apert's syndrome	• Prematurity
• Athyrotic hypothyroidism	• Pyknodysostosis
• Cleidocranial dysostosis	• Rubella syndrome
• Hallerman Streiff syndrome	• Russell silver syndrome
• Hydrocephaly	• Trisomies 13,18,21
• Hypophosphatasia	• Vitamin D deficiency rickets
• IUGR	

486. The number of fontanelles present in a newborn child is:

A. 1 **B.** 2
C. 5 **D.** 6

The number of fontanelles present in a newborn child is 6.	
• Anterior fontanelles	1
• Posterior fontanelles	1
• Sphenoid fontanelles	2
• Mastoid fontanelles	2
Total	**6**

487. Most indicative sign of *pneumonia* in 12 months old child with cough and fever is:
- **A.** Temperature 39.5°C and respiratory rate is 60/min
- **B.** Intercostal retraction and fever
- **C.** Temperature 39.5°C
- **D.** Grunting and respiration rate is 60/min

(JIPMER 1995)

Features that indicate severity of acute respiratory infection are:
1. Increased respiratory rate
2. Indrawing of lower chest wall
3. Inability to drink
4. Lethargy or unconsciousness
5. Convulsions
6. Nasal flaring and grunting
7. Head nodding
8. Central cyanosis

Note: Crepitations are a common auscultatory finding in bronchopneumonia but they are difficult to hear in small children and upper airway noises or rhonchi may be confused with them.

488. Obesity is associated with:
- **A.** Laurence Moon Biedl syndrome
- **B.** Prader Willi syndrome
- **C.** Carpenter's syndrome
- **D.** All of the above

Causes of Obesity

Endocrine causes	**Genetic causes**	**Other**
Cushing's syndrome	Laurence-Moon-Biedl syndrome	Cohen's syndrome
Hypothyroidism	Turner's syndrome	Carpenter's syndrome
Hyperinsulinemia	Alstrom-Hallgren syndrome	
Prader-Willi syndrome		
Growth hormone deficiency		
Hypothalamic dysfunction		
Stein Leventhal syndrome (Polycystic ovary)		
Pseudohypoparathyroidism type I		

489. Murmur heard in Eisenmenger syndrome is:
- **A.** Carey Coomb murmur
- **B.** Austin-Flint murmur
- **C.** Graham Steell murmur
- **D.** None

(CMC VELLORE 2002)

490. A child with VSD developed *Eisenmenger syndrome*. Correct sequence of events which leads to this change is:

A. Pulmonary hypertension, right to left shunt, right ventricular hypertrophy, left to right shunt
B. Pulmonary hypertension, right ventricular hypertrophy, left to right shunt, right to left shunt
C. Pulmonary hypertension, left ventricular hypertrophy, left to right shunt, right to left shunt
D. Left to right shunt, right ventricular hypertrophy, pulmonary hypertension, right to left shunt *(AIIMS 2000)*

Eisenmenger syndrome is a term used to designate a condition in which there is a large communication between the two circulations at the aortopulmonary, ventricular, or atrial levels and bidirectional or **predominantly right to left shunts** because of high-resistance and obstructive pulmonary hypertension. The principal physiological abnormality is an elevation of pulmonary vascular resistance. In VSD the pulmonary hypertension occurs as a result of high pulmonary blood flow due to **left to right shunt**. A few patients may develop elevated pulmonary vascular resistance (**pulmonary hypertension**) if the defect is not repaired in time. This pulmonary hypertension is responsible for reversal of shunt (**right to left shunt**), a condition known as *Eisenmenger syndrome.* Symptoms may not occur till 2nd or 3rd decade of life. Cyanosis, dyspnea, fatigue and tendency to develop dysrhythmias begin to occur. CHF, chest pain, syncope and hemoptysis are features of late stage of disease. *On examination* there is a right ventricular heave and a loud narrowly split second heart sound. A soft ejection systolic murmur may be audible along the left sternal border. Functional incompetence of pulmonary valve produces a blowing diastolic murmur along the left sternal border (**Graham Steell murmur**).

- **Carey-Coombs murmur** is a soft mid-diastolic murmur sometimes heard in patients with acute rheumatic fever.
- **Austin-Flint murmur** is heard in severe, chronic aortic regurgitation, and it may be either mid-diastolic or pre-systolic.

491. The clinical sign of hyaline membrane disease generally *first* appears:

A. In the first 6 hours of life
B. After 48 hr of life
C. Between 12 and 24 hr of life
D. Between 36 and 48 hr of life

Respiratory distress syndrome (RDS or hyaline membrane disease) is the most important pulmonary disorder of newborn infants. The syndrome is more common in premature infants weighing less than 1.5 kg, infants of diabetic mothers, infants delivered by cesarean section, and infants with a history of birth asphyxia. The lungs of these infants are immature and unable to secrete the surfactant that normally reduces the surface tension and prevents atelectasis. Hyaline membrane disease is characterized by a **triad of tachypnea, expiratory grunt and inspiratory retractions in a prematurely born asphyxiated infant**. The **symptoms may begin at birth or within 6 hours of delivery**.

492. X-ray appearance in hyaline membrane disease is:

A. Homogenous ground glass appearance
B. Air bronchogram
C. Reticulonodular shadow
D. Normal X-ray

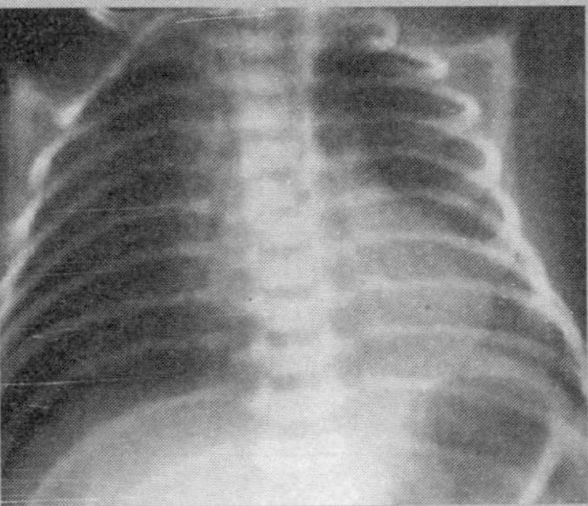

A chest X-ray film in a newborn with HMD reveals uniform minute reticulogranular densities, producing a so called **'ground glass' picture**. The radiological findings are fairly constant.

493. Which of the following is *true* of Hyaline membrane disease of newborn:

A. Maternal steroid exposure increases severity of disease
B. Surfactant increases the surface tension of alveoli
C. Phosphatidyl glycerol estimation is a reliable method of diagnosis
D. Prematurity provides relative protection to occurrence

The pulmonary immaturity of the fetal lungs can be assessed by determination of lecithin/sphingomyelin ratio in the amniotic fluid. Lecithin/sphingomyelin ratio of 2 or more indicates adequate lung maturity, while a ratio of less than 1.5 is associated with HMD. Amniotic fluid 'shake test' is a simple bedside test for assessment of lung maturity. Estimation of **phosphotidyl glycerol** is a more specific indicator of lung maturity (especially in diabetic mothers), and its absence is invariably associated with development of HMD.

494. In physiological jaundice in term infants, serum bilirubin *does not* generally exceed:

A. 20 mg% **B.** 5 mg%
C. 15 mg% **D.** 10 %

Physiological Jaundice: About 60-70% of healthy newborn babies are likely to develop physiological jaundice. Physiological jaundice appears between 24 and 72 hr of age, its maximum intensity is seen on the 4th and 5th day of life, and the peak serum **bilirubin level does not exceed 15 mg/dl.** This type of jaundice usually disappears before 14 days of life and does not need any specific therapy.

495. Convulsions in infants can be caused by:

A. Hypocalcemia **B.** Anoxia
C. Hypoglycemia **D.** All of the above

Important Causes of Neonatal Seizure

Hypoxic ischemic encephalopathy	Intracranial hemorrhage	Molybdenum cofactor deficiency
Hypoglycemia	Hypocalcemia	Hypomagnesemia
Hyponatremia	Hypernatremia	Pyridoxine dependency
Maple syrup urine disease	Phenylketonuria	Isovaleric acidemia
Urea cycle disorders	Beta alanine abnormalities	Methylmalonic acidemia
Propionic acidemia	Congenital lactic acidosis	Glutaric aciduria type II
Fructose intolerance	Menke's kinky hair disease	CNS trauma
Bacterial meningitis	Brain abscess	Cerebral dysgenesis
Phakomatoses	Narcotic withdrawal	Familial neonatal seizure
Hypertensive encephalopathy	Local anesthesia	Unknown causes (25%)

496. Which of the following is *true* regarding a 1-year-old child with PDA:

A. Indomethacin may help in closure
B. Chances of spontaneous closure is high
C. Symptoms similar to aorto-pulmonary window
D. Endocarditis is rare

(AIIMS 1995)

Unlike PDA in preterm infants **spontaneous closure of PDA does not occur in term infants** and anatomical existence of PDA regardless to its size is an indication for surgical ligation. Surgical procedure may be performed anytime between 6 months to 2 years. Subacute **endocarditis** is a frequent complication seen with small PDA. **Indomethacin** is effective only in preterm newborns and has no role, what so ever, in term infants and grown up children.

497. *Most common* cause of convulsions in a child with fever is:

A. Hypothyroidism **B.** Febrile convulsions
C. Meningitis **D.** Epilepsy

Febrile seizure is the most common neurological disease of childhood. It usually occurs between the age of 5 months to 5 years. The child while having high grade fever due to some other common childhood infection develops seizure which is generalized, tonic clonic, brief (less than 15 minutes) and self limiting. Reduction in fever by hydrotherapy and paracetamol along with short-term prophylaxis with diazepam is all that is required.

498. Dyslexia is characterized by all *except*:
A. Mental retardation
B. Inability to interpret written language
C. Male preponderance
D. Retardation reading

Dyslexia: An imprecise term concerning a condition in which an individual with normal vision is **unable to interpret written language**. **The condition is more common in males** and is noticed in children with **reading difficulty** in the first grade. These individuals can see and recognize letters but are unable to spell and write words. They have no difficulty recognizing the meaning of objects and pictures. **Dyslexia is unrelated to intelligence**.

499. Hyaline membrane seen in lung is composed of:
A. Polysaccharide
B. Mucoprotein
C. Globulin
D. Fibrin

Hyaline membranes are largely made up of fibrinogen and fibrin admixed with cell debris derived chiefly from necrotic alveolar lining pneumocytes. The sequence of events that leads to the formation of hyaline membranes is given below.

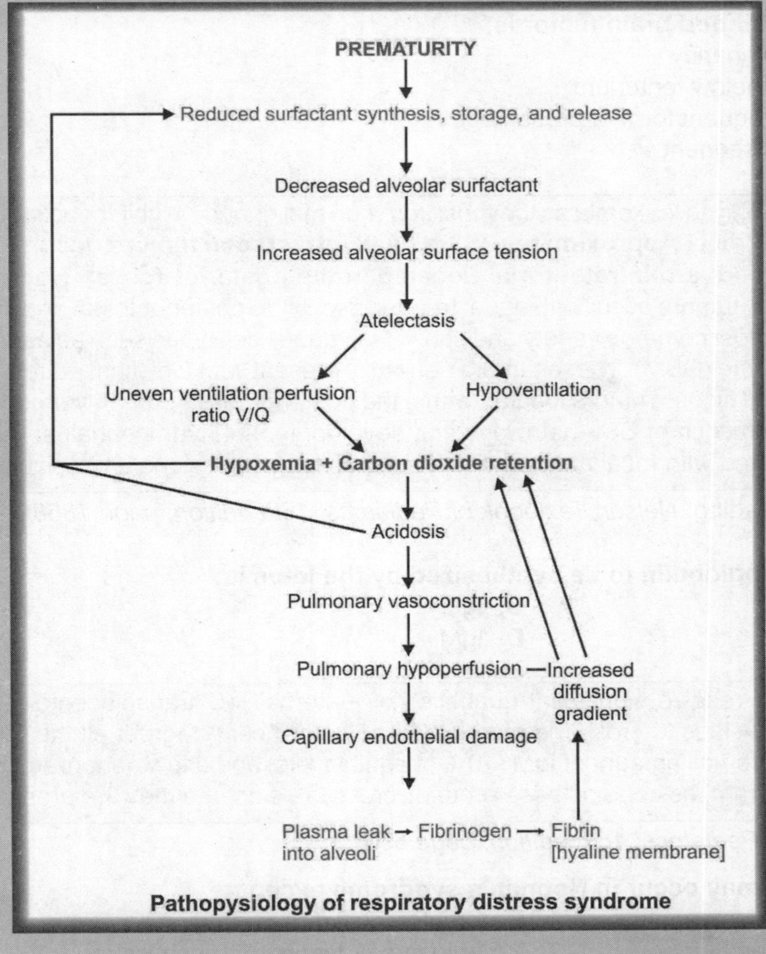

Pathopysiology of respiratory distress syndrome

500. The characteristics of caput succedaneum *do not* include:

A. A diffuse edematous swelling of the soft tissues of scalp
B. Crosses the suture line
C. Does not disappear within 2-3 days
D. Crosses midline

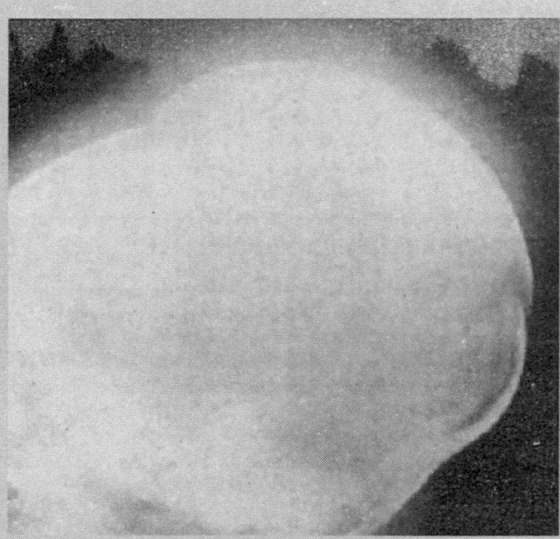

Caput succedaneum: **Diffuse edema of the fetal scalp** that **crosses the suture lines**. Head compression against the cervix impedes venous return, forcing serum into the interstitial tissues. **The swelling reabsorbs within 1 to 3 days.**

501. *True* regarding childhood brain tumor is:

A. Rare form of malignancy
B. Most tumors are below tentorium
C. Hemiparesis is frequent form of presentation
D. Papilledema is infrequent *(SGPGI 1999)*

Brain tumors are second only to leukemia as the *most common* malignancy in childhood, and they are *most common* 'solid' tumors in this age group. **Approximately 2/3rd of all intracranial tumors occurring in children between the ages of 2 and 12 years are infratentorial (located in the posterior fossa).** However, in adolescents and children less than 2 years, tumors occur with equal frequencies in the posterior fossa and the supratentorial region. Glial cell tumors are the *most common* variety and consist of various cell types such as astrocytoma, ependymoma, and glioblastoma multiforme (GBM). These tumors generally present with 2 distinct patterns, viz. features of raised ICT and focal neurological signs. Tumors located within the posterior fossa primarily produce symptoms and signs of raised ICT due to obstruction of CSF pathways and development of hydrocephalus. Supratentorial tumors are more likely to be associated with focal abnormalities, such as long-tract signs and seizures.

Reference and further reading: *Nelson Textbook of Pediatrics; 16th edition; page 1858*

502. The *earliest* immunoglobulin to be synthesized by the fetus is:

A. IgA
B. IgG
C. IgE
D. IgM *(AI 2003)*

A human fetus begins to receive significant quantities of maternal IgG transplacentally at around 12 weeks of gestation. IgG is the only class to cross the placenta at any significant degree; all the four subclass do this, but IgG_2 does so least well. A small amount of IgM (10% of adult levels) and a few nanograms of IgA, IgD, and IgE are normally found in cord serum; as none of these proteins cross the placenta they are presumed to be of fetal origin.

Ref: *Nelson Textbook of Pediatrics; 16th edition; page 593*

503. All of the following may occur in Noonan's syndrome *except*:

A. Hypertrophic cardiomyopathy
B. Cryptorchidism
C. Infertility in females
D. Autosomal dominant transmission *(AI 2003)*

The term **Noonan syndrome** has been applied to males and females that have certain phenotypic features that also occur in females with Turner syndrome. These children have normal karyotypes and Noonan syndrome occurs once in 2000 live births.[1] It is an autosomal dominant disorder in both sexes.
[2] Most common abnormalities are short stature, webbing of the neck, pectus carinatum (chest protrusion) or pectus excavatum (chest depression), cubitus valgus, right-sided congenital heart disease and characteristic facies. Hypertelorism (abnormal distance between two paired organs, esp. the eyes), epicanthus (a vertical fold of skin extending from the root of the nose to the median end of the eyebrow, covering the inner canthus and caruncle) and downward slanted palpebral fissures, ptosis, micrognathia, and ear abnormalities are common. Clinodactyly (hypoplasia of the middle phalanx of one or more of the fingers resulting in these fingers curving inward), hernias and vertebral anomalies occur less frequently. Moderate mental retardation occurs in 1/4th of patients and sensorineural deafness is common. Cardiac defect is *most often*-pulmonary valvular stenosis, hypertrophic cardiomyopathy, or ASD. Hepatosplenomegaly, several hematological diseases, ALL, and CML have been described in patients with Noonan syndrome. Males frequently have cryptorchidism and small testes; they may be hypogonadal or normal. Puberty is delayed 2 years on average; adult height is achieved by the end of the second decade and usually reaches the lowest limit of the normal population.
[3] Girls with Noonan syndrome show certain anomalies that also occur in girls with 45, X Turner syndrome, but they have normal 46, XX chromosomes. Mental retardation is often present, cardiac defect is most often pulmonary valvular stenosis or an atrial septal defect rather than an aortic defect, normal sexual maturation usually occurs but is delayed 2 years on average and premature ovarian failure has been reported.

Ref: [1] *Harrison's Principles of Internal Medicine*
[2] *Nelson Textbook of Pediatrics; 16th edition; page 1747*
[3] *Nelson Textbook of Pediatrics; 16th edition; page 1756*

504. The *treatment of choice* for primary grade-V vesicoureteral reflux involving both kidneys in a 6-month-old boy is:

A. Antibiotic prophylaxis
B. Ureteric reimplantation
C. Cystoscopy followed by subureteric injection of Teflon
D. Bilateral ureterostomy

(AIIMS May 2003)

Vesicoureteral reflux may be defined as **retrograde flow of urine from the bladder to the ureter and renal pelvis**. Reflux severity is graded using the international study classification of I to V and is based on the appearance of the urinary tract on a contrast voiding cystourethrogram (VCUG). The more severe the reflux, the higher the rates of renal injury. Reflux may be primary or secondary. Primary vesicoureteral reflux results from an anatomic deformity of the ureterovesical junction. The goals of treatment are to prevent pyelonephritis, renal injury, and other complications. Open surgical repair is generally performed in children with breakthrough UTI, un-resolving reflux, and grade IV or V reflux.[1] Surgery (**ureteral reimplantation**) is the definitive method of correcting primary reflux, especially in the setting of anatomic abnormalities. Surgical principles of successful reimplantation include (1) creating a long submucosal tunnel to provide a 5:1 tunnel-to-diameter ratio, (2) providing good detrusor muscle backing, (3) avoiding ureteric kinking, and (4) creating a tunnel in the fixed area of the bladder.[2]

Ref: *Nelson Textbook of Pediatrics; 16th edition; page 1625–1629* [1]
http://www.emedicine.com [2]

505. Which of the following maternal antibody causes heart block in newborn?

A. Anti ds DNA
B. Anti Jo
C. Anti-Ro antibodies
D. Anti-histone antibodies

(SGPGI 2002)

Lupus in newborns results from maternal transfer of IgG auto-antibodies (usually anti-Ro). Manifestations include congenital heart block, cutaneous lesions, liver disease, thrombocytopenia, neutropenia, and pulmonary and neurological disorders. Most manifestations resolve spontaneously; however, congenital heart block is a permanent phenomenon and often requires cardiac pacing.

Ref: *Nelson Textbook of Pediatrics; 16th edition; page 716*

506. There is a high risk of renal dysplasia in:

A. Posterior urethral valves
B. Bladder extrophy
C. Anorectal malformation
D. Neonatal sepsis
(AIIMS May 2003)

About 50% of children with anorectal anomalies have a urological problem. The more serious and complex the anorectal defect, the more frequently it is associated with a urological anomaly.

Ref: *Nelson Textbook of Pediatrics; 16th edition; page 1146*

507. Which one of the following is the *most common* cause of abdominal mass in neonates?

A. Neuroblastomas
B. Wilms' tumor
C. Distended bladder
D. Multicystic dysplastic kidneys
(AI 2003)

Multicystic dysplastic kidney is the *most common* cause of an abdominal mass in the newborn.

Ref: *Nelson Textbook of Pediatrics; 16th edition; page 1620*

508. *True* regarding ectopia cordis is:

A. Is seen between the ribs
B. The heart is seen projecting from a defect in the lower thorax and the upper abdominal wall
C. Projects from the whole of defect arising from the abdominal wall
D. Projects from the upper thoracic region
(SGPGI 2003)

The 'thoracic form' is the *most common* type of **ectopia cordis**. In this condition the sternum is split and the heart protrudes outside the chest. In other forms the heart protrudes through the diaphragm into the abdominal cavity or may be situated in the neck. Associated intracardiac anomalies are common and death occurs in the first few days of life in most of the cases usually due to infection, cardiac failure, or hypoxemia. Surgical therapy for neonates without severe cardiac anomalies consists of covering the heart with skin without compromising venous return or ventricular ejection. Occasional patients with 'abdominal type' have survived to adulthood.

Ref: *Nelson Textbook of Pediatrics; 16th edition; page 1408*

509. 8-year-old boy presents with swelling in left eye of 3 months duration. Examination revealed proptosis of left eye with preserved vision. Right eye is normal. CT scan revealed intraorbital extra coneal mass lesion. Biopsy revealed embryonal rhabdomyosarcoma. Metastatic work up was normal. The standard line of treatment is:

A. Chemotherapy only
B. Wide local incision
C. Enucleation
D. Chemotherapy and radiotherapy
(AIIMS Nov 2002)

[1] **Rhabdomyosarcoma** is the *most common* pediatric soft tissue sarcoma accounting for 5–8% of childhood cancers. These tumors occur virtually at any anatomic site but are most often found in the head and neck (40%), genitourinary tract (20%), extremities (20%) and trunk (10%); retroperitoneal and other sites account for the remainder. Rhabdomyosarcoma occurs with increased frequency in patients of Neurofibromatosis and has been associated with maternal cancer in Li-Fraumeni syndrome suggesting a genetic influence. The *most common* presenting feature is a mass that may or may not be painful and symptoms are due to displacement or obstruction of normal structures. Orbital primaries are usually diagnosed early in their course because of associated proptosis, periorbital edema, ptosis, change in visual acuity and local pain. Treatment is based on the primary tumor location and the disease stage. Unresectable tumor localized to certain favorable sites such as the orbit has a high likelihood of cure. The treatment of rhabdomyosarcoma of orbit is a combination of chemotherapy and radiotherapy. [2]

Ref: [1] *Nelson Textbook of Pediatrics; 16th edition; page 1556-1558*
[2] *Parsons' Diseases of the Eye; 18th edition; page 385*

510. Kernicterus is caused by:

A. Bilirubin monoglucuronide
B. Albumin bound bilirubin
C. Unbound bilirubin
D. Bilirubin diglucuronide
(MANIPAL 2002)

Kernicterus is a neurologic syndrome resulting from deposition of unconjugated bilirubin (UCB) in brain cells. The risk of kernicterus in *erythroblastosis fetalis* is directly related to serum bilirubin levels but this relationship is uncertain in *healthy term neonates*. Lipids soluble unconjugated bilirubin may cross the blood-brain-barrier and enter the brain by diffusion if the bilirubin binding capacity of albumin and other plasma proteins is exceeded. *Alternatively*, bilirubin may enter the brain after damage to the blood-brain-barrier by asphyxia or hyperosmolality. The precise serum bilirubin level above which unconjugated bilirubin will be toxic for an individual infant is unpredictable, but kernicterus is *rare* in healthy term infants and in the absence of hemolysis if the serum level is under 25 mg/dL. Less mature the infant, the greater the susceptibility of kernicterus. Kernicterus develop at lower bilirubin levels in preterm infants and in the presence of asphyxia, intraventricular hemorrhage (IVH), hemolysis or drugs that displace bilirubin from albumin. Signs and symptoms of kernicterus usually appear 2–5 days after birth in term infants and as late as the 7th day in the preterm infants. The early signs are subtle and indistinguishable from those of sepsis, asphyxia, hypoglycemia, intracranial hemorrhage and other acute systemic illnesses in a newborn. Poor feeding, lethargy and loss of Moro reflex are initial signs; subsequently the infant may appear gravely ill with diminished tendon reflexes and respiratory distress; opisthotonos, bulging fontanel, twitching of face or limbs and shrill high-pitched cry may follow. In advanced cases convulsions and spasm occur with the newborn stiffly extending his/her arms in inward rotation with fists clinched. Most of them die; the survivors are seriously disabled.

Ref: *Nelson Textbook of Pediatrics; 16th edition; page 517*

511. All of the following are seen in atrial septal defect *except*:

A. There may be no murmurs audible **B.** Right ventricular hypertrophy
C. Wide split 2nd heart sound **D.** Pulmonary oligemia *(SGPGI 2003)*

In chest X-ray of patients of *ostium secundum* ASD there is varying degree of enlargement of right ventricle and atrium depending upon the size of the shunt. The pulmonary artery is large, and pulmonary vascularity is increased.

Ref: *Nelson Textbook of Pediatrics; 16th edition; page 1366*

512. Karyotype in Klinefelter syndrome:

A. XY **B.** XXY
C. XO **D.** XX *(MANIPAL 2001)*

Approximately 1 in 500 or 1 in 1000 newborn males has a 47, XXY chromosome complement. The incidence is 1% among the mentally retarded. The **47, XXY chromosome complement** is the *most common* chromosomal pattern in persons with **Klinefelter syndrome** (80%); some have mosaic patterns.

Reference and further reading: *Nelson Textbook of Pediatrics; 16th edition; page 1747*

513. Transient myeloproliferative disorder of the newborn is seen in association with:

A. Turner syndrome **B.** Down syndrome
C. Neurofibromatosis **D.** Ataxia telangiectasia *(AI 2003)*

Patients of Down syndrome have 10–30 times greater risk of developing leukemia than the general population. Neonates and infants with **Down syndrome** may develop a condition known as **transient myeloproliferative syndrome** that mimics *congenital leukemia*. These children may have hepatosplenomegaly, anemia, thrombocytopenia, and a significant leukemoid reaction. These features usually resolve spontaneously but a close follow-up is indicated as these children have a higher risk of subsequent development of leukemia (especially the acute megakaryocytic subtype of AML-FAB M_7). Children who have Down syndrome and who develop AML have a *much better* prognosis than other children due to unknown reasons.

Ref: *Nelson Textbook of Pediatrics; 16th edition; page 1547*

514. A 2-year-old presented with leukocoria in the right eye since 2 months. On examination, a total retinal detachment was present in the same eye. Ultrasound B scan revealed a heterogeneous subretinal mass with calcification, associated with a retinal detachment. The *most likely* clinical diagnosis is:

A. Coats disease **B.** Retinoblastoma
C. Toxocariasis **D.** Retinal tuberculoma *(AIIMS Nov 2002)*

515. A 1 year old child having leukocoria was detected to be having a unilateral, large retinoblastoma filling half the globe. Current therapy would involve:

A. Enucleation
B. Chemotherapy followed by local dyes
C. Direct laser ablation using photodynamic cryotherapy
D. Scleral radiotherapy followed by chemotherapy *(AIIMS Nov 2002)*

516. A 1 year old child having leukocoria was detected to be having a unilateral, large retinoblastoma filling half the globe. Current therapy would involve:

A. Enucleation
B. Chemotherapy followed by local dyes
C. Direct laser ablation using photodynamic cryotherapy
D. Scleral radiotherapy followed by chemotherapy *(AI 2003)*

517. Hereditary retinoblastomas develop the following chromosomal deletion:

A. 13q14 **B.** 13p14
C. 14p13 **D.** 14q13 *(AI 2003)*

Retinoblastoma occurs ones in 18,000 live births in USA and bilateral involvement is seen in 20–30% of cases. The **retinoblastoma gene (RBI) is located on the long arm of chromosome 13** and acts as a tumor suppressor gene. Familial cases are generally multifocal and bilateral, whereas non-familial cases tend to have unifocal and unilateral involvement. Retinoblastoma may arise in any of the 'nucleated' layers of the retina exhibiting various degrees of differentiation. It tends to 'outgrow' its blood supply resulting in necrosis and subsequent calcification. Retinoblastoma classically presents with a **white papillary reflex** (leukocoria). Strabismus is commonly the initial presenting complaint, whereas orbital inflammation, hypemia or papillary irregularity occurs with advancing disease. Pain is usually a feature if secondary glaucoma is present. The diagnosis is made by ophthalmoscopy under general anesthesia by an ophthalmologist. Orbital ultrasonography and CT-scan are used to evaluate intra-ocular extent and extra-ocular spread and MRI is not intended for routine examination. Bone scan, CSF evaluation and bone-marrow sampling are necessary only if indicated by other clinical, laboratory or imaging studies. Differential diagnosis includes hyperplastic primary vitreous, Coat disease, cataract, visceral larva migrans, choroidal coloboma, and retinopathy of prematurity (ROP). The *primary aim* of treatment is cure with a *secondary goal* of preserving vision. Primary enucleation is no longer routinely undertaken. For **unilateral disease enucleation is undertaken** if there is no potential for useful vision. If possible, small tumors can be treated with laser photocoagulation or cryosurgery with careful follow-up for recurrence or new tumor growth. Larger tumors often respond to multi-drug chemotherapy involving carboplatin, vincristine, and etoposide. if this approach fails external beam irradiation or brachytherapy should be considered, although it may result in significant orbital deformity and a high incidence of 'second' malignancy. After primary enucleation of unilateral intraocular tumors, the cure rate exceeds 90%. In **bilateral disease** the traditional approach involves enucleation of the more severely affected eye and irradiation of the other eye in hope of saving some useful vision.

Malignancy	Chromosomal region affected
• Ewing's sarcoma	11q24 and 22q12
• Alveolar rhabdomyosarcoma	2q35-37 and 13q14
• Small cell carcinoma of lung	3p13-23
• Liposarcoma, myxoid	12q13 and 16p11
• Sarcoma, synovial	Xp11 and 18q11
• Neuroblastoma	1p31 to 3p36
• Retinoblastoma	13q14
• Wilms tumor	11p13

Ref *Nelson Textbook of Pediatrics; 16th edition; page 1561*

518. While working in the neonatal ICU your team delivers a premature infant at 27 weeks of gestation and weighing 1,500 grams. How soon will you request fundus examination by an ophthalmologist?

A. Immediately **B.** 3-4 weeks after delivery
C. At 34 weeks gestational age **D.** At 40 weeks gestation period *(AIIMS Nov 2002)*

Systemic ophthalmologic examination of infants at risk of retinopathy of prematurity (ROP) is recommended. Although the guidelines vary but generally include infants weighing less than 1,500 gm at birth and those born before 28 weeks of gestational age. Infants born weighing over 1,500 gm and having an unstable clinical course and thought to be at risk should also be examined for ROP. **The initial examination should be performed between 4 and 6 weeks of chronological age or at 31–33 weeks of postconceptional age**. ROP is diagnosed most often at 32–44 week postconception.

Ref: *Nelson Textbook of Pediatrics; 16th edition; page 1926*

519. Osler's nodes are *typically* seen in which 1 of the following:

A. Chronic candida endocarditis **B.** Acute staphylococcal endocarditis
C. *Pseudomonas* endocarditis **D.** Libman-Sack's endocarditis *(AI 2003)*

Serious neurological complications such as emboli, cerebral abscesses, mycotic aneurysm, and hemorrhage are *most often* associated with **staphylococcal infective endocarditis**. These complications are manifested by meningismus, increased intracranial pressure, altered sensorium, and focal neurological signs. Myocardial abscesses may occur with staphylococcal disease and may rupture into the pericardium producing purulent pericarditis. The embolic phenomenon are enumerated as under:

- Roth spots;
- Petechiae;
- Splinter nail-bed hemorrhages;
- Osler's nodes; and
- CNS or ocular lesions

Ref: *Nelson Textbook of Pediatrics; 16th edition; page 1425*

520. Rotaviruses are responsible for:

A. Acute non-bacterial gastroenteritis **B.** Infantile diarrhea
C. Teratogenic effects **D.** Respiratory tract infection *(KARNATAKA 2001)*

Diarrhea is the leading cause of childhood mortality in the world accounting for about 10 million deaths per year. **In early childhood, the single most important cause of severe dehydrating diarrhea is rotavirus infection**. Rotavirus, astrovirus, adenovirus, and calciviruses such as Norwalk agent, are medically important pathogens of human viral gastroenteritis. Rotavirus infection typically begins after an incubation period of less than 2 days with fever and vomiting followed by the onset of frequent watery stools. Vomiting and fever *typically* abate during the second day of illness but diarrhea continues for 5 to 7 days. Isotonic dehydration with acidosis is the most common finding in children with severe viral enteritis and stools are free of blood and leukocytes. Differential diagnosis includes other infectious causes of enteritis such as bacteria and protozoa; occasionally appendicitis, bowel obstruction and intussusception may initial mimic viral gastroenteritis. Avoiding and treating dehydration are the main goals in treatment of viral enteritis. There is no role of antiviral drugs and controlled studies have shown no benefit from anti-emetics or anti-diarrheal drugs, and there is a significant risk of serious side effects. Antibiotics are similarly of no benefit. Rehydration can be accomplished via the oral route (ORS) in most patients.

Ref: *Nelson Textbook of Pediatrics; 16th edition; page 996*

521. An 8-month-old child presented with itchy, exudative lesions on the face, palms and soles, the siblings also have similar complaints. The treatment of choice in such a patient is:

A. Systemic ampicillin **B.** Topical betamethasone
C. Systemic prednisolone **D.** Topical permethrin *(AI 2003)*

Application of **permethrin** 5% cream or 1% lindane cream or lotion to the entire body from neck down, with particular attention to intensely involved areas, is standard therapy of scabies in children. Scabies is frequently found above the neck in infants also necessitating treatment of the scalp. The medication is left on the skin for 12 hours and if required it may be reapplied after 1 week.

Ref: *Nelson Textbook of Pediatrics; 16th edition; page 2042*

522. The syndrome of inappropriate antidiuretic hormone is characterized by the following:

A. Hyponatremia and urine sodium excretion >20 mEq/liter
B. Hypernatremia and urine sodium excretion < 20 mEq/liter
C. Hyponatremia and hyperkalemia
D. Hypernatremia and hypokalemia *(AI 2003)*

Diseases of CNS are frequently associated with disturbances in sodium concentration. Patients with diverse diseases such as brain injury, encephalitis, brain abscess, brain tumor, Guillain-Barré syndrome, bulbar poliomyelitis, cerebrovascular accident, tumors of 4th ventricle, subdural hematoma, and meningitis may present with hyponatremia. Hyponatremia in this setting is associated with normal body sodium and is almost entirely the result of retention of water. The diagnosis of **syndrome of inappropriate antidiuretic hormone** (SIADH) should be considered in the absence of hypovolemia, edema, endocrine dysfunction, renal failure and drugs impairing water excretion. The condition represents a defect in osmoregulation of vasopressin and the diagnosis is established by measuring 'inappropriate' secretion of ADH under hypotonic conditions. Patients with this syndrome generally have concentrated urine despite the presence of hyponatremia and a urinary sodium concentration greater than 20 mEq/liter. Along with CNS caused mentioned above neonatal hypoxia, hydrocephalus, pneumonia, tuberculosis, asthma, positive pressure ventilation and certain carcinomas can also result in this condition.

Ref: *Nelson Textbook of Pediatrics; 16th edition; page 220*

523. All of the following are associated with low C_3 levels *except*:

A. Post-streptococcal glomerulonephritis
B. Membranoproliferative glomerulonephritis
C. Goodpasture's disease
D. Systemic lupus erythematous *(AI 2003)*

Goodpasture's disease consists of pulmonary hemorrhage and glomerulonephritis associated with antibodies against lung and against glomerular basement membrane (GBM). It is rare in childhood; hemoptysis is usually the presenting complaint and pulmonary hemorrhage is a potential cause of death. In days to weeks, proteinuria, hematuria, and progressive renal failure develops. **Complement C_3 level is normal.** Diagnosis is suggested by kidney biopsy. Prognosis is poor and patients who survive pulmonary hemorrhage progress to end stage renal failure (ESRF). Rates of survival and recovery of renal function have improved with pulse methylprednisolone, oral cyclophosphamide, and plasmapheresis therapy.

Ref: *Nelson Textbook of Pediatrics; 16th edition; page 1586*

524. In 'asymmetrical' IUGR which organ is *not* affected:

A. Subcutaneous fat **B.** Muscle
C. Liver **D.** Brain *(BHU 1996)*

IUGR is often classified as reduced growth that is symmetric (head circumference, length, and weight are equally affected) or **asymmetric** (with relative **head growth sparing**).

Ref: *Nelson Textbook of Pediatrics; 16th edition; page 478*

525. IUGR is characterized by all *except*:

A. Polycythemia
B. Meconium aspiration syndrome
C. HMD
D. Hypocalcemia *(PGI May 2001)*

526. Full-term, small-for-date infants (IUGR) are predisposed to which of the following condition:

A. PDA
B. Hypercalcemia
C. CNS infections
D. Hypoglycemia *(AIIMS 1995)*

Complications related to small-for-date (IUGR) infants

• Congenital anomalies	• Perinatal depression
• **Meconium aspiration**	• Pulmonary hemorrhage
• Persistent pulmonary hypertension	• Hypothermia
• Hypoglycemia	• **Hypocalcemia**
• Hyponatremia	• **Polycythemia**

Ref: *Manual of neonatal care; John P. Cloherty and Ann R. Stark; 4th edition; page 48*

527. All are *true* of 'cartilage hair hypoplasia syndrome' *except*:

A. Short-limbed dwarf
B. Sparse hair
C. Neutropenia
D. T-cell dysfunction

(AIIMS 1997)

Cartilage hair hypoplasia (CHH) is an unusual form of **short-limbed dwarfism** with frequent and severe infections. It occurs commonly among Pennsylvania Amish although non-Amish patients have been described. Features include short,[1] pudgy hands;[2] redundant skin, hyper-extensible joints of hands and feet but an inability to extend the elbows completely; and **fine, sparse, light hair** and eyebrows. Three patterns of immune dysfunction have been observed viz. defective antibody-mediated immunity, CID (*most common*) and SCID. *In vitro* studies have shown decreased number of T-cells and defective T-cell proliferation. *However,* NK-cells are increased in number and function.

- *Pudgy means chubby, chunky, stout, plump* [1]
- *Redundant means needless superfluous, irrelevant, excessive* [2]

Ref: *Nelson Textbook of Pediatrics; 16th edition; page 602*

528. A 2-year-old boy has vitamin D 'refractory' rickets. Investigations show serum calcium to 9-mg/dl, phosphate 2.4-mg/dl, alkaline phosphatase 1040 IU. Parathyroid hormone level and bicarbonate levels are normal. The most probable diagnosis is:

A. Distal renal tubular acidosis
B. Hypophosphatemic rickets
C. Vitamin D dependent rickets
D. Proximal renal tubular acidosis

(AIIMS Nov 2002)

The *most commonly* encountered non-nutritional form of rickets is **familial hypophosphatemia** (vitamin D resistant rickets or X-linked hypophosphatemia). The usual mode of inheritance is X-linked dominant; although autosomal recessive and sporadic forms has been reported. Pathogenic mechanism involves defects in the proximal tubular reabsorption of phosphate and in conversion of 25(OH) D to 1,25$(OH)_2$ D. Serum calcium levels are usually normal, with low intestinal absorption and renal excretion of calcium. Children with familial hypophosphatemia present with bowing of the lower extremities related to weight bearing at the age of walking. Tetany is not present, and profound myopathy, rachitic rosary, and Harrison groove (pectus deformity) characteristic of calcium deficient rickets are not evident. These children develop a waddling gait, smooth (rather than angular) bowing of lower extremities, coxa vera, genu varum, genu valgum and short stature. Pulp deformities and 'intraglobular dentin' are characteristic tooth abnormalities. *By contrast* calcium deficient rickets usually results in enamel defects. **The patients have normal or slightly raised calcium levels (9–9.4 mg%); a moderately reduced phosphate level (1.5 -3 mg%); elevated alkaline phosphatase activity and no evidence of secondary hyperparathyroidism.** Urinary phosphate excretion is large (despite hypophosphatemia) indicating a defect in renal tubular phosphate reabsorption. Oral phosphate supplements coupled with a vitamin D analogue to 'offset' the secondary hyperparathyroidism that may accompany an oral phosphate load is the preferred treatment.

Ref: *Nelson Textbook of Pediatrics; 16th edition; page 2136*

529. Failure to pass meconium within 48 hrs of birth in a newborn with no obvious external abnormality should lead to suspicion of:

A. Anal atresia
B. Congenital pouch colon
C. Congenital aganglionosis
D. Meconium ileus

(AIIMS Nov 2002)

Clinical symptoms of **Hirschsprung disease** usually begin at birth with the delayed passage of meconium. Ninety-nine percent of full-term infants pass the meconium within 48 hours of birth and Hirschsprung disease (congenital aganglionic megacolon) should be suspected in any full-term infant with delayed passage of stool (the disease is unusual in preterm infants).

Ref: *Nelson Textbook of Pediatrics; 16th edition; page 1139*

530. SSPE (subacute sclerosing panencephalitis) is associated with:

A. Mumps
B. Chickenpox
C. Herpes
D. Measles

(PGI May 2001)

Subacute sclerosing panencephalitis (SSPE) or Dawson's encephalitis caused by persistent **measles virus infection** of the central nervous system. The mean interval between measles and onset of SSPE was formerly of about 7 years but recently it has increased to 12 years.

Ref: *Nelson Textbook of Pediatrics; 16th edition; page 949*

531. Pure gonadal dysgenesis will be diagnosed in the presence of:

A. Bilateral streak gonads
B. Bilateral dysgenetic gonads
C. One side streak and other dysgenetic gonads
D. One side streak and other normal looking gonad

(AI 2003)

Some phenotypically and genetically normal females have gonadal lesions identical to 45, X patients but without somatic features of Turner syndrome; this condition is termed as **pure gonadal dysgenesis** or **pure ovarian dysgenesis.** This disorder is rarely recognized in children because the external genitals are normal, no other abnormalities are visible, and growth is normal. At pubertal age, sexual maturation fails to take place. Plasma gonadotropin levels are elevated. Delay of epiphyseal fusion results in a eunuchoid habitus. **Pelvic USG reveals streak ovaries**. Tumors of gonads have not been reported in these patients. Treatment consists of estrogen replacement therapy.

Ref: *Nelson Textbook of Pediatrics; 16th edition; page 1755*

532. A 10-year-old 'girl' presents with swelling of one knee joint. All of the following conditions can be considered in the differential diagnosis, *except*:

A. Tuberculosis
B. Juvenile rheumatoid arthritis
C. Hemophilia
D. Villonodular synovitis

(AI 2003)

- Knee is a common site of **tuberculosis**. The patient, usually in the age group of 10–25 years, presents with pain and swelling in the knee, which is gradual in onset without any preceding history of trauma. Thereafter the pain increases and the knee takes an attitude of flexion. The child starts limping and there is severe stiffness of the knee.
- **Juvenile rheumatoid arthritis** is one of the *most common* rheumatic diseases of children and is a major cause of chronic disability. There is idiopathic synovitis of the peripheral joints associated with soft tissue swelling and effusion.
- **Hemophilia** occurs in about 1 in 5000 'males' with 85% having factor 8 deficiency and 10–15% having factor 9 deficiency.
- **Pigmented villonodular synovitis** is characterized by exuberant proliferation of synovial cells, usually involving a single joint. It occurs most often in young adults and affects both sexes equally. The cause of this disorder is unknown.

533. A patient has diarrhea. Stool examination reveals no RBC or pus cells. Identify the organism:

A. *Balantidium coli*
B. *Entamoeba histolytica*
C. *Giardia*
D. *E. intestinalis*

(AI 2000)

534. An anxious mother brought her 4-year-old daughter to the pediatrician. The girl was passing loose bulky stools for the past 20 days. This was often associated with pain in abdomen. The pediatrician ordered the stool examination, which showed the following organisms. Identify the organism:

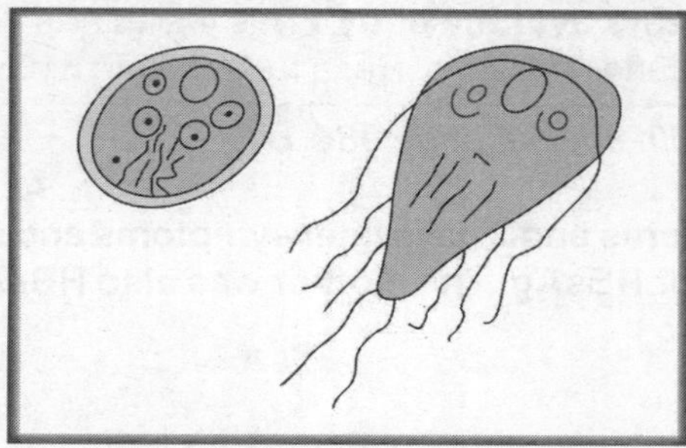

A. *Entamoeba histolytica* **B.** *Giardia lamblia*
C. *Cryptosporidium* **D.** *Escherichia coli* *(AI 2003)*

Giardia lamblia is a flagellated protozoan, which infects the duodenum and small intestine. The clinical manifestations range from asymptomatic colonization to acute or chronic diarrhea and malabsorption. Infection is more prevalent in children than in adults. *Giardia* is a particularly significant pathogen in people with malnutrition, immunodeficiencies and cystic fibrosis. The incubation period is usually 1–2 weeks but may be longer. Most symptomatic children have a limited period of acute diarrheal disease with or without low-grade fever, nausea and anorexia. Initially the stools may be profuse and watery and later become greasy and foul smelling. **Blood, mucus and leukocytes are not present in stool**. A definitive diagnosis of giardiasis is established by documentation of trophozoites, cysts, or *Giardia* antigen in stool specimen or duodenal fluid. Children with acute diarrhea in whom *Giardia* organisms are identified should receive therapy. In addition children who manifest with failure to thrive or exhibit malabsorption or GI tract symptoms such as chronic diarrhea should be treated.

Metronidazole	15 mg per kg per 24 hours in 3 divided doses for 5 days
Furazolidone	6 mg per kg per 24 hours in 4 divided doses for 10 days

Ref: *Nelson Textbook of Pediatrics; 16th edition; page 1036*

535. Social smile appears by:

A. 2 months **B.** 3 months
C. 5 months **D.** 9 months *(SGPGI 2003)*

The infant smiles on social contact at 8 weeks of age.

Ref: *Nelson Textbook of Pediatrics; 16th edition; page 35*

536. *Most common* solid tumor in children and infants is:

A. Neurofibroma **B.** Neuroblastoma
C. Sacrococcygeal teratoma **D.** Wilms' tumor

Neuroblastoma accounts for 8% of childhood cancers and is the *most common* solid tumor of childhood outside the central nervous system. Neuroblastoma is the most frequently diagnosed neoplasm in infants.

Ref: *Nelson Textbook of Pediatrics; 16th edition; page 1552*

537. Roseola infantum is caused by:

A. Herpes virus type 6 **B.** Parvovirus
C. Coxsackie virus **D.** *Escherichia coli* *(JIPMER 2002)*

538. Fever stops and rash begins is diagnostic of:

A. Fifth disease **B.** Roseola infantum
C. Measles **D.** Toxic shock syndrome *(JIPMER 1995)*

Roseola infantum is also known as exanthem subitum. In 90% of cases **human herpes virus 6** causes it. Onset of illness is sudden with high-grade fever, bulging anterior fontanelle. Seizures are seen in 5-35% of cases. Child looks relatively well despite high-grade fever. **Fever falls by 3-4th day and 'as the temperature returns to normal a macular or maculopapular rash appears over the body'.** This rash starts from the truck and then spread to arms and neck and sometimes involves face and neck also. Rash fades within 3 days. There is no residual pigmentation.

Ref: *Nelson Textbook of Pediatrics; 16th edition; page 984*

539. A 45-day-old infant developed icterus and 2 days later symptoms and signs of acute liver failure appeared. Child was found to be positive for HBsAg. The mother was also HBsAg carrier. The mother's hepatitis B serological profile is likely to be:

A. HBsAg positive only
B. HBsAg and HBeAg positive
C. HBsAg and anti-Hbe antibody positive
D. Mother infected with mutant HBV *(AI 2003)*

540. In a patient immunized with hepatitis B vaccine, which of the following is seen in serum:

A. HBsAg **B.** HBeAg
C. Anti-HBsAg **D.** Anti-HBcAg *(AIIMS May 2002)*

541. A person vaccinated with hepatitis B will present with the following markers in the blood:

A. IgG-Anti-HBV **B.** Anti-HBsAg
C. Anti-HBeAg **D.** IgM Anti-HBV *(SGPGI 2003)*

HBsAg is the first serological marker of hepatitis B infection to appear and is found in almost all infected persons. Rise of HBsAg closely coincides with the onset of symptoms. **HBeAg is often present during the acute phase and indicates a highly infectious state**. Anti-HBcAg is the most valuable single serological marker of acute hepatitis B infection because it is present almost as early as HBsAg and continues to be present later in the course of disease when HBsAg has disappeared. **Only anti-HBsAg is present in persons immunized with hepatitis-B vaccine** whereas anti-HBsAg and anti-HBcAg are detected in persons with resolved infection.

Ref: *Nelson Textbook of Pediatrics; 16th edition; page 772*

542. Poststreptococcal glomerulonephritis is associated with all of the following *except*:

A. Associated with decreased complement
B. ASLO titers are specific disease markers
C. Endo-capillary proliferation
D. Has good prognosis *(SGPGI 2003)*

Acute poststreptococcal glomerulonephritis is the classical example of acute nephritic syndrome, which consists of sudden onset of gross hematuria, edema, hypertension, and renal insufficiency. It was the *most common* cause of gross hematuria in children but IgA nephropathy is now the *most common* cause of hematuria. **The serum C3 level is usually reduced;** to document streptococcal infection properly, an elevated antibody titer to streptococcal antigen(s) should be confirmed. **Although most commonly obtained, determination of the ASO titer may not be helpful because it rarely rises after streptococcal skin infection.** The best *single* antibody titer to measure is that to the deoxyribonuclease B-antigen. Complete recovery occurs in more than 95% of children with acute poststreptococcal glomerulonephritis.

Ref: *Nelson Textbook of Pediatrics; 16th edition; page 1581–1582*

543. *True* about diphtheria is:

A. Causes cranial nerve palsies in the 2nd and 3rd week
B. Treatment is with erythromycin
C. It is Gram-negative organism
D. Passive immunization is harmful and should not be tried *(SGPGI 2003)*

Corynebacterium diphtheriae is an aerobic, nonmotile, nonsporulating, irregularly staining, **Gram-positive rod**. The primary goal of antibiotic therapy for patients or carriers is therefore to eradicate *Corynebacterium diphtheriae* and prevent its transmission from the patient to susceptible contacts. Acutely or **2–3 weeks after onset of oropharyngeal inflammation, hyperesthesia and local paralysis of the soft palate occur commonly**. Weakness of the posterior pharyngeal, laryngeal, and facial nerves may follow causing a nasal quality in the voice, difficulty in swallowing and risk of death due to aspiration. Most authorities recommend erythromycin, penicillin G, rifampin, or clindamycin. *In children* penicillin is the drug of choice and should be given for 7–10 days. **Diphtheria immunoglobulin** (DIG) should be given in a dose of 0.6-ml/kg-body weight.

Further reading: *Nelson Textbook of Pediatrics; 16th edition; page 817*

544. A 3-year-old boy is detected to have bilateral renal calculi. Metabolic evaluation confirms the presence of marked hypercalciuria with normal blood levels of calcium, magnesium, phosphate, uric acid and creatinine. A diagnosis of idiopathic hypercalciuria is made. The dietary management includes all, *except*:

A. Increased water intake **B.** Low sodium diet
C. Reduced calcium intake **D.** Avoid meat proteins *(AIIMS May 2003)*

Idiopathic hypercalciuria is possibly an autosomal dominant disorder. It may present as recurrent gross hematuria, persistent microscopic hematuria, or dysuria in the absence of stone formation. Hypercalciuria (without hypercalcemia) results from excessive GI absorption of normal dietary calcium or a defect in renal tubular calcium reabsorption. Diagnosis is confirmed by finding a 24-hour urinary calcium excretion more than 4 mg/kg. Hypercalciuria may lead to nephrolithiasis. Oral thiazide diuretics can normalize urinary calcium excretion by stimulating calcium reabsorption in the distal tubule (DT). In patients with persistent gross hematuria or dysuria, treatment is started with chlorothiazide at a dosage of 10–20 mg/kg/day as a single morning dose. The dosage is titrated upward until the urinary calcium excretion approaches 4 mg/kg/24 hour and the clinical manifestations resolve. Chlorothiazide treatment is discontinued after 1 year. **Dietary calcium restriction is not recommended because of the obligate requirement of growth.**

Ref: *Nelson Textbook of Pediatrics; 16th edition; page 1580*

545. A 3-year-old boy presents with poor urinary stream. *Most likely* cause is:

A. Stricture urethra **B.** Neurogenic bladder
C. Urethral calculus **D.** Posterior urethral valves *(AIIMS May 2003)*

The *most common* cause of severe obstructive uropathy in children is **posterior urethral valves**. This is seen only in boys; incidence is 1 in 8000 boys. These urethral 'valves' are tissue leaflets fanning distally from the posterior urethra to the external urinary sphincter. Typically the leaflets are separated by a slit like opening. About 30% of patients develop end stage renal disease (ESRD) or chronic renal insufficiency; posterior urethra dilates and the bladder muscle undergoes hypertrophy. Vesicoureteral reflux (VUR) occurs in 50% of patients. Prenatal maternal USG reveals bilateral hydronephrosis; a distended bladder; and if obstruction is severe, oligohydramnios. In the male neonates, posterior urethral valves should be suspected when there is a palpable distended bladder and the urinary stream is weak. If the obstruction is severe and goes unnoticed during the neonatal period the infants present later in life with failure to thrive (FTT) due to uremia or sepsis caused by infection in the obstructed urinary tract. Lesser degree of obstruction presents with difficulty in achieving diurnal urinary continence or UTI. The diagnosis is established by voiding cystourethrography or perineal USG. After the diagnosis is established the anatomy of upper renal tract and renal function should be carefully evaluated. In healthy newborn a small feeding tube (5 or 8 FG) is inserted in the bladder and left *in situ* for several days. If serum creatinine remains normal or returns to normal, transurethral ablation of the valve leaflets is the treatment of choice. This is done under general anesthesia. However, if the serum creatinine level remains high or increases despite bladder drainage by a small catheter, secondary urethral obstruction, irreversible renal damage, or renal dysplasia should be suspected. A vesicostomy should be done in such cases.

- At 16 weeks of gestation and thereafter, fetal urine is the major source of amniotic fluid, and fluid is "consumed" by means of fetal swallowing and gastrointestinal absorption. Fetal anomalies affecting these organ systems will cause abnormalities of amniotic fluid volume. Fetal causes of *polyhydramnios* include anencephaly, presumably due to impaired swallowing on a neurologic basis, and gastrointestinal tract obstruction (e.g. esophageal or duodenal atresia). Maternal diabetes is also associated with a high incidence of polyhydramnios. Genitourinary tract anomalies that diminish fetal urine output, such as bilateral renal agenesis or posterior urethral valves, lead to *oligohydramnios*. Other causes of oligohydramnios include IUGR and ruptured membranes.

Ref: *Nelson Textbook of Pediatrics; 16th edition; page 1636–1637*

546. Posterior urethral valves are *most commonly* situated:

A. At verumontanum
B. Above verumontanum
C. Just distal to verumontanum
D. Near bladder neck

(UP 2003)

547. One year old male child is presented with poor urinary stream since birth. The investigation of choice for evaluation is:

A. Voiding cystourethrography (VCUG)
B. USG bladder
C. Intravenous urography
D. Uroflowmetry

(AIIMS May 2003)

Congenital valves of the posterior urethra are the symmetrical folds of urothelium, which can cause obstruction of the urethra of boys. **They are usually found just distal to the verumontanum** but they may be within the prostatic urethra. As they behave as flap valves, a urethral catheter can be passed without difficulty although urine does not flow normally. These valves are difficult to see on urethroscopy, but if the bladder is filled with contrast medium, the dilatation of urethra above the valves can be demonstrated on a **voiding cystogram**. A suprapubic catheter should be inserted to relieve the bag pressure and allow the effects of renal failure to subside before definitive treatment by **transurethral resection** of the valves using a pediatric resectoscope can be done.

Ref: *Bailey and Love's Short Practice of Surgery; 23rd edition; page 1257*

548. All of the following are characteristic features of Kwashiorkor, *except:*

A. High blood osmolarity
B. Hypoalbuminemia
C. Edema
D. Fatty liver

(AIIMS May 2003)

Kwashiorkor is a clinical syndrome that results from a severe deficiency of protein and an inadequate calorie intake. Kwashiorkor is characterized by pitting edema. The child is listless, lethargic, **apathetic** and miserable. Hairs are thin, dry, brittle and lusterless. They become straight and hypopigmented grayish white or reddish brown in color. During recovery growing part of hair are pigmented giving appearance of a flag (the **flag sign**). The skin lesions appear as large areas of erythema followed by hyperpigmentation. Skin becomes dry and hyperkeratotic. Alternate areas of hypo- and hyperpigmentation give a resemblance to pavement (pavement dermatosis). Mosaic pattern may also be seen (**mosaic dermatosis**). Liver is enlarged and fatty.

Features	Marasmus	Kwashiorkor
• **Muscle wasting**	Present	Hidden by edema and fat
• **Fat wasting**	Severe	Fat is retained
• **Edema**	None	Present
• **Weight for height**	Very low	Low
• **Mental changes**	Quite and apathetic	Irritable
• **Appetite**	Good	Poor
• **Skin changes**	None	Diffused pigmentation
• **Hair changes**	Rare	Sparse, easily pluckable
• **Diarrhea**	Common	Common
• **Fatty liver and hepatomegaly**	Never	Sometimes

Diagnostic criteria of kwashiorkor

Essential criteria

- **Growth retardation**
- Muscle wasting with retention of subcutaneous fat
- Psychomotor changes such as **mental apathy** and lack of interest in surroundings
- Hypoalbuminemic pitting **edema** with serum albumin < 2.5 gm/dL

Nonessential criteria

- Hair changes, skin changes, mineral and vitamin deficiency
- Hepatomegaly, clubbing and non-specific ECG changes
- Diarrhea, vomiting, anorexia
- Superadded infections such as tuberculosis, bronchopneumonia, pyoderma, etc.

The causes of mortality include dehydration and electrolyte imbalance, hypoglycemia, hypothermia, fulminant systemic infections and congestive cardiac failure.

Dietary management of severe PEM can be divided into 3 phases:

- In **initial phase** 80 calorie per kg per day and 0.7 gm of protein per kg per day with the calculation being based on the actual weight should be started. The intake can be gradually 'stepped up' so that by the end of 7 days the child is able to take about 100 calories per kg per day and 1 gm of protein per kg per day.
- After the child passes through the initial phase and shows sign of improvement one can gradually increase the calorie intake to about 150–180 calories per kg per day and 1.5–2 gm of protein per kg per day.
- Once the child is able to tolerate a high dose of therapeutic nutrition and has started gaining weight, solid or semisolid family foods containing cereals, pulses, vegetables rich in calories can be given. Bengal gram, groundnuts and dark green leafy vegetables should be added to regular family foods. Oils, sugar and fruits should also be given and minerals and vitamins should be continued for 5–6 weeks.

549. Which one of the following *does not* produce cyanosis in the first year of life?

A. Atrial septal defect **B.** Hypoplastic left heart syndrome
C. Truncus arteriosus **D.** Double outlet right ventricle *(AIIMS May 2003)*

A child with an ostium secundum ASD is most often asymptomatic and the lesion is discovered during a routine physical examination. Atrial septal defect is an acyanotic congenital heart disease with left to right shunt.

Ref: *Nelson Textbook of Pediatrics; 16th edition; page 1366*

550. A 9-year-old boy has steroid dependent nephrotic syndrome for the last 5 years. He had received corticosteroids almost continuously during this period and has cushingoid features. The blood pressure is 120/86 mmHg and there are bilateral sub-capsular cataracts. The *treatment of choice* is:

A. Levamisole **B.** Cyclophosphamide
C. Cyclosporine A **D.** Intravenous pulse corticosteroids *(AIIMS May 2003)*

If the age of child is between 1-8 years it is most likely that the child is having **minimal change disease** and oral steroid therapy should be started as prednisolone 2 mg/kg/day (maximum 60 mg/kg/day) in 3 divided doses without further investigation. Renal biopsy is indicated if the age of child is <1 years or >8 years. A combination of furosemide (1-2 mg/kg/day) and spironolactone is useful in reducing edema. Average time required for response of prednisolone is about 2 weeks and response is defined as the point at which the urine becomes free of protein. If the child continues to have proteinuria of 2+ or more after one-month prednisolone therapy then the nephrotic syndrome is termed as steroid resistant and is an indication of renal biopsy. Five days after the urine becomes free of protein (negative, trace or 1 +) the total dose of prednisolone is given as a single dose with breakfast on alternate day for 3-6 months. After such a period prednisolone is discontinued abruptly.

A relapse is defined as recurrence of edema and not merely proteinuria, which may occur intermittently and resolves spontaneously. **Repeated relapse and severe corticosteroid toxicity are indication of cyclophosphamide** therapy (3 mg/kg/day OD) along with alternate day prednisolone for 3 months. TLC must be monitored during cyclophosphamide therapy and it should be withheld if TLC falls below 5000.

Further reading: *Nelson Textbook of Pediatrics; 16th edition; page 1592–1595*

551. Visceromegaly, microcephaly with blood sugar below 20 mg/dl with sinusitis is:

A. Prader Willi syndrome **B.** Beckwith-Wiedemann syndrome
C. Alport's syndrome **D.** Cockayne syndrome *(ORRISA 1998)*

A group of disorders associated with excessive somatic growth and growth of specific organs are collectively known as **overgrowth syndromes**. These disorders are caused by excessive availability of insulin-like-growth-factor-II (IGF-II), encoded by the gene *Igf2*.[1] **Beckwith-Wiedemann syndrome** (BWS) is the best described of these syndromes. It is an overgrowth-malformation syndrome that occurs with an incidence of about 1 in 14,000 live births. It is characterized by exophthalmos, gigantism, macroglossia, microcephaly and visceromegaly. Distinctive lateral earlobe fissures are present, and hemi-hypertrophy occurs in many of these infants. Patients with Beckwith-Wiedemann syndrome may acquire tumors, including Wilms' tumor, hepatoblastoma, adrenal carcinoma and rhabdomyosarcoma.[2]

Ref: [1] *Nelson Textbook of Pediatrics; 16th edition; page 1687*
[2] *Nelson Textbook of Pediatrics; 16th edition; page 445*

552. All of the following methods are used for the diagnosis of HIV infection in a 2-month-old child, *except*:

A. DNA-PCR
B. Viral culture
C. HIV ELISA
D. p24-antigen assay

(AIIMS May 2003)

In any children older than 18 months, demonstration of IgG antibody to HIV by a repeatedly reactive enzyme immunoassay (ELISA) and confirmatory test (western immunoblot or immunofluorescence assay) establishes the diagnosis of HIV infection. **All infants born to HIV-infected mothers have positive ELISA test at birth due to 'passive' transfer of maternal IgG antibody across the placenta; that is why, positive IgG antibody tests cannot be used for a definitive diagnosis of HIV infection in infants younger than 18 months.** Several viral detection assays are available, including HIV-DNA or RNA by PCR, HIV-culture, HIV p24-antigen, and immune-complex-dissociated p24-antigen (ICD-p24). These are very useful in young infants allowing a definitive diagnosis in most infected infants by 1 to 6 months of age. HIV-DNA-PCR is the preferred virologic assay. For infants born to HIV infected mothers, viral diagnostic testing should be performed within first 2 days of life, 1 to 2 month of age, and at 4 to 6 months of age.

Reference and further reading: *Nelson Textbook of Pediatrics; 16th edition; page 1028*

553. In a child immunized with BCG, all of the following can later develop *except*:

A. Miliary tuberculosis
B. Increases generalized immune response
C. *Cannot* protect against tuberculosis
D. Mantoux positive

(BHU June 2002)

The type of tuberculosis seen in BCG vaccinated children is commonly intrathoracic tuberculosis (particularly mediastinal lymph node tuberculosis and its local complications). This is due to the fact that intradermal BCG vaccination cannot prevent lodgment of natural virulent tubercle bacilli in the lungs and development of primary infection and its progressive local complication. However, BCG vaccination reduces the hematogenous dissemination of infection in vaccinated children. Hence **miliary tuberculosis, tuberculous meningitis and protracted hematogenous tuberculosis are much more common in non-vaccinated than in vaccinated children.**

Ref: *IAP Textbook of Pediatrics; 2nd edition; page 205*

554. A married middle-aged female gives history of repeated abortions for the past 5 years. The given below is conceptions pre-natal karyogram.

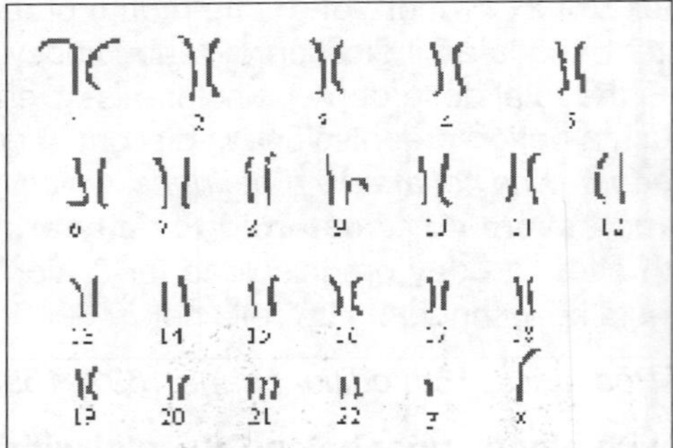

This karyogram suggests the following:

A. Klinefelter's syndrome
B. Turner's syndrome
C. Down's syndrome
D. Patau's syndrome

(AI 2003)

Down syndrome is one of the best-recognized and the *most common* serious chromosomal disorder which is usually caused by an **extra copy of chromosome 21**.
Women at high risk of giving birth to a child with **Down syndrome** are:

- **Those over 40**
- Those who have had a previous child with the syndrome
- Those who themselves have Down syndrome.

The overall incidence of Down syndrome is 1 in 600. The incidence rises with advancing age of the mother, reaching a peak in about 1 in 25 by the age of 45.

Maternal age (years)	Estimated rate	Maternal age (years)	Estimated rate
• 20	1 in 1925	• 35	1 in 365
• 21	1 in 1695	• 36	1 in 285
• 22	1 in 1540	• 37	1 in 225
• 23	1 in 1410	• 38	1 in 175
• 24	1 in 1300	• 39	1 in 140
• 25	1 in 1205	• 40	1 in 110
• 26	1 in 1125	• 41	1 in 85
• 27	1 in 1050	• 42	1 in 67
• 28	1 in 990	• 43	1 in 53
• 29	1 in 935	• 44	1 in 41
• 30	1 in 885	• 45	1 in 32
• 31	1 in 825	• 46	1 in 25
• 32	1 in 725	• 47	1 in 20
• 33	1 in 590	• 48	1 in 16
• 34	1 in 465	• 49	1 in 12

Further reading: *IAP Textbook of Pediatrics; 2nd edition; page 628*

555. A 3-year-old boy is brought to casualty by his mother with progressive shortness of breath for 1 day. The child has a history of bronchial asthma. On examination, the child is gasping and unresponsive. What will you do first?

A. Intubate
B. Administer 100% oxygen by mask
C. Ventilate with bag and mask
D. Administer nebulised salbutamol *(AIIMS Nov 2002)*

Asthma and bronchiolitis are the 2 common causes of the lower respiratory tract obstruction in children. *Almost without exception*, bronchiolitis is confined to the infants and asthma is much more commonly diagnosed in those above 1-year of age. **Emergency treatment of asthma is as under:**

- **Give high flow oxygen via a face mask with reservoir bag;**
- Attach pulse oximeter;
- Give salbutamol (2.5 mg for children under 5 years and 5 mg for children over 5 years) and ipratropium bromide (250 microgram for children under 5 years and 500 microgram for children over 5 years) nebulised with oxygen to any child with respiratory distress known to have asthma, or if this is their first wheeze episode, over the age of 9-months;
- If the patient is clearly in respiratory failure, depressed conscious level and poor saturation (SpO_2) despite maximum oxygen therapy, attempt to support ventilation with bag-valve-mask.

Ref: *Advanced Pediatric Life Support; 3rd edition; page 87–88*

556. *Not* beneficial in management of 'acute' attacks of bronchial asthma:

A. Nebuliser
B. IV hydrocortisone
C. Sodium cromoglycate
D. Salbutamol *(SGPGI 1996)*

Cromolyn inhalation is indicated as 1st-line anti-inflammatory medication, either alone or as an adjunct to bronchodilator therapy, for the 'prevention' of airway inflammation and bronchoconstriction in patients with mild to moderate asthma who require daily therapy. **Cromolyn inhalation is not indicated for the reversal or relief of acute asthma attacks**, especially in status asthmaticus; cromolyn has no immediate bronchodilating activity.

Ref: *1998 United States Pharmacopeial Convention*

557. A two-year-old child presented with respiratory distress, cough and wheezing. On examination breadth sound diminished on left side. Chest X-ray revealed homogenous opacity in left side. *Most likely* cause of this condition is:

A. Aspiration
B. Pleural effusion
C. Foreign body
D. Pneumothorax *(AIIMS 2000)*

558. A child has hoarseness of voice, croupy cough and asthmatic wheeze. *Most* likely he is suffering from:

A. Foreign body larynx
B. Retropharyngeal abscess
C. Bronchopneumonia
D. Asthmatic bronchitis

(JIPMER 1990)

Aspiration of foreign bodies is common in 'toddler' age group and the *most common* aspirated material is the omnipresent peanut (groundnut); but a plethora of small objects that the youngsters put into their mouth exist that can be aspirated. A solid 'foreign body' causes air trapping with hyperlucency of the affected lobe or lung. Oil from the peanut is very irritating and may cause pneumonia. The delay in diagnosis can lead to atelectasis and infection. The *most common* anatomical location for a foreign body is the *right main stem bronchus* or *the right lower lobe*. Symptoms start immediately with the child coughing or chocking during eating and may range from total respiratory obstruction (with tracheal foreign bodies) to mild respiratory distress or no symptoms at all except for a *unilateral* wheeze. This wheeze often leads to the wrong diagnosis of 'asthma' leading to delayed and inappropriate treatment. CXR will show a radio opaque foreign body but in case of nuts and sunflower seeds the only clue may be the non-deflation of the affected lobe in an expiratory film. **Bronchoscopy will confirm the diagnosis and allow the removal.**

559. Opsoclonus-myoclonus is seen in which of the following:

A. Astrocytoma
B. Wilms tumor
C. Meningioma
D. Neuroblastoma

(PGI 1998)

A syndrome of **opsoclonus**, **myoclonus**, and ataxia ("dancing eyes-dancing feet syndrome") occurs in both children and adults. **About 50% of affected children have differentiated neuroblastomas**, usually in the thorax.

Ref: *Harrison's Principles of Internal Medicine; 14th edition*

560. Useful for diagnosis of Down syndrome all *except*:

A. hCG (increased)
B. AFP (decreased)
C. Unconjugated estriol (decreased)
D. Progesterone

(MANIPAL 2001)

561. Which of the following is included in triple test for Down syndrome?

A. Ultrasound
B. Karyotyping
C. Human placental lactogen
D. Estriol estimation

(UP 1999)

562. Which of the following is *not* included in triple-test for Down syndrome?

A. Estriol estimation
B. Alpha fetoprotein
C. Serum HPL level
D. Beta HCG

(AI 1999)

Low levels of maternal serum alpha-fetoprotein (MSAFP) may be associated with chromosomal abnormalities. Altered levels of human chorionic gonadotropin (hCG) and unconjugated estriol (UE3) may also be associated with fetal chromosomal abnormalities. **A fetus with Down syndrome results in hCG levels that are higher than expected and UE3 levels that are decreased.** A **triple-panel-screen** in combination with maternal age can be used to estimate the risk of fetal trisomy 21.

Ref: *Manual of Neonatal Care by John P. Cloherty; 4th edition; page 1–2*

563. All the following are features of diarrhea + hemolytic uremic syndrome *except*:

A. Negative Coombs' test
B. Low platelet count
C. Low complement level
D. Fall in hematocrit

(JIPMER 2002)

Hemolytic uremic syndrome (HUS) is the *most common* cause of acute renal failure in young children. HUS most frequently follows an episode of gastroenteritis caused by enterohemorrhagic stain of *Escherichia coli* (0157: H7). The organism elaborates a toxin (**verotoxin**), which is absorbed from the intestine and initiates endothelial cell injury. The 'primary event' in pathogenesis of HUS is endothelial cell injury; capillary and arteriolar endothelial injuries in the kidneys lead to localized clotting. The microangiopathic hemolytic anemia results from mechanical damage to the RBCs as they pass through 'altered' vasculature. Thrombocytopenia is due to intrarenal platelet adhesion or damage. Damaged platelets and RBCs are removed from circulation by liver and spleen. **Hemoglobin is common in the range of 5–9 gm%** and GBP reveals helmet cells, burr cells and fragmented RBCs. 'Plasma' hemoglobin is elevated and haptoglobin diminished; reticulocyte count is moderately elevated and **Coombs' test is negative**. TLC may rise to 30,000 per mm^3; **thrombocytopenia** (20,000–1, 00,000) occurs in more than 90% of patients. PTT and PT are usually normal.

Reference and further reading: *Nelson Textbook of Pediatrics; 16th edition; page 1586–1587*

564. *True* regarding transient tachypnea of newborn (TTN) is:
A. Interlobular fissure effusion
B. Respiratory distress resolves in 6-10 days
C. Air bronchogram is seen
D. Common in preterm infant
(PGI 1999)

565. All the following are seen in transient tachypnea of newborn *except*:
A. Seen in early neonatal period
B. May be associated with grunting and cyanosis
C. May be associated with crepitation and wheezes
D. Interlobar effusion is present
(JIPMER 2002)

Transient tachypnea of newborn (TTN) is also known as **wet lung disease** or **RDS type-II**. It is a common, mild, self-limited disorder, affecting near-term or term infants. It is characterized by tachypnea with mild retractions and mild cyanosis with a FiO_2 requirement of less than 0.4. The infant is usually near-term or at term and develops tachypnea (more than 80 breaths per minute) within 2–6 hours of birth. The symptoms typically persist for 12–24 hours in mild TTN, but may persist for more than 72 hours in severe TTN. There is cyanosis, slight subcostal and intercostal retractions, increased AP-diameter of the upper thorax, nasal flaring, and intermittent expiratory grunting. **These infants usually have good air exchange without crackles or rhonchi.** Fluid may be seen in the minor fissures, the pleural space, or both. Widening of the interlobar fissures and prominence of the right-lung minor fissures are occasional findings.

Ref: *Manual of neonatal care; John P. Cloherty and Ann R. Stark; 4th edition; page 369–371*

566. A 2-months old child is brought with a complaint of intermittent stridor. The *most likely* diagnosis in this case is?
A. Foreign body
B. Laryngomalacia
C. Croup
D. Carcinoma larynx
(JHARKHAND 2003)

Laryngomalacia or **congenital laryngeal stridor** is the *most common* congenital abnormality of the larynx. **It is the *most common* condition causing an inspiratory stridor at or shortly after birth**, which may persist throughout infancy. It is due to abnormal flaccidity of laryngeal cartilage, which causes the laryngeal structures to vibrate like a small-elongated reed. Stridor increases when the child cries but gets relieved by placing the child in a prone position. This condition usually disappears by 2 years of age. Direct laryngoscopy demonstrates elongated epiglottis, which is curled upon itself (omega shaped), floppy aryepiglottic folds and prominent arytenoids. Treatment is symptomatic with early antibiotic therapy for upper respiratory tract infection and reassurance to the parents.

567. The *most specific* abnormality associated with diabetes mellitus is:
A. Omphalocele
B. Neural tube defects
C. Heart defects
D. Sacral agenesis
(SGPGI 2003)

Congenital anomalies are found more frequently in **infants of diabetic mothers** (IDMs) than in infants of non-diabetic mothers. The central nervous system and cardiac anomalies make up two-thirds of the malformations seen in IDMs. Although there is a general increase in anomaly rate in IDMs, no anomaly is specific for IDMs, although **half of all cases of 'caudal regression syndrome' are seen in IDMs**. Caudal regression syndrome involves sacral agenesis, partial absence or underdevelopment of the lower extremities, and genitourinary and gastrointestinal abnormalities.

Ref: *Manual of Neonatal Care by John P. Cloherty; 4th edition; page 19*

568. Hypoglycemia in newborn is defined as the blood sugar level below (in mg%):
A. 30
B. 40
C. 50
D. 55
(MANIPAL 2001)

Hypoglycemia is defined as a blood glucose level < 40 mg/dL in any infant, regardless of gestational age and whether symptomatic or not. The pathogenesis of neonatal hypoglycemia in IDMs is explained by Pederson's maternal hyperglycemia-fetal **hyperinsulinism** hypothesis.

569. All of the following complications are seen in diabetes mellitus in neonates *except*:

A. Hypomagnesemia　**B.** Hypercalcemia
C. Hypocalcemia　**D.** Hypoglycemia　*(SGPGI 2003)*

Common complications in infants of diabetic mother (IDM)

- Poor feeding
- Polycythemia
- Congenital anomalies
- Macrosomia
- Renal vein thrombosis
- Hypoglycemia
- Hypocalcemia
- Jaundice
- Poor feeding
- Myocardial dysfunction
- Small left colon syndrome
- Respiratory distress

Further reading: *Manual of Neonatal Care by John P. Cloherty; 4th edition; page 11 onwards*

570. Erythroblastosis fetalis occurs in:

A. Rh-negative mother with Rh-positive in the 2nd child
B. Rh-positive mother with Rh-negative in the 2nd child
C. Rh-negative mother with Rh-positive in the 1st child
D. Rh-positive mother with Rh-negative in the 1st child　*(SGPGI 2003)*

Hemolytic disease of the newborn or **erythroblastosis fetalis** results from *transplacental* passage of maternal antibodies active against the red cell antigens of the infant, leading to an increased rate of RBC destruction. **Erythroblastosis fetalis** continues to be an important cause of *anemia* and *jaundice* in newborn infants despite the development of a method of prevention of maternal isoimmunization by Rh antigens. There are more than 60 different red cell antigens, which are capable of eliciting an antibody response in a suitable recipient; *significant* disease is associated primarily with the D antigen of the Rh group and with incompatibility of ABO group. **Rh incompatibility may develop when an Rh-negative woman carries an Rh-positive fetus.** At the time of delivery, fetal red blood cells may enter maternal circulation, stimulating antibody production against the Rh factor. In a **subsequent** pregnancy, these antibodies cross the placenta to the fetal circulation and destroy fetal red blood cells.

Reference and further reading: *Nelson Textbook of Pediatrics; 16th edition; page 521*

571. All of the following groups of newborns are at an increased risk of hypoglycemia *except*:

A. Birth asphyxia　**B.** Respiratory distress syndrome
C. Maternal diabetes　**D.** Post-term infant　*(AIIMS Nov 2002)*

Some Common Causes of Neonatal Hypoglycemia

Increased utilization	*Decreased production or store*	*Increased utilization and / or decreased production or other causes*
• Diabetic mother • Erythroblastosis • Islet-cell hyperplasia or hyperfunction • Backwith-Weidemann syndrome • Insulin producing tumor • Maternal tocolytic therapy with beta agonist agents • Maternal chlorpropamide therapy • After exchange transfusion	• Prematurity • Intrauterine growth retardation • Inadequate caloric intake	• Perinatal stress • Shock • Asphyxia • Hypothermia • Septicemia • Defects in carbohydrate metabolism • Defects in amino acid metabolism • Endocrine deficiency

Further reading: *Manual of Neonatal Care by John P. Cloherty; 4th edition; page 545*

572. *Best* parameter for estimation of fetal age by ultrasound in 3rd trimester is:

A. Femur length
B. Biparietal diameter
C. Abdominal circumference
D. Interocular distance

(AIIMS Nov 2002)

During the 2nd and 3rd trimesters measurement of the biparietal diameter (BPD) and the fetal femur length are useful in estimating gestational age. The length of calcified fetal femur is measured and used in validating BPD measurements or used alone in circumstances where BPD cannot be measured (deeply engaged fetal head) or is inadequate (hydrocephalus).

Ref: *Manual of Neonatal Care by John P. Cloherty; 4th edition; page 1*

573. In 'pediatric advanced life support' intraosseous access for drug and fluid administration is recommended for pediatric age of:

A. <1-year age
B. <5-years age
C. <6-years age
D. Any age

(AIIMS Nov 2002)

Intraosseous infusion (IOI) is an easily achieved alternative to an intravenous line when vascular access is imperative and a peripheral IV line cannot be rapidly placed in children **6-year of age and younger**. An IOI can be established by inserting a 15 or 18 gauge bone marrow needle into the marrow cavity of the proximal tibia.

Reference and further reading: *Nelson Textbook of Pediatrics; 16th edition; page 242*

574. Which of the following is 'most suggestive' of neonatal small-bowel obstruction:

A. *Generalized* abdominal distension
B. Failure to pass meconium in the first 24 hours
C. Bilious vomiting
D. Refusal of feed

(AI 2003)

Duodenal atresia in 70% of infants is associated with other congenital anomalies, including Down syndrome, CVS anomalies and other GI anomalies such as annular pancreas, esophageal atresia, malrotation of small intestine, small bowel atresia, and imperforate anus. There may be a history of polyhydramnios. **Vomiting of bile-stained material usually starts a few hours after birth.** Abdominal distention is 'limited' to the upper abdomen. The infant may 'pass' meconium in the first 24 hours of life and then bowel movements seize. Aspiration of the stomach by a nasogastric tube returns more than 30 ml of gastric contents prior to feeding. A plain X-ray film of abdomen will demonstrate air in the stomach and upper part of the abdomen (**double-bubble sign**) with no air in the small or large intestine. Neonate may develop icterus in the presence of intestinal obstruction. Preoperative management consists primarily of nasogastric suction.

Ref: *Manual of Neonatal Care by John P. Cloherty; 4th edition; page 623*

575. A 31 weeks pregnant lady delivered a child. After 6 hours the baby develops dyspnea and cyanosis. Chest X-ray and bronchogram showed ground glass appearance. *Most likely* diagnosis is:

A. Pulmonary edema
B. Meconium aspiration syndrome
C. Hyaline membrane disease
D. Consolidation

(AIIMS 1999)

The primary cause of **respiratory distress syndrome (RDS)** or **hyaline membrane disease** is inadequate pulmonary surfactant. Factors that affect the state of lung development at birth include prematurity, maternal diabetes and genetic factors (white race, history of RDS in siblings, male sex). Thoracic malformations that cause lung hypoplasia, such as diaphragmatic hernia, may also increase the risk for surfactant deficiency. Factors that may acutely impair surfactant production, release or function include perinatal asphyxia in premature infants and cesarean section without labor. Maternal glucocorticoid treatment is recommended if delivery of an infant with severe RDS seem imminent. This applies to pregnancies shorter than 34 weeks regardless of gender or race or those in which lung immaturity is shown by amniotic fluid analysis and when delivery can be postponed to allow the glucocorticoid to take effect. The premature infant with RDS will have clinical signs shortly after birth. These include tachypnea, retractions, flaring of the nasal alae, grunting and cyanosis. The classic radiographic appearance is of low volume lungs with a diffuse reticulogranular pattern and air bronchograms. The keys to management of RDS are:

- To prevent hypoxia and acidosis;
- To optimize fluid management;

- To reduce metabolic demands;
- To prevent worsening atelectasis and pulmonary edema; and
- To minimize lung injury due to barotrauma or oxygen.

Surfactant replacement therapy has been shown in numerous clinical trials to ameliorate RDS. Delivery of oxygen should be sufficient to maintain PaO_2 between 50–80 mmHg because this range is generally sufficient to meet metabolic demands. Higher than necessary fraction of oxygen in inspired air (FiO_2) level should be avoided because of the danger of potentiating the development of lung injury and retinopathy of prematurity (ROP). The indications for starting mechanical ventilation are $PaCO_2$ > 50 mmHg, PaO_2 < 50 mmHg or oxygen saturation < 90% with a FiO_2 above 0.5, or severe apnea. A continuous flow, pressure limited, time cycle ventilator is useful for ventilation newborns. The initial setting generally consists of PIP = 20–25 cmH_2O; PEEP = 4–6 cmH_2O; frequency 20–30 breaths/minute; time of inspiration (Ti) of 0.5 second and the previously required FiO_2 (0.5–1).

Ref: *Manual of Neonatal Care by John P. Cloherty; 4th edition; page 329*

576. Which of the following condition is *not* associated with 'unconjugated' hyperbilirubinemia in a newborn?

A. Septicemia
B. Breast milk jaundice
C. Crigler-Najjar syndrome
D. Hypothyroidism *(SGPGI 1996)*

577. Neonatal jaundice persisting for 2-weeks after birth is *not* seen in:

A. Rh incompatibility
B. Hypothyroidism
C. Galactosemia
D. Breast milk jaundice *(AI 1992)*

Jaundice is an important manifestation of infection in newborn babies and occurs due to hemolysis and hepatitis. Systemic features of **septicemia** and the occurrence of jaundice usually dominate the clinical picture after the age of 3-days. The **conjugated bilirubin is often elevated to 2.0 mg/dl or more**, and jaundice often persists beyond 14 days of life. The neonatal jaundice, whether physiological or pathological, usually disappears by the second week of life. **The important causes of persistent neonatal jaundice are as under:**

Unconjugated hyperbilirubinemia	Conjugated hyperbilirubinemia
• Breast milk jaundice • Hypothyroidism • Crigler-Najjar syndrome • Intestinal obstruction or stasis • Ongoing hemolysis (Rh, ABO)	• Neonatal hepatitis • Extrahepatic biliary atresia • Inborn errors of metabolism • Total parenteral nutrition

Ref: *IAP Textbook of Pediatrics; 2nd edition; page 71*

578. *Not* seen in hypophosphatemic vitamin D resistant rickets:

A. X linked inheritance
B. Hypocalcemia
C. Reduced tubular reabsorption of phosphate
D. Lower limb deformity *(SGPGI 1999)*

The *most commonly* encountered non-nutritional form of rickets is **familial hypophosphatemia** (**vitamin D resistant rickets** or **X-linked hypophosphatemia**). The usual mode of inheritance is **X-linked dominant**; although autosomal recessive and sporadic forms has been reported. Pathogenic mechanism involves **defects in the proximal tubular reabsorption of phosphate** and in conversion of 25(OH) D to $1,25(OH)_2$ D. **Serum calcium levels are usually normal**, with *low intestinal absorption* and renal excretion of calcium. Children with familial hypophosphatemia *present with* bowing of the lower extremities related to weight bearing at the age of walking. Tetany is not present, and profound myopathy, rachitic rosary, and Harrison groove (pectus deformity) characteristic of calcium deficient rickets are not evident. These children develop a waddling gait, smooth (rather than angular) **bowing of lower extremities**, coxa vera, genu varum, genu valgum and short stature. Pulp deformities and 'intraglobular dentin' are characteristic tooth abnormalities. *By contrast* calcium deficient rickets usually results in enamel defects. The patients have normal or slightly raised calcium levels (9–9.4 mg%); a moderately reduced phosphate level (1.5 -3 mg%); elevated alkaline phosphatase activity and no evidence of secondary hyperparathyroidism. Urinary phosphate excretion is large (despite hypophosphatemia) indicating a defect in renal tubular phosphate reabsorption.

Oral phosphate supplements coupled with a vitamin D analogue to 'offset' the secondary hyperparathyroidism that may accompany an oral phosphate load is the preferred treatment.

Reference and further reading: *Nelson Textbook of Pediatrics; 16th edition; page 2136–2137*

579. *False* regarding an infant of a woman with HIV infection:

A. Diagnosis of HIV in newborn cannot be made with routinely available test
B. Failure to thrive may be presenting symptom
C. Risk of HIV infection in infants is greater than 50%
D. Transmission of HIV infection may take place during parturition *(SGPGI 1999)*

- Reported rates of transmission of HIV from mother to child have varied but most large studies in the USA and Europe have documented **transmission rates in untreated women between 12–30%**. However, reported vertical transmission rates in Africa and Haiti are 25–52%. [1]
- The rate of mother to child transmission (vertical) of HIV-1 evaluated epidemiologically in several surveys has varied from **13–42%** with 65% of newborns infected during final 6 weeks of pregnancy and at delivery. [2]

Reference and further reading: *Nelson Textbook of Pediatrics; 16th edition; page 1023* [1] and *IAP Textbook of Pediatrics; 2nd edition; page 259* [2]

580. Which of the following is a cyanotic congenital heart disease?

A. TOF
B. AS
C. Patent ductus arteriosus
D. Ventricular septal defect *(SGPGI 1999)*

Common Cyanotic Congenital Heart Diseases

- Tetralogy of Fallot (*most common*)
- Transposition of great vessels with VSD and PS
- Pulmonary atresia with VSD
- Pulmonary atresia with intact ventricular septum
- Tricuspid atresia
- Double output right ventricle (DORV) with pulmonary stenosis
- Ebstein anomaly of the tricuspid valve
- Double output right ventricle (DORV) without pulmonary stenosis
- DORV with TGA
- Total anomalous pulmonary venous return
- Truncus arteriosus
- Single ventricle
- Hypoplastic left heart syndrome
- Abnormal position of heart and heterotaxy syndromes (asplenia, polysplenia)

Reference and further reading: *Nelson Textbook of Pediatrics; 16th edition; page 1384 onwards*

581. An 18-month-old child has gastroenteritis with dehydration. Blood urea is 80 mg/dL and Creatinine is 1.1 mg/dL. Measurement of fractional excretion of which of the following solutes is most helpful in evaluating renal functions:

A. Potassium
B. Sodium
C. Phosphate
D. Bicarbonate *(SGPGI 1999)*

582. A 3-day-old child presents with 22-25 stools per day and pneumonitis. He has *not* passed urine for 36 hours. Blood pressure is low, pH is 7.21, urine Na^+ 18 mEq/L and serum urea is 120, and creatinine is 1.2. This indicates:

A. Acute cortical necrosis
B. Acute medullary necrosis
C. Acute tubular necrosis
D. Prerenal azotemia *(AIIMS 1995)*

Prerenal azotemia is the *most common* form of ARF and represents a physiologic response to mild to moderate renal hypoperfusion. It is rapidly reversible upon restoration of renal blood flow and glomerular ultra-filtration pressure. Renal parenchymal tissue is not damaged in this condition. More severe hypoperfusion may lead to ischemic injury of renal parenchyma and 'intrinsic' renal azotemia. Analysis of urine and blood biochemistry is particularly useful for distinguishing prerenal azotemia from ischemic or nephrotoxic intrinsic renal azotemia. The **fractional excretion of sodium** (FeNa) is most useful in this regard.

$$\text{Fractional excretion of sodium (\%)} = \frac{\text{Urinary Na x plasma Cr}}{\text{Plasma Na x urinary Cr}} \times 100$$

Patients with prerenal azotemia typically have a FeNa of <1.0% (frequently <0.1%, whereas the FeNa in patients with ischemic or nephrotoxic ARF is usually >1.0%.

583. Calculate the 24-hour fluid requirement of a 6 kg child:

A. 1500 ml **B.** 1000 ml
C. 800 ml **D.** 600 ml *(AIIMS 1991)*

Maintenance fluid requirement

Body weight in kg	Fluid requirement in ml per 24 hour
• **Up to 10**	100 ml per kg
• **11–20**	1000 ml + 50 ml per kg for each kg above 10 kg
• **Above 20**	1500 ml + 20 ml per kg for each kg above 20 kg

Ref: *Nelson Textbook of Pediatrics; 16th edition; page 211*

584. *Not* a feature of tetanus:

A. Normal sensorium **B.** Bulging fontanelle
C. Increased tone **D.** Spasm of muscle *(AIIMS 1991)*

Tetanus (lockjaw) is an acute, spastic paralytic disease caused by tetanospasmin, the neurotoxin produced by *Clostridium tetani*. The *most common* form, neonatal tetanus (umbilical tetanus) kills about 5 lakh infants every year. Tetanus may be either localized or generalized, the later being more common form. In *generalized tetanus*, trismus (**spasm** of masseter muscle or lockjaw) is the presenting feature in about 50% of cases. Headache, restlessness and irritability are early symptoms, often followed by stiffness, difficulty in chewing, dysphagia and neck muscle spasm. The patient may be febrile, although many have no fever; **mentation is unimpaired**. **Markedly increased tone** in central muscles (face, neck, chest, back, and abdomen) with superimposed generalized spasms and relative sparing of the hands and feet strongly suggests tetanus.

Ref: *Nelson Textbook of Pediatrics; 16th edition; page 878 and Harrison's Principles of Internal Medicine; 14th edition*

585. Which of the following treatment should *not* be done in a child with pruritic lesion in axilla and groin?

A. Treatment of contacts **B.** Benzyl benzoate application
C. Clothes are to be boiled **D.** Systemic steroid *(AI 1992)*

Scabies should be treated with an application of either 25% **benzyl benzoate** or 1% gamma benzene hexachloride (GBH). 1% GBH is less irritant and more effective and should be applied to the whole skin from neck downward ideally with a brush. It is essential that the *whole skin* be completely covered and is quite *useless* to treat only areas with active lesion. Two applications are required at 24-hour interval and after another 24 hours of 2nd, application bath should be taken because for the treatment to be effective the drug must remain on the skin for a total of 48 hours. The patient should be *strictly* told *not* to wash *any* part of his body before the final bath. Washing of clothes, dishes and even hands must be forbidden because scabies will not be cured until these instructions are strictly followed. Sulphur ointment (2.5–10%) daily for 4 days is a cheap remedy. Due to prolonged incubation period of the disease and impossibility of recognizing the disease during this period **all the members of the family must be treated** simultaneously. Unless this is done the disease will remain *endemic* within the family for months or years. *Finally* it is *not* necessary to disinfect clothing or bedclothes and a change of clothing and **ordinary laundering** is all that is required after the final bath.

586. In simple partial seizure the *drug of choice* is:
- **A.** Phenobarbitone
- **B.** Carbamazepine
- **C.** Valproic acid
- **D.** Phenytoin

(AI 1997)

587. In petit-mal (absence) seizures the *drug of choice* is:
- **A.** Valproate
- **B.** Diazepam
- **C.** Phenytoin
- **D.** Clonazepam

(AI 1995)

Antiepileptic Drugs of Choice

Focal onset seizure	Generalized tonic-clonic	Absence	Myoclonic	Atonic
• Carbamazepine • Phenytoin • Valproic acid	• Valproic acid • Carbamazepine • Phenytoin	• Ethosuximide • Valproic acid	• Valproic acid	• Valproic acid

Ref: *Harrison's Principles of Internal Medicine; 14th edition*

588. Which of the following is a feature of typical febrile seizures in children?
- **A.** Focal neurological deficits
- **B.** Diagnostic EEG changes
- **C.** Positive family history in 30% of cases
- **D.** Mental retardation

(AI 1991)

589. Which of the following is *true* regarding febrile seizure?
- **A.** Status epilepsy is common
- **B.** 50% recurrence is common
- **C.** Interictal EEG is normal
- **D.** Long term treatment is required

(AI 1993)

590. *Not* a characteristic feature of febrile seizure:
- **A.** Occurs with sudden rise in temperature
- **B.** Male children are more prone
- **C.** Phenobarbitone prevents further attacks
- **D.** Manifests with generalized seizure

(KARNATAKA 2000)

Febrile seizures are the *most common* seizure disorder during childhood, with a uniformly excellent prognosis. They are rare before 9 months and after 5 years of age. **A strong family history of febrile convulsions in siblings and parents suggests a genetic predisposition.** The seizure is **typically generalized**, tonic clonic of a few seconds to 10 minutes in duration followed by a brief period of drowsiness. An EEG is not required after a simple febrile seizure. Although sodium valproate is effective in management of febrile seizure, the potential risks of the drug do not justify its use in a disorder with an excellent prognosis irrespective of treatment. **Phenobarbital has been ineffective in preventing recurrent febrile seizures.** Short-term anticonvulsant prophylaxis is **not recommended.**

Ref: *Nelson Textbook of Pediatrics; 16th edition; page 1818*

591. Absence seizure in children is seen in:
- **A.** Psychogenic disorder
- **B.** Petit mal epilepsy
- **C.** Grand mal epilepsy
- **D.** Attention deficit disorder

(AIIMS 1998)

Absence seizures: Simple (typical) absence (**petitmal**) seizures are characterized by a sudden cessation of motor activity or speech with a blank facial expression and flickering of the eyelids. These seizures are not common before 5 years of age; more common in girls; never associated with an aura; *rarely* persist longer than 30 seconds; and not associated with a postictal state. Children may experience 'countless' seizures daily, whereas CPS are usually less frequent. Children do not loose body tone, but their head may fall forward slightly. Immediately after the absence seizure patient resumes pre-seizure activity with no indication of any postictal impairment. Simple absence seizure is frequently accompanied by automatic behavior. Hyperventilation for 3–4 minutes routinely 'produces' an absence seizure. The EEG demonstrates a typical 3-second spike and generalized wave discharge. Complex (atypical) absence seizures have an associated motor component consisting of myoclonic movement of the face, fingers or extremities and sometimes loss of body tone.

Ref: *Nelson Textbook of Pediatrics; 16th edition; page 1815*

592. Unilateral renal agenesis is associated with:

A. Single umbilical artery **B.** Polycystic disease of pancreas
C. Hiatus hernia **D.** Hypogonadism *(AIIMS 1995)*

The umbilical cord contains 2 umbilical arteries, 1 umbilical vein, the rudimentary allantois, remnant of omphalomesenteric duct, and a gelatinous substance called Wharton's jelly. The 'muscular' umbilical arteries contract readily, but the vein does not. The umbilical vein retains a fairly large lumen after birth. The blood vessels are 'functionally' closed but are patent 'anatomically' for the first 10–20 days of life. Umbilical cord usually sloughs within 2 weeks of life. Delayed separation of cord (> 1 month) has been associated with neutrophil chemotactic defect and overwhelming bacterial infection. **Single umbilical artery** is found in about 5–10 per 1000 live births; 35–70 per thousand twin births. 33% of newborns with a single umbilical artery have congenital abnormalities, usually more than 1, and many such infants are stillborn or die shortly after birth. Trisomy 18 (Edward's syndrome) is one of the most frequent abnormalities. It is important that at every delivery the cut cord and the maternal and fetal surfaces of the placenta be inspected and the number of arteries present should be recorded. Renal USG is recommended for infants with a single umbilical artery. **Unilateral renal agenesis is found with increased frequency in newborns with a single umbilical artery**. Bilateral renal agenesis is incompatible with extra-uterine life and death occurs shortly after birth (Potter syndrome).

593. A baby delivered at 32 weeks is on ventilator. X-ray shows white out lesions. ABG shows SpO_2 75, and ventilator settings are FiO_2=70, rate 50 per minute. Next step in management of this newborn should be:

A. Wean off the ventilator **B.** Continue with the same settings
C. Increase FiO_2 to 80 **D.** Increase rate to 60 *(AI 2001)*

Arterial Oxygenation improves when either the fraction of inspired oxygen concentration (FiO_2) and/or mean airway pressure (MAP) are increased. To increase oxygenation: Increase FiO_2, or increase PEEP, or increase tidal volume.

594. In which of the following condition, bacterial endocarditis is *rarely* seen:

A. Ostium secundum ASD **B.** MVP
C. PDA **D.** VSD *(UP 2000)*

Patients of **congenital heart disease** (CHD) having a high velocity of blood ejected through a 'hole' or stenotic orifice are more susceptible to endocarditis. Therefore children with VSD, *left* sided valvular disease and systemic pulmonary arterial communication (including palliative shunts) are at the highest risk. Tetralogy of Fallot (TOF), **VSD**, AS, **PDA**, TGV and palliative shunts are the 'most frequent' structural lesions associated with endocarditis. In older children congenital bicuspid aortic valves and mitral valve prolapse (**MVP**) pose additional risks for endocarditis. Surgical 'repair' of CHD *may reduce* but *does not eliminate* the risk of endocarditis except the repair of a simple ASD or PDA.

595. In which of the following condition, decreased serum iron and decreased iron-binding capacity is seen:

A. Sideroblastic anemia **B.** Thalassemia
C. Chronic infection **D.** Iron deficiency anemia *(AI 1991)*

In **anemia of chronic disease levels of both serum iron and iron-binding capacity (transferrin) are reduced**, and the percentage saturation of transferrin is reduced. In contrast to the markedly reduced serum ferritin level in iron deficiency anemia, the low serum iron level in the anemia of chronic disorders is accompanied by a normal or elevated serum ferritin level.

Ref: *de Gruchy's Clinical Hematology in Medical Practice; 5th edition; page 103*

596. Raised intracranial pressure in a 9-month-old infant is diagnosed by all *except*:

A. Bulging fontanelle **B.** Papilledema
C. Diplopia **D.** Increased head size *(AIIMS 1991)*

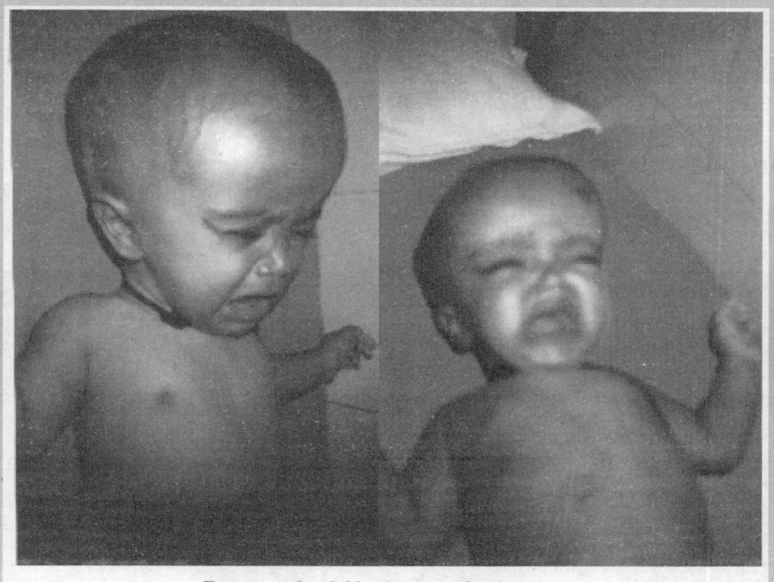

Congenital Hydrocephalus
note the prominent scalp veins
Photograph Courtesy: Dr. Sharad Chandra, MBBS, DCH, MIAP; Consultant Pediatrician; Fatima Hospital; Lucknow, India

Papilledema rarely occurs in infancy, as the skull sutures are capable of separating to 'accommodate' the expanding intracranial contents.

Reference and further reading: *Nelson Textbook of Pediatrics; 16th edition; page 1795*

597. What is the content of sodium in ORS solution, in mEq/L?
A. 90 mmol **B.** 60 mmol
C. 40 mmol **D.** 20 mmol *(CUPGME 2003)*

598. In ORS solution, the benefit of adding glucose to it is:
A. Increases absorption of Na^+ **B.** Provides calories
C. Increases absorption of K^+ **D.** Increases absorption of Cl^- *(MAHE 2001)*

Composition of WHO/UNICEF recommended ORS

Ingredient	Composition (gm/l)	Concentration	mEq/l
Sodium chloride	3.5	Sodium	90
Potassium chloride	1.5	Chloride	80
Trisodium citrate	2.9	Citrate	10
Glucose	20	Glucose	111 (mmol/l)

- Osmolality should be 311.

Oral rehydration is possible if glucose is added with salt. It capitalizes on glucose facilitated sodium ion absorption.

Ref: *IAP Textbook of Pediatrics; 2nd edition; page 416*

599. All the following are features of CCF in an infant *except*:
A. Diaphoresis
B. Failure to gain weight
C. Pedal edema
D. Tachypnea *(JIPMER 2002)*

Heart failure may be difficult to identify in infants. Important features include **tachypnea**, difficulty in feeding, **poor weight gain**, **excessive perspiration**, irritability, weak cry and noisy-labored respiration with intercostal and subcostal retractions as well as flaring of the alae nasi. Hepatomegaly usually occurs and cardiomegaly is invariably present.

Reference and further reading: *Nelson Textbook of Pediatrics; 16th edition; page 1441*

600. *Not* present in congenital rubella syndrome:

A. Blindness B. IUGR
C. Renal anomalies D. Deafness *(AIIMS 1999)*

Classically, **congenital rubella syndrome** (CRS) is characterized by the constellation of cataracts, sensorineural deafness, and congenital heart disease. The *most common* manifestation of CRS is intrauterine growth retardation (IUGR). The *most common* cardiac defects are PDA, and pulmonary artery stenosis.

Reference and further reading: *Nelson Textbook of Pediatrics; 16th edition; page 952*

601. Which of the following age group is *most severely* affected by rubella infection?

A. Females aged 25-35 years B. Young girls
C. Adolescent girls D. Unborn child *(JIPMER 2002)*

Complications of rubella are relatively uncommon in childhood. **The *most important* consequence of rubella in a pregnant woman is congenital rubella syndrome.**

Reference and further reading: *Nelson Textbook of Pediatrics; 16th edition; page 952*

602. Narrow anterior fontanelle in children is seen in which of the following conditions:

A. Hydrocephalus B. Vitamin deficiency rickets
C. Craniosynostosis D. Cleidocranial dysostosis *(MAHE 2001)*

Persistently small fontanels suggest microcephaly, **craniosynostosis**, congenital hyperthyroidism or wormian bones.

Reference and further reading: *Nelson Textbook of Pediatrics; 16th edition; page 455*

603. *Bad* prognostic indicator for ALL is:

A. Hypoploidy B. TLC < 50000
C. Female sex D. Age > 1 year *(AIIMS May 2002)*

The overall 'cure rate' for childhood ALL is estimated to be about 80%. In general, a **poor prognosis is associated with onset at an age under 2 years or over 10 years**, with a WBC count > 1 lakh/mm^3 at the time of diagnosis, with the presence of mediastinal mass, with early involvement of the CNS, and with leukemia in a black patient. Common ALL antigen (CALLA) has the *most favorable* prognosis; no more than a few patients with T-cell ALL can expect long-term control. The *FAB classification* also permits some prognostic predictions. Those patients with L_1 morphology have a better prognosis as a group than do patients with L_2 morphology. Patients with L_3 morphology have the poor prognostic characteristics of B-cell leukemias and non-Hodgkin lymphomas.

Reference and further reading: *Nelson Textbook of Pediatrics; 16th edition*

604. A 2-month-old baby with acute icteric viral hepatitis like illness slips into encephalopathy after 48 hours. The mother is a known hepatitis B carrier. Mother's hepatitis B virus serological profile is *most likely* to be:

A. HBsAg positive only B. HBsAg and HBeAg positive
C. HBsAg and HBe antibody positive D. HBV DNA positive *(AI 2003)*

HBsAg-positive serum containing HBeAg is more likely to be highly infectious and to be associated with the presence of hepatitis B virions than HBeAg-negative or anti-HBe-positive serum. **HBsAg carrier mothers who are HBeAg positive almost invariably transmit hepatitis B infection to their children**, while HBsAg carrier mothers with anti-HBe *rarely* infect their offspring.

605. All of the following are causes of seizures in the 'neonate' *except*:

A. Hypoxia
B. Pertussis vaccine
C. Septicemia
D. Meningitis

(BHU June 2002)

Important Causes of Neonatal Seizure

• Hypoxic ischemic encephalopathy	• Intracranial hemorrhage	• Molybdenum cofactor deficiency
• Hypoglycemia	• Hypocalcemia	• Hypomagnesemia
• Hyponatremia	• Hypernatremia	• Pyridoxine dependency
• Maple syrup urine disease	• Phenylketonuria	• Isovaleric acidemia
• Urea cycle disorders	• Beta alanine abnormalities	• Methylmalonic acidemia
• Propionic acidemia	• Congenital lactic acidosis	• Glutaric aciduria type II
• Fructose intolerance	• Menke's kinky hair disease	• CNS trauma
• Bacterial meningitis	• Brain abscess	• Cerebral dysgenesis
• Phakomatoses	• Narcotic withdrawal	• Familial neonatal seizure
• Hypertensive encephalopathy	• Local anesthesia	• Unknown causes (25%)

606. In neonatal resuscitation to be done is:

A. Suction nose *then* mouth
B. Place the baby on the back
C. Wipe with *wet* towel
D. All of the above

(BHU June 2002)

Resuscitation of babies at birth is different from resuscitation of all other age groups. The *majority* of newborns will establish normal respiration and circulation *spontaneously*. The 1st breath usually occurs within 60–90 seconds of clamping or obstructing the umbilical cord in a healthy term newborn. Clamping of cord leads to the onset of asphyxia, which is the 'major stimulant' to start respiration although the physical stimuli such as cold air or physical discomfort may also provoke respiratory efforts. The 1st breaths are especially important, as the lungs are initially full of fluid. Labor causes the fluid producing cells within the lungs of the fetus to stop secretion and begin reabsorption of that fluid. The 1st spontaneous breaths generate a negative pressure between–40 cmH_2O and–100 cmH_2O, which inflates the lung for the 1st time. This pressure is 10–15 greater than that is needed for later breathing. These powerful chest movements cause fluid to be displaced from the airway into the lymphatics. That is why, a caesarean section before onset of labor may slow the clearance of pulmonary fluid from the lungs and reduce the initial functional reserve capacity (FRC). Surfactant is produced by type-2 (granular) pneumocytes in the alveolar epithelium and it reduces alveolar surface tension and prevents alveolar collapse on expiration. Surfactant can be demonstrated from 20 weeks of gestational age, but the increase is slow until a 'surge' in production at 30–34 weeks. Its half-life is about 12 hours and its production is reduced by hypothermia (<35°C), hypoxia and acidosis (pH < 7.25). When the placental O_2 supply is interrupted, the fetus initiates **breathing movements**. If these breathing movements fail to provide an 'alternative' O_2 supply (as they will obviously fail to do *in-utero*) the baby loses consciousness. If hypoxia continues then the *respiratory centre* becomes unable to continue initiating breathing and breathing stops, usually within 2–3 minutes (**primary apnea**). Babies have a number of **automatic reflex responses** to such a situation, conserving energy by shutting down the circulation to non-vital organs. Bradycardia starts but BP is maintained primarily by peripheral vasoconstriction but also by an increased stroke volume. After a latent period of apnea (**primary apnea**), which may vary in duration, the *primitive spinal centers* are no longer 'suppressed' by the respiratory center and they exert an effect by initiating **primitive gasping breaths**. These deep spontaneous gasps can be easily distinguished from normal respiration as they occur 6–12 times/minute and involve all 'accessory' muscles in a maximal inspiratory effort. After a while (if hypoxia continues) even this activity ceases (**terminal apnea**). The time taken for such activity to stop is longer (up to 20 minutes) in newborn babies than in later life. **The circulation is almost always maintained until all respiratory activity stops and this resilience is a feature of all newborn term mammals, largely due to the reserve of glycogen in the heart**. Resuscitation is therefore relatively easy if started before 'all' respiratory activity has stopped. Once the lungs are inflated, O_2 will be carried to the heart and then to the brain followed by rapid recovery. *Most* newborns who have not progressed to the stage of terminal apnea, will resuscitate themselves provided their airway is patent. However, once gasping stops the circulation starts to fall and these infants are likely to require extensive resuscitation. Hypoxia *in-utero* in a term infant (> 37 weeks), leads to vasoconstriction in gut vessels, increased peristalsis, and a relaxation of the sphincters. This may result in passage of meconium *in-utero*. If fetal hypoxia is severe enough it may initiate gasping and aspiration of amniotic fluid with meconium before birth. Once the baby is delivered, meconium causes problem due to complete or partial airway obstruction.

Practical aspects of neonatal resuscitation: Most babies (even those born apneic) will resuscitate themselves given a clear airway.

- Dry the baby immediately and then wrap in a dry towel because a 'cold' baby has an increased O_2 consumption and is more likely to become hypoglycemic and acidotic with resultant increased mortality. Most of the heat loss is by latent heat of evaporation–hence the need to dry and wrap the baby. Babies have a large surface area to weight ratio and therefore heat can be lost very quickly. Ideally the baby should be put under a radiant warmer (He/she should be given a warm welcome in the world!).
- The Apgar score was proposed as a tool for evaluating a baby's condition at birth but it is not used to guide resuscitation. Acute assessment is made by assessing the following parameters:
  - Color (pink, blue, or white)
  - Respiration (rate and quality)
  - Heart rate (fast, slow, or absent)
  - Tone (unconscious and apneic babies are 'floppy')

This will categorize the baby into 1 of the following 3 groups:

- **Pink, regular respiration and fast heart rate (>100/minute)**: These are healthy babies and they should be kept warm and given to the mothers.
- **Blue, irregular or inadequate respiration and slow heart rate (60/minute or less)**: If gentle stimulation does not induce effective breathing, the airway should be opened and cleaned. If the baby responds then no further resuscitation is required. If not, then lung inflation should be started.
- **Blue or white, apneic and slow (<60/minute) or absent heart rate**: Whether the baby is in primary or terminal apnea, the initial management is the same. Airway should be opened and lungs then inflated. A reassessment of response to heart rate should direct further resuscitation. White color, apnea and low or absent heart rate suggests *terminal apnea*.

Depending upon the above assessment the resuscitation follows **a**irway, **b**reathing, **c**irculation and use of drugs in selected cases.

- **Airway:** Baby should be positioned with the head in 'neutral' position as over extension may collapse the newborn baby's pharyngeal airway just as the flexion will. A folded towel placed under the neck and shoulder may help to maintain the airway in a neutral position and a '**jaw thrust**' may be required to bring the tongue forward and open the airway if the baby is floppy. Gentle suction of nares and oropharynx with a soft suction catheter may stimulate respiration. Blind deep pharyngeal suction should be avoided as it may cause bradycardia and laryngospasm by stimulating the vagus nerve. Meconium stained babies should be intubated and meconium should be aspirated from trachea using the endotracheal tube as a suction catheter. However, while attempting to clear the airway, if the heart rate falls below 60 beats per minute then airway clearance should be stopped and lung inflation should be started.
- **Breathing:** The first 5 breaths should be **inflation breaths**. These should be 2–3 seconds sustained breaths using a continuous oxygen supply, a pressure limiting device and a mask. Mask should be transparent, circular, soft and big enough to cover the nose and mouth of the baby. If no system is available then **a 500 ml self inflating bag** and a blow of valve set at 30–40 cmH_2O can be used. The chest may not move during the first 1–3 breaths as the fluid is displaced. Once the chest is inflated heart rate should be reassessed. Air entry should be assessed by chest movement and not by auscultation because in fluid filled lungs, breath sounds may be heard without lung inflation. It is safe to assume that the chest has been inflated successfully if the heart rate increases. The ventilation should be continued at a rate of 30–40 breaths per minute. Most babies can be resuscitated using a mask system and only 1 in 500 babies actually need endotracheal intubation. *However*, endotracheal intubation remains the gold standard in airway management. A normal full term newborn usually requires a 3.5 mm endotracheal tube, but 3.0 and 2.5 mm tubes should also be available.

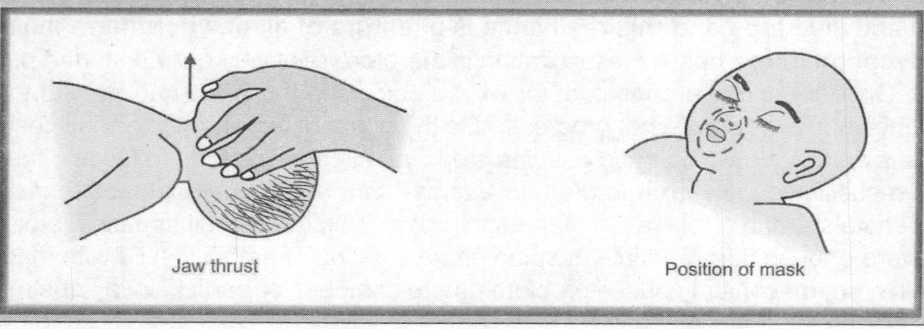

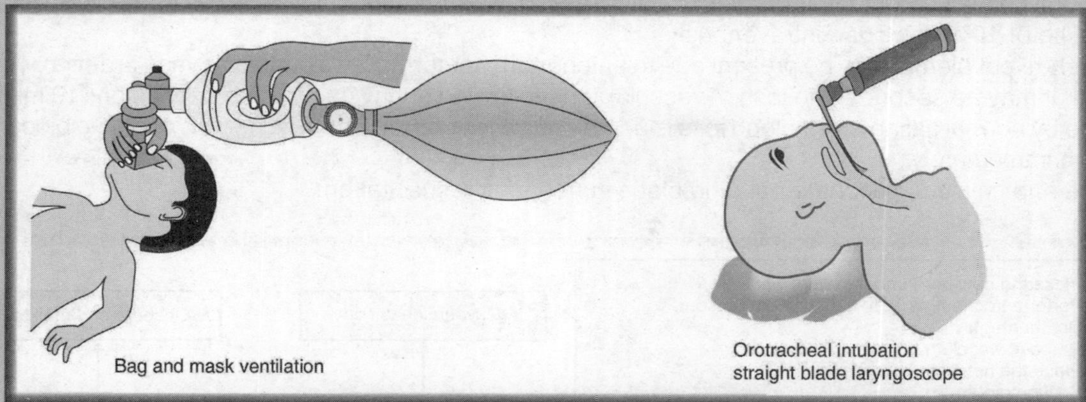

- **Circulation:** If the heart rate remains below 60 per minute (once the lungs are inflated), cardiac compression should be started. The most efficient way of doing this in a neonate is to encircle the chest with both ends, so that the fingers lie behind the baby and the thumbs are apposed on the sternum just below the inter-nipple line. Compress the chest briskly, by one third of its depth. Current advice is to perform 3 cardiac compressions for each inflation of the chest. Once the heart rate is above 60 and rising, cardiac compression can be discontinued.

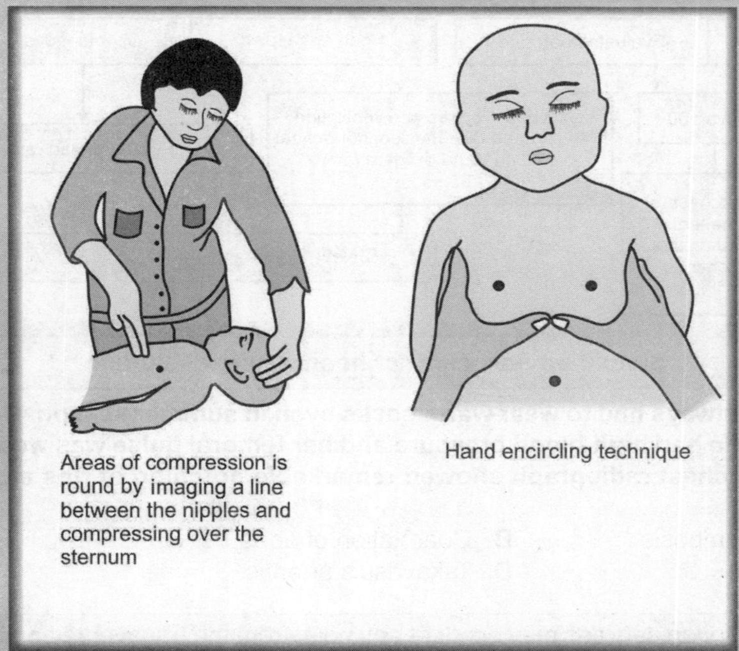

- **Drug therapy:** It should be considered only if after adequate lung inflation and cardiac compression, the heart rate has not responded. However, the *most common* reason for failure of the heart rate to respond is failure to achieve proper lung inflation. Airway and breathing must be reassessed before proceeding to drug therapy. Venous access will be required via an umbilical venous catheter as drugs should be given 'centrally'. The outcome is poor if drugs are required for resuscitation.
  - In the presence of profound unresponsive bradycardia or cardiac standstill, 10 microgram per kg (0.1 ml/kg; 1: 10,000) **adrenaline** may be given intravenously or via endotracheal tube. Further doses of 0.1–0.3 ml/kg of 1: 10,000 adrenaline may be tried at 5-minute intervals if there is no response.
  - Babies with terminal apnea will have a significant metabolic acidosis. Acidosis depresses cardiac function and prevents binding of adrenaline to the receptors. **Sodium bicarbonate** 1 mmol/kg (2 ml/kg of 4.2% solution) is used to raise the pH and enhance the effects of oxygen and epinephrine. However, bicarbonate use remains controversial and should only be used in the absence of apparent cardiac output, or in profound or unresponsive bradycardia.

- Hypoglycemia is a 'potential' problem for all stressed or asphyxiated babies and is treated by a slow bolus of 5 ml/kg of **10% dextrose** intravenously.
- *Rarely* hypovolemia may be present due to antepartum hemorrhage, placenta or vasa praevia or unclamped cord. It may be secondary to loss of vascular tone following asphyxia. Volume expansion (10 ml/kg) can be done by normal saline and if blood loss is acute and severe *non-cross matched 'O' negative* blood should be given immediately.

Atropine and calcium gluconate have no place in neonatal resuscitation.

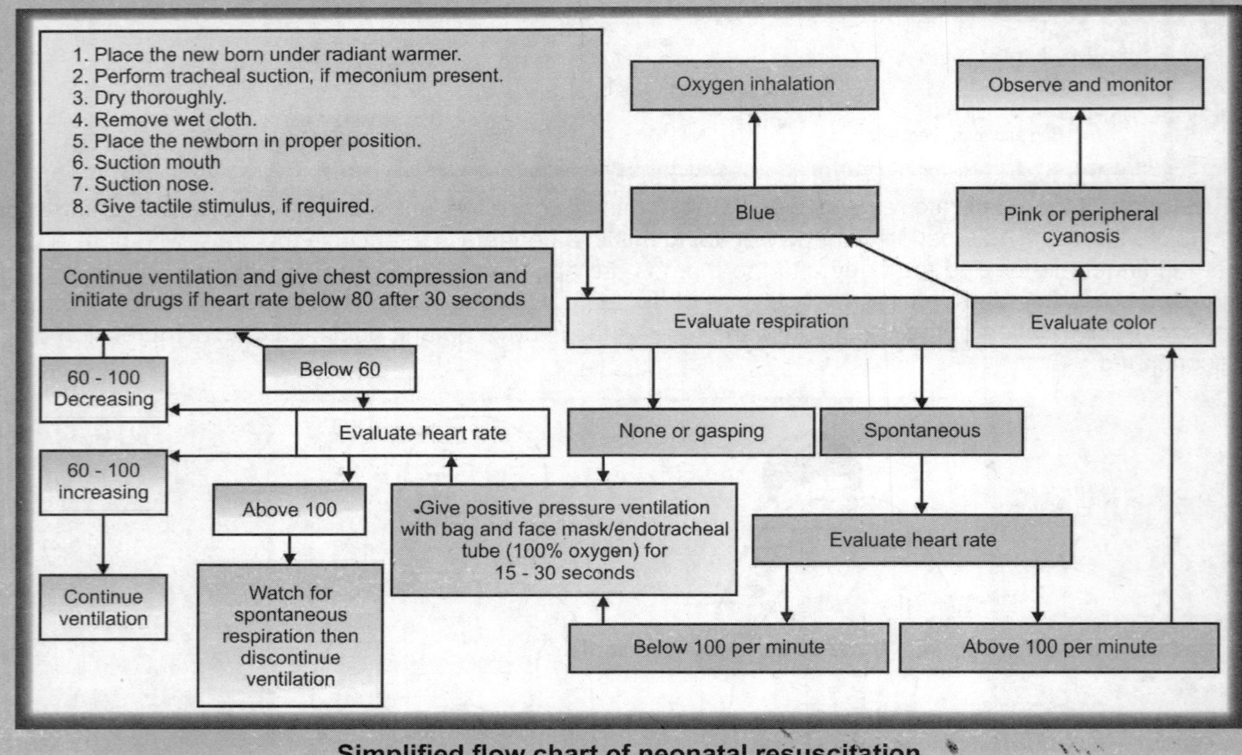

Simplified flow chart of neonatal resuscitation

607. A 4 ½-year girl child always had to wear warm socks even in summer season. On physical examination, it was noticed that she had high blood pressure and her femoral pulse was weak as compared to radial and carotid pulse. A chest radiograph showed remarkable notching of ribs along their lower borders. This was due to:

A. Femoral artery thrombosis **B.** Coarctation of aorta
C. Raynaud's disease **D.** Takayasu's arteritis *(AIIMS Nov 2002)*

Coarctation of aorta of varying degrees may occur at any point from the transverse aortic arch to the iliac bifurcation but **98% occur just below the origin of left subclavian artery** at the junction of ductus arteriosus (juxtaductal coarctation).

608. ***Most common*** **cause of neonatal sepsis is:**

A. *Staphylococcus aureus* **B.** Group B *Streptococcus*
C. *Klebsiella pneumoniae* **D.** *Listeria monocytogenes* *(UP 2003)*

609. ***Most common*** **cause of neonatal meningitis is:**

A. *Escherichia coli*
B. *Clostridia*
C. *Listeria monocytogenes*
D. *Streptococcus pneumoniae* *(SGPGI 2003)*

Bacterial sepsis and **meningitis** continue to be a major cause of morbidity and mortality in the newborn infants. Sepsis neonatorum can be devastating and surviving infants can have significant neurological sequelae as a consequence of CNS involvement, septic shock, or hypoxemia secondary to severe parenchymal lung disease or persistent pulmonary hypertension of newborn (PPHN). The overall incidence of sepsis neonatorum varies between 1 to 8 cases per 1000 birth. About 1/3rd of the septic newborns develop meningitis. The 'risk factors' can be divided between *maternal* and *neonatal* factors. The maternal risk factors are premature onset of labor, premature rupture of membranes (PROM), and maternal peripartum infection. The single most important neonatal risk factor is low birth weight (LBW). **Group B streptococcus (GBS) is the *most common* cause of neonatal sepsis and meningitis** in USA. *Escherichia coli* K_1 has been recognized as the *2nd most* prevalent cause of neonatal sepsis and meningitis in previous decades. *Listeria monocytogenes* is another important cause of neonatal sepsis and meningitis. [1] However in India *Klebsiella pneumoniae* (30%), *Staphylococcus aureus* (13%) and *Escherichia coli* (12.2%) are the main organisms responsible for neonatal sepsis. If the disease occurs within the first week it is known as **early onset sepsis** and if it occurs between 8-28 days it is known as **late onset sepsis**. Mortality is 15 - 50% in early onset sepsis and 10 -15% in late onset sepsis. Microbiological etiology of neonatal sepsis varies in different parts of the world and often changes over the years.

[1] Neonatal morbidity and mortality. Report of the National Neonatal Perinatal Database. *Indian Pediatr 1999;* **36:** 167-169.

610. The umbilical cord contains:

A. 1 umbilical artery and 2 veins
B. 1 umbilical artery and 1 vein
C. 2 umbilical arteries and 1 vein
D. 2 umbilical arteries and 2 veins

(SGPGI 2003)

The **umbilical cord contains 2 umbilical arteries, 1 umbilical vein**, the rudimentary allantois, remnant of omphalomesenteric duct, and a gelatinous substance called Wharton's jelly. The 'muscular' umbilical arteries contract readily, but the vein does not. The umbilical vein retains a fairly large lumen after birth. The blood vessels are 'functionally' closed but are patent 'anatomically' for the first 10–20 days of life. Umbilical cord usually sloughs within 2 weeks of life. Delayed separation of cord (> 1 month) has been associated with neutrophil chemotactic defect and overwhelming bacterial infection. Single umbilical artery is found in about 5–10 per 1000 live births; 35–70 per thousand twin births. 33% of newborns with a single umbilical artery have congenital abnormalities, usually more than 1, and many such infants are stillborn or die shortly after birth. Trisomy 18 (Edward's syndrome) is 1 of the most frequent abnormalities. It is important that at every delivery the cut cord and the maternal and fetal surfaces of the placenta be inspected and the number of arteries present should be recorded. Renal USG is recommended, by some authors, for infants with a single umbilical artery. Unilateral renal agenesis is found with increased frequency in newborns with a single umbilical artery. Bilateral renal agenesis is incompatible with extra-uterine life and death occurs shortly after birth (Potter syndrome).

611. Which one of the following statements is *false* with regard in Xanthogranulomatous pyelonephritis in children?

A. Often affects those younger than 8 years of age
B. It affects the kidney focally more frequently than diffusely
C. Boys are affected more frequently
D. Clinical presentation in children is same as in adults

(AI 2003)

Xanthogranulomatous pyelonephritis (XGP) is a serious, debilitating illness characterized by an infectious renal phlegmon. This disease process shares many characteristics with a true neoplasm in terms of its radiographic appearance and ability to involve adjacent structures or organs. Patients are often immunocompromised. XGP is defined as a chronic inflammatory disorder of the kidney characterized by **a mass originating in the renal parenchyma**. The condition has a common association with *Proteus* or *Escherichia coli* infection. *Pseudomonas* species have also been implicated. The kidney is usually nonfunctional. Although **most cases of XGP are unilateral**, bilateral disease has been reported. XGP occurs in approximately 1% of all renal infections. Although it is **rare in the pediatric population**, its incidence in pediatric nephrectomy specimens is approximately 16%. **XGP is 4 times more common in women than men** and is usually noted in the fifth and sixth decades of life.

612. Role of glucose in ORS is:

A. Energy source
B. Taste to ORS
C. Non-specific
D. Carries Na^+ into cell

(MANIPAL 2001)

Oral rehydration is only possible if glucose is added to the salts because there is absorption of sodium ions along with glucose due to glucose facilitated sodium ion absorption (co-transport).

Ingredients	Bicarbonate ORS	Citrate ORS
• **Glucose**	111mmol/L	111 mmol/L
• **Sodium ions**	90 mmol/L	90 mmol/L
• **Chloride ions**	80 mmol/L	80 mmol/L
• **Bicarbonate ions**	30 mmol/L	Nil
• **Potassium ions**	20 mmol/L	20 mmol/L
• **Citrate**	Nil	10 mmol/L

613. A boy presents with bilateral nasal polyps. X-ray shows opacity in the para-nasal sinus region. All the following can be given as treatment *except*:

A. Antihistamines
B. Intranasal corticosteroids
C. Amphotericin B
D. Epinephrine

(AIIMS May 2002)

Local or systemic **decongestants** are usually not effective in shrinking the polyps although they may provide some symptomatic relief from associated mucosal edema. Intranasal **steroid sprays** and systemic steroids may bring about dramatic shrinkage of nasal polyps and have proved useful in children with cystic fibrosis. Polyps should be removed surgically if complete obstruction, uncontrolled rhinorrhea, or deformity of nose appears. If the underlying pathogenic mechanism cannot be eliminated (as is the case with cystic fibrosis) the polyps soon return. Functional endoscopic sinus surgery may provide more complete polyp removal and reduce the need of frequent surgeries. Antrochoanal polyps must be surgically removed and they do not respond to medical measure.

Further reading: *Nelson Textbook of Pediatrics; 17th edition; page 1388 - 1389*

614. A five-day-old, full term male infant was severely cyanotic at birth. Prostaglandin E was administered initially and later balloon atrial septostomy was done which showed improvement in oxygenation. The *most likely* diagnosis of this infant is:

A. Tetralogy of Fallot
B. Transposition of great vessels
C. Truncus arteriosus
D. Tricuspid atresia

(AI 2004)

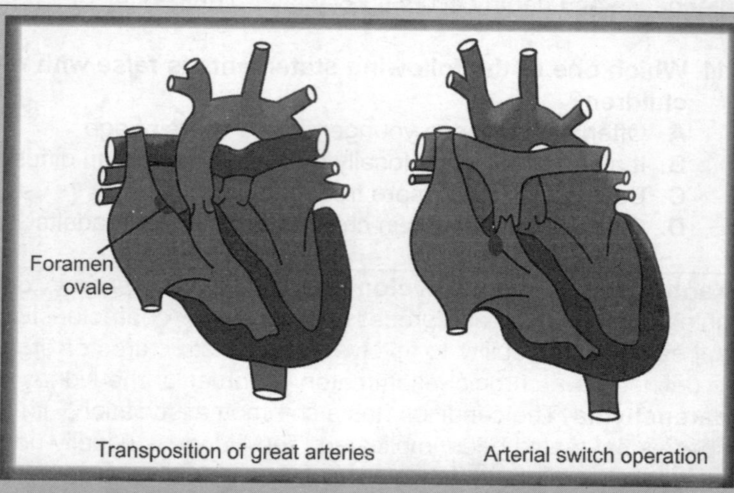

In **transposition of great arteries** (TGA) the aorta arises from right ventricle and pulmonary artery from left ventricle. 50% of patients have an associated VSD (leading to ejection systolic murmur). In patients with an intact interventricular septum a communication is *must* either as PDA or as patent foramen ovale (PFO). The **newborn is clinically cyanosed within few hours of life** due to mixing of oxygenated and deoxygenated blood. Initial management consists of:

1. Make certain that there is adequate mixing between 2 parallel circuits (PGE_1 infusion).
2. Maximization of mixed venous oxygen saturation.

Foramen ovale

Transposition of great arteries

Arterial switch operation

If the patient does not respond to the above measures foramen ovale should be enlarged by balloon atrial septostomy (Rashkind procedure). In this procedure a deflated balloon is inserted into a vein, passed through the foramen ovale, and then inflated and pulled vigorously through the atrial septum to enlarge the opening and improve oxygenation of the blood. Definitive management consists of surgical correction with an **arterial switch operation** (Jatene procedure) in early neonatal period.

615. Webbing of neck, increased carrying angle, low posterior hair line and short fourth metacarpal are characteristics of:

A. Noonan syndrome
B. Cri du chat syndrome
C. Turner syndrome
D. Klinefelter syndrome *(AI 2004)*

Gonadal dysgenesis (**Turner syndrome**) is characterized by primary amenorrhea, sexual infantilism, short stature, multiple congenital anomalies, and bilateral streak gonads in phenotypic women with any of several defects of the X chromosome. The associated anomalies involve the skeleton and connective tissue. Lymphedema of the hands and feet, webbing of the neck, low hairline, redundant skin folds on the back of the neck, a shield-like chest with widely spaced nipples, and growth retardation are features that suggest the diagnosis in infancy.

Ref: *Harrison's Principles of Internal Medicine; 14th edition*

616. A 10-month-old child presents with 2 weeks' history of fever, vomiting and alteration of sensorium. Cranial CT scan reveals basal exudates and hydrocephalus. The *most likely* etiological agent is:

A. *Mycobacterium tuberculosis*
B. *Streptococcus pneumoniae*
C. *Listeria monocytogenes*
D. *Cryptococcus neoformans* *(AI 2004)*

Tuberculosis of the CNS is the *most serious* complication of *Mycobacterium tuberculosis* infection in children and is fatal without effective treatment. Tuberculous meningitis (TBM) arises from the formation of a metastatic caseous lesion in the cerebral cortex or meninges which develop during lympho-hematogenous dissemination of the primary infection. This initial lesion increases in size and discharges small numbers of *Mycobacterium tuberculosis* into the subarachnoid space. This results in gelatinous exudate formation infiltrating the cortico-meningeal blood vessels, producing inflammation, obstruction and subsequent infarction of the cerebral cortex. Brainstem is the site of 'greatest' involvement resulting in dysfunction of third, sixth and seventh cranial nerves. These exudates also block the normal flow of CSF in and out of the ventricular system at the level of basilar cisterns producing communicating hydrocephalus. This combination of vasculitis, infarction, cerebral edema and hydrocephalus results in severe damage to the CNS leading to profound impairment.

Ref: *Nelson Textbook of Pediatrics; 17th edition; page 965*

617. All are the features of absence seizures *except*:

A. Usually seen in childhood
B. 3 Hz spike wave in EEG
C. Postictal confusion
D. Precipitation by hyperventilation *(AI 2004)*

Absence seizures: Simple (typical) absence (petit-mal) seizures are characterized by a sudden cessation of motor activity or speech with a blank facial expression and flickering of the eyelids. These seizures are not common before 5 years of age; more common in girls; never associated with an aura; rarely persist longer than 30 seconds; and **not associated with a postictal state**. Children may experience 'countless' seizures daily, whereas CPS are usually less frequent. Children do not loose body tone, but their head may fall forward slightly. Immediately after the absence seizure patient resumes pre-seizure activity with no indication of any postictal impairment. Simple absence seizure is frequently accompanied by automatic behavior. Hyperventilation for 3 – 4 minutes routinely 'produces' an absence seizure. The EEG demonstrates a typical 3 second spike and generalized wave discharge. Complex (atypical) absence seizures have an associated motor component consisting of myoclonic movement of the face, fingers or extremities and sometimes loss of body tone.

618. A 5-year-old girl came with history of progressively increasing pallor since birth and hepatosplenomegaly. Which of the following is the *most relevant* test for achieving diagnosis?

A. Hemoglobin electrophoresis
B. Bone marrow examination
C. Osmotic fragility test
D. Peripheral smear examination *(AI 2004)*

The newborn infant with **beta thalassemia major** is not anemic and the onset of anemia is insidious. The pallor is obvious within the first year of life. The child fails to thrive, and anorexia, diarrhea, loss of body fat, and recurrent episodes of fever are common. The severe anemia usually results in cardiac dilatation. Splenomegaly is obvious by the age of 3-years. Moderate to marked hepatomegaly is also present. In **hemoglobin electrophoresis**, the predominant hemoglobin is fetal hemoglobin, constituting 10 – 98% of the total.

Ref: *de Gruchy's Clinical Hematology in Medical Practice; 5th edition; page 157*

619. A 5-year-old child presents with history of fever off and on for past 2 weeks and petechial spots all over the body and increasing pallor for past 1 month. Examination reveals splenomegaly of 2 cm below costal margin. The most likely diagnosis is:

A. Acute leukemia
B. Idiopathic thrombocytopenic purpura
C. Hypersplenism
D. Aplastic anemia *(AI 2004)*

About 66% of children with ALL have signs and symptoms of their disease for <1month at the time of diagnosis; first symptoms are usually nonspecific and may include anorexia, irritability and lethargy. Progressive **bone marrow failure** leads to pallor, bleeding, petechiae and fever. *On examination* the child is pale and about 50% having petechiae or mucus membrane bleeding. About 25% have fever; which may be 'falsely' ascribed to an URTI or otitis media. Lymphadenopathy is occasionally prominent; splenomegaly is found in 60% of patients, whereas hepatomegaly is less common. 25% of patients present with significant bone pain and arthralgias cause by infiltration of the perichondral bone or joints by leukemic cells or by leukemic expansion of the marrow cavity. *Rarely* signs of increased intracranial pressure such as headache and vomiting indicate leukemic meningeal involvement. Children with **T-cell ALL** are likely to be older and are more often males; may have an **anterior mediastinal mass** (a feature that is strongly associated with this subtype of disease).

620. All of the following are neural tube defects except:

A. Holoprosencephaly
B. Encephalocele
C. Anencephaly
D. Myelomeningocele *(AI 2004)*

Neural tube defects (dysraphism) account for *most* congenital anomalies of the CNS. The major NTDs include spina bifida occulta, meningocele, myelomeningocele, encephalocele, anencephaly, dermal sinus, tethered cord, syringomyelia, diastematomyelia and lipoma involving the conus medullaris.

Ref: *Nelson Textbook of Pediatrics; 17th edition; page 1983*

621. Bone marrow transplantation can be used as a treatment for all *except*:

A. Hemochromatosis
B. Hurler's syndrome
C. Adrenoleukodystrophy
D. Osteopetrosis *(AI 2004)*

Indications of bone marrow transplant	
Acquired disorders	**Inherited disorders**
• Aplastic anemia • Acute myelogenous leukemia • Acute lymphocytic leukemia • Myelodysplatic and myeloproliferative disorders • Lymphomas • Neuroblastoma • Brain tumor • Solid tumors	• Immunodeficiency disorders • Fanconi anemia • Storage diseases (adrenoleukodystrophy, Hurler syndrome) • Thalassemia • Sickle cell disease • Other congenital anemias
Ref: *Nelson Textbook of Pediatrics; 17th edition; page 732*	
Allogeneic bone marrow transplantation should be a successful therapy for any genetic disorder involving the immunologic or hematopoietic system. Examples include the reversal of infantile malignant osteopetrosis, Gaucher's disease, infantile metachromatic leukodystrophy, and X-linked adrenoleukodystrophy.	

Ref: *Harrison's Principles of Internal Medicine; 14th edition*

622. The *most common* underlying anomaly in a child with recurrent urinary tract infection is:

A. Posterior urethral valves
B. Vesicoureteral reflux
C. Neurogenic bladder
D. Renal calculi *(AIIMS Nov 2003)*

The *most common* cause of severe obstructive uropathy in children is posterior urethral valves. This is seen only in boys; incidence is 1 in 8000 boys. These urethral 'valves' are tissue leaflets fanning distally from the posterior urethra to the external urinary sphincter. Typically the leaflets are separated by a slit like opening. About 30% of patients develop end stage renal disease (ESRD) or chronic renal insufficiency; posterior urethra dilates and the bladder muscle undergoes hypertrophy. Vesicoureteral reflux (VUR) occurs in 50% of patients.

623. Retardation of skeletal maturity can be caused by all *except*:

A. Chronic renal failure
B. Congenital adrenal hyperplasia
C. Protein energy malnutrition (PEM)
D. Hypothyroidism

(AI 2004)

- Bone age correlates well with stage of pubertal development and can be helpful in predicting adult height in adolescence. In familial short stature, the bone age is normal (comparable to chronological age). In constitutional delay, endocrinologic short stature (growth hormone deficiency and hypothyroidism), and under nutrition, the bone age is low and comparable to the height age. Bone age is assessed by X-rays of wrist and elbow.
- In **congenital adrenal hyperplasia** the excessive androgen levels result in accelerated growth, so that **bone age exceeds chronologic age.** Since epiphyseal closure is hastened by excessive androgens, growth stops, but truncal development continues, the characteristic appearance being a short child with a well-developed trunk.

Endocrine causes of proportionate short stature of post-natal onset

- Hypopituitarism
- Hypothyroidism
- Hypogonadism
- Diabetes mellitus
- Cushing's syndrome

624. A 7-year-old boy presented with generalized edema:

A. Fusion of foot processes of the glomerular epithelial cells
B. Rarefaction of glomerular basement membrane
C. Deposition of electron dense material in the basement membrane
D. Thin basement membrane

(AIIMS Nov 2003)

About 90% of children with nephrotic syndrome have 'idiopathic' nephrotic syndrome which includes 3 histological subtypes. Minimal change disease accounts for 85% of these cases and the glomeruli appear normal or show a minimal increase in mesangial cells and matrix. Electron microscopy reveals effacement of the epithelial cell foot processes

Ref: *Nelson Textbook of Pediatrics; 17th edition; page 1755*

625. A 2-month-old child is able to:

A. Show a positive parachute protective reflex
B. Hold head steady in a seated position
C. Sustain head level with the body when placed in ventral suspension
D. Lift head and chest off a flat surface

(AI 2004)

Behavior pattern at 8 week	
Prone	Raises head slightly farther; head sustained in plane of body on ventral suspension
Supine	Tonic neck posture predominates; head lags on pull to sitting position
Visual	Follows moving object 180 degrees
Social	Smiles on social contact; listens to voice and coos

Ref: *Nelson Textbook of Pediatrics; 17th edition; page 34*

626. A 7-year-old boy with left renal mass had bone pain and was detected to have bone metastatic deposits. The *most likely* renal tumor is:

A. Favorable histology Wilms' tumor
B. Renal cell carcinoma
C. Clear cell sarcoma
D. Rhabdoid tumor

(AIIMS Nov 2004)

Clear cell sarcoma of the kidney (CCSK), an uncommon renal neoplasm of childhood, represents one of the most common tumors with "unfavorable histology" listed in the National Wilms Tumor Study Group (NWTSG) clinical protocols. CCSK is extremely rare in infants younger than 6 months and in young adults. Most patients are aged 1 to4 years. A male predominance exists. Fifty percent of cases are diagnosed in children aged 2 to 3 years. **Age of presentation ranges from 2 months to 14 years**, with a mean age of 36 months. Using the Fifth National Wilms Tumor Study (NWTS-5) criteria for tumor staging, 25% of patients had localized stage I tumors, most patients presented with stage II (37%) or stage III (34%) disease, and only 4% of patients presented with distant metastases. The most common site of metastasis at the time of presentation in patients with CCSK is the ipsilateral renal hilar lymph nodes. Skip metastases to periaortic lymph nodes have been reported in patients with CCSK in the presence of hilar lymph nodes that were histologically confirmed with negative results. Only 4% of patients present with distant metastases. **Bone is the *most common* site of metastases** (15%), followed closely by lung, abdomen, retroperitoneum, brain, and liver. Unusual soft tissue sites (scalp, epidural, nasopharynx, neck, paraspinal, ovary, abdominal wall, axilla) and other sites (orbit) have been reported. Approximately 20% of documented CCSK metastases occurred at least 3 years after diagnosis; some occurred as long as 10 years later. Manifestations in patients with CCSK are similar to those in patients with Wilms tumor. Patients present with an abdominal mass, which usually is identified by a caregiver or family relative who has not seen the child for a while. Often, abdominal swelling or the presence of an abdominal mass is noticed by a parent while bathing or dressing the child. Abdominal pain, gross hematuria, fever, and hypertension are other frequent findings.

Ref: *http://www.emedicine.com/ped/topic3018.html*

627. A 10-days-old neonate is posted for pyloric stenosis surgery. The investigation report shows a serum calcium level of 6 mg/dl. What information would you like to know before you supplement calcium to this neonate?

A. Blood glucose
B. Serum protein
C. Serum bilirubin
D. Oxygen saturation

(AIIMS Nov 2004)

In general, the total calcium provides a satisfactory assessment of physiologic calcium. However, there are a few clinical situations in which the total serum calcium is not an adequate substitute for the ionized calcium concentration. The *most common* and severe problem is in the presence of hypoalbuminemia, such as patients with nephrotic syndrome, liver disease, capillary leak, or protein-loosing enteropathy. Each 1 gm/dl of albumin in the serum binds about 0.8 mg/dl of calcium.

$_{(Corrected)}$ calcium = Total calcium $_{(measured)}$ + [0.8 x (decrease in albumin concentration below normal in g/dL)]

Ref: *Nelson Textbook of Pediatrics; 17th edition; page 208 and 209*

628. Deficiency of enzyme α-ketoacid dehydrogenase leading to a block in the metabolism of branch amino acids is observed in:

A. Maple syrup urine disease
B. Hartnup's disease
C. Alkaptonuria
D. Phenylketonuria

(AIIMS May 2005)

Decarboxylation of leucine, isoleucine, and valine is accomplished by a complex enzyme system (branched-chain **alpha-ketoacid dehydrogenase**). Deficiency of this enzyme system causes **maple syrup urine disease**.

Ref: *Nelson Textbook of Pediatrics; 17th edition; page 409*

629. All of the following are features of absence seizures, *except*:

A. Usually seen in childhood
B. 3-Hz spike wave in EEG
C. Postictal confusion
D. Precipitation by hyperventilation

(AIIMS May 2005)

A sudden cessation of motor activity or speech with a blank facial expression and flickering of eyelids characterize **typical absence seizures**. These seizures are uncommon before the age of 5 years and are more common in girls. They are never associated with an aura and rarely persist longer than 30 seconds. **They are *not* associated with a postictal state.** Hyperventilation for 3 to 4 minutes routinely produces absence seizure. The EEG shows a typical 3 per second spike and generalized wave discharge.

Ref: *Nelson Textbook of Pediatrics; 17th edition; page 1997*

630. A continuous murmur is heard in all of the following conditions, *except:*

A. Ventricular septal defect with aortic regurgitation
B. Patent ductus arteriosus
C. Coronary arteriovenous fistula
D. Venous hum *(AIIMS May 2005)*

Some causes of continuous murmur

- *Patent ductus arteriosus*
- Surgically produced connections
- Small atrial septal defect with a high left atrial pressure
- Subclavius-pulmonary artery anastomosis
- Pulmonary arteriovenous fistulas
- Congenital or acquired systemic arteriovenous fistula
- *Coronary arteriovenous fistula*
- Anomalous origin of the left coronary artery from the pulmonary artery
- Cervical *venous hum*
- Communications between the sinus of Valsalva and the right side of the heart

631. All of the following are *true* about manifestations of vitamin E deficiency, *except*:

A. Hemolytic anemia
B. Posterior column abnormalities
C. Cerebellar ataxia
D. Autonomic dysfunction *(AI 2005)*

Patient with malabsorption and **vitamin E deficiency** secondary to biliary atresia develop a degenerative, potentially reversible, neurological syndrome consisting of **cerebellar ataxia**, peripheral neuropathy, and **posterior column abnormalities**. Some premature infants with low serum levels of tocopherol develop **hemolytic anemia** between 6 to10 weeks of age that is correctable by administration of vitamin E.

Ref: *Nelson Textbook of Pediatrics; 17th edition; page 189*

632. The *most common* malignant neoplasm of infancy is:

A. Malignant teratoma
B. Neuroblastoma
C. Wilms' tumor
D. Hepatoblastoma *(AI 2005)*

Neuroblastoma comprises 8 to 10% of all childhood cancers and is the *most common* extracranial solid tumor in children and ***most common* solid tumor in infants**. Peak incidence is at 2 years of age and is very rare after 10 years of age. Sometimes it is congenital with metastases to placenta.

Ref: *IAP Textbook of Pediatrics; 2nd edition; page 564*

633. The *most common* presentation of a child with Wilms' tumor is:

A. An asymptomatic abdominal mass
B. Hematuria
C. Hypertension
D. Hemoptysis due to pulmonary secondary *(AI 2005)*

Wilms' tumor is the *most common* primary malignant renal tumor of childhood comprising 5 to 6% of childhood cancers. It is slightly more frequent in girls than in boys. The median age of presentation is 4 years for unilateral tumors and 2 ½ years for bilateral tumors. An abdominal tumor appears which grows rapidly while the general well being of the child deteriorates. Fever, hematuria are other important features.

Ref: *IAP Textbook of Pediatrics; 2nd edition; page 562 and Bailey and Love's Short Practice of Surgery; 23rd edition; page 1196*

634. The *most common* site of leak in CSF rhinorrhea is:

A. Sphenoid sinus
B. Frontal sinus
C. Cribriform plate
D. Tegmen tympani *(AI 2005)*

Cerebrospinal fluid also may leak through the **cribriform plate** or the adjacent sinus and present as a watery discharge from the nose (CSF rhinorrhea).

Ref: *Harrison's Principles of Internal Medicine; 14th edition*

635. The *most common* type of total anomalous pulmonary venous connection is:

A. Supracardiac **B.** Infracardiac
C. Mixed **D.** Cardiac *(AI 2005)*

Total anomalous pulmonary venous connection occurs when all pulmonary veins drain into the systemic venous system with complete mixing of pulmonary and systemic venous return, usually in the right atrium. The systemic blood flow is therefore dependent on an *obligate* shunt through the patent foramen oval (PFO) into the left side of the heart. The anomalous connections of the pulmonary veins may be **supracardiac, cardiac, subdiaphragmatic or mixed.**

Ref: *Manual of Neonatal Care by John P Cloherty MD; 4th Edition; page 427*

Site of connection	Percentage
Supracardiac	50
o Left superior vena cava	40
o Right superior vena cava	10
Cardiac	25
o Coronary sinus	20
o Right atrium	05
Infracardiac	20
Mixed	05

Ref: *Nelson Textbook of Pediatrics; 17th edition; page 1539*

636. Diagnosis of beta thalassemia is established by:

A. NESTROFT test **B.** Hemoglobin A1C estimation
C. Hemoglobin electrophoresis **D.** Target cells in peripheral smear *(AI 2005)*

Thalassemias are the *most common* genetic disorder on worldwide basis. The infant is born only with Hb F or in some cases Hb F and Hb E. [1] **Hemoglobin electrophoresis is diagnostic.**[2]

[1]Ref: *Nelson Textbook of Pediatrics; 17th edition; page 1630*
[2]Ref: *IAP Textbook of Pediatrics; 2nd edition; page 506*

637. Blood specimen for neonatal thyroid screening is obtained on:

A. Cord blood
B. 24 hours after birth
C. 48 hours after birth
D. 72 hours after birth *(AI 2005)*

Obtaining early TSH measurements has increased the false-positive rate for congenital hypothyroidism (CH) screening. Since T_4 is also elevated on day one and two of life, mild cases of CH may be missed. It is recommended by Massachusetts State Newborn Screening Program to test at 3 to 4 days of life.

Ref: *Manual of Neonatal Care by John P Cloherty MD; 4th Edition; page 23*

638. The appropriate approach to a neonate presenting with vaginal bleeding on day 4 of life is:

A. Administration of vitamin K
B. Investigation for bleeding disorder
C. No specific therapy
D. Administration of 10 ml/kg of fresh frozen plasma over 4 hours *(AI 2005)*

About 20 to 25% female babies may develop menstruation like withdrawal **vaginal bleeding** after 4 to 5 days of birth. The bleeding is usually mild and lasts for 2 to 4 days. It does not need any specific therapy apart from local aseptic cleaning of genitals.

Ref: *IAP Textbook of Pediatrics; 2nd edition; page 59*

639. A child with recurrent urinary tract infections is *most likely* to show:

A. Posterior urethral valves
B. Vesicoureteric reflux
C. Neurogenic bladder
D. Renal and ureteric calculi *(AI 2005)*

640. The *most common* cause of renal scarring in a 3-year-old child is:

A. Trauma
B. Tuberculosis
C. Vesicoureteral reflux-induced pyelonephritis
D. Interstitial nephrites *(AI 2005)*

Urinary tract infections are common during childhood and are often associated with congenital anomalies of urinary tract and vesicoureteric reflux (VUR), which together constitute an important cause of CRF in children. During micturition **VUR** allows the rise in intravesical pressure to be transmitted to the ureter and renal pelvis, which enables urine to enter papillary collecting ducts and renal tubules (intrarenal reflux). Thus, pathogenic organisms present in the bladder urine reach the renal parenchyma and initiate inflammation with **subsequent scar formation**.

Ref: *IAP Textbook of Pediatrics; 2nd edition; page 480*

641. Which one of the following is the *common* cause of congenital hydrocephalus?

A. Craniosynostosis
B. Intrauterine meningitis
C. Aqueductal stenosis
D. Malformations of great vein of Galen *(AI 2005)*

Obstructing or noncommunicating hydrocephalus develops *most commonly* in children because of an **abnormality of the aqueduct** or a lesion in the 4th ventricle.

Ref: *Nelson Textbook of Pediatrics; 17th edition; page 1190*

642. Which one of the following drugs is used for *fetal therapy* of congenital adrenal hyperplasia?

A. Hydrocortisone
B. Prednisolone
C. Fludrocortisone
D. Dexamethasone *(AI 2005)*

In families with an affected infant with **congenital adrenal hyperplasia**, prenatal treatment is useful in subsequent pregnancies. The aim of prenatal treatment is to prevent external genital deformity in the female fetus due to virilization. As soon as pregnancy is confirmed, the mother is commenced on **oral dexamethasone 20 micrograms/kg/day in 3 divided doses**, even prior to the fetal diagnosis being established.

Ref: *IAP Textbook of Pediatrics; 2nd edition; page 601*

643. The coagulation profile in a 13-year-old girl with menorrhagia having von Willebrand's disease (vWD) is:

A. Isolated prolonged PTT with a normal PT
B. Isolated prolonged PT with a normal PTT
C. Prolongation of both PT and PTT
D. Prolongation of thrombin time *(AI 2005)*

Patients with **vWD** *were said to* have a long bleeding time and **a long PTT**. However these tests are frequently normal in patient with type I disease.

Ref: *Nelson Textbook of Pediatrics; 17th edition; page 1662*

644. Differential expression of same gene depending on parent of origin is referred to as:

A. Genomic imprinting **B.** Mosaicism
C. Anticipation **D.** Nonpenetrance *(AI 2005)*

Genomic imprinting means that phenotype expression depends on the parent of origin for certain genes and chromosome segments.

Ref: *Nelson Textbook of Pediatrics; 17th edition; page 390*

645. The chances of having an unaffected baby, when both parents have achondroplasia, are:

A. 0% **B.** 25%
C. 50% **D.** 100% *(AI 2005, AIIMS May 2004))*

All patient with typical **achondroplasia** have mutations at *FGFR3* codon 380. Achondroplasia is an autosomal dominant trait; most cases arise from a fresh mutation to normal parents. Due to high incidence of achondroplasia among dwarfs, it is relatively common for adults with achondroplasia to marry. **Such couples have 50% risk of transmitting their condition**, heterozygous achondroplasia, to each offspring, as well as a 25% risk for homozygous achondroplasia.

Ref: *Nelson Textbook of Pediatrics; 17th edition; page 2330*

646. All of the following therapies may be required in a 1 hour old infant with severe birth asphyxia, *except*:

A. Glucose **B.** Dexamethasone
C. Calcium gluconate **D.** Normal saline *(AI 2005)*

- Blood glucose level should be kept at 75 to 100 mg/dl to provide adequate substrate for the brain.
- Calcium level should be kept in a normal range because hypocalcemia is common metabolic problem.

Ref: *Manual of Neonatal Care by John P Cloherty MD; 4th Edition; page 523*

There is no role of dexamethasone, atropine, calcium and respiratory stimulants like nikethamide, lobeline, etc. in resuscitation.

Ref: *IAP Textbook of Pediatrics; 2nd edition; page 49*

647. Eisenmenger's syndrome is characterized by all, *except*:

A. Return of left ventricle and right ventricle to normal size
B. Pulmonary veins not distended
C. Pruning of peripheral pulmonary arteries
D. Dilatation of central pulmonary arteries *(AI 2005)*

The term **Eisenmenger's syndrome** is used for patients with a large communication between the two circulations at the aortopulmonary, ventricular, or atrial levels and bidirectional or predominantly right-to-left shunts due to high-resistance and obstructive pulmonary hypertension.

Ref: *Harrison's Principles of Internal Medicine; 14th edition*

648. The *best* time to do chorionic villus sampling is

A. Between 6 to 8 weeks **B.** Between 7 to 9 weeks
C. Between 9 to 11 weeks **D.** Between 11 to 13 weeks *(AIIMS May 2005)*

Chorionic villus sampling (CVS): A sample of placental tissue is obtained via catheter placed under ultrasonic guidance either transcervically or transabdominally. **Performed at 10 to 12 weeks' gestation, CVS provides the earliest possible detection of a genetically abnormal fetus through analysis of trophoblast cells.**

Ref: *Manual of Neonatal Care by John P Cloherty MD; 4th Edition; page 3*

649. All of the following are biochemical markers included for triple test, *except*:

A. Alfa-fetoprotein (AFP) **B.** Human chorionic gonadotropin (hCG)
C. Human placental Lactogen (HPL) **D.** Unconjugated estriol *(AIIMS Nov 2004, AIIMS May 2005)*

Low levels of **maternal serum alpha-fetoprotein (MSAFP)** may be associated with chromosomal abnormalities. Altered levels of **human chorionic gonadotropin (hCG)** and **unconjugated estriol (UE3)** also may be associated with fetal chromosomal abnormalities. A fetus with trisomy 21 results in hCG levels that are higher than expected and UE3 levels that are decreased. A **triple panel screen** in combination with maternal age can be used to estimate the risk of fetal trisomy 21 for an individual woman.

Ref: *Manual of Neonatal Care by John P Cloherty MD; 4th Edition; page 1 and 2*

650. When does 'switchover' from fetal to adult hemoglobin synthesis begin?

A. 14 weeks gestation
B. 30 weeks gestation
C. 36 weeks gestation
D. 7 to 10 days postnatal

(AIIMS Nov 2004, May 2005)

Hemoglobin A (Hb-A) comprises 97% of the hemoglobin of adult red cells. Small amounts of Hb-A are detected in the fetus as early as the 8th week of life. During the first few months of postnatal life, hemoglobin A completely replaces hemoglobin F, and the adult pattern is fully established by 6 months.

Hemoglobin F (Hb-F) is the major respiratory pigment from early intrauterine life up to term. It has a structural formula $\alpha_2\gamma_2$, with each gamma chain containing 146 amino acids and each alpha chain containing 141 amino acids. Gamma chains are of 2 types and are designated as $^G\gamma$ and $^A\gamma$ depending on whether they have glycine or alanine at position 136. **At term, Hb-F accounts for 70 to 90% of the total hemoglobin. It then falls rapidly to 25% at 1 month, and 5% at 6 months**. The adult level of about 1% is not reached in some children until puberty.

Ref: *de Gruchy's Clinical Hematology in Medical Practice; 5th edition; page 138*

651. Epiglottitis in a 2-year-old child occurs *most commonly* due to infection with:

A. Influenza virus
B. *Staphylococcus aureus*
C. *Haemophilus influenzae*
D. Respiratory syncytial virus

(AIIMS May 2005)

In the past, *Haemophilus influenzae* type b was the *most common* identified etiological agent of acute epiglottitis. Since the widespread use of HIB vaccine in USA, invasive disease due to *Haemophilus influenzae* type b in pediatric patients has been reduced by 80 to 90%. Therefore, other agents such as *Streptococcus pyogenes, Streptococcus pneumoniae,* and *Streptococcus aureus*, now represent a larger proportion of pediatric cases of epiglottitis.

Ref: *Nelson Textbook of Pediatrics; 17th edition; page 1405*

Acute epiglottitis is a serious condition and effects children 2 to 7 years of age. *Haemophilus influenzae* type b is the *most common* organism responsible for it in children.

Ref: *Diseases of Ear, Nose and Throat; PL Dhingra; 2nd edition; 5th impression 2001; page 283 and 284*

652. Which one of the following is the leading cause of mortality in under five children in developing countries?

A. Malaria
B. Acute lower respiratory tract infections
C. Hepatitis
D. Prematurity

(AIIMS May 2005)

UNICEF defines **under-5 mortality rate** as *annual number of deaths of children age less than five years, expressed as rate per 1000 live birth.*

Cause of death in 1000 in developing countries	1993
Acute respiratory infections	4110
Neonatal and Perinatal causes	3715
Diarrhea alone	2740
Malaria	940
Pertussis	360
Neonatal tetanus	290
Measles	290
Tuberculosis	280
Malnutrition	190
Accidents	170
HIV related	100

Ref: *Park's Textbook of Preventive and Social Medicine; 17th edition; page 397*

653. In which of the following conditions, aniridia and hemihypertrophy are *most likely* present?

A. Neuroblastoma **B.** Wilms' tumor
C. Non-Hodgkin's lymphoma **D.** Germ cell tumor *(AIIMS May 2004)*

Several syndromes, congenital abnormalities and chromosomal aberrations are associated with Wilms' tumor. **WAGR syndrome** comprises **W**ilms' tumor, **a**niridia, **g**enitourinary abnormalities and mental **r**etardation. The Beckwith-Wiedemann syndrome comprises hemihypertrophy, macroglossia and visceromegaly, with a risk of developing Wilms' tumor of 3 to 5 percent.

Ref: *Nelson Textbook of Pediatrics; 17th edition; page 1712*

654. The following cardiac defects are characterized by ductus dependent blood flow, *except*:

A. Transposition of great arteries with intact septum
B. Interrupted aortic arch
C. Truncus arteriosus
D. Hypoplastic left heart syndrome *(AIIMS May 2005)*

Transposition of great arteries is defined as an aorta arising from right ventricle and pulmonary artery from left ventricle. Fifty percent of these patients have an associated VSD. Following separation from the placenta, neonates with TGA are dependent on mixing between the parallel systemic and pulmonary circulations in order for them to survive. **In patients with an intact ventricular septum, this communication exists through the PDA and PFO.**

Ref: *Manual of Neonatal Care by John P Cloherty MD; 4th Edition; page 425*

Interrupted aortic arch consist of complete atresia of a segment of aortic arch. Three anatomical subtypes have been described; distal to subclavian artery (type-A), between left subclavian artery and left carotid artery (type-B), and between innominate artery and the left carotid artery (type-C). Type-B is the *most common* variety. Over 99% of these patients have a VSD. **Infants with interrupted aortic arch are completely dependent on a patent ductus arteriosus for the lower body blood flow**; thus they become critically ill when the ductus closes.

Ref: *Manual of Neonatal Care by John P Cloherty MD; 4th Edition; page 414 and 415*

Truncus arteriosus consists of a single 'great' artery arising from the heart that gives rise to (in order) the coronary arteries, the pulmonary arteries, and the brachiocephalic arteries. The coexisting VSD is present in more than 98% of cases. Extracardiac anomalies are present in 20 to 40% of cases and DiGeorge syndrome in one-third.

Ref: *Manual of Neonatal Care by John P. Cloherty MD; 4th Edition; page 427*

Hypoplastic left heart syndrome represents a heterogenous group of anatomical abnormalities in which there is a small or absent left ventricle with hypoplastic or atretic mitral and aortic valves. Resuscitation of these neonates involves pharmacological maintenance of ductual patency with PGE_1.

Ref: *Manual of Neonatal Care by John P Cloherty MD; 4th Edition; page 417*

655. Which of the following syndromes is *best* associated with congenital heart disease?

A. Lesch-Nyhan syndrome **B.** Rasmussen syndrome
C. Holt-Oram syndrome **D.** LEOPARD syndrome *(AIIMS May 2005)*

Syndromes associated with CHD

- CATCH 22 (DiGeorge syndrome, velocardiofacial syndrome)
- Familial ASD with heart block
- Alagille syndrome (bile duct hypoplasia, right sided cardiac lesions)
- **Holt-Oram syndrome** (limb defects and ASD)
- Trisomy 21 (AV septal defect)
- Familial TAPVR
- Noonan syndrome (PS, ASD, hypertrophic CMP)
- Ellis-van Creveld syndrome (polydactyly and ASD)
- Char syndrome (craniofacial, limb defects; PDA)
- Williams' syndrome (supravalvular AS, branch PS, hypercalcemia)
- Marfan syndrome (connective tissue weakness, aortic root dilation)
- Familial laterality abnormalities (situs inversus and complex CHD)

Ref: *Nelson Textbook of Pediatrics; 17th edition; page 1501*

656. Characteristic radiological feature of transient tachypnea of newborn is:

A. Reticulogranular appearance **B.** Low volume lungs
C. Prominent horizontal fissure **D.** Air bronchograms *(AIIMS May 2005)*

Transient tachypnea of newborn (TTN) or RDS type II usually follows uneventful normal preterm or term normal delivery or LSCS. It is characterized by early onset of tachypnea, sometimes with retractions, or expiratory grunting and, sometimes, cyanosis that is relieved by minimal oxygen (less than 40%). Child usually recover rapidly within 72 hours. Lung fields are clear without rales or rhonchi, and the CXR shows prominent pulmonary vascular markings, **fluid lines in the fissures**, over-inflation, flat diaphragm, and sometimes, pleural fluid. The distinctive features of TTN from HND are sudden recovery and absence of reticulogranular pattern or air bronchograms in CXR.

Ref: *Nelson Textbook of Pediatrics; 17th edition; page 583*

657. Which mechanism in phototherapy is *chiefly* responsible for reduction in serum bilirubin?

A. Photo-oxidation **B.** Photo-isomerization
C. Structural isomerization **D.** Conjugation *(AIIMS May 2005)*

Structural isomerization is the intramolecular cyclization of bilirubin to lumirubin. Lumirubin makes up to 2 to 6% of serum concentration of bilirubin during phototherapy and is rapidly excreted in the bile and urine without conjugation. Unlike photoisomerization, the conversion of bilirubin to lumirubin is irreversible, and it cannot be reabsorbed. **It is the most important pathway for the lowering of serum bilirubin levels** and is strongly related to the dose of phototherapy used in the range of 6 to 12 u W/cm^2/nm.

Ref: *Manual of Neonatal Care by John P Cloherty MD; 4th Edition; page 195*

658. Which of the following is *true* regarding mumps?

A. Salivary gland involvement is limited to the parotids
B. The patient is not infectious prior to clinical parotid enlargement
C. Meningoencephalitis can precede parotitis
D. Mumps orchitis frequently leads to infertility *(AIIMS May 2005)*

Mumps is an acute viral infection characterized by painful enlargement of the salivary glands, chiefly the parotids, as the usual presenting sign. Although, the parotid glands alone are affected in the majority of patients, swelling of the submandibular glands occur frequently and usually accompanies or closely follows that of the parotid glands. In 10 to 15 % of patients only the submandibular gland(s) may be swollen. The virus has been isolated from saliva as long as 6 days before and up to 9 days after the appearance of swelling in salivary glands. **Transmission *does not* seem to occur more than 24 hours before the appearance of swelling or later than 3 days after it has subsided.** Meningoencephalomyelitis is the *most frequent* complication of mumps in childhood. The pathogenesis of mumps meningoencephalitis may be either a primary infection of neurons or a postinfectious encephalitis with demyelination. In the first type, parotitis frequently appears at the same time or following the onset of encephalitis. In the later type, encephalitis follows parotitis by an average of 10 days. Parotitis may be in some cases absent. Aquaductal stenosis and hydrocephalus has been associated with mumps infection. Infertility is rare even with bilateral orchitis.

Ref: *Nelson Textbook of Pediatrics; 17th edition; page 1035 and 1036*

659. Bag and mask ventilation is *contraindicated* in:

A. Cleft lip **B.** Meconium aspiration
C. Diaphragmatic hernia **D.** Multicentric bronchogenic cyst *(AIIMS May 2004)*

Infants with diaphragmatic hernia and thickly meconium stained babies are electively incubated because bag and mask ventilation is contraindicated in these situations.

Ref: *IAP Textbook of Pediatrics; 2nd edition; page 49*

660. *Most appropriate* management for maintaining patency of ductus arteriosus in a neonate is:

A. Prostaglandin E_1 **B.** Nitric oxide
C. Oxygen **D.** Indomethacin *(AIIMS May 2004)*

Prostaglandin E_1 (PGE_1) has been used since the late 1970s to pharmacologically maintain patency of the ductus arteriosus in patients with duct-dependent systemic or pulmonary circulation. Most cyanotic and congestive lesions will benefit from distal blood flow. Some lesions will be made worst with the prostaglandins and these include TAPVR with obstruction, mitral atresia, and PGA with intact ventricular and atrial septum. Since apnea may be a side effect of PGE_1 the newborn should be first intubated. Usual starting dose is 0.05 to 0.10 microgram per kg per minute and once a therapeutic effect has been achieved dose may be decreased to as low as 0.025 microgram per kg per minute without loss of therapeutic effects. The response is immediate if the patency of the ductus is important for the hemodymanic state of the infant. Failure to respond to PGE_1 means that initial diagnosis was incorrect, the ductus is unresponsive to PGE_1 (usually only in older infants), or the ductus is absent.

Ref: *Manual of Neonatal Care by John P Cloherty MD; 4th Edition; page 439*

661. A 2-year-old child comes with seborrheic dermatitis, polyuria and hepatosplenomegaly. Which of the following is the *most likely* diagnosis?

A. Leukemia
B. Lymphoma
C. Langerhans cell histiocytosis
D. Germ cell tumor

(AIIMS May 2004)

The name **Langerhans cell histiocytosis (LCH)** has been applied to class I histiocytosis. LCH has an extremely variable presentation. The skeleton is involved in 80% of patients and may be the only affected site, especially in children above 5 years of age. Lesions may be single or numerous and are *most common* in the skull. They may be asymptomatic or associated with pain and local swelling. Skin involvement occurs in 50% of patients at sometime during the course of the disease (usually a seborrheic dermatitis of the scalp or diaper region). Hepatosplenomegaly occurs in 20% of patients. Pituitary dysfunction or hypothalamic involvement may result in growth retardation. In addition, patients may have diabetes insipidus (this is state of excessive water intake and hypotonic polyuria).

Ref: *Nelson Textbook of Pediatrics; 17th edition; page 1728 and 1729*

662. A 13-year-old boy has bilateral gynecomastia. His height is 148 cm, weight 58 kg, the sexual maturity rating is stage 2. The gynecomastia is *most likely* due to:

A. Prolactinoma
B. Testicular tumor
C. Pubertal gynecomastia
D. Chronic liver disease

(AIIMS Nov 2004)

Any visible or palpable development of the breast in boys or men is called gynecomastia. It is attributed to transient hormone imbalances, and resolves as the adolescent develops usually within 2 years. Sometimes it causes considerable loss of self-esteem in the boy and in cases where assurance does not work, plastic surgery is the only answer. However, before deciding on surgery, a thorough physical examination including testicular size and neurological and hormonal evaluation should be done.

Ref: *IAP Textbook of Pediatrics; 2nd edition; page 771*

663. A 9-year-old boy has steroid dependent nephrotic syndrome for last five years. The patient is markedly cushingoid with BP of 120/86 mm Hg and small sub-capsular cataracts. The *most appropriate* therapy of choice is:

A. Long-term frusemide with enalapril
B. Cyclophosphamide
C. IV immunoglobulin
D. IV pulse corticosteroids

(AIIMS Nov 2004)

Cyclophosphamide is indicated as an immunosuppressant in the treatment of steroid-resistant or frequently relapsing steroid-sensitive *biopsy proven* minimal-change nephrotic syndrome in children.

Ref: *US Pharmacopoeia*

664. A male infant presented with distension of abdomen shortly after birth with passing of less meconium. Subsequently a full thickness biopsy of the rectum was performed. The rectal biopsy is likely to show:

A. Fibrosis of submucosa
B. Lack of ganglion cells
C. Thickened muscularis propria
D. Hyalinization of the muscular coat

(AIIMS Nov 2004)

Aganglionic megacolon (Hirschsprung's disease) is a congenital disorder due to **absence of enteric neurons (ganglions) in the distal colon and rectum**. This aganglionic segment loses its neural inhibition and remains contracted.

Ref: *Harrison's Principles of Internal Medicine; 14th edition*

665. In a child, non-functioning kidney is *best* diagnosed by:

A. USG **B.** IVU
C. DTPA renogram **D.** Creatinine clearance *(AI 2005)*

Radionucleotide imaging methods are fast replacing conventional radiocontrast studies such as IVP and renal angiography, which now have limited indications. Radionucleotide procedures are noninvasive, highly selective and expose the patient to a much smaller amount of radiation. Various radionuclear techniques are renal perfusion study (renography), renal static imaging, clearance studies and radionucleotide cystography. Renography monitors the arrival uptake and elimination of a radiopharmaceutical by the kidney. **DTPA is the most commonly used agent.**

Ref: *IAP Textbook of Pediatrics; 2nd edition; page 465*

666. *Most appropriate* method for obtaining a urine specimen for culture in an 8-month-old girl is:

A. Suprapubic aspiration **B.** Indwelling catheter sample
C. Clean catch void **D.** Urinary bag sample *(AIIMS May 2004)*

The urine specimen should be fresh and relatively concentrated. A mid stream urine specimen is generally adequate. In infants, a specimen obtained by suprapubic aspiration or transurethral catheterization is preferred.

Ref: *IAP Textbook of Pediatrics; 2nd edition; page 464*

667. An 8-year-old boy during a routine checkup is found to have *Escherichia coli* 1,00,000 cc/ml on a urine culture. The urine specimen was obtained by midstream clean-catch void. The child is asymptomatic. Which is the *most appropriate* next step in the management?

A. Treat as an acute episode of UTI
B. No treatment
C. Prophylactic antibiotics for 6 months
D. Administer long-term urine alkalinizer *(AIIMS May 2004)*

In toilet-trained children, a midstream urine sample is usually satisfactory. If the culture shows greater than 1,00,000 colonies of a single pathogen, or if there are 10,000 colonies and the child is symptomatic, it is considered to be a urinary tract infection.

Ref: *Nelson Textbook of Pediatrics; 17th edition; page 1787*

668. A 15 year old girl was admitted to the infectious disease hospital with a provisional diagnosis of rabies. The *most suitable* clinical sample that can confirm the *antemortem* diagnosis is:

A. Serum for antirabies IgG antibody
B. Corneal impression smear for immunofluorescence stain
C. CSF sample for viral culture
D. Giemsa stain on smear prepared from salivary secretion *(AIIMS Nov 2004)*

Laboratory diagnosis of rabies is possible before death. The **virus may be demonstrated by florescent antibody stain or reverse transcriptase polymerase-chain reaction (RT-PCR) of smears of corneal epithelial cells or sections of skin from the neck at the hairline**. The virus can also be isolated or identified in saliva. Serological diagnosis is also possible if the patient survives beyond the acute phase. Neutralizing antibodies develop eventually in both serum and CSF and rapidly increase to extremely high levels, usually more than 100 IU per ml. Even the most potent vaccine is unlikely to raise the titers above 20 IU per ml.

Ref: *Nelson Textbook of Pediatrics; 17th edition; page 1103*

669. A 2-month-old girl has failure to thrive, polyuria and medullary nephrocalcinosis affecting both kidneys. Investigations show blood pH 7.48, bicarbonate 25 mEq/l, potassium 2 mEq per liter, sodium 126 mEq per liter and chloride 88 mEq per liter. The *most likely* diagnosis is:

A. Distal renal tubular acidosis
B. Primary hyperaldosteronism
C. Bartter's syndrome
D. Pseudohypoaldosteronism *(AIIMS Nov 2004)*

Hypokalemia secondary to renal potassium wasting, metabolic alkalosis, high urine chloride and normal to low blood pressure are the clinical features of **Bartter's syndrome**. Most cases are diagnosed during childhood, with the presenting symptoms, such as **polyuria** and weakness, being attributable to hypokalemia. **Growth and developmental retardation** may be associated with Bartter's syndrome. Bartter's syndrome is associated with hypercalciuria, often with **nephrocalcinosis**.

Further reading: *Nelson Textbook of Pediatrics; 17th edition; page 207, 218, 236 and 1763*

670. A 6-month-old child with TOF develops cyanotic spell initiated by crying. Which one of the following drugs you would like to avoid?

A. Sodium bicarbonate
B. Propranolol
C. Phenylephrine
D. Isoprenaline *(AIIMS Nov 2004)*

Isoprenaline is contraindicated in **tetralogy of Fallot** with RV outflow tract obstruction as may constrict pulmonary vasculature exacerbating pre-existing pulmonary hypertension or right ventricular dysfunction.
Ref: http://www.perfusion.com.au/CCP/Pharmacology/isoprenaline.html

ANSWERS

1 D 2 B 3 C 4 B 5 A 6 A 7 C 8 C 9 B 10 A
11 D 12 B 13 C 14 B 15 D 16 B 17 C 18 D 19 C 20 D
21 C 22 B 23 C 24 A 25 C 26 B 27 C 28 D 29 C 30 A
31 D 32 B 33 D 34 B 35 B 36 D 37 C 38 D 39 C 40 D
41 D 42 C 43 D 44 B 45 B 46 A 47 C 48 C 49 B 50 A
51 D 52 A 53 D 54 A 55 C 56 D 57 C 58 A 59 B 60 A
61 D 62 C 63 A 64 D 65 C 66 C 67 C 68 C 69 C 70 D
71 C 72 B 73 B 74 A 75 D 76 D 77 B 78 B 79 D 80 A
81 C 82 A 83 C 84 C 85 C 86 C 87 A 88 A 89 C 90 B
91 B 92 C 93 C 94 C 95 B 96 C 97 B 98 D 99 C 100 B
101 B 102 C 103 A 104 C 105 D 106 D 107 B 108 C 109 B 110 C
111 B 112 D 113 C 114 B 115 D 116 C 117 B 118 D 119 B 120 A
121 C 122 B 123 A 124 A 125 A 126 A 127 D 128 D 129 C 130 B
131 D 132 C 133 D 134 A 135 A 136 A 137 D 138 A 139 C 140 B
141 D 142 A 143 D 144 B 145 C 146 B 147 B 148 D 149 A 150 B
151 B 152 C 153 C 154 D 155 C 156 B 157 D 158 D 159 C 160 B
161 B 162 D 163 C 164 C 165 B 166 A 167 D 168 D 169 B 170 A
171 D 172 D 173 D 174 A 175 B 176 A 177 B 178 B 179 A 180 A
181 B 182 B 183 C 184 D 185 A 186 C 187 B 188 C 189 C 190 D
191 B 192 A 193 D 194 A 195 D 196 D 197 A 198 B 199 C 200 D
201 B 202 D 203 B 204 C 205 C 206 D 207 B 208 D 209 B 210 D
211 A 212 C 213 C 214 B 215 B 216 C 217 C 218 D 219 D 220 B
221 C 222 C 223 A 224 C 225 A 226 B 227 A 228 B 229 A 230 B
231 B 232 B 233 A 234 B 235 A 236 A 237 B 238 D 239 B 240 A
241 C 242 A 243 A 244 A 245 D 246 C 247 B 248 D 249 B 250 C
251 C 252 C 253 B 254 A 255 B 256 A 257 C 258 C 259 C 260 D
261 A 262 B 263 D 264 D 265 D 266 A 267 C 268 D 269 D 270 C
271 C 272 B 273 D 274 B 275 A 276 A 277 A 278 C 279 B 280 C
281 B 282 C 283 C 284 C 285 C 286 D 287 C 288 C 289 B 290 C
291 A 292 B 293 C 294 B 295 C 296 B 297 C 298 C 299 A 300 D
301 D 302 D 303 C 304 D 305 B 306 A 307 C 308 B 309 C 310 A
311 D 312 A 313 A 314 C 315 B 316 A 317 A 318 A 319 A 320 D
321 A 322 A 323 A 324 C 325 A 326 A 327 C 328 B 329 B 330 A
331 A 332 D 333 C 334 C 335 D 336 B 337 D 338 C 339 B 340 D
341 A 342 C 343 A 344 D 345 C 346 A 347 B 348 A 349 B 350 D
351 B 352 A 353 D 354 B 355 C 356 B 357 A 358 C 359 B 360 C
361 B 362 C 363 A 364 D 365 A 366 A 367 C 368 A 369 C 370 C
371 B 372 D 373 A 374 D 375 A 376 B 377 B 378 C 379 A 380 B
381 C 382 B 383 D 384 B 385 D 386 C 387 B 388 C 389 A 390 C
391 A 392 D 393 D 394 D 395 D 396 B 397 D 398 A 399 C 400 A
401 D 402 D 403 B 404 C 405 D 406 B 407 C 408 A 409 A 410 C
411 B 412 B 413 C 414 B 415 C 416 A 417 C 418 C 419 A 420 B

421 C 422 A 423 B 424 C 425 D 426 C 427 A 428 B 429 A 430 A
431 A 432 B 433 B 434 D 435 D 436 A 437 D 438 A 439 C 440 A
441 A 442 A 443 D 444 C 445 B 446 C 447 A 448 D 449 C 450 C
451 B 452 C 453 A 454 D 455 A 456 A 457 B 458 C 459 D 460 A
461 D 462 A 463 B 464 B 465 D 466 C 467 A 468 B 469 C 470 D
471 D 472 A 473 A 474 B 475 D 476 A 477 A 478 C 479 C 480 B
481 B 482 B 483 C 484 D 485 C 486 D 487 D 488 D 489 C 490 D
491 A 492 A 493 C 494 C 495 D 496 C 497 B 498 A 499 D 500 C
501 B 502 D 503 C 504 B 505 C 506 C 507 D 508 D 509 D 510 C
511 D 512 B 513 B 514 B 515 A 516 A 517 A 518 C 519 B 520 B
521 D 522 A 523 C 524 D 525 C 526 D 527 C 528 B 529 C 530 D
531 A 532 C 533 C 534 B 535 A 536 B 537 A 538 B 539 B 540 C
541 B 542 B 543 A 544 C 545 D 546 C 547 A 548 A 549 A 550 B
551 B 552 C 553 A 554 C 555 B 556 C 557 C 558 A 559 D 560 D
561 D 562 C 563 C 564 A 565 C 566 B 567 D 568 B 569 B 570 A
571 D 572 B 573 C 574 C 575 C 576 A 577 C 578 B 579 C 580 A
581 B 582 D 583 D 584 B 585 D 586 B 587 A 588 C 589 C 590 C
591 B 592 A 593 C 594 A 595 C 596 B 597 A 598 A 599 C 600 C
601 D 602 C 603 D 604 B 605 B 606 B 607 B 608 B 609 A 610 C
611 A,C 612 D 613 C 614 B 615 C 616 A 617 C 618 A 619 A 620 A
621 A 622 A 623 B 624 A 625 C 626 C 627 B 628 A 629 C 630 A
631 D 632 B 633 A 634 C 635 A 636 C 637 D 638 C 639 B 640 C
641 C 642 D 643 A 644 A 645 C 646 B 647 A 648 C 649 C 650 D
651 C 652 B 653 B 654 C 655 C 656 C 657 C 658 C 659 C 660 A
661 C 662 C 663 B 664 B 665 C 666 B 667 A 668 B 669 C 670 D

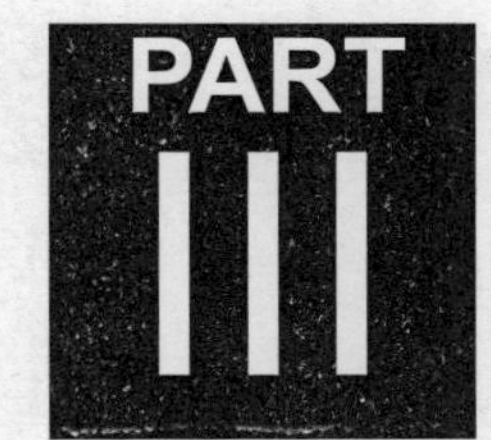

Dermatology and Venereal Diseases

Dermatology and Venereal Diseases

1. **Pinta is caused by:**
   A. *Treponema pertenue* **B.** *Treponema pallidum*
   C. *Treponema carateum* **D.** *Borrelia burgdorferi* *(JIPMER 2001)*

Pinta is caused by ***Treponema carateum*** and involves the skin alone.

2. **In which of the following condition, erythema marginatum is seen:**
   A. Rheumatic fever **B.** Enteric fever
   C. Typhus **D.** Drug reaction *(KERALA 1990)*

There are 5 criteria termed *major* because they are most commonly found in patients with **rheumatic fever.** They are carditis, migratory polyarthritis, Sydenham's chorea, subcutaneous nodules, and **erythema marginatum**.

3. **Necrobiosis lipoidica diabeticorum is more marked on:**
   A. Back of legs **B.** Front of legs
   C. Face **D.** Trunk

Necrobiosis lipoidica diabeticorum is a plaque-like lesion with a central yellowish area surrounded by a brownish border and is usually found over the **anterior surfaces of the legs.**

4. **Chancroid is caused by:**
   A. *Haemophilus ducreyi* **B.** *Chlamydia trachomatis*
   C. *Leishmania donovani* **D.** *Treponema pallidum* *(AI 1999)*

5. **In chancroid, the drug of choice is:**
   A. Streptomycin
   B. Tacrolimus
   C. Tetracycline
   D. Trimethoprim-sulfamethoxazole

Haemophilus ducreyi is the etiologic agent of **chancroid**, a STD characterized by genital ulceration and inguinal adenitis. *Haemophilus ducreyi* is a highly "choosy" coccobacillary gram-negative bacterium whose growth requires X factor (hemin). Chancroid is a common cause of genital ulcers in developing countries. Infection is acquired due to a break in the epithelium during sexual contact with an infected person. After an incubation period of 4 to 7 days, the initial lesion—a papule with surrounding erythema—is seen. In 2 to 3 days, the papule changes into a pustule, this spontaneously ruptures and forms a sharply circumscribed ulcer that is generally not indurated. The ulcers are painful and bleed easily; little or no inflammation of the surrounding skin is seen. Approximately 50% patients develop enlarged, tender inguinal lymph nodes, which commonly become fluctuant and spontaneously rupture. Gram's staining of a swab of the lesion may reveal a predominance of characteristic gram-negative coccobacilli, but an accurate diagnosis of **chancroid** relies on cultures of *Haemophilus ducreyi* from the lesion. Chancroid can be treated *effectively* with several regimens, including (1) **ceftriaxone**, 250 mg IM as a single dose; (2) **erythromycin**, 500 mg orally 4 times daily for 7 days; (3) **trimethoprim-sulfamethoxazole**, one double-strength tablet twice daily for 7 days (in regions where resistant strains are not prevalent); and (4) **ciprofloxacin**, 500 mg orally BD for 3 days.

6. **Hydradenitis suppurativa is an infection of:**
   A. Hair follicle **B.** Apocrine sweat glands
   C. Eccrine sweat glands **D.** Sebaceous glands *(AIIMS 1999)*

Hydradenitis suppurativa is a chronic disease of the scent or **apocrine glands** which causes chronic scarring and pus formation of the axillae and groin areas. It usually starts as one or more red, tender, swellings in the groin or axilla. Over a period of hours to days the lesions enlarge and often open to the skin surface draining clear to yellow fluid. The involved area then heals with scarring. The condition usually continues for years with periods of flare and remission. *Apocrine sweat glands are sweat glands located in the axillae and pubic region that open into hair follicles rather than directly onto the surface of the skin as do eccrine sweat glands.*

7. Non-specific urethritis is *most commonly* caused by:
A. Gonococcus
B. *Mycoplasma*
C. *Chlamydia*
D. Fungus

Non-gonococcal urethritis (non-specific urethritis) is an urethral inflammation caused by organisms **other than** *Neisseria gonorrhoeae*. **NGU is the** most common **STD in men**. Symptoms generally develop within 7-14 days. The major symptoms are dysuria and a urethral discharge. The 2 organisms most commonly associated with NGU are ***Chlamydia trachomatis*** and *Ureaplasma urealyticum*. Other causes of NGU are herpes simplex virus (HSV), *Trichomonas vaginalis*, *Haemophilus influenzae*, *Gardnerella vaginalis*, and *Clostridium difficile*.

8. *Most common* cause of non-gonococcal urethritis (NGU) is:
A. *Chlamydia trachomatis*
B. *Trichomonas vaginalis*
C. *Mycoplasma*
D. Virus

(UP 1996)

Non-gonococcal urethritis (NGU) is a diagnosis of exclusion that is applied to men with symptoms and/or signs of urethritis who *do not* have gonorrhea. ***Chlamydia trachomatis* causes 20 to 40 % of the cases of NGU.**

9. A smear from a genital lesion shows Donovan bodies. The diagnosis is:
A. Lymphogranuloma venereum
B. Chancroid
C. Granuloma inguinale
D. Syphilis

(JIPMER 2000)

10. Pseudobubo is seen in which of the following:
A. Donovanosis
B. LGV
C. Syphilis
D. Chancroid

(AI 1996)

11. "Safety pin" appearance is shown by:
A. *Haemophilus ducreyi*
B. *Chlamydia*
C. *Calymmatobacterium granulomatis*
D. *Mycoplasma*

12. The treatment of granuloma inguinale is:
A. Tetracycline
B. Streptomycin
C. Sulphonamide
D. Penicillin

13. Lymphadenopathy is *not* seen in:
A. Chancroid
B. LGV
C. Donovanosis
D. Primary syphilis

(UP 1994, AI 1995)

14. Donovanosis is caused by:
A. *Haemophilus ducreyi*
B. *Chlamydia trachomatis*
C. *Treponema pertenue*
D. *Calymmatobacterium granulomatis*

(AI 1997)

Donovanosis or **granuloma inguinale** is a mildly contagious, chronic, indolent, progressive, autoinoculable, ulcerative disease of the skin and lymphatics of the genital or perianal regions. The disease is associated with the presence, in affected tissues, of an intracellular microorganism, identified morphologically as the **Donovan body**. It is caused by ***Calymmatobacterium granulomatis.*** Donovan bodies are rounded coccobacilli of 1 by 2 μm lying within cystic spaces in the cytoplasm of large mononuclear cells. The capsule stains as a dense acidophilic zone surrounding the bacterium, which resembles a closed **"safety pin"** due to bipolar condensation of chromatin. The pathognomonic mononuclear cell is 25 to 90 μm in diameter and has many cystic areas containing Donovan bodies. Extension to the inguinal region by autoinoculation, by continuity, or via the lymphatics leads to a diffuse intradermal and subcutaneous swelling or suppuration known as a **pseudobubo** because **involvement of the underlying lymph nodes is minimal.** Drugs effective in the treatment of donovanosis in various parts of the world include trimethoprim-sulfamethoxazole, **tetracycline**, erythromycin, newer quinolones, gentamicin, and chloramphenicol. Streptomycin, once commonly used for this condition, is *not* widely used nowadays.

15. Which of the following is *not* sexually transmitted:

A. *Entamoeba histolytica* B. *Giardia lamblia*
C. *Trichomonas vaginalis* D. *Leishmania braziliensis* *(JIPMER 2000)*

16. *Not* an STD:

A. *Molluscum contagiosum* B. *Echinococcus*
C. *Candida* D. Group B *streptococcus* *(AIIMS 2000)*

17. *Not* a sexually transmitted disease:

A. Candidiasis B. Gonorrhea
C. Endemic syphilis D. Syphilis *(AI 1993)*

Some Sexually Transmitted Pathogens

Bacteria	
• *Neisseria gonorrhoeae*	• *Calymmatobacterium granulomatis*
• *Treponema pallidum*	• *Ureaplasma urealyticum*
• *Haemophilus ducreyi*	• *Chlamydia trachomatis*
• *Mycoplasma hominis*	• *Shigella* spp.
• *Campylobacter* spp.	• Group B *Streptococcus*
• Bacterial vaginosis–associated organisms	
Viruses	
• HIV (types 1 and 2)	• Hepatitis B virus
• Human T cell lymphotropic virus type I	• Cytomegalovirus
• Herpes simplex virus type 2	• Molluscum contagiosum virus
• Human papilloma virus (multiple genotypes)	
Protozoan	
• *Trichomonas vaginalis*	• *Giardia lamblia*
• *Entamoeba histolytica*	
Fungal	
• *Candida albicans*	
Ectoparasites	
• *Phthirus pubis*	• *Sarcoptes scabiei*

18. Tinea capitis is caused by all *except*:

A. *Epidermophyton*
B. *Microsporum audouini*
C. *Microsporum canis*
D. *Trichophyton tonsurans*

Tinea capitis is a fungal infection of the scalp in which dermatophytes invade the hair shafts. Dermatophytes commonly causing tinea capitis include *Microsporum canis, Microsporum audouini,* and *Trichophyton tonsurans*.

19. Tinea capitis in children is caused by:

A. *Trichophyton mentagrophytes*
B. *Trichophyton rubrum*
C. *Microsporum audouini*
D. *Trichophyton verrucosum*

(JIPMER 2000)

The ringworm of scalp or **tinea capitis** is most common in children before puberty and is usually caused by *Microsporum audouini, Microsporum canis or Trichophyton sulphureum.* In adults, tinea capitis is usually *caught* from a horse or cow (*Trichophyton mentagrophytes* or *Trichophyton verrucosum*). The **1st sign is a fairly well-defined patch of hair loss in which the remaining hairs are broken, lusterless and lie at various angles to each other.** The patch may be single or multiple and usually lies where the hairs are short (at the sides or back of skull).

20. Kerion is caused by:

A. Dermatophytes
B. Human papilloma virus
C. Candida
D. None

(PGI 1998)

A **kerion** is a *nodular, inflammatory, pustular lesion due to a fungus infection*. ***Tinea capitis*** is a fungal infection of the scalp with invasion of the hair shafts by a **dermatophyte**. In the cases *caught* from horses or cattle, kerion formation usually occurs. Kerions indicate an intense host immune response typically against *Trichophyton verrucosum* or *T. mentagrophytes*.

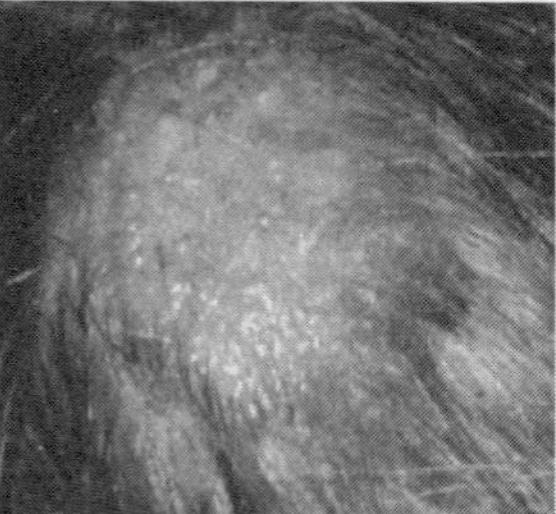

21. Wavelength of light produced by Wood's lamp is:

A. 320 nm
B. 360 nm
C. 400 nm
D. 480 nm

22. Tinea capitis caused by *Microsporum* appears in Wood's lamp as:

A. Greenish blue fluorescence
B. Yellow fluorescence
C. Coral red fluorescence
D. Pink fluorescence

(JIPMER 2002)

23. Use of Wood's light includes:

A. Erythrasma
B. Examination of hair in tinea capitis
C. Tinea versicolor
D. All of the above

24. Wood's lamp is *not* useful in diagnosing:

A. Tuberous sclerosis
B. Certain porphyria
C. Tinea rubra
D. Erythrasma

(KERALA 1999)

25. Pinkish red fluorescence of urine with Wood's lamp is seen in:

A. Acrocyanosis
B. Porphyria cutanea tarda
C. Lead poisoning
D. Erythromelalgia

26. Coral red fluorescence Wood's lamp seen in:

A. Porphyria cutanea tarda
B. Hypomelanosis
C. Livedo reticularis
D. Erythrasma

Wood's Light: A Wood's lamp generates **360-nm ultraviolet** (or "**black**") light that is used to aid the evaluation of certain skin disorders. For example	
• **Erythrasma**	Coral red color
• **Wounds colonized by *Pseudomonas***	Pale blue
• **Tinea capitis (*Microsporum canis* or *M. audouini*)**	Yellow fluorescence
• **Freckles**	Get accentuated
• **Post-inflammatory hyperpigmentation**	Fades
• **Vitiligo**	Totally white
• **Tuberous sclerosis**	Blue white
• **Porphyria cutanea tarda**	Pinkish red (urine)
• **Tinea versicolor**	Dull yellow

27. 8-year-old male child with recurrent scaly hypopigmented macules on the cheek. The diagnosis is:
A. Pityriasis alba
B. Leprosy
C. Tinea versicolor
D. Pityriasis rosea
(AI 1998, AIIMS 1999)

28. A boy aged 8 from Tamil Nadu has a white non-anesthetic, scaly hypopigmented macule on his face:
A. Pityriasis alba
B. Indeterminate leprosy
C. Pityriasis versicolor
D. Pure neuritic leprosy
(AIIMS 1999, 2000, AI 2001)

Pityriasis alba is typically found on the face, particularly the cheeks and chin, of children. Patches of oval macular skin lesions with fine adherent scales are seen. These patches are the sites of a mild eczematous process, resulting in poor melanin transfer to keratinocytes, as well as desquamation of the previously tanned skin. The lesions are virtually painless. They may disappear spontaneously. The treatment of choice is a mild topical steroid such as 1% hydrocortisone cream.

Pityriasis alba

29. Patch test is read after:
A. 2 hours
B. 2 days
C. 2 weeks
D. 2 months
(AI 1999)

Patch testing is used to detect sensitivity to a specific antigen. In this test, a battery of suspected allergens is applied to the patient's back under occlusive dressings and allowed to remain in contact with the skin for **48 hours.** The dressings are then removed, and the area is examined for delayed hypersensitivity reactions (such as erythema, edema, or papulovesicles). This test is helpful in the evaluation of patients with chronic dermatitis.

30. All of the following are true about psoriasis *except*:
A. Scalp is commonly involved
B. Nails are involved
C. May be associated with arthritis
D. It commonly occurs in flexer areas
(SGPGI 2002)

31. Characteristic feature of psoriasis is:
A. Pitting of nail
B. Köebner phenomenon or isomorphic response
C. Silvery scales
D. All of the above
(UP 1994)

32. In psoriasis, the site *least* commonly involved is:
A. Arthritis
B. CNS involvement
C. Nail involvement
D. Scalp involvement
(AI 1998)

33. Nails are involved in:
A. Dermatitis herpetiformis
B. Psoriasis
C. Pemphigoid
D. Pemphigus

34. The important feature of psoriasis is:
A. Crusting
B. Scaling
C. Oozing
D. Erythema

35. Psoriasis is characterized by all *except*:
A. Definite pink plaque with clear margin
B. Men and women are equally affected
C. Always associated with nail infection
D. Commonly involves knees and elbows

36. Psoriasis is exacerbated by:
A. Lithium
B. Antimalarials
C. β blockers
D. All of the above

37. Psoriasis is *not* caused by:
A. Lithium
B. Calcium channel blocker
C. Propranolol
D. Chloroquine
(UP 2001)

38. Psoralen + UV A is used for treating:
A. Porphyria
B. Psoriasis
C. Pemphigus
D. Tinea versicolor

39. Photochemotherapy is used in:
A. Psoriasis
B. Scabies
C. Erythroderma
D. Pityriasis rosea
(AI 1993)

40. *False* regarding psoriasis is:
A. Oncholysis and pitting of nails are seen
B. Red scaly lesions are seen in natal cleft and sub-mammary area
C. Oligoarticular is seen with nail involvement in 50% of cases
D. Does *not* involve skin of head, neck and face
(AI 2000)

41. A patient with psoriasis was started on systemic steroids. After stopping treatment, the patient developed generalized pustules all over his body. The cause is *most likely* to be:
A. Drug induced reaction
B. Septicemia
C. Bacterial infections
D. Pustular psoriasis
(AIIMS Nov 2001, AI 2002)

42. Thimble pitting nails are seen in:
A. Psoriasis
B. Tinea versicolor
C. Lichen planus
D. Tuberculosis
(JIPMER 2001)

Psoriasis, parapsoriasis, pityriasis lichenoides, pityriasis rosea and seborrhoeic dermatitis are grouped together under the heading **"erythematosquamous eruptions"** because in each condition the *cardinal* physical signs are **erythema** *(a form of macula showing diffused redness of the skin)* and **scaling** and are frequently mistaken for each other. Psoriasis, seborrhoeic dermatitis and pityriasis rosea are among the most common dermatological disorders although their cause remains obscure. **Psoriasis** is a chronic disease characterized by **sharply defined patches of erythema covered by silvery scales**. It may occur at any age although it is rare in infancy and old age. The *most common age of onset is between 5–15 years.* There is hereditary tendency in 30% of cases and it is not an infectious disease. Men and women are equally affected and it is more common in colder northern Europe. The disease is rare in tropics and is more common in fair haired than in dark haired people. The attack of psoriasis may be precipitated by emotional stress or by an intercurrent infection. Local trauma sometimes determines the site of the lesion and the patches are seen in healing cuts, abrasions or even after some other skin disease such as contact dermatitis. This characteristic feature is known as **Köebner phenomenon** or **isomorphic response**. **This phenomenon is also seen in lichen planus and plain warts.** It is due to this phenomenon that psoriasis is commonly seen in areas such as knee and elbow which are constantly subjected to mild trauma. Other external factors which may exacerbate psoriasis are infections, stress, and drugs such as **lithium, beta blockers, and antimalarials**. Two **pathological changes** are seen in skin. There is marked elongation and coiling of dermal capillaries with irregular fusiform dilatation of their walls. The second aspect of psoriatic lesion is related to the epidermis. Normally it takes 27 days to replace the epithelium, i.e. from basal cell to fully keratinized horny cell. In psoriasis this process takes only 3-4 days and as a result the horny layer is immature and **parakeratotic** with nuclear fragments still present in horn cells. **It is this parakeratosis which is responsible for silvery scaling.** The lesions may vary in size from minute papules to sheets covering large area of the body. Often lesions are disc shaped half to several inches in diameter, which are more or less circular or sometimes irregular in outline. Occasionally the lesions heal in the center leaving the "rings". In *every* case the lesions are *exceeding* well-defined, i.e. the **transition from psoriatic patch to normal skin is abrupt,** the lesions are slightly raised and reddish; covered with easily detachable scales which become silvery on scrapping. If the process of scrapping is continued and all the scales come off, a smooth red surface with numerous small bleeding points is left. The lesions of psoriasis are *always* dry and they *seldom* irritate much. The most common site is on the **extensor surfaces**; the sites of election being scalp, elbows, knees and lumbosacral region. In its mildest form there is nothing more than the odd "scaly pink patch" on the elbow or knee but more commonly the disease begin to spread widely over the trunk and limbs with individual patches spreading at their margins to blend with other patches producing a bizarre geographic pattern. The face is only *rarely* affected. Such attacks last for weeks or months and thereafter the disease remits leaving only a few lesions at the sites of election. Such episodes are an "annual event" in most severe cases but in other it occurs only once or twice in the life time. **Flexural psoriasis** is seen in a minority of cases in which the lesions are found in the "body folds". This type of disease is more common in middle-aged obese women and the lesions are well-demarcated, nonscaly and frequently itchy. **Guttate psoriasis** is seen in children and young adults often after 2-3 weeks of acute tonsillitis. β hemolytic *Streptococci* have been clearly implicated in may patients and recurrent episodes may be aborted by antibiotics or tonsillectomy. Small lesions <1cm in diameter appear abruptly covering much of skin of trunks and limbs. Sometimes the psoriasis may spread to involve the *whole* skin including the face and the skin becomes *thick, red* and *scaly* (**erythroderma**). The nails are involved in half of the cases and may show multiple small pits resembling a **thimble** or the nail may becomes detached from its bed over its distal half; the affected portion being opaque, friable and discolored. Sometimes the nail may become thickened, rough and pigmented. **Arthropathic psoriasis** is the form of psoriasis which is associated with some type of erosive arthritis. In **pustular psoriasis** sterile pustule formation is seen. This type of psoriasis is usually localized and most commonly superficial "lakes" of pus appear in crops on a background of erythema; most commonly on the thenar or hypothenar eminence or the center or inner aspect of the sole. Individual pustules *dry up*, turn brown and exfoliate. The pustules may also *sometimes* be seen in the ordinary lesions of psoriasis when the disease is acute and severe. *Finally* pustules may be widespread and associated with sheets of *bright* erythema (**generalized pustular psoriasis**). This is the most severe form of psoriasis and death occurs in 1/4th of the cases. Psoriasis is usually **easy to diagnose** and points to be looked out are **dryness**, **silvery scales** and **sharp edges**. The skin lesions are variably pruritic. Treatment of psoriasis depends on the type, location, and extent of disease and all patients should be instructed to avoid excess drying or irritation of their skin and to maintain adequate cutaneous hydration. *Most* patients with localized plaque-type psoriasis can be managed with mid-potency topical steroids, although their long-term use is often accompanied by loss of effectiveness (*tachyphylaxis*). Crude coal tar is a useful method of treatment along with ultraviolet light therapy. A topical vitamin D analogue (calcipitriol) is also effective in the treatment of psoriasis. Ultraviolet light is an effective therapy for patients with *widespread* psoriasis. The ultraviolet B (UV-B) spectrum is effective alone or may be combined with coal tar (*Goeckerman regi-*

men) or anthralin (*Ingram regimen*). Natural sunlight or an artificial light source may be used. The combination of the UV-A spectrum and either oral or topical psoralens (**PUVA**) is also extremely effective for the treatment of psoriasis, but long-term use is associated with an increased incidence of squamous cell cancer of the skin. Methotrexate is useful in patients with associated **psoriatic arthritis** but liver toxicity from long-term use limits its use to patients with widespread disease *not* responsive to less aggressive methods of treatment. The synthetic retinoid, etretinate, has been shown to be effective in some patients with severe psoriasis, but it is a potent teratogen.

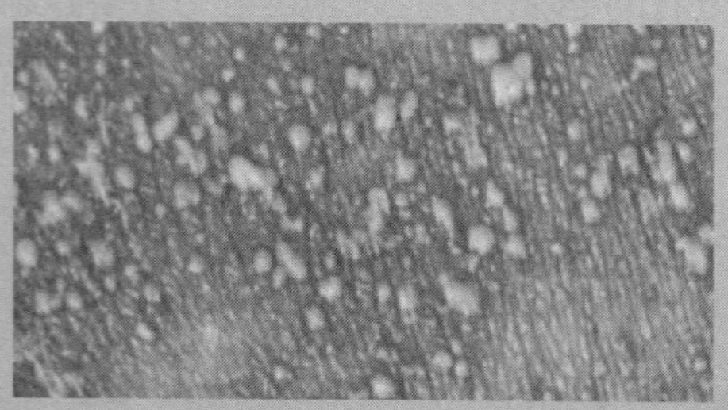

Generalized pustular psoriasis

Silvery scales of psoriasis

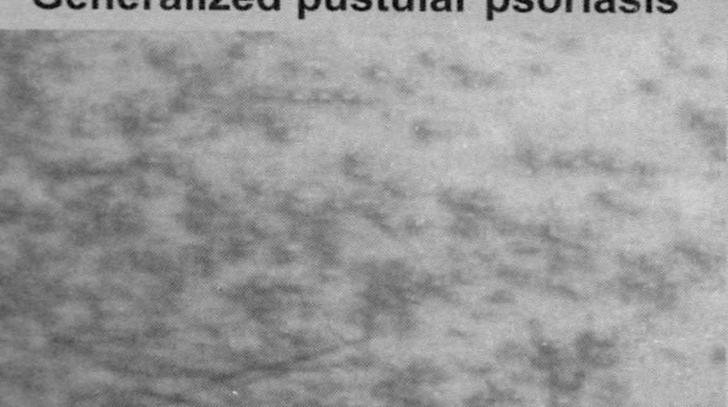

Guttate psoriasis

Flexural psoriasis

43. "Pitting" of nails is seen in:
A. Lichen planus
B. Psoriasis
C. Pemphigus
D. Arsenic poisoning

44. "Oil drop" phenomenon is seen in:
A. Clubbing
B. Psoriasis of nails
C. Lichen planus of nails
D. Tinea unguium

(AP 1996)

Psoriasis of the nails may be an isolated phenomenon or it can be a part of a generalized psoriasis. Appearance of translucent areas, in the nail the so called **"oil-drop" phenomenon,** is the typical manifestation of psoriasis of nails. **Nail pits** are arranged longitudinally on the nail and appear 1/3-2/3 of the way down the nail. Psoriatic nails can also be thickened. **Oncholysis** is common.

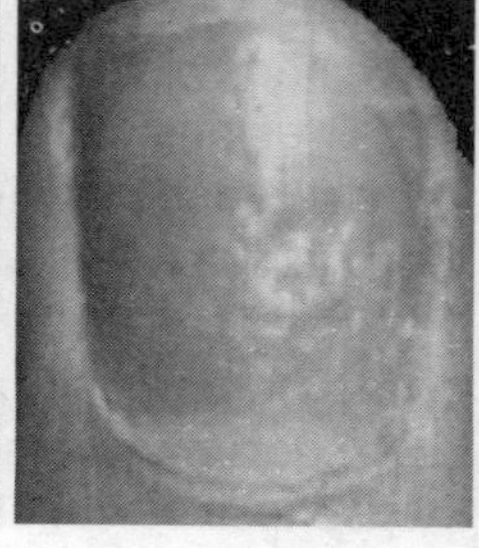

PSORIASIS—NAIL PITS

45. Munro's microabscesses are characteristic of:
A. Psoriasis
B. Lichen planus
C. Sezary syndrome
D. Streptococcal infection

(JIPMER 2002)

46. Munro's microabscesses are seen in:
A. Stratum granulosum
B. Stratum corneum
C. Basal layer
D. Papillary tips

(PGI 1999)

In **psoriasis** the increased rate of proliferation (to replace the damaged, exfoliated keratin) is reflected in epidermal thickening (acanthosis), down growth of elongated epidermal ridges, and increased mitotic activity. The stratum granulosum is thin or absent, and there is extensive overlying parakeratotic scale. The dermal papillae are elongated and contain dilated capillaries; these extend close to the parakeratotic scale due to thinning of the overlying epidermis. When the psoriatic scale is removed, this results in minute points of bleeding (**Auspitz's sign**). Within the epidermis are focal areas of slight edema (**spongiosis**); collections of neutrophils in the **stratum corneum** produce the characteristic **Munro's microabscesses**.

47. Pustular psoriasis is treated with:

A. Psoralen
B. Methotrexate
C. Systemic corticosteroids
D. Coal tar with ultraviolet rays

48. In pustular psoriasis, the treatment of choice is:

A. Etretinate
B. Methotrexate
C. Systemic corticosteroids
D. Psoralen + UV therapy *(AI 1994)*

Pustular psoriasis of the palms and soles is extremely resistant to therapy. Treatment generally involves the use of **potent topical steroids** but occasionally, systemic agents such as cyclosporine or **methotrexate** are necessary. Generalized pustular psoriasis responds usually quite well to bland therapy. It is very important to avoid any irritants such as anthralin for generalized pustular psoriasis. 1 % hydrocortisone ointment applied topically may result in good improvement. Systemic cyclosporine and methotrexate may be needed if the disease does not respond well to such topical therapy. When more stable plaque-type psoriasis is present, treatment with PUVA can be considered. Hospitalization is often necessary.

49. Chloroquine causes exacerbation of:

A. Malaria
B. Psoriasis
C. Rheumatoid arthritis
D. DLE

Chloroquine may precipitate severe attacks of **psoriasis**. It may cause exacerbation of porphyria.

50. For erythrodermic psoriasis the *treatment of choice* is:

A. Topical corticosteroids
B. Coal tar topically
C. Methotrexate
D. Corticosteroids *(SGPGI 1999)*

An important point in treatment of erythrodermic psoriasis is *not* to irritate the skin further and therefore anthralin and other irritating compounds are relatively contraindicated in erythrodermic psoriasis. **Bland topical steroids such as 1% hydrocortisone in an ointment base applied *liberally* can be useful.** If there is not a reasonably rapid improvement, consideration should be given to the use of cyclosporine 2 to 5 mg/kg/per dose or methotrexate 5 mg, 12 hourly for 3 doses, once a week. When the acute episode has subsided, UVB or PUVA can be restarted.

51. "Wickham's striae" are seen in:

A. Lichen sclerosis
B. Lichen planus
C. Lichen simplex chronicus
D. Psoriasis *(AI 2002)*

52. Itchy, polygonal violaceous (violet) papular lesion is seen in:

A. Pityriasis rubra
B. Pityriasis rosea
C. Psoriasis
D. Lichen planus *(AI 1998, UP 2000)*

53. Mouth lesion is seen in which of the following:

A. Basal cell carcinoma
B. Icthyosis vulgaris
C. Lichen planus
D. Psoriasis *(AI 1994)*

54. Which of the following is *true* of lichen planus:

A. Affects skin only
B. Affects skin, oral and genital areas
C. Affects skin and nails
D. Affects skin, nails and mucous membranes *(JIPMER 2002)*

55. Which of the following is pruritic:
A. Lichen planus
B. Psoriasis
C. Icthyosis
D. Secondary syphilis

56. Mucosal lesion is common in:
A. Pemphigoid
B. Psoriasis
C. Lichen planus
D. Pityriasis rubra

57. A 30-year-old male presents with pruritic flat topped polygonal, shiny violaceous papules with flexural distribution. *Most probable* diagnosis is:
A. Psoriasis
B. Pityriasis rosea
C. Lichen planus
D. Lichenoid dermatitis

58. Autoimmune pathology is seen in:
A. Pityriasis rosea
B. Pemphigus vulgaris
C. Psoriasis
D. Lichen planus
(AI 2000)

59. *False* regarding lichen planus is:
A. Hypopigmentation is seen in previously involved areas
B. Lymphocytes aggregate in subepidermal region
C. Involves skin, mucous membranes and nails
D. Polygonal, pruritus, papule
(AI 2000)

60. Lacy white papules in oral cavity and pterygium of nail are seen in:
A. Pemphigus
B. Candida
C. Lichen planus
D. Psoriasis
(AIIMS 1999)

61. The characteristic nail finding in lichen planus is:
A. Pitting
B. Beau's lines
C. Hyperpigmentation of the nails
D. Pterygium
(AIIMS May 2001)

62. Basal cell degeneration is characteristic of:
A. Pemphigus
B. Lichen planus
C. Pemphigoid
D. Psoriasis
(JIPMER 2002)

63. Degeneration of basal cells occurs in:
A. Pemphigoid
B. Psoriasis
C. Lichen planus
D. Pemphigus
(JIPMER 1993)

64. In which of the following condition basal cell degeneration is seen:
A. Viral warts
B. Lichen planus
C. Psoriasis
D. Atopic dermatitis
(PGI 1999)

Lichen is the designation given to **an aggregation of *similar* papules** while **papules** are **small superficial raised abnormalities**. Physical signs of **lichen planus** consist of aggregations of *flat topped* papules. The cause of disease is unknown but predominance of T cell infiltrate at the epidermo-dermal junction and association with diseases such as thymoma, myasthenia gravis and lupus erythematous **point towards an altered immune function** state. It mainly occurs between the ages of 30 and 60 years and women are affected 3 times more often than men. Lichen planus like lesions may appear in graft versus host disease and in patients treated for rheumatoid arthritis with drugs that alter immune function (gold and antimalarials). In **chronic type of lichen planus** a number of **small,**

flat topped, polygonal, shiny papules; a millimeter or 2 in diameter; bluish pink or violet in color are present on the anterior surface of forearms, front of the legs and the inner sides of the thighs. **Köebner phenomenon** may be present. Some of the papules are discrete while some have coalesced to form slightly raised scaly plaques. These small flat-topped papules show a white lacy network on their surface, the "**Wickham's striae**". The eruptions may be severely pruritic or hardly at all. **In 50% cases of lichen planus lace like white spots and streaks are present on the inner surface of the cheeks which cause no symptoms**. "Bald areas" sometimes occur on the tongue leading to a *false* diagnosis of leukoplakia. Nose, larynx, urethra, colon, rectum and anus may also be involved. Involvement of **nails is seen in 10% of cases** and the appearance varies from a diffuse pitting or vertical ridging to progressive thinning and finally complete loss of the nail plate. *Rarely* the matrix can be permanently destroyed with prominent **pterygium** formation. Histologically there is **hyperkeratosis,** a prominent granular layer, **basal cell degeneration** (forming *colloid* or *Civatte bodies* in the epidermis), *liquefactive degeneration* or the basal cell layer and heavy T lymphocyte infiltration in the upper dermis. Spontaneous resolution occurs in 6 to 24 months and topical glucocorticoids are the mainstay of treatment if needed at all. Antihistaminic drugs are used for pruritus and oral lichen planus is more difficult to treat and typically lasts longer than skin lichen planus.

65. Köebner phenomenon is seen in:

A. Erythema marginatum
B. Pemphigus
C. Lichen planus
D. Pityriasis rosea

(AI 1993, SGPGI 2002)

66. Köebner phenomenon is seen in:

A. Lichen planus
B. Psoriasis
C. Plain warts
D. All of the above

67. Köebner phenomenon is seen in:

A. Psoriasis
B. Lupus vulgaris
C. Syphilis
D. Lupus erythematous

(AI 1991)

Köebner's phenomenon was defined by German dermatologist, Heinrich Köebner as "*the appearance of a skin lesion due to nonspecific trauma such as sunlight, burn, operative wound. It appears at the site of trauma and may be of a type found elsewhere on the skin. It may be seen in* ***lichen planus*** *or* ***plain warts*** *but is particularly characteristic of* ***psoriasis****. The lesion will appear in and must be sufficient to act on the papillary and epidermal layers of the skin*".

68. "Sign of groove" is found in:

A. Chancroid
B. LGV
C. Granuloma inguinale
D. Syphilis

69. Lymphogranuloma venereum is caused by:

A. *Treponema pallidum*
B. *Haemophilus ducreyi*
C. *Leishmania donovani*
D. *Chlamydia trachomatis*

(AIIMS 1999)

70. Buboes with multiple sinuses discharging into inguinal lymph node are seen in:

A. Syphilis
B. Lymphogranuloma venereum
C. Granuloma inguinale
D. Chancroid

(AI 1994)

71. Frei test is done for:

A. Leprosy
B. Syphilis
C. Donovanosis
D. Lymphogranuloma venereum

(AI 1996)

72. For lymphogranuloma venereum the *drug of choice* is:

A. Ceftriaxone
B. Erythromycin
C. Doxycycline
D. Ampicillin

(KERALA 1990)

Lymphogranuloma venereum is a STD caused by *Chlamydia trachomatis* strains of the L_1, L_2, and L_3 serovars. A *primary genital lesion* develops from 3 days to 3 weeks after exposure which is a small, painless vesicle or nonindurated ulcer or papule located on the penis in males and on the labia, posterior vagina, or fourchette in females. The primary lesion is noticed by less than 33% of men with LGV and only rarely by women. It heals in a few days without scarring. LGV strains of *Chlamydia trachomatis* have occasionally been recovered from genital ulcers and from the urethra of men and the endocervix of women who present with inguinal adenopathy. Most common presenting picture in heterosexual men is the *inguinal syndrome*, which is characterized by **painful inguinal lymphadenopathy** starting 2 to 6 weeks after *presumed* exposure. These enlarged glands are called **buboes**. Extensive involvement of chains of inguinal nodes above and below the inguinal ligament (**the sign of the groove**) is nonspecific and, although common, is documented in only a *minority* of cases. The diagnosis of LGV may be confirmed by the **Frei intradermal test**, by a complement fixation test, or by recovery of chlamydiae from the blood, feces, or buboes. One week of treatment with **doxycycline** or tetracycline should be given for *uncomplicated* genital infections caused by *Chlamydia*, but a 2-week course of therapy is recommended for *complicated* chlamydial infections (e.g., pelvic inflammatory disease, epididymitis) and **at least a 3-week course for lymphogranuloma venereum**.

73. Tinea incognito occurs with:

A. Griseofulvin
B. Gamma benzyl hexachloride
C. Permethrin
D. Topical corticosteroids

(PGI 1999)

74. Tinea "incognito" is due to inappropriate use of systemic and topical:

A. Antibiotics
B. Antifungals
C. Steroids
D. Antivirals

(JIPMER 2002)

Tinea incognito is an extensive ringworm which is caused by **inappropriate use of topical corticosteroids.**

75. Tinea cruris common by affects:

A. Adult females
B. Adult males
C. Male child
D. Female child

Dermatophytes are a group of fungi which infect skin, hair, and nails and include members of the genera *Trichophyton*, *Microsporum*, and *Epidermophyton*. Infection of the foot (**tinea pedis**) is *most common*; it is characterized by erythema and edema, scaling, pruritus, and occasionally vesiculation. Involvement may be widespread or localized, but *almost invariably the web space between the 4th and 5th toes is affected*. **Infection of the nails (tinea unguium)** occurs in many patients with tinea pedis and is characterized by opacified, thickened nails and subungual debris. Groin is the *next* most commonly involved area (**tinea cruris**), **with males affected much more often than females**. It presents as a scaling erythematous eruption that spares the scrotum. Microscopic examination of either untreated tinea pedis or tinea cruris scale after digestion with **KOH preparation** will demonstrate hyphae.

76. An adult male presents with oval scaly hypopigmented macules over the chest and the back. The diagnosis is:

A. Leprosy
B. Lupus vulgaris
C. Pityriasis versicolor
D. Lichen planus

(AIIMS May 2001)

77. Causative agent of tinea versicolor is:

A. *Tinea schoenleinii*
B. *Tinea rubrum*
C. *Malassezia furfur*
D. *Epidermophyton* floccosum

(AI 1993)

Malassezia furfur is part of the normal flora of the human skin but may cause **tinea (pityriasis) versicolor** or catheter-acquired sepsis. Tinea versicolor appears as café au lait colored patches or sheets usually on the upper part of trunk. In dark races or after sun bathing the **patches appear paler than the surrounding skin**. The affected skin may show wrinkling and scales readily on light scratching. A fine "branny" scale or folliculitis is sometimes visible. Symptoms are usually absent and it should be distinguished from vitiligo, leprosy, Addison's disease and arsenical pigmentation. Any sulfur containing solution will cure the disease but the most affective is **2.5% selenium sulfide suspension** (Selsun®) applied widely on trunk and limbs and there after left on for 20 minutes for 14 days.

78. The treatment of tinea versicolor:

A. Ketoconazole **B.** Imidazoles
C. Selenium sulfide **D.** All of the above

- **Ketoconazole** 400 mg a day for 3 days is highly effective in **Tinea versicolor**. However, it is important that the ketoconazole should be taken well away from a bath, as removal of ketoconazole, which is secreted in sweat, may cause the treatment failure.
- Topical treatment by zinc pyrithione 1% or **selenium sulfide** 1% used daily for 1-4 weeks.
- Daily use of solutions containing sulfur, salicylic acid, or selenium sulfide for a week will clear the infection.
- Topical **imidazoles** are also effective.

79. Tinea unguium affects:

A. Inter-digital spaces **B.** Joints
C. Nail fold **D.** Nail plate *(AI 1995)*

80. For tinea unguium the *drug of choice* is:

A. Nystatin **B.** Griseofulvin
C. Miconazole **D.** Amphotericin B *(AI 1993)*

Ringworm of the nail is known as tinea unguium and is a common infection especially in the great toes. It is usually caused by *Trichophyton rubrum*, *Trichophyton mentagrophytes* or *Epidermophyton floccosum.* The fungus "gets under" the free edge of the nail and grows back in the nailbed eventually **attacking the nail *itself***. The affected nail is *opaque*, *rough*, and friable. It has an accumulation of keratinous debris under it. Certain diagnosis can be made by finding the fungus in the shavings from the nail which should be soaked in a small quantity of 20% KOH. The organism can also be grown on Sabouraud's medium. **Griseofulvin is the specific antimicrobial for the ringworm fungus and is active against all varieties except *Candida***.

81. Griseofulvin is *not* used in:

A. Tinea unguium **B.** Tinea corporis
C. Tinea capitis **D.** Tinea versicolor

Griseofulvin is indicated in the treatment of tinea barbae, **tinea capitis**, **tinea corporis**, tinea cruris, tinea pedis, and **tinea unguium** (onychomycosis) caused by *Trichophyton rubrum*, *T. tonsurans*, *T. mentagrophytes*, *T. interdigitale*, *T. verrucosum*, *T. megninii*, *T. gallinae*, *T. schoenleinii*, *Microsporum audouinii*, *M. canis*, *M. gypseum*, and *Epidermophyton floccosum*.

82. Wood's lamp examination is helpful in the diagnosis of:

A. Lichen planus **B.** Psoriasis
C. Tinea versicolor **D.** Varicella *(AIIMS May 2002)*

Wood's Light: A Wood's lamp generates **360-nm ultraviolet** (or "**black**") light that is used to aid the evaluation of certain skin disorders. For example

• **Erythrasma**	Coral red color
• **Wounds colonized by *Pseudomonas***	Pale blue
• **Tinea capitis (*Microsporum canis* or *M. audouini*)**	Yellow fluorescence
• **Freckles**	Get accentuated
• **Post-inflammatory hyperpigmentation**	Fades
• **Vitiligo**	Totally white
• **Tuberous sclerosis**	Blue white
• **Porphyria cutanea tarda**	Pinkish red (urine)
• **Tinea versicolor**	Dull yellow

83. Discharging sinus is seen in:

A. Molluscum contagiosum **B.** Actinomycosis
C. Herpes genitalis **D.** Syphilis *(AI 1996)*

Actinomycosis is a slowly progressive bacterial infection caused by a variety of gram + ve, non-spore-forming anaerobic or microaerophilic rods, most of which belong to the genus *Actinomyces.* **Actinomycosis is most commonly caused by *Actinomyces israelii.* Actinomycosis occurs most frequently at an oral, cervical, or facial site**, as a soft tissue swelling, abscess, or mass lesion that is often misjudged as a neoplasm. Actinomycotic **sulfur granules** consist of aggregated microorganisms; are yellow; can be oval, round, or U-shaped; and, if sought after, can be identified macroscopically and/or microscopically in drainage from **sinus tracts** or other purulent material. IV administration of 18 to 24 million units of penicillin for 2 to 6 weeks, followed by oral therapy with penicillin or amoxicillin for 6 to 12 months is the treatment of choice.

84. Fordyce spots are ectopic:
A. Mucosal glands
B. Apocrine glands
C. Eccrine glands
D. Sebaceous glands
(AI 1995)

In **Fordyce's disease**, enlarged **ectopic sebaceous glands** in the mucosa of the mouth and genitals are present. They appear as small yellow spots, called *Fordyce's spots.* They are usually asymptomatic.

85. A 25-year-old woman has palatal ulcers and blisters. The diagnosis is:
A. Pemphigoid
B. Dermatitis herpetiformis
C. Pemphigus foliaceus
D. Pemphigus vulgaris
(AI 1997)

86. In pemphigus vulgaris, antibodies are present against:
A. Epidermal keratin
B. Intercellular substance
C. Basement membrane
D. None of the above
(PGI 2000)

87. Intraepithelial bulla is a feature of:
A. Polymorphous light eruption
B. Dermatitis herpetiformis
C. Pemphigoid
D. Pemphigus
(AI 1991)

88. Acantholysis is seen in:
A. Psoriasis
B. Steven Johnson syndrome
C. Pemphigus
D. Pemphigoid

89. Acantholysis is seen in:
A. Subcutaneous tissue
B. Dermoepidermis junction
C. Dermis
D. Epidermis
(AI 1995)

90. Mucous membrane lesions are seen in:
A. Dermatitis herpetiformis
B. Impetigo
C. Pemphigoid
D. Pemphigus

91. In pemphigus the acantholytic cells have:
A. Hyperchromatic nuclei and perinuclear halo
B. Hypochromatic nuclei and perinuclear halo
C. Multinucleated cells
D. None of the above
(PGI 1996)

92. *Most common* variety of pemphigus:
A. Pemphigus vulgaris
B. Pemphigus foliaceus
C. Pemphigus neonatorum
D. Pemphigus cutanea tarda

Pemphigus vulgaris* is the most common variant of pemphigus. Pemphigus vulgaris is a chronic and *potentially* fatal disease which is characterized by appearance of bullae upon *apparently* normal skin. The blister is **intra-epidermal and separation of epidermal cells is known as acantholysis.** Autoantibodies against **intercellular material** of the epidermal cells are present both in serum and bound to the intercellular material of the epidermal cells suggesting the autoimmune etiology of the disease. It occurs most commonly between 40 and 60 years of age and affects females more frequently than males. The bullae *usually* appear first in the mouth and subsequently spread to the skin. Even when the skin is the site of primary involvement the mouth is *almost always* affected *sooner or later*. The bullae are flaccid and arise on normal looking skin (without previous erythema). The contents are first sterile, clear, and serous fluid which later become infected and purulent giving rise to a red areola around the bulla. Bullae may be of large size and keep on arising in new locations. As they rupture, they leave behind tender raw areas which may eventually extend over a large proportion of the skin. Smaller bullae may "dry up" and form crust. If the tip of the finger is pressed on the skin of a patient the horny layer of the epidermis is felt to slide on the underlying layers (**Nikolsky's sign**). The mouth may become extremely painful and septic due to loss of epithelium from the large part of its surface and other **mucous membranes** such as that of upper respiratory passages or genitalia may also be affected. Conjunctival involvement may produce acute but transient conjunctivitis. The general condition of the patient deteriorates slowly or rapidly due to pyrexia and septic infection of mouth and skin surface. Diarrhea, vomiting and albuminuria may be present. If left untreated the disease is invariably fatal with the average time from onset of disease to death being 14 months. Before diagnosing the disease it must be kept in mind that it is a *rare* disorder and the bullous eruptions may be confused with those of *pemphigoid*, *dermatitis herpetiformis*, *erythema multiforme*, *bullous impetigo*, *bullous drug eruptions* and *bullous reaction to mosquito bites.* The characteristic degenerated cells or acantholytic cells may be found in scarping from the floor of a fresh bulla and are helpful in diagnosis as they are not found in any other bullous eruption. Acantholytic epidermal cells are round homogeneous cells containing **hyperchromatic nuclei**. The patient should be kept in bed preferably on air mattress or water bed and steroid treatment can be life saving. Sometimes very **high dosages of steroids** (up to 250 mg of prednisolone per day) have to be given to control the disorder but it is then possible to *gradually* reduce the dose. **Azathioprine** is also helpful but it takes 2 months to show its full effect.

*** Vulgaris means common or ordinary.**

93. An old man in good health has tense bullous lesion over thigh and abdomen with itching lesion *without* involvement of mucosa of mouth. *Most likely* diagnosis is:

A. Dermatitis herpetiformis
B. Pemphigus foliaceus
C. Pemphigus vulgaris
D. Bullous pemphigoid *(AI 2000)*

94. Subepidermal bulla is found in:

A. Pityriasis alba
B. Psoriasis
C. Pemphigoid
D. Pemphigus

95. An 85 years old female with *negative* Nikolsky's sign has blisters on thigh and trunk which come on and off. *Most likely* diagnosis is:

A. Dermatitis herpetiformis
B. Lichen planus
C. Pemphigoid
D. Pemphigus vulgaris *(PGI 2000)*

96. A 60-year-old man has a tense hemorrhagic blister found in thigh region with no oral involvement. The *most likely* diagnosis is:

A. Erythema multiforme
B. Dystrophic epidermolysis
C. Bullous pemphigoid
D. Pemphigus vulgaris

Pemphigoid is a bullous disease of old people in which large, tense and sometimes hemorrhagic blisters are seen widely on limbs, trunk and occasionally mucous membrane. **The blister is always sub-epidermal.** They arise on normal skin or on a sheet of edematous erythema that precede them by days or weeks and can cause severe itching. The cause is unknown. It can be differentiated from pemphigus by the following points:

	Pemphigus vulgaris	**Pemphigoid**
Age of onset	40–60 years	60–80 years
Most common site of primary involvement	Mucous membranes	Legs, arms, head and trunk *in that order*
Most common initial lesion	Localized cutaneous crusting or ulceration of mucosa	Groups of tense bullae which may be hemorrhagic
Mucosal involvement	Early and common	Late and rare
Prognosis	Always poor	Poor in old people
Course	Slow evolution and deterioration	Varied; recurrent attacks and spontaneous remissions

Glucocorticoids are used similarly as in pemphigus although dosage in excess of 40 mg/day of prednisolone is *only rarely* required. Immunosuppressants are also useful and dapsone will rarely control the disease alone or may allow a reduction in dose of systemic corticosteroids.

97. Nikolsky's sign is *not* seen in:

A. Pemphigus vulgaris
B. Toxic epidermal necrolysis
C. Bullous pemphigoid
D. Staphylococcal scalded skin syndrome (SSSS) *(AIIMS 2000)*

Conditions Associated with Positive Nikolsky's Sign

- Pemphigus
- Porphyria
- Staphylococcal scalded skin syndrome
- Steven Johnson's syndrome
- Toxic epidermal necrolysis

98. In which of the following condition, herald patch is seen:

A. Psoriasis
B. Scarlet fever
C. Tinea versicolor
D. Pityriasis rosea *(AI 1991, SGPGI 1999, JIPMER 2000)*

99. In a patient, annular erythematous lesions on the trunk were seen circumscribed by collarette scales. The diagnosis is *most likely* to be:

A. Pityriasis versicolor
B. Pityriasis rosea
C. Pityriasis rubra
D. Lichen planus *(AI 2002)*

Pityriasis rosea is a *common* disease characterized by an eruption of **oval pink macules** on the trunk and upper parts of the limbs which tend to scale from the centre outwards. Most probably it is a viral infection although the virus is yet to be identified. General symptoms are absent *except* in the most severe cases where slight pyrexia, sore throat and lymphadenitis may be seen. Most of the patients are between 6 and 30 years of age and maximum incidence is in the first 3 months of the years. Case to case transmission is unusual but when it occurs incubation period is between 2 and 3 weeks. The first lesion (**herald patch**) is a **red scaly macule of up to 4 cm in diameter situated on some part of the trunk or upper part of the limbs**. After a week the general eruption appear *suddenly* all over the trunk and over the upper parts of the limbs. *Exceptionally* the lesions may spread *up* the neck, on to the scalp and sides of the face or extend *down* on the forearms and legs. The general eruption consists of 2 types of lesions viz. small red follicular papules and pink oval macules. These are oval, 1-2 cm in length and their long axis is parallel to the underlying ribs. After a few days they become wrinkly in the centre and buff (fawn) colored and then begin to peel off from centre outwards. A **ring of scales** is *typically* formed whose free edges are *towards* the centre and attached edges towards the periphery of the lesion (**collarette of trailing scales**). The disease is self limiting and usually lasts for 6-8 weeks. Second attacks are very rare. **Itching is the only symptom** and is never very severe. It may be absent altogether. The disease clears without treatment and treatment is only required to suppress itching when it is present. 1% hydrocortisone cream is very effective and bath should be restricted to twice a week because excessive soap and water irritate the lesions.

100. Gluten free diet is beneficial in which of the following condition:

A. Pemphigoid **B.** Dermatitis herpetiformis
C. Exfoliative dermatitis **D.** Psoriasis *(KARNATAKA 1996)*

101. For dermatitis herpetiformis the drug of choice is:

A. Psoralen **B.** Zinc cream
C. Dapsone **D.** Steroids *(AI 1991)*

102. In dermatitis herpetiformis the drug of choice is:

A. Psoralen **B.** Zinc cream
C. Tetracycline **D.** Dapsone *(UP 1997)*

103. HLA associated with Dermatitis herpetiformis is:

A. HLA A5 **B.** HLA B27
C. HLA B8 **D.** HLA A28

Dermatitis herpetiformis is a disease characterized by erythematous vesicular or bullous lesions and severe itching. The disease most commonly occurs between 20-40 years of age and men are more commonly affected. IgA is deposited in the reticular dermis of the uninvolved skin suggesting an immune etiology. **More than 90% of patients express the HLA B8**/DRW3 and HLA DQW2. It is also associated with gluten sensitive enteropathy. Polymorphism of the eruption (erythematous blotches or stain, grouped vesicle or bullae) and intense itching are characteristic features of the disease. The attacks last for weeks or months with intervals of partial remission over a period of years. General health of the patient is unaffected except due to sleeplessness caused by irritation or secondary infection. Although any part of the body may be involved but mucous membranes are involved only in 1% of the cases. Distribution is usually bilateral and symmetrical and forearms, thighs, inter-scapular region and buttocks beings most commonly involved. **Dapsone** is the drug of choice and is given 50 mg 1–4 times a day orally. Most of the patients are controlled by 100 mg daily dose but the requirement varies from time to time. The affect of dapsone is *dramatic* and *rapid* with all signs disappearing in 48 hours. However, the treatment must be continued indefinitely as it is *suppressive* and *not curative*. It is also necessary to treat the patient with a **gluten free diet** because this reduces the dose of drug required to suppress the eruption.

104. Berloque dermatitis is due to contact with which of the following:

A. Plants
B. Food
C. Cosmetics
D. Metal

Berloque dermatitis is a skin condition in which patients develops a brownish to reddish discoloration of the neck and sometimes the arms **due to applying perfume or cologne to the skin**. Sometimes the skin 1st turns red before changing to a brownish color. This condition can persist for years or even be permanent. Many perfumes and colognes contain **oil of bergamot**, an extract of the peel of a specific orange grown in the South of France and the *Calabria* district of Italy. When this oil comes in contact with the skin and the skin is exposed to sunlight, the oil of bergamot causes the skin to discolor. With repeated exposures to sunlight, the discoloration becomes permanent.

105. Growing phase of hair is:

A. Catagen and telogen
B. Telogen
C. Anagen
D. Catagen *(PGI 1997)*

- **Telogen** is the resting stage of the hair growth cycle.
- **Anagen** is the growth stage of hair development.
- **Catagen** is the intermediate phase of the hair-growth cycle, between the growth or anagen stage and the resting or telogen phase.

106. Acrodermatitis enteropathica responds dramatically to:
A. Corticosteroids **B.** Zinc
C. Dapsone **D.** Ciprofloxacin

Acrodermatitis enteropathica is an autosomal recessive disease. **Zinc deficiency** is due to a defect in zinc absorption. The symptoms begin when an affected infant is weaned from human to cow's milk. It is **treated with oral zinc 2 mg/kg/day**.

107. "Flaky paint" appearance of skin is seen in:
A. Kwashiorkor **B.** Marasmus
C. Psoriasis **D.** Pellagra *(AI 1995)*

The skin lesions in **kwashiorkor** appear as large areas of erythema, followed by hyperpigmentation. The skin becomes dry and hyperkeratotic. The epidermis peels off in large scales, exposing a raw area below. This area is prone to infection. It resembles old paint flaking off (*so called* **flaky paint appearance**) the surface of the wood.

108. Phrynoderma is a cutaneous manifestation of severe deficiency of vitamin:
A. A **B.** B
C. C **D.** D

Phrynoderma or the **toad skin** is caused by the deficiency of **vitamin A** and essential fatty acids.

109. Pseudopelade is also known as:
A. Cicatricial alopecia **B.** Traction alopecia
C. Premature alopecia **D.** Alopecia totalis *(PGI 1990)*

Cicatricial alopecia is also known as folliculitis decalvans or **pseudo pelade**. This disease usually attacks the upper part of scalp and is of insidious onset and slow evolution. Small bald patches from which the hair follicles have disappeared appear on the scalp which is converted into a depressed atrophic scar. *To begin with* the patches are small and irregular but they often run together to form large bald areas leaving a few tufts of hair "here and there". No treatment is effective and prognosis is unfavorable.

110. *Not* a characteristic feature of Melkersson-Rosenthal syndrome:
A. Plication of tongue **B.** Black hairy tongue
C. Labial edema **D.** Recurrent VII nerve palsy *(DELHI 1993)*

Melkersson-Rosenthal syndrome consists of a triad of:
- **Recurrent facial paralysis** (recurrent and eventually permanent)
- **Facial** (particularly labial) **edema**;
- **Plication of the tongue**.

111. Toxic shock syndrome is caused by:
A. *Escherichia coli* **B.** *Pseudomonas*
C. *Streptococcus* **D.** *Staphylococcus* *(AI 1993)*

112. Scalded skin syndrome in infancy is caused by:
A. *Corynebacterium*
B. *Pseudomonas*
C. *Streptococcus*
D. *Staphylococcus* *(UP 1997)*

Staphylococcal scalded skin syndrome (SSSS) is caused by *Staphylococcus aureus* phase group II and is most common in children *under 10 years of age*. It is termed as **Ritter's syndrome** in neonates and **toxic epidermal necrolysis** (TEN) in older patients. There is diffused tender erythema with bullae and desquamation. Nikolsky's sign may be present.

113. Staphylococcus causes all *except*:

A. Scarlet fever
B. Toxic shock syndrome
C. SSSS
D. Carbuncle

(PGI 1999)

Scarlet fever consists of *streptococcal* infection, usually pharyngitis, associated with a characteristic rash.

114. *Most common* etiology of erythema multiforme is:

A. Viral
B. Bacterial
C. Food
D. Drugs

Erythema multiforme represents a **hypersensitivity reaction** to drugs or infections. The most *severe* form of erythema multiforme is known as *toxic epidermal necrolysis.* It is generally idiopathic but the ***most common* cause is infection of herpes simplex virus**, with the erythema multiforme forming 1-3 weeks after development of a typical herpes simplex lesion.

115. A 60-year-old man has severe bullous lesions for last three days. Each bulla was surrounded by and erythematous halo. There were multiple "target" lesions and the patient also has oral erosions. Diagnosis is:

A. Steven Johnson syndrome
B. Herpes gestationis
C. Herpes simplex
D. Chicken pox

(SGPGI 1999)

116. *False* regarding erythema multiforme is:

A. Associated with adverse drug reaction
B. Target lesion with bull's eye lesion is seen over hand and soles
C. Associated with internal malignancy
D. Vesicle and bullae are *not* seen

(AI 2000)

117. "Target iris" lesion is seen in:

A. Lichen planus
B. Scabies
C. Erythema multiforme
D. Urticaria

(AI 1998)

Erythema multiforme is an eruption consisting of circular or irregular erythematous blotches which are bilateral and symmetrical and usually occur on the backs of the hands and forearm. Other common sites are dorsal surfaces of the feet, legs, knees, sides of neck, face and mucous membrane of the mouth. The disease has strong tendency to reoccur and is *probably* caused by circulating immune complexes. It may occur after vaccination, herpes simplex infection, *Mycoplasma pneumoniae* infection or can be caused by drugs (mainly sulphonamides and barbiturates). It may be associated with internal malignancy or its treatment with radiotherapy. Erythema multiforme is more common in children and young adults. Either general symptoms are absent or the eruption is preceded by malaise, fever and joint pain. Sore throat, diarrhea, high fever and severe pain in large joints may be present. In **local maculopapular type** of erythema multiforme the lesions are red or violaceous macules or papules on the backs of hands, forearms, dorsal surfaces of feet, legs, knees and sides of neck. Backs of hands and wrists are the most common site. The size varies from 1–5 cm and a common lesion (**erythema iris or bull's eye lesion**) consists of circular lesions resembling **targets**. In the centre of this circular lesion is a purpuric spot surrounded by concentric rings of shades of red or violet. In **vesicular and bullous type** of disease the lesions appear first as red macules which soon develops a vesicle in the centre. **Steven Johnson's syndrome is a severe type of bullous erythema multiforme involving skin, respiratory tract, mucous membranes (usually those of eyes, mouth and urethral meatus) associated with a high continuous fever. Kidneys may be involved leading to nephritis.** No drug has any specific affect in erythema multiforme but when mucous membranes are involved local or systemic antibiotics may be required to control secondary infection.

118. Skin doubling time is..........weeks:

A. 12
B. 8
C. 4
D. 1

Skin is the boundary between man and his environment and its paramount function is protection. It may be divided into 3 layers viz. the epidermis, dermis and subcutaneous tissue. Although they arise in the dermis, glands, hairs and nails are epidermal structures. Epidermis is an avascular cellular tissue consisting of 2 main layers of cells viz. **stratum Malpighii**, and **stratum corneum** (horny layer). Stratum Malpighii is further subdivided into the **basal layer**, **prickle layer** and the **granular layer** *from within outwards*. The principal function of epidermis is constant replacement of the stratum corneum which is being continuously shed and the differing cell types found within stratum Malpighii represents the stages in conversion of the epithelial cells into horn cells. **It takes about 28 days from the division of basal cells to the formation of mature horn cells.**

119. Saber tibia is seen in:
- **A.** Syphilis
- **B.** Leprosy
- **C.** Rickets
- **D.** Scurvy

(AI 1993, UP 1997)

Saber-shaped tibia is the deformity of the tibia caused by gummatous periostitis due to syphilis, in which it curves outward.
**Saber means a heavy cavalry sword with a slightly curved blade.*

120. A 9-month-old infant has itchy papules on face and papulo-vesicular lesions on palms and soles and trunk. *Most likely* diagnosis is:
- **A.** Insect bite
- **B.** Seborrheic dermatitis
- **C.** Scabies
- **D.** Atopic dermatitis

121. Characteristic lesion of scabies is:
- **A.** Burrow
- **B.** Fissure
- **C.** Vesicle
- **D.** Papule

122. Scabies in infants differs from that in adults in that it affects:
- **A.** Web space
- **B.** Face
- **C.** Genitalia
- **D.** Axilla

(JIPMER 2000)

Scabies is a highly communicable skin disease caused by *Sarcoptes scabiei*, variety *hominis*, commonly called, the **itch mite.** The impregnated females live in burrows that appear as dark wavy lines in the epidermis measuring 3 to 15 mm and end in a small pearly bleb which contains the female mite. Scabies manifests as papules, vesicles, pustules, and **burrows** and causes **intense itching** resulting in eczema. The body parts most commonly involved are the hands, between the fingers, the wrists, axillae, genitalia, beneath the breasts, and the inner aspect of the thighs. **Except in infants, the lesions do *not* develop on face, scalp, neck, palms, and soles.** Female mite deposits eggs within the tunnel and they hatch within 3 to 5 days. The larvae molt into nymphs on the skin surface and mature in 14–21 days. Mature insects mate, and the gravid female invades the skin to begin a new cycle. Scabies is transmitted by direct contact with infected persons, and rarely by fomites. **Norwegian or crusted scabies is a rare condition characterized by extensive crusting and scaling; involvement of face; enormous numbers of acari even beneath the finger nails.** It is due to neglect of scabies and is common among mentally retarded people in whom the condition appears to cause *little* itching. Scabies should be treated with an application of either **25% benzyl benzoate** or **1% gamma benzene hexachloride** (GBH). 1% GBH is less irritant and more effective and should be applied to the **whole skin from neck downward** ideally with a brush. It is essential that the *whole skin* be completely covered and is quite *useless* to treat only areas with active lesion. Two applications are required at 24 hour interval and after another 24 hours of second application bath should be taken because for the treatment to be effective the drug must remain on the skin for a total of 48 hours. The patient should be *strictly* told *not* to wash *any* part of his body before the final bath. Washing of clothes, dishes and even hands must be forbidden because scabies will not be cured until these instructions are strictly followed. Due to prolonged incubation period of the disease and impossibility of recognizing the disease during this period **all the members of the family must be treated simultaneously.** Unless this is done the disease will remain *endemic* within the family for months or years. *Finally* it is *not* necessary to disinfect clothing or bedclothes and a change of clothing and *ordinary* laundering is all that is required after the final bath.

123. Most severe form of scabies is:

A. Norwegian scabies
B. Neular scabies
C. Animal scabies
D. Genital scabies

Crusted or **Norwegian scabies is a hyperinfestation with thousands or millions of mites** and may result from glucocorticoid use, immunodeficiency diseases (e.g. AIDS), and neurologic and psychiatric illnesses that interfere with itching and scratching.

124. Burrows of scabies are in:

A. Stratum corneum
B. Stratum germinativum
C. Dermis
D. Stratum Malpighii

(KERALA 1990)

The female mite **burrows horizontally in the deeper part of horny layer (stratum corneum)** advancing at a rate of 0.5–5 mm/day and leaving behind in the burrow a trail of eggs and feces.

125. Latest systemic oral medication for scabies is:

A. Gamma benzene hexachloride
B. Carbaryl
C. Benzyl benzoate
D. Ivermectin

(PGI 2000)

126. Permethrin is useful in:

A. Leishmaniasis
B. Body louse
C. Leprosy
D. Scabies

(AI 1999, UP 2000)

- The **treatment of choice of scabies for children 8 weeks and older is permethrin 5% cream** which should be **applied once to the entire skin area**, *avoiding the eyes, nose, and mouth*. The cream should be thoroughly washed off after **8 to 10 hours of application**.
- The fingernails should be trimmed to prevent the harboring of mites.
- For adults, permethrin, 5% cream or lindane 1% lotion is applied thinly and thoroughly behind the ears and from the neck down after bathing and left on overnight for 8 to 14 hr and are then removed with soap and water. **Lindane** is absorbed through the skin, and its overuse may cause seizures and aplastic anemia.
- Alternatives include **topical crotamiton cream, benzyl benzoate, and sulfur ointments.**
- Pregnant women and infants less than 2 months of age should be treated with 6% to 10% precipitated sulfur in petrolatum daily for 3 days.
- Successful treatment of crusted scabies requires the application first of a keratolytic agent such as 6% salicylic acid which improve the penetration of scabicides and then followed by application of scabicides to the scalp, face, and ears.
- **A single oral dose of ivermectin (200 µg/kg) effectively treats scabies in otherwise healthy individuals.**

127. Melanocytes are present in:

A. Stratum spinosum
B. Stratum basalis
C. Stratum corneum
D. Stratum granulosum

(PGI 1999)

128. Pigmentation of skin is due to:

A. ACTH
B. Keratin
C. Melanin
D. Pigmentin

(UP 1999)

Scattered in the **basal layer of epidermis** and in the hair matrix are the cells which do not stain with H&E and are referred as "clear cells". These clear cells are the **melanocytes** and are the *only* cells in the *normal* human skin which are capable of synthesizing **melanin**. These melanocytes have long branching processes known as dendrites which form a network by anastomosing with other melanocytes. The melanin is injected into the basal cells and the suprabasal keratinocytes in the form of granules. The amount of melanin depends on the *activity* of melanocytes and not on their number which is same in both Negro and Albino races. Melanin protects the skin from UV radiation. Intensity of skin pigmentation is governed by the pituitary hormones α and β MSH, ACTH, estrogens and progesterone. MSH and ACTH cause generalized hyperpigmentation with accentuation over the buccal mucosa and palmer creases (Addison's disease) while estrogen and progesterone increase pigmentation over specific areas.

129. "Cradle cap" is a special form of:

A. Down's syndrome
B. Cephalhematoma
C. Seborrheic dermatitis
D. Alopecia steatoides

Seborrheic dermatitis may become evident within the first few weeks of life. It occurs in the scalp "**cradle cap**", face, or groin. It is rarely seen in children beyond infancy but becomes evident again during adult life. The majority of individuals with seborrheic dermatitis have no underlying disorder, although it is frequently seen in patients suffering from Parkinson's disease, and HIV infection or those who have had cerebrovascular accidents. It is treated with low-potency topical glucocorticoids in addition to shampoos containing coal tar and/or salicylic acid.

130. Alopecia aerate is:

A. Inflammatory
B. Fungal
C. Non-cicatricial
D. Cicatricial scar

(UP 1996)

131. Alopecia areata is due to:

A. Lichenoid reaction
B. Autoimmune disease
C. Estrogen stimulation
D. Androgen stimulation

132. Exclamation mark hair is a characteristic feature of:

A. Tinea capitis
B. Telogen effluvium
C. Androgenic alopecia
D. Alopecia areata

(SGPGI 1999)

133. Alopecia areata totalis is treated by:

A. Minoxidil
B. Tranquilizers
C. Diphencyprone
D. Parenteral penicillin

Alopecia areata is a disease characterized by a **sudden loss of hair over circumscribed patches** on the scalp, beard or elsewhere. In *alopecia totalis* the whole scalp becomes bald while in *alopecia universalis* the whole body is affected. They are varieties of alopecia areata. The alopecia areata occurs mainly between the ages of 5–25 years and is uncommon over 45 years. There is some evidence that it is an **autoimmune disease**. The patient complains that the hairs are "coming out" suddenly, i.e. over night or gradually. The **patches** are **completely bald** and the skin surface is smooth. A few **exclamation mark stumps** may be seen at the edges of the patches. These are the hairs broken off about 6mm from the scalp whose free ends are of normal colored and thickened while the inserted ends are depigmented and very thin. The course of disease is very unpredictable but in 80% of cases the first attack makes a complete recovery. **Multiple patches and rapid extension are the bad prognostic signs and the prognosis is less good if the condition begins before puberty.** Vigorous brushing, combing, massage or rubbing of lotions and ointments must be avoided. In early cases having only 1–2 small patches a **vigorous reassurance along with a simple lotion such as salicylic acid lotion is all that is required.** The systemic steroids will make the hair grow but relapse will occur when they are stopped. Alopecia areata *totalis* gives excellent response to topical **diphencyprone.**

134. Condyloma lata occurs in:

A. Late syphilis
B. Latent syphilis
C. Secondary syphilis
D. Primary syphilis

(AIIMS 1999, UP 2000)

In **secondary syphilis** scattered red-brown papules with thin scale are found. The palms and soles are involved often. Other findings include annular plaques on the face, nonscarring alopecia, **condyloma lata** which are broad-based and moist, mucous patches and lymphadenopathy, malaise, fever, headache, and myalgias. The interval between the primary chancre and the secondary stage is 4 to 8 weeks.

135. Multidrug therapy is commonly given in:

A. Leprosy
B. Syphilis
C. Icthyosis vulgaris
D. Herpetiformis

(AI 1994)

136. For *Mycobacterium leprae*, the most potent drug is:

A. Clofazimine
B. Ofloxacin
C. Rifampicin
D. Dapsone

The drugs used in **WHO-MDT are a combination of rifampicin, clofazimine and dapsone for MB leprosy patients and rifampicin and dapsone for PB leprosy patients.** Among these **rifampicin is the most important antileprosy drug** and therefore is included in the treatment of both types of leprosy. Treatment of leprosy with *only* one antileprosy drug will *always* result in development of drug resistance to that drug. *Treatment with dapsone or any other antileprosy drug used as monotherapy should be considered as an unethical practice.*

Rifampicin: The drug is given once a month. No toxic effects have been reported in the case of monthly administration. The urine may be colored slightly reddish for a few hours after its intake; this should be explained to the patient while starting MDT.

Clofazimine: It is most active when administered daily. The drug is well-tolerated and virtually non-toxic in the dosage used for MDT. The drug causes brownish black discoloration and dryness of skin. However, this disappears within few months after stopping treatment. This should be explained to patients while starting MDT regimen for MB leprosy.

Dapsone: The drug is very safe in the dosage used in MDT and side effects are rare. The main side effect is allergic reaction, causing itchy skin rashes and exfoliative dermatitis. Patients known to be allergic to any of the sulpha drugs should not be given dapsone.

137. Borderline tuberculoid leprosy should be treated with:

A. Clofazimine
B. Dapsone + clofazimine
C. Dapsone + rifampicin
D. Dapsone

(UP 1996)

Paucibacillary leprosy	**Multibacillary leprosy**
Smear negative intermediate (I)	Lepromatous (L)
Smear negative tuberculoid (T)	Borderline lepromatous (BL)
Smear negative **borderline tuberculoid** (BT)	
Smear negative pure neuritic (N)	

138. In a single lesion of paucibacillary leprosy, the single dose treatment is:

A. Dapsone, clofazimine
B. Rifampicin, ofloxacin, minocycline
C. Dapsone, rifampicin, clofazimine
D. Rifampicin, ofloxacin, clarithromycin

(PGI 2000, AIIMS 2000)

139. WHO regime for paucibacillary leprosy is:

A. Rifampicin + clofazimine daily
B. Dapsone + rifampicin + clofazimine daily
C. Dapsone daily + clofazimine daily
D. Dapsone daily + rifampicin monthly

(AI 1996)

140. According to WHO recommendation the duration of treatment of multibacillary leprosy is:

A. 7 years
B. 5 years
C. 2 years
D. 1 year

(SGPGI 1999)

141. The first line antileprosy drugs include all *except*:
- **A.** Dapsone
- **B.** Thiacetazone
- **C.** Clofazimine
- **D.** Rifampicin

WHO-recommended MDT Regimens for Adults

Multibacillary leprosy	Paucibacillary leprosy	Single Skin Lesion Paucibacillary leprosy
• Rifampicin: 600 mg once a month • Dapsone: 100 mg daily • Clofazimine: 300 mg once a month and 50 mg daily	• Rifampicin: 600 mg once a month • Dapsone: 100 mg daily	• Rifampicin: 600 mg • Ofloxacin: 400 mg • Minocycline: 100 mg
Duration= 24 months	Duration= 6 months	***(single dose)***

142. Most sensitive index to assess the drug effectiveness in skin smears of leprosy patient is:
- **A.** Culture of lesion
- **B.** Granuloma index
- **C.** Morphological index
- **D.** Bacteriological index

(KARNATAKA 1994)

Two indices which depend on observation of *Mycobacterium leprae* in smears from skin or nasal smears are useful in assessing the amount of infection, and the viability of the organisms and also the progress of the patient under treatment. They are the morphological index and the bacteriological index.

1. **The bacteriological index (BI) is an expression of the extent of bacterial loads.** It is calculated by counting 6 to 8 stained smears under the 100 x oil immersion lens in a smear made by nicking the skin with a sharp scalpel and scraping it; the fluid and tissue obtained are spread fairly thickly on a slide and stained by the Ziehl-Neelsen method and decolorized (but not completely) which 1% acid alcohol. The results are expressed on a logarithmic scale.

- 1+ At least 1 bacillus in every 100 fields.
- 2+ At least 1 bacillus in every 10 fields.
- 3+ At least 1 bacillus in every field.
- 4+ At least 10 bacilli in every field.
- 5+ At least 100 bacilli in every field.
- 6+ At least 1000 bacilli in every field.

The **bacteriological index is valuable** because it is simple and is representative of many lesions but is affected by the depth of the skin incision, the thoroughness of the scrape and the thickness of the film. A more accurate and reliable index of the bacillary content of a lesion is given by the *logarithmic index of biopsies* (LIB). **These indices help to assess the state of patients at the beginning of treatment and to assess progress.**

2. **The morphological index (MI) is calculated by counting the numbers of solid-staining acid-fast rods.** Only the solid-staining bacilli are viable. It is not unusual for solid-staining *Mycobacterium leprae* to reappear for short periods in patients being successfully treated with drugs. It is important to recognize that measurement of MI is liable for observer variations and therefore *not always reliable*.

143. Thalidomide is the *drug of choice* for:
- **A.** Nerve excision
- **B.** Nerve abscess
- **C.** Lepra type II reaction
- **D.** Lepra type I reaction

(AI 1999)

144. The drug of choice for type 2 lepra reaction is:
- **A.** Clofazimine
- **B.** Chloroquine
- **C.** Thalidomide
- **D.** Steroids

(JIPMER 2000)

145. Reversal lepra reaction *does not* respond to:
- **A.** Thalidomide
- **B.** Glucocorticoids
- **C.** Clofazimine
- **D.** NSAIDs

(DELHI 1993)

146. In a patient of tuberculoid leprosy, type 1 lepra reaction occurs, the treatment is:
A. No change in treatment **B.** Stop dapsone permanently
C. Continue dapsone and start steroid **D.** Stop dapsone immediately *(AIIMS 1999)*

147. For leprosy and lepra reaction which of the following antileprosy drug is used:
A. Dapsone **B.** Dexamethasone
C. Clofazimine **D.** L dapsone

148. ENL is seen in:
A. Indeterminate leprosy **B.** Borderline tuberculoid leprosy
C. Lepromatous leprosy **D.** Tuberculoid leprosy

The general course of leprosy is indolent but may be interrupted by 2 types of reaction. Both reactions *can* occur in untreated patients but more often occur as complications of chemotherapy.

- **Erythema nodosum leprosum (ENL), or type 2 lepra reaction**, develops in **lepromatous** and **borderline lepromatous** patients. Tender, inflamed subcutaneous nodules usually develop in crops. Each nodule lasts for a week or 2, but new crops *may* continue to appear. Fever, lymphadenopathy, and arthralgias can be present in severe ENL. Mild ENL is managed with antipyretics and anti-inflammatory agents and severe cases can be rapidly controlled with high dosages of **prednisone**. **Antimicrobial therapy should be continued. Thalidomide is the most effective drug for ENL. Clofazimine** has anti-inflammatory properties *as well as* antimycobacterial activity and can be valuable in the treatment of chronic ENL. Other anti-inflammatory agents, including **chloroquine, cyclosporine**, and cytotoxic drugs.
- The **reversal reaction, or type 1 lepra reaction**, may complicate all 3 borderline categories. Mild episodes may be managed with NSAIDs, but **glucocorticoids are essential in severe reversal reactions.** Prolonged maintenance therapy is often required. **Reversal reactions *do not* respond to thalidomide.**

149. Koenen's periungual fibromas are seen in cases of:
A. Tuberous sclerosis **B.** Sturge-Weber's syndrome
C. Ataxia telangiectasia **D.** Neurofibromatosis *(JIPMER 2002)*

In patients of *tuberous sclerosis* **Koenen's tumors** (subungual or periungual fibromas) usually first appear in adolescence; toes are more commonly involved than fingers.

150. *Not* a feature of lepromatous leprosy:
A. Gynecomastia **B.** Madarosis
C. Collapse of bridge of nose **D.** Perforating ulcer

151. Virchow cells are seen in:
A. Leprosy **B.** Congenital syphilis
C. Toxic epidermal necrolysis **D.** Henoch-Schönlein purpura *(PGI 1992)*

152. *Maximum* numbers of lepra bacilli are seen in:
A. BL **B.** TT
C. BT **D.** LL *(PGI 1993)*

153. *Maximum* suppression of cell-mediated immunity occurs in:
A. Indeterminate leprosy **B.** Tuberculoid leprosy
C. Lepromatous leprosy **D.** Borderline leprosy

In **lepromatous leprosy** there is extensive cutaneous involvement and is *roughly* bilaterally symmetric across the midline of the patient. Individual skin lesions are variable and can include macules, nodules, plaques, or papules. The borders of the lesions are ill defined, and the centers of raised lesions are indurated and convex. There is diffuse infiltration of the dermis between discrete lesions, and *apparently* normal skin usually contains bacilli which are demonstrable by staining. The sites of preference are the face (cheeks, nose, and brows), ears, wrists, elbows, buttocks, and knees. Loss of the lateral portions of the eyebrows (**madarosis**) is common and later on the skin of the face and forehead becomes thickened and corrugated (**leonine facies**), and the earlobes become pendulous. Nasal "stuffiness," epistaxis, and obstructed breathing are common early symptoms. Complete nasal obstruction, laryngitis, and hoarseness may also develop. Septal perforation and nasal collapse leads to **saddlenose** and invasion of the anterior portion of the eye can result in keratitis and iridocyclitis. Painless inguinal and axillary lymphadenopathy occurs. In men, infiltration and scarring of the testes lead to sterility. **Gynecomastia** is common. Involvement of the major nerve trunks is less prominent in the lepromatous than in the tuberculoid form, but diffuse hypesthesia involving the peripheral portions of the extremities is common in advanced disease. Pathologic studies demonstrate that the **peripheral nerves are heavily infected** but often better preserved than in the tuberculoid form. Histological examination reveals a diffuse granulomatous reaction with macrophages, large foam (**Virchow or lepra**) cells, and many intracellular bacilli, frequently in spheroidal masses (**globi**) but epithelioid cells and giant cells are *not* found.

**Loss of eyelashes or eyebrows is known as madarosis.*

154. Single skin lesion is seen in which of the following type of leprosy:

A. Lepromatous leprosy
B. BT
C. BL
D. TT

(AI 1993)

155. *False* regarding tuberculoid leprosy is:

A. Body immunity is high
B. Prognosis is good
C. Negative lepromin test
D. It is non-infective

(KARNATAKA 1996)

156. Acid-fast bacilli in slit smear are *absent* in ....leprosy:

A. Neuritic type
B. Tuberculoid type
C. Indeterminate type
D. Lepra reaction

Leprosy is a chronic infectious disease caused by *Mycobacterium leprae*. It mainly affects the **skin**, **mucus membrane** and **peripheral nerves**. The spread requires *prolonged* human to human contact. Transmission is via nasal lesions in lepromatous leprosy while the mode of spread in other forms is not known. **The disease is found in 2 polar type's viz. lepromatous and tuberculoid.** All forms are dependent on the **immune status** of the patient. **Lepromatous type** represents the state of **minimal resistance** to the disease and the **bacteria are present in large numbers in all lesions.** The patient is highly infectious and histopathological picture consists of a dense widespread dermal infiltrate *crowded* with bacilli. Lepromatous leprosy is a progressive disease. In **tuberculoid leprosy** there is **maximum host resistance** and the **bacteria is very difficult to find in the lesions**. The patient is **almost or completely *noninfectious*** and the histopathological picture is that of a sarcoid granuloma. Tuberculoid leprosy has a tendency of spontaneous limitation. The **intermediate types** include *borderline lepromatous (BL), borderline (BB) and borderline tuberculoid (BT)*. In early stages one intermediate type show various characteristics of the other two types but later on evolve into either lepromatous or tuberculoid leprosy. The **lepromin test** consists of injecting 0.1 ml of an emulsion of killed lepra bacilli *intradermally* into the skin of the front of forearm. A positive result consists of a small nodule that appears within 48 hours (**Fernandez reaction**). **The reaction is positive in tuberculoid leprosy** and also in large individuals living in endemic area. The **tuberculoid leprosy** presents as **one** or more asymmetrical, acutely defined slightly scaly areas of pale skin in which the pigmentation is not completely lost. There is **always loss of sensation in these lesions** usually of light touch and temperature but sometimes also of pain. There is frequent involvement of peripheral nerves and peroneal, ulnar and great auricular nerves may be become palpable. The symptoms of polyneuritis may develop producing foot drop or ulnar palsy. In **lepromatous leprosy** there is insidious onset and vagueness of the margins of the skin lesions which are ill defined erythematous macules. These **macules may be widespread** and symmetrical. The more characteristic nodules and plaques appear later and develop gradually. There is diffuse infiltration of skin and mucosa. The **borderline leprosy** consists of a mixture of clinical features.

157. A male patient presents with multiple nodulocystic lesions on the face with multiple sinuses. The *treatment of choice* is:

A. Retinoids
B. Antibiotics
C. Antituberculous drugs
D. Steroids

(AIIMS May 2002)

Acne vulgaris can affect both adolescents and adults. The pathogenesis of acne is multifactorial and involves overproduction of sebum, an abnormal follicular keratinization process, proliferation of Propionibacterium acnes, and hormonal and immunologic factors. Clinical manifestations of acne range from noninflammatory comedones to inflammatory papules, pustules and cysts. Current therapy allows the physician to select a variety of topical and/or systemic antibiotics, retinoids, and hormone agents aimed at specific pathogenic factors.

When choosing a treatment regimen and evaluating the response to treatment, it is sometimes helpful to grade acne in a particular patient on the basis of the following severity scale.

- Type 1: Comedonal, few lesions (fewer than 10) on face only, without scarring.
- Type 2: Papular, moderate number of lesions (10 to 25) on face and trunk, with mild scarring.
- Type 3: Pustular, many lesions (more than 25), moderate scarring.
- Type 4: Nodulocystic, extensive scarring.

Acne conglobata, an atypical and severe form of acne, is characterized by numerous inflamed cystic lesions, sinuses and extensive scarring over the face and upper trunk.

Treatment options include isotretinoin, steroid injections and hormone therapy. Isotretinoin or oral **13-cis-retinoic acid** is a derivative of vitamin A. It is the only systemic drug that decreases sebum production and reverses the abnormal epithelial desquamation process. It also can decrease the population of P acnes in the sebaceous follicle. These actions make it the treatment of choice for patients with severe nodulocystic acne.

158. A patient presented with single hypopigmented anesthetic patch and satellite lesions on forearm. He is suffering from which type of leprosy:

A. Lepromatous **B.** Neuritic
C. Tuberculoid **D.** Indeterminate

159. Satellite lesions are seen in:

A. Historic leprosy **B.** Borderline tuberculoid leprosy
C. Lepromatous leprosy **D.** Tuberculoid leprosy *(AIIMS 1999, AI 1999, UP 2000)*

This picture demonstrates an infiltrated, well-demarcated, anesthetic scaly lesion of borderline tuberculoid leprosy on the knee. Small **"satellite"** lesions help to classify this lesion **clinically as borderline tuberculoid**.

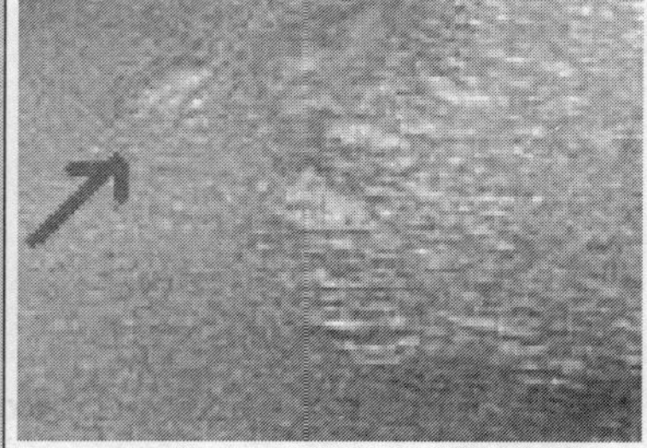

160. Negative smear is seen in...........leprosy:

A. Borderline **B.** Lepromatous
C. Neuritic type **D.** Indeterminate *(AI 1997)*

In pure neuritic type there is nerve involvement but no skin lesion. These cases are bacteriologically negative.

161. Ridley-Jopling classification includes all *except*:

A. Lepromatous leprosy **B.** Borderline
C. Tuberculoid **D.** Neuritic *(JIPMER 2001)*

Leprosy is bedevilled by classifications and many classifications are available such as the Indian classification, the Madrid classification, Ridley-Jopling classification, etc. The **Ridley-Jopling classification** divides cases of leprosy into 5 groups according to their position in an immunohistological scale viz. tuberculoid (TT), borderline tuberculoid (BT), borderline (BB), borderline lepromatous (BL) and lepromatous (LL). Neuritic type does not find a place in this classification. An overview of other classification is as under:

Indian classification	**Madrid classification**
• Indeterminate	• Indeterminate
• Tuberculoid	• Tuberculoid
• Borderline	• Borderline
• Lepromatous	• Lepromatous
• Pure neuritic	

162. *Not* a feature of lesion of leprosy:

A. Flat and raised
B. Hypopigmented
C. Vesicle
D. Erythematous

(AI 1997)

According to WHO the **diagnosis of leprosy** is most commonly based on the clinical signs and symptoms. These are easy to observe and elicit by any health worker after a short period of training. In an endemic country or area, an individual should be regarded as having leprosy if he or she shows **one** of the following **cardinal signs**:

- Skin lesion consistent with leprosy and with definite sensory loss, with or without thickened nerves
- Positive skin smears

The **skin lesion can be single or multiple, usually less pigmented than the surrounding normal skin.** *Sometimes* the lesion is **reddish** or copper-colored. **A variety of skin lesions may be seen but macules (flat), papules (raised), or nodules are common. Sensory loss is a *typical* feature of leprosy.** The skin lesion may show loss of sensation to *pin pick* and/or *light touch*. **Thickened nerves**, mainly peripheral nerve trunks constitute another feature of leprosy. A thickened nerve is often accompanied by other signs as a result of damage to the nerve. These may be loss of sensation in the skin and weakness of muscles supplied by the affected nerve. In the absence of these signs, nerve thickening by itself, without sensory loss and/or muscle weakness is often not a reliable sign of leprosy.

Positive skin smears: In a small proportion of cases, rod-shaped, red-stained leprosy bacilli, which are diagnostic of the disease, may be seen in the smears taken from the affected skin when examined under a microscope after appropriate staining.

A person presenting with skin lesions or with symptoms suggestive of nerve damage, in which the cardinal signs are *absent* or *doubtful* should be called a '**suspect case**' in the absence of any immediately obvious alternate diagnosis.

163. Multidrug therapy is employed in leprosy in order to:

A. Decrease relapse rate
B. Cost-effective
C. Decrease side effects
D. To prevent drug resistance

(MAHE 1999)

The main objectives of MDT for leprosy are:

- To interrupt the transmission of infection in community by sterilizing the infectious patient as early as possible by bactericidal drugs;
- To prevent drug resistance;
- To ensure early detection and treatment of cases and prevent deformities.

164. Clofazimine is associated with all the following side effects *except*:

A. Pigmentation of skin
B. Gastrointestinal intolerance
C. Icthyosis
D. Pseudoporphyria

(JIPMER 2002)

165. One of the following is a side effect of clofazimine used in leprosy therapy:

A. Constipation
B. Erythema
C. Discoloration of body secretions
D. Macular rash

Common side effects of **clofazimine** used in leprosy therapy are:

- Loss of appetite
- Diarrhea
- Nausea and vomiting
- Dry skin and
- **Discoloration (from pink to brownish-black) of the skin, stools, urine, saliva, sweat, tears or lining of the eyelids.** Reversible pink or red to **brownish-black discoloration of the skin** may occur in majority of patients within a few weeks of treatment with **clofazimine**. This may take several months or years to completely disappear after discontinuation of clofazimine.

166. Skin pigmentation is a side effect of:

A. Steroid
B. Dapsone
C. Clofazimine
D. Rifampicin

(AI 1996)

Reversible pink or red to brownish-black discoloration of the skin may occur in 75 to 100% of patients taking clofazimine within a few weeks. It also produces an **ichthyosis like scaling** which is more pronounced over leprosy lesions. These changes may require several months or years to completely disappear after discontinuation of clofazimine.

167. Dose of dapsone is:

A. 1-2 mg/kg
B. 5 mg/kg
C. 10 mg/kg
D. 20 mg/kg

Dapsone is used in the treatment of leprosy, dermatitis herpetiformis, and mycetoma secondary to actinomyces.
Dosage:
- Leprosy-100 mg (2mg/kg) daily for one or more years.
- Dermatitis herpetiformis-50 to 200 mg daily for months to years.
- Mycetoma-200 mg bid for at least a few months after clinical clearing.

168. Daily dose of thalidomide for controlling ENL is:

A. 100 mg
B. 200-400 mg
C. 500 mg
D. 1000 mg only

The most effective drug for ENL is **thalidomide**. For patients with chronic ENL the usual initial dosage of **200 mg twice a day**. It can be gradually tapered to a maintenance dosage of 50 to 100 mg/day.

169. Half life of dapsone is:

A. 12 hours
B. 36 hours
C. 24 hours
D. 6 hours

Dapsone is a folate antagonist, and is used in the treatment of leprosy. The daily dosage is 50 to 100 mg in adults. Dapsone is safe in pregnancy, and has a long serum half-life of about 24 hours.

170. *Most common* nerve involved in leprosy is:

A. Ulnar
B. Median
C. Radial
D. Musculocutaneous

Intense bacillemia is frequent in lepromatous leprosy and in most advanced cases destructive lesions are limited to the skin, peripheral nerves, anterior portions of the eyes, upper respiratory passages above the larynx, testes, and structures of the hands and feet. Two sites which are most commonly involved are **the ulnar nerves** near the elbow and **the peroneal nerves.**

171. Mitsuda reaction in lepromin test indicates:

A. Hypersensitivity to antigen
B. Strong immunity
C. Does not indicate anything
D. Cell-mediated immunity

Lepromin test is performed by injecting intradermally 0.1 ml of lepromin into the inner aspect of the forearm of the patient. The reaction is read at 48 hours and 21 days. There are 2 types of positive reaction:

- Early reaction is also known as **Fernandez reaction.**
- Late reaction is the classical **Mitsuda reaction**. The reaction develops late, becomes apparent in 7-10 days following injection and reaching its maximum in 3 or 4 weeks. The test is read at 21st day. At the end of 21st day, if there is a nodule more than 5 mm in diameter at the site of inoculation, the reaction is positive. The late reaction is induced by the bacillary component of the antigen. **It indicates cell-mediated immunity.**

172. *Treatment of choice* in nerve abscess in leprosy is:

A. Systemic corticosteroid
B. Clofazimine
C. Thalidomide
D. Incision and drainage

173. *Drug of choice* in type I lepra reaction with severe neuritis is:

A. Chloroquine
B. Thalidomide
C. Clofazimine
D. Systemic steroid

(AI 1995)

Patients having pustular or ulcerative ENL, **acute neuritis**, orchitis, iritis or arthritis should be treated with a high dose of **corticosteroids**.

174. Ichthyosis vulgaris is inherited as:

A. X-linked recessive
B. X-linked dominant
C. Autosomal recessive
D. Autosomal dominant *(AI 1993)*

Ichthyosis is characterized by **roughness, dryness and scaling of the skin.** It may be subdivided into three subtypes on genetic and clinical grounds viz. **ichthyosis vulgaris (autosomal dominant),** a more severe form **ichthyosis nigricans** (X-linked recessive) and the most severe form **Harlequin fetus** (autosomal recessive). The essential defect in ichthyosis is one of keratinization in which the horny layer is not normally shed. As a result it becomes thicker and drier than normal. Ichthyosis vulgaris begins at the ages of 1-4 years and gets worse during the next few years. In its mildest form (**xeroderma**) there is only drying and slight scaling of skin. There may be hyperkeratosis at the mouths of hair follicles (*ichthyosis follicularis*) at the extensor surfaces of limbs and buttocks producing a **goose skin** appearance. In severe cases there is "heaping up" of grayish brown scales.

175. Ichthyosis is associated with:

A. Lymphogranuloma venereum
B. Hypothyroidism
C. Hodgkin's disease
D. AIDS *(TN 1996)*

Acquired ichthyosis may develop in association with some other diseases. The **most common disease to be associated with acquired ichthyosis is Hodgkin's disease** but it has also been reported with other forms of malignancies, malabsorption syndromes and leprosy.

176. Dhobi itch is:

A. Tinea versicolor
B. Tinea capitis
C. Tinea barbae
D. Tinea cruris

Tinea cruris is also known as **jock itch** or **dhobi itch** and is a fungal infection of the groin. It is caused by species of *Trichophyton* or *Epidermophyton floccosum*. It is most common in the tropics and among males.

177. Rhinophyma is:

A. Glandular form of acne rosacea
B. Form of acne vulgaris
C. Affects the scalp
D. A form of dermatofibroma *(PGI May 2001)*

Rhinophyma is a benign, slow growing *tumor* due to **hypertrophy of the sebaceous glands** of the tip of the nose. **It is glandular form of acne rosacea**. A pink lobulated mass is seen over the nose with superficial vascular dilation commonly in men past middle age. Bulk of tumor should be removed with a sharp knife or CO_2 laser.

178. The treatment of pustular psoriasis is:

A. Steroids
B. Thalidomide
C. Retinoids
D. Hydroxy urea *(AIIMS May 2002)*

Pustular psoriasis of the palms and soles is extremely resistant to therapy. **Treatment generally involves the use of potent topical steroids** but *occasionally*, systemic agents such as cyclosporine or methotrexate are necessary. Generalized pustular psoriasis responds usually quite well to bland therapy. It is very important to avoid any irritants such as anthralin for generalized pustular psoriasis. 1% hydrocortisone ointment applied topically may result in good improvement. Systemic cyclosporine and methotrexate may be needed if the disease does not respond well to such topical therapy. When more stable plaque-type psoriasis is present, treatment with PUVA can be considered. Hospitalization is often necessary.

179. Rose spots are seen in:

A. Malaria
B. Typhus fever
C. Typhoid fever
D. Rheumatic fever

"**Rose spots**" appear as small, pale red, blanching, slightly raised macules and are frequently seen on the chest and abdomen during the 1st week in **typhoid fever**. They evolve into non-blanching small hemorrhages.

180. For *pediculosis corporis* the treatment of choice is:

A. Disinfection of clothes
B. Four applications of benzyl benzoate
C. One application of benzyl benzoate
D. Three applications of gamma benzene hexachloride

Pediculosis corporis *(Pediculosis vestimentorum)* "lives" on the undersurface of clothing and to which it attaches its eggs. Sometimes the eggs are fastened to the lanugo hairs of the midline of the back and, if infestation is heavy, even to the pubic and axillary hairs. The "necks" of the garments and their seams are the most favored sites. The life of the adult is about 4 weeks and during this time a female will lay 200–300 eggs. It lives on the underclothing and "visits" the skin only for food. That is why it tends to bite those areas which are in close contact with underclothes (upper part of shoulders and upper part of buttocks). At the site of the bite there is a visible minute red macule which irritates greatly. The linear scratch marks caused by itching are very characteristic and are sufficient for diagnosis. With time the *Pediculosis corporis* and the itching caused by it produces thickening and pigmentation of skin (**Vagabond's disease**). Treatment is directed towards **disinfecting all the clothes and beddings of the patient.** The clothes should be either boiled or insufflated with 5% DDT powder or 1% gamma benzene hexachloride or 0.25% malathion. The excoriations on the trunk should be treated with application of calamine lotion or topical corticosteroids with an antibiotic along with a systemic antihistaminic for pruritus.

181. In systemic candidiasis the drug of choice is:

A. Ketoconazole
B. Nystatin
C. Amphotericin
D. Griseofulvin

(JIPMER 1993)

Intravenous **amphotericin B** is the drug of choice in **disseminated candidiasis.**

182. Crystalline miliaria occurs due to obstruction of:

A. Accessory sweat gland
B. Hair roots
C. Sweat glands
D. Sebaceous glands

(JIPMER 1993)

The important, troublesome and most common example of decreased sweating is **miliaria** in which the **sweat ducts are blocked** by keratotic plugs. In **miliaria crystallina** the "block" is situated at the orifice of sweat ducts producing minute glassy vesicles containing sweat on the trunk of the patient with an acute febrile illness. Miliaria crystallina produces no symptoms and disappears in a few days. However, when the block appears in the epidermis, it results in a widespread eruption on the trunk of severely itching and erythematous papulovesicles. This condition is very common in Europeans visiting the tropics and is known as **miliaria rubra** (*prickly heat*). Spontaneous resolution occurs within 14 days on returning to a cool environment. Management consists of avoiding unnecessary sweating and because plugging of sweat ducts is increased by mild cutaneous injury too frequent bathing, rough clothing, excessive use of soap and application of "medicines" should be avoided. Local application of any drug is of little use and best thing is a simple dusting powder. Vitamin C (1 gm OD) helps in some cases.

183. A child has fever for three days followed by appearance of maculopapular rash which disappeared in 48 hours without any pigmentation. The diagnosis is:

A. Fifth disease
B. Typhoid
C. Roseola infantum
D. Measles

(AIIMS 2000)

Roseola infantum is also known as exanthem subitum. In 90% of cases it is caused by human herpes virus 6. Onset of illness is sudden with high grade fever and bulging anterior fontanelle. Seizures are seen in 5-35% of cases. Child looks relatively well despite high grade fever. Fever falls by 3-4th day and *as the temperature returns to normal a macular or maculopapular rash appears over the body.* This rash starts from the trunk and then spread to arms and neck and sometimes involves face and neck also. Rash fades within 3 days. There is no residual pigmentation.

184. Ringworm infection affects:

A. Papillary layer
B. Dermis
C. Stratum corneum
D. Prickle cell layer of epidermis

The characteristic feature of ringworm group of fungi is their ability to "invade" keratinized structures *without* being able to penetrate the deeper living cells. The diseases caused by them are therefore limited to hair, nails and the horny layer (stratum corneum) of the epidermis.

185. Which of the following presents as umbilicated papules:
A. Plain warts
B. Chickenpox
C. Molluscum contagiosum
D. Herpes genitalis
(AIIMS 1999)

186. Which of the following is *true* of molluscum contagiosum:
A. Is an STD
B. Central umbilication
C. Viral infection
D. All of the above

187. Causative organism of molluscum contagiosum is:
A. Papovavirus
B. Poxvirus
C. Parvovirus
D. Orthomyxoviruses

188. Umbilicated pearly white asymptomatic skin lesion, diagnosis is:
A. HSV
B. Molluscum contagiosum
C. EBV
D. None

Molluscum contagiosum is a benign disease and is characterized by pearly, flesh-colored, **umbilicated** skin lesions which are 2-5 mm in diameter. The infection can be transmitted by close contact, including sexual intercourse. Lesions can be found *anywhere* on the body *except* the palms and the soles but they *typically* occur in the genital region. Molluscum contagiosum develops in advanced stages of HIV infection, frequently involving the face and upper body. The diagnosis is made by histological demonstration of cytoplasmic eosinophilic inclusions characteristic of **poxvirus** replication. This condition is generally self limiting and there is no specific systemic treatment but a variety of techniques for physical ablation are used.

189. *Most common* fungal infection of the female genitalia in diabetes:
A. Cryptococcal
B. Candidiasis
C. Maduromycosis
D. Aspergillosis

In diabetic women, vaginal moniliasis may become troublesome during hyperglycemic-glycosuric period. **Vulvovaginal candidiasis** is especially common in the 3rd trimester of pregnancy.

190. Etiology of epidermolysis bullosa is:
A. Genetic
B. Infection
C. Senile
D. Malignant

Epidermolysis bullosa is a group of disorders in which the skin and related epithelial tissues break and blister due to minor trauma. It is a **heritable disorder** of connective tissues.

191. "Honey colored" crusts are characteristic of:
A. Nummular eczema
B. Impetigo
C. Herpes zoster
D. Cutaneous diphtheria

Impetigo is a skin infection caused by *Streptococcus* spp but by 1 week time most lesions are also growing *Staphylococci*, which may become the predominant organism. Primary lesion is a thin-walled vesicle which easily breaks. There is lateral extension of the superficial lesion with **a honey colored crust** at the edge. Satellite lesions appear and spread to remote areas of the skin. Streptococcal impetigo is a major cause of post-streptococcal acute glomerulonephritis. Topical mupirocin (Bactroban or T bact ointment) or fusidic acid (Fusiwal ointment) is very effective for the *streptococcal* lesion, with or without *staphylococcal* overgrowth.

192. *Most common* site of affection of herpes simplex:
A. Thorax
B. Oral mucosa
C. Abdomen
D. Extremities

Gingivostomatitis and pharyngitis are the most common clinical presentations of 1st episode of HSV-1 infection. The recurrent herpes labialis is the most common clinical presentation of reactivation HSV infection. HSV pharyngitis and gingivostomatitis are generally due to primary infection and are commonly seen in children and young adults.

193. *Most common* site of herpes gestationis:

A. Infraorbital
B. Periumbilical region
C. Thorax
D. Vulva

Pemphigoid gestationis is also known as **herpes gestationis**. It is a rare, non-viral, sub-epidermal blistering disease of pregnancy and the puerperium. Pemphigoid gestationis may begin during any trimester of pregnancy or shortly after delivery. Lesions are generally distributed over the abdomen, trunk, and extremities. Early lesions include urticarial papules, wheals and finally blisters appearing at the **umbilicus**. Subsequent pregnancies produce an earlier onset than the preceding pregnancy. The lesions consist of urticarial plaques and annular wheals, surrounded by multiple small tense vesicles. Severe pruritus is common. Prednisolone in a dose of about 40 mg/day suppresses the eruption.

194. Incubation period of syphilis is..........days:

A. 9–90
B. 20–30
C. 7–14
D. 2–5

(UP 1996)

Incubations Periods of Some STDs

Incubation period	Disease
• Syphilis	9–90 days
• Herpes	2–7 days
• Chancroid	1–14 days
• Lymphogranuloma venereum	3 days to 6 weeks
• Donovanosis	1–4 weeks (up to 6 months)

195. Rash of secondary syphilis is usually:

A. Unaccompanied by lymphadenopathy
B. Not seen in palms and soles
C. Asymptomatic
D. Vesicular

(AI 1991, UP 1996)

196. *Not* a skin manifestation of secondary syphilis:

A. Vesicle
B. Pustular syphilides
C. Papule
D. Bilaterally symmetrical

The **skin rash** in secondary syphilis consists of macular, papular, papulosquamous, and occasionally pustular syphilides; often more than 1 form is present at the same time. The eruption may be very *subtle*. About **25 % of patients with a discernible rash of secondary syphilis may be unaware that they have dermatologic manifestations**. Initial lesions are **bilaterally symmetric**, pale red or pink, nonpruritic, discrete, round **macules** that measure 5 to 10 mm in diameter and are distributed on the trunk and proximal extremities. After several days or weeks, red papular lesions 3-10 mm in diameter also appear. These lesions, may progress to necrotic lesions in association with increasing endarteritis and perivascular mononuclear infiltration, are distributed widely, frequently involve the palms and may occur on the face and scalp.

197. Which of the following is an early feature of congenital syphilis:

A. Vesicles
B. Microcephaly
C. Interstitial keratitis
D. Saber skin

(PGI 1999)

198. Vesicular lesion is seen in:

A. Primary syphilis
B. Secondary syphilis
C. Tertiary syphilis
D. Congenital syphilis *(JIPMER 2001)*

199. Primary bullous lesion is seen in:

A. Congenital syphilis
B. Tertiary syphilis
C. Secondary syphilis
D. Primary syphilis *(AI 1994)*

The earliest sign of **congenital syphilis** is usually **rhinitis** (snuffles), which is soon followed by other mucocutaneous lesions. These may include **bullae** (syphilitic pemphigus), **vesicles**, superficial desquamation, petechiae, and later papulosquamous lesions, mucous patches, and condylomata lata. The most common early manifestations are osteochondritis and osteitis, particularly involving the metaphyses of long bones, which progress in severity during the first 6 months of life and then spontaneously subside, and periostitis, which continues to progress after the first 6 months. Hepatosplenomegaly, lymphadenopathy, anemia (usually hypoproliferative but may be hemolytic), jaundice, thrombocytopenia, and leukocytosis are commonly seen.

200. A 20-year-old man presented with penile ulcer which is indurated and painless inguinal lymphadenopathy. *Most likely* diagnosis is:

A. AIDS
B. Lymphogranuloma venereum
C. Chancroid
D. Primary syphilis

201. A 30-year-old male, with a history of sexual exposure comes with a painless indurated ulcer over the penis. The diagnosis is:

A. Syphilis
B. Chancroid
C. Lymphogranuloma venereum
D. Granuloma inguinale *(AIIMS May 2001)*

The typical primary chancre of **primary syphilis** begins as a **single painless papule** that rapidly becomes eroded and usually becomes **indurated**, with a characteristic cartilaginous consistency on palpation of the edge and base of the ulcer. In heterosexual men the chancre is usually located on the penis, while in homosexual men it is often found in the anal canal or rectum, in the mouth or on the external genitalia and in women, common primary sites are the cervix and labia. Regional lymphadenopathy usually accompanies the primary syphilitic lesion, appearing within a week of the onset of the lesion. The nodes are firm, nonsuppurative, and painless. **Inguinal lymphadenopathy** is bilateral and may occur with anal as well as with external genital chancres.

202. Which is a *non*venereal form of treponemal infection:

A. Yaws
B. Chancroid
C. Syphilis
D. GV

203. Yaws is cause by:

A. *Treponema pallidum*
B. *Treponema pertenue*
C. *Treponema carateum*
D. *Treponema endemicum*

Yaws, pinta, and endemic syphilis are caused by **nonvenereal treponemes**. They do *not* have significant morphologic or genetic differences from *Treponema pallidum* which is the causative organism of venereal syphilis.

- The endemic syphilis is caused by *Treponema pallidum* spp. *endemicum*. It involves the skin, bones, and mucous membranes.
- Yaws is caused by *Treponema pallidum* spp. *pertenue*. It affects skin and bones.
- Pinta is caused by *Treponema carateum* .It involves the skin alone.

204. Which of the following is an example of nonvenereal disease:

A. Endemic syphilis
B. Gonorrhea
C. Chancroid
D. LGV

Endemic syphilis also known as bejel, siti, dichuchwa, njovera, or skerljevo is a chronic nonvenereal treponemal infection of *childhood* which is characterized by early mucous membrane or mucocutaneous lesions, a latent period of indeterminate duration, and late complications including gummas of bone and skin.

205. *Not* useful in diagnosing syphilis is:

A. TPHA
B. Reagin test
C. Frei test
D. VDRL

(AI 1993)

Common Serologic Tests for Syphilis

Nontreponemal (reagin) tests		Treponemal tests	
Microscopic flocculation	Venereal disease research laboratory (VDRL) test	Immunofluorescence	Absorbed fluorescent treponemal antibody-absorbed (FTA-ABS) test; 19S IgM FTA-ABS test
Macroscopic flocculation	Rapid plasma reagin (RPR) test Toluidine red unheated serum test (TRUST)	Hemagglutination	*T. pallidum* hemagglutination assay (MHA-TP, TPHA)
** Frei test is done for LGV.*			

206. In primary syphilis the *treatment of choice* is:

A. Benzathine penicillin
B. Crystalline penicillin
C. Oral penicillin
D. Corticosteroid

(AI 1993)

Primary, secondary, or early latent syphilis should be treated with **penicillin G benzathine** (**single dose of 2.4 million units IM**, 1.2 million units in each buttock) and patients with *confirmed* penicillin allergy should be treated with *tetracycline* hydrochloride (500 mg PO 6 hourly) or *doxycycline* (100 mg PO 12 hourly) for 2 weeks.

207. Dennie Morgan fold is seen in:

A. Atopic dermatitis
B. Seborrheic dermatitis
C. Mastocytosis
D. Sarcoidosis

(KARNATAKA 1996)

Atopic dermatitis is the cutaneous expression of the atopic state and is characterized by a family history of asthma, hay fever, or dermatitis in up to 70 % of patients. *Pruritus* is an important characteristic of atopic dermatitis. Other cutaneous features are perioral *pallor* (cheilitis); an extra fold of skin beneath the lower eyelid known as **Dennie Morgan folds**; increased palmar markings; and increased incidence of cutaneous infections, mainly with *Staphylococcus aureus*.

208. In which of the following condition, intraepidermal blisters are seen:

A. Pemphigus foliaceus
B. PCT
C. Dermatitis herpetiformis
D. Erythema marginatum

(PGI 1999)

In **pemphigus foliaceus**, acantholytic blisters are located high **within the epidermis**, just below the stratum corneum. Pemphigus foliaceus is a more superficial blistering disease than pemphigus vulgaris. In pemphigus vulgaris mucous membrane lesions are *rare*. **Patients *rarely* demonstrate intact blisters but *rather* exhibit shallow erosions** associated with erythema, scale, and crust formation.

209. Drug induced pemphigus is *not* seen with:

A. Frusemide
B. Phenobarbital
C. Rifampin
D. Penicillin

(AI 1994)

The most frequently implicated agent for pemphigus is **penicillamine**; other offenders are captopril, cefadroxil, phenylbutazone, **rifampin**, piroxicam, **penicillin**, and phenobarbital.

210. Cause of acne vulgaris is:
A. Obstruction to sebaceous duct
B. Sweat gland hyperplasia
C. Diphtheroids
D. *Staphylococcus aureus* *(JIPMER 1991)*

211. A 19-year-old girl has multiple papulopustular erythematous lesions on face and neck. She has:
A. Lupus vulgaris
B. Pityriasis versicolor
C. Acne vulgaris
D. Acne rosacea

212. Acne vulgaris is due to involvement of:
A. Sebaceous glands
B. Eccrine glands
C. Sweat glands
D. Apocrine glands *(AIIMS Nov 2001)*

213. Comedones are seen in:
A. Acne vulgaris
B. Adenoma sebaceum
C. Seborrheic keratosis
D. Acne rosea

Acne vulgaris is caused by overproduction of sebum and **sebaceous duct blockage. The clinical hallmark of acne vulgaris is the comedone**, which may be closed (*whitehead*) or open (*blackhead*). Comedones, **erythematous papulopustular lesions**, and, in some patients, cysts develop due to increased production of oil in adolescence. The lesions are situated chiefly on cheeks, forehead, chin, nose and the temporal regions. The predisposing factors include hereditary tendencies and disturbances in the androgen-estrogen balance. Acne begins typically at puberty, when there is increased secretion of androgen in both sexes. Androgens **increase the size and activity of the pilosebaceous glands**. Other factors include food allergies, endocrine disorders, therapy with adrenal corticosteroid hormones, and psychogenic factors.

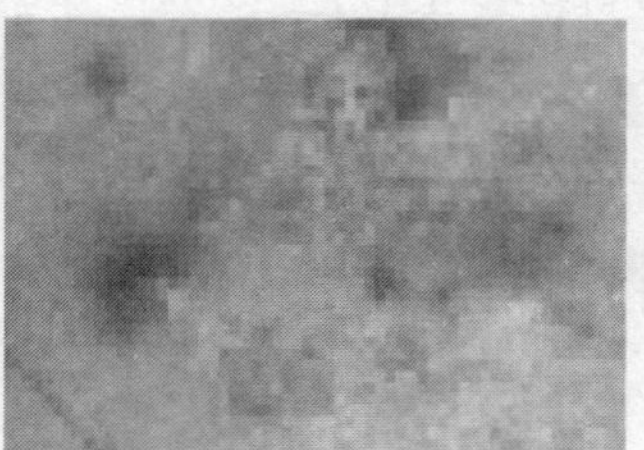

214. A girl aged 22 has light brown pigmentation macular lesions over the bridge of nose and cheek after exposure to light. *Most likely* diagnosis is:
A. Photodermatitis
B. Chloasma
C. SLE
D. Air borne contact dermatitis *(AIIMS 1999, AI 2001)*

215. 30-year-old woman presents with light brown lesions involving both her cheeks. The lesions had never been erythematous. Which of the following is the *most probable* diagnosis:
A. Chloasma
B. Air borne contact dermatitis
C. Photodermatitis
D. SLE *(AIIMS May 2000)*

216. Light brown macules over the cheeks of a woman for the past 5 years, never been erythematous. *Most likely* diagnosis is:
A. SLE
B. Chloasma
C. Photodermatitis
D. Malingering *(AIIMS May 2000)*

Chloasma or melasma or seborrheic melanosis is characterized by asymptomatic, very superficial looking macular areas of **brownish pigmentation**. The skin does not show any other change. Lesions are usually located on one or more of the following sites, the **bridge of nose, both cheeks, upper lip and the forehead**. On the forehead a linear area just above the eyebrows is frequently involved, while an area of upper lip below the nose and skin around the eyes are *as a rule* spared. It does not occur anywhere else on the body. Most commonly the lesions appear during pregnancy but they have also been seen in unmarried girls as well as males. Women taking oral contraceptive pills may also develop chloasma, which is **augmented by exposure to the sun.**

217. Slapped cheeks appearance is seen in:
A. Erythema infectiosum
B. Erythema subitum
C. Erythema multiforme
D. Roseola infantum

218. A child presents with slapped cheek appearance of face, diagnosis is:

A. Pityriasis alba
B. Leprosy
C. Tinea versicolor
D. Erythema infectiosum *(PGI May 2001)*

The initial cutaneous manifestation of **erythema infectiosum** (**5th disease**) is a *malar flush*, giving the appearance of "**slapped cheeks**" and circumoral pallor. It occurs during the recovery phase of the infection and is immunologically mediated.

219. Lupus like picture is *not* caused by:

A. INH
B. Hydralazine
C. Chloroquine
D. Procainamide *(AI 1991)*

Drugs Causing Drug Induced Lupus Erythematosus

- Acebutolol
- Asparaginase
- Barbiturates
- Bleomycin
- Cephalosporins
- **Hydralazine**
- Iodides
- **Isoniazid**
- Methyldopa
- Phenolphthalein
- Phenytoin
- **Procainamide**
- Quinidine
- Sulfonamides
- Thiouracil

220. Chloroquine is used in treatment of:

A. Discoid lupus erythematosus
B. Lichen planus
C. Psoriasis
D. Pemphigoid *(AI 1991)*

Chloroquine is also used in the treatment of following skin conditions:

- Discoid lupus erythematosus
- Polymorphous light eruption
- Solar urticaria
- Systemic lupus erythematosus
- Porphyria cutanea tarda
- Chronic cutaneous vasculitis

221. Tuberculosis of skin is known as:

A. Lupus pernio
B. Spina tuberculid
C. Lupus vulgaris
D. Lupus acne *(UP 2000)*

Lupus vulgaris is a belligerent **cutaneous form of tuberculosis** in a patient with moderate to good host resistance. There are many clinical variants including a plaque form, an ulcerating form, a vegetating form, and papulonodular and tumor-like forms. Typical skin lesion is a plaque composed of nodules with an "**apple-jelly**" color. As lesions expand peripherally, central scarring usually results.

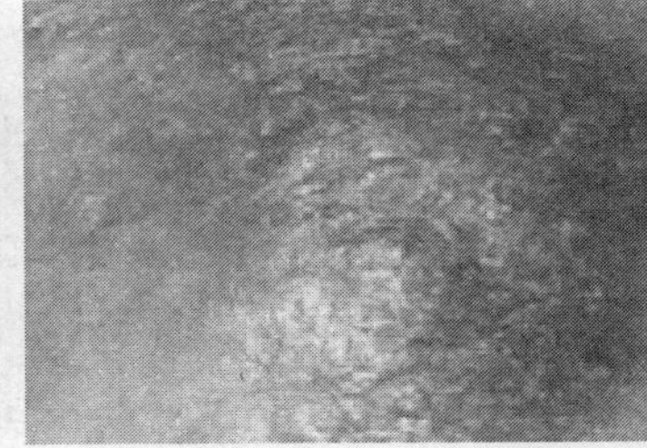

* *Lupus* means any chronic, progressive, usually ulcerating, skin disease and *vulgaris* means ordinary or common.

222. Tzanck cell is a:

A. Lymphocyte
B. Monocyte
C. Neutrophil
D. Keratinocyte

Tzanck cell is a degenerated cell from the **keratin** layer of the skin, which is disconnected from adjacent cells. It is seen in *pemphigus*.

223. Underlying internal malignancy is shown by all *except*:

A. Erythema gyratum repens
B. Bullous pemphigoid
C. Bullous pyoderma
D. Acanthosis nigricans

(AI 1996)

Cutaneous Markers of Internal Malignancy

- **Acanthosis nigricans**
- Dermatomyositis
- Acquired icthyosis
- **Bullous pemphigoid**
- Cowden's disease
- Pyoderma gangrenosum
- Necrolytic migratory erythema
- **Erythema gyratum repens**
- Thrombophlebitis migrans
- Sudden appearance of lanugo hair
- Bowen's disease
- Paraneoplastic acrokeratosis

224. Drug of choice for herpes zoster:

A. Acyclovir
B. Idoxuridine
C. Actinomycin
D. Vidarabine

Oral **acyclovir** is indicated in the treatment of herpes zoster infections caused by varicella-zoster virus in adult patient with herpes zoster. Therapy should be started within 48 hours of the onset of rash.

225. Acyclovir resistant herpes is treated with:

A. Foscarnet
B. Lamivudine
C. Ganciclovir
D. Valacyclovir

(JIPMER 2002)

Foscarnet is used in the treatment of acyclovir-resistant mucocutaneous herpes simplex virus (HSV-1 and HSV-2) infections in human immunodeficiency virus (HIV)-positive patients.

226. Lagophthalmos is seen in:

A. Leprosy
B. Syphilis
C. Peripheral neuritis
D. HZV infection

(JIPMER 2001)

Lagophthalmos is incomplete closure of the palpebral fissure when an attempt is made to shut the eyelids. This results in exposure and injury to the bulbar conjunctiva and cornea. It is caused by contraction of a scar of the eyelid, facial nerve injury, atony of the orbicularis palpebrarum, or exophthalmos. In **tuberculoid leprosy** when the facial nerves are involved, there may be **lagophthalmos**, exposure keratitis, and corneal ulceration leading to blindness.

227. Painful penile ulcer with inguinal adenitis is seen in infection with:

A. Chlamydia
B. *Haemophilus ducreyi*
C. *T. pallidum*
D. Gonococcus

Haemophilus ducreyi is the etiologic agent of chancroid, a sexually transmitted disease characterized by **genital ulceration** and **inguinal adenitis**. After an incubation period of 4-7 days, a papule with surrounding erythema appears. In 2-3 days, the papule evolves into a pustule, which spontaneously ruptures and forms a sharply circumscribed ulcer that is generally **not indurated**. The ulcers are **painful** and bleed easily; little or no inflammation of the surrounding skin is evident. About 50% of patients develop enlarged, tender inguinal lymph nodes, which frequently become fluctuant and spontaneously rupture.

228. In Tzanck smear, multinucleated giant cells are seen in:

A. Herpes simplex
B. Pemphigoid
C. Molluscum contagiosum
D. Pemphigus

(PGI 1998)

A **Tzanck smear** is a cytologic technique commonly used in the diagnosis of herpes virus infections (simplex or varicella-zoster). An early vesicle, not a pustule or crusted lesion, is unroofed, and the base of the lesion is scraped gently with a scalpel blade. The material is then placed on a glass slide, air-dried, and stained with Giemsa or Wright's stain. **Multinucleated giant cells suggest the presence of herpes**.

229. Hypercholesterolemia occurs in:

A. Tuberous xanthoma
B. Lupus
C. Xanthelasma
D. None of the above

(DELHI 1992)

Increased β-lipoproteins (primarily types II and III) result in one or more of the different types of xanthoma, viz. *xanthelasma, tendon xanthomas,* and *plane xanthomas.*

- **Xanthelasma** are found on the eyelids
- **Tendon xanthomas** are frequently associated with the Achilles and extensor finger tendons
- **Plane xanthomas** are flat and favor the palmar creases, face, upper trunk, and scars.

Tuberous xanthomas are frequently associated with hypertriglyceridemia, but they are also seen in patients with **hypercholesterolemia (type II)** and are found most frequently over the large joints or hand.

230. The term "tuberculid" includes which of the following:

A. Lichen scrofulaceum
B. Lichen planus
C. Erythema nodosum
D. Tuberculous gumma

(PGI Dec 2000)

231. Multidrug therapy is employed in tuberculosis in order to:

A. Prevent drug resistance
B. Decrease adverse effects
C. Broader spectrum
D. Synergistic effect

(MAHE 1999)

Papulonecrotic tuberculid (PNT) is a recurrent, chronic and symmetric eruption of necrotizing skin papules arising in crops and primarily involving the arms and the legs. Individual lesions heal with varioliform scarring. The eruption represents a hypersensitivity reaction to tuberculosis antigens released from a *distant* focus of infection. Most patients display a markedly positive Mantoux skin test (PPD) and have evidence of active or past tuberculosis infection. **The tuberculids represent a form of cutaneous hypersensitivity reaction to tuberculosis antigens. Papulonecrotic tuberculid and lichen scrofulosorum are accepted by most authors as representing *true* tuberculids.** The characteristic lesions of tuberculids are small erythematous inflammatory papules that undergo central ulceration and heal *spontaneously* within weeks leaving a varioliform scar. Lesions arise in symmetric crops typically with an acral predilection. Typically, lesions develop over the extensor surfaces, particularly the knees, elbows, and dorsum of the hands and feet, though widespread involvement may be present. New lesions form as older lesions resolve giving the eruption a *polymorphous* appearance. Lesions of PNT have been reported to coexist with lesions of erythema induratum and in several studies both types of lesions resolved with appropriate ATT. **Treatment of tuberculid** is directed towards eradicating the underlying mycobacterial infection. Tuberculosis treatment guidelines vary from region to region. Currently, for patients with active tuberculosis, 4-drug therapy (4D ATT) with isoniazid, rifampin, pyrazinamide and ethambutol is recommended **to avoid development of resistance**. A minimum of 6 months of ATT is recommended.

232. Dyskeratosis is a feature of:

A. Darier's disease
B. Pemphigus vulgaris
C. Psoriasis
D. Lichen planus

(PGI Dec 2000)

Faulty and premature keratinization of individual keratinocytes is called **dyskeratosis.** Dyskeratotic cells are usually intensely eosinophilic and may contain a small, dense, basophilic nuclear remnant. Dyskeratotic cells may also be densely basophilic as seen in **Darier's disease**.

233. Skin tuberculosis which involves skin after involving lymph nodes is:

A. Lupus erythematosus
B. Scrofuloderma
C. Lupus pernio
D. Lupus vulgaris

(AI 1999)

Scrofuloderma or *tuberculosis colliquativa* is a more active form of tuberculosis of skin and consists of a diffuse infiltration with tubercle bacilli and cells. It starts as a bluish red, swollen, painless area situated over "broken down" tuberculous lymph node.

234. Exfoliative dermatitis is seen in all the following *except*:
- **A.** Pityriasis rosea
- **B.** Atopic eczema
- **C.** Psoriasis
- **D.** Drug reaction

(AI 2002)

The 4 cardinal features of erythroderma or exfoliative dermatitis are redness, desquamation, thickening and universal distribution. The condition is uncommon below 50 years and men are affected 3 times more than women. In 50% of cases it "evolves" from a preceding skin disease most common being the **psoriasis**, contact dermatitis, **drug eruption**, seborrheic dermatitis, **atopic eczema** and varicose dermatitis. Thirty percent cases are "primary" or "idiopathic" and 15% are caused by a "lymphoreticulosis" such as mycosis fungoides or CLL.

235. Palpable purpura is *not* seen in:
- **A.** Polyarteritis nodosa
- **B.** Idiopathic thrombocytopenic purpura
- **C.** Rocky Mountain spotted fever
- **D.** Ecthyma gangrenosum

Non-palpable purpura	Palpable purpura
Thrombocytopenia (including ITP)	Leukocytoclastic vasculitis
Abnormal platelet function	Polyarteritis nodosa
Clotting factor defects	Acute meningococcemia
Amyloidosis	Disseminated gonococcal infection
Ehlers-Danlos syndrome	Rocky Mountain spotted fever
Scurvy	Ecthyma gangrenosum
Disseminated intravascular coagulation	
Monoclonal cryoglobulinemia	
Thrombotic thrombocytopenic purpura	
Warfarin reaction	
Emboli of cholesterol	
Emboli of fat	
Gardner-Diamond syndrome (auto-erythrocyte sensitization)	
Waldenström's hypergammaglobulinemic purpura	

236. Vasodilatation of skin does *not* occur with:
- **A.** Substance P
- **B.** Vasopressin
- **C.** Bradykinin
- **D.** Hyperthermia

(UP 1999)

High concentrations of vasopressin acting on V_1 receptors can also cause **vasoconstriction**, as in response to severe hypotension or after infusion of **vasopressin** for treatment of bleeding esophageal varices.

237. Tzanck smear in a patient of bullous lesions shows:
- **A.** Absence of melanin pigment
- **B.** Leukocytosis
- **C.** Acantholysis
- **D.** Langerhans' cells

(AI 1996)

The diagnosis of pemphigus can be confirmed by a skin biopsy and demonstration of acantholytic cells in the Tzanck smear from the lesions. **Acantholysis** is the loss of cohesion *between* epidermal or adnexal keratinocytes.

238. In contact dermatitis the diagnostic method of choice is:
- **A.** Patch test
- **B.** Skin biopsy
- **C.** Intradermal test
- **D.** Tzanck test

(AI 1993)

Patch testing is used to document sensitivity to a specific antigen. In this procedure, a *battery* of suspected "allergens" is applied to the patient's back under occlusive dressings and allowed to remain in contact with the skin for **48 hours**. The dressings are then removed, and the area is examined for evidence of delayed hypersensitivity reactions such as erythema, edema, or papulovesicles. This test is best performed by physicians with special expertise in patch testing and is often helpful in the evaluation of patients with *chronic dermatitis*.

239. In urticaria pigmentosa, the cell *most commonly* seen in skin on microscopy is:
- **A.** Mast cell
- **B.** Langerhans' cell
- **C.** Melanocytes
- **D.** Lymphocytes

(JIPMER 2001)

240. Darier's sign is seen in:
- **A.** Xeroderma pigmentosa
- **B.** Urticaria pigmentosa
- **C.** Herpes zoster
- **D.** Glucagonoma

Mastocytosis is a relatively uncommon disease, characterized by **abnormal accumulation of mast cells** in skin and / or other organs. The disease can manifest at any time from infancy to middle age with a *variety* of cutaneous manifestations. The **most common manifestation seen in 65% of cases is called urticaria pigmentosa** which starts during infancy and consists of multiple, irregular, hyperpigmented macules on trunk and extremities. Mast cells degranulate by, stimuli such as rubbing or heat and this leads to the formation of localized urticaria **(Darier's sign).**

241. Oral hairy leukoplakia and whitish plaque on the tongue and palate seen gives clue to *most likely* diagnosis of:
- **A.** HIV infection
- **B.** HTLV–1
- **C.** Infectious mononucleosis
- **D.** *Candida albicans*

(KARNATAKA 1996, JIPMER 2001)

In a patient of **HIV**, thrush due to *Candida* infection, and **oral hairy leukoplakia** due to Epstein-Barr virus, is usually indicative of fairly advanced immunologic decline, generally occurring in patients with less than 300 CD4+ T cells per μliter.

242. Disease *not* caused by *Staphylococcus* is:
- **A.** Scalded skin syndrome
- **B.** Ecthyma
- **C.** Erysipelas
- **D.** Impetigo

(AI 1997)

One form of **streptococcal cellulitis is known as erysipelas** and is characterized by a bright red appearance of the involved skin, which forms a plateau sharply demarcated from the surrounding normal skin. The lesions typically develop over a few hours and are associated with chills and fever. Erysipelas tends to occur in certain characteristic locations, i.e. the malar area of the face (often with extension over the bridge of the nose to the contralateral malar region) and the lower extremities. Classic cases of erysipelas, with the typical features described above, are almost always due to group A *streptococci*.

243. A tuberculous patient treated with 4 drugs, presented with neuropathy. The treatment should be:
- **A.** Change the drug and start second line
- **B.** Continue treatment
- **C.** Stop isoniazid and give pyridoxine
- **D.** Stop ATT

(UP 2000)

Isoniazid (INH) is a synthetic, bactericidal antitubercular drug, which is active against many mycobacteria, **primarily those that are actively dividing**. About 75-95% is excreted by kidneys within 24 hours. Isoniazid has been reported to cause severe hepatitis which is more prevalent in patients over 50 years of age. If signs and symptoms of hepatotoxicity occur, rifampin, isoniazid, and pyrazinamide combination should be *discontinued* immediately. **Peripheral neuritis due to isoniazid usually can be prevented by administration of pyridoxine (10 to 25 mg per day).** Pyridoxine is recommended for patients at risk of neuritis, such as patients over 65 years of age, pregnant women, patients with diabetes mellitus, chronic renal failure, alcoholism, or malnutrition, and patients taking anticonvulsant medications. Corticosteroids have been used for therapy in children with tuberculous meningitis to reduce vasculitis, inflammation, and intracranial pressure. Data indicate that dexamethasone may lower mortality rates and reduce long-term neurologic impairment. The administration of corticosteroids should be considered in all children with *tuberculous meningitis*, and also may be considered in children with *pleural and pericardial effusions* (to hasten reabsorption of fluid), *severe miliary disease* (to mitigate alveolocapillary block), and *endobronchial disease* (to relieve obstruction and atelectasis). *Corticosteroids should be given only when accompanied by appropriate antituberculosis therapy.*

244. *Not* used in androgenic alopecia:

A. Minoxidil
B. Spironolactone
C. Cyproterone acetate
D. Testosterone

(AI 2000)

Treatment of **androgenic alopecia** is required only for cosmetic reasons and they include *antiandrogens* such as **spironolactone**, **cimetidine** and **cyproterone acetate**. **Minoxidil** which is an antihypertensive drug may also be effective.

245. Podophyllin is used in the treatment of:

A. Plantar wart
B. Palmar wart
C. Genital wart
D. Pemphigus vulgaris

(MAHE 1999)

246. Podophyllin is used in:

A. Condyloma acuminate
B. Condyloma lata
C. Palmar warts
D. Plantar warts

Condyloma acuminate or genital wart is a wart of the genitalia. It is caused by human papillomavirus (HPV). Treatment is as under:

- Topical application of **podophyllin**
- Laser therapy
- Surgery
- Recombinant interferon α-2a,

Although there is no completely safe and effective treatment currently available for genital warts, the above mentioned therapies are used with varying degrees of success.
Podophyllum is the dried rhizome and roots of *Podophyllum peltatum*.

247. Mycosis fungoides is treated with:

A. Intravenous adriamycin
B. Electron beam radiation
C. Radiotherapy
D. 5 FU cream

248. Mycosis cells are altered:

A. T lymphocytes
B. Monocytes
C. B lymphocytes
D. Eosinophils

The cutaneous **T cell lymphomas** are diseases of middle-aged people. Its major variants include **mycosis fungoides** and the Sézary syndrome, characterized by peripheral blood involvement. These diseases present with cutaneous manifestations and lymphadenopathy and follow an *indolent* course. Later, patients will develop hepatic, splenic, GIT, pulmonary, and renal involvement. Infiltration of the bone marrow and circulating leukemia cells (*Sézary cells*), usually in the presence of generalized erythroderma, and are late manifestations. The median survival from diagnosis is about 10 years, and infection is the most common cause of death. **Local and systemic therapies are used in the treatment of mycosis fungoides. Patients with disease limited to the skin may be cured with electron beam radiation therapy.** Topical treatment of skin lesions with drugs such as nitrogen mustard can induce remissions in up to 90 % of patients with disseminated disease. Systemic therapy with either drugs alone or combined modality therapy can induce high response rates (up to 80). Interferon α is an effective 2nd line *palliative* therapy. Monoclonal antibodies, extracorporeal phototherapy, and the adenosine deaminase inhibitor *pentostatin* are still investigational while fludarabine and cladribine may also be active.

249. *Gonococcus* is:

A. Extracellular gram-positive
B. Intracytoplasmic gram-positive
C. Intracellular gram-negative
D. Intranuclear gram-positive

Neisseria gonorrhoeae is the causative organism of gonorrhea; it is **a gram-negative intracellular** *Diplococcus.* This bacterium may be found in or on the genitals and in blood, joints, heart, eyes, urine, feces, and boils.

250. Main feature of gonorrhea is:

A. Purulent discharge per urethra
B. Rashes
C. Inguinal adenitis
D. Ulcer over glans penis

Purulent urethral discharge develops in almost 95 % of men with urethral gonococcal infection. It is associated with dysuria and meatal erythema.

251. In gonorrhea the *drug of choice* is:

A. Benzyl penicillin
B. Phenoxymethylpenicillin
C. Ceftriaxone
D. Benzathine penicillin

Although long-acting forms of penicillin (such as benzathine penicillin G) are effective in therapy for syphilis, they have *no place* in the treatment of gonorrhea. 1993 **centre for disease control** *guidelines* recommend a regimen combining a **single dose** of any of the 4 most effective drugs for gonorrhea, i.e. **ceftriaxone**, cefixime, ciprofloxacin, or ofloxacin + 7-day course of doxycycline (for potential coinfection with chlamydiae).

252. The rash in measles occurs first in the .... region:

A. Head
B. Chest
C. Post auricular
D. Neck

Measles or rubeola is an acute highly infectious disease of children caused by a specific RNA paramyxovirus. Incubation period is commonly 10 days from exposure to onset of fever and 14 days from exposure to appearance of rash. Prodromal stage begins 10 days after the exposure and lasts until 14th day. It is characterized by fever, sneezing, and nasal discharge, and cough, redness of eyes, lacrimation and photophobia. A day or two before appearance of rash, Koplik's spots appear in the buccal mucosa opposite the first and second upper molar. These are pathognomic of measles. **Eruptive phase is characterized by a typical red macular and maculopapular rash which starts from behind the ears** and spreads rapidly in a few hours to the face and neck. Thereafter it extends down the body and reaches lower extremities in 3 days. It may remain discrete but it often becomes confluent.

253. Toxic epidermal necrolysis is *not* caused by:

A. Penicillin
B. Phenytoin
C. Barbiturates
D. Insulin

Drugs are the primary cause of toxic epidermal necrolysis (TEN). Most common drugs causing TEN are phenytoin, barbiturates, sulfonamides, penicillins, and NSAIDs. It is characterized by bullae that arise on widespread areas of erythema and then slough. As a result large areas of skin get denuded.

254. Erythema toxicum in a neonate indicates:
- **A.** Staphylococcal sepsis
- **B.** Meningococcemia
- **C.** Drug hypersensitivity
- **D.** Is not of any significance

Erythema neonatorum or **erythema toxicum neonatorum** or **toxic erythema** or **urticaria neonatorum** is a minor developmental peculiarity seen in 33% of term healthy newborn babies. The newborn develops and erythematous rash with a central pale papule on the 2nd or 3rd day of life. The rash usually starts on the face and spreads to the trunk and extremities in 24 hours. The exact cause is not known but some authors consider it to be an early marker of atopy. The rash should be differentiated from *pyoderma* and skin lesions of *congenital syphilis*. The rash disappears spontaneously after 2-3 days without any specific treatment.

255. Reliable test for chancroid detection:
- **A.** Skin test
- **B.** Biopsy
- **C.** Culture
- **D.** Clinical examination

Clinical diagnosis in case of **chancroid** is inaccurate, and laboratory confirmation should be made in suspected patients. Gram's staining of a swab of the lesion show a predominance of typical gram-negative coccobacilli, but the other bacteria present makes it difficult to reach any definitive conclusion. **An accurate diagnosis of chancroid is made by cultures of *Haemophilus ducreyi* from the lesion.**

256. The *pathognomonic* sign of neurofibromatosis is:
- **A.** Café au lait macules
- **B.** Axillary freckling
- **C.** Shagreen patch
- **D.** None

The presence of at least 6 **café au lait** spots of > 1.5 cm in diameter is **diagnostic** of **neurofibromatosis**.

257. Lisch nodules are seen in:
- **A.** Albright's syndrome
- **B.** Neurofibromatosis
- **C.** Tuberous sclerosis
- **D.** Piebaldism

Neurofibromas are soft papules or nodules and they invaginate into the skin with pressure in a manner similar to a hernia (*the button hole sign*). Multiple neurofibromas, usually in combination with 6 or more café au lait spots measuring >1.5 cm and multiple Lisch nodules, are seen in von Recklinghausen's disease (NF type I). **Lisch nodules are 1-mm yellow-brown spots within the iris and are best seen on slit-lamp examination.** Other manifestations include axillary freckling and peripheral and CNS tumors.

258. Ocular hallmark of pseudoxanthoma elasticum is:
- **A.** Retinal hemorrhage
- **B.** Iritis
- **C.** Angioid streak
- **D.** Keratitis

Pseudoxanthoma elasticum is characterized by *abnormal* deposition of calcium on the elastic fibers of the skin, eye, and blood vessels. In the skin, the neck, axillae, antecubital fossae, and inguinal area are the primary sites of involvement. The yellow papules coalesce to form reticulated plaques. In severely affected skin, hanging, redundant folds develop. Biopsy specimens of involved skin reveal swollen and irregularly clumped elastic fibers with deposits of calcium. **In the eye, the calcium deposits in Bruch's membrane lead to angioid streaks and choroiditis.**

259. Porphyria cutanea tarda can be treated by:

A. High dose of systemic steroids **B.** Hemoglobin
C. Low dose chloroquine **D.** Metronidazole

Porphyria cutanea tarda is a group of disorders which are characterized by raised porphyrins in the plasma, urine and feces. Although it is usually acquired, it can also be inherited as an autosomal dominant trait .When the disease is acquired, it is generally secondary to liver damage, most typically from alcohol abuse. Alcohol and estrogens may also precipitate autosomal dominant porphyria cutanea tarda. Patients typically have increased hair on the sides of the face and periorificial violaceous discolorations and blisters on the dorsum of the hands that leave scar after healing. Sclerotic plaques can also develop. There is marked skin fragility in sun-exposed skin areas. Urine of these patients show a pink fluorescence under Wood's light. Lesions similar to porphyria cutanea tarda are seen in some dialysis patients and this condition is known as "pseudo-porphyria". If the disease is secondary to alcohol or estrogens, their ingestion should be stopped. Patient should avoid exposure to direct sun light. Venisection, the removal of 500 ml of blood every 2 weeks, results in remission. **Chloroquine**, starting at very low doses to avoid an acute exacerbation of symptoms, is also very effective. Patients with pseudo-porphyria secondary to dialysis are treated with erythropoietin in combination with venisection.

260. Swimming pool granuloma is caused by:

A. *Mycobacterium bovis* **B.** *Mycobacterium ulcerans*
C. *Mycobacterium kansasii* **D.** *Mycobacterium marinum*

Mycobacterium marinum can cause cellutitis or granulomas on skin surfaces exposed to the water in aquariums or injured in swimming pools.

261. "Shagreen patch" is usually found in:

A. Face **B.** Cervical region
C. Lumbosacral region **D.** Limbs

Tuberous sclerosis is characterized by cutaneous lesions, mental retardation and seizures. The cutaneous lesions include facial angiofibromas, **ash leaf**-shaped hypopigmented macules, **Shagreen patches** which are **yellowish thickenings of the skin over the lumbosacral region of the back** and depigmented nevi. Rhabdomyomas of the myocardium and angiomyomas of the kidney, liver, adrenals, and pancreas can occur. Neurologic features include seizures, mental retardation, and hydrocephalus.

SHAGREEN PATCH

262. Mongolian spots are usually seen at............region:

A. Cervicofacial **B.** Lumbosacral
C. Deltoid **D.** Thoracolumbar

"Mongolian" blue spots are irregular blue patches of skin pigmentation especially over the **sacral region** or **buttocks** of *almost* all newborn babies of African and Asian origin. These patches have *no relationship* with *Down syndrome (Mongolism)*. Mongolian spots are benign skin markings, and are not associated with any illnesses, complications or risk factors. There is no known prevention and they *generally* fade in a few years and disappear by puberty. Though occasionally they persist into adulthood, there is no need for treatment.

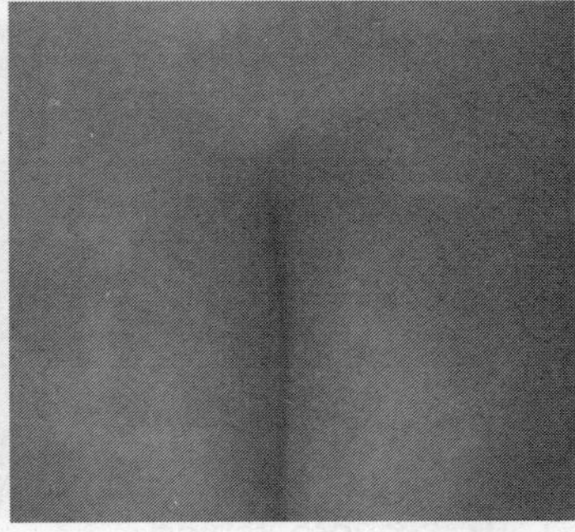

263. ***Most common*** **skin infection in children is:**

A. Scabies **B.** Impetigo contagiosa
C. Molluscum contagiosa **D.** Warts

Impetigo is the **most common** bacterial skin infection in children and manifests as thin, superficial vesiculopustules which soon rupture to form a **honey colored** crusts with a **stuck on** appearance. Bullous lesions can also occur in neonates and infants (**bullous impetigo**) which on rupture spread peripherally causing annular lesions.

264. Hailey-Hailey disease is inherited as:

A. Autosomal dominant **B.** Autosomal recessive
C. X-linked dominant **D.** X-linked recessive

Benign familial chronic pemphigus or **Hailey-Hailey disease** is an **autosomal dominant disorder**. It is characterized by recurrent vesicles, bullae and erosions typically on the axillae, neck and groin. It frequently gets worse in warm weather. Treatment is by topical potent glucocorticoids, such as clobetasol 0.05% cream .Patients should avoid heat. Lesions of Hailey-Hailey disease are prone to overgrowth with bacteria. Therefore appropriate broad spectrum antibiotics should also be used.

265. In treatment of which of the following disease Psoralen A (PUVA) is used:

A. Icthyosis **B.** Vitiligo
C. Pemphigus **D.** Pityriasis *(JIPMER 1991)*

266. Psoralen + ultraviolet therapy is useful in:

A. Vitiligo **B.** Mycosis fungoides
C. Psoriasis **D.** All of the above *(KARNATAKA 1994)*

- **Psoriasis**: PUVA is a combination of oral or topical psoralen and ultraviolet A and is used if the disease does not respond to ultraviolet B. Treatments twice a week for several months are required for resolution of severe systemic psoriasis.
- **Generalized vitiligo** occasionally responds to PUVA therapy. It may take 30 weeks of twice weekly treatments to achieve the response.
- **Mycosis fungoides**: Ultraviolet B or PUVA is helpful in producing improvement in parapsoriasis en plaque and early patch or plaque stage mycosis fungoides. If lesions are less than a few mm thick PUVA may also produce good response.

267. Quincke's disease is *popularly* known as:

A. Norwegian scabies **B.** Angioneurotic edema
C. Seborrheic dermatitis **D.** Saddle nose

Quincke's disease (**angioedema**) is also known as **angioneurotic edema.** It is marked by development of urticaria and edematous areas of skin, mucous membranes, or viscera and is a benign condition *when limited to the skin.* The reaction is dependent on IgE and may be associated with specific antigen sensitivity to foods, drugs, stings, or molds, atopic diathesis, or it may be a physical reaction of the skin to cold, light, pressure, or exercise or may also be complement mediated.

268. Castellani's paint contains all of the following *except*:

A. Basic fuchsin **B.** Phenol
C. Benzene hexachloride **D.** Boric acid

Castellani's paint is used to disinfect skin and to treat fungus infections of the skin. Its components are **phenol**, resorcinol, **basic fuchsin**, **boric acid**, and acetone.

269. Regarding "athlete's foot" which is correct:

A. 4th toe web commonly involved
B. Severe itching
C. Caused by *Trichophyton rubrum*
D. All of the above

Tinea pedis is a dermatophyte infection of the feet (**athlete's foot**) most commonly caused by *Trichophyton rubrum*. Dermatophytes generally grow in humid areas, such as on the foot inside a shoe. **Tinea pedis** is characterized by erythema and edema, scaling, **pruritus**, and vesiculation. Involvement may be widespread or localized. **The web space between the 4th and 5th toes is almost invariably affected.**

270. Acanthosis nigricans is indicative of:
- **A.** Internal malignancy
- **B.** Endocrine disorder
- **C.** Cushing's syndrome
- **D.** All of the above

Acanthosis nigricans is also known as keratosis nigricans and is a rare, chronic, inflammatory disease of the skin in adults. It is characterized by symmetrically distributed hard and soft papillary growths accompanied by velvety hyperpigmentation and hyperkeratosis usually present in the posterior and lateral folds of the **neck**, the axilla, groin, umbilicus, and other areas. **Acanthosis nigricans may be a sign of occult malignancy**. In the majority of patients, acanthosis nigricans is associated with obesity, but it may be a reflection of an **endocrinopathy** such as acromegaly, the polycystic ovarian disease, **Cushing's syndrome**, or insulin-resistant diabetes mellitus (type A, type B, and lipoatrophic forms).

271. Acrodermatitis enteropathica is due to deficiency of:
- **A.** Zinc
- **B.** Copper
- **C.** Selenium
- **D.** Magnesium

(UP 1997)

Acrodermatitis enteropathica is an autosomal recessive disease. **Zinc deficiency** is due to a defect in zinc absorption. The symptoms begin when an affected infant is weaned from human to cow's milk. It is **treated with oral zinc 2 mg/kg/day**.

272. Erythrasma is caused by:
- **A.** *Corynebacterium minutissimum*
- **B.** *Corynebacterium diphtheriae*
- **C.** *Corynebacterium vaginalis*
- **D.** *Corynebacterium ulcerans*

Erythrasma is a superficial infection of the skin, most typically in the skin folds and is caused by *Corynebacterium minutissimum*. A well demarcated brown discoloration with fine superficial scale is located in the skin folds, such as the submammary skin and groin. When examined under Wood's light, it shows an orange red fluorescence. Erythrasma responds well to topical azoles, e.g. clotrimazole and miconazole, as well as topical erythromycin cream.

273. Gottron's papules or sign is seen in:
- **A.** Dermatomyositis
- **B.** Acute myeloid leukemia
- **C.** Psoriasis
- **D.** Multiple myeloma

Dermatomyositis is a collagen vascular disease and myositis is its predominant feature. It is manifested in the skin by a pink-violaceous heliotrope hue of the periorbital skin, dilations of nail fold capillaries, erythema over small joints, erythematous 2-4 mm papules with some central scarring also over the joints, called **Gottron's papules**.

274. In a patch of vitiligo:
- **A.** Melanin synthesis is inhibited
- **B.** Melanosomes are absent
- **C.** Melanocytes are absent
- **D.** Melanocytes are reduce

In vitiligo there is complete loss of melanocytes from a circumscribed patch of skin. It is sometimes inherited as an autosomal dominant.

275. The *treatment of choice* of sweet syndrome is:
- **A.** Antibiotic
- **B.** Antifungals
- **C.** Corticosteroids
- **D.** UV light

Sweet's syndrome is characterized by fever; raised painful red-brown plaques on the limbs, face, and neck; neutrophil leukocytosis and dense dermal infiltration with mature neutrophil polymorphs. The cause is not known but 10% of the cases have an associated malignancy, mostly acute non-lymphocytic leukemia. Sweet's syndrome also has been reported with lymphoma, chronic leukemia, myeloma, myelodysplastic syndromes and solid tumors of the genitourinary tract. Extracutaneous sites of involvement are joints, muscles, eye, kidney and lung. The idiopathic form of Sweet's syndrome is generally seen in women, following a respiratory tract infection. **Treatment with adrenal cortical hormone is very effective.**

276. A patient has silver scaly lesions on the elbow and knee joint. Which of the following is a bedside test for provisional diagnosis of the illness?

A. KOH preparation
B. Auspitz's sign
C. Tzanck smear
D. Split skin smear

(AIIMS May 2002)

- **Auspitz's sign** is positive when slight scratching or curetting of a scaly lesion reveals punctate bleeding points within the lesion which suggests of *psoriasis*.
- *Darier's sign* is positive when a brown macular or papular lesion of urticaria pigmentosa becomes palpable wheal after being rubbed with the blunt end of an instrument.
- *Nikolsky's sign* is positive when a new blister is generated with ease by applying shearing force to skin.

277. Ciclopirox olamine is used in:

A. Dermatophytosis
B. Psoriasis
C. Acne
D. Lichen planus

Dermatophytosis or **ringworm** or **tinea**, is a chronic fungal infection of the skin, hair, or nails. Non-inflammatory lesions of the trunk, groin, hands, and feet are treated with twice-daily applications of clotrimazole, miconazole, ketoconazole, econazole, naftifine, terbinafine, or **ciclopirox olamine** cream. Hyperkeratotic lesions of the palms and soles should be first treated with the application of Whitfield's ointment to thin the keratin.

278. *Most common* site for zoster involvement is:

A. Sacral area
B. Limbs
C. Thoracic area
D. Cervical area

Herpes zoster also known as **shingles** is characterized by a unilateral vesicular eruption within a dermatome. It causes severe pain. The **dermatomes from T_3 to L_3 are most frequently involved.** Zoster ophthalmicus results due to involvement of ophthalmic branch of the trigeminal nerve.

279. Which of the following is Burow's solution:

A. Aluminum acetate
B. Potassium permanganate
C. Sodium thiosulfate
D. Silver nitrate

Burow's solution is a solution of **aluminum acetate** and is used in dermatology as a drying agent for weeping skin lesions.

280. Pyoderma gangrenosum is seen in all *except*:

A. Ulcerative colitis
B. Carcinoma colon
C. Sweet syndrome
D. Crohn's disease

Pyoderma gangrenosum is an idiopathic necrotizing skin disease and the primary lesion is a pustule with a deeply violaceous rim. The central area becomes necrotic forming a deep ulcer, with a broad violaceous rim and an overhanging edge. The lesion is very tender and expands peripherally. Pyoderma gangrenosum is also seen in patients with **ulcerative colitis**, **Crohn's disease**, collagen vascular disease and **sweet syndrome**.

281. Crocodile skin or *sauroderma* is seen in:

A. Toxic epidermal necrolysis
B. Darier's syndrome
C. Psoriasis
D. Ichthyosis vulgaris

Ichthyosis vulgaris is a hereditary form of ichthyosis and it includes 2 genetically distinct types:
- Dominant ichthyosis vulgaris is produced by an autosomal dominant gene. It is characterized by **dry, rough, scaly skin**. It is not present at birth and is usually noticed between the ages of 1 and 4 years.
- The second type is sex-linked ichthyosis vulgaris and only males are affected. It is transmitted by the female as a recessive gene. Onset of scattered large brown scales is seen in early infancy. The scalp is involved, but the face is spared *except* for the sides and in front of the ear.

282. In congenital erythropoietic porphyria, enzyme deficient is:
- **A.** Ferrochelatase
- **B.** Uroporphyrinogen co-synthetase I
- **C.** Uroporphyrinogen III synthase
- **D.** Uroporphyrinogen decarboxylase

Type of porphyria	Deficient enzyme
• ALA dehydratase deficiency	ALA dehydratase
• Acute intermittent porphyria (AIP)	HMB synthase
• Hereditary coproporphyria (HCP)	COPRO oxidase
• Variegate porphyria (VP)	PROTO oxidase
• Porphyria cutanea tarda (PCT)	URO decarboxylase
• X-linked sideroblastic anemia (XLSA)	ALA synthase
• **Congenital erythropoietic porphyria (CEP)**	**Uroporphyrinogen III synthase**
• Erythropoietic protoporphyria (EPP)	Ferrochelatase

283. The mechanism of action of psoralen is:
- **A.** Inhibits keratinization
- **B.** Inhibits angiogenesis
- **C.** Inhibiting protein synthesis
- **D.** Binding to DNA

In photochemotherapy the topically applied or systemically administered psoralens are combined with UV-A (PUVA) **Psoralens are tricyclic furocoumarins that, when intercalated into DNA and exposed to UV-A, form adducts with pyrimidine bases and eventually forms DNA cross-links.** These structural changes decrease DNA synthesis and are related to improvement that occurs in patients of psoriasis. PUVA photochemotherapy also stimulates melanin synthesis.

284. Pruritus is seen in all *except*:
- **A.** Pemphigus
- **B.** Psoriasis
- **C.** Contact dermatitis
- **D.** Lichen simplex chronicus *(AI 1991)*

- **Lichen simplex chronicus** (LSC) is thickening of the skin with variable scale that arises secondarily to repetitive scratching or rubbing. LSC is *not* a primary process. Rather, a person *senses* **pruritus** in a specific area of skin (with or *without* underlying pathology) and causes mechanical trauma to the point of lichenification.
- Lesions of **psoriasis** are variably **pruritic**.
- Allergic **contact dermatitis** is a cutaneous delayed hypersensitivity reaction to the application of an external allergen. Erythema, vesicles, bullae and associated **pruritus** is present.

285. *Most common* side effect of dapsone is:
- **A.** Hemolytic anemia
- **B.** Thrombocytopenia
- **C.** Bone marrow depression
- **D.** Cyanosis

More frequent side effects of dapsone are hemolytic anemia, pain in back, leg, or stomach, loss of appetite, pale skin, unusual tiredness ,fever, skin rash, methemoglobinemia.

286. Cells cultured from patients with this disorder exhibit low activity for the nucleotide excision *repair* process. This autosomal recessive genetic disease includes marked sensitivity to sunlight, ultraviolet light, with subsequent formation of multiple skin cancer and premature death, the disorder is:

A. Acute intermittent porphyria
B. Xeroderma pigmentosa
C. Ataxia telangiectasia
D. Alkaptonuria

Xeroderma pigmentosa is rare, progressive, **autosomal recessive**, degenerative disease. It is characterized by **severe photosensitivity** which develops in the 1st years of life. Disease is manifested by rapid onset of erythema, bullae, pigmented macules, hypochromic spots, and telangiectasia. Skin becomes atrophic, dry, and wrinkled. **A variety of benign and malignant growth appear early in life.**

287. A flat discoloration on skin of less than 1 cm in diameter is called:

A. Macule
B. Papule
C. Boil
D. Plaque

Erythema	It is due to vasodilatation and results in various shades of redness.
Purpura	It results from extravasation of blood into the surrounding skin; small patches are called petechiae while the large areas are called ecchymoses; its color is not obliterated by pressure as it is in erythema.
Pigmentation	Change in color of skin other than that brought about by variation in vascular tone. **Most common pigment is melanin** and the most common color is various shades of brown.
Macules	Small (less than 1 cm in diameter) areas of abnormal color.
Papules	Small superficial raised abnormalities.
Nodules	Deeper and larger raised lesions.
Weals	Well defined, slightly raised flat lesions which are pink at the margin and white in the centre. They are caused by liberation of histamine and other vasoactive substances.
Vesicles	Tiny serous blisters not bigger than a pinpoint.
Bullae	Blisters varying in size from one to many centimeters containing serum.
Pustules	Vesicles or small bullae containing pus.
Crusts	Result from dried exudates and may be yellow (serum), blackish (blood) or grey green (pus); usually they consist of varying mixture of these "ingredients" and is brown in color.
Scales	Accumulation of *horn cells*; yellow or greasy in seborrheic dermatitis; silvery in psoriasis and grey in eczema.
Atrophy	Thinning and depigmentation of skin.
Ulcers	Well defined areas in which epidermis and superficial portion of dermis has been destroyed.
Telangiectasias	Tiny, permanently dilated blood vessels.
Lichen	An aggregation of similar papules.
Lichenification	Thickening of prickle cell layer of epidermis; result in brown or violet patches in which lozenge shaped areas between the normal creases of skin stand as flat topped papules.

288. Atopic dermatitis can be *best* diagnosed by:

A. Clinical evaluation
B. Biopsy
C. Patch test
D. IgE level *(AI 1999)*

Clinical Criteria for the Diagnosis of Atopic Dermatitis

- Pruritus and scratching
- Course marked by exacerbations and remissions
- Lesions typical of eczematous dermatitis
- Personal or family history of atopy (asthma, allergic rhinitis, food allergies, or eczema)
- Clinical course lasting longer than 6 weeks

289. "Liver" spots are signs of:

A. Cirrhosis
B. Hepatoma
C. Echinococcosis
D. Senility

In **lentigo senilis** flat, brown spots appear on the exposed skin of aged white people. They commonly occur on the back of the hands, due to the accumulation of lipofuscin in tissues during the aging process. They are uniformly tan to dark brown and range from 1 mm to more than 1 cm in size. Although these spots are commonly known as "**liver spots**," they are *not* related to liver disease.

290. Medically important form of UV radiation is:

A. UV-A
B. UV-B
C. UV-C
D. None

Pyrimidine dimers are produced as a result of the absorption of UV-B by DNA. These structural changes are repaired by mechanisms that result in their recognition, excision, and the re-establishment of normal base sequences. The repair of these structural changes is crucial, because individuals with defective DNA repair are at high risk for the development of cutaneous cancer. **Patients with xeroderma pigmentosum are characterized by decreased repair of UV-induced photoproducts**, as a result their skin develop the xerotic appearance of photo-aging as well as basal cell and squamous cell carcinomas and melanoma in the first two decades of life.

291. Treatment of psoriatic erythroderma consists of all *except*:

A. Methotrexate
B. PUVA
C. Etretinate
D. Chloroquine

In **psoriatic erythroderma** the pink-red, sharply demarcated silvery scale are found over elbows, knees, scalp, pre-sacral area. Nail dystrophy, arthritis, pustules may occur. It is diagnosed by skin biopsy and treated with **etretinate, PUVA and methotrexate.**

292. Lichenoid drug eruption is seen in................. therapy:

A. Rifampicin
B. Gold
C. Streptomycin
D. Tetracycline

Lichenoid drug eruptions are associated with a variety of drugs and chemicals. **Gold** and antimalarials are most commonly associated with this eruption although antihypertensive agents, such as β blockers and captopril can also cause it.

293. "Black dot" ring worm is caused by:

A. *Microsporum*
B. *Epidermophyton*
C. *Candida*
D. *Trichophyton*

In endothrix, a ***Trichophyton* infection**, the hair shaft breaks off at the skin surface, leaving the hairs visible as **black dots** in the scalp.

294. Lilac colored, heliotrope, pigmentation over the face is characteristic of:

A. Dermatomyositis
B. Polymyositis
C. SLE
D. Systemic sclerosis

Primary idiopathic dermatomyositis comprises over 1/3rd of all cases of myositis. The skin changes precede or follow the muscle syndrome and include a localized or diffuse erythema, maculopapular eruption, scaling eczematoid dermatitis, or an exfoliative dermatitis. **The typical lilac-colored, heliotrope, rash is seen on the eyelids, bridge of the nose, cheeks (butterfly distribution), forehead, chest, elbows, knees and knuckles, and around the nailbeds.** Periorbital edema is frequent in acute cases. Subcutaneous calcification occurs, especially in children.

295. Which of the following are premalignant conditions of skin:

A. Bowen's disease
B. Actinic keratosis
C. Both
D. None

Squamous cell carcinoma has many premalignant forms (**actinic keratosis**, actinic cheilitis, and some cutaneous horns) and *in situ* forms (such as **Bowen's disease**) that are confined to the epidermis.

296. Vesicles are *never* seen in:

A. Herpes simplex
B. Herpes zoster
C. Chickenpox
D. Measles

The typical erythematous, nonpruritic, **maculopapular rash** of **measles** begins at the hairline and behind the ears. It spreads down the trunk and limbs to include the palms and soles, and becomes confluent.

297. Amongst the connective tissue disorders, malignancy is *most frequently* associated with:

A. Rheumatoid arthritis
B. SLE
C. Scleroderma
D. Dermatomyositis

In **polymyositis or dermatomyositis with neoplasia** the incidence of neoplasia is higher in patients over 40 years and is particularly high in patients over 60 years of age. The common malignancies are of lung, ovary, breast, gastrointestinal tract, and lymphoproliferative disorders. The myositis is a paraneoplastic syndrome, which may be due to an altered immune status, cross-reactive antigens between tumor and muscle, or an occult viral infection of the muscle.

298. Which one of the following is associated with CREST (calcinosis, Raynaud's phenomenon, esophageal dysmotility, sclerodactyly and telangiectasia) syndrome:

A. SLE
B. Dermatomyositis
C. Polyarteritis nodosa
D. Limited cutaneous variety of progressive systemic sclerosis

Limited cutaneous scleroderma generally has features of the **CREST syndrome, an acronym for *c*alcinosis, *R*aynaud's phenomenon, *e*sophageal dysmotility, *s*clerodactyly, and *t*elangiectasia.**

299. Nail involvement is *not* a feature of:

A. Dermatophytosis
B. DLE
C. Psoriasis
D. Lichen planus

Psoriasis of the nails can be a separate phenomenon or it can be a part of a generalized psoriasis. Typical manifestation in nails is the appearance of the "*oil-drop*" phenomenon, i.e. translucent areas in the nail. Nail pits are also present. These pits are arranged longitudinally on the nail and generally appear one-third to two-thirds of the way down the nail. Psoriatic nails can also be thickened. Onycholysis is common.

Lichen planus of the nails can occur alone, or in association with other types of lichen planus. The typical nail changes are marked thinning of the nail plate, enhancement of longitudinal lines, and pterygium formation. There may be complete destruction of the nail. All nails can be affected.

Dermatophytosis or tinea, is a chronic fungal infection of the skin, hair, or **nails**. Tinea unguium involves nails. There is a white crumbling nail. The nail may be thickened.

Nail involvement occurs in some patients of alopecia and pitting is the most common finding. Other findings are trachyonychia, Beau's lines, onychorrhexis, koilonychias, leukonychia and red lunulae.

300. Ballooning is a characteristic feature of:

A. Insect bite
B. Pemphigoid
C. Herpes zoster
D. Pemphigus

(JIPMER 1992)

Viremia in patients with chickenpox is reflected by the diffuse and scattered nature of the skin lesions and can be ascertained in selected cases by the recovery of **varicella zoster virus** from the blood. Vesicles are found in the corium and dermis, with degenerative changes characterized by **ballooning**, the presence of multinucleated giant cells, and eosinophilic intranuclear inclusions. Infection may also involve localized blood vessels of the skin, resulting in necrosis and epidermal hemorrhage.

301. A 24-year-old female has flaccid bullae in the skin and oral erosions. Histopathology shows intraepidermal acantholytic blister. The *most likely* diagnosis is:

A. Pemphigoid
B. Erythema multiforme
C. Pemphigus vulgaris
D. Dermatitis herpetiformis

(AIIMS 11 May 2003)

302. A 40-year-old male developed persistent oral ulcers followed by multiple flaccid bullae on trunk and extremities. Direct examination of a skin biopsy immunofluorescence showed intercellular IgG deposits in the epidermis. The *most probable* diagnosis is:

A. Pemphigus vulgaris
B. Bullous pemphigoid
C. Bullous lupus erythematosus
D. Epidermolysis bullosa acquisita

(AI 2003)

303. Acantholysis is characteristic of:

A. Pemphigus vulgaris
B. Pemphigoid
C. Erythema multiforme
D. Dermatitis herpetiformis

(AI 2003)

304. Mucous membrane is involved in:

A. Donovanosis
B. Bullous impetigo
C. Pemphigoid
D. Pemphigus

(UP 1996)

305. Pruritus is *not* seen in:

A. Contact dermatitis
B. Psoriasis
C. Pemphigus
D. Lichen simplex chronicus

(JIPMER 1995)

Pemphigus produces blistering due to a 'loosening' of desmosomal links between the epidermal cells, caused by immunological 'attack'. There are several types of pemphigus and all are *rare*. **Pemphigus vulgaris is the least rare variety**. In pemphigus vulgaris, the split occurs within the epidermis just above the basal layer (supra-basal). The lesions produced are thin-walled, delicate blisters, which rapidly rupture and erode. Although they may occur anywhere on the skin, they occur very frequently within the mouth and throat causing much discomfort and disability. It is a persistent and fluctuating disorder and before adequate treatment became available it was usually fatal. In more than 90% of patients there is a circulating antibody directed to the area between epidermal cells. Biopsy reveals the intra-epidermal split, with rounded up epidermal cells (acantholysis). Direct immunofluorescence examination of the skin around the lesion will show the presence of antibody of the IgG class and the complement component C_3 between epidermal cells. Patient should be treated with large doses of systemic steroids and immunosuppressive therapy with azathioprine or methotrexate should be started simultaneously.

Ref: *Roxburgh's Common Skin Diseases; 17th edition; page 91 – 92*

306. *Rarest* variety of pemphigus is:

A. Pemphigus vulgaris
B. Pemphigus vegetans
C. Pemphigus foliaceus
D. Pemphigus erythematodes

(UP 1992)

Pemphigus vegetans is a variant of pemphigus vulgaris in which there is more inflammatory component. It is a **very rare** intra-epidermal blistering condition in which the lesions are usually limited in extent.

Ref: *Roxburgh's Common Skin Diseases; 17th edition; page 92*

307. Podophyllum resin is indicated in the treatment of:

A. Psoriasis
B. Pemphigus
C. Condyloma acuminata
D. Condyloma lata

(AIIMS 11 May 2003)

Podophyllum is indicated for the treatment of **condylomata acuminatum** (venereal warts).

Further reading: *Roxburgh's Common Skin Diseases; 17th edition; page 53 – 55*

308. The following drug is indicated in the treatment of pityriasis versicolor:

A. Ketoconazole
B. Metronidazole
C. Griseofulvin
D. Chloroquine

(AIIMS 11 May 2003)

A yeast-like microorganism *Pityrosporum ovale* causes **pityriasis versicolor**. Pale and scaling macules develop insidiously over the skin of the chest and back in young adults, although rarely other sites can also be affected. These pale areas are left even when the condition resolves. Diagnosis is established by microscopic identification of grape-like clusters of spores and a meshwork of pseudomycelium in skin scrapings made transparent by soaking the scales for 20 minutes in 20% KOH. A more elegant and permanent slide can be made by a technique known as *skin surface biopsy*. In this method 'crazy' glue (cyanoacrylate adhesive) is used to remove a strip of superficial *stratum corneum* from the skin surface on a glass slide. The slide is rolled off the skin after 20 seconds and then stained with periodic acid-Schiff (PAS) reagent. Skin patches fluoresce in apple green color when examined under long-waved UVR (Wood's light). Topical imidazoles creams (miconazole, clotrimazole, econazole) applied once daily for 6 weeks or **Ketoconazole** shampoo to wash the affected area once daily for 5-days are usually sufficient. Old medicines such as 20% sodium thiosulphate solutions, selenium disulphide shampoo, and oral itraconazole (for 7 – 15 days) are also effective.

Ref: *Roxburgh's Common Skin Diseases; 17th edition; page 37 – 39*

309. A 5-year-old boy has multiple, asymptomatic, oval and circular faintly hypopigmented macules with fine scaling on his face. The most probable clinical diagnosis is:

A. Pityriasis versicolor
B. Indeterminate leprosy
C. Pityriasis alba
D. Acrofacial vitiligo

(AI 2003)

310. The test likely to help in diagnosis of a patient who presents with an itchy annular plaque on the face is:

A. Gram stain
B. KOH mount
C. Tissue smear
D. Wood's lamp examination

(AI 2003)

311. *False* about pityriasis alba:

A. No active treatment required
B. Common in children
C. Variant of vitiligo
D. Common over the face

(PGI May 2001)

Pityriasis alba occurs mainly in children. The lesions are hypopigmented, round or oval, macular or slightly elevated patches with fine adherent scales. Sometimes they may be mildly erythematous and relatively well defined but lack a sharply marginated border. Lesions occur on the face, neck, upper trunk, and proximal arms. Itching is minimal or absent. Etiology is unknown but the eruption is exacerbated by dryness and is often regarded as a mild form of eczema. It is often 'misdiagnosed' as tinea versicolor or corporis, each of which can be readily excluded by KOH examination of surface scales. Lesions wax and wane and eventually disappear. Application of a lubricant may be helpful and if pruritus is troublesome a topical 1% hydrocortisone cream applied 8 or 6 hourly may be useful. Normal pigmentation reappears in weeks to months.

Ref: *Nelson Textbook of Pediatrics; 17th edition; page 2190*

312. An 11-year-old boy is having tinea capitis on his scalp. The *most appropriate* line of treatment is:

A. Oral griseofulvin therapy
B. Topical griseofulvin therapy
C. Shaving of the scalp
D. Selenium sulphate shampoo

(AI 2003)

313. *Most common* organism causing tinea capitis:

A. *Trichophyton tonsurans*
B. *Microsporum*
C. Epidermophyton
D. *Candida albicans*

(AI 2001)

314. The *most common* organism causing *tinea capitis* is:

A. *Epidermophyton*
B. *Trichophyton tonsurans*
C. *Microsporum rubrum*
D. *Trichophyton rubrum*

(JHARKHAND 2003)

315. An 8-year-old boy has localized non-cicatricial alopecia over scalp with itching and scales. *Most likely* diagnosis is:

A. Lichen planus
B. Tinea capitis
C. Alopecia areata
D. Tinea barbae

Tinea capitis or **ringworm of the scalp** occurs exclusively in children and is mainly due to *Microsporum canis.* It invades the stratum corneum of the scalp and the hair cuticle causing pink, scaling patches on the scalp and areas of hair loss due to breakage of hair shafts.[1]

The predominant organism of tinea capitis is *T. tonsurans.*[2]

Tinea capitis is a dermatophyte infection of scalp **most often caused by *Trichophyton tonsurans,*** occasionally *Microsporum canis,* and much less commonly by other *Microsporum* and *Trichophyton* species. Oral administration of griseofulvin (15-20 mg/kg/24 hour) is the recommended treatment for all forms of tinea capitis. It may be necessary for 2 – 3 months and should be terminated only after fungal culture results are negative.[3]

Ref: *Roxburgh's Common Skin Diseases; 17th edition; page 41* [1] *and Harrison Principles of Internal Medicine; 14th edition;* [2] *and Nelson Textbook of Pediatrics; 17th edition; page 2231 – 2232* [3]

316. Herald patch is seen in which of the following conditions:

A. Pemphigus vulgaris
B. Pityriasis versicolor
C. Pityriasis rosea
D. Lichen planus

(SGPGI 2003)

Pityriasis rosea is a papulosquamous eruption of unknown cause. Its first manifestation is the development of a 2 to 6 cm annular lesion known as the '**herald patch**'.

Ref: *Harrison's Principles of Internal Medicine; 14th edition*

317. Photochemotherapy is indicated in which of the following:

A. Erythema nodosum
B. Psoriasis
C. Lichen planus
D. Pemphigus

(SGPGI 2003)

318. All of the following are seen in psoriasis *except*:

A. Auspitz's sign present
B. 10% associated with arthritis
C. It is premalignant disease
D. Worsening of disease during winter

(SGPGI 2003)

Psoriasis is a common inflammatory skin disease of unknown cause, which is genetically determined. It is characterized by well demarcated, raised, red, scaling patches that are localized preferentially to the extensor surfaces. When the psoriatic scale is removed, this results in minute points of bleeding (**Auspitz's sign**). There is a higher prevalence of rheumatoid-like arthritis with symmetrical involvement of the small joints of the hand and feet, wrists and ankles in patients with psoriasis (5-6%) compared to a matched control population (1-2%). Ultraviolet radiation has long been known to have therapeutic effects in a number of skin disorders including psoriasis. PUVA (**Photochemotherapy** with ultraviolet radiation of type A) is mainly used for treatment of psoriasis.

Ref: *Roxburgh's Common Skin Diseases; 17th edition; page 128 – 148*

319. A patient of severe psoriasis for 15 years is taking methotrexate. Now he developed abnormal LFT and jaundice. He should be managed with:

A. Stop methotrexate and start dapsone
B. Stop methotrexate and start steroid
C. Continue methotrexate and start cyclosporine
D. Stop methotrexate and start cyclosporine *(UP 1998)*

- **Methotrexate** is an antimetabolite because it is competitive antagonist of tetrahydrofolate reductase, blocking the formation of thymidine and thus DNA. It is highly effective treatment for patients with severe psoriasis. It is quite toxic producing hepatotoxicity in most patients who stay on the drug for long time.
- **Cyclosporine** is an immunosuppressant used in organ transplantation. It is dramatically effective in psoriasis in a dose of 3-5 mg/kg/day. Toxic side effects include severe renal damage and hypertension.

Ref: *Roxburgh's Common Skin Diseases; 17th edition; page 139 – 141*

320. Granules coming out of the multiple discharging sinuses in mycetoma foot contain:

A. Fungus colonies **B.** Pus cells
C. Inflammatory cells **D.** Granules *(AIIMS May 2002)*

Actinomycetoma refers to infection by actinomycetes of the genera *Nocardia*, *Nocardiopsis*, *Streptomyces*, and *Actinomadura*. True fungi of many different genera cause *Eumycetoma*. **Mycetoma** is a chronic suppurative infection of subcutaneous tissue and characterized by the presence of **'grains'**, which are **tightly clumped colonies of the causative agent.**

Ref: *Harrison's Principles of Internal Medicine; 14th edition*

321. A 28-year-old patient has multiple grouped papulovesicular lesions on elbows, knees, buttocks and upper back associated with severe itching. The *most likely* diagnosis is:

A. Pemphigus vulgaris **B.** Bullous pemphigoid
C. Dermatitis herpetiformis **D.** Herpes zoster *(AIIMS Nov 2002)*

Dermatitis herpetiformis is an intensely pruritic, chronic papulovesicular skin condition characterized by lesions symmetrically distributed over extensor surfaces (elbows, knees, buttocks, back, scalp, and posterior neck).

Ref: *Harrison's Principles of Internal Medicine; 14th edition*

322. A 45-year-old male has multiple grouped vesicular lesions present on the T_{10} segment dermatome associated with pain. The *most likely* diagnosis is:

A. Herpes zoster **B.** Dermatitis herpetiformis
C. Herpes simplex **D.** Scabies *(AIIMS Nov 2002)*

Herpes zoster (shingles) is characterized by a unilateral vesicular eruption within a dermatome and it is often associated with severe pain. The dermatomes from T_3 to L_3 are most frequently involved.

Ref: *Harrison's Principles of Internal Medicine; 14th edition*

323. Drug of choice for herpes zoster is:

A. Actinomycin **B.** Idoxuridine
C. Vidarabine **D.** Acyclovir *(UP 1992)*

For most patients of herpes zoster, no specific treatment is required; apart from keep the lesion clean and applying antimicrobial preparations to prevent secondary infection. **Acyclovir**, administered by mouth in a dose of 800 mg 5 times a day shortens the disease and decreases its severity.

Ref: *Roxburgh's Common Skin Diseases; 17th edition; page 53*

324. A child has multiple itchy papular lesions on the genitalia and fingers. Similar lesions are also seen in the younger brother. Which of the following is *most possible* diagnosis:

A. Papular urticaria
B. Scabies
C. Atopic dermatitis
D. Allergic contact dermatitis *(AIIMS Nov 2002)*

Scabies is a highly communicable skin disease caused by *Sarcoptes scabiei*, variety hominis, commonly called, the itch mite. Scabies manifests as papules, vesicles, pustules, and burrows and causes intense itching resulting in eczema. The body parts most commonly involved are the hands, between the fingers, the wrists, axillae, genitalia, beneath the breasts, and the inner aspect of the thighs. Except in infants, the lesions do not develop on face, scalp, neck, palms, and soles.

Ref: *Roxburgh's Common Skin Diseases*

325. All of the following are used in treatment of scabies *except*?

A. BHC
B. Permethrin
C. Pyrimethos
D. Benzyl benzoate *(CUPGME 2003)*

Scabies should be treated with an application of either 25% benzyl benzoate or 1% gamma benzene hexachloride (GBH). 1% GBH is less irritant and more effective and should be applied to the whole skin from neck downward ideally with a brush.

Treatment used for scabies	
• Crotamiton (10%)	Claimed to be antipruritic as well
• Malathion (0.5%)	Second line treatment
• Monosulfiram (25%)	May cause disulfiram-like alcohol reaction
• Permethrin (1%)	New effective agent

Ref: *Roxburgh's Common Skin Diseases; 17th edition; page 62*

326. A man presents to a STD clinic with urethritis and urethral discharge. Gram stain shows numerous pus cells but no microorganism. The culture is negative on the routine laboratory media. The *most likely* agent is:

A. *Chlamydia trachomatis*
B. *Haemophilus ducreyi*
C. *Treponema pallidum*
D. *Neisseria gonorrhoeae* *(AIIMS Nov 2002)*

327. All are *true* about *Neisseria gonorrhoeae except*:

A. Gram-positive cocci
B. Causes stricture urethra
C. Involves seminal vesicles and spreads to epididymis
D. Drug of choice is ceftriaxone *(AIIMS May 2001)*

Urethritis is the most commonly recognized STD syndrome in men. About 30 to 40% of non-gonococcal urethritis cases are caused by *Chlamydia trachomatis*. Gonorrhea is diagnosed by the demonstration of typical **gram-negative diplococci** within neutrophils, and a preliminary diagnosis of NGU is acceptable if gram-negative diplococci are not found.

Ref: *Harrison's Principles of Internal Medicine; 14th edition*

328. A 32-year-old male, Kallu, who recently visited a seacoast, presented with an ulcer over the left leg. The probable cause is:

A. *Pasturella multocida*
B. *Micrococcus catarrhalis*
C. *Vibrio vulnificus*
D. *Neisseria catarrhalis* *(AIIMS May 2001)*

Vibrio vulnificus is a marine Vibrio of medical importance. It causes 2 types of illnesses. The first is **wound infection following contact of open wounds with seawater**; the second type occurs in compromised hosts particularly those with liver disease.

Ref: *Textbook of Microbiology by R. Ananthanarayan and C. K. J. Paniker; 6th edition; page 293*

329. In an 8-day-old child with no history of consanguinity in the parents, the mother reports blisters and peeling off of the skin at the site of handling and pressure. There was a similar history in the previous child, which proved to be fatal. The diagnosis is:

A. Bullous pemphigoid
B. Letterer-Siwe disease
C. Congenital syphilis
D. Congenital epidermolysis bullosa *(AIIMS May 2001)*

Diseases characterized under the general term **epidermolysis bullosa** are a heterogeneous group of hereditary blistering disorders. All of them are characterized by induction of blisters by trauma and exacerbation of blistering in warm weather. Disorders can be categorized in 3 main headings, viz. epidermolysis bullosa simplex, junctional epidermolysis bullosa and dystrophic epidermolysis bullosa. **Junctional epidermolysis bullosa** is an autosomal recessive condition which is life-threatening. Affected infant is usually blistered at birth or develops lesions during the neonatal period.

Ref: *Nelson Textbook of Pediatrics; 17th edition; page 2184 – 2185*

330. Scabies, an infection of the skin caused by *Sarcoptes scabiei*, is an example of:

A. Water-borne diseases
B. Water-washed disease
C. Water-based disease
D. Water-related disease *(AIIMS Nov 2002)*

Classification of Diseases

I	Fecal-oral
II	Water-washed
III a	Water-based (Penetrating skin)
III b	Water-based (Ingested)
IV	Water-related insect vectors

Category	Disease	Category	Disease
I	Cholera	II	Scabies
I	Typhoid	II	Yaws
I	Leptospirosis	II	Leprosy
I	Tularaemia	II	Tinea
I	Paratyphoid	II	Louse-borne fevers
I	Infective hepatitis	II	Diarrheal diseases
I	Some enteroviruses	II	Ascariasis
I, II	Bacillary dysentery	III a	Schistosomiasis
I, II	Amoebic dysentery	III b	Guinea worm
I, II	Gastroenteritis	IV	Gambian sleeping sickness
II	Skin sepsis and ulcers	IV	Onchocerciasis
II	Trachoma	IV	Yellow fever
II	Conjunctivitis		

Water-washed disease occurs when water is not available for washing and personal hygiene. Without enough water, skin and eye infections are easily spread.

331. A patient gets recurrent urticaria while doing exercising and on exposure to sunlight. Which of the following is the *most likely* cause?

A. Cholinergic urticaria
B. Chronic idiopathic urticaria
C. Universal dermographism
D. Pressure urticaria *(AIIMS May 2000)*

Cholinergic urticaria is a very common form of hives. It manifests as multiple, small, 2 to 3 mm red hives on the upper trunk and arms, although it can occur from the neck to the thighs. These hives appear in response to a rise in body temperature from exercise, overheating, or stress. Usually the hives develop within 2 to 20 minutes after the body temperature rises, although they can take up to an hour to occur. They cause itching, tingling, burning, and warmth of the skin. The hives last for minutes to hours with an average of 30 minutes. It is believed that histamine is released in response to stimulation by the parasympathetic nervous system. Cholinergic urticaria is diagnosed by history and reproducing the hives under certain conditions. Many times the patient is asked to exercise by jogging in place or riding a stationary bike and the time it takes for hives to develop is noted. Cholinergic urticaria can be treated by limiting strenuous exercise. It responds well to hydroxyzine. Showering with hot water may cause a release of histamine throughout the body depleting histamine stores and causing a 24-hour refractory period.

332. Koenen's periungual fibromas are seen in >50% of cases of:

A. Tuberous sclerosis
B. Sturge-Weber syndrome
C. Ataxia telangiectasia
D. Neurofibromatosis *(JIPMER 2002)*

Periungual fibromas or Koenen's tumors develop in 50% of the cases of tuberous sclerosis.

333. Epididymoorchitis is seen in which of the following:

A. Measles
B. Tuberculosis
C. Leprosy
D. Syphilis *(AI 1993)*

Chronic tuberculous epididymoorchitis begins insidiously. There is a firm discrete swelling of the lower pole of epididymis, which aches a little. In neglected cases a tuberculous 'cold' abscess form, which may discharge. In two-thirds of cases there is evidence of renal tuberculosis or previous disease. Treatment with ATT is less effective in genital tuberculosis than in urinary tuberculosis and if resolution does not occur within 2 months, epididymectomy or orchidectomy is advised. However, a full course of ATT should be completed.

Ref: *Bailey and Love's Short Practice of Surgery; 23rd edition; page 1277*

334. A 20-year-old male patient, from Jaipur, has erythematous lesion with central crusting, on cheek; diagnosis:

A. SLE
B. Lupus vulgaris
C. Cutaneous leishmaniasis
D. Chilblains *(AI 2001)*

Cutaneous leishmaniasis used to occur in the Northwestern states of India extending from Amritsar to Kutch and Gujrat plains. One focus of zoonotic cutaneous leishmaniasis (ZCL) has been discovered in Rajasthan. Most skin lesions evolve from papular to nodular to ulcerative, with a central depression surrounded by a raised indurated border; some lesions persist as nodules or plaques.

Ref: *Park's Textbook of Preventive and Social Medicine; 17th edition; page 234 and Harrison's Principles of Internal Medicine; 14th edition*

335. Cicatricial alopecia is seen in:

A. Alopecia areata
B. Discoid lupus erythematosus
C. Psoriasis
D. Tinea capitis *(AI 1999, UP 2000)*

In **chronic discoid lupus erythematosus** (CDLE), irregular red plaques appear on light exposed skin of the face, scalp, neck, hands and arms. These plaques develop patchy atrophy with patchy hypopigmentation and hyperpigmentation. On the scalp, **scarring alopecia** occurs in the affected areas. The condition may be aggravated or initiated by the exposure to the sun.

Ref: *Roxburgh's Common Skin Diseases; 17th edition; page 79*

336. *Most common* precipitant of contact dermatitis is:

A. Silver
B. Copper
C. Nickel
D. Gold *(AI 1993)*

Allergic contact dermatitis is an eczematous condition that develops after contact with an agent to which delayed hypersensitivity has developed. An enormous number of substances are capable of causing allergic contact dermatitis and **nickel dermatitis** is one of the *most common* examples. About 5% of women in UK are nickel 'sensitive'.

Ref: *Roxburgh's Common Skin Diseases; 17th edition; page 123*

337. Treatment of alopecia areata includes:

A. Whitfield's ointment
B. Minoxidil
C. Tranquilizers
D. Parenteral penicillin *(JIPMER 1992)*

Alopecia areata is an autoimmune disease of hair follicles, which causes hair loss in sharply defined areas of skin. Patients with a solitary patch of hair loss or a few patches usually do not require treatment. When patches coalesce to produce a cosmetic problem or when there is alopecia totalis, patients often demand treatment, which is not often affective. The following 'treatments' have been used:

- Potent topical steroids or systemic steroids;
- Photochemotherapy with PUVA;
- Dithranol;
- Diphencyprone; and
- Topical minoxidil.

Ref: *Roxburgh's Common Skin Diseases; 17th edition; page 271 – 273*

338. Pyoderma gangrenosum is seen in:

A. Carcinoma colon
B. Ulcerative colitis
C. Binswanger's disease
D. Diverticulosis *(TN 1997)*

Pyoderma gangrenosum is a *rare* but serious ulcerative disorder, which is often due to a serious underlying systemic disease. An acutely inflamed purple nodule develops, which rapidly becomes an ulcer. This ulcer spreads with a frightening speed. The ulcers may become 'dinner plate' sized or even larger. Finally they become static and may then spontaneously heal. A few patients have multiple lesions and may succumb to the disorder. Lesions may reoccur after a dormant phase. **The disorder may occur in the course of ulcerative colitis, Crohn's disease, rheumatoid arthritis or myeloma**, although in about 50% of cases no predisposing cause if found. It has been suggested that the tissue destruction is due to vasculitis. Cyclosporine, minocycline and dapsone have been reported as promoting the healing of these lesions.

Ref: *Roxburgh's Common Skin Diseases; 17th edition; page 180*

339. Which of the following causes painful ulcers?

A. Chancroid
B. LGV
C. Syphilis
D. Granuloma inguinale *(CUPGME 2003)*

Haemophilus ducreyi is the causative agent of chancroid, a sexually transmitted disease characterized by genital ulceration and inguinal adenitis. The ulcers are painful and bleed easily; little or no inflammation of the surrounding skin is evident.

Ref: *Harrison's Principles of Internal Medicine; 14th edition*

340. Erythema nodosum does *not* occur in:

A. Sarcoidosis
B. Giant cell arteritis
C. Sulfonamides
D. Primary tuberculosis *(AI 1999)*

341. Erythema nodosum is seen in:

A. Syphilis
B. Tuberculosis
C. Typhoid
D. Salicylate poisoning *(UP 1999)*

Erythema nodosum is a painful inflammatory disorder in which 'crops' of tender nodules occur in response to antigenic stimuli. Common causes are as under:

- Tuberculosis
- Brucellosis
- Crohn's disease
- Oral contraceptives
- Penicillins
- Sarcoidosis
- Ulcerative colitis
- Leprosy
- Sulfonamides

Ref: *Roxburgh's Common Skin Diseases; 17th edition; page 77*

342. Soft chancre is caused by:
A. *Neisseria gonorrhoeae* **B.** *Calymmatobacterium granulomatis*
C. *Haemophilus ducreyi* **D.** *Treponema pallidum* *(UP 2001)*

343. *Haemophilus ducreyi* is the causative agent of:
A. Hard chancre **B.** Urethritis
C. Soft sore **D.** Granuloma inguinale *(KARNATAKA 2001)*

Chancroid (simple chancre; soft chancre) is a highly infectious non-syphilitic venereal ulcer. It is caused by *Haemophilus ducreyi*.

344. Nail involvement is *not* a feature of:
A. Eczema **B.** DLE
C. Psoriasis **D.** Lichen planus

Psoriasis, lichen planus and eczema may affect the nails producing characteristic clinical appearances.

Ref: *Roxburgh's Common Skin Diseases; 17th edition; page 276*

345. Isomorphic phenomenon is *not* seen in:
A. Discoid lupus erythematosus **B.** Lichen planus
C. Pityriasis rosea **D.** Psoriasis *(KERALA 1999)*

Psoriasis sometimes appears at the site of minor injury such as a graze or a scratch. This reaction is known as **Köebner phenomenon** or **isomorphic response**. This phenomenon is characteristic of psoriasis but is also seen in lichen planus and discoid lupus erythematosus. Its cause is unknown.

Ref: *Roxburgh's Common Skin Diseases; 17th edition; page 130*

346. *Not* seen in internal malignancy:
A. Acquired ichthyosis **B.** Acanthosis nigricans
C. Lichen planus **D.** Dermatomyositis *(KERALA 1999)*

Skin markers of internal malignant diseases

- Acquired ichthyosis
- Dermatomyositis
- Necrolytic migratory erythema
- Skin metastases
- Acanthosis nigricans
- Erythema gyratum repens
- Bullous pemphigoid

Ref: *Roxburgh's Common Skin Diseases; 17th edition; page 282*

347. Which among the following is a sign of internal malignancy:
A. Granuloma annulare **B.** Acanthosis nigricans
C. Granuloma atrophicans **D.** Erythema migrans *(SGPGI 2003)*

Acanthosis nigricans also can be a reflection of an internal malignancy, *most commonly* of the gastrointestinal tract, and it appears as velvety hyperpigmentation.

348. Vesiculobullous lesions are *not* seen in:

A. Pemphigoid
B. Pemphigus
C. Scabies
D. Dermatitis herpetiformis

(KERALA 1995)

Vesiculobullous lesions characterize many diseases. Some of these disorders are enumerated below:

- Hand-foot-and-mouth syndrome
- Rickettsial pox
- Staphylococcal scalded-skin syndrome
- Disseminated *Vibrio vulnificus* infection
- Toxic epidermal necrolysis
- Ecthyma gangrenosum
- Erythema multiforme
- Stevens-Johnson syndrome
- Epidermolysis bullosa
- Pemphigus
- Bullous pemphigoid
- Dermatitis herpetiformis
- Linear IgA dermatosis (chronic bullous dermatosis of childhood)

Ref: *Harrison's Principles of Internal Medicine; 14th edition; and Nelson Textbook of Pediatrics; 17th edition; page 2181-2187*

349. A 30-year-old male had severely itchy papulo-vesicular lesions on extremities, knees, elbows, and buttocks for one year. Direct immunofluorescence staining of the lesions showed IgA deposition at dermoepidermal junction. The *most probable* diagnosis is:

A. Pemphigus vulgaris
B. Bullous pemphigoid
C. Dermatitis herpetiformis
D. Nummular eczema

(AI 2004)

In **dermatitis herpetiformis** (DH) intensely itchy vesicles, papulovesicles and utricarial papules appear in crops on the knees, elbows, scalp, buttocks and around the axilla. Most patients of DH have a mild GI absorptive defect due to gluten enteropathy. Thyrotoxicosis, rheumatoid arthritis, myasthenia gravis and ulcerative colitis are more common in patients of DH. It is a persistent disorder which fluctuates in intensity. Small intestine mucosal biopsy demonstrates partial villous atrophy in 70 – 80% of patients. Biopsy of new lesions reveals that the vesicle forms sub-epidermally and develops from a collection of inflammatory cells in the papillary tips (*papillary tip abscess*). Direct immunofluorescent examination demonstrates the presence of IgA in the papillary tips in the skin around the lesion in *all* patients.

Ref: *Roxburgh's Common Skin Diseases; 17th edition; page 89 – 90*

350. Maculae ceruleae are caused by:

A. Pubic lice
B. Head lice
C. Body lice
D. Mites

(KARNATAKA 2001)

The 'cosmopolitan crab' or 'pubic louse' (*Phthirus pubis*) is transmitted by sexual contact but can infest eyelashes, axillary hair, and hair in other sites as well as pubic hair. Intensely 'pruritic' lesions and 2 to 3 mm blue macules (**maculae ceruleae**) develop at the site of bites. Blepharitis commonly accompanies infestations of the eyelashes.

351. A 5-year-old male child has multiple hyperpigmented macules over the trunk. On rubbing the lesions with the rounded end of a pen, he developed urticarial wheal, confined to the border of the lesion. The *most likely* diagnosis is:

A. Fixed drug eruption
B. Lichen planus
C. Urticaria pigmentosa
D. Urticarial vasculitis

(AI 2004)

Urticaria pigmentosa is the *most common* form of mastocytosis which occurs primarily in infants and children. It may be present at birth but more often erupt in crops during the first several months to 24 months of age. Sometimes early bullous or urticarial lesions fade, only to reoccur at the same site, immediately becoming fixed and hyperpigmented. Rapid appearance of erythema and whealing in response to vigorous stroking of a lesion can usually be elicited.

Ref: *Nelson Textbook of Pediatrics; 17th edition; page 2209 - 2210*

352. A 25-year-old man presents with recurrent episodes of flexural eczema, contact urticaria, recurrent skin infections and severe abdominal cramps and diarrhea upon taking sea foods. He is suffering from:

A. Seborrheic dermatitis
B. Atopic dermatitis
C. Airborne contact dermatitis
D. Nummular dermatitis

(AI 2004)

Atopic dermatitis is a very common, extremely itchy disorder of unknown cause which characteristically, but not always, affects the face and flexures of infants, children, adolescents and young adults. Foods, inhaled allergens, bacterial infection, reduced humidity; excessive sweating and irritants can exacerbate pruritus and scratching.

Ref: *Roxburgh's Common Skin Diseases; 17th edition; page 105*
Ref: *Nelson Textbook of Pediatrics; 17th edition; page 774*

353. Characteristic skin lesion in Peutz-Jeghers syndrome is:

A. Freckles
B. Lentigines
C. *Café au lait* spots
D. Adenoma sebaceum

(MANIPAL 2002)

The **lentigines** in patients with **Peutz-Jeghers syndrome** are located primarily around the nose and mouth, on the hands and feet, and within the oral cavity.

354. Characteristic lesion in tuberous sclerosis is:

A. *Café au lait*
B. Adenoma sebaceum
C. Lentigines
D. Melanoma

(MANIPAL 2002)

In **tuberous sclerosis**, the earliest cutaneous sign is an ash leaf spot. These lesions are often present at birth and are usually multiple. Examination of the patient for additional cutaneous signs such as **adenoma sebaceum** (multiple angiofibromas of the face), ungual and gingival fibromas, fibrous plaques of the forehead, and connective-tissue nevi (shagreen patches) should be done.

355. The *most effective* drug against *Mycobacterium leprae* is:

A. Dapsone
B. Rifampin
C. Clofazimine
D. Prothionamide

(AI 2003)

Dapsone, a folate antagonist, is the mainstay of therapy. The daily dosage is 50 to 100 mg in adults. **Rifampin is the most rapidly acting mycobactericidal drug known for use against *Mycobacterium leprae*.** Clofazimine, a compound derived from a phenazine dye, is highly lipophilic and accumulates in the skin, the gastrointestinal tract, and macrophages and monocytes. The several older agents with limited activity against *M. leprae* include ethionamide, prothionamide, thiambutosine, and amithiozone.

Ref: *Harrison's Principles of Internal Medicine; 14th edition*

356. Causative organism in chancroid is:

A. LGV
B. Gonococci
C. *Calymmatobacterium granulomatis*
D. *Haemophilus ducreyi*

(BHU June 2002)

Haemophilus ducreyi is the etiologic agent of ***chancroid***, a sexually transmitted disease characterized by genital ulceration and inguinal adenitis.

357. The Tzanck cell is a:

A. Mast cell
B. Keratinocyte
C. Melanocyte
D. Lymphocyte *(SGPGI 2003)*

358. Tzanck test is used in the diagnosis of:

A. Epidermolysis Bullosa
B. Bullous Impetigo
C. Pemphigus vulgaris
D. Tinea Corporis *(KARNATAKA 2001)*

Tzanck cell is a degenerated cell from the ***keratin layer*** of the skin, which is disconnected from adjacent cells. It is seen in ***pemphigus***.

359. Tzanck smear is useful for diagnosis of:

A. Herpes infection
B. CMV
C. EBV
D. Chlamydia *(MANIPAL 2001)*

Both clinical and laboratory criteria are useful for establishing the diagnosis of ***herpes simplex*** virus infections. Staining of scrapings from the base of the lesions with Wright's, Giemsa's (**Tzanck preparation**), or Papanicolaou's stain demonstrates characteristic giant cells or intranuclear inclusions of herpesvirus infection.

360. A 16-year-old student reported for the evaluation of multiple hypopigmented macules on the trunk and limbs. All of the following tests are useful in making a diagnosis of leprosy, *except*:

A. Sensation testing
B. Lepromin test
C. Slit smears
D. Skin biopsy *(AIIMS Nov 2004)*

Lepromin test is not a diagnostic test but is of great value in estimating the prognosis in cases of leprosy of all types.

Ref: *Park's Textbook of Preventive and Social Medicine; 17th edition; page 247*

361. A 30-year-old male patient has a large, spreading and exuberant ulcer with bright red granulation tissue over the glans penis. There was no lymphadenopathy. The *most likely* causative organism is:

A. *Treponema pallidum*
B. Herpes simplex virus type 1
C. Herpes simplex virus type 2
D. *Calymmatobacterium granulomatis* *(AIIMS Nov 2004)*

Donovanosis or granuloma inguinale is a contagious, chronic, indolent, progressive, auto-inoculable, ulcerative disease involving the skin and lymphatics of the genital or perianal areas. It is caused by bacteria, which are known as ***Calymmatobacterium granulomatis***, measure 1.5 by 0.7 micrometers. The incubation period for donovanosis ranges from 8 days to 12 weeks, but most lesions appear within 30 days after exposure. In men, the lesions are usually located on the glans, prepuce, or shaft of the penis or in the perianal area, while infection of the labia is most common in women. Extension to the inguinal region by autoinoculation, by continuity, or via the lymphatics produces a diffuse intradermal and subcutaneous swelling or suppuration known as a *pseudobubo* because involvement of the underlying lymph nodes is minimal.

Ref: *Harrison's Principles of Internal Medicine*; *14th edition*

362. A 12-year-old boy had a gradually progressive plaque on a buttock for the last 3 years. The plaque was 15 cm in diameter, annular in shape, with crusting and indurations at the periphery and scarring at the center. The *most likely* diagnosis is:

A. Tinea corporis
B. Granuloma annulare
C. Lupus vulgaris
D. Borderline leprosy *(AIIMS Nov 2004)*

Lupus vulgaris is a cutaneous variety of tuberculosis seen in previously infected and sensitized individuals. There is often underlying active tuberculosis elsewhere, usually in the lungs or lymph nodes. About 90 % of the lesions occur in the head and neck area and are red-brown plaques with a yellow-brown color on diascopy. Secondary scarring and squamous cell carcinomas can develop within the plaques.

Ref: *Harrison's Principles of Internal Medicine*; *14th edition*

363. A 24-year-old man had multiple, small hypopigmented macules on the upper chest and back for the last three months. The macules were circular, arranged around follicles and many had coalesced to form large sheets. The surface of the macules showed fine scaling. He had similar lesions one year ago which subsided with treatment. The *most appropriate* investigation to confirm the diagnosis is:

A. Skin biopsy of coalesced macules
B. Tzanck test
C. Slit skin smear from discrete macules
D. Potassium hydroxide preparation of scales

(AIIMS Nov 2004)

A **potassium hydroxide** preparation is performed on scaling skin lesions when a fungal etiology is suspected.

Ref: *Harrison's Principles of Internal Medicine*; *14th edition*

364. A 22-year-old woman developed small itchy wheals after physical exertion, walking in the sun, eating hot spicy food and when she was angry. The *most likely* diagnosis is:

A. Cholinergic urticaria
B. Solar urticaria
C. Heat urticaria
D. Chronic idiopathic urticaria

(AIIMS Nov 2004)

Cholinergic urticaria is characterized by pruritic wheals that are of small size (1 to 2 mm) and are surrounded by a large area of erythema; attacks are precipitated by fever, a hot bath or shower, or exercise and are presumptively attributed to a rise in core body temperature.

Ref: *Harrison's Principles of Internal Medicine*; *14th edition*

365. A 45-year-old male had multiple hypoanesthetic mildly erythematous large plaques with elevated margins on trunk and extremities. His ulnar and lateral popliteal nerves on both sides were enlarged. The *most probable* diagnosis is:

A. Lepromatous leprosy
B. Borderline leprosy
C. Borderline tuberculoid leprosy
D. Borderline lepromatous leprosy

(AIIMS Nov 2004)

The early lesion of **tuberculoid leprosy** is often a hypopigmented macule that is sharply demarcated and hypesthetic. Slowly the lesions enlarge by peripheral spread, and the margins become elevated and circinate or gyrate. Then the central area becomes atrophic and depressed. Fully developed lesions are densely anesthetic and have lost the normal skin organs (sweat glands and hair follicles). Although any peripheral nerve may be enlarged, most commonly affected are ulnar, posterior auricular, peroneal and post-tibial.

Ref: *Harrison's Principles of Internal Medicine*; *15th edition; page 1036*

366. A 6-month-old infant presented with multiple papules and exudative lesions on the face, scalp, trunk and few vesicles on the palms and soles for 2 weeks. His mother had history of itchy lesions. The *most likely* diagnosis is:

A. Scabies
B. Infantile eczema
C. Infantile seborrheic dermatitis
D. Impetigo contagiosa

(AIIMS May 2005)

Scabies is due to infestation with human scabies mite, which is an obligate parasite and has no separate existence outside the human body. The disorder is notorious for the intensity of itch that it causes, even in the presence of relatively minor physical signs. Physical signs are essentially those of eczema and the effects of scratching vesicle are seen, but excoriations and prurigo-like papules are more common.

Ref: *Roxburgh's Common Skin Diseases; 17th edition; page 58 to 62*

367. Which of the following is the *treatment of choice* for dermatitis herpetiformis:

A. Dapsone
B. Corticosteroids
C. Methotrexate
D. Retinoids

(AIIMS May 2005)

The skin lesion of dermatitis herpetiformis can be suppressed with **dapsone** (50 – 200 mg per day) in most patients. A gluten free diet will improve the GI lesion and improves the skin disorder in many patients after some months.

Ref: *Roxburgh's Common Skin Diseases; 17th edition; page 90*

368. Migratory necrolytic erythema is seen in:

A. Glucagonoma syndrome
B. Peutz-Jeghers syndrome
C. Sarcoidosis
D. Amyloidosis

(AIIMS May 2005)

In 1966, a rare syndrome of diabetes mellitus and **necrolytic migratory erythema** in association with a pancreatic islet cell tumor was described. The observation that these tumors secrete high levels of glucagon suggested a cause for the diabetes. Although these tumors frequently synthesize and secrete additional peptides, including pancreatic polypeptide, somatostatin, insulin, and gastrin, the common link is hyperglucagonemia. **Glucagonomas** are characteristically single, large, and slow growing.

Ref: *Harrison's Principles of Internal Medicine; 14th edition*

369. A 25-year-old male had pigmented macules over the palm, sole and oral mucosa. He also had anemia and pain in abdomen. The *most probable* diagnosis is:

A. Albright's syndrome
B. Cushing's syndrome
C. Peutz-Jeghers syndrome
D. Incontinentia pigmenti

(AIIMS May 2005)

Multiple polypoid tumors may occur throughout the small bowel (and occasionally the stomach and colorectum) in the **Peutz-Jeghers syndrome**. The polyps are usually hamartomas (juvenile polyps) having a low potential for malignant degeneration. **Mucocutaneous melanin deposits** as well as tumors of the ovary, breast, pancreas, and endometrium are also associated with this autosomal dominant disease.

Ref: *Harrison's Principles of Internal Medicine; 14th edition*

370. "Pinch purpura" is diagnostic of:

A. Primary systemic amyloidosis
B. Secondary systemic amyloidosis
C. Idiopathic thrombocytopenic purpura
D. Drug induced purpura

(AIIMS May 2005)

The cutaneous lesions associated with **primary systemic amyloidosis** are pink in color and translucent. Petechiae and purpura develop in clinically normal skin as well as in lesional skin following minor trauma, hence the term "**pinch purpura**."

Ref: *Harrison's Principles of Internal Medicine; 14th edition*

371. A 27-year-old male had burning micturition and urethral discharge. After 4 weeks he developed joint pains involving the knees and ankles, redness of the eye and skin lesions. The *most probable* clinical diagnosis is:

A. Psoriasis vulgaris
B. Reiter's syndrome
C. Behcet's syndrome
D. Sarcoidosis

(AIIMS May 2005)

Reiter's syndrome is a syndrome of reactive arthritis associated with rash, urethritis, conjunctivitis, uveitis, and oral ulcers develops several weeks after about 1% of cases of nongonococcal urethritis and 2% of enteric infections, particularly with those due to *Yersinia enterocolitica*, *Shigella flexneri*, *Campylobacter jejuni*, and *Salmonella* species. Reactive arthritis is most common among young men.

Ref: *Harrison's Principles of Internal Medicine; 14th edition*

372. A 10-year-old schoolgirl has recurrent episodes of boils on the scalp. The boils subside with antibiotic therapy but recur after some time. The *most likely* cause of the recurrences is:

A. Primary immunodeficiency syndrome
B. Juvenile diabetes mellitus
C. *Pediculus capitis*
D. HIV infection

(AIIMS May 2005)

Head lice (Pediculus capitis): Infestation with *Pediculus capitis* is extremely common. It is more often seen in poorer section of society and longhaired school children regardless to their social background. The louse is passed among children by casual contact and by sharing combs and brushes. Itching is the predominant complaint and scratching that results can cause secondary infection with exudation and crusting.

Ref: *Roxburgh's Common Skin Diseases; 17th edition; page 63*

373. A 40-year-old man had multiple blisters over the trunk and extremities. Direct immunofluorescence studies showed linear IgG. Which of the following is the *most likely* diagnosis?

A. Pemphigus vulgaris **B.** Pemphigus foliaceus
C. Bullous pemphigoid **D.** Dermatitis herpetiformis *(AIIMS Nov 2004)*

Bullous pemphigoid is a subepidermal blistering skin disorder generally seen in the old people. Lesions *typically* consist of tense blisters on either normal-appearing or erythematous skin. The *lesions are usually distributed over the lower abdomen, groin, and flexor surface of the extremities*; oral mucosal lesions are found in 10 to 40% of patients. **Direct immunofluorescence microscopy of normal-appearing perilesional skin shows linear deposits of IgG** and/or C3 in the epidermal basement membrane.

Ref: *Harrison's Principles of Internal Medicine; 14th edition*

374. A 40-year-old woman presented with an 8 month history of erythema and swelling of the periorbital region and papules and plaques on the dorsolateral aspect of forearms and knuckles with ragged cuticles. There was no muscle weakness. The *most likely* diagnosis is:

A. SLE **B.** Dermatomyositis
C. Systemic sclerosis **D.** Mixed connective tissue disorder *(AIIMS Nov 2004)*

Dermatomyositis comprises over 33% of all cases of myositis. The skin changes may precede or follow the 'muscle-syndrome' and include a localized or diffuse erythema, maculopapular eruption, scaling eczematoid dermatitis, or rarely, an exfoliative dermatitis. The classic lilac-colored (*heliotrope*) rash is on the eyelids, bridge of the nose, cheeks (so called *butterfly distribution*), forehead, chest, elbows, knees and knuckles, and around the nail beds. Itching may be troublesome in some cases. Periorbital edema is frequent. The skin lesions may occasionally ulcerate.

Ref: *Harrison's Principles of Internal Medicine; 14th edition*

375. A 56-year-old man has painful weeping rashes over the upper eyelid and forehead for the last two days along with ipsilateral acute punctate keratopathy. One-year back, he had chemotherapy for non-Hodgkin's lymphoma. There is no other abnormality. Which of the following is the *most likely* diagnosis?

A. Impetigo **B.** SLE
C. Herpes zoster **D.** Pyoderma gangrenosum *(AIIMS Nov 2004)*

Herpes zoster mostly afflicts those past 50 years of age, but also affects immunocompromised individuals. It is due to reactivation of a virus that has been sitting latent in a posterior root ganglion of a spinal nerve. It starts with pain or parasthesiae in the distribution of one or more dermatomes. Involvement of one of the branches of trigeminal ganglion, with lesions in the distribution of maxillary, mandibular or ophthalmic sensory nerves, is common, as is involvement of dermatomes of thoracic and cervical regions. For most people no specific treatment is required apart from keeping the lesions clean and application of antibiotic creams to prevent secondary infection. Acyclovir administered PO 800 mg 5 times daily on day one of the disorder shortens the disease and decreases its severity.

Ref: *Roxburgh's Common Skin Diseases; 17th edition; page 52 and 53*

376. A 16-year-old boy presented with asymptomatic multiple, erythematosus, annular lesions with a collarette of scales at the periphery of the lesions present on the trunk, the *most likely* diagnosis is:

A. Pityriasis versicolor
B. Pityriasis alba
C. Pityriasis rosea
D. Pityriasis rubra pilaris *(AI 2005)*

Pityriasis rosea is a papulosquamous eruption of unknown cause, which occurs more commonly in the spring and fall. Its 1st feature is the development of a 2 to 6 cm annular lesion (*herald patch*). Herald patch is followed in a few days to a few weeks by the appearance of many smaller annular or papular lesions with a predilection to occur on the trunk. The lesions are generally oval with their long axis parallel to the skin fold lines. The individual lesions may range in color from red to brown and have a trailing scale. Treatment is generally directed at alleviating pruritus and consists of oral antihistamines, topical glucocorticoids, and sometimes, the use of UV-B phototherapy.

Ref: *Harrison's Principles of Internal Medicine; 14th edition*

377. A 40-year-old woman presents with a 2-year history of erythematosus papulopustular lesions on the convexities of the face. There is a background of erythema and telangiectasia. The *most likely* diagnosis in this patient is:

A. Acne vulgaris **B.** Acne rosacea
C. Systemic lupus erythematosus **D.** Polymorphic light eruption *(AI 2005)*

Acne rosacea is an inflammatory disorder mainly affecting the central face. It is seen almost exclusively in adults, **only rarely affecting patients less than 30 years of age**. Rosacea is seen more often in **women**. It is characterized by the presence of **erythema, telangiectases**, and superficial pustules but is not associated with the presence of comedones.

Ref: *Harrison's Principles of Internal Medicine; 14th edition*

378. An 8-year-old boy from Bihar presents with a 6 months history of an ill-defined hypopigmented slightly atrophic macule on the face. The *most likely* diagnosis is:

A. Pityriasis alba **B.** Indeterminate leprosy
C. Morphoca **D.** Calcium deficiency *(AI 2005)*

The first signs of *leprosy* usually appear in skin. The lesions of **indeterminate leprosy** are very subtle and are *most commonly* diagnosed during the examination of contacts of known leprosy patients. One or more hypopigmented or hyperpigmented macules or plaques may occur. Often an anesthetic or paresthetic patch is the 1st symptom noted by the patient. Sensation is often relatively preserved in these early lesions, particularly those on the face. The lesions may clear spontaneously in a year or 2, but specific treatment is required.

Ref: *Harrison's Principles of Internal Medicine; 14th edition*

379. A 27-year-old sexually active male develops a vesiculobullous lesion on the glans soon after taking tablet paracetamol for fever. The lesion healed with hyperpigmentation. The *most likely* diagnosis is:

A. Behcet's syndrome **B.** Herpes genitalis
C. Fixed drug eruption **D.** Pemphigus vulgaris *(AI 2005)*

Localized hyperpigmentation is seen as a side effect of several *systemic medications*, including those that produce **fixed drug reactions** (phenolphthalein, tetracyclines, sulfonamides, barbiturates, and analgesics) and those that can complex with melanin (antimalarials). Fixed drug eruptions recur in the same location as circular areas of erythema that can become bullous and then resolve as brown macules. The eruption **usually appears within hours of administration of the offending agent, and common locations include the genitalia**, extremities, and perioral region.

Ref: *Harrison's Principles of Internal Medicine; 14th edition*

380. All of the following drugs are effective in the treatment of pityriasis versicolor, *except*:

A. Selenium disulphide **B.** Ketoconazole
C. Griseofulvin **D.** Clotrimazole *(AI 2005)*

Pityriasis versicolor is caused by yeast-like microorganism *Pityrosporum ovale*. Pale, scaling macules develop insidiously over the skin of the chest and back in young adults. Tropical imidazole creams (miconazole, clotrimazole, econazole) applied once daily for 6 weeks or use of ketoconazole shampoo to wash the affected areas once daily for 5 days are usually sufficient. Older medicines such as 20% sodium thiosulfate solution and selenium disulphide shampoo are also effective, as is the oral itraconazole for 7 to 15 days.

Ref: *Roxburgh's Common Skin Diseases; 17th edition; page 37 to 39*

381. A 36-year-old factory worker developed itchy, annular scaly plaques in both groins. Application of a corticosteroid ointment led to temporary relief but the plaques continued to extend at the periphery. The *most likely* diagnosis is:

A. Erythema annulare centrifugum **B.** Granuloma annulare

C. Annular lichen planus **D.** Tinea cruris *(AI 2005)*

Tinea cruris (groin ring worm) is a very itchy condition and is a disorder of young men. Well-defined, itchy, red scaling patches are found asymmetrically on the medial aspect of both groins. T. rubrum and E. floccosum are the causative fungi. These gradually extend down the thigh and on to the scrotum unless treated. For ordinary ringworm of hairy skin, an imidazole-containing preparation (such as miconazole, clotrimazole, econazole) used twice daily for one month period is usually adequate. When multiple areas are affected and when topical treatment has failed for some reason one of the following systemic drugs can be used.

Griseofulvin (500 mg bid); ketoconazole (200 mg daily), itraconazole (100 mg daily); and terbinafine (250 mg daily). These drugs are administered for 2 to 6 weeks *except* griseofulvin which when given for tinea ungium of toe nail may be given for 6 to 12 months.

Ref: *Roxburgh's Common Skin Diseases; 17th edition; page 40*

ANSWERS

1 C   2 A   3 B   4 A   5 D   6 B   7 C   8 A   9 C   10 A
11 C   12 A   13 C   14 D   15 D   16 B   17 C   18 A   19 C   20 A
21 B   22 B   23 D   24 C   25 B   26 D   27 A   28 A   29 B   30 D
31 D   32 B   33 B   34 B   35 C   36 D   37 B   38 B   39 A   40 D
41 D   42 A   43 B   44 B   45 A   46 B   47 B   48 B   49 B   50 A
51 B   52 D   53 C   54 D   55 A   56 C   57 C   58 D   59 A   60 C
61 D   62 B   63 C   64 B   65 C   66 D   67 A   68 B   69 D   70 B
71 D   72 C   73 D   74 C   75 B   76 C   77 C   78 D   79 D   80 B
81 D   82 C   83 B   84 D   85 D   86 B   87 D   88 C   89 D   90 D
91 A   92 A   93 D   94 C   95 C   96 C   97 C   98 D   99 B   100 B
101 C   102 D   103 C   104 C   105 C   106 B   107 A   108 A   109 A   110 B
111 D   112 D   113 A   114 A   115 A   116 D   117 C   118 C   119 A   120 C
121 A   122 B   123 A   124 A   125 D   126 D   127 B   128 C   129 C   130 C
131 B   132 D   133 C   134 C   135 A   136 C   137 C   138 B   139 D   140 C
141 B   142 D   143 C   144 C   145 A   146 C   147 C   148 C   149 A   150 D
151 A   152 D   153 C   154 D   155 C   156 B   157 A   158 C   159 B   160 C
161 D   162 C   163 D   164 D   165 C   166 C   167 A   168 B   169 C   170 A
171 D   172 A   173 D   174 D   175 C   176 D   177 A   178 A   179 C   180 A
181 C   182 C   183 C   184 C   185 C   186 D   187 B   188 B   189 B   190 A
191 B   192 B   193 B   194 A   195 C   196 A   197 A   198 D   199 A   200 D
201 A   202 A   203 B   204 A   205 C   206 A   207 A   208 A   209 A   210 A
211 C   212 A   213 A   214 B   215 A   216 B   217 A   218 D   219 C   220 A
221 C   222 D   223 C   224 A   225 A   226 A   227 B   228 A   229 A   230 A
231 A   232 A   233 B   234 A   235 B   236 B   237 C   238 A   239 A   240 B
241 A   242 C   243 C   244 D   245 C   246 A   247 B   248 A   249 C   250 A
251 C   252 C   253 D   254 D   255 C   256 A   257 B   258 C   259 C   260 D
261 C   262 B   263 B   264 A   265 B   266 D   267 B   268 C   269 D   270 D
271 A   272 A   273 A   274 C   275 C   276 B   277 A   278 C   279 A   280 B
281 D   282 C   283 D   284 A   285 A   286 B   287 A   288 A   289 D   290 B
291 D   292 B   293 D   294 A   295 C   296 D   297 D   298 D   299 B   300 C
301 C   302 A   303 A   304 D   305 C   306 B   307 C   308 A   309 C   310 B
311 C   312 A   313 A   314 B   315 B   316 C   317 B   318 C   319 D   320 A
321 C   322 A   323 D   324 B   325 C   326 A   327 A   328 C   329 D   330 B
331 A   332 A   333 B   334 C   335 B   336 C   337 B   338 B   339 A   340 B
341 B   342 C   343 C   344 B   345 C   346 C   347 B   348 C   349 C   350 A
351 C   352 B   353 B   354 B   355 B   356 D   357 B   358 C   359 A   360 B
361 D   362 C   363 D   364 A   365 C   366 A   367 A   368 A   369 C   370 A
371 B   372 C   373 C   374 B   375 C   376 C   377 B   378 B   379 C   380 C
381 D

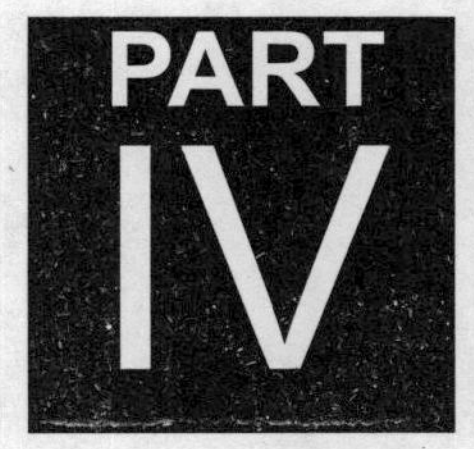

Radiology

Radiology

1. **The *best* view to visualize a small *left* sided pneumothorax is:**
   A. Right lateral **B.** Left lateral
   C. Right lateral decubitus **D.** Left lateral decubitus *(JIPMER 2002)*

2. **Pneumothorax is *best* demonstrated by taking a radiograph, with the patient in:**
   A. Inspiration **B.** Full inspiration
   C. Expiration **D.** Prone

An **expiratory film** will make a close pneumothorax easier to see since on full expiration the lung volume is at its smallest while the volume of pleural air is unchanged. In infants a **lateral decubitus film with the affected side upper-most** is more useful. Decubitus is patient's position in bed. When a *suggested* pneumothorax is not definitively observed on an inspiratory film, an expiratory film may be helpful. At end expiration, the constant volume of the pneumothorax gas is accentuated by the reduction of the hemithorax, and the pneumothorax is recognized more easily. Similar accentuation can be obtained with lateral decubitus studies of the appropriate side (**for a possible *left* pneumothorax, a *right* lateral decubitus film of the chest should be obtained**, with the beam centered over the left lung).

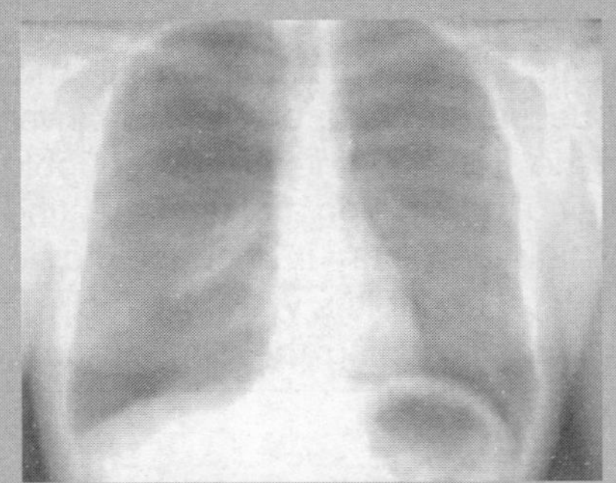

• **Andral's decubitus**	To lie on the sound side during the early stages of pleurisy
• **Dorsal decubitus**	To lie on the back
• **Ventral decubitus**	To lie on the stomach
• **Lateral decubitus**	To lie on the side

- **Lateral decubitus views** are useful in demonstrating the gravitational shift of free flowing **pleural effusion** and in demonstrating the hyperexpanded lung anatomy when the underlying lung is in the uppermost position. The decubitus view (and ultrasound) may detect pleural fluid accumulations that are much smaller than the **300 ml minimum that is usually detectable with erect radiographs**. Decubitus views can also aid in the detection of **pneumothorax** at the bedside.

3. ***Minimal* pleural effusion is best detected by X-ray.....view:**
   A. AP **B.** PA
   C. Oblique **D.** Lateral

4. **The *best* view of the chest to show minimal pleural effusion is:**
   A. PA view **B.** AP view
   C. Lateral decubitus view **D.** Oblique view *(AI 1992)*

5. ***Best* view to diagnose *minimal* amount of fluid in pleural space:**
   A. AP view
   B. PA view
   C. Apical view
   D. Lateral decubitus view *(PGI May 2001)*

6. **The chest X-ray view best suited for pleural effusion detection is:**
   A. AP view **B.** PA view
   C. Lateral decubitus view **D.** Lateral view

7. **The *best* view to visualize a *right* pleural effusion in chest X-ray is:**
   A. Right lateral **B.** Left lateral
   C. Right lateral decubitus **D.** Left lateral decubitus *(AI 1993)*

8. **A patient presents with *minimal* pleural effusion on the right side. The best method to detect this would be:**
   A. Right side chest X-ray **B.** Left side chest X-ray
   C. Left lateral decubitus chest X-ray **D.** Right lateral decubitus chest X-ray *(AIIMS May 2001)*

- If there is a doubt about the presence of **pleural fluid** or one wants to quantify the volume, **a lateral decubitus X-ray with the patient lying on the side of the effusion should be obtained.** Lateral decubitus films are helpful in determining *whether* the effusion is free flowing *and* to decide whether there is enough fluid to sample by thoracentesis.
- Up to 75 ml of pleural fluid can collect in a subpulmonic location, before it is radiographically apparent on the *lateral* radiograph. Up to 175 ml of fluid is needed before it is radiographically apparent of the *PA radiograph*. On both views, an effusion is identified by "blunting" of the normally sharply triangular costophrenic margin. *On decubitus views as little as 10 ml of fluid can be identified as it layers between the rib margin and the lung*. If the patient is supine when a frontal view is obtained, the fluid may only be appreciated as a hazy increase in density of the involved hemithorax. Because a large effusion can invert the diaphragm, it is difficult to quantify a right-sided effusion. If there is air in the stomach (the stomach bubble) a left-sided effusion can be quantified. Decubitus views are helpful in quantifying the effusion and documenting that it is free-flowing. Loculated effusion can appear mass-like. Occasionally, fluid may stay in a subpulmonic location and cause the appearance of an elevated hemidiaphragm. An ipsilateral decubitus view will document that fluid is present. Sometimes fluid will collect in the major or minor fissures, causing the appearance of a "pseudotumor".

9. **All the following calcify *except*:**
   A. Medulloblastoma **B.** Ependymoma
   C. Oligodendroglioma **D.** Meningioma *(JIPMER 2002)*

Tumor	Calcification
• **Ependymoma**	About 50% of cases
• **Medulloblastoma**	Rare; 1%-2%
• **Oligodendroglioma**	Common heterogeneous enhancement
• **Meningioma**	Focal calcification may be present but massive calcification and spontaneous hemorrhage are rare

10. **The *earliest* USG finding in pregnancy is:**
    A. Gestational sac **B.** Fetal cardiac activity
    C. Placenta **D.** Fundal thickening *(JIPMER 2002)*

The **earliest consistent finding** on transvaginal sonography in early pregnancy is a small (2 to 5 mm), rounded, anechoic structure eccentrically located within the thickened decidua, representing the developing **gestational sac**.

11. **Half-life of ^{99m}Tc is:**
    A. 2 hours **B.** 4 hours
    C. 6 hours **D.** 8 hours *(AI 1993, JIPMER 2002)*

The advent of ^{99m}Tc scanning allowed a marked reduction in radiation dose to the patient because of its **6-hour half-life** and favorable decay scheme *without* particulate emission.

12. Which of the following is a *naturally occurring* radioactive substance in the body found in small quantities:

A. Radium^{226} **B.** Bismuth^{60}
C. Iodine^{131} **D.** Potassium^{40} *(JIPMER 2002)*

Radiation originating in the body comes *mainly* from **radioactive potassium**, which emits β and γ rays.

13. Residual mediastinal and retroperitoneal lymphoma is best assessed by:

A. Bipedal lymphangiogram **B.** Technetium 99m pyrophosphate scans
C. Restaging procedure **D.** Gallium scan *(JIPMER 2002)*

The staging evaluation of a patient with Hodgkin's disease involves history and physical examination; CBC, ESR, serum chemistry; CXR, CT-scan of chest, abdomen, pelvis and bone-marrow biopsy. A bipedal lymphangiogram can be helpful. **Gallium scans are most useful at the completion of therapy to document remission.**

Ref: *Harrison's Principles of Internal Medicine; 15th edition; page 726*

14. Atomic number corresponds to:

A. Number of protons **B.** Number of electrons
C. Number of neutrons **D.** Electrons + protons *(PGI May 2001)*

Atomic number is the number of **protons** in an atomic nucleus.

15. Bilateral "spider leg" sign in IVP is indicative of:

A. Renal stone **B.** Hypernephroma
C. Hydronephrosis **D.** Polycystic kidney *(AI 1991)*

Autosomal dominant polycystic kidney (*syn.* **congenital cystic kidneys**) disease has a prevalence of 1:300 to 1:1000 and accounts for approximately 10% cases of end-stage renal disease in the USA. 90% of cases are inherited as an autosomal dominant trait, and approximately 10% are spontaneous mutations. **In 18% of cases there is an associated congenital cystic liver** and occasionally the pancreas and lung are also affected. It is slightly more common in women and 6 important clinical features are as under:

- Renal enlargement
- Hematuria **(25%)**
- Hypertension **(75%)**
- Pain
- Infection (*most common complication*)
- Uremia

Patients pass abundant urine of low specific gravity (1.010 or less) which neither contains cast nor cells. One kidney is larger than the other. Severe anemia is common. Ultrasonography and CT scan demonstrate multiple cysts in both kidneys. *Typical* **"spider leg appearance"** is seen in **excretory urography**. Rovsing's operation is done for polycystic kidney. *Renal transplant* is done if renal failure occurs.

Infantile polycystic kidney is an unrelated, *autosomal recessive* and rare condition in which the kidneys are large and many cases are stillborn; rest of the patient die of renal failure in early life.

Mnemonic: *"Adults are dominant so are their polycystic kidneys"*

16. Calcification of meniscal cartilage is a feature of:

A. Pseudogout **B.** Reiter's syndrome
C. Hyperparathyroidism **D.** Acromegaly *(AI 1991)*

Pyrophosphate-related arthropathy (*calcium pyrophosphate deposition disease*) is often radiologically *distinctive*. It *resembles* osteoarthritis in that the cartilage space is reduced and there is associated subchondral sclerosis with varying degrees of osteophyte formation. The distribution of affected joints *differs* from osteoarthritis in that there is a predilection for the metacarpophalangeal joints, particularly the 2nd and 3rd, often with noticeable sparing of the interphalangeal joints. **Calcification of fibrocartilages, especially in the wrists and knees, is common in elderly individuals who do not have a history of clinically significant arthropathy.** The clinical picture often associated with this arthropathy has been termed "**pseudogout syndrome**" because of the episodic character of acute joint inflammation that mimics that of gout.

17. Ideal imaging method to diagnose hydrocephalus in infant is:
A. MRI **B.** USG
C. CT scan **D.** Plain X-ray *(AI 1991)*

18. Neurosonography of neonates is preferred *over* CT scan because:
A. Open fontanelle **B.** Inexpensive
C. Children more cooperative **D.** Better resolution

The absences of radiation, low cost, lack of need for contrast agents, **an open fontanelle** and ease to performance are the factors that have popularized **neurosonography.**

19. Excretory urography should be *cautiously* performed in:
A. Leukemia **B.** Neuroblastoma
C. Bone secondaries **D.** Multiple myeloma *(AI 1991)*

20. IVP is contraindicated in:
A. Multiple myeloma **B.** Kidney stones
C. Transplanted kidney **D.** Renal cyst

IVP is contraindicated in patient with **multiple myeloma** as ARF may be precipitated.

21. *Most important* investigation for pericardial effusion is:
A. Lateral view of X-ray chest **B.** Echocardiography
C. USG **D.** Cardiac catheterization *(AI 1997)*

22. *Best* method for diagnosing pericardial effusion is:
A. Echocardiography **B.** Gallium scan
C. Angiography **D.** USG *(AI 1993)*

Echocardiography is the **most effective** diagnostic laboratory technique available for diagnosing **pericardial effusion**, since it is sensitive, specific, simple, noninvasive, and may be performed at the bedside.

23. 'Tram line' calcification is seen in:
A. Ependymoma **B.** Thrombosed cerebral vein
C. Sturge-Weber syndrome **D.** Meningioma

24. 'Tram track' appearance on X-ray of the head is seen in:
A. Sturge-Weber syndrome **B.** von Hippel-Lindau disease
C. Tuberous sclerosis **D.** Neurofibroma *(AIIMS May 2001)*

Sturge-Weber syndrome or encephalotrigeminal angiomatosis was first described in 1879 by *W. Allen Sturge*, who described a child with sensorimotor seizures *contralateral* to a facial "port-wine stain". *Weber* provided the first radiographic demonstration of an important component of the disorder- intracerebral meningeal angiomatous calcification (characteristic **tram line calcification** seen in simple X-ray) ipsilateral to a trigeminal nevus.

- **Port**- after *Oporto*, city in Portugal (a sweet, usually **dark-red**, fortified wine).

25. Which *one* of the following is the contrast used in MRI scan:
A. Iodine **B.** Gadolinium
C. Rose Bengal **D.** Strontium *(PGI Dec 2000)*

The sensitivity of **MRI** for the diagnosis of pituitary tumors depends on the types of tumors, sizes of tumors, MR equipment standards, and the use of **gadolinium**. *Gadolinium* occurs with other rare earth elements in many minerals, such as samarskite, gadolinite, monazite, and some varieties of Norwegian ytterspar. It is the 41st element in order of abundance in the crust of the earth.

26. "Egg shell" calcification is seen in:
A. Silicosis
B. Sarcoidosis
C. Tuberculosis
D. Histoplasmosis *(SGPGI 1999, JIPMER 2000, PGI May 2001)*

Some of the *unusual* chest X-ray findings in **sarcoidosis** include **"egg shell" calcification** of hilar nodes, pleural effusions, cavitation, atelectasis, pulmonary hypertension, pneumothorax and cardiomegaly.

27. Radiological sign characteristic of ischemic colitis is:
A. Inverted 3 appearance
B. Cobra head sign
C. Craggy popcorn appearance
D. Thumb print appearance

28. Radiological feature of ischemic colitis is:
A. Saw tooth appearance
B. Nose pipe appearance
C. Thumb printing
D. Cobble stone appearance *(UP 1999, KARNATAKA 2001)*

The term **ischemic colitis** describes the structural changes in colon which result due to deprivation of blood supply. Such episodes occur mainly in the region of **splenic flexure of colon** where blood supply is precarious. Clinical features are *lower abdominal pain of acute onset, vomiting, fever, and* **passage of bright red blood per rectum.** Plain films of the abdomen often show a mild or moderate increase in bowel gas. In the sub-acute phase, the developing edema and hemorrhage in the sub-mucosa cause thickening of the bowel wall that is evident on the plain film in approximately 20% of patients with ischemic colitis. If sufficiently focal, this thickening will cause soft-tissue indentations into the air-filled colonic lumen **("thumb-printing")**.

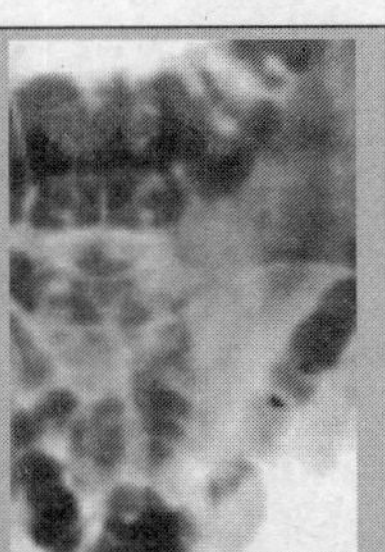

29. Half-life of cobalt^{60} is..............years:
A. 2.3
B. 1.2
C. 5.7
D. 3.4 *(MP 2001)*

30. Radioactive cobalt emits:
A. Neutrons
B. Alpha rays
C. Gamma rays
D. Beta rays *(PGI 1990)*

Radioactive cobalt-60 is the most important among the several known isotopes of cobalt. **It has a half-life of 5.7 years** and produces **intense gamma radiation**.

31. The half-life of Co^{57} is:
A. 2.6 years
B. 5.2 years
C. 270 days
D. 3200 years

The half-life of Co^{57} is 270 days.

32. Which of the following investigations are to be done for the diagnosis of carcinoma head of pancreas:
A. Plain X-ray abdomen
B. CT
C. USG
D. Hypotonic duodenography *(PGI Dec 2000)*

33. *Best* diagnosis for pancreatic disease is:
A. PTC
B. ERCP
C. CT scan
D. USG *(UP 1993)*

34. *Most sensitive* investigation of pancreatic carcinoma is:
A. Angiography
B. ERCP
C. CT scan
D. Ultrasound

While more costly than ultrasonography, **CT is technically simpler, more reproducible, provides better definition of the body and tail of the pancreas, and requires less interpretive skill.** Magnetic resonance imaging (MRI) has *not* been shown to be better than CT in the evaluation of pancreatic lesions.

35. Looser's zone is characteristic of:
A. Hyperparathyroidism **B.** Scurvy
C. Hyperparathyroidism **D.** Milkman's pseudofractures *(UP 1994)*

36. Pseudofracture or Looser's zone is seen in:
A. Vitamin C deficiency **B.** Thyroiditis
C. Osteoporosis **D.** Osteomalacia *(MAHE 2000)*

Rickets and osteomalacia are the different expressions of the same pathology i.e. inadequate mineralization of the bone. The bones throughout the skeleton are incompletely calcified and softened (osteo*malacia*). In children this process also affects the physeal growth and ossification resulting in the deformities of the endochondral skeleton (*rickets*). Inadequacy may be due to calcium deficiency, hypophosphatemia, defects along the metabolic pathway of vitamin D; nutritional rickets, under exposure to sunlight, malabsorption, decreased 25 hydroxylation due to liver disease or phenytoin and reduced 1 α hydroxylation in renal disease, nephrectomy, or 1 α hydroxylase deficiency. The infant with rickets may present with tetany or convulsions and there is listlessness, muscle flaccidity and failure to thrive. **Earliest sign of rickets is craniotabes** which may be defined as an abnormal softening of the skull bones. Bones of the occipital region are more severely affected and may become almost thin like paper. There is enlargement of costochondral junction (*rickety rosary*), lateral indentation of chest (*Harrison's sulcus*) and genu varum or valgum. In severe rickets coxa vera, spinal curvature and fractures of long bone may occur. The **X-ray findings of osteomalacia** are more difficult to diagnose. **The most specific feature of osteomalacia is the presence of Looser transformation zones, also referred to as Milkman's pseudofractures or umbauzonen.**

37. *Best* investigation for cardiac tamponade is:
A. M mode ECG **B.** USG
C. Real time ECG **D.** 2 D echocardiography *(AI 1994)*

In **cardiac tamponade** pericardiocentesis may be carried out without cardiac catheterization but, whenever possible, after confirmation of the clinical diagnosis by **echocardiography**.

38. Half-life of I^{131} is:
A. 10 days **B.** 4 days
C. 8 days **D.** 4 hours *(AI 1994)*

The half-life of I^{131} is 8 days.

39. Renal GRF can be estimated by:
A. Tc^{99m} + gallium^{121} **B.** Tc^{99m} DSMA
C. Tc^{99m} DTPA **D.** Tc^{99m} DMSA *(AI 1995, UP 1995)*

^{99m}Tc -diethylenetriamine-penta-acetic acid (**^{99m}Tc-DTPA**) is cleared from the kidneys by means of glomerular filtration without tubular reabsorption or secretion. This agent is therefore **used for the evaluation of filtration function, and obstruction as well as the measurement of glomerular filtration rate**. Since ^{99m}Tc -DTPA is rapidly cleared from the renal cortex, scars or space occupying parenchymal lesions, which may be transiently evident on early images, are more readily defined with other renal agents, in particular dimercaptosuccinic acid (DMSA) or glucoheptonate (GHA).

40. Safe *maximum* dose of radiation per year in human beings is:
A. 20 rads **B.** 10 rads
C. 5 rads **D.** 1 rads *(AI 1992)*

Maximum dose of radiation per year is **5 rads.**

41. Kerley B-lines are seen when pulmonary venous pressure is:
- **A.** 5 mm Hg
- **B.** 10 mm Hg
- **C.** 22 mm Hg
- **D.** 40 mm Hg

42. Pulmonary Kerley B-lines are seen in all the following *except*:
- **A.** Pulmonary edema
- **B.** Mitral valve disease
- **C.** Interstitial fibrosis
- **D.** Bronchoalveolar carcinoma

(AIIMS May 2001)

When the mean pulmonary venous pressure exceeds the osmotic colloid pressure (22 mm Hg to 25 mm Hg), the lymphatic channels of the interlobular septa in the base of the lung becomes prominent. The fluid that has entered the interlobular septa is reflected radiographically as thin, dense, horizontal streaks, often termed **Kerley B-lines**. This sign indicates a moderate to severe degree of **pulmonary venous hypertension** (left ventricular failure and **mitral stenosis**) with the mean left atrial or venous pressure at 22 mm Hg or more. These lines are also seen in lymphatic obstruction caused by **pneumoconiosis** and lymphangitis carcinomatosa.

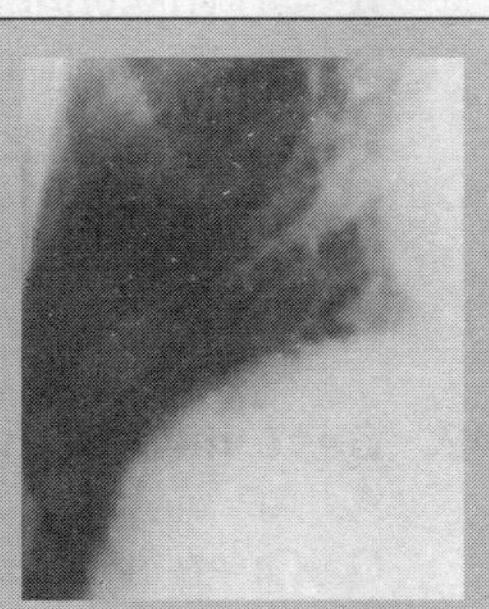

43. *Contraindication* for the use of NMR imaging is:
- **A.** Psychotic patients
- **B.** Patients on lithium
- **C.** Intracranial *metallic* aneurysm clips
- **D.** Patients receiving radiotherapy

44. Radiation exposure does *not* occur in:
- **A.** Plain X-ray
- **B.** Fluoroscopy
- **C.** MRI scan
- **D.** CT scan

(AI 1993)

When used for medical applications, NMR is now referred to as magnetic resonance imaging (MRI), in order to avoid the "negative" connotations of the word "nuclear". **MRI does not, in fact, involves radioactivity or other ionizing radiation.** MRI is excellent as an imaging technique for scans of the brain, head, and neck. **People with metal implants should not be scanned by MRI.**

TYPES OF RADIATIONS USED IN RADIOLOGY

Electromagnetic and Ionizing	Electromagnetic but nonionizing	Nonelectromagnetic and nonionizing
• X-rays • Gamma rays	• Radiofrequency radiation • Infrared light • Visible light	• Ultrasound

Fluoroscope is a device consisting of a fluorescent screen, mounted either separately or in conjunction with an **X-ray tube**, which shows the images of objects interposed between the tube and the screen. It has been largely replaced by the image intensifier for performing fluoroscopic studies.

45. Which is *not* mutagenic:
- **A.** Ultraviolet rays
- **B.** β-rays
- **C.** X-ray
- **D.** Ultrasound

(PGI 1993)

Mutation is produced only by ionizing radiations; as **ultrasound** is *not* an ionizing radiation it is not mutagenic.

46. Investigation of choice for acute subarachnoid hemorrhage is:
- **A.** Angiography
- **B.** CT scan
- **C.** Enhanced MRI
- **D.** MRI

(AI 1998)

47. *Noninvasive* procedure for CVA is:
A. EEG
B. Echoencephalography
C. Angiography
D. CT scan
(UP 1994)

Atherosclerotic CVS disease (including cerebrovascular accident, myocardial infarction, and peripheral vascular disease) is the leading cause of mortality in the United States and western Europe. **CT scanning is an important noninvasive diagnostic tool for assessment and management of patients with acute intracranial hemorrhage.**

48. Congenital malformation that can be detected *earliest* on USG:
A. Down syndrome
B. Sacral agenesis
C. Hydrocephalus
D. Anencephaly
(AI 1994)

Obstetric ultrasonography performed in the 1st trimester of pregnancy can detect a fetus without a brain (anencephaly). Polyhydramnios may result from either *failure* of the fetus to swallow amniotic fluid or the formation of choroid plexuses because the exposed plexus secretes cerebrospinal fluid directly into the amniotic cavity.

49. *Best* view for visualizing sella turcica in X-ray is:
A. AP view
B. Lateral view
C. Open mouth view
D. Dorsal view
(AI 1994)

Frontal and **lateral plain films of the skull** have been traditionally used to evaluate the bony anatomy of the **sella turcica** and pituitary fossa in order to diagnose an intrasellar expansion of the pituitary gland or a parasellar / suprasellar mass originating in contiguous soft tissues.

50. In pancreatic scanning isotope *most commonly* used is:
A. I^{131}
B. Tc^{99}
C. Se^{75}
D. Cr^{51}

51. Technetium labeled red blood cells are used for:
A. Splenic disease
B. Pulmonary embolism
C. Renal disease
D. Biliary tree
(AI 1995)

Specific Mechanisms of Localization of Radiopharmaceuticals

Active Transport
^{131}I or ^{125}I iodine, or ^{99m}Tc pertechnetate for thyroid gland ^{99m}Tc -glucoheptonate and ^{131}I orthoiodohippurate for kidneys ^{131}I rose Bengal and ^{99m}Tc HIDA for liver ^{75}Se selenomethionine for pancreas ^{43}K or ^{201}Tl for myocardial perfusion
Phagocytosis
^{99m}Tc sulfur colloid, ^{113}mIn colloid for liver, spleen, and bone marrow Labeled leukocytes for thrombus or abscess localization
Cell Sequestration
Heat damaged ^{51}Cr or **^{99m}Tc red blood cells for spleen**
Capillary Blockage
^{131}I macroaggregated albumin, ^{99m}Tc MAA ^{99m}Tc albumin microspheres for lungs
Simple or Exchange Diffusion
^{18}F, ^{85}Sr, ^{87m}Sr, for bone Agents for brain lesion localization

^{99m}Tc DTPA for glomerular filtration studies ^{133}Xe for gas inhalation studies
Physiochemical Adsorption
^{99m}Tc phosphates for bone studies ^{131}I or ^{99m}Tc labeled fibrinogen in thrombi
Compartmental Localization
^{131}I albumin, ^{99m}Tc albumin, ^{113m}In transferrin for cardiovascular blood pool ^{113m}In or ^{99m}Tc albumin, ^{113m}In transferrin for placental localization

52. Gold standard for pulmonary embolism is:

A. ECG
B. Venous USG
C. Lung scanning
D. Pulmonary angiography *(PGI 1997)*

53. In pulmonary embolism the investigation of choice is:

A. Ventilation perfusion scan
B. Contrast MRI
C. MRI
D. CT *(AI 1998)*

54. Pulmonary embolism is *best* diagnosed by:

A. CT scan
B. Ventilation perfusion scan
C. USG
D. X-ray chest PA view *(AI 1996, 1998)*

Radiologic studies for **pulmonary thromboembolism** (PTE) include the plain chest X-ray, the perfusion and ventilation lung scan, and pulmonary angiography. **The only *absolute* way of establishing the diagnosis in life is by pulmonary angiography.** However, the use of the less invasive methods in appropriate clinical settings may provide a sufficient degree of certainty of pulmonary embolism to justify anticoagulant therapy *without* angiography. **Lung scanning is the principal imaging test for the diagnosis of PTE** and in this technique small particulate aggregates of albumin labeled with a γ-emitting radionuclide are injected IV. They are trapped in the pulmonary capillary bed and a perfusion scan defect indicates absent or decreased blood flow, *possibly* due to PTE. Ventilation scans, obtained with radiolabeled inhaled gases such as xenon or krypton, improve the specificity of the perfusion scan.

55. Radio sensitive stage is:

A. G_2M stage
B. G_2 stage
C. G_1 stage
D. S phase *(AI 1996, 1998)*

Cells are most sensitive to radiation at the **G_2M interface.**

56. "Popcorn" calcification is seen in:

A. Tuberculosis
B. Metastasis
C. Fungal infection
D. Pulmonary hamartoma *(AI 1997)*

57. "Popcorn" calcification in lung is *virtually* diagnostic of:

A. Tuberculoma
B. Carcinoid
C. Hamartoma
D. Teratoma

Hamartomas are typically round, smooth, slightly lobulated peripheral masses < 4 cm in size without lobar predominance. Calcification is present in < 5% of cases. The typical pattern of **"popcorn" calcification** seen in chest X-ray is pathognomonic of hamartoma.

58. Best method of detecting *minimal* bronchiectasis is:

A. Chest X-ray
B. Radionuclide lung scan
C. CT scan (HRCT)
D. Bronchography *(AI 1992, KARNATAKA 2001)*

59. In bronchiectasis the *investigation of choice* was:

A. USG **B.** Bronchography
C. Bronchoscopy **D.** X-ray

Plain X-rays usually suffice to define pulmonary processes, but in difficult cases the lungs can be shown exquisitely by high-resolution computed tomography (CT), which is particularly useful for interstitial processes and in generalized pulmonary illnesses. **CT has also superseded bronchography in the study of bronchiectasis.**

60. Which of the following is seen in Pindborg tumor:

A. Sunray appearance **B.** Onion peel appearance
C. Driven snow appearance **D.** Cherry Blossom appearance *(AI 2002)*

The *most common* odontogenic tumors are the ameloblastoma and the calcifying epithelial odontogenic tumor (**Pindborg tumor**), both of *ectodermal* origin, and the mesodermal odontogenic myxoma (fibromyxoma or myxofibroma). Like the ameloblastoma, Pindborg tumor occurs more frequently in the mandible than the maxilla, but tends to occur, on the average, somewhat later in life. Like the ameloblastoma, Pindborg tumor is a benign lesion but is locally invasive. It is readily distinguishable from the ameloblastoma under the microscope. The Pindborg tumor is variable in radiographic presentation. When presenting in its least distinctive form it appears as a unilocular radiolucency, but *typically* the lesion contains multiple calcifications and many small trabeculations, giving an "**driven snow appearance**" or a honeycomb pattern.

61. Multiple punched out lytic lesions in X-ray are seen in:

A. Eosinophilic granuloma **B.** Multiple myeloma
C. Craniopharyngioma **D.** Paget's disease *(AI 2001, MP 2001)*

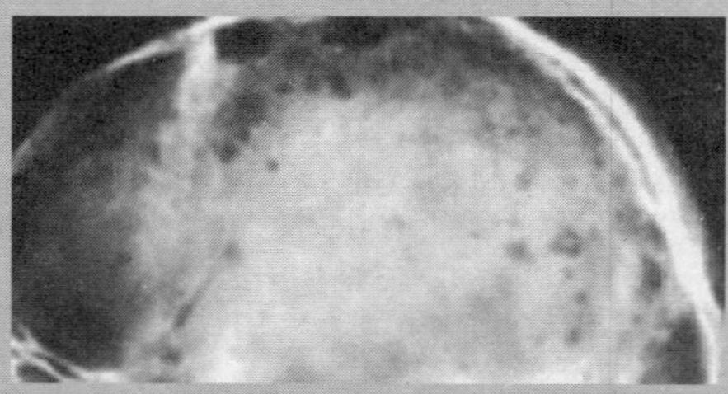

Multiple myeloma usually produces small, mostly discrete round holes of variable size, sometimes referred to as **punched out lesions**.

62. "Chain of lakes" appearance is seen in:

A. Ductal adenoma **B.** Carcinoma head of pancreas
C. Acute pancreatitis **D.** Chronic pancreatitis *(AI 1996)*

In **chronic pancreatitis**, early changes at endoscopic retrograde cholangiopancreatography (ERCP) include ectasia and strictures of the main pancreatic duct and the branch ducts. With disease progression, the side branches increasingly dilate as does the main pancreatic duct. Ultimately, the main pancreatic duct either appears as a "**chain of lakes**" (alternating dilatation and stenosis) or is uniformly widely dilated with both calcified and non-calcified proteinaceous deposits.

63. "Marble bone appearance" is characteristic of:

A. Achondroplasia **B.** Fluorosis
C. Osteogenesis imperfecta **D.** Osteopetrosis *(DNB 1990)*

Osteopetrosis or marble bone disease or Albers-Schönberg disease is a rare idiopathic condition of bone. A feature of this disease is a high susceptibility to osteomyelitis. This is a particular problem in the jaws, because infective organisms may be introduced by caries and periodontal disease.

64. Investigation of *choice* for gallstone is:

A. CT scan **B.** Oral cholecystography
C. USG **D.** X-ray

Real-time sonography of the gallbladder has largely replaced conventional oral cholecystography **for diagnosis of gallbladder stone**. Its advantages include lack of dependence on absorption of the oral contrast medium from the bowel, or excretion into the biliary system, or concentration by the gallbladder. As it involves no exposure to ionizing radiation, ultrasonography can be used in situations in which oral cholecystography may be less useful and should be avoided.

65. "Bull's eye lesion" is seen in:
- **A.** Metastatic tumor of breast
- **B.** Leiomyoma
- **C.** Carcinoma lung
- **D.** Malignant melanoma

(UP 1998)

Ulceration into a submucosal mesenchymal tumor such as a **leiomyoma** or a submucosal metastasis produces a variably shaped crater, but because the epithelium is not primarily involved its edges are often sharply defined. This is the basis for terms such as **bull's eye,** target, and buttercup to describe these lesions.

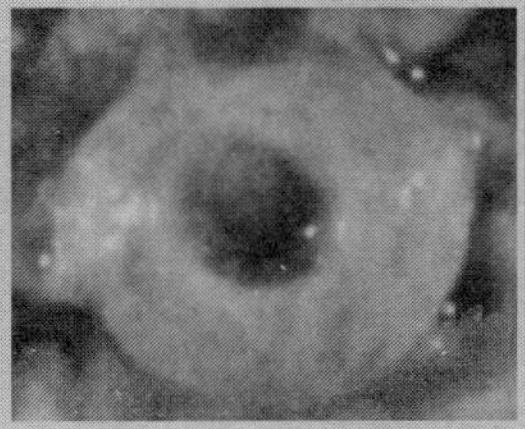

66. *Most common* calcifying brain tumor in a child is:
- **A.** Meningioma
- **B.** Glioma
- **C.** Craniopharyngioma
- **D.** Medulloblastoma

Suprasellar calcification in a flocculent, granular, or curvilinear pattern is present on skull X-rays in *most* children and in *some* adults with **craniopharyngioma**. But calcification is evident on CT in most of these adults.

67. Radioisotope used for myocardial scanning is:
- **A.** Indium
- **B.** Gallium
- **C.** Technetium^{147h}
- **D.** Thallium

The information gained from an exercise test can be enhanced by stress myocardial perfusion scanning after the intravenous administration of a radioisotope such as **thallium^{201}** or **technetium^{99m}** sestamibi during exercise or a pharmacologic stress.

68. NMR is based on:
- **A.** Electrical movement of nucleus
- **B.** Magnetic movement of nucleus
- **C.** Nuclear fission
- **D.** Charge of nucleus

69. In MRI the images are produced due to:
- **A.** K^+
- **B.** N_2O
- **C.** H^+
- **D.** CO_2

70. NMR (MRI) is based on principle of:
- **A.** Electron
- **B.** Neutron
- **C.** Proton
- **D.** Microwaves

MRI (NMR) is a versatile, powerful, and sensitive tool that can generate thin section images of any part of the body from any angle and direction, without surgical invasion and in a relatively short period of time. MRI is possible in the human body because the body is filled with small biological *magnets*, the most abundant and responsive of which is the **proton (H^+)**. The principles of MRI take advantage of the *random distribution of protons*, which possess fundamental magnetic properties. Once the patient is placed in the cylindrical magnet, the diagnostic process follows three basic steps. 1st, MRI creates a steady state within the body by placing the body in a steady magnetic field that is 30,000 times stronger than the Earth's magnetic field. Then MRI stimulates the body with radiowaves to change the steady-state orientation of protons. It then stops the radiowaves and *listens* to the body's electromagnetic transmissions at a selected frequency. These transmitted signals are used to construct internal images of the body using principles similar to those developed for computerized axial tomography, or CAT scanners.

71. Characteristic of benign lesion on chest X-ray is:
A. Concentric dense calcification
B. Peripheral location
C. Cavitation
D. > 5 cm in diameter
(PGI 1997)

72. *Not* included in the differential diagnosis of *solitary* pulmonary nodule:
A. Neurofibroma
B. Hamartoma
C. Bronchial adenoma
D. Tuberculoma

Solitary pulmonary nodule (SPN) is defined as an X-ray density completely surrounded by normal aerated lung, with circumscribed margins, of any shape, usually 1 to 6 cm in *greatest* diameter. About 35 % of all such lesions in adults will be malignant, most being primary lung cancer, while less than 1 % are malignant in *non*smoking patients under 35 years of age. Only two radiographic criteria are *reliable* predictors of the benign nature of a solitary pulmonary nodule viz. **lack of growth over a period > 2 years** and *certain* **characteristic patterns of calcification**. Calcification alone *does not* exclude malignancy. But a *dense central nidus*, *multiple punctate foci*, and *bull's eye* (**granuloma**) and *popcorn ball* (**hamartoma**) calcifications are all highly *suggestive* of a benign lesion.

73. Radioactive material used for ventriculography is:
A. Tc^{99m}
B. K^{9}
C. Th^{201}
D. Co^{60}

Radionuclide ventriculography is also known as *equilibrium gated blood pool imaging*; MUGA (the name of an early *computer software processing package*), or *radionuclide angiography*. All of these names refer to the technique in which **^{99m}Tc labeled red blood cells** are injected into the patient where they equilibrate within the intra-vascular space and define the great vessels and the four chambers of the heart. The images should be *gated* using the ECG signal to identify the beginning of each cardiac cycle to accumulate a sufficient number of beats and identify discrete time intervals or frames in the heart cycle to assess global parameters such as ejection fraction, filling, and emptying rates or regional contraction analysis.

74. Dye used for myelography is:
A. Iopanoic acid
B. Metrizamide
C. Dianosil
D. Conray (Iothalamate)

- **Myelography** is the radiography of the spinal cord and associated nerves after intrathecal injection of a radiopaque, water-soluble contrast medium (**metrizamide**). This technique has limited use nowadays due to availability of computed tomography and magnetic resonance imaging. Metrizamide is indicated in adults and pediatric patients for lumbar, thoracic, cervical, and total columnar myelography to determine the presence of abnormalities in the spinal column, spinal canal, and CNS.
- *Oral cholecystographic agents* such as **iopanoic acid** are indicated for radiographic delineation of the gallbladder.
- **Iothalamate** meglumine and iothalamate sodium injection are indicated to visualize lesions or *malformations of the heart* and *obstructions or anomalies of the major thoracic blood vessels.*
- **Dianosil** (propyl-iodine) is used for bronchography.

75. Cell which is *most* sensitive to radiation is:
A. Platelet
B. Basophil
C. Lymphocyte
D. Neutrophil

Chromosomal changes can be observed in human cells exposed to much lower doses of radiation. A significant increase in the background level of chromosomal aberrations has been observed in **peripheral lymphocytes** of some patients exposed to diagnostic X-ray examinations.

76. Investigation of *choice* in parathyroid pathology is:
A. Thallium technetium isotope subtraction scan
B. Thallium scan
C. Gallium scan
D. CT scan
(AI 1995)

Thallium technetium isotope subtraction scan can locate about 95% of **parathyroid** adenomas.

77. Investigation *not* done in brain tumor is:
A. X-ray skull
B. MRI
C. Lumbar puncture
D. CT scan
(AI 1997)

Lumbar puncture is contraindicated in patients with papilledema or cerebral edema, especially due to **tumors in posterior fossa**, for fear of producing a cerebellar pressure cone. Unilateral space occupying lesion (SOL) may result in herniation through the tentorial hiatus. Lumbar puncture is contraindicated in *suspected spontaneous subarachnoid hemorrhage* unless a CT scan has been performed. *Relative* contraindications are blood dyscrasia, patients on anticoagulant therapy, skin sepsis and spinal deformity.

78. Chemotherapeutic agent of *choice* in carcinoma pancreas is:
A. Streptomycin
B. Adriamycin
C. 5-FU
D. Mitomycin C

The median survival for patients whose pancreatic cancers are surgically unresectable is about 6 months. Management of such individuals should be directed at *palliation* of symptoms. However, the addition of chemotherapy with **5-FU** to external beam irradiation has increased the survival time for these patients, perhaps because fluorouracil acts as a radiosensitizing agent.

79. "String sign" is indicative of:
A. Irritable bowel syndrome
B. Ulcerative colitis
C. Hypertrophic pyloric stenosis
D. Toxic mega colon

Hypertrophic pyloric stenosis is the *most common* acquired obstruction of the young infants. It is more common in males and develops usually between the 3rd and 6th weeks of life. The clinical features of projectile vomiting, visible gastric peristaltic waves, and a palpable pyloric mass are frequently diagnostic while the radiologic findings are *confirmatory* and consist of gastric dilatation with a deficiency of small-bowel gas. Positive fluoroscopic and radiographic signs include a *pyloric beak*, *elongated pyloric canal* (**string sign**), flattening of the pre-pyloric area of the lesser curvature (*shoulder sign*), and usually, active gastric peristalsis. Ultrasound examination is also a reliable method of diagnosis of hypertrophic pyloric stenosis by an experienced sonographer. Longitudinal measurements of > 16 mm and a wall thickness in the axial view of > 3.5 to 4 mm are *diagnostic*.

80. Vertebra plana is seen in:
A. Eosinophilic granuloma
B. Tuberculosis
C. Malignancy
D. Fracture of spine

Eosinophilic granuloma is the mildest form of histiocytosis X. Pathological changes are predominantly bony although sometimes pulmonary involvement can occur. Solitary lesions of spine can collapse presenting the classical appearance of **vertebra plana** or Calvé's vertebral compression or vertebral osteochondritis.

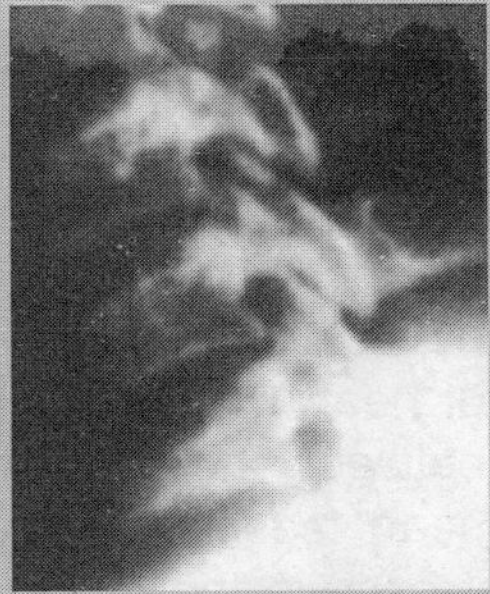

81. 'Rim sign' in IVP is characteristic of:
A. Hypernephroma
B. Chronic pyelonephritis
C. Infantile polycystic kidney
D. Hydronephrosis

In severe **hydronephrosis**, the enlarged kidney may appear as a mass on the plain film. If the parenchyma has been markedly thinned by obstructive atrophy, the nephrogram consists of nothing more than a thin border of opacified tissue giving the typical appearance known as a **rim or shell nephrogram**.

82. ***Most common*** **radiological feature in pulmonary embolism is:**
A. Rat tail configuration of vessels
B. Westermark's sign
C. Normal X-ray
D. Pleural effusion
(UP 1999)

A normal or near-normal chest X-ray in a dyspneic patient suggests pulmonary thromboembolism. Well-established abnormalities in CXR include focal oligemia (Westermark's sign), a peripheral wedged-shaped density above the diaphragm (Hampton's hump), or an enlarged right descending pulmonary artery.

83. **Cobra head deformity is characteristic of:**
A. Cystitis
B. Ureterocele
C. Posterior urethral valve
D. Bladder tumor

The term **ureterocele** denotes a *cystic or aneurysmal ectasia of the subepithelial segment of the intravesical ureter protruding into the bladder*. Ureteroceles are of two types, ectopic and simple. Simple ureteroceles represent a congenital prolapse of the dilated distal ureter and its orifice into the bladder lumen. Acquired *pseudo*ureteroceles may occasionally result from any inflammatory, traumatic, or neoplastic process that produces stenosis of the ureteral orifice.

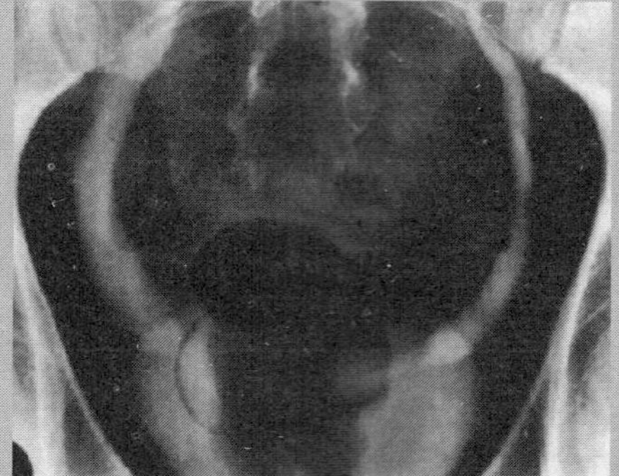

Simple ureteroceles are common in children and may present in the newborn. Urographically, early filling of the bulbous terminal ureter is noted, a finding that has been referred as a "**spring onion**" or "**cobra head**" appearance.

84. **Radiofrequency ablation treatment is most useful in:**
A. Ventricular premature complex
B. WPW syndrome
C. Atrial fibrillation
D. Ventricular fibrillation

Wolff-Parkinson-White syndrome is a *hereditary* condition and although present from birth it is not usually diagnosed until adolescence. The electrical signal controlling the heart beat should pass over the atria and flow through the atrioventricular (AV node) before passing over the ventricles. In Wolff-Parkinson-White syndrome the electrical signal *bypasses* the AV node and triggers the ventricles *too soon*. The presence of this electrical bypass (*short circuit*) causes **atrioventricular reentry tachycardia** (AVRT). The bypass consists of an extra piece of heart muscle, which is present from birth. The bypass allows the electrical signal to pass in *both* directions between the atria and the ventricles allowing the electrical signal to continue to circulate (reentry) around the heart muscles. Because the signal is able to pass from the atria to the ventricles faster via the bypass than it can via the correct path through the AV node there is a change to the QRS section of the ECG waveform. The delta wave formed in the QRS complex is described as the WPW abnormality. WPW syndrome may cause tachycardia but this does not normally occur until the teens or early twenties. This tachycardia is caused by the bypass allowing signals to pass at between 250 and 300 beats per minute to the ventricles. This causes fibrillation of the ventricles to arise; this affects the pumping efficiency of the heart causing low blood pressure and possible loss of life. A patient with AVRT may experience a fast heart beat, weakness, light-headedness, syncope and shortness of breath. If tachycardia occurs, this can normally be controlled by medication. **It may become necessary to have the abnormal electrical path (bypass) treated by radiofrequency ablation. Radiowaves are used to 'burn away' the tissue that provides the path for the short circuit.**

85. In cerebral angiography the dye is injected through:

A. Radial artery
B. Axillary artery
C. Brachial artery
D. Femoral artery *(AI 1999)*

At one time, direct carotid puncture was the most common approach to angiography. It has been replaced in most institutions by the **femoral cerebral approach** and is now usually reserved for those patients in whom catheterization is difficult or impossible.

86. On USG finding of cystic hygroma is suggestive of:

A. Klinefelter syndrome
B. Marfan's syndrome
C. Down syndrome
D. Turner's syndrome

Bilateral **cystic hygroma of the neck** is caused by a developmental abnormality of vascular channels and is characteristic (but *not* specific) for **Turner's syndrome**.

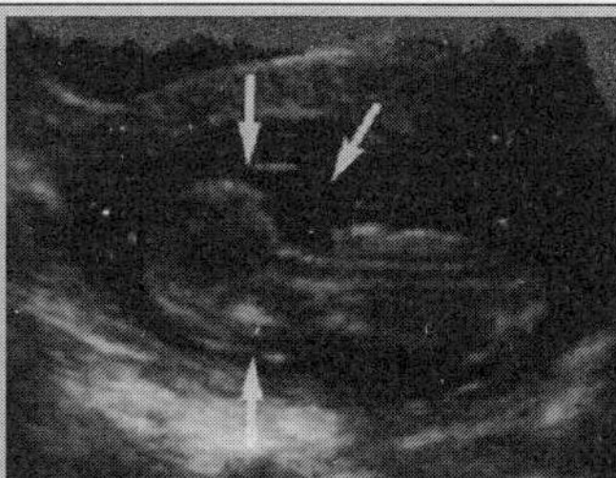

87. X-ray view for supraorbital fissure is:

A. Basal
B. AP
C. Caldwell
D. Towne's

Plain radiographs such as Water's view and the Caldwell view, were once the mainstay of diagnosis of sinus disease, but have now been replaced by high-resolution CT (HRCT) for the evaluation of sinus inflammatory disease. The frontal sinuses are evaluated best in the Caldwell and Water's projections. The ethmoid sinuses are evaluated best on the Caldwell view. The maxillary sinuses are nearly symmetric sinuses and are best visualized on the Water's view. On a **Caldwell view**, the foramen rotundum, which contains the maxillary division of the trigeminal nerve, is projected through the superomedial portion of the antrum. **The superior orbital fissure can easily be recognized, as well.**

88. Half-life of Rn^{222} is:

A. 3.8 days
B. 4 days
C. 6 days
D. 5 days

89. *Longest* half-life is of:

A. Cesium
B. Uranium
C. Radon
D. Radium

Isotopes Used in Brachytherapy

Isotope	Half-life
• Caesium-137	30 years
• Cobalt-60	5.26 years
• Gold-198	2.7 days
• Iridium-192	74 days
• Radium-226	1640 years
• **Radon-222**	**3.8 days**
• Strontium-90	28 years
• Tantalum-182	11.5 days
• Yttrium-90	64 hours

90. Microwaves cause:

A. Retinal detachment
B. Heating up of tissues
C. Microscopic hemorrhages
D. Convulsions

Exposure to **microwaves** is dangerous mainly when high densities of microwave radiation are involved, as with MASERS. They can cause **burns**, cataracts, damage to the nervous system and sterility. The possible danger of long-term exposure to low-level microwaves is not yet well established.

91. Ultrasound waves are produced by means of a .... crystal:

A. Ferromagnetic
B. Piezoelectric
C. Ferro electric
D. Paramagnetic

Piezoelectric effect is defined as appearance of an electric potential across certain faces of a crystal when it is subjected to mechanical pressure. Conversely, when an electric field is applied on certain faces of the crystal, the crystal undergoes mechanical distortion. Pierre Curie and his brother Jacques discovered the phenomenon in quartz and Rochelle salt in 1880 and named the effect piezoelectricity (from Greek *piezein,* "to press").The piezoelectric effect occurs in several crystalline substances, such as barium titanate and tourmaline. Because of their capacity to convert mechanical deformation into electric voltages, and electric voltages into mechanical motion, **piezoelectric crystals are used in such devices as the transducer in ultrasonography**, record-playing pickup elements, and the microphone. Piezoelectric crystals are also used as resonators in electronic oscillators and high-frequency amplifiers, because the mechanical resonance frequency of adequately cut crystals is stable and well-defined.

92. Noble prize for 1998 was given for discovery of:

A. Nitric oxide
B. Super oxide
C. Nitrous oxide
D. H_2O_2

Ferid Murad was an American physician, pharmacologist, and Nobel laureate who **shared the 1998 Nobel Prize in physiology or medicine with colleagues Louis Ignarro and Robert Furchgott. Murad determined that NO is a signaling molecule** - a molecule that transmits messages from one cell to another. Murad investigated the action of NO in the blood vessels of the cardiovascular system.

93. Nucleus of an atom contains:

A. Neutrons
B. Protons
C. Both A and B
D. Positrons

The **nucleus** is composed of nucleons, that is, **protons and neutrons**, and it accounts for *nearly* all the mass of the atom.

94. The theory of nuclear magnetic resonance was elucidated by:

A. Branwald
B. Richard Wolf
C. Edward Purcell
D. Goldman

Nuclear Magnetic Resonance or **NMR** is the technique developed separately in 1945 by American physicists **Felix Bloch** and **Edward Mills Purcell** for the spectroscopic analysis of substances.

95. Nuclear medicine is the term used for:

A. Treatment by radiation
B. Using radium for diagnosis
C. Nucleic acid analysis
D. X-rays

Nuclear medicine is the medical specialty that uses radioactive substances, or radiopharmaceuticals, combined with imaging techniques to diagnose and treat injury or disease, such as sports injuries, heart disease, cancer, and Alzheimer's disease.

96. Hertz is a unit of:
A. Loudness
B. Intensity
C. Power
D. Frequency

Hertz is derived SI unit of **frequency** and its symbol is Hz. It is named after the German physicist *Heinrich Hertz*. The hertz is equal to 1 repetition or cycle per second.

97. Ultrasound refers to sound waves with a frequency of:
A. 20/sec
B. 20-200/sec
C. 200/sec
D. More than 20,000/sec

Sound can be divided into 3 categories based upon frequency or pitch - **infrasound**, **audible sound**, and **ultrasound**. Human beings can hear sounds having frequencies between about 20 cycles per second and 20,000 cycles per second. This is the audible range; it is the range of frequencies produced by most stereo speakers. Sounds having frequencies below 10 cycles per second are termed infrasound, and **those having frequencies above 20,000 cycles per second are termed ultrasound.** The frequencies associated with diagnostic ultrasound instruments are about 50 to 1000 times greater than the highest frequency we hear. (The diagnostic ultrasound frequency range is about 1 million to 20 million cycles/second).

98. In ultrasound machine the piezoelectric crystal is made of:
A. Silicon
B. Lead zirconate titanate
C. Tungsten
D. Molybdenum

The piezoelectric effect occurs in several crystalline substances, such as barium titanate and tourmaline. The crystal in most modern transducers of ultrasound machines is actually a **polarized ceramic made of lead zirconate titanate (PZT).** This ceramic is permanently polarized in the manufacturing process by heating it to above its Curie temperature (365°C) and placing it in a strong electric field as it cools. Some advantages of using ceramic elements instead of crystalline elements in a transducer are that they are far more efficient at transmitting sound, nearly as efficient at receiving sound, and better suited for creating the very short sound pulses used in ultrasound imaging. Although the piezoelectric element of an ultrasound transducer is usually a ceramic, it is traditionally referred to as a crystal.

99. Neutron emitting radioisotope, which is used in radiotherapy, is:
A. Californium
B. Polonium
C. Helium
D. Strontium

Californium^{252}, with a half-life of 2.6 years, has an unusually high rate of spontaneous fission, with an **abundant emission of neutrons**. It has practical application as a high-intensity neutron source in electronic systems and in medical research.

100. Which radioisotope is capable of *displacing* calcium from the body:
A. Radium
B. Strontium
C. Plutonium
D. Iridium

Radio **strontium** is similar to calcium in its chemical behavior, including its **deposition in human bone**. Most biological systems *prefer* calcium to strontium; therefore, the amount of ^{90}Sr absorbed by plant roots and by animals depends on the availability of calcium.

101. The stethoscope was invented by:
A. William Harvey
B. Laënnec
C. Lister
D. Robert Koch

The **stethoscope was invented by** the French physician René-Théophile-Hyacinthe **Laënnec in 1819**. The *modern* stethoscope was invented by the American physician George Philip Cammann.

102. The ophthalmoscope was invented by:

A. Tachernig
B. Honarda
C. Coldmann
D. Helmholtz

From 1856 to 1866, as a professor of anatomy at the University of Heidelberg, Helmholtz studied the eye. The result of this extensive research was his multivolume 'Physiological Optics', a work that remained for many decades the definitive study on the physiology and physics of vision. During these studies **Helmholtz** also **invented the ophthalmoscope** (an instrument used to view the interior of the eye) and developed a theory of color vision.

103. Posterior iliac horn is seen in:

A. Marfan's syndrome
B. Hurler's syndrome
C. Ankylosing spondylitis
D. Nail patella syndrome *(AIIMS May 2002)*

The patella may be absent or hypoplastic in association with the **nail patella syndrome**. Other features of this syndrome are hypoplasia and splitting of the nails, elbow abnormalities and bony **"spurs"** on the ileum.

* *Spur* is a spine like process, as on the wings or legs of certain birds; a *spine like outgrowth of bone*, as on the human heel, resulting from injury, disease, etc.

104. Chondrocalcinosis is seen in:

A. Rickets
B. Hypoparathyroidism
C. Ochronosis
D. Hyperthyroidism *(AIIMS May 2002)*

Chondrocalcinosis is a descriptive term that may apply to any type of cartilage calcification *without* specifying its etiology. A 5 to 7% incidence is seen in the general population. When the cartilagenous calcifications occur with sudden onset of polyarticular swelling and redness, the syndrome is referred to as *pseudogout*. Chondrocalcinosis may also be observed in a variety of unrelated conditions such as vitamin D intoxication, hemochromatosis, rheumatoid arthritis, lupus erythematosus, and **ochronosis**. It may also be seen after trauma.

105. Right heart border in a chest X-ray PA view is formed by all *except*:

A. IVC
B. SVC
C. Ascending aorta
D. Right atrium *(MP 2001)*

106. In X-ray chest right border of mediastinum is formed by all *except*:

A. Right brachiocephalic vein
B. Right ventricle
C. Right atrium
D. Superior vena cava *(PGI 1997, AI 1998)*

107. In a chest X-ray PV view, the right border of heart is *not* formed by:

A. Aorta
B. Superior vena cava
C. Right atrium
D. Inferior vena cava *(SGPGI 1999)*

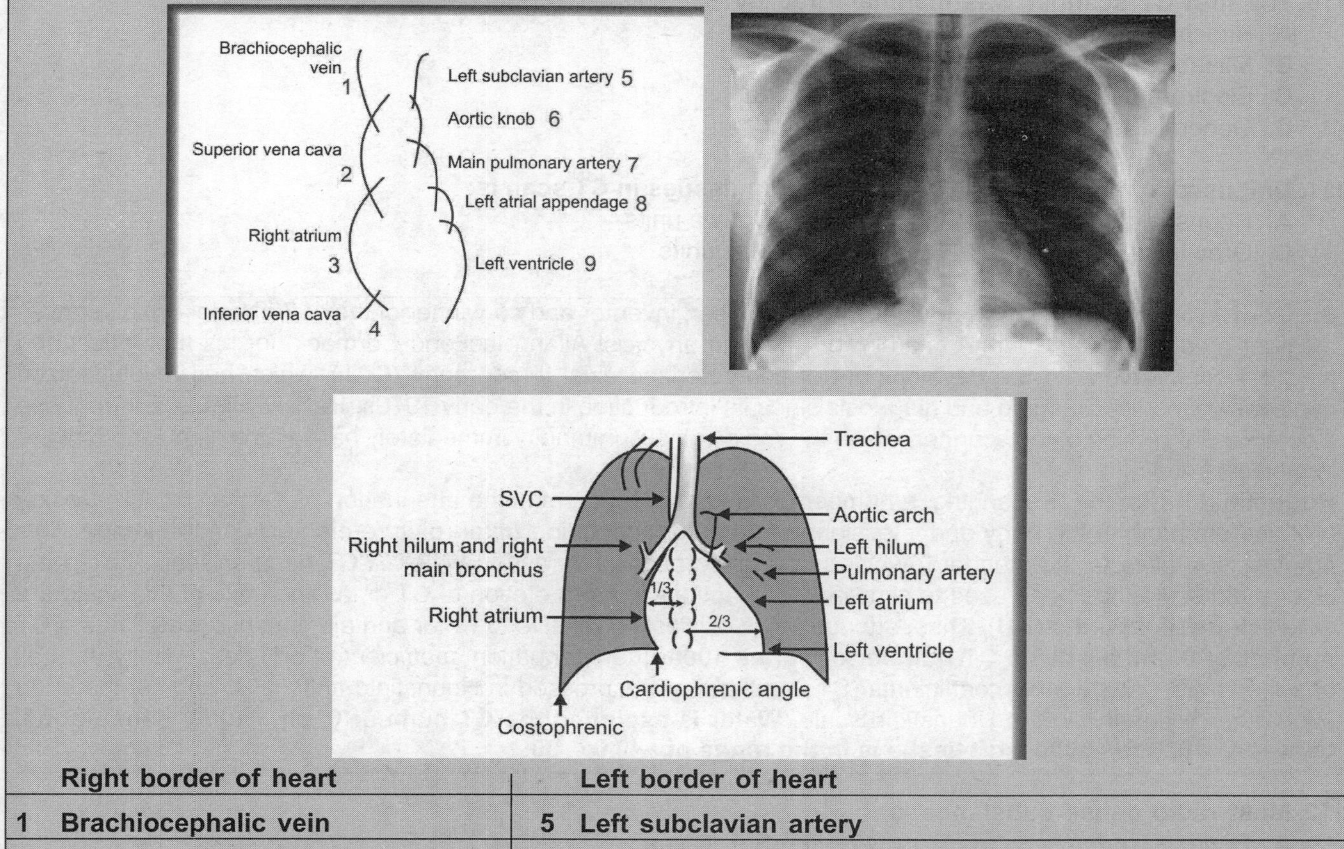

	Right border of heart		Left border of heart
1	**Brachiocephalic vein**	5	**Left subclavian artery**
2	**Superior vena cava**	6	**Aortic knob**
3	**Right atrium**	7	**Main pulmonary artery**
4	**Inferior vena cava**	8	**Left atrial appendage**
		9	**Left ventricle**

In the frontal projection, the straight upper half of the **right cardiac border** is formed by the *superior vena cava* and the lower half by the *convex curve of the right atrium*. A convex bulging of the upper right border of the cardiac silhouette is usually caused by outward displacement of the superior vena cava by a dilated ascending aorta. The **left border** of the cardiac silhouette is composed of a series of convex arcs. The uppermost bulge is formed by the *aortic knob*. This is not a specific anatomical structure but represents the most distal portion of the aortic arch, where it turns downward to become the descending aorta. The *prominence of the main pulmonary artery* and a small portion of the *outflow tract of the right ventricle* lie immediately beneath the aortic knob. The lowest portion of the left cardiac contour, reaching the diaphragm, is formed by the broad sweeping curve of the *anterolateral wall of the left ventricle*.

108. For splenic rupture the *investigation of choice* is:

A. Peritoneal lavage **B.** MRI
C. USG **D.** CT

Splenic injuries are the *most common* serious intraabdominal injury. **Ultrasound** of spleen is of value in determining its size and consistency and whether or not a cyst is present. It can be used for diagnosing a rupture.

109. CT scan was invented by:

A. Godfrey Hounsfield **B.** Eric Honda
C. John Snow **D.** Suzuki Kobe *(SGPGI 1999)*

110. The first CT scanner was manufactured by:

A. Hitachi, Japan
B. Mitsubishi, Japan
C. Electro-musical instruments (EMI), England
D. General Electric, USA

111. Unit used in measuring the density of body tissues in CT scan is:

A. Hounsfield units
B. Ogawa units
C. Gray units
D. Mac units

Sir Godfrey Newbold Hounsfield is a British engineer, inventor and co-winner of the 1979 Nobel Prize in physiology or medicine, with South African-born American physicist Allan MacLeod Cormack, for his theoretical and practical contributions to the development of computerized axial tomography (CAT), which has revolutionized noninvasive medical imaging and diagnosis since its introduction in the early 1970s. In 1972 **EMI Ltd.** introduced a commercial version of the scanner, which the radiological community immediately hailed as a giant leap forward in medical imaging.

Hounsfield units: In CT scanning, a number or value that represents the attenuation of X-rays through a **voxel** (**vo**lume **el**ement) in the body and is assigned to the corresponding **pixel** (**pi**cture **el**ement) on the image. This number is relative to the standard, which is the absorption of X-rays in water. A CT number scale, called the Hounsfield scale, has been used to simplify the quantitative interpretation of CT data. The units of this scale are called **Hounsfield units (HU).** Thus, attenuation is expressed relative to water and air, because **water has a CT number of 0 and air has a CT number of *minus* 1000** (the attenuation *coefficient* of air is essentially 0) at all beam energies. Attenuation coefficients (CT numbers) are expressed in Hounsfield units (HU) and compared to each other according to the Hounsfield scale. **Water is assigned the CT number 0; air, –1000; dense bone, between +1000 to +3000; soft tissue is in the range of +40 to +80.**

112. Most radio dense substance is:

A. Bone
B. Soft tissue
C. Brain
D. Fluid

113. On usual CT scale of densities (–1000 to +1000), brain tissue measures:

A. –10 to +10
B. 0 to + 20
C. +10 to +30
D. +22 to +46

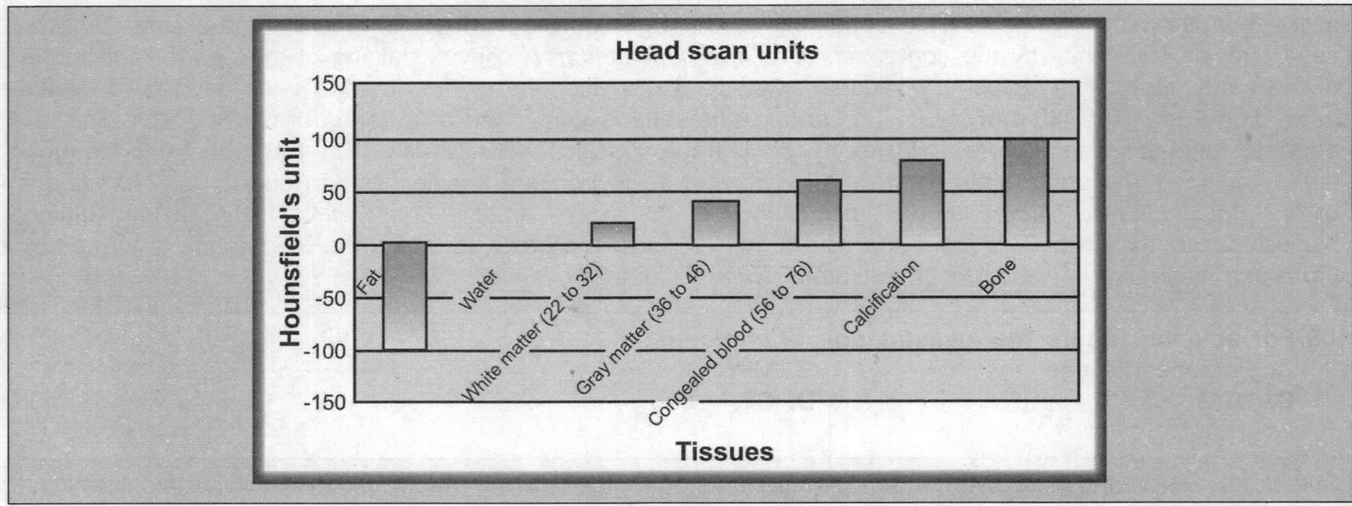

114. X-rays are:

A. Neutrons
B. Electromagnetic waves
C. Electrons
D. Protons

(JIPMER 1992)

115. Target material used for generating X-ray:

A. Tungsten
B. Cadmium
C. Cobalt
D. Palladium

116. X-ray with shorter wavelengths:

A. Are produced by lower KV
B. Have more penetrating power
C. Travel slower
D. Travel faster
(SGPGI 1999)

117. X-rays are generated when .... strike tungsten:

A. Protons
B. Electrons
C. Electromagnetic waves
D. Neutrons

X-rays are penetrating **electromagnetic radiation** having a *shorter* wavelength than light (ranging in wavelength from about 100 A to 0.01 A). They are produced by bombarding a target, usually made of **tungsten**, with high-speed **electrons**. *The shorter the wavelength of the X-ray, the greater is its energy and its penetrating power.* Longer wavelength X-rays, near the ultraviolet-ray band of the electromagnetic spectrum, are known as "soft" X-rays, while the shorter wavelengths, closer to and overlapping the gamma-ray range, are called "hard X-rays". A mixture of many different wavelengths is known as "white" X-rays, as opposed to "monochromatic" X-rays, which represent only a *single* wavelength.

118. Time sector scanning of neonates is preferred because of which of the following practical reason:

A. Better resolution
B. Neonates are more cooperative
C. Inexpensive
D. Open fontanelle
(PGI 1995)

Almost any available ultrasound machine can be used to examine the neonatal brain. The **real-time sector scanner** is *advantageous* from a number of standpoints. **Foremost is its ability to use the anterior fontanelle as an acoustic window.** Although the neonatal skull is very thin, it degrades the ultrasound image considerably. The sector scanner has a wide field of view and requires *only* a small acoustic window. One can therefore optimally visualize almost all portions of the brain without the image degradation inherent in transcranial methods.

119. Notching of ribs on X-ray is *not* seen in:

A. Aortitis
B. Neurofibromatosis
C. Coarctation of aorta
D. AV fistula
(SGPGI 1999)

120. Rib notching is *not* seen in:

A. Neurofibromatosis
B. Hypoparathyroidism
C. Coarctation of aorta
D. Blalock-Taussig operation shunt
(AIIMS 2000)

Causes of Inferior Rib Notching

• **Aortic**	Coarctation, occlusion.
• **Subclavian**	Takayasu disease, Blalock-Taussig operation (unilateral).
• **Reduced Pulmonary blood flow**	Pulmonary atresia and stenosis, TOF, truncus type 4.
• **Venous**	SVC, IVC obstruction.
• **Shunts**	Pulmonary or intercostal AV fistula, intercostal pulmonary fistula.
• **Other causes**	Hyperparathyroidism, neurogenic tumor, idiopathic.

121. In coarctation of aorta the rib changes are seen from:

A. 1-12th
B. 3-6th
C. 8-12th
D. 4-9th
(KARNATAKA 1995)

Erosions of the ribs due to adjacent structures result in the appearance of rib notching. In coarctation of aorta the notching is due to enlargement of the intercostal arteries which extends from the **4th to 9th ribs** and is asymmetrical.

☺ Both upper and lower 3 ribs are spared.

122. ***Not*** **a radiological feature of mitral stenosis:**

A. Kerley B-lines **B.** Pulmonary hemosiderosis
C. Oligemia of upper lung field **D.** Straight left heart border *(AIIMS 2000)*

The earliest changes in **mitral stenosis** are **straightening of the left border of the cardiac silhouette**, prominence of the main pulmonary arteries, dilatation of the upper lobe pulmonary veins, and backward displacement of the esophagus by an enlarged left atrium. In patients with mild or moderate mitral stenosis, the heart is not grossly enlarged. In severe mitral stenosis, however, all chambers and vessels upstream to the narrowed valve are prominent, including the atria, pulmonary arteries and veins, right ventricle, and superior vena cava. **Kerley B-lines** are fine, dense, opaque, horizontal lines that are most prominent in the lower and mid lung fields and that result from distention of interlobular septa and lymphatics with edema when the resting mean left atrial pressure exceed approximately 20 mmHg. In patients who have had multiple hemoptyses, hemosiderin containing macrophages fill the air spaces, and if they become confluent, they result in a fine, diffuse nodulation most prominent in the lower lung fields (**pulmonary hemosiderosis**)

123. "Ehrlenmeyer flask" appearance is seen in:

A. Thrombocytopenia **B.** Sickle cell anemia
C. Chronic anemias **D.** Gaucher's disease

"**Ehrlenmeyer flask**" appearance of the femurs is seen in **Gaucher's disease.**

124. The amount of I^{131} used for a thyroid scan is:

A. 5 microcuries **B.** 50 millicuries
C. 50 microcuries **D.** 500 millicuries

The amount of I^{131} used for a thyroid scan is 0.005 millicuries (5 microcuries).

125. The number of carpel bones seen in a radiograph of an infant is:

A. 0 **B.** 2
C. 3 **D.** 4

In the newborn, radiographic evaluation of the feet, rather than the hands, is more helpful since **the carpal bones are normally not ossified**; however, after the neonatal period the hands may be most helpful in determining bone age.

126. Isotope use in bone scans:

A. Technetium **B.** Gallium
C. Selenium **D.** Chromium

With the advent of **better bone uptake agents (Tc^{99m}** MDP and PYP) and more refined cameras, bone scintigraphy is now mainly used in staging of prostatic carcinoma. Bone scintigraphy series have demonstrated that, at the time of diagnosis, approximately 5% of patients with clinical stage I disease will have positive scans.

127. Beheaded Scottish terrier sign is seen in:

A. Spondylosis
B. Fracture rib
C. Spondylolisthesis
D. Fracture scaphoid

128. Scottish terrier sign is seen in:

A. AP view
B. PA view
C. Lateral view
D. Oblique view *(JIPMER 1990)*

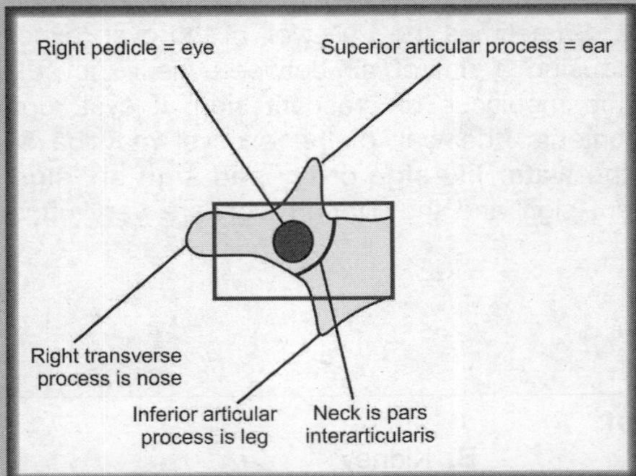

Spondylolisthesis is a forward "slip" of one lumbar vertebra on another. Normally this kind of movement is prevented by resistance to forward thrust but the integrity of the anterior part of neural arch made up of the pedicle, the pars interarticularis and the inferior articular process. The inferior articular process is held in position by the superior articular processes of the vertebra below. In the **oblique projection** the shape of the neural arch can be compared to the silhouette of a Scots terrier; the transverse process representing the nose, the superior articular process representing the ear and the inferior articular process representing the front leg. The defect of the pars interarticularis breaks the *neck* of the dog. The majority of these lesions are due to stress fractures of one or both sides of the neural arch through the *relatively* weak **pars interarticularis.**

129. Bronchorrhea is characteristically seen in:

A. Sarcoidosis
B. Scleroderma
C. Bronchioloalveolar carcinoma
D. Goodpasture's syndrome

Bronchorrhea is an abnormal offensive secretion from the bronchial mucous membrane. **Bronchioloalveolar carcinoma** comprises about 5% of all bronchogenic carcinomas. As with other tumors, cough, chest pain, weight loss, and dyspnea occurs. The **classic manifestation of massive bronchorrhea**, up to 4 liters daily, is rare and may result in electrolyte disturbance and severe hypovolemia. Hemoptysis is also less common than with other bronchogenic carcinomas.

130. Renal papillary necrosis is associated with:

A. Sickle cell disease
B. Tuberculosis
C. Diabetes mellitus
D. All of the above

Papillary necrosis is the necrosis of all or part of the papilla of renal pyramid and is the result of a number of diseases that mainly affect the renal medulla. Many causes of interstitial nephritis may bring about papillary necrosis. These include bacterial nephritis, analgesic abuse, diabetes mellitus, sickle cell disease, and tuberculosis.

131. Neural tube defect is *best* detected by:

A. Placentography
B. Amniocentesis
C. Chromosomal analysis
D. USG

(AI 1995)

Neural tube defects, including anencephaly, encephalocele, and spina bifida, are among the *most common* fetal anomalies (1.5:1000 live births). The incidence is considerably higher when the **mother is diabetic**, when there is a **family history of neural tube defects**, or when the **maternal serum** α**-fetoprotein level is elevated**. Increased level of APF in amniotic fluid along with presence of acetylcholinesterase (AChE) signifies presence of neural tube defect (NTD) with 98% accuracy.

132. Water lily sign is found in:

A. Fungal granuloma
B. Actinomycosis
C. Hydatid cyst of liver
D. Hydatid cyst of lung

(PGI 1997)

Pulmonary echinococcosis manifests in X-ray usually by a single pulmonary mass or by multiple pulmonary masses. Sometimes the true wall of the cyst (exocyst) may retract from the pericyst, causing a rim of air between the exocyst and pericyst. This has been called the meniscus or crescent sign. If cyst rupture occurs with expulsion of cyst contents, the wall of the exocyst may be seen floating within the cyst, causing the **water lily sign** or **lily-pad sign** or **"sign of the Camalote."** Both the crescent sign and the lily-pad sign are very unusual findings in **hydatid disease**.

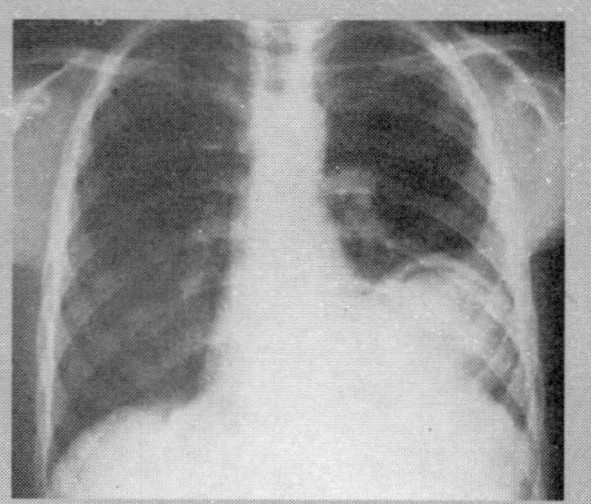

Meniscus or crescent sign

133. Phrygian cap is a feature of:

A. Stomach
B. Kidney
C. Gallbladder
D. Pancreas

The **gallbladder** is frequently folded upon itself, but the position of the fold may not be fixed. A fold or septated compartment near the fundus of the gallbladder produces a so-called **phrygian cap**.

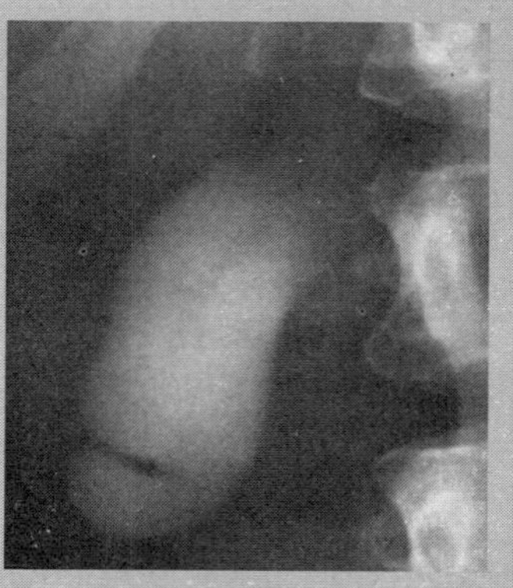

Phrygian cap

134. Calcification of heart wall is suggestive of:

A. Endomyocardial fibrosis
B. Fibroelastosis
C. Carcinoid syndrome
D. Scleroderma

(JIPMER 1992)

The **carcinoid syndrome** includes diarrhea, abdominal pain, skin flushes, asthma, and cardiac **valvular lesions, usually of the right heart**. The symptoms are due to serotonin and other hormonally active compounds (histamine, kinin peptides) produced by the tumor and the presence of the syndrome is a good indicator of liver metastases. Carcinoid confined to the small bowel and mesentery *does not* produce the *syndrome* because serotonin released into the mesenteric veins from an intestinal carcinoid is metabolized as it passes through the liver. Almost all patients with carcinoid syndrome have primary tumors in the small bowel, but only a minority of the small bowel lesions present with the endocrine syndrome. This syndrome can also occur with primary carcinoid tumors of other organs.

135. Thickness of stomach in USG is:

A. 10 mm
B. 7 mm
C. 5 mm
D. 2 mm

(JIPMER 1995)

The normal pyloric channel is 0.8 cm to 1.0 cm long and has a wall thickness of 4 mm to 8 mm, with **a mean of 5 mm**. In hypertrophic pyloric stenosis the channel is 2 cm to 4 cm long and its thickness exceeds 1 cm.

136. "Double bubble" sign on plain X-ray of abdomen is seen in:

A. Ileal atresia
B. Jejunal atresia
C. Duodenal atresia
D. Pyloric stenosis

(AIIMS 1999)

Congenital obstructive lesions of the duodenum are common and are usually secondary to atresia, annular pancreas, and stenosis. The technique of examining duodenal obstructions consists of using air as the contrast medium rather than liquid contrast material, which only enhances the danger of vomiting and aspiration. In **duodenal atresia**, annular pancreas, and duodenal stenosis, the duodenal bulb is usually markedly dilated. An upright film of the abdomen shows air-fluid levels in the stomach and duodenum ("**double bubble**" sign). In duodenal atresia there is complete absence of air distal to the obstruction, whereas in annular pancreas and duodenal stenosis, air is usually identified in small amounts distal to the obstruction. Down's syndrome is frequently associated with duodenal stenosis.

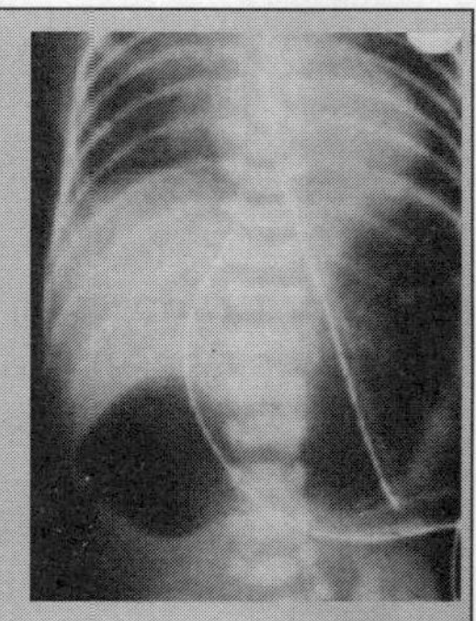

137. For small intestine tumor the *investigation of choice* is:

A. CT scan with contrast
B. X-ray abdomen
C. Echocardiography
D. Barium meal swallow

(JIPMER 1992)

Tumors of the small intestine comprise almost 5% of all alimentary tract tumors. Computed tomography (CT) and ultrasound are of relatively *low* yield as primary diagnostic modalities, especially in the absence of a palpable mass. However, **CT has become an increasingly common method to evaluate patients with vague abdominal symptoms, and it may provide an initial opportunity to detect and characterize a small bowel tumor.**

138. Cardiac catheterization was *first* attempted by:

A. Philip Bozzini
B. Gustav Killian
C. Dulius Bruck
D. Warner Forssmann

Werner Forssmann (1904-1979), German physician and Nobel laureate performed innovative experiments in **cardiac catheterization,** i.e. the passage of a thin tube into the heart through a vein or artery to measure blood pressure within the heart and major blood vessels.

139. Monge's disease is seen in:

A. Lowlanders in highland
B. Highlander in lowland
C. Highlanders in highland
D. None

Secondary polycythemia: Traveling at high altitudes leads to decreased saturation of arterial blood with oxygen and stimulates the production of more red blood cells. The oxygen saturation, rather than oxygen tension, is more important determinant of the erythropoietic response to chronic hypoxia. A condition known as **chronic mountain sickness** or **soroche** (**Monge's disease**) may develop insidiously after several years of continued residence at high altitude.

140. 'Champagne glass' pelvis is seen in:

A. Congenital dislocation of hip
B. Down syndrome
C. Achondroplasia
D. Cretinism

In **achondroplasia** rhizomelic limb shortening is seen. On plain film short tubular bones with normal width and shortening of humerus compared to radius and ulna with flared metaphyses are seen. Pelvis has a "**champagne glass**" appearance with square iliacs bones, broad flat acetabular roofs, and a small sciatic notch. Decreased distance between pedicles in lumbar spine is noted. The pedicles are shortened. Vertebral bodies are of normal height but have concave posterior border. There is a large calvarium with prominent frontoparietal and occipital regions with a short skull base and mid face hypoplasia.

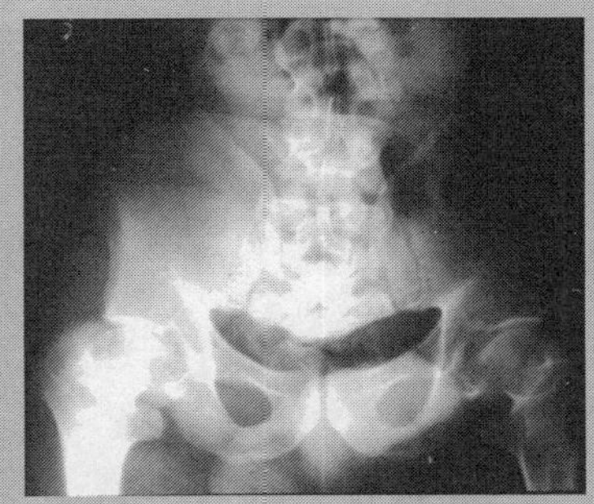

141. Optical activity of organic substances is measured by:

A. Spectrometer
B. Polarimeter
C. Photometer
D. Multimeter

Substances that are optically active rotate the plane of linearly polarized light. A sugar crystal or a solution of sugar, for example, may be optically active. If a solution of sugar is placed between a crossed polarizer and analyzer, some of the light is able to pass through. The amount of rotation of the analyzer required to restore extinction of the light determines the concentration of the solution. The **polarimeter** is based on this principle.

142. *True* regarding Hydatid cyst of the lung in a chest X-ray:
A. Is seen on a calcified ring shadow **B.** Shows spackled calcification
C. Calcification is rare **D.** A and B are correct

Hydatid cyst is seen as smooth, spherical and homogenous density in X-ray chest PA view and may grow to the size of grape fruit. There is seldom significant reaction in the surrounding lung so that **calcification is rare**. Rupture or infection may occur.

143. Deleterious effect of ultrasound on small organism is:
A. Ionization **B.** Vacuolation
C. Cavitation **D.** Disintegration

It can not be said with any amount of certainty that ultrasound has no effect on the tissues of patients and embryos. In fact, because the ultrasound beam consists of traveling pressure waves, it obviously places some stress and strain on tissue components though which it travels. Some mechanisms for producing **biologic effects** with ultrasound that have been observed at therapy intensity levels include significant **local heating, cavitation, (bubble formation, collapse, and oscillation) and micro-streaming (flow of bubbles).**

144. Radioactivity was discovered by:
A. Marie Curie **B.** Pierre Curie
C. Rutherford **D.** Henri Becquerel

145. Radioactivity was discovered by Becquerel in:
A. 1796 **B.** 1896
C. 1901 **D.** 1946

Radioactivity is defined as spontaneous disintegration of atomic nuclei by the emission of subatomic particles called alpha particles and beta particles, or of electromagnetic rays called X-rays and gamma rays. **The phenomenon was discovered in 1896 by the French physicist Antoine Henri Becquerel when he observed that the element uranium can blacken a photographic plate, although separated from it by glass or black paper.** In 1898 the French chemists **Marie Curie and Pierre Curie** deduced that radioactivity is a phenomenon associated with atoms, independent of their physical or chemical state.

146. Basal ganglia calcification is seen in:
A. Hypoparathyroidism **B.** Fahr's syndrome
C. Mitochondria cytopathy **D.** All of the above

Causes of Calcification in the Basal Ganglia

Major	Minor or atypical
• Idiopathic (**most common**) • Familial • Hypoparathyroidism • Pseudohypoparathyroidism	• Fahr's syndrome • Cockayne's syndrome • CO poisoning • Lead poisoning • Toxoplasmosis • Mineralizing microangiopathy • Secondary hyperparathyroidism • Mitochondria cytopathy

147. Xeroradiography is used in ....cancer detection:
A. Stomach **B.** Breast
C. Colonic **D.** Pancreatic

Xeroradiography is a method of photo-reproduction used in radiography. It is a dry process involving the use of metal plates covered with a powdered substance, such as selenium; electrically and evenly charged. The X-rays alter the charge of the substance to varying degrees, depending on the tissues they have traversed. This produces the image. This procedure has been replaced by film and screen **mammography** because of its high radiation dose. It was widely used for breast imaging for early diagnosis of **carcinoma breast**.

148. Radiation protection shields are made up of:

A. Copper
B. Silver
C. Lead
D. Tin

Because **lead** absorbs high-energy radiation, lead glasses are used in shields to protect personnel in nuclear installations.

149. Raised intracranial tension in *adults* is seen as:

A. Silver beaten appearance
B. Separation of sutures
C. Erosion of sella
D. All of the above

Erosion of the dorsum sellae is the cardinal sign of **raised intracranial pressure in adults**. Erosion commences as slight porosis of the anterior cortex of the dorsum and of the sellar floor cortex, best seen in a lateral film. It progresses to loss of definition of the cortex and eventually to frank erosion.

150. Onion peel appearance is seen in:

A. Osteoclastoma
B. Chondrosarcoma
C. Osteosarcoma
D. Ewing's sarcoma

Ewing's sarcoma constitutes about 10 to 15 % of all bone sarcomas, is common in adolescence and has a peak incidence in the 2nd decade of life. The plain radiograph may show a characteristic **"onion-peel"** periosteal reaction with a generous soft tissue mass, which is better demonstrated by CT or MRI.

151. Stryker view is used in shoulder joint to visualize:

A. Recurrent subluxation
B. Subacromial calcification
C. Bicipital groove
D. Muscle calcification

After an *initial* dislocation, the shoulder may return to functional stability or it may fall victim to *recurrent glenohumeral instability*. While intermediate forms of recurrent instability do occur, the great majority of recurrently unstable shoulder may be thought of as being either atraumatic or traumatic in origin. Radiographs frequently help to provide confirmation of *traumatic* glenohumeral instability. In **Stryker notch view** the patient is supine on the table with the cassette placed under his shoulder. The palm of the hand of the affected shoulder is placed on top of the head, with the fingers directed toward the back of the head. The elbow of the affected shoulder should point straight upward. The X-ray beam tilts 10° toward the head, centered over the coracoid process. This technique was developed by William S. Stryker and reported by Hall and coworkers. They stated that they could demonstrate the humeral head defect in 90 % of 20 patients with a history of **recurring anterior dislocation of the shoulder**.

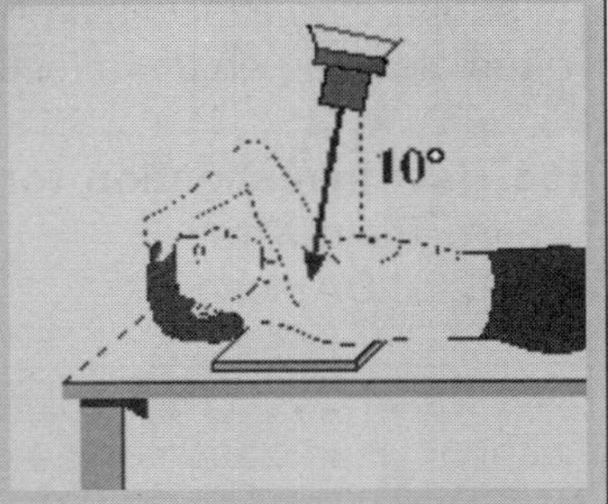

152. Suprasellar calcification is seen in:

A. Craniopharyngioma
B. Meningioma
C. Calcified pineal gland
D. Pituitary adenoma

Suprasellar calcification in a flocculent, granular, or curvilinear pattern is present on skull X-rays in most children and in some adults with **craniopharyngioma**.

153. Radium emits:

A. Electrons
B. X-ray
C. Alpha rays
D. Gamma rays

Of the isotopes of **radium**, ranging in mass number from 206 to 232, the most abundant and most stable is the isotope of mass 226. Radium-226 is formed by the radioactive disintegration of the thorium isotope of mass 230, which is the fourth successive isotope in the decay series starting with uranium-238. The half-life of radium-226 is 1620 years. **It emits alpha particles**, forming the gas radon.

154. *Best* diagnostic procedure in acute pancreatitis is:

A. CT scan **B.** MRI scan
C. Ultrasound scan **D.** Pipida scan

A **CT scan** will confirm the clinical impression of **acute pancreatitis** even if the serum amylase levels are normal.

155. Centenary year for X-ray is:

A. 1995 **B.** 1997
C. 1999 **D.** 2001

X-rays were discovered accidentally in **1895** by the German physicist Wilhelm Conrad Roentgen while he was studying cathode rays in a high-voltage, gaseous-discharge tube.

156. Medical thermography is based on the principle of man emitting:

A. X-ray **B.** Ultrasonic rays
C. Ultraviolet radiation **D.** Infrared radiation

Thermography should be considered an experimental technique. Various thermographic techniques are available, but all basically measure the superficial skin temperature **(infrared rays).** Although the technique is *totally* without risk because it is a passive measurement, wavelengths that are measured have very poor tissue penetration and consequently heat generated deep within the breast may be insulated from the skin by the intervening breast tissue. Some cancers, particularly rapidly growing lesions, appear to be hypermetabolic and produce an asymmetric thermographic pattern.

157. Which is the *most common* sign of subphrenic abscess:

A. Basal consolidation **B.** Tented diaphragm
C. Pleural effusion **D.** Subdiaphragmatic calcification

In subphrenic abscess a plain X-ray sometimes shows the presence of gas or pleural effusion. The diaphragm is often elevated on the affected side (so called **tented diaphragm**) which is quite specific for this condition.

158. *Best* investigation for acute cholecystitis is:

A. Plain X-ray **B.** PIPIDA scan
C. HIDA scan **D.** Technetium scan *(KARNATAKA 1991)*

The radionuclide (e.g. HIDA) biliary scan may be confirmatory for acute cholecystitis if bile duct imaging is seen without visualization of the gallbladder.

HIDA: **D**imethylimminodiacetic **A**cid

159. 'Figure of 3' appearance is seen in:

A. Coarctation of aorta **B.** TOF
C. TGV **D.** All of the above

Coarctation of the Aorta: Chest radiograph demonstrates rib notching. There is a **'figure of 3' sign** in the left upper mediastinum secondary to hypoplasia of the aortic arch with poststenotic dilation of the aorta infra-coarctation.

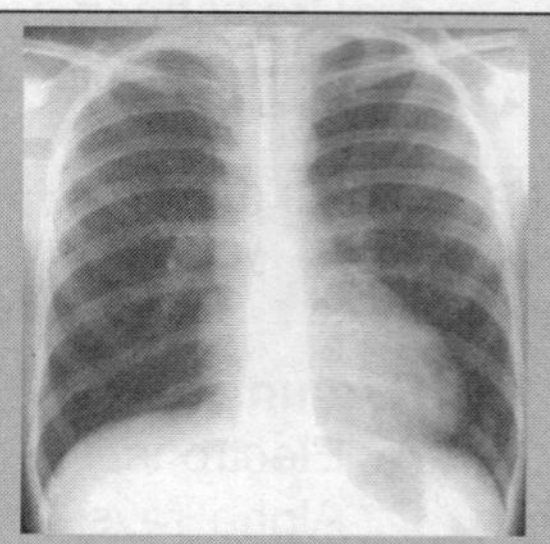

160. Thesaurosis is a disease said by some to be related to:
A. Molding of copper tube **B.** Resins in hairspray
C. Inhalation of barium dust **D.** In eosinophilia

Thesaurosis or hair spray pneumonitis is a rare disease. In the lungs a granulomatous infiltration similar to sarcoid has been found.

161. "Reverse 3 sign" of Frostberg in barium study indicates:
A. Reversed midgut rotation **B.** Periampullary carcinoma
C. Annular pancreas **D.** Duodenal atresia *(KARNATAKA 2000)*

Duodenal Signs of Pancreatic Enlargement

- Mass impression
- Widened loop
- Inverted three sign of Frostberg nodularity

Frostberg's inverted 3 sign is an uncommon but distinctive sign of pancreatic head enlargement occurring because the duodenal wall is focally fixed at the major papilla owing to the insertion of the biliary and pancreatic ducts. This *too* is *non*specific as to etiology.

162. Gold standard in insulinoma is:
A. Arteriography **B.** MRI
C. USG **D.** CT scan *(PGI 2000)*

Success rates for insulinoma localization range from 25% to 60%. **Intraoperative ultrasound, especially when combined with surgical palpation, can detect 85% to 100% of islet cell tumors.** Successful arteriographic localization rates vary between 63% and 90% for insulinomas and 15% to 88% for gastrinomas.

163. A break in Shenton's line is seen in:
A. Cretinism **B.** Developmental displasia of hip
C. Down syndrome **D.** All of the above

The **break in Shenton's line** seen in **developmental displasia of hip** (DDH) represents hip subluxation or dislocation as opposed to acetabular dysplasia. *However* in pure dyplasia, this line remains intact.

164. Echoencephalography is *most useful* for detecting:
A. Ventricular dilatation **B.** Midline shift
C. Epilepsy **D.** Vascular lesions

Ultrasound is presently used in the evaluation of almost every form of intracranial pathology that occurs *prior* to the closing of the anterior fontanelle. It is now considered to be the primary imaging modality for a wide range of intracranial diseases, including intracranial congenital anomalies (**ventricular dilatation** in congenital hydrocephalus) and inflammatory, hemorrhagic, neoplastic, and ischemic diseases.

165. Osteoporosis is diagnosed by all *except*:
A. Dual energy X-ray densitometry
B. Dual-photon absorptiometry
C. Plain X-ray
D. CT scan

In the absence of fractures, **standard roentgenograms** are **insensitive indicators of bone loss**, since a decrease by as much as 30% in bone mass may *not* be appreciated. **Dual energy X-ray densitometry** [DEXA] is an excellent technique because of its sensitivity, ability to scan the entire skeleton, low radiation exposure, and short scanning time. Single and dual-photon absorptiometry and quantitative **computed tomography (CT)** also can detect small (1 to 2%) changes in the bone mineral density of the hip and lumbar spine.

166. String sign of Kantor is seen in:

A. Crohn's disease
B. TB of the ileocaecal region
C. Idiopathic hypertrophic pyloric stenosis
D. All of the above

String sign of Kantor is a greatly narrowed terminal ileum seen in X-ray examination of the abdomen in regional enteritis (**Crohn's disease**). The earliest manifestation of Crohn's disease in barium enema are aphthoid ulcers which appear as small collection of barium surrounded by radiolucent halo producing a *Bull's eye* or *target lesion*.

167. Signs of increased intracranial tension in a child in a skull X-ray:

A. Separation of sutures
B. Tense anterior fontanelle
C. Silver beaten appearance of bones
D. All of the above

The radiological signs of raised intracranial pressure are:

- Suture diastasis
- Sellar erosion
- Beaten silver appearance
- Pineal displacement

The skull bones are joined together by sutures. In the infant there is a fairly wide separation between the bones and large midline openings or fontanelles (one frontal, the largest, and one occipital), which ordinarily close by the time the child reaches 24 months. In the child the sutures become progressively smaller. Between 2 and 3 years of age the sutures, measured at the upper aspect of the **coronal suture** on lateral views, should not measure more than 2 mm on the films. **A width larger than that suggests increased intracranial pressure. Pineal displacement** is another important sign seen in adults and is of little use in children. Increased convolutional markings sometimes referred as '**copper beaten appearance'** were thought to be due to raised ICT in past but now it is clear that they are not necessarily pathological and are found in normal children between 4 to 10 years of age. In chronically elevated intracranial pressure as the so-called "**beaten silver appearance**" of accentuated digital markings attributed to the imprint of the gyral surface of the brain.

168. "Lead pipe" appearance in barium enema is seen in:

A. Crohn's disease
B. Ulcerative colitis
C. Schistosomiasis
D. Carcinoma colon

In **ulcerative colitis** fibrosis and longitudinal retraction result in shortening of the colon. Loss of the normal haustral pattern leads *radiologically* to a smooth, "**lead-pipe" appearance** of the colon.

169. Intracranial calcification in skull X-ray may be seen in:

A. Pineal calcification
B. Cockayne's syndrome
C. Cysticercosis
D. All of the above

Causes of Pathological Intracranial Calcification

NEOPLASTIC	VASCULAR	INFECTION & INFESTATION	METABOLIC & MISCELLANEOUS
Craniopharyngioma	Atheroma	Toxoplasmosis	Idiopathic basal ganglion calcification
Glioma	Aneurysm	CMV inclusion disease	Hypoparathyroidism
Meningioma	Angioma	Herpes	Pseudo-hypoparathyroidism
Ependymoma	Subdural hematoma	Rubella	Tuberous sclerosis
Papilloma of choroid plexus	Intracranial hematoma	Tuberculoma	Sturge-Weber syndrome
Pinealoma		Pyogenic abscess	Neurofibromatosis
Chordoma		Cysticercosis	Lissencephaly (smooth brain)
Hamartoma		Hydatid cyst	Fahr's syndrome
Lipoma		*Paragonimus westermani* abscess	X-ray radiation and methotrexate
Pituitary adenoma		Trichinosis	Cockayne's syndrome
Metastasis		Torulosis	Hemodialysis
Dermoid epidermoid and teratoma		*Coccidioides*	Lead and carbon monoxide poisoning

170. Radioactive gold is used in:

A. Bladder　**B.** Malignant ascites
C. Glioma　**D.** None

Ascites due to carcinomatosis of peritoneum **(malignant ascites)** can be considerably *ameliorated* by instillation of **radioactive gold** and chemocytotoxic agent such as methotrexate.

171. Hot nodule is seen in:

A. Adenolymphoma　**B.** Mixed parotid
C. Adenocystic carcinoma　**D.** All of the above

Radionuclide imaging of the salivary glands provides much *functional* information in the study of abnormalities of these glands associated with systemic diseases such as Sjögren's syndrome. On the other hand, this method has provided little additional useful information in the study of mass lesions *except* Warthin's tumor (**adenolymphoma**) and oncocytomas that manifest *increased* uptake (**hot spots**) of pertechnetate ^{99m}TC.

172. Oligemic lung fields are seen in:

A. TOF　**B.** Pulmonary stenosis
C. ASD　**D.** Both A and B

Oligemic lung fields are seen when pulmonary blood flow is *reduced* such as in **pulmonary stenosis** and **tetralogy of Fallot** with consist of VSD, over riding of aorta, pulmonary stenosis and right ventricular hypertrophy.

173. Contrast material used in the diagnosis of esophageal atresia is:

A. Barium swallow　**B.** Gastrografin
C. Conray　**D.** Propyliodone (Dianosil®)

On *no* account should the barium emulsion be given in cases of suspected esophageal atresia. Injection of 1 ml of **propyliodone (Dianosil®)** down the catheter will demonstrate the obstruction. In *all* cases it should be aspirated after radiograph has been taken.

174. Hair on end appearance in skull X-ray is characteristic of:

A. Sickle cell anemia　**B.** Megaloblastic anemia
C. Hemochromatosis　**D.** Thalassemia

In **thalassemia major (Cooley's anemia)** the vault is greatly thickened and has the typical "**hair on end**" appearance. CT scan demonstrates the thickening with very little inner or outer table bone due to the greatly expanded erythropoietic dipole.

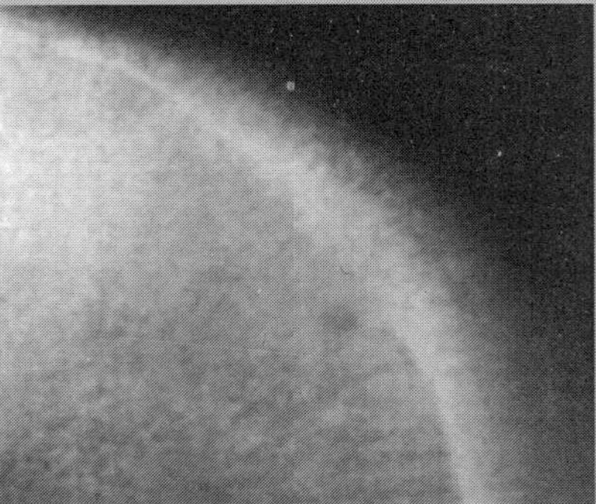
Hair on end appearance

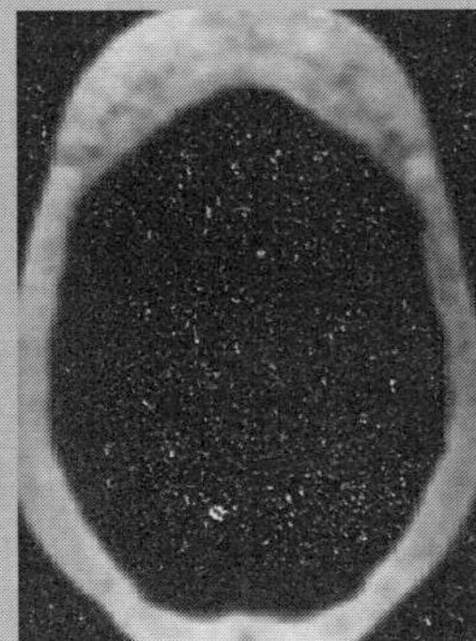

175. Chest X-ray of a newborn with respiratory distress shows multiple air containing lesions in left hemithorax and mediastinal shift. *Likely* diagnosis is:

A. Pneumatoceles　**B.** Neonatal emphysema
C. Diaphragmatic hernia　**D.** Congenital lung cysts

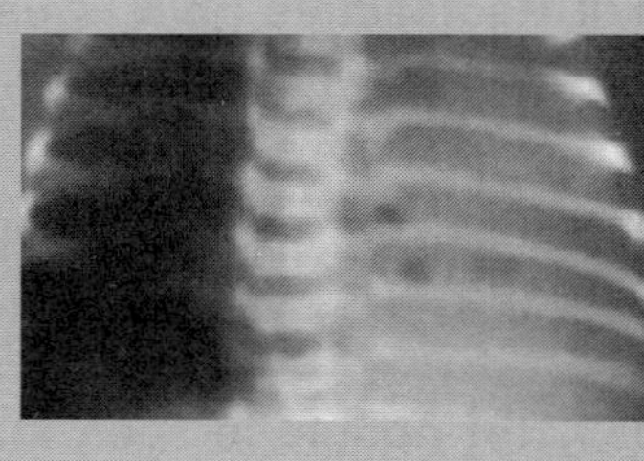

The large diaphragmatic hernias that compromise lung growth are posterolateral in position and are caused by *defective closure of the pleuroperitoneal canal.* The remnant of this canal in the normally developed diaphragm is the foramen of Bochdalek. **Infants with congenital diaphragmatic hernias are severely distressed at birth**, and because the abdomen contains fewer contents than normal, it appears **scaphoid**. *Radiographically*, the abdominal contents, which may include stomach, bowel, spleen, and liver, can be identified within the thorax. **About 85% of congenital hernias are left-sided.** The ipsilateral lung is the more severely hypoplastic, but because of mediastinal shift, a *lesser degree* of *contralateral* hypoplasia is also present.

176. *Investigation of choice* for spinal cord tumor is:

A. Myelography
B. CT scan
C. Plain X-ray
D. MRI

With or without Gadolinium enhancement **MRI is now the investigation of choice for spinal cord tumors.**

177. 'Doughnut' sign seen on a brain scan usually suggests:

A. Osteoid osteoma
B. Metastases
C. Fibrous dysplasia
D. All of the above

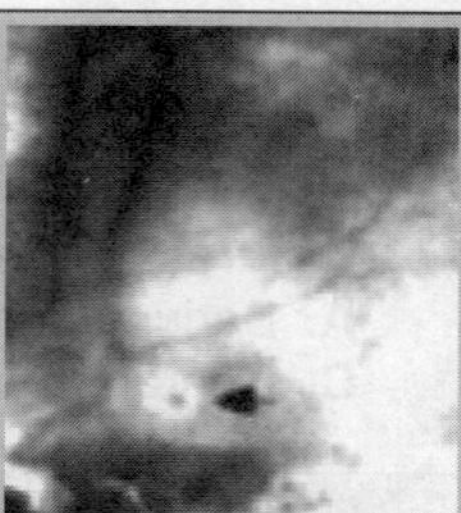

Doughnut lesions are tiny dense lesion with a lucent center was found incidentally in a patient with non-focal headaches. Similar lesions when explored surgically have been histologically nonspecific, showing bone and fibrous tissue, but could represent tiny versions of a variety of specific abnormalities such as **osteoid osteoma**, epidermoid inclusion, **fibrous dysplasia, metastasis,** etc.

- (Doughnut is a small, usually ring-shaped cake of sweetened, leavened dough, fried in deep fat)

178. The *treatment of choice* for anaplastic carcinoma thyroid is:

A. External radiation
B. Surgery
C. Radiotherapy
D. Thyroxin

Radiotherapy should be given to all the cases of anaplastic carcinoma of thyroid.

179. Splenic calcification occurs in:

A. Tuberculosis
B. Malaria
C. Gaucher's disease
D. Celiac disease

Causes of Splenic Calcifications

• Tuberculosis (*most common*)	• Old hematoma
• Histoplasmosis	• Old hemorrhage
• Splenic artery aneurysm	• Sickle cell anemia

180. The photosensitive material used in X-ray films consists of:

A. Zinc sulphate
B. Silver bromide
C. Cadmium bromide
D. Cellulose

The most common film used in radiology is film on blue-tinted polyester base coated with **silver *halide*** emulsion on both sides. X-ray film is coated on both sides so that the X-ray beam absorption can be increased by using two intensifying screens.

181. In color Doppler the color depends upon:
A. Strength of returning echo
B. Relation of transducer to blood flow
C. Frequency of Doppler used
D. Type of Doppler machine used

The *apparent* variation in frequency of any emitted wave, such as a wave of light or sound, as the source of the wave approaches or moves away, relative to an observer is known as Doppler's effect. **Red-shifts** occur due to Doppler effect. The Doppler effect occurs when a wave-emitting object moves toward *or* away from an observer, and the observer sees or hears the waves differently than he or she *would if the object were stationary* relative to the observer. If a sound reflecting (**blood**) object is moving away from an observer, each wave leaves the object from a point slightly farther away from the observer than the previous wave did. *Therefore*, **the distance between waves (called the wavelength)** is longer than it would be if the object *were* stationary.

182. When bones show a "bone within bone" appearance this is indicative of:
A. Chronic myelogenous leukemia
B. Bone infarction
C. Osteopetrosis
D. Sickle cell anemia

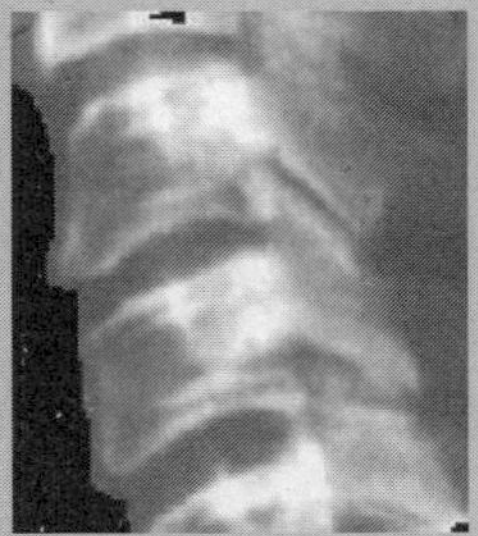

In **osteopetrosis (Albers-Schönberg's Disease)**, sclerosis is more prominent at the base of the skull, while in the spine it marks the vertebral end-plates with a characteristic "sandwiched" or broad-striped ("rugby jersey") appearance. Foci of sclerosis, yielding the impression of "bone **in bone**," may be a distinctive feature (in young patients).

183. Soft tissues calcification can be seen around the hip joint on a plain radiograph in all *except*:
A. Poliomyelitis
B. Melorheostosis
C. Polyostotic fibrous dysplasia
D. Tumor calcinosis

Soft tissues calcification around hip joint is seen in the following 3 conditions:
- Poliomyelitis
- Metastatic calcification of tumor
- Melorheostosis (Leri's Disease)

184. Convolutional markings in a child usually disappear by the age of....:
A. 3 months
B. 6 months
C. 3 years
D. 12 years

The pulsating brain produces very shallow depressions on the inner table of the skull usually referred to as **convolutional markings**. These are commonly observed in **normal children up to age 12 years** and tend to disappear after that age. Persistence or increased prominence of these may be related to increased intracranial pressure or to craniosynostosis.

185. Regarding syringomyelia all are *true except*:
A. Is associated with Dandy-Walker malformation
B. Is *commonly* associated with Arnold-Chiari syndrome
C. Is associated with a scoliosis
D. Is associated with Klippel-Feil syndrome

- In cases of **syringohydromyelia**, an abnormal cavity containing CSF-*like* fluid is present *within* the spinal cord. Syringohydromyelia is a combination of the terms syringomyelia and hydromyelia; 2 entities that frequently coexist and can be difficult to differentiate radiologically. Classically, however, **syringomyelia** refers to a glial-lined cavity within cord substance. **Hydromyelia**, on the other hand, implies persistent dilatation of the central canal of the spinal cord; this channel is lined by ependymal tissue. The central canal eventually closes normally; in fact, it has been shown to have been obliterated in 70% to 80% of neonates.
- In a series of patients with syringohydromyelia, researches reported an 80% association of Chiari 1, but only 1 case of the Chiari 2 malformation (or **Arnold-Chiari**). Other associated anomalies include the Dandy-Walker malformation, diastematomyelia, Klippel-Feil syndrome, and other spinal segmentation defects.
- In the Chiari type 1 malformation, there is protrusion of the cerebellar tonsils through the foramen magnum and into the cervical spinal canal; when this abnormality is associated with protrusion of meninges (*meningocele*) or meninges and cord (*meningomyelocele*) through a spinal canal that has *incompletely* closed, it is designated a Chiari type 2 (or Arnold-Chiari) malformation.

186. *Massive* splenomegaly is seen in the following conditions *except*:

A. Hairy cell leukemia
B. Sarcoidosis
C. Celiac disease
D. Polycythemia rubra vera

Diseases Associated with Massive Splenomegaly

- Chronic myelogenous leukemia
- Lymphomas
- **Hairy cell leukemia**
- Myelofibrosis with myeloid metaplasia
- **Polycythemia rubra vera**
- Gaucher's disease
- Chronic lymphocytic leukemia
- **Sarcoidosis**
- Autoimmune hemolytic anemia
- Diffuse splenic hemangiomatosis

***Massive* splenomegaly is said to be present when the spleen extends > 8 cm below left costal margin *and/or* weighs more than 1000 g.**

187. Which of the following is *false* regarding "J shaped sella":

A. Normal variant in 30% of cases
B. Seen in optic glioma
C. Associated with Hurler's syndrome
D. Associated with low grade hydrocephalus

J shaped Sella (omega shaped, shoe shaped, hourglass sella) is an elongated sella with shallow anterior convexity. It is rarely seen in films of adult skull but present in **5% normal children**. Also found in 3 pathological conditions:

- Chronic hydrocephalus
- Gargoylism (Hurler's syndrome)
- Glioma

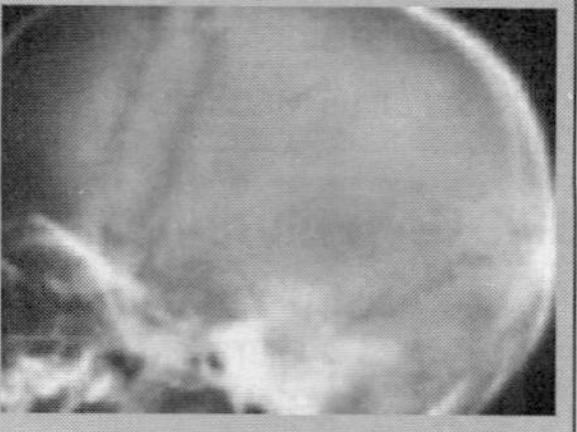

188. "Sunray" appearance on X-ray is seen in:

A. Ewing's sarcoma
B. Osteogenic sarcoma
C. Osteomyelitis
D. Chondrosarcoma

The typical X-ray appearance of **osteogenic sarcoma** of the mandible is that of an expansile sclerosing lesion. In some cases bone deposition at the periphery of a lesion will occur in a radial linear pattern, said to resemble that of **sunrays** on radiographs.

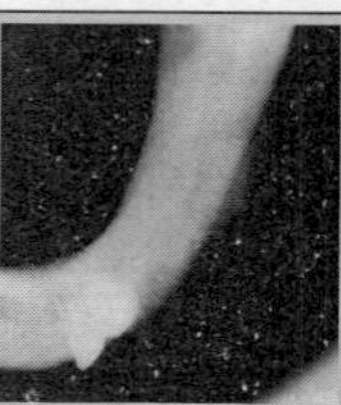

189. *Most common* site of spina bifida is:

A. Cervical
B. Lumbosacral
C. Sacral
D. Dorsal

In **spina bifida** there is congenital defect in posterior bony wall of spinal canal through which the contents may protrude out. It is mostly seen in **lumbosacral region**.

190. Pantomography is done for all *except*:

A. TM joint
B. Dental cyst
C. Dental caries
D. Transverse fracture of atlas

Pantomography or panoramic radiograph is a type of extra-oral curved surface X-ray that shows the **entire upper and lower jaws** in a continuous single film.

191. *Most common* cause of spontaneous pneumothorax:

A. Tuberculosis
B. Bronchogenic carcinoma
C. Rupture of sub-pleural blebs
D. Bronchial adenoma

Primary spontaneous pneumothorax is *most commonly* caused by the rupture of apical pleural blebs which are the small cystic spaces that lie within or immediately under the visceral pleura. Primary spontaneous pneumothoraces occur *exclusively* in smokers.

192. Hydrocephalus in children, *first* seen is:

A. Sutural diastasis
B. Sellar erosion
C. Large head
D. Thinned out vault

In infant and children sutural diastasis is the first and most prominent feature of raised intracranial tension. The younger the child more marked the sign. It may be the *only* sign of raised intracranial tension in children. Sellar erosion may occur but is a *late sign* and implies long standing chronic raised ICT. In children < 10 years if sellar erosion without sutural diastasis is found, it is more likely to be due to local erosive lesion rather than raised ICT.

193. Seldinger needle is used for:

A. Arteriography
B. Ureterography
C. Arthrography
D. Sonography

In 1953, **Seldinger** introduced the "catheter replacement technique" for the percutaneous introduction of catheters into blood vessels. Seldinger modified the technique of *Peirce* by passing a flexible wire through the needle; the needle was then withdrawn over the wire and replaced with a flexible catheter that was passed into the vessel. The introduction of this excellent technique resulted in a dramatic increase in the number of angiographic procedures performed for a variety of indications, and it **remains the standard method for performing most angiographic studies** nowadays.

194. Epiphyseal dysgenesis is a *pathognomonic* feature of:

A. Hyperthyroidism
B. Hyperparathyroidism
C. Hypothyroidism
D. Hypoparathyroidism

In addition to delayed epiphyseal ossification, the epiphyses of children with **hypothyroidism** may also have irregular ossification at multiple centers, a finding termed epiphyseal **dysgenesis**.

195. *All* are associated with greenhouse effect *except*:

A. CO_2
B. N_2
C. CH_4
D. O_3

Greenhouse effect is also known as global warming. The atmosphere is largely transparent to incoming short-wave solar radiation, which is absorbed by the Earth's surface. Much of this radiation is then reemitted at infrared wavelengths, but it is reflected back by gases such as **carbon dioxide, methane**, nitrous oxide, halocarbons, and **ozone** in the atmosphere. This heating effect is the basic cause of global warming.

196. "Round pneumonia" occurs in:

A. Children
B. Adult males
C. Adult females
D. Elderly

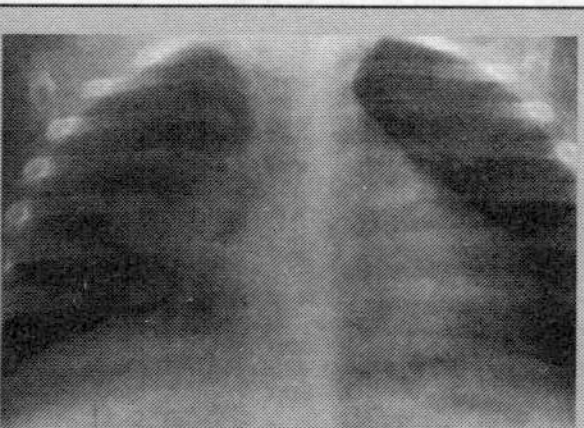

Pneumococcal pneumonia cause rapid consolidation of an entire lobe, due to filling of the alveoli with hemorrhagic edema fluid, white blood cells and fibrin. Sometimes in **children**, the pneumonia has a rounded, mass-like appearance. This has been called **"round pneumonia"** and is due to the centrifugal spread of infection via pores of Kohn and canals of Lambert from a small primary focus of infection in the lung.

197. Stenver's view is used to visualize:

A. Temporomandibular joint
B. Optic foramina
C. Mastoid air cells
D. Internal auditory meatus

Structures best visualized in Stenver's view:

- Internal auditory canal
- Vestibule
- Lateral semicircular canal
- **Mastoid air cells**
- Mastoid process
- Jugular fossa

198. Cavitating lesions in lung are found in:

A. Squamous cell carcinoma
B. Adenocarcinoma
C. Small cell carcinoma
D. Large cell carcinoma

Squamous cell carcinoma is the most common lung tumor to cavitate. **Cavitation** occurs in about 7% of all cases of squamous cell carcinoma.

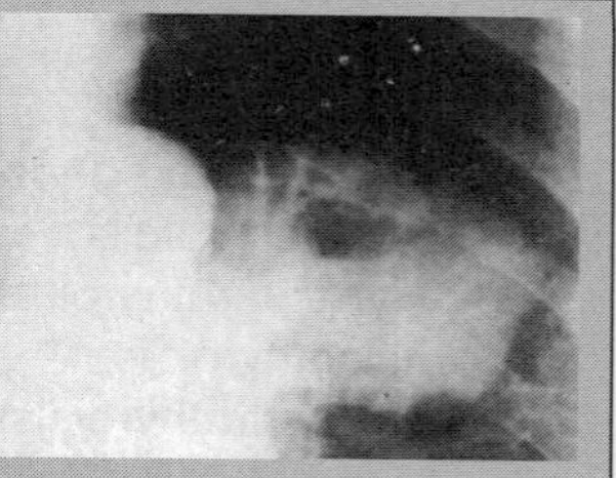

199. In urinary schistosomiasis, calcification is commonly seen in:

A. Bladder
B. Entire ureter
C. Lower half of the ureters
D. Upper half of the ureters

Urinary schistosomiasis is produced by *Schistosoma hematobium*. Schistosomiasis involves mainly the bladder. Since the lesions tend to heal by fibrosis, contraction of the bladder and bladder neck is seen. **Calcifications in the bladder** have been reported to occur in 5 to 50% of patients.

200. *Most common* cause of intracranial calcification is:

A. Pineal calcification **B.** Intracranial aneurysm
C. Meningioma **D.** Tuberculoma

Calcification of the pineal body is common and occurs in *approximately* 50% of all adults. On plain films it is visible less than half of the time but on CT a higher incidence of pineal calcification is seen.

201. Calcification and sclerosis of the fibrous cardiac skeleton is suggestive of:

A. Lev's disease **B.** Lenegre's disease
C. Both **D.** None

- In **Lev's disease**, there is **calcification** and **sclerosis** of the fibrous cardiac skeleton.
- *Lenegre's disease* is a primary *sclerodegenerative* disease within the conducting system itself with no involvement of the myocardium or the fibrous skeleton of the heart.

202. A neonate presents with history of not having passing meconium. On examination there is no anal opening. Investigation of choice is:

A. Invertogram **B.** Gastrograffin study
C. X-ray erect posture **D.** X-ray supine posture *(JIPMER 1990)*

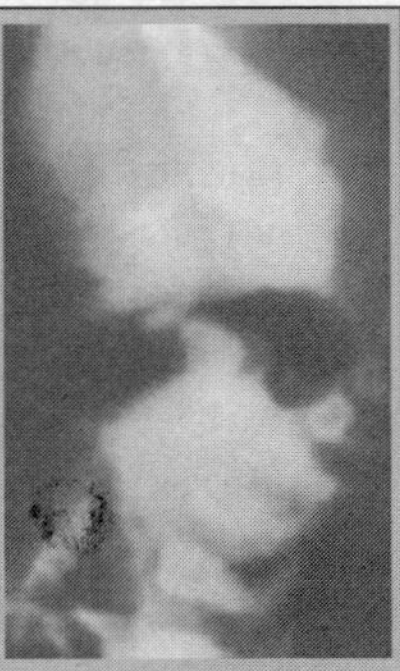

Imperforate anus (anal atresia/agenesis) has an incidence of 1 in 4500 births. It is of 2 types viz. high and low; depending on the level at with bowel terminates either above or below the pelvic floor. A radiograph of the infant's abdomen in an inverted position with a metal marker, or coin (**invertogram**) at the site of the imperforate anus is the **investigation of choice**. It should be taken 6 hours *after* birth so that sufficient amount of air is collected in large intestine to cast the shadow in X-ray .If the distance between metal indicator and blind end rectum is more than 2.5 cm the abnormality is of "high variety" and if less than 2.5 cm it is of "low variety". If gas can be identified below this level, injection of one or two milliliters of non-ionic water-soluble iodine contrast media is helpful in more accurately determining the position of the obstruction and in identifying rectourethral or rectovesical fistulas.

203. Curie is the unit for:

A. Radiation emitted **B.** Radiation absorbed
C. Radioactivity **D.** None of the above *(DELHI 1996)*

Curie is a unit of measurement of **radioactivity**. The rate of decay of a radioactive sample is described by its activity, *the number of atoms that disintegrate per unit time*. An activity of 3.7 × 1010 s-1 is defined as 1 Curie (Ci), this being the decay rate of 1 g of radium-226.

204. *Most important* investigation for posterior urethral valve is:

A. Micturating cystogram **B.** Retrograde cystogram
C. IVP **D.** Plain X-ray

Male babies with **posterior urethral valve** present with difficulty in passing urine, dribbling of urine, failure to thrive, poor feeding, sepsis and renal failure. Diagnosis is based on ultrasonography, **micturating cystogram**, and cystoscopy. Treatment consists of valve fulguration. In sick babies with severe urinary sepsis initial urinary diversion followed by valve fulguration may be necessary; diversion may be either as vesicostomy or ureterostomy. Later reimplantation of the ureters may be necessary in few cases where reflux persists.

205. Dye used for bronchography is:
- **A.** Iopanoic acid
- **B.** Sodium diazotize
- **C.** Meglumine Iothalamate
- **D.** Propyliodone (Dianosil)

Bronchography is radiography of the tracheobronchial tree after instillation of an oil-based contrast medium. The major indication for bronchography is for the detection of localized bronchiectasis in patients considered for operative resection. Propyliodone **(Dianosil)** bronchography has a limited place in evaluating selected patients presenting with hemoptysis, chronic right middle lobe atelectasis (children), and congenital abnormalities.

206. The substance used for oral cholecystography is:
- **A.** Iopanoic acid
- **B.** Sodium diazotize
- **C.** Meglumine iothalamate
- **D.** Dianosil

Telepaque® or **Iopanoic acid** is the *most common* medium used for oral cholecystography. IV cholangiography and oral cholecystography should *not* be used if patient has plasma bilirubin above 3 mg%.

207. Contrast used in liver scan is:
- **A.** TechneColl® (technetium^{99m})
- **B.** I^{131} Rose Bengal
- **C.** Gallium^{238}
- **D.** Thallium^{201}

Technetium **(Tc^{99m} sulfur colloid)**, administered intravenously, is indicated for imaging the functioning reticuloendothelial cells of the liver in the evaluation of metastatic disease, primary liver tumors, abscesses, and other focal hepatic lesions; and in the evaluation of patients with cirrhosis, hepatitis, and other hepatic disorders. **Liver scan** is also known as technetium scan; Liver-spleen scan; Liver technetium sulfur colloid scan; Liver-spleen radionuclide scan. It is a scan that uses a radioactive isotope to help determine liver and/or spleen function. A radioisotope is injected into a vein. After the liver has had sufficient time to absorb the radioisotope, patient is asked to lie on a table under the scanner. The scanner is able to detect where the radioisotope material is located, and images are displayed on a computer. This test is probably the best way to study the liver without surgery. It is particularly valuable because it can provide information about liver function. It is also used to help confirm other test results. The liver and spleen should appear normal in size, shape, and location. The radioisotope is absorbed evenly.

208. Dye used in intravenous cholangiography is:
- **A.** Dianosil®
- **B.** Conray®
- **C.** Cholografin®
- **D.** Myodil®

Iodipamide (Cholografin®) is indicated for **intravenous cholangiography** and cholecystography for the visualization of the gallbladder and biliary ducts in acute abdominal conditions in which rapid diagnosis is required; for the visualization of the biliary ducts in patients with post-cholecystectomy symptoms; for visualization of the gallbladder in patients unable to take oral contrast media or to absorb contrast media from the gastrointestinal tract. It should be remembered that, because of the potential for systemic toxicity with intravenous cholangiography, sonography and hepatobiliary scintigraphy are usually the preferred methods for evaluation of the gallbladder and the bile ducts.

209. While doing renal scan, hippuran (orthoiodohippurate) is attached to:
- **A.** Iodine^{125}
- **B.** Iodine^{131}
- **C.** Iodine^{132}
- **D.** Iodine^{113}

	Organ or tissue of interest	Radio nucleotide
•	Tumors	$Gallium^{67}$
•	Thyroid	$Iodine^{123}$ iodide scan
•	Thyroid	$Iodine^{131}$ iodide(uptake)
•	Kidney	$Iodine^{131}$ iodohippurate
•	Heart	$Thallium^{201}$ chloride
•	Brain	$Technetium^{99m}$ pertechnetate
•	Brain, kidney	DTPA
•	Cardiovascular	HAS
•	Lung	MAA microspheres
•	Blood pools	Red blood cells
•	Liver, spleen	Sulfur colloid
•	Bone, heart	Diphosphonate

^{131}I-orthoiodohippurate or ^{131}I-hippuran (^{131}I-OIH) is cleared by glomerular filtration as well as tubular excretion. The extraction efficiency of this agent is similar to paraaminohippurate (PAH). Tubular function and effective renal plasma flow can also be accurately assessed with this agent.

210. "Target sign" in CT scan means:

A. Ovarian carcinoma
B. Ectopic kidney
C. Intussusception
D. Liver metastasis

Ultrasound and CT demonstrate a target or concentric ringed mass (**"target sign"**) that can have either a reniform or round configuration in patients of **intussusception**.

211. Lymphangiomyomatosis is characterized by all of the following *except*:

A. Postmenopausal women
B. Recurrent chylous pleural effusions
C. Miliary densities
D. Recurrent spontaneous pneumothorax

Lymphangiomyomatosis (lymphangioleiomyomatosis) is a *rare disorder* of **women of reproductive age**, the major symptom being dyspnea but the chest X-ray may be abnormal for a long time before symptoms appear. Pathologically there is a widespread infiltration of pleura, septa and alveolar walls by proliferating muscle and lymphatics. *Radiographically* there is a fine reticulation with **miliary densities** distributed widely and not sparing the lung bases in contrast to eosinophilic granuloma which it otherwise resembles closely. Other features are progressively enlarging lung volumes, small emphysematous cysts, **pneumothorax**, interstitial edema, septal lines and **chylous pleural effusions**.

212. In colitis cystica profunda:

A. Cysts may be up to 2 cm in diameter
B. On a barium enema the appearance is indistinguishable from adenomatous polyps
C. Benign condition
D. All of the above

In **colitis cystica profunda** there are large mucous epithelium-lined cysts measuring **up to 2 cm in diameter** present in the submucosal layer of the colon, most commonly in the rectum and sigmoid. The disorder *most frequently* affects young adults and presents with recurrent rectal bleeding, mucous discharge, and diarrhea. Colitis cystica profunda appears in X-ray as multiple, irregular colonic filling defects **suggesting adenomatous polyps. Colitis cystica profunda is a benign condition with no malignant potential**; surgery is indicated only in patients in whom there is significant bleeding or associated rectal prolapse.

213. An aneurysm of the sinus of valsalva usually ruptures into:

A. Right atrium
B. Left atrium
C. Posterior aortic sinus
D. Left ventricle

Persons with a congenital deficiency in the elastic continuity between the aorta and the aortic valve ring are predisposed to the development of **sinus of valsalva aneurysms**. Aneurysms usually do not cause cardiac dysfunction, as they enlarge, they may cause following complications:

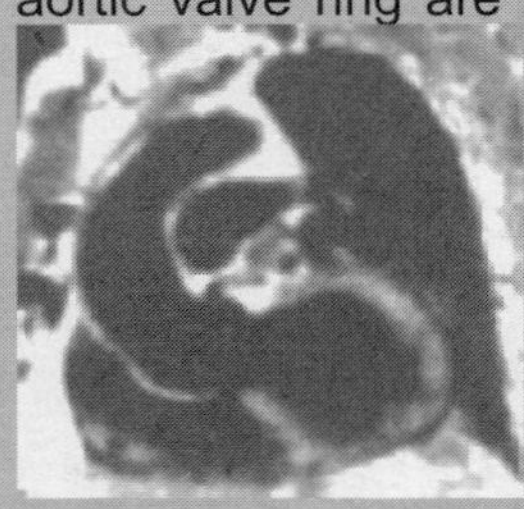

- Coronary insufficiency and occlusion leading to myocardial infarction.
- Aortic insufficiency, secondary to aneurysm-displaced aortic valve leaflets, may be present with or without rupture.
- Rupture of a sinus of valsalva aneurysm occurs more commonly in men than women. When this occurs, it is more commonly into the **right atrium** or right ventricle.

214. Pneumomediastinum can be seen in:

A. Valsalva maneuver
B. Ketoacidosis
C. Asthma
D. All of the above

Pneumomediastinum or mediastinal emphysema is the presence of air within the mediastinal space. Air can enter the mediastinum by 4 routes:

- By way of the interstitial tissues of the lungs (spontaneous);
- Along the fascial planes of the neck;
- As a result of perforations of the trachea, bronchus, or esophagus;
- By dissection along the retroperitoneal spaces.

Clinical conditions that cause an increase in intra-alveolar pressure, resultant alveolar rupture, and possible pneumomediastinum include:

- Forceful inhalation during anesthesia or resuscitation
- Valsalva maneuvers
- Coughing
- Vomiting
- Asthma
- Diabetic ketoacidosis
- Mechanical ventilation (barotrauma)

215. Unit of one dose of radiation absorbed is:

A. Gray
B. Roentgen
C. Curie
D. Becquerel

A flow of ionizing radiation through matter will deposit energy in that matter. This quantity is known as the absorbed dose. Its units are the **rad**, defined as 100 ergs/gram, and the **Gray**, defined as 1 joule/kg in the new SI system of units (1 gray = 100 rad).

216. In aortic dissection the *investigation of choice* is:

A. ECG
B. Aortography
C. CT scan
D. MRI scan

CT is now the investigation of choice for aortic dissection.

217. Estimation of fetal maturity by biparietal sonic measurement at 20-28 weeks of gestation is accurate to within +/–:

A. 7 days
B. 14 days
C. 10 days
D. 20 days

Using BPD as a yardstick for measurements made at 14-20 weeks of gestation, the variation is +/- 10-11 days; at 20-28 weeks, it is +/- 14 days; and at 29-40 weeks, the variation is +/- 21 days.

218. Investigation of choice for acute subarachnoid hemorrhage:

A. Enhanced MRI
B. MRI
C. CT scan
D. Angiography

The *most common* cause of spontaneous SAH is a ruptured saccular aneurysm. CT scanning is an important diagnostic tool for assessment and management of patients with acute intracranial hemorrhage.

219. Diagnostic of rickets on X-ray is:

A. White line of Frankel
B. Epiphyseal widening
C. Periosteal elevation
D. Cupping and flaring

The pathologic alterations in rickets that occur within the growth plate are characteristic. The zones of resting and proliferative cartilage are normal. However, the cartilaginous columns in the zone of maturation are elongated and increased in height. In some cases, these abnormal changes extend far into the metaphyses. This increases the axial height of the growth plate as well as its transverse diameter, producing the **classic cupping** or **flaring** of the epiphyseal-metaphyseal area.

220. A characteristic of benign tumor of lung in X-ray is:

A. Size > 5 cm diameter
B. Peripheral location
C. Cavitation
D. Calcification

Calcification of a pulmonary nodule generally indicates benign disease. *However*, both primary and metastatic malignancies *do sometimes* calcify.

221. The following is a radiolucent renal stone:

A. Cystine
B. Calcium phosphate
C. Uric acid
D. Calcium oxalate

Uric acid calculi, when pure, are radiolucent.

222. Fish mouth vertebra occurs in the:

A. Osteogenesis imperfecta
B. Ehler-Danlos syndrome
C. Gaucher's disease
D. Marfan's syndrome

In **Gaucher's disease** biconcave deformities of the vertebral bodies result from herniation of the nucleus pulposus. This pattern, called "cod fish" or "fish mouth" vertebra, is *also* seen in osteoporosis or osteomalacia.

223. Coffee bean sign indicates:

A. Toxic megacolon
B. Volvulus of cecum
C. Strangulation of incompletely obstructed loop of small bowel
D. Mesenteric artery embolism

In **strangulated bowel occlusion** a closed-loop obstruction may remain gas filled, with the lucency appearing as a featureless shadow that could be mistaken for a dilated sigmoid colon, a cecal or sigmoid volvulus, a gas-containing abscess, or a gas-filled giant duodenal or sigmoid diverticulum. Due to its typical ovoid appearance it is also known as **"the coffee bean sign"**.

224. Chickenpox pneumonia is characterized by:

A. Nodular infiltrate
B. Basilar infiltrate
C. Pulmonary edema
D. Linear pattern

In **varicella (chickenpox)** chest X-ray shows **patchy alveolar nodules** that can vary from a few nodules to very extensive disease that involves almost the entire lung. The diagnosis can be made with confidence on the basis of the radiographic appearance in the presence of the skin changes of chickenpox or zoster.

225. Candle wax appearance is seen in:
- **A.** Osteogenesis imperfecta
- **B.** Melorheostosis
- **C.** Diaphyseal dysplasia
- **D.** Exostosis

Melorheostosis (Leri's disease): The "flowing" cortical hyperostosis characteristic of melorheostosis resembles wax dripping down one side of a candle producing so called "**candle wax appearance**".

226. Primary anomaly in Klippel-Feil syndrome is:
- **A.** Torticollis
- **B.** Fusion
- **C.** Absence
- **D.** Segmentation

Klippel-Feil syndrome is characterized by **congenital fusion of the cervical spine**, short neck, low posterior hairline, and painless limitation of cervical movement.

227. Loss of lamina dura is observed in:
- **A.** Cushing's disease
- **B.** Legg-Calvé -Perthe's disease
- **C.** Hyperparathyroidism
- **D.** Osteopetrosis

There are some diseases affecting the metabolism of bone and causing a **loss of lamina dura**. Severe arterial hypertension, **hyperparathyroidism** (primary and secondary), and severe nutritional problems as seen in alcoholics, with involvement of the metabolic process of bone, are examples.

228. Hamman-Rich syndrome is:
- **A.** Fibrosing alveolitis
- **B.** Idiopathic pulmonary fibrosis
- **C.** Recurrent spontaneous pneumothorax
- **D.** Central mediastinal adenopathy

Idiopathic pulmonary fibrosis is also known as Hamman and Rich syndrome.

229. Batwing pattern of pulmonary edema is typical of:
- **A.** Renal failure
- **B.** Congestive cardiac failure
- **C.** ILD
- **D.** Sarcoidosis

Advanced **cardiogenic** pulmonary edema gives a central **batwing** appearance on chest X-ray.

230. Differential diagnosis of honeycomb lung includes:
- **A.** Eosinophilic granuloma
- **B.** Sarcoidosis
- **C.** Both
- **D.** None

"Honeycomb" lung is not specific for interstitial pneumonitis *and* may result from **eosinophilic granuloma** or other interstitial diseases. In **sarcoidosis** varying degrees of fibrosis may occur, causing distortion of alveolar and bronchiolar architecture and eventually end-stage "honeycomb" lung.

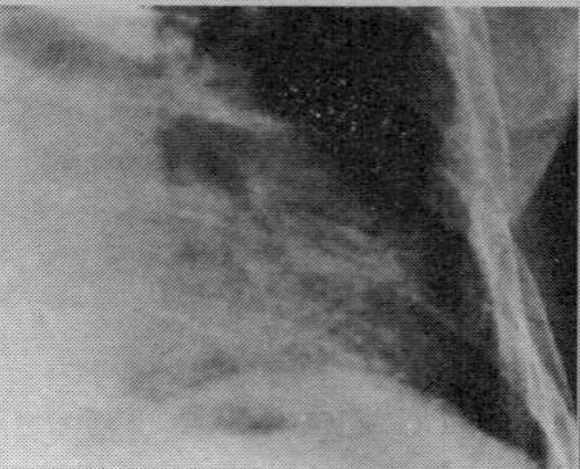

231. Pancoast tumor is *most commonly* due to which cell type:
- **A.** Squamous
- **B.** Columnar
- **C.** Adenocarcinoma
- **D.** Pseudo-stratified

If the primary tumor of lung involves the superior sulcus (4%) then the Pancoast syndrome may result. **Squamous cell carcinoma is most commonly associated with this syndrome**.

232. Ulcer crater on barium X-ray examination indicates the diagnosis of:
A. Gastric carcinoma
B. Duodenal ulcer
C. Duodenal diverticulum
D. Duodenal stricture

The most important X-ray feature of the **giant duodenal ulcer** is constant size and shape of the ulcer on barium meal, **ulcer crater,** and prolonged retention of barium in the crater.

233. *Best* diagnostic modality for subphrenic abscess is:
A. Plain X-ray
B. Ultrasound
C. CT scan
D. Diagnostic laparotomy

More than 80% of **subphrenic abscesses** follow intra-abdominal surgeries. Gastric, duodenal, or appendiceal perforation, diverticulitis, cholecystitis, pancreatitis, and trauma can all lead to the formation of a subphrenic abscess. **Abdominal CT is the most accurate method in the diagnosis of subphrenic abscess.**

234. Latest source of neutrons for radiotherapy is:
A. Strontium 90
B. Iodine 131
C. Californium 252
D. Radium 226

Neutron activation analysis (NAA) consists of irradiating a part or whole of a subject's body with fast neutrons (average energy typically 4 MeV-14 MeV) produced by a D-T-type neutron generator, cyclotron, or arrays of neutron-producing isotopic sources, such as plutonium-238-beryllium or californium-252.

235. Terminal phalangeal sclerosis is associated with:
A. Rheumatoid arthritis
B. Normal variation
C. Sarcoidosis
D. All of the above

Terminal phalangeal sclerosis (**acral sclerosis**) is seen as a normal variation and in association with **scleroderma**, **dermatomyositis**, **rheumatoid arthritis**, and **sarcoidosis**.

236. Round, smooth, slightly lobulated peripheral opacity in the lung with calcification is a feature of:
A. Hamartoma
B. Hydatid cyst
C. Amoebic abscess
D. Carcinoma lung

Hamartomas are *typically* round, smooth, slightly lobulated peripheral masses less than 4 cm in size without lobar predominance. On X-ray they show the typical pattern of **"popcorn" calcification** which is *almost* pathognomonic of hamartoma.

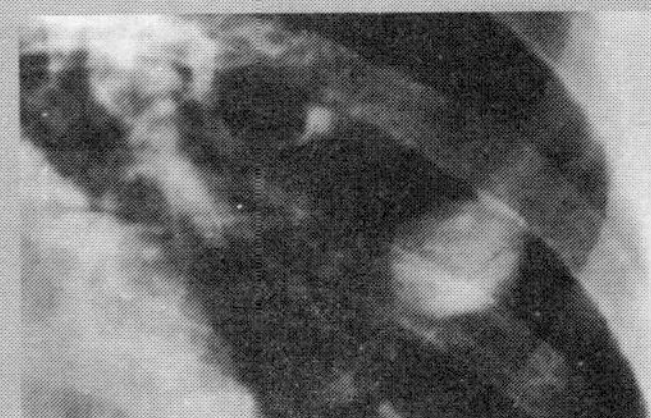

237. Wimberger's ring is seen in:
A. Scurvy
B. Rickets
C. Osteomalacia
D. Osteopetrosis

(KARNATAKA 2001)

In scurvy there often are characteristic signs such as Wimberger's ring, the white line of Frankel, the Truemmerfeld zone, and subperiosteal hemorrhage, which aid in distinguishing this condition.

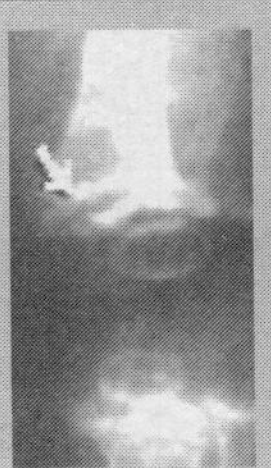

238. Brachytherapy means:

A. Irradiation by radiopharmaceuticals
B. Irradiation of tissue at 3 cm from the surface
C. Irradiation of tissue by placing radioactive sources into the tissue
D. Irradiation of tissue from a distance

(SGPGI 1999)

Brachytherapy is the radiation therapy in which there is use of implants of radioactive materials such as radium, cesium, iridium, or gold **at the site**. It is in contrast to teletherapy.

239. Type of radiation used in radiotherapy is:

A. Photons
B. Infrared rays
C. Ionizing radiation
D. UV rays

240. Which of the following is provided by linear accelerator:

A. Infrared rays
B. Neutrons
C. Electrons
D. Protons

A **linear accelerator** (LINAC) is the device most commonly used for external beam radiation (*teletherapy*) treatments for patients with cancer. It delivers a uniform dose of high-energy X-ray to the region of the patient's tumor. These X-rays can destroy the cancer cells, while sparing the surrounding normal tissue.

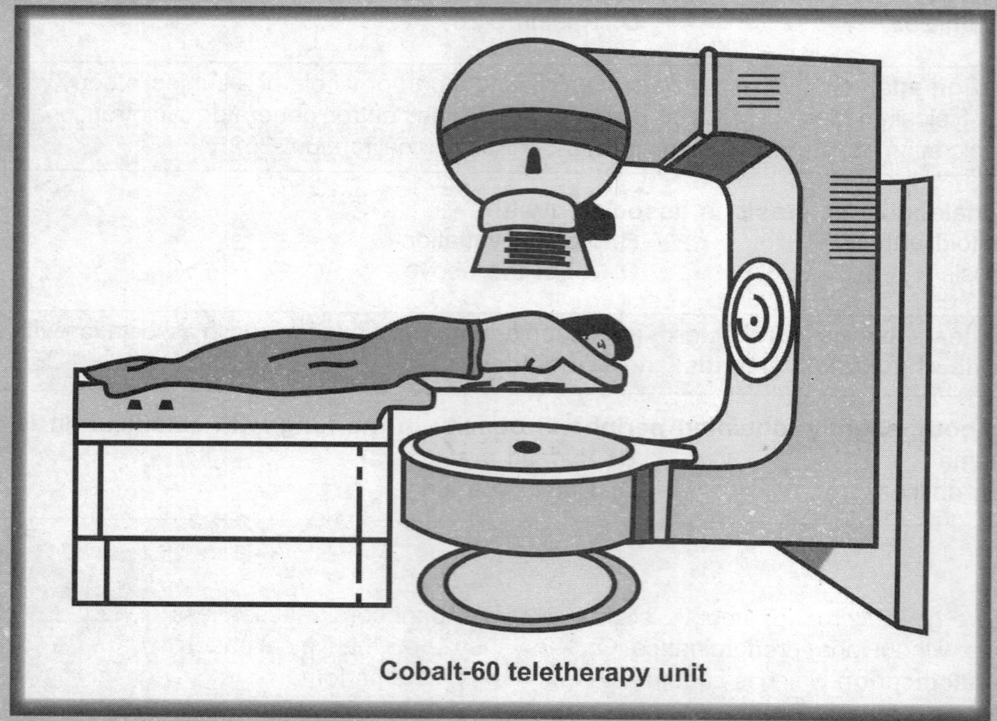

Cobalt-60 teletherapy unit

The linear accelerator uses microwave technology to **accelerate electrons** and then allows these electrons to collide with a heavy metal target. As a result of these collisions, high energy X-rays are scattered from the target. A portion of these X-rays is collected to form a beam that matches the size and shape of the patient's tumor. The beam comes out of a part of the accelerator called a gantry, which rotates around the patient. The patient lies on a movable treatment couch and lasers are used to make sure the patient is in the proper position. Radiation can be delivered to the tumor from any angle by rotating the gantry and moving the treatment couch.

241. Atomic weight is equal to the number of:

A. Neutrons
B. Protons and neutrons
C. Electrons
D. Protons

(DELHI 1996)

Atomic weight is equal to the number of protons and neutrons. The unit of atomic mass *in physics* is defined in terms of the carbon^{12} atom, which is 12 atomic mass units (amu). The actual mass of an atom can be calculated on the basis that one gram atomic weight of any element contains 6.02×10^{23} atoms (Avogadro's number, *N*a). Thus, 12 g of carbon contain 6.02×10^{23} atoms, and therefore 1 amu is a mass of $1/12 \times 12/ 6.02 \times 10^{23}$ g, or 1/ *N*ag. Similarly, the actual mass of a molecule can be calculated, and the number of molecules per gram, on the basis of the gram molecular weight (one mole) containing *N*a molecules.

242. ***Normal* metacarpal index is:**

A. > 10.4 **B.** > 5.4
C. 5.4-7.9 **D.** 8.4-10.4

Metacarpal index can be determined by dividing the length of each of the last four metacarpals by the width of its midpoint and averaging the values. Patients of Marfan's syndrome have the metacarpal index (MCI) > 8.4 (**normal MCI is less than 8**).

243. Tear drop sign is seen in:

A. Posterior cranial fossa fracture **B.** Maxillary sinus
C. Zygoma fracture **D.** Blow-out fracture of orbit *(UP 1998)*

Blow-out fractures occur when a blow to the eye increases pressure in the orbit, causing the weak floor or lamina papyracea to "blow-out" into the maxillary sinus or ethmoid bone. This results in a fracture, though it often prevents globe rupture and loss of the eye. Periorbital fat and extra-ocular muscles can become entrapped in the fracture, leading to problems of ocular movement. When the medial wall (lamina papyracea) is fractured, the medial rectus becomes entrapped, leading to lateral gaze dysfunction. If patient is immobilized on a backboard when film is taken, blood layers in the posterior of the sinus, making it appear clouded. Another sign of orbital blow-out fracture is the **tear drop sign**, an opacification in the upper maxillary sinus, which represents periorbital fat and possibly an entrapped extra-ocular muscle in the maxillary sinus.

244. Which of the following is differential diagnosis for miliary shadow in chest X-ray:

A. Tuberculosis **B.** Pulmonary hemosiderosis
C. Histoplasmosis **D.** All of the above *(PGI Dec 2000)*

Nodular miliary shadow in chest X-ray means numerous discrete, tiny (< 5 mm), uniform densities; evenly distributed throughout the lungs; quite uniform in size. They are seen in miliary tuberculosis, other fungal diseases (histoplasmosis), pneumoconiosis, histiocytosis X (early stage), pulmonary hemosiderosis (late stage) and primary amyloidosis.

245. Figure of '8' features are seen in which of the following:

A. TOF **B.** Abnormal origin of aorta
C. TAPVC **D.** Partial APVC *(AI 2000)*

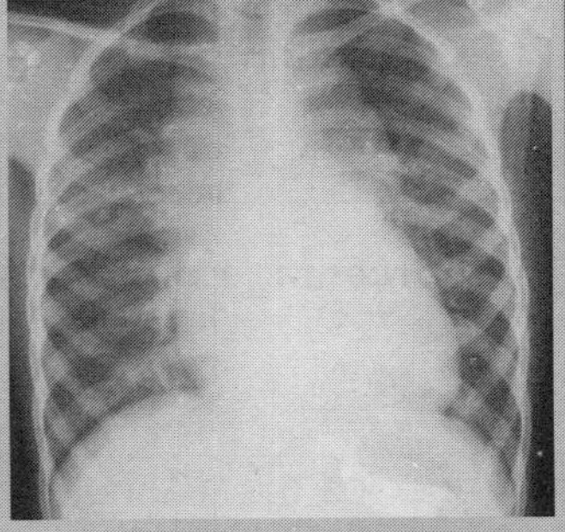

Total anomalous pulmonary venous connection is preferable to anomalous venous return as one may have anomalous drainage in the absence of anomalous connection. Anomalous pulmonary venous connection is classified as *either* partial or total. In TAPVC all the pulmonary veins drain into the right atrium either directly or via a venous channel. In all cases there is an ASD or patent foramen ovale which allows right to left atrial shunting in order to maintain survival. About 33% of patients with TAPVC have other *associated* cardiac lesions including single ventricle, atrioventricular septal defect, transposition of the great arteries; hypoplastic left heart syndrome or PDA. Many of these patients have heterotaxy syndrome with atriovisceral situs abnormalities and polysplenia / asplenia (Ivemark syndrome). TAPVC accounts for less than 1% of all cardiac defects. There is a 3:1 male preponderance in infants with infra-diaphragmatic TAPVC. It is of 4 types viz. type 1: supra-cardiac connection (55%); type 2: cardiac connection (30%); type 3: infra-cardiac connection (13%) and type 4: mixed pattern (2%);

In supra-cardiac connection there is cardiomegaly with increased pulmonary arterial markings. There is dilation of both the left and right innominate veins and the right superior vena cava producing the classical **"snowman" or "figure of 8" appearance**. The superior mediastinum is enlarged secondary to dilation of the right vena cava, innominate vein and ascending vertical vein.

246. *Best* conductor of electricity is:

A. Diamond
B. Coke
C. Coal
D. Graphite

Graphite is one of the allotropes of carbon. *Unlike* diamond, **graphite is a conductor**, and can be used, for instance, as the material in the electrodes of an electrical arc lamp. The pi orbital electrons delocalized across the hexagonal atomic sheets of carbon contribute the graphite's conductivity. In an oriented piece of graphite, conductivity parallel to these sheets is greater than that perpendicular to these sheets. The loose coupling among the sheets in graphite contributes to another industrially-important property—graphite powder is used as a dry lubricant.

247. Which of the following is a *characteristic* radiological finding in neonatal necrotizing enterocolitis:

A. Gas in the portal system
B. Gas in the intestinal wall
C. Pneumoperitoneum
D. Air fluid levels

(JIPMER 2000)

Necrotizing enterocolitis (NEC) is the most common gastrointestinal emergency in the newborn infant. Although it is predominately a disease of **preterm infants**, about 10% cases occur in term babies. **Prematurity is the single most important risk factor for development of NEC**. Abdominal X-rays are the mainstay for the diagnosis and following the course of NEC. A left lateral decubitus film (baby lying on the side with right side *up*) may be required to exclude a perforation as an air leak on an AP film (supine) may be missed. Other than perforation X-ray findings include dilated bowel loops with thickened bowel wall, fixed and dilated loop. **Intramural gas seen as "train track" lucency (pneumatosis intestinalis) is pathognomic of NEC.** Abdominal free air (*football sign*) over the liver with *outlining* of the *falciform ligament* suggests perforation and requires surgical intervention. Gas in the portal venous system may also be seen. Ascites is a late feature and is seen in children with perforation. Severity of NEC has been classified by **Bell** *et al* into 3 stages with stage 1 corresponding to non-specific symptoms; stage 2 signifying definite disease with clinical signs and symptoms and pneumatosis intestinalis in X-ray and stage 3 corresponding to advanced disease with critically ill newborn with perforation or *near* perforation.

248. In the diagnosis of pheochromocytoma one of the following radionuclide scan is useful:

A. MIBG scan
B. MIDA scan
C. DTPA scan
D. DMSA scan

(KARNATAKA 2001)

When a **pheochromocytoma** is suspected, metaiodobenzylguanidine (**MIBG**) labeled with iodine^{131} is used. MIBG is an analogue of guanethidine that is concentrated in catecholamine storage granules of sympathetic nerve endings.

249. Radiological investigation in female of reproductive age should be restricted to:

A. First 10 days of menstrual cycle
B. Period of menstruation
C. 10-20th day of the cycle
D. Last 10 days of the cycle

(AI 1993)

Ten days rule is that X-ray should be carried out within 10 days of LMP.

250. Percentage of cold thyroid nodule likely to be malignant is:

A. 72%
B. 20%
C. 40%
D. 30%

(PGI 1990)

All nodules that cannot be demonstrated to function are considered "cold". All thyroid carcinomas will be cold, as will lymphoma and metastatic disease. Many benign thyroid abnormalities will *also* be "cold," including adenomas, nodular goiter, focal involvement of thyroiditis, and cysts. Because of the relative frequencies of these abnormalities, the vast majority of "cold" nodules are benign. **The true incidence of carcinoma in nonfunctioning nodules is difficult to determine but probably lies somewhere near the 6% to 20% range.**

251. The test, which is both sensitive and specific for diagnosis of renal artery hypertension, is:

A. Captopril-enhanced radionucleotide renal scan
B. Angiography
C. CT
D. MRI

(AIIMS Nov 2001)

The standard approach to screen for renovascular hypertension was previously rapid-sequence IVP but now one of the 3 noninvasive techniques is used. These 3 techniques are the captopril-enhanced radionucleotide renal scan (the preferred choice), a duplex Doppler flow study, or magnetic resonance angiography. However, the most sensitive and 'screening' test is the spiral computerized tomography (CT) scan, which gives a three-dimensional view. The **'definitive' test for surgically correctable renal disease is the combination of a renal angiogram and renal vein renin determinations.**

Ref: *Harrison's Principles of Internal Medicine; 15th edition; page 1419*

252. Stereotactic radiosurgery is a form of:

A. Radiotherapy
B. Radio-iodine therapy
C. Robotic surgery
D. Cryosurgery

(AIIMS 11 May 2003)

Stereotactic radiosurgery is the very precise delivery of radiation to a brain tumor with sparing of the surrounding normal brain. To achieve this precision, special procedures for localization of the brain tumor are required. These tools include the stereotactic frame, the CT or MRI scanner, a computerized system for calculating the radiation dose to the brain tumor, and a precise system for delivering the radiation to the brain tumor. Stereotactic radiosurgery offers an important alternative to more invasive treatments for many brain tumors.

Ref: *http://www.hopkinsmedicine.org/radiosurgery/treatmentoptions/stereotacticradiosurgery.cfm*

253. Which one of the following radioisotope is commonly used as a source for external beam radiotherapy in the treatment of cancer patients?

A. Strontium-89
B. Radium-226
C. Cobalt-59
D. Cobalt-60

(AI 2003)

External beam therapy (EBT) is a method for delivering a beam of high-energy X-rays to the location of the tumor. The beam is generated outside the patient (usually by a linear accelerator) and is targeted at the tumor site. These X-rays can destroy the cancer cells and careful treatment planning allows the surrounding normal tissues to be spared. No radioactive sources are placed inside the patient's body. X-rays for external beam radiotherapy are produced by special machines called linear accelerators and are much higher in energy than those used for normal X-ray imaging. The higher the energy, the deeper the X-rays can penetrate, therefore the radiation can be delivered to cancers deep in the body. In addition to X-rays, some other forms of radiation are gamma rays (emitted from **cobalt-60** or radium sources) and particulate radiation such as electrons, protons, and neutrons.

254. "Bracket" calcification of skull in X-ray is seen in:

A. Meningioma
B. Sturge-Weber syndrome
C. Corpus callosum lipoma
D. Tuberous sclerosis

(JIPMER 2002)

Lipomas usually occur in relation to the **corpus callosum**, and a large lesion may show a highly characteristic marginal calcification ('**bracket sign**'). Less specific calcification may also be seen.

Ref: *http://www.sums.ac.ir/~semj/vol3/jul2002/ricc.htm*

255. A male patient presents with abdominal pain and distension. On barium enema examination, there is a "bird's beak" deformity. Which of the following is the likely diagnosis?

A. Intussusception
B. Volvulus of the sigmoid colon
C. Enteric perforation
D. Crohn's disease

(JHARKHAND 2003)

A confirmatory X-ray of the abdomen shows the closed-loop type of obstruction. In the case of a **sigmoid volvulus** there is a classical picture on barium enema X-ray that includes a "**bird's-beak**" appearance or sign, whereby the proximal rectum narrows down toward the point of the obstruction, thus creating a beaklike projection.

Ref: *http://www.hemorrhoid.net/volvulus.htm*

256. Thickness of lead apron to prevent radiation is:

A. 0.5 mm
B. 7 mm
C. 3 mm
D. 1 mm

(JIPMER 1995)

The lead equivalency of most **lead aprons** today is **0.5 mm**; these attenuate the primary beam by about 96-97 percent. The lead thickness in most standard diagnostic X-ray walls is 1-1.5 mm so at least 99 percent of the primary beam is stopped.

Ref: *http://hps.org/publicinformation/ate/q301.html*

257. A young patient presents with history of dysphagia more to liquids than solids. The first investigation you will do is:

A. Barium swallow
B. Esophagoscopy
C. Ultrasound of the chest
D. CT scan of the chest

(AIIMS 11 May 2003)

Dysphagia may be defined as *a sensation of sticking or obstruction of the passage of food through the mouth, pharynx or esophagus*. Difficulty only with solids implies mechanical dysphagia with a lumen that is not severely narrowed. Classically, **structural lesions result in dysphagia for solids; on the other hand, motility disorders cause difficulty with liquids**. **Achalasia** is *most common* in middle life, but can occur at any age. It typically presents with dysphagia. Achalasia may be suspected by **endoscopy** by finding a tight cardia and food residue in the esophagus.

Ref: *Bailey and Love's Short Practice of Surgery; 23rd edition; page 883*

258. Fraying and cupping of metaphyses of long bones in an child *does not* occur in:

A. Rickets
B. Lead poisoning
C. Metaphyseal dysplasia
D. Hypophosphatasia

(AI 2003)

Rickets is characterized by diminished or absent calcification in the cartilage of the growth plate of bone. The pathologic alterations that occur within the growth plate are characteristic. The zones of resting and proliferative cartilage are normal. However, the cartilaginous columns in the zone of maturation are elongated and increased in height. In some cases, these abnormal changes extend far into the metaphyses. This increases the axial height of the growth plate as well as its transverse diameter, producing the **classic cupping or flaring of the epiphyseal-metaphyseal area**. Other zones are also irregular. The bones undergoing rapid growth are predominantly affected, and the findings are therefore best seen in the long bones, ribs, skull, and scapula.

Schmid type is the *most common* form of **metaphyseal chondrodysplasia**. It is inherited as autosomal dominant. Patients are usually normal at birth. After the second year of life, affected children present moderately short stature with relatively short limbs, bowed legs with a waddling gait, and exaggerated lumbar lordosis. Radiographic findings involve primarily the metaphyses of the long and tubular bones, with cupping, fraying, and splaying especially noted in the lower extremities. The proximal femoral metaphyses are more severely affected than the distal femoral metaphyses. There is varus deformity of the hips and knees. All long and tubular bones are shortened, and their curvatures accentuated.

Rickets is a feature of a deficiency of alkaline phosphatase in infants and children termed **hypophosphatasia.**

259. High resolution computed tomography of the chest is the ideal modality for evaluating:

A. Pleural effusion
B. Interstitial lung disease
C. Lung mass
D. Mediastinal adenopathy

(AI 2003)

High resolution computed tomography (HRCT) is superior to the plain CXR for early detection and confirmation of suspected interstitial lung disease.

Ref: *Harrison's Principles of Internal Medicine; 15th edition; page 1501*

260. Extensive pleural thickening and calcification especially involving the diaphragmatic pleura are classical features of:

A. Coal worker's pneumoconiosis
B. Asbestosis
C. Silicosis
D. Siderosis
(AI 2003)

CXR can be used to detect a number of manifestations of **asbestos** exposure. Past exposure is 'specifically' indicated by pleural plaques, which are characterized by thickening or calcification along the parietal pleura, particularly along the lower lung fields, diaphragm, and the cardiac border.

Ref: *Harrison's Principles of Internal Medicine; 15th edition; page 1469*

261. Modality of choice for detection of acute subarachnoid hemorrhage is:

A. MRI
B. X-ray computed tomography
C. USG
D. Plain X-ray of skull
(SGPGI 1999)

The *most common* cause of spontaneous subarachnoid hemorrhage is a ruptured saccular aneurysm. The hallmark of aneurysmal rupture is blood in the cerebrospinal fluid. About 80% have enough blood to be visualized on a non-contrast CT scan obtained within 72 hours.

Ref: *Harrison's Principles of Internal Medicine; 15th edition; page 2389*

262. A 40-year-old man presented with acute episode of GI bleeding. Initial management was given for 6 hours. Which is important procedure for diagnosis is:

A. Radiolabeled RBC
B. Barium meal
C. Endoscopy
D. USG
(AIIMS 1999)

The initial treatment of esophageal varices is endoscopic sclerotherapy using 5% ethanolamine oleate.

Ref: *Bailey and Love's Short Practice of Surgery; 23rd edition; page 940*

263. A patient has ARF but normal USG report. Next most useful investigation is:

A. DTPA scan
B. IV pyelography
C. Retrograde pyelography
D. Renal angiography
(AIIMS 1999)

Radioisotope scanning is used to obtain information about 'function' in individual renal units. Diethyltriamine-pentacetic acid (**DTPA**) behaves in the kidney like inulin (filtered by glomeruli and not absorbed by the tubules). DTPA labeled with technetium-99m can be followed during its transit through individual kidneys to give dynamic representation of renal function.

Ref: *Bailey and Love's Short Practice of Surgery; 23rd edition; page 1168*

264. Which of the following isotopes is used to assess renal function?

A. DTPA
B. DMSA
C. Gallium
D. Thallium
(JHARKHAND 2003)

265. Impaired renal function is assessed by:

A. MAGS
B. Iodohippurate
C. DMSA scan
D. DTPA
(AI 1999)

DMSA, MAG-3, and Hippuran labeled with suitable radioactive isotopes have been used to investigate **renal 'function'**.

Ref: *Bailey and Love's Short Practice of Surgery; 23rd edition; page 1168*

Gamma camera scanning following the injection of technetium-99m labeled **DMSA** (dimercaptosuccinic acid) will give information about the renal plasma flow and its handling in the glomerulus; the majority being reabsorbed in the proximal tubules. Therefore, a comparative value of renal contribution can be obtained. Similarly technetium-99m **DTPA** (diethylene triamine pentacetic acid) is excreted earlier giving a good image of the renal outline.

Ref: *Bailey and Love's Short Practice of Surgery; 20th edition; page 1200 – 1201*

266. A patient has renal cell carcinoma with thrombus in IVC and renal vein. *Best* investigation for diagnosis is:

A. IVP
B. Color Doppler imaging
C. CT scan
D. Angiography *(AIIMS 1999)*

Definitive diagnosis of renal vein thrombosis can only be established through selective renal venography with visualization of the occluding thrombus. Without angiography, MRI often provides definitive evidence of thrombus.

Ref: *Harrison's Principles of Internal Medicine; 15th edition; page 1611*

267. A young girl presented with pain in chest. Pain is *not* associated with exercise. On auscultation there was multiple non-ejection clicks with murmur. Most important investigation for diagnosis is:

A. ECG
B. Tc pyrophosphate scan
C. Thallium scan
D. EEG *(AIIMS 1999)*

Mitral valve prolapse is more common in females and has been noted in a wide age range but most commonly between the ages of 14 and 30 years. Many patients have chest pain that is difficult to evaluate. The most important finding is the mid- or late systolic click, which occurs 0.14 second or more after the S_1. Systolic clicks may be multiple and may be followed by a high-pitched late systolic crescendo-decrescendo murmur. The ECG most commonly is normal but may show biphasic or inverted T waves in leads II, III, and aVF and occasionally supraventricular or ventricular premature contractions. 2D-echo is particularly useful in identifying the abnormal position and prolapse of the mitral valve leaflets.

Ref: *Harrison's Principles of Internal Medicine; 14th edition*

268. A 50-year-old man who is a chronic smoker presents with single lymph node enlargement and hoarseness of voice. Next investigation should be:

A. FNAC
B. IDL with chest X-ray
C. Percutaneous biopsy
D. Advise him to stop smoking *(AIIMS 2000)*

There are about 800 lymph nodes in the body and not less than 300 of them lie in the neck. **Chronic-painless cervical lymphadenopathy** may either be tuberculous (in children or young adults) or due to secondary malignant metastases, most commonly from squamous cell carcinoma in older people. Lymphoma also commonly presents in cervical lymph nodes in young adults. **Fine needle aspiration (FNAC) of enlarged cervical lymph nodes is preferable to any form of open biopsy.**

Ref: *Bailey and Love's Short Practice of Surgery; 23rd edition; page 704*

269. In aortic dissection the investigation of choice is:

A. Digital segmental angiography
B. MRI
C. CT-scan
D. USG *(AI 1996)*

CT and MRI are both highly accurate in identifying the intimal flap and extent of the dissection; each has a sensitivity and specificity exceeding 90%. These non-invasive tests are now becoming the diagnostic procedures of choice for aortic dissection.

Ref: *Harrison's Principles of Internal Medicine; 15th edition; page 1433*

270. At birth first paranasal sinus to develop is:

A. Sphenoid
B. Frontal
C. Maxillary
D. Ethmoidal *(AIIMS 1998)*

The maxillary and ethmoid sinuses are present at birth; the frontal and sphenoid sinuses develop after ages of 2 and 7 years respectively.

Ref: *Harrison's Principles of Internal Medicine; 15th edition; page 188*

271. An 8-year-old boy presents with back pain and mild fever. His plain X-ray of the dorsolumbar vertebra with preserved disc spaces. There was no associated soft tissue shadow. The *most likely* diagnosis is:

A. Ewing's sarcoma **B.** Tuberculosis
C. Histiocytosis **D.** Metastasis *(AI 2003)*

Histiocytosis-X is an *unusual* group of disorders in which cells of RE-system (histiocytes and eosinophils) form granulomatous collections, which may cause osteolytic lesions resembling bone tumors. **Eosinophilic granuloma** is *most common* of these conditions and the only one presenting as a 'pure' bone lesion. The marrow containing bone is resorbed and 1 or more 'lytic' lesions may appear in the flat bones or the metaphyses of long bones. Eosinophilic granuloma usually occurs during the first 3 decades of life and is *most common* in boys between 5 and 10 years of ages. There is seldom any complaint of pain and usually the condition is discovered incidentally or after a pathological fracture. X-ray demonstrates a well-demarcated oval area of radiolucency within a bone, sometimes associated with marked 'reactive' sclerosis. Multiple lesions may be present and in the skull they have a characteristic punched out appearance. Collapse of vertebra may result in a flat wedge (**vertebra plana**), which is pathognomic of this condition. It usually heals spontaneously. Operation is usually done to obtain a biopsy. If the lesion is easily accessible it may be completely excised or curetted; if not radiotherapy should be done.

Ref: *Apley's System of Orthopedics and Fractures; 8th edition; page 182 and Nelson Textbook of Pediatrics; 17th edition; page 1722*

The spine is the *most common* site of **skeletal tuberculosis** and the most dangerous. Blood-borne infection usually settles in a vertebral body adjacent to the Intervertebral disc followed by bone destruction and caseation. Thereafter the infection spreads to disc space and to adjacent vertebrae. When the vertebral bodies collapse into each other, a sharp angulation (kyphos) develops. Caseation and cold abscess formation may extend to neighboring vertebrae or escape into the paravertebral soft tissues. Pott's paraplegia is the most feared complication of the spinal tuberculosis. **The earliest X-ray signs are local osteoporosis of 2 adjacent vertebrae and narrowing of the intervertebral disc space.**

Ref: *Apley's System of Orthopedics and Fractures; 8th edition; page 387 – 389*

272. Which one of the following is a recognized X-ray feature of rheumatoid arthritis?

A. Juxta-articular osteosclerosis **B.** Sacroiliitis
C. Bone erosions **D.** Peri-articular calcification *(AI 2003)*

273. All the following are X-ray features of rheumatoid arthritis *except*:

A. Soft tissue swelling **B.** Osteoporosis
C. Periosteal new bone formation **D.** Bony erosions *(JIPMER 2002)*

Early in the course of **rheumatoid arthritis**, X-rays show only the features of synovitis (soft-tissue swelling and periarticular osteoporosis). Later stages are marked by appearance of marginal **bony erosions** and narrowing of the articular space. In advanced disease, articular destruction and joint deformity are obvious.

Ref: *Apley's System of Orthopedics and Fractures; 8th edition; page 55*

274. Which of the following is the *best* choice to radiological evaluation of a posterior fossa tumor?

A. CT scan **B.** MRI
C. Angiography **D.** Myelography *(AI 2003)*

In general, **MRI is more sensitive than CT-scan** for the valuation of most lesions affecting the CNS, particularly those in the spinal cord, cranial nerves and **posterior fossa**. However, CT is more sensitive than MRI for visualizing fine osseous details, such as temporal bone anatomy and fractures.

Ref: *Harrison's Principles of Internal Medicine; 15th edition; page 2337*

275. Treatment of carcinoma thyroid using radioactive iodine is:

A. I^{131} **B.** I^{125}

C. I^{133} **D.** I^{140} *(JIPMER 2001)*

Well-differentiated **thyroid cancers** still incorporate radioiodine, though less efficiently than normal thyroid follicular cells. After near-total thyroidectomy, substantial thyroid tissue remains, particularly in the thyroid bed and surrounding the parathyroid glands. Therefore, **^{131}I ablation** is necessary to eliminate remaining normal thyroid tissue may treat residual tumor cells.

Ref: *Harrison's Principles of Internal Medicine; 15th edition; page 2081*

276. Most suitable radioisotope of iodine for treating hyperthyroidism is:

A. I^{123} **B.** I^{125}

C. I^{131} **D.** I^{132} *(AI 2003)*

Radioiodine causes progressive destruction of thyroid cells and can be used as initial treatment of hyperthyroidism or for relapses after a trial of antithyroid drugs. ^{131}I dose generally ranges between 185 MBq and 555 MBq.

Ref: *Harrison's Principles of Internal Medicine; 15th edition; page 2072*

277. Radioiodine is *not* used in the treatment of which of the following:

A. Anaplastic carcinoma **B.** Follicular carcinoma

C. Medullary carcinoma **D.** Papillary carcinoma *(AI 1992)*

Anaplastic thyroid cancer (ATC) is a poorly differentiated and aggressive malignancy. **Due to the undifferentiated state of these tumors, radioiodine uptake is usually negligible** but can be used therapeutically *if there is residual uptake*. Although chemotherapy has been attempted with multiple agents, it is usually futile. External radiation therapy can be attempted and continued if tumors are responsive.

Ref: *Harrison's Principles of Internal Medicine; 15th edition; page 2082*

278. *Non*-caseating granulomas are seen in all the following *except*:

A. Tuberculosis **B.** Byssinosis

C. Hodgkin's lymphoma **D.** Metastatic carcinoma of lung *(AIIMS May 2001)*

Tuberculosis is the prototype granulomatous disease of humans. Other granulomatous conditions are sarcoidosis, brucellosis, tularemia, syphilis, leprosy, glanders, LGV, cat-scratch fever, berylliosis, and some of the mycosis.

Ref: *Robbins Pathologic Basis of Disease; 4th edition; page 376*

Caseous necrosis is a 'distinctive' type of necrosis, which is a combination of coagulative and liquefactive necrosis found principally in the center of tuberculous infections.

Ref: *Robbins Pathologic Basis of Disease; 4th edition; page 19*

279. Pleural involvement in sarcoidosis is:

A. Unilateral **B.** Bilateral

C. Very common **D.** Very rare *(AI 1992)*

In **sarcoidosis** the pleura is involved in 1 to 5% of cases, almost always manifesting as a **unilateral pleural effusion** with characteristics of an exudate containing lymphocytes.

Ref: *Harrison's Principles of Internal Medicine; 14th edition*

280. X-rays are produced when:

A. Electron beam strikes the nucleus of the atom

B. Electron beam strikes the anode

C. Electron beam reacts with the electromagnetic field

D. Electron beam strikes the cathode *(AIIMS Nov 2002)*

Electrode is a component of an electric circuit that connects the conventional wiring of the circuit to a conducting medium such as an electrolyte or a gas. The **electrically positive electrode is called the anode** and the negative electrode the cathode.

X-rays are penetrating electromagnetic radiation having a *shorter* wavelength than light (ranging in wavelength from about 100 A to 0.01 A). Bombarding a target, usually made of tungsten, with high-speed electrons, produces them.

281. For the treatment of deep-seated tumors, the following rays are used:
- **A.** X-rays and gamma rays
- **B.** Alpha rays and beta rays
- **C.** Electrons and positrons
- **D.** High power laser beams

(AIIMS 11 May 2003)

282. Ionization radiation act on tissue depending upon:
- **A.** Thermal injury
- **B.** Formation at pyrimidine dimmers
- **C.** Excitation of electron from orbit
- **D.** Linear acceleration energy

(AI 1998)

283. Principle used in radiotherapy is:
- **A.** Low dose causes tissue neurosis
- **B.** DNA damage
- **C.** Ionizing the molecule
- **D.** Cytoplasmic coagulation

(AI 1997)

X-rays and **gamma rays** are the forms of radiation *most commonly* used to treat cancer. They are electromagnetic and non-particulate waves that cause the ejection of an orbital electron when absorbed. This orbital ejection is known as **ionization**. X-rays are produced by linear accelerators while gamma rays are generated from decay of atomic nuclei in the radioisotopes such as cobalt and radium.

Ref: *Harrison's Principles of Internal Medicine; 15th edition; page 532*

284. The maximum penetration among the following is seen with which ray:
- **A.** Alpha
- **B.** Beta
- **C.** Gamma
- **D.** Electron beam

(AI 2002)

285. Which of the following has the maximum penetrating power?
- **A.** Alpha rays
- **B.** Beta rays
- **C.** Gamma rays
- **D.** Electron beam

(JHARKHAND 2003)

Alpha particles are helium nuclei, consisting of 2 protons and 2 neutrons. The mass and charge are great enough that these particles do not penetrate far enough through matter unless they have tremendous energy. Even a piece of paper is enough to protect against most alpha particles.

Electrons or **beta particles** are small and negatively charged and can be accelerated to close to the speed of light. They decelerate quite rapidly in the tissue and penetrate it to only a limited depth. Therefore, electron beams are often used to treat superficial lesions.

Rutherford discovered that at least 2 components are present in the radioactive radiations: alpha particles, which penetrate into aluminum only a few thousandths of a centimeter, and beta particles, which are nearly 100 times more penetrating. Subsequent experiments in which radioactive radiations were subjected to magnetic and electric fields revealed the presence of a third component, gamma rays, which were found to be much more penetrating than beta particles.

Further reading: *Harrison's Principles of Internal Medicine; 15th edition; page 2586*

286. *Characteristic* finding in CT-scan of a TBM case is:
- **A.** Exudates seen in basal cistern
- **B.** Hydrocephalus is commonly seen
- **C.** Ventriculitis
- **D.** Calcification of cerebellum

(AI 2001)

In **tuberculous meningitis** (TBM) imaging studies (CT and MRI) may show hydrocephalus and **abnormal enhancement of basal cisterns** or ependyma.

Further reading: *Harrison's Principles of Internal Medicine; 15th edition; page 1028*

287. What is the diagnostic radiological finding in skeletal fluorosis?
A. Sclerosis of sacroiliac joint
B. Interosseous membrane ossification
C. Osteosclerosis of vertebral body
D. Ossification of ligaments of knee joint
(JIPMER 2000)

Fluorine in very low concentration (1 ppm or less) has been used to reduce incidence of dental carries. At slightly higher levels (2 to 4 ppm) it may produce mottling of the teeth. In some parts of India where fluorine concentration in drinking water may be above 10-ppm chronic fluorine intoxication (**fluorosis**) is endemic and wide spread skeletal abnormalities are encountered. Fluorine directly stimulates osteoblastic activity and fluoroapatite crystals are laid down in bone and these are unusually 'resistant' to osteoclastic resorption. Other effects are due to calcium retention, impaired mineralization and secondary hyperparathyroidism. The characteristic pathological features are sub-periosteal new bone accumulation and osteosclerosis, most marked in the vertebrae, ribs, pelvis and the forearm and leg bones, together with hyperostosis at the bony attachments of ligaments, tendons and fascia in these areas. Although the bones appear 'thick-and-dense', their tensile strength is reduced and they fracture easily. Patients complain of backache, bone pain, and joint stiffness. **Typical X-ray features are osteosclerosis, osteophytosis and ossification of ligamentous and fascial attachments. These changes are most marked in the spine and pelvis.** There is no specific treatment.

Ref: *Apley's System of Orthopedics and Fractures; 8th edition; page 125 – 126*

288. On CT-scan, all are seen as hypodense area *except*:
A. Cerebral hemorrhage
B. Glioblastoma
C. Cerebral edema
D. Cerebral infarct
(JIPMER 2001)

Subdural hematomas are the *most common* intracranial mass-lesions resulting from head injury. Most of them result from torn **bridging veins** draining blood from cerebral cortex and dura. Blood follows the subdural space over the convexity of the brain and appears as a concave, **hyperdense lesion**.

Ref: *Bailey and Love's Short Practice of Surgery; 23rd edition; page 550 – 551*

289. Pneumoperitoneum can be used to visualize peritoneal / retroperitoneal structures. The gas that is best for use in pneumoperitoneum is?
A. Oxygen
B. Nitrogen
C. CO_2
D. N_2O
(JHARKHAND 2003)

Laparoscopic examination of pelvic organs is a well established procedure in cases of obscure pelvic pain; evaluation of pelvic mass; suspected ectopic pregnancy; testing the patency and assessing the pathology of fallopian tubes; and in diagnosing endometriosis. It is done under general anesthesia. The patient is put in Trendelenburg and lithotomy position and **pneumoperitoneum is created by using CO_2** with *Veer's* needle. Trocar with cannula is now inserted and laparoscope is passed after withdrawing the trocar. Optic fiber illumination is used to visualize pelvic organs.

290. Investigation of choice to demonstrate vesicoureteral reflex is:
A. Cystoscopy
B. IVP
C. Contrast MCU
D. Isotope cystogram
(AI 1992)

Voiding cystourethrography is of great value in the diagnosis of **vesicoureteral reflux** and bladder neck and urethral obstructions.

Ref: *Harrison's Principles of Internal Medicine; 14th edition*

291. Radiation therapy is given to a carcinoma patient. After 2 days the *most common* skin manifestation is:
A. Dermatitis
B. Hyperpigmentation
C. Atopy
D. Erythema
(AI 1998)

292. Earliest skin change noticed after irradiation is:
A. Erythema
B. Hyperpigmentation
C. Ulceration
D. Dryness
(SGPGI 1999)

Skin reaction can be seen within 2 weeks of radiotherapy. **Erythema** is observed, soon followed by desquamation.

Ref: *Harrison's Principles of Internal Medicine; 15th edition; page 2588*

293. *Most common* presentation of radiation carditis is:
- **A.** Pyogenic pericarditis
- **B.** Myocardial fibrosis
- **C.** Atheromatous plaques
- **D.** Pericardial effusion

(AI 1997)

Exposure of a large heart volume to high-dose radiation therapy accelerates the development of coronary artery disease. Acute pericarditis may result from cardiac irradiation. It is usually self-limited and manifests itself a few months after treatment. **Asymptomatic pericardial effusion is the *most common* manifestation of radiation-induced heart disease.**

Ref: *Harrison's Principles of Internal Medicine; 15th edition; page 2588 – 2589*

294. *Best* diagnostic test for deep vein thrombosis is:
- **A.** MRI
- **B.** Venography
- **C.** Impendence phlebography
- **D.** Duplex USG

(PGI 1997)

The only reliable way to detect deep vein thrombosis is by using an imaging investigation. **The test of choice is duplex ultrasonography as it is a noninvasive and hazard-free method of investigation.** For diagnosis of pulmonary embolism, enhanced helical CT-scanning is considered the standard test and is replacing isotope-imaging studies.

Ref: *Bailey and Love's Short Practice of Surgery; 23rd edition; page 253*

295. X-ray chest with reticular pattern, air bronchogram sign is seen in:
- **A.** Septicemia
- **B.** Bronchopulmonary dysplasia
- **C.** Pulmonary hypertension
- **D.** Respiratory distress syndrome

(PGI 1997)

The premature infant with **respiratory distress syndrome** will have clinical signs shortly after birth. These include tachypnea, retractions, flaring of the nasal alae, grunting and cyanosis. The classic radiographic appearance is of low volume lungs with a diffuse reticulogranular pattern and **air bronchograms**.

296. Intracavitary radiation is given in:
- **A.** Oral cavity carcinoma
- **B.** Esophageal carcinoma
- **C.** Lung carcinoma
- **D.** Cervix carcinoma

(AIIMS 1999)

Brachytherapy may consist of **intracavitary inserts**, used in the treatment of gynecologic malignancies such as **cervical** or vaginal carcinomas, or interstitial implants, such as those used for prostate carcinoma.

Ref: *Harrison's Principles of Internal Medicine; 14th edition*

297. On X-ray all the following renal calculi can be seen *except*:
- **A.** Calcium oxalate
- **B.** Triple phosphate
- **C.** Uric acid
- **D.** Cystine stones

(SGPGI 2002)

Pure uric acid stones are radiolucent and appear on an excretion urogram as a 'filling-defect'.

Ref: *Bailey and Love's Short Practice of Surgery; 23rd edition; page 1184*

298. In bone-scan, hot spots are seen in all the following *except*:
- **A.** Osteoblastic metastasis
- **B.** Multiple myeloma
- **C.** Osteomyelitis
- **D.** Bony lesions of hyperparathyroidism

(JIPMER 2002)

Radionucleotide scintigraphy provides useful information regarding the metabolic status of bone and is well suited for total-body assessment of the extent and distribution of musculoskeletal involvement. It is very sensitive but poorly specific means of detecting inflammatory or metabolic alterations in bone or periarticular soft tissue structures.

Ref: *Harrison's Principles of Internal Medicine; 15th edition; page 1983*

Increased activity in the bone phase could be due either to excessive isotope uptake in the osseous extracellular fluid or to more avid incorporation into newly forming bone tissue. Either can be seen in fracture, infection, a local tumor or healing after necrosis.

Ref: *Apley's System of Orthopedics and Fractures; 8th edition; page 20*

299. In a patient with solitary nodule of thyroid, investigation of choice is:

A. FNAC **B.** USG
C. CT **D.** Radioisotope scan *(JIPMER 2001)*

Fine needle aspiration cytology (FNAC) has become established as the *investigation of choice* in discrete **thyroid swellings**.

Ref: *Bailey and Love's Short Practice of Surgery; 23rd edition; page 716*

300. Which of following is the most radiosensitive phase of cell cycle?

A. G_1 **B.** S
C. G_2 **D.** M *(PGI 1997, JIPMER 2001, AIIMS Nov 2002)*

The cell cycle for mammalian cells can be divided into 4 phases: mitosis (M), followed by G_1, followed by the DNA synthetic phase (S), then G_2, and into mitosis again. In general, cells are most radiosensitive in late M and G_2 phases and most resistant in late S.

Ref: http://www.uic.edu/com/uhrd/manual/section3/section3.html

"The use of neo-adjuvant chemotherapy in patients with Stage II/III breast cancer allows us to analyze potential biological parameters, which may predict for response to therapy. Pre-clinical data has shown that paclitaxel leads to cell cycle arrest in M-phase and subsequent inhibition of tumor growth. Since **M-phase is the most radiosensitive portion of the cell cycle**, it is postulated that these changes could be used as potential markers of clinical outcome to neo-adjuvant paclitaxel/RT."

Ref: http://www.asco.org/ac/1,1003,_12-002326-00_18-002002-00_19-00271-00_29-00A,00.asp?cat=Adjuvant%20Therapy

For most cell lines, cells that have a short G_1 period are **most sensitive at the G_2/mitosis interface**, less sensitive in G_1, and most resistant toward the end of the synthesis (S) period.

Ref: *Harrison's Principles of Internal Medicine; 14th edition*

301. MRI rooms are shielded completely by a continuous sheet or wire mesh of copper or aluminum to shield the image from external electromagnetic radiations, etc., it is called:

A. Maxwell cage **B.** Faraday cage
C. Edison's cage **D.** Ohm's cage *(AIIMS Nov 2003)*

Mu-copper foil is used for electromagnetic shielding of rooms, buildings, tempest applications computer-rooms, EMC-test-sites, susceptibility measurements hospitals, MRI rooms, anechoic chambers, shielded enclosures, Faraday chambers, and other EMI/RFI appliances. With this material, which can be applied as wallpaper, an existing room can be transformed easily into a Faraday-cage with an attenuation level of 40 to 80 dB. For magnetic shielding, monitor protection and shielding of transformers and cable-trunks, mu-ferro plates are available.

Ref: *http://www.emishieldinggaskets.com/faraday_cage.htm*

302. A 45-year-old coal mine worker presents with:

A. Sjögren's syndrome **B.** Caplan's syndrome
C. Silicosis **D.** Wegener's granulomatosis *(AIIMS Nov 2003)*

A variety of pulmonary manifestations of rheumatoid arthritis can occur, including pleural disease (pleural effusion and subpleural nodules), parenchymal nodular infiltrates associated with pneumoconiosis in *miners* (**Caplan's syndrome**), and diffuse interstitial fibrosis.

Ref: *Harrison's Principles of Internal Medicine; 14th edition*

303. A patient is suspected to have vestibular schwannoma, the *investigation of choice* for its diagnosis is:

A. Contrast enhanced CT scan **B.** PET Scan
C. SPECT **D.** Gadolinium enhanced MRI *(AI 2004)*

MRI with gadolinium contrast is superior to CT-scan in diagnosing acoustic neuroma (8th nerve schwannoma or neurilemmoma).

Ref: *Diseases of Ear, Nose and Throat by PL Dhingra; 2nd edition; page 117*

304. In which of the following, a Coer-en-Sabot' shape of the heart is seen?

A. Tricuspid atresia **B.** Tetralogy of Fallot
C. Transposition of great arteries **D.** Ventricular septal defect *(AI 2004)*

RADIOGRAPHIC APPROACH

Characteristic configurations	
Coer en sabot	Right ventricular enlargement (tetralogy of Fallot)
Egg on a string	Anterior/posterior relationship of great vessels in transposition complexes
Snowman, figure 8	Anomalous drainage chamber in superior mediastinum of total anomalous pulmonary venous return

Ref: *http://www.indyrad.iupui.edu/rtf/teaching/medstudents/pedcard.htm*

305. In scurvy all of the following radiological signs are seen, *except*:

A. Zone of demarcation near epiphysis **B.** Soap bubble appearance
C. Frenkel's line **D.** Pelican spur *(AI 2004)*

Osteoclastoma or giant cell tumor is a common bone tumor with variable growth potential. The characteristic radiological feature of this tumor is **soap-bubble appearance.**

Ref: *Essential Orthopedics by J Maheshwari; 3rd edition; page 216*

306. A 50-year-old smoker male presents with pain along the left arm and ptosis:

A. Adenocarcinoma lung **B.** Bronchial carcinoid
C. Pancoast's tumor **D.** Bronchoalveolar carcinoma *(AIIMS Nov 2003)*

Pancoast's (or superior sulcus tumor) syndrome results from local extension of a tumor (usually epidermoid) growing in the apex of the lung with involvement of the 8th cervical and first and second thoracic nerves, with shoulder pain which characteristically radiates in the ulnar distribution of the arm, often with radiologic destruction of the first and second ribs.

Ref: *Harrison's Principles of Internal Medicine; 14th edition*

307. Sunray appearance on X-ray is suggestive of:

A. A chondrosarcoma **B.** A metastatic tumor in the bone
C. An osteogenic sarcoma **D.** An Ewing's sarcoma *(AIIMS May 2004)*

The typical X-ray appearance of **osteogenic sarcoma** of the mandible is that of an expansile sclerosing lesion. In some cases bone deposition at the periphery of a lesion will occur in a radial linear pattern, said to resemble that of **sunrays** on radiographs.

308. The *investigation of choice* for imaging of urinary tract tuberculosis is:

A. Plain X-ray **B.** IV urography
C. USG **D.** CT *(AIIMS May 2004)*

Tuberculosis of the urinary tract arises from hematogenous infection from a distant focus which is often 'impossible' to identify and the lesions are usually confined to one kidney. Renal tuberculosis usually occurs between 20 to 40 years of age and is 2-times more common in men than in women. Surprisingly right kidney is affected more often than the left. Frequency is the earliest symptom and may be the only one. **Intravenous urography: In the very earliest stages of the disease the normally clear-cut outline of a renal papilla may be rendered indistinct by the presence of ulceration.**

Ref: *Bailey and Love's Short Practice of Surgery; 23rd edition; page 1194 and 1195*

309. Which of the following technique uses piezoelectric crystals?

A. USG **B.** NMR imaging
C. X-ray diffraction **D.** Xeroradiography *(AIIMS Nov 2004)*

Piezoelectric effect is defined as appearance of an electric potential across certain faces of a crystal when it is subjected to mechanical pressure. Conversely, when an electric field is applied on certain faces of the crystal, the crystal undergoes mechanical distortion. Pierre Curie and his brother Jacques discovered the phenomenon in quartz and Rochelle salt in 1880 and named the effect piezoelectricity (from Greek *piezein,* "to press").The piezoelectric effect occurs in several crystalline substances, such as barium titanate and tourmaline. Because of their capacity to convert mechanical deformation into electric voltages, and electric voltages into mechanical motion, **piezoelectric crystals are used in such devices as the transducer in ultrasonography**, record-playing pickup elements, and the microphone. Piezoelectric crystals are also used as resonators in electronic oscillators and high-frequency amplifiers, because the mechanical resonance frequency of adequately cut crystals is stable and well-defined.

310. In which of the following conditions the lead pipe appearance of the colon on a barium enema is seen?

A. Amebiasis **B.** Ulcerative colitis
C. Tuberculosis of colon **D.** Crohn's involvement of the colon *(AIIMS Nov 2004)*

In **ulcerative colitis** fibrosis and longitudinal retraction result in shortening of the colon. Loss of the normal haustral pattern leads *radiologically* to a smooth, **"lead-pipe" appearance** of the colon.

311. The EEG cabins should be completely shielded by a continuous sheet of wire mesh of copper to avoid the picking up of noise from external electromagnetic disturbances. Such a shielding is called as:

A. Maxwell cage **B.** Faraday cage
C. Edison's cage **D.** Ohm's cage *(AIIMS Nov 2004)*

Electromagnetic interference particularly plays a role in areas where sensitive neurophysiological recordings are made for example electromyography, various types of evoked potential recordings and electroencephalograms (EEG). It is very important to shield such areas against electromagnetic interference from outside. This can be protected by the use of **Faraday's cage.**

312. The technique employed in radiotherapy to counteract the effect of tumor motion due to breathing is known as:

A. Arc technique **B.** Modulation
C. Gating **D.** Shunting *(AI 2005)*

A better solution in many cases has been **respiratory gating**, which involves tracking the patient's natural breathing cycle via computer and determining an algorithm to control radiation administration at the optimum moments—the "gate"—to deliver dose. The computer synchronizes the beam to switch on only when the target area is within the calculated parameters. The patient's respiration is continuously monitored and the beam switches off as the tumor moves out of the target range.

Ref: *http://www.radiologytoday.net/archive/rt_110804p33.shtml*

313. Gamma camera in 'Nuclear Medicine' is used for:

A. Organ imaging **B.** Measuring the radioactivity
C. Monitoring the surface contamination **D.** RIA *(AI 2005)*

The gamma camera is a device to scan patients who have been injected with small amounts of radioactive materials.

Ref: *http://www.umm.edu/radiology/nucmed.html*

314. In which one of the following conditions, the sialography is *contraindicated*?

A. Ductal calculus **B.** Chronic parotitis
C. Acute parotitis **D.** Recurrent sialadenitis *(AI 2005)*

Acute suppurative parotitis (ASP) is a bacterial infection of the parotid gland that occurs when decreased salivary flow allows for retrograde ascension of bacteria from Stenson's duct into the gland parenchyma. ASP is distinguished from viral parotitis, *most commonly* caused by the mumps virus, and chronic parotitis, which may be due to infectious, neoplastic, autoimmune, or systemic processes. *Sialography is contraindicated* in acute disease because the contrast can cause rupture of the duct as well as exacerbate the infection by pushing bacteria back into the gland.

Ref: *http://www.urmc.rochester.edu/smd/Rad/neurocases/Neurocase111.html*

315. Which of the following ultrasound marker is associated with greatest increased risk for trisomy 21 in fetus?

A. Echogenic foci in heat **B.** Hyperechogenic bowel
C. Choroid plexus cysts **D.** Nuchal edema *(AI 2005)*

There are a number of **ultrasound markers of Down's syndrome** at 15 to 22 weeks, of which **nuchal fold thickness is the most discriminatory on its own**, but not discriminatory enough for screening. The markers could be used in combination with the serum markers but no studies assessing this have been completed to date.

Ref: *http://www.ncchta.org/execsumm/summ201.html*

316. In computed tomography (CT), the attenuation values are measured in Hounsfield units (HU). An attenuation value of '0' (zero) HU corresponds to:

A. Water **B.** Air
C. Very dense bone structures **D.** Fat *(AIIMS Nov 2004)*

In CT scanning, a number or value that represents the attenuation of X-rays through a voxel (volume element) in the body and is assigned to the corresponding pixel (picture element) on the image. This number is relative to the standard, which is the absorption of X-rays in water. A CT number scale, called the Hounsfield scale, has been used to simplify the quantitative interpretation of CT data. The units of this scale are called **Hounsfield units** (HU). Thus, attenuation is expressed relative to water and air, because **water has a CT number of 0** and air has a CT number of –1000 (the attenuation coefficient of air is essentially 0) at all beam energies. Attenuation coefficients (CT numbers) are expressed in Hounsfield units (HU) and compared to each other according to the Hounsfield scale. Water is assigned the CT number 0; air, –1000; dense bone, between +1000 to +3000; soft tissue is in the range of +40 to +80.

317. The *most sensitive* imaging modality for diagnosing uretreic stones in a patient with acute colic is:

A. X-ray KUB region
B. Ultrasonogram
C. Noncontrast CT scan of the abdomen
D. Contrast enhanced CT scan of the abdomen *(AI 2005)*

Most urinary calculi are radiodense and visible on a plain abdominal radiograph. An IV urogram performed while the patient has pain can confirm the diagnosis. If the urogram is normal during an attack, the patient does not have renal colic.

Ref: *Bailey and Love's Short Practice of Surgery; 23rd edition; page 1189*

318. Which of the following is the *investigation of choice* for assessment of depth of penetration and perirectel nodes in rectal cancer?

A. Transrectal USG
B. CT scan of pelvis
C. MRI
D. Double contrast barium enema *(AIIMS Nov 2004)*

Evaluation of the pelvis by **magnetic resonance imaging** has been effective due to the absence of biologic motions and the superb tissue contrast afforded by pelvic fat. In addition, although the anatomic detail as seen on transaxial images is similar to CT, the multiplanar abilities of MRI for sagittal and coronal images are a distinct advantage when evaluating the rectum, especially for staging of rectal carcinoma. T_1-weighted spin echo (SE) images with repetition times (TR) of 500 millisecond and echo delay (TE) of 30 millisecond (SE 500/30) give the best contrast between tumor, tumor extension, fat, and lymph nodes when evaluating rectal cancer. Although neither modality (CT and MRI) can effectively evaluate the degree of bowel wall penetration or of tumor-containing lymph nodes MRI, like CT, can identify invasion into the perirectal fat as irregular, medium-signal-intensity areas extending directly from the primary tumor or as discrete foci surrounded by perirectal fat. Lymph nodes appear as round or oval low-signal-intensity areas in the perirectal fat. However, there is no difference in tissue characteristics that discriminates tumor-containing lymph nodes from hyperplastic lymph nodes.

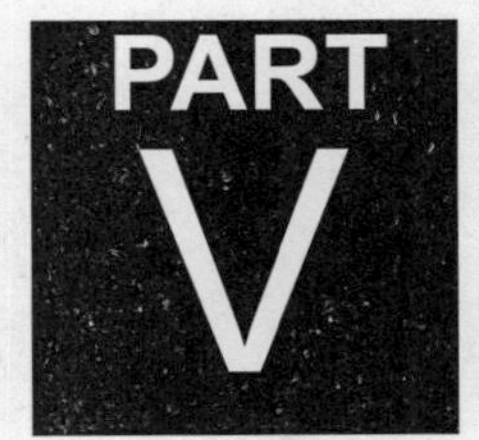

Psychiatry

Psychiatry

1. **An 18-year-old boy hears voices discussing him in third person. He is suffering from:**
   A. Schizophrenia
   B. Mania
   C. Depression
   D. TLE

2. ***Not* a classical 4 'As' of Bleuler in schizophrenia:**
   A. Affective blunting
   B. Automatism
   C. Autism
   D. Ambivalence
   (AI 1991)

3. ***Not* a feature of Schizophrenia:**
   A. Anhedonia
   B. Autochthonous delusion
   C. Elated mood
   D. Hallucination

4. **Neologism is a characteristic feature of:**
   A. OCN
   B. Mania
   C. Schizophrenia
   D. All of the above

5. **Loss of insight occurs in:**
   A. Somatoform disorder
   B. OCN
   C. Schizophrenia
   D. Hysteria

6. ***Not* a first order rank symptom of schizophrenia:**
   A. Somatic passivity
   B. Primary delusion
   C. Running commentary
   D. Depersonalization
   (AI 1998)

7. **Delusions are characteristically seen in which of the following condition:**
   A. Depression
   B. Dementia
   C. Delirium
   D. Schizophrenia
   (AI 1993)

8. **A 25-year-old man who lives alone has developed suspicious behavior towards his neighbor. He also has "auditory hallucinations" and lodges a FIR which he himself was not able to prove. Symptoms are present for last two years. *Most likely* diagnosis is:**
   A. Acute psychosis
   B. Mania
   C. Schizophrenia
   D. Depression
   (AIIMS 2001)

9. **Ambivalence is associated with which of the following condition:**
   A. Schizophrenia
   B. Hysteria
   C. Depression
   D. OCN
   (PGI 1999)

10. **A 22-year-old single unmarried man is suffering from sudden onset of *3rd person hallucinations* for the past 2 weeks. He is suspicious of his family members and had decreased sleep and appetite. The diagnosis is:**
    A. Schizophrenia
    B. Acute psychosis
    C. Acute mania
    D. Delirium
    (AIIMS May 2001)

Schizophrenia has puzzled philosophers, physicians and people alike for centuries. 1% of world's population suffers from schizophrenia. In 1896 *Emil Kraepelin* classified major psychiatric diseases into two groups' viz. **dementia precox** and **manic depressive psychosis (MDP).** Under the dementia precox he put various psychiatric diseases which were earlier thought to be distinct diseases having poor outcome and recognized *delusions, hallucinations, disturbances of affect and motor disturbances.* **Eugen Bleuler (1857–1939) was a Swiss psychiatrist who renamed dementia precox as schizophrenia (mental splitting).** He further noticed that this disorder *did not always* have a poor prognosis. The **fundamental symptoms** or the **classical 4 As** described by Bleuler are as under:

Ambivalence	Severe inability to decide for or against something
Autism	Withdrawal into self
Affect disturbances	Inappropriate affect
Association disturbances	Thought disorder

Accessory symptoms *as described by Bleuler* are delusions, hallucinations, negativism, etc. The fundamental symptoms were thought to be diagnostic of schizophrenia.

Kurt Schneider described certain symptoms which, *although not specific,* are of great help in making a clinical diagnosis of schizophrenia. These are described as under:

First rank symptoms (FRS) of schizophrenia

- **Hallucinations of 3 types**: Audible thoughts or "thought echoes"; voices are heard arguing something, i.e. *2 or more hallucinatory voices discussing the subject in third person;* and voices commenting on the patient's action.
- **Delusion of 6 types**: Thought withdrawal (*thoughts stop and patient experiences them as being removed by some external force); thought insertion (patient experiences thoughts imposed by some external force on his passive mind)*; thought diffusion or "broadcasting" *(patient experiences that his thoughts are escaping the confines of his self and are being known to others around him)*; "made" feelings (affect), impulses or volition of acts *(patient experiences that feelings, impulses or actions are imposed by some external force and in "made" volition he thinks that his own acts are under the control of some external force and the subject is like a robot.*
- **Delusional perception**
- **Somatic passivity,** i.e. body sensation (sensory symptoms) imposed on body by external force.

Second rank symptoms (SRS) of schizophrenia

Other forms of hallucinations, affect disturbances and perplexity (to make a *person* uncertain, doubtful, or hesitant; confused; puzzled).

Clinical features: One of the most important symptoms of schizophrenia is that the thinking is governed by private and illogical rules (**autistic thinking**). The patient with *autistic thinking* may consider the two different things identical if they have identical predicates or properties (*Von Domarus law*). For example *Bill Gates has got a computer, I have also got a computer, and therefore I am Bill Gates or Amir Khan drinks coca cola, I also drink coca cola, therefore I am Amir Khan.* There is **loosening of associations,** i.e. things said in juxtaposition lack a meaningful relation with each other and this type of speech is often described as *disjointed*. If this *loosening* becomes severe speech becomes incomprehensible and is known as **incoherence.** There is a sudden interruption of speech *before the thought is completed* (**thought blocking**) although this can be seen in complex partial seizure (temporal lobe epilepsy). After *the pause* the patient *can not recall* what he meant to say. The patient *creates* new words and phrases to express a *concept* for which he has no dictionary words (**neologism**). *Sometimes* "normal" words are used in a distorted or unconventional fashion (**word approximation or paraphasias**), although the meaning can be understood; for example *describing stomach as a fuel tank.* There may be no speech production at all (**mutism**); decreases speech production (**poverty of speech**); amount of speech is adequate but it conveys *little* information (**poverty of ideation**); repetition or "echoing" of words or phrases of the psychiatrists by the patient (**echolalia**); *persistent* repetition of words beyond any relevance (**perseveration**) or senseless repetition of same word or phrases again and again (**verbigeration**). **Delusions** may be defined as *false and firm believes which is not in line with patient's socioculture and educational background.* Delusions may be of two types viz. primary and secondary. **Primary delusions are also known as autochthonous** (indigenous) **delusions and are characteristic of schizophrenia.** They are seen in *early* stages of the disorder and arise *de novo,* i.e. cannot be explained on the basis of other experiences or perceptions. **Secondary delusions are the most common delusions seen in clinical practice and are *not* diagnostic of schizophrenia.** The common secondary delusions are delusions of persecution (*being persecuted*);

delusions of reference (*being referred to by other people*); delusions of grandeur; delusions of control (*controlled by known or unknown external forces*) and hypochondrial (*abnormal anxiety over one's health, often with imaginary illnesses*) or somatic delusions. **Over-inclusion** (*inclusion of irrelevant items in speech*); **impaired abstract** (*loss of ability to generalize things*); **ambivalence** (simultaneous conflicting feelings toward a person or thing, as love and hate); **perplexity** (the condition of being perplexed; bewilderment; confusion) are other **thought and speech disorders** associated with schizophrenia. **Disorder of perception** seen in schizophrenia is hallucination which means *perception without stimulus.* **Auditory hallucination is the most common hallucination seen in schizophrenia.** *Only the third person hallucinations* (voices heard arguing) *are characteristic of schizophrenia.* Visual hallucinations can also occur along with the auditory hallucination but tactile, gustatory and olfactory hallucinations are far less common. **Disorders of affect** include emotional blunting and shallowness, apathy, anhedonia (*inability to experience pleasure*) and inappropriate emotional response. This inability of the patient to establish emotional contacts with others leads to **lack of rapport with the psychiatrist. Disorders of motor behavior** may manifest as *either* a decrease in psychomotor activity (stupor, inertia) *or* an increase (*aggression, agitation, restlessness, excitement*). Mannerisms, grimacing, stereotypes (*repetitive strange behavior*), reduced self care and poor grooming are common features. There is decreased functioning in work place, loss of ego boundaries (between self and environment), uncertainty about ones own identity and existence. **Insight into the illness is absent but there is no disturbance of consciousness, orientation, attention, memory and intelligence.**

Clinical types of schizophrenia		
• **Catatonic**	• **Paranoid**	• **Hebephrenic**
• **Residual**	• **Undifferentiated**	• **Others**

Catatonic and hebephrenic schizophrenia together are known as *nuclear schizophrenia*. Catatonic schizophrenia is characterized by disturbance of motor behavior (*cata means disturbed; tonic means tone*). PFROPF SCHIZOPHRENIA occurs in presence of mental retardation (IQ < 70).
Catatonic-type describes patients whose clinical presentation is dominated by profound changes in motor activity, negativism, and echolalia or echopraxia.
Paranoid-type describes patients who have a prominent preoccupation with a specific delusional system and who otherwise do not qualify as having *disorganized-type* disease, in which disorganized speech and behavior are accompanied by a superficial or silly affect.
In **residual-type** disease, negative symptomatology exists in the absence of delusions, hallucinations, or motor disturbance.
The diagnosis of **schizophreniform disorder** is reserved for patients who meet the symptom requirements but not the duration requirements for schizophrenia, and that of *schizoaffective disorder* is used for those whose symptoms of schizophrenia are independent of associated periods of mood disturbance.
Positive symptoms of schizophrenia are those symptoms which are *added* to the clinical picture, i.e. delusion, hallucination, agitation, etc.
Negative symptoms of schizophrenia are those symptoms which are *subtracted* from the clinical picture, i.e. social withdrawal, apathy, anhedonia, poverty of thoughts, etc.

11. In schizophrenia, bad prognostic factor is:
A. Presence of depression
B. Fat patient
C. Family history
D. Late onset
(UP 1996)

12. Good prognostic factor for schizophrenia is:
A. Chronic course
B. Catatonic features
C. Early onset
D. Gradual onset
(SGPGI 1999)

13. *Not* a bad prognostic factor of schizophrenia:
A. Early onset
B. Family history
C. Presence of precipitating factor
D. Insidious onset
(KERALA 1999)

Prognosis of Schizophrenia

Favorable prognostic features	Poor prognostic features
Acute onset	Gradual onset
Onset after 35 years of age	Onset before 25 years of age
Short duration (less than 6 months)	Long duration (more than 2 years)
Precipitation by environmental or physical factors	Absence of precipitating factors
Good pre-disease adjustment	Poor pre-disease adjustment
Depression present	Depression absent
Fat physique	Thin physique
History of previous attacks from which recovery has occurred	Family history of schizophrenia
Catatonic or paranoid subtypes	Undifferentiated, hebephrenic or chronic catatonic subtypes

14. *Absolute* contraindication for ECT is:
A. Heart disease
B. Raised ICT
C. Very ill patient
D. Pregnancy
(AI 1992, UP 1997))

15. *Most common* side effect of modified ECT is:
A. Convulsions
B. Body aches
C. Amnesia
D. Arrhythmia
(AI 1992)

16. ECT causes:
A. Retrograde amnesia
B. Anterograde amnesia
C. Both
D. None

17. ECT is most effective in:
A. Parkinsonism
B. OCN
C. Paranoid syndrome
D. Neurotic depression

18. ECT is *not* indicated in:
A. Catatonic schizophrenia
B. Acute depression
C. Obsessive compulsive neurosis
D. Acute mania
(UP 1995)

19. Memory disturbance of ECT recovers after:
A. Few days-few weeks
B. They are permanent
C. Few weeks–few months
D. Few months–few years

20. ECT is useful in treatment of all of the following *except*:
A. Acute psychosis
B. Endogenous depression
C. Chronic schizophrenia
D. Catatonic schizophrenia
(AI 1993)

21. A 36-year-old girl has no interest in anything, nihilistic attitude, sad appearance with suicidal ideas and plans. She should be managed with:
A. ECT
B. Antidepressants
C. Behavior therapy
D. Haloperidol
(AIIMS 2001)

22. Treatment of choice in a patient of depression with suicidal tendency:
A. ECT
B. MAO inhibitors
C. Tricyclic antidepressant
D. Fluoxetine
(AI 1994)

23. A 26-year-old female diagnosed to be suffering from depression, now for the past 2 days had suicidal tendencies, thoughts and ideas. The best treatment is:

A. Amitryptiline **B.** Selegiline
C. Haloperidol + Chlorpromazine **D.** ECT *(AIIMS May 2001)*

24. Absolute contraindication for ECT is:

A. Myocardial disease **B.** Aortic aneurysm
C. Glaucoma **D.** Brain tumor

Cerletti and Bini used **electro convulsive therapy** (ECT) for the first time in 1938. In 1976 American Psychiatric Association (APA) task force on ECT declared it to be a safe and effective method of treatment by professionals trained in the technique and gave guideline for its use. **Unilateral ECT is safer than the bilateral ECT and carries much less side effects mainly those of memory impairment** *but* the bilateral ECT is superior to unilateral ECT in *effectiveness*. **Direct ECT** is given in the *absence* of muscle relaxant and GA and is only *rarely* used. **Modified ECT** is given with drug (suxamethonium) induced muscle relaxation and anesthesia (thiopentone sodium).

Indications of ECT

1. **Major severe depression**
   - With suicidal risk **(first and most important indication for ECT)**
   - With stupor
   - With poor intake of fluids and food
   - With melancholia
   - With psychotic features
   - With unsatisfactory response to drug therapy
   - When drugs are contraindicated or have serious side effects
   - When fast recovery is needed
2. **Severe catatonia (functional)**
   - With stupor
   - With poor intake of fluids and food
   - With unsatisfactory response to drug therapy
   - When drugs are contraindicated or have serious side effects
   - When fast recovery is needed
3. **Severe psychosis (schizophrenia or mania)**
   - With risk of suicide, homicide or danger of physical assault
   - With unsatisfactory response to drug therapy
   - When drugs are contraindicated or have serious side effects
   - With very prominent depressive features
4. **Organic mental disorders**
   - Organic mood syndrome
   - Organic psychotic syndrome
   - Delirium
5. **Medical disorders**
   - Organic catatonia
   - Hypopituitarism
   - Intractable seizure disorders
   - Neuroleptic malignant syndrome
   - Parkinsonism

Contraindications of ECT

Absolute contraindications	**Relative contraindications**
• Raised intracranial tension	• Recent myocardial infarction • Cerebrovascular accident (CVA) • Severe hypertension • Severe lung disease • Retinal detachment • Pheochromocytoma

Adverse effects of ECT
• Death • Memory disturbances (both anterograde and retrograde) are **very common** and **recovery occurs within 1–6 months of ECT** • Confusion is much common with bilateral ECT • Headache, apnea, prolonged seizures, CVS dysfunctions, mania, muscle pains and apprehension for further ECT are other side effects

* **ECT does not cause brain damage.**

25. *Not* seen in attention deficit hyperactivity disorder (ADHD):
A. Mental retardation **B.** Impulsivity
C. Less attention in study **D.** Hyperactivity *(UP 1997)*

26. *Not* seen in hyperkinetic child:
A. Soft neurological signs **B.** Left to right disorientation
C. Decreased attention span **D.** Aggressive out burst *(AI 1991)*

27. *Not* a feature of hyperkinetic child:
A. Amphetamine is the drug of choice **B.** Right to left dissociation
C. Low attention span **D.** Difficulty in completing tasks *(JIPMER 1991)*

28. Attention deficiency disorder is seen with which of the following drug:
A. Phenobarbitone **B.** Amphetamine
C. Low doses benzodiazepine **D.** Cocaine *(JIPMER 1991)*

29. An 11-year-old child was found to be very restless and hyperactive in the classroom making it difficult for the other students in the classroom to concentrate. He runs round the class all the day cannot sit at one place for a long time. He gets very agitated when the toy in his hand is taken away. The *most probable* diagnosis is:
A. Autism
B. Conduct disorder
C. Attention deficit hyperactivity disorder
D. Conversion *(AI 2002)*

The main symptoms of **attention deficit hyperactivity disorder (ADHD)** are short attention span, difficulty in concentration, impulsivity, distractibility, excitability and hyperactivity. *Hyperactivity* is defined as *an increase in motor activity to a level which interferes with the child's functioning at school, at home and in society.* It is important to remember that *the symptoms of ADHD may exist with or without hyperactivity.* The *Diagnostic and Statistical Manual of Mental Disorders 4th edition* (DMS–IV) divides it into 3 subtypes:
- ADHD–predominantly inattentive type;
- ADHD–predominantly hyperactive-impulsive type;
- ADHD–combined type.

Diagnostic criteria for ADHD

Inattention	Hyperactivity	Impulsivity
Lack of attention to details	Excessive talking	Answering without raising hand
Difficulty in *sustaining* attention for prolonged period	Difficulty in performing "non action" activities	Answering before the end of the question
Not listening	Difficulty in remaining in seat and sitting quietly	Difficulty with "turn taking" activities
Difficulty in completing tasks	Restlessness	Interruption or intrusion into other peoples conversations or activities.

Disorganization	Developmentally excessive activity level
Forgetfulness	
Marked distractibility	
Tendency to loose personal belongings	
Avoidance of activity that require sustained attention	
Some symptoms should be present before 7 years of age and must be causing significant functional impairment.	
Sedative and hypnotic drugs (*paradoxical effect*), depression, anxiety, head injury, serious CNS disease, constitutional hyperactivity, intolerant parent, teacher or supervisor, specific language disabilities, language disorders and Tourette syndrome can all lead to ADHD.	
Any underlying disorder should be treated and stimulant medications such as methylphenidate, dextroamphetamine and pemoline are effective. Clonidine, desipramine and bupropion are alternative effective drug in some children. Behavior modification programs, psychotherapy and environmental engineering are all beneficial.	
Due to normal developmental activity, diagnosis may be difficult in children under 5 years of age. In children at least 5 years old, "soft signs" may appear early and suggest the presence of ADHD. These soft signs of the neurological system include the following: • Coordination difficulty • Impaired motor skills • Nystagmus (i.e. constant, involuntary movement of eyes) • Visual motor problem (e.g. hand eye coordination) When observed collectively, these symptoms can suggest a diagnosis of ADHD.	

30. *Most common* complication of obsessive compulsive disorder is:
- **A.** Mania
- **B.** Dissociation of symptoms
- **C.** Persecutory delusions
- **D.** Depression

31. *False* regarding obsessive compulsive neurosis is:
- **A.** Insight is present
- **B.** Ego syntonic
- **C.** Patient tries to resist against ego
- **D.** Ego alien

(AI 1995)

32. *Not* a characteristic feature of obsessive compulsive neurosis:
- **A.** Excessive slowness
- **B.** Sexual thoughts
- **C.** Repeated hand washing
- **D.** Elaborate checking

(PGI 1993)

33. Drug *not* used in obsessive compulsive neurosis is:
- **A.** Lithium
- **B.** Haloperidol
- **C.** Fluoxetine
- **D.** Clomipramine

(UP 2001)

34. *Not* a feature of obsessive compulsive neurosis:
- **A.** Persistence
- **B.** Resisting the idea
- **C.** Ego-syntonic
- **D.** Irrational thoughts

(AI 1993)

35. In obsessive compulsive neurosis, the *drug of choice* is:
- **A.** Lithium
- **B.** Fluphenazine
- **C.** Clomipramine
- **D.** Chlorpromazine

(UP 1994, AI 1994, 1995, 1996, 1998)

36. A woman complains that she feels like abusing god and slap a gentleman. The thoughts persist in spite of her not willing to do so. She is suffering from:

A. Conversion disorder
B. Hypochondriasis
C. Somatization
D. Obsessive compulsive disorder *(AI 2000)*

37. Delusions are seen in all the following *except*:

A. Obsessive compulsive disorder
B. Depression
C. Mania
D. Schizophrenia *(AI 2002)*

Obsessive compulsive disorder (OCD): An obsession may be defined as an "idea", "impulse", or an "image" which intrudes into the conscious awareness time and again. The idea is patient's own but is **ego alien,** i.e. foreign to the patient's personality and is **recognized as absurd and irrational by the patient** (**insight is present**) who tries to resist against it but is unable to do so. This failure to resist leads to marked distress. *In contrast* the *delusion* is ones own idea but is not "recognized" as ego alien, hence the patient never thinks it to be irrational and is never resisted. The "**obsession**" is associated with "**compulsion**" which is a form of *behavior* that *follows* the obsession. The aim of compulsion is to prevent or *neutralize* the distress or fear aroused by obsession. The behavior caused by compulsion is unrealistic and is *irrational* or *excessive*. As the insight is present the patient *also realizes the irrationality of compulsion.* In our country OCD is common in unmarried men of upper social strata with high intelligence and the average age of onset is in late twenties. *Insel* in 1985 described **4 clinical syndromes**, although "mixture" is common than pure syndromes. **The *most common* type of patients of OCD are "washers".** There is obsession of *contamination* with dirt, germs, and body secretions and, naturally, the compulsion is *washing* of hands or whole body several times in a day. As the condition progresses it "spreads" to washing of clothes, bathroom, bedroom, door knobs and even any article, although the patient tries to avoid "contamination" but is unable to do so and the washing becomes a *ritual.* The SECOND types of patients are "**checkers**" who have multiple *doubts* about lock in the door, kitchen gas knob, and counting of money. The *compulsion*, naturally, is repeated *checking* to "clear" the *doubt.* Any attempt to stop the *checking* leads to *anxiety*. The tragedy is that even before one *doubt* is *cleared* the other creeps in. The THIRD syndrome is "**pure obsession**" characterized by repeated intrusive thoughts, impulses or even images *not* associated with compulsion. The distress caused by these obsessions is *dealt* with *counter thoughts.* A variant of this syndrome is *thought rumination* in which there is **preoccupation with thoughts**. The FOURTH and relatively rare syndrome is that of *primary obsessive slowness* characterized by severe obsession and extensive compulsion *without anxiety* leading to marked slowness in daily activities. **Depression is commonly associated with obsessive compulsive disorder and at least 50% of patients have major depressive episode while the others have mild depression.**

Behavior therapy has a success rate of 80% for compulsive acts. **Anti-depressants such as clomipramine and selective serotonin reuptake inhibitors (SSRIs) are affective in OCD even in absence of co-existing depression.**

- **Ego-syntonic means something that is consistent with the individual's self-image.**

38. Best use of lithium is in:

A. Treatment of schizophrenia
B. Treatment of recurrent depression
C. Treatment of first depressive episode
D. Prophylaxis of bipolar mood disorders *(SGPGI 1999)*

39. In bipolar manic disorder, the drug used is:

A. Amitriptyline
B. Pimozide
C. Phenytoin
D. Lithium *(UP 1996)*

40. In manic depressive psychosis, prophylaxis is:

A. Haloperidol
B. Sodium valproate
C. Chlorpromazine
D. Lithium carbonate *(AI 1996)*

Lithium is indicated as the **primary drug in the treatment of acute manic and hypomanic episodes in bipolar disorder**, and for *maintenance therapy* to help reduce the intensity and frequency of subsequent manic episodes in patients with a history of mania.

41. A woman has a car accident in which she suffered minor injuries but the driver of the car died on spot. Six months after this accident she still feels afraid of cars and avoids traveling in cars. She is suffering from:
A. Schizophrenia
B. Delusion
C. Traveling phobia
D. Post-traumatic stress disorder *(AI 2000)*

42. Post traumatic stress syndrome is because of:
A. Vascular accident
B. Major life threatening events
C. Minor stress
D. Head injury *(AI 1998)*

43. A 40-year-old woman had an accident while traveling in a bus. She has a fracture of pelvis and remained in the hospital for a long time. Now she refuses to sit in a bus. Diagnosis is:
A. Phobia
B. Conversion disorder
C. Post-traumatic stress disorder
D. Anxiety neurosis *(AI 2001)*

Post-traumatic stress disorder (PTSD) is seen after a catastrophic event in a person's or a close friend or relative's life which is usually life threatening or potentially fatal (war, robbery, accident, earthquake, riot, etc.). It is essential for diagnosing the PTSD that symptoms must be of more than one month duration. 50% patients recover completely within 3 months while others may have symptoms for years. Features of PTSD are as under:

Avoidance	**Intrusion**	**Hyperarousal**
Detachment	Recurrent distressing dreams	Irritability
Survivor's guilt	"Flash backs"	Insomnia
Low interest in activities	Difficulty in recalling stressful events at will	Persistent anxiety
Inability to feel emotions		Poor coordination
Avoidance of reminder of events		

44. In delirium tremens, the *drug of choice* is:
A. Diazepam **B.** Morphine
C. Disulfiram **D.** Chlordiazepoxide *(AI 1993, 1995)*

45. *Not* a feature of alcohol withdrawal:
A. Hallucination **B.** Restlessness
C. Epileptic seizure **D.** Hypersomnolence *(AI 1998)*

46. A 42-year-old alcoholic man has an accident. After that he suddenly stops drinking. 24 hours after this he developed tremors, irritability, poor attention span and inability to identify his family members. Most likely diagnosis is:
A. Acute psychosis **B.** Alcohol intoxication
C. Delirium tremens **D.** Wernicke's encephalopathy *(AIIMS 2001)*

47. A known alcoholic stops taking alcohol for 2 days. After which he develops insomnia, altered sensorium, restlessness. The diagnosis is most likely to be:
A. Delirium tremens
B. Korsakoff's psychosis
C. Conversion
D. Schizophrenia *(AI 2002)*

Sudden decrease in alcohol intake may cause symptoms of withdrawal from the central nervous system depressant effects. Clinical features include a tremor of the hands (*shakes or jitters*); autonomic nervous system abnormalities such as tachycardia, tachypnoea, and fever; insomnia, may be accompanied by bad dreams; feelings of generalized anxiety or panic attacks; and GI upset. Symptoms start within 5 to 10 hours of decreasing ethanol intake, peak in intensity on day 2 or 3, and improve by day 4 or 5. Anxiety, insomnia, and mild levels of autonomic dysfunction may persist for even 6 months or more as a **protracted abstinence syndrome**, which may result in the tendency to return to drinking. A small number of alcoholics also demonstrate one or two generalized seizures (**"rum fits"**), usually within 48 hours of stopping drinking. About 5 % or less of alcoholics in withdrawal show severe symptoms such as **delirium tremens** which is **a state of confusion sometimes accompanied by visual, tactile, or auditory hallucinations.** The **benzodiazepines** (diazepam) have the highest margin of safety and are, therefore, the preferred class of drugs in the treatment of alcohol withdrawal.

48. *Not* a feature of morphine withdrawal:
- **A.** Increased nasal secretion
- **B.** Constipation
- **C.** Insomnia
- **D.** Piloerection

49. *Not* a feature of opioid withdrawal:
- **A.** Miosis
- **B.** Rhinorrhea
- **C.** Lacrimation
- **D.** Diarrhea

(AI 1993)

Symptoms of Opioid Withdrawal

- **Lacrimation**
- Sweating
- Tachycardia
- Fever
- Severe anxiety
- **Rhinorrhea**
- **Diarrhea**
- Mild hypertension
- Muscle cramps
- **Piloerection**
- **Pupillary dilatation**
- Yawning
- **Insomnia** and anorexia
- Generalized body ache
- Nausea and vomiting

50. Epileptic fits are distinguished from hysterical fits by:
- **A.** Amnesia
- **B.** Sleep convulsion
- **C.** Incontinence
- **D.** Injury

(UP 1996)

Difference Between Generalized Seizure and Hysterical Fits

	Generalize seizure	**Hysterical fit**
Pattern of attack	Known clinical patterns	No pattern
Place of event	Any where	Outdoors or safe places
Warning sign	Aura may be present	Variable
Time	Anytime	**Never during sleep**
Tongue bite	Present	Absent
Urinary and fecal incontinence	Can occur	Very rare
Injury	Can occur	Very rare
Speech	Not present	May be present
Duration	Usually short	Prolonged
Neurological sign	Present	Absent
Amnesia	Complete	Partial
Post ictal confusion	Present	Absent
Stress	Seen in 25% cases	Much more common
Head turning	Unilateral	Side to side
Eye gaze	Staring	Avoidant gaze

51. Mini mental scale is:
A. Method to investigate common psychiatric problem
B. 30 questions for cognitive function
C. To evaluate schizophrenia
D. Instrument to measure delirium *(JIPMER 2002)*

I. **Indications of minimental scale**
   A. Cognitive Function Assessment
   B. Documentation of subsequent cognitive function decline
II. **Questions (Total of 30 points)**
   A. Orientation (10 points)
      1. Year, Season, Date, Day of week, and Month
      2. State, County, Town or City
      3. Hospital or clinic, Floor
   B. Registration (3 points)
      1. Name three objects: Apple, Table, Penny
      2. Each one spoken distinctly and with brief pause
      3. Patient repeats all three (one point for each)
      4. Repeat process until all three objects learned
      5. Record number of trials needed to learn all 3 objects
   C. Attention and Calculation (5 points)
      1. Spell WORLD backwards: DLROW
      2. Points given up to first misplaced letter
      3. Example: DLORW scored as 2 points only
   D. Recall (3 points)
      1. Recite the 3 objects memorized in Registration above
   E. Language (9 points)
      1. Patient names two objects when they are displayed
         a. Example: Pencil and Watch (1 point each)
      2. Repeat a sentence: 'No ifs ands or buts'
      3. Follow three stage command
         a. Take a paper in your right hand
         b. Fold it in half
         c. Put it on the floor
      4. Read and obey the following
         a. Close your eyes
         b. Write a sentence
         c. Copy the design (picture of 2 overlapped pentagons)
III. **Interpretation of Mini-mental State Score (Maximum: 30)**
   A. Normal score: 24 or higher
   B. Educational and Age Norms
      1. Fourth Grade Education
         a. Ages 18 to 69: Median MMSE Score 22-25
         b. Ages 70 to 79: Median MMSE Score 21-22
         c. Age over 79: Median MMSE Score 19-20
      2. Eighth Grade Education
         a. Ages 18 to 69: Median MMSE Score 26-27
         b. Ages 70 to 79: Median MMSE Score 25
         c. Age over 79: Median MMSE Score 23-25
      3. High School Education
         a. Ages 18 to 69: Median MMSE Score 28-29
         b. Ages 70 to 79: Median MMSE Score 27
         c. Age over 79: Median MMSE Score 25-26
      4. College Education
         a. Ages 18 to 69: Median MMSE Score 29
         b. Ages 70 to 79: Median MMSE Score 28
         c. Age over 79: Median MMSE Score 27

52. All are *false* regarding schizophrenia *except*:
A. Seen in affluent society
B. Seen in old people
C. Seen in primitive society
D. Common in low socioeconomic strata *(PGI 2000)*

Schizophrenia is more common in lower socioeconomic status. CT scan of brain demonstrates enlarged ventricles in chronic schizophrenia probably due to functional increase in dopamine at the post synaptic receptor.

53. Psychoanalysis was founded by which of the following scientist:
A. Eysenck
B. Freud
C. Jung
D. Adler *(KARNATAKA 2000)*

Psychoanalysis is a specific method of investigating unconscious mental processes and is a form of psychotherapy. The term also refers to the systematic structure of psychoanalytic theory, which is based on the relation of conscious and unconscious psychological processes. The technique of psychoanalysis and much of the psychoanalytic theory based on its application was developed by **Sigmund Freud.**

54. In which of the following disorder 'La belle indifférence' is seen:
A. Depersonalization disorder
B. Obsessive compulsive disorder
C. Phobia
D. Conversion disorder

55. *False* regarding conversion reaction is:
A. Symbolic relationship with stress
B. Patient does not consciously produce sign, symptom
C. Onset is late
D. Secondary gain

In **conversion disorder** there is unconscious *conversion* of a psychological conflict into a loss of physical function *suggesting* a neurological or other disease. The symptom is *temporary* and related to a psychological *stressor.* An additional psychiatric diagnosis such as adjustment disorder, schizophrenia or personality disorder can be made in 50% of patients. Conversion disorders are also seen in patients with *real* physical diseases. **'La belle indifférence'** in which the patient shows *little* concern for the symptoms is sometimes present. However, 'La belle indifférence' alone is not a reliable sign of conversion because a patient with a physical illness may be unmoved about his condition. **Modeling,** in which the patient unconsciously imitates the symptoms observed in *important* individuals in their life is common. Although most of the times it is a *transient* disorder sometimes it can have a chronic course resulting in significant disability. The symptoms are *inconsistent* with known diseases and patient classically presents with **an acute loss of function** suggesting a neurological disease. The symptoms are bizarre but the common symptoms are given below:

- Anesthesias and paresthesias
- "Paralysis"
- Aphonia
- Fainting
- Gait disturbances
- Unconsciousness and "seizures"
- Vomiting
- Blindness and tunnel vision

Conversion disorder is more common in low socioeconomic classes and the *usual* age group is around adolescence *but* it can occur at any age. It commonly occurs in girls although boys are sometimes also affected. It is purely a psychological disorder and two mechanisms have been described to explain the **"gains"** experienced by the patients. The **primary gain** is that the internal conflict is kept from consciousness and the **secondary gain** is reinforcement from the environment (*avoiding unpleasant duties due to "symptoms"*). Other "advantage" is that the less powerful individual (patient) gains "control" over her environment by the *display* of "symptoms". The symptoms are **learned** and then **reinforced** by the **reaction of the caretakers and parents.** A good prognosis is associated with an acute onset after an *obvious* stressful precipitant and good pre morbid functioning.

Treatment: The stressful events in the patient's life should be *evaluated* followed by appropriate *intervention* (psychotherapy or family therapy). Any associated psychiatric illness (such as depression), *if present*, should be treated by drugs or psychotherapy. Telling the patient that the symptoms are psychological is *not* helpful. *Some* patients understand the symbolic aspect of the symptom and gain conscious mastery of the conflict but *most* of them are receptive to the explanation that *the disorder is a reaction to stress* and the reassurance that *the condition will resolve over time*. These interventions allow the patient to let go off symptoms without losing face.

56. Déjà vu is seen in:
A. Temporal lobe epilepsy
B. Normal person
C. Psychosis
D. All of the above
(KERALA 1994)

57. Unfamiliarity of familiar things is seen in:
A. Déjà vu
B. Jamais vu
C. Déjà entendu
D. Déjà pence
(KERALA 1999, JIPMER 2002)

- **Déjà vu feelings are defined as those in which unfamiliar situations feel 'strangely' familiar.** It may occur as a normal phenomenon and is also associated with several forms of epilepsy and schizophrenia.
- **Jamais vu** are those feelings in which the familiar situations are perceived unfamiliar. Apart from schizophrenia it also occurs in epilepsy.
- **Déjà entendu** is the illusion that what one is hearing was heard previously.

58. Methadone is indicated in:
A. Opioid overdose
B. Opioid dependence
C. Opioid withdrawal
D. Alcohol withdrawal
(UP 1999)

59. *False* regarding opiate withdrawal syndrome:
A. Characterized by body pain
B. Characterized by dilatation of pupils
C. Treated with naltrexone
D. Treated with methadone
(SGPGI 1999)

Detoxification is the **mode of treatment of opioid withdrawal** in which the addicted person is *taken off* opioids by abrupt withdrawal and use of **substitution drugs** like **methadone.**

60. *True* regarding confabulation is:
A. Making stories to fill up gaps in memory loss
B. Perception in the absence of stimuli
C. Misinterpretation of stimulus
D. Conversion with imaginary person
(AI 1991)

61. Confabulation is a defect of:
A. Concentration
B. Attention
C. Intelligence
D. Memory

Confabulation is a behavioral reaction to **memory loss** in which the patient fills in memory "gaps" with inappropriate words.

62. All are the features of Korsakoff psychosis *except*:
A. Confabulation of memory
B. Loss of immediate memory
C. Loss of recent memory
D. Normal sensorium

63. In Korsakoff psychosis, the site of lesion is:
A. Cingulate gyrus
B. Corpus striatum
C. Mammillary bodies
D. Frontal lobe

Amnestic syndrome or dysmnesic syndrome or Korsakov's (Korsakoff) psychosis or syndrome is characterized by impairment of memory due to *organic disease*. There is no disturbance of conscious, attention, global intellectual function, abstract thinking or personality. **Recent or short term memory is more severely disturbed.** There may be impairment of remote or long-term memory but there is **no impairment of immediate memory.** Loss of recent memory leads to disorientation in time and place. To fill in the memory gaps the patient *uses* imaginary events in the early phase of the disease (**confabulation**). **Confabulation disappears with progression of disease**. Any lesion involving the inner core of limbic system (**mammillary body,** fornix, hippocampus and parahippocampal structures of medial temporal lobe, posterior hypothalamus and dorsal thalamic nuclei), bilaterally, like head injury, bilateral temporal lobectomy, hypoxia, stroke, herpes simplex encephalitis, SOL in region of 3rd ventricle may result in this condition.

64. In enuresis, most useful drug is:

A. Chlorpromazine **B.** Trimipramine
C. Diazepam **D.** Haloperidol

65. A child becomes dry by day and night by the age of 6. Before this age which of the following condition is commonly seen:

A. Diurnal diuresis **B.** Nocturnal diuresis
C. Both **D.** None *(KERALA 1999)*

A child suffering from *enuresis* continues to urinate at "inappropriate" *time* and *places* after the time when he should have been "toilet trained" (between ages of 2 and 4 years). This disorder is much more common in boys. Enuresis is said to be *primary* when there has been no period of good bladder control since birth. **"Nocturnal"** enuresis is a *parasomnia* which occurs during **stage 3 and 4 of sleep.** "Diurnal" enuresis occurs during waking hours. Juvenile diabetes mellitus, sickle cell anemia or sickle cell trait, diabetes insipidus, frontal lobe tumor, spina bifida, spina bifida occulta, peripheral nerve injury, posterior urethral valve and proximal genitourinary malformations can all lead to enuresis. Urinary tract infection and delayed CNS maturation are other causes. *Psychological factors* such as acute stress, over ambition, hostilities, family reaction may also cause enuresis. As enuresis is a self limiting disorder, sometimes no treatment is required. Parents should be reassured that it is a *normal* developmental variant (especially primary nocturnal enuresis). **Tricyclic antidepressants** (Imipramine) or desmopressin nasal spray may be sometimes useful.

66. Lithium is used in treatment of:

A. Acute mania **B.** Schizophrenia
C. Bipolar MDP prophylaxis **D.** Unipolar MDP prophylaxis

67. Prophylactic maintenance serum level of lithium is...........mEq/L:

A. 2–2.5 **B.** 1.2-2
C. 0.7–1.2 **D.** 0.5–1.5 *(AI 1994)*

- **Lithium carbonate is a mood stabilizer (antimanic).**
- It inhibits hydrolysis of inositol-1-phosphate.
- Leukocyte count is increased by lithium therapy.
- Lithium is handled by kidney in much the same way as Na^+.
- **0.5-1.0 mEq/L is considered optimum for maintenance therapy in MDP while 0.8-1.3 mEq/L is required for episodes of mania. Toxicity symptoms occur frequently when serum levels exceed 1.5 mEq/L.**
- Mothers on lithium should not breastfeed.
- Side effects include CNS toxicity, cardiac arrhythmias, and renal diabetes insipidus (on long term use).
- Hypothyroidism is a rare side effect. Thyroxine administration inhibits TSH and reverses thyroid enlargement.
- Lithium is *contraindicated* during pregnancy. Fetal goiter and other congenital abnormalities especially cardiac can occur.

68. *Not* a "learning" disability of childhood:

A. Ataxia **B.** Dyslexia
C. Agraphia **D.** Apraxia *(UP 1997)*

Ataxia is a common and important "neurologic sign" and patients manifest symptoms and signs of ataxia with gait impairment, unclear speech, blurred vision, altered hand coordination, and tremor with movement.

69. "Flash backs" are seen in which of the following:

A. Opiates
B. Cocaine
C. Amphetamine
D. LSD

Although no withdrawal syndrome is described with **LSD** use but sometimes there is a spontaneous recurrence of LSD use **experience** in a drug free state known as "**flash back**". This phenomenon is also described with cannabis use.

70. In alcohol withdrawal, the drug of choice is:

A. Chlordiazepoxide
B. LSD
C. Lithium
D. Haloperidol

Chlordiazepoxide, clorazepate, diazepam, lorazepam and oxazepam are indicated for the relief of **acute alcohol withdrawal symptoms** such as acute agitation, tremor, impending or acute delirium tremens, and hallucinosis.

71. Hypochondriasis means:

A. Abnormal preoccupation with normal body function
B. Normal preoccupation with normal body function
C. Normal preoccupation with abnormal body function
D. Abnormal preoccupation with abnormal body function *(AI 1994)*

72. Preoccupation with disease is known as:

A. Conversion reaction
B. Hypochondriasis
C. Obsession
D. Somatization *(AI 2000)*

73. A patient presents with a history of continuous headache for the past 8 years. Repeated examinations had failed to reveal any lesion. The patient is not convinced and is sure that he has a tumor in his brain. He is referred to a psychiatrist, who, after examination of his case comes to a conclusion. The diagnosis is most probably:

A. Hypochondriasis
B. Somatization
C. Somatoform pain disorder
D. Obsessive compulsive disorder *(AI 2002)*

Hypochondriasis is defined as *a preoccupation with a fear or belief of having a serious disease, based on person's own interpretation of normal body function or a minor physical abnormality.* However the complete physical examination and investigations do not show presence of any significant abnormality and the fear or belief persists despite assurance to the contrary by showing normal reports to the patient. Repeated change of physicians is common. Treatment is very difficult and consists of psychotherapy and treatment of underlying depression, if present.

74. Cataplexy is seen in:

A. Catatonic schizophrenia
B. Narcolepsy
C. Chronic depressing
D. Neuro-malignant syndrome *(JIPMER 2002)*

The **classical tetrad of narcolepsy** consists of **sleep attacks** (most common), **cataplexy, hypnagogic hallucination and sleep paralysis** (least common). Abrupt, complete, or partial paralysis (**cataplexy**) occurs in response to a variety of stimuli.

- Hypnagogic hallucinations are vivid perceptions, usually dream like, which occur at the onset of sleep and are associated with fearfulness. When these occur at awakening, they are called hypnopompic hallucinations.

75. Lithium is useful in:

A. Hyperkinetic disorder
B. Acute depression
C. Acute mania
D. All of the above

76. Lithium is *not* indicated in:
A. Drug induced leucopenia **B.** Seizures
C. Prophylaxis in bipolar mood disorder **D.** Acute mania *(UP 1999)*

Indications of Lithium

- Acute mania
- Recurrent neuropsychiatric illness
- SIADH
- Prophylaxis of vascular headache
- Prophylaxis of MDP
- Chemotherapy induced leucopenia and agranulocytosis

77. The family members of a 56-year-old man reported that he has become increasingly irritable, decreased sleep and has started spending large amount of money. *Most likely* diagnosis is:
A. OCN **B.** Mania
C. Impulse control disorder **D.** Depression *(AIIMS 2001)*

78. *Not* seen in mania:
A. Disorientation **B.** Pressure of speech
C. Elation **D.** Delusions of grandeur *(AI 1991)*

Mania and depression are **mood disorders**. The disturbances of mood in mood disorders may be of 3 types viz. mania, major depression, and mixed type.

In a persons life the life time risk of **mania** is 1% and the episodes last for 3–4 months followed by complete recovery. Each episode is characterized by:

- **Stage I**: **Euphoria** (enhanced sense of psychological wellbeing and happiness not in line with ongoing life events);
- **Stage II**: **Elation** (feeling of confidence and joy);
- **Stage III**: **Exaltation** (intense elation with delusion of grandeur) and
- **Stage IV**: **Ecstasy** (intense sense of blissfulness or spiritual joy).

Sometimes *irritable mood* may predominate if the person is stopped from doing what he wants to do. There is *increased psychomotor activity* ranging from restlessness to maniac excitement, i.e. the person is *on the toes* and involved in ceaseless activities which are goal oriented and based on external environment. The person is *unusually talkative* with *thoughts racing in mind*. **There is pressure of speech** and *uses playful language with joking, teasing, rhyming, punning and speaks very loudly*. There is **flight of ideas,** i.e. rapid speech which shifts from topic to topic taking clues from environment. There are **delusions of ideas or delusion of grandeur** with inflated self esteem. *Delusions of persecution* (harassment) secondary to delusion of grandeur, i.e. the patient thinks that he is so great that people are against him. The person is unusually alert and tries to do so many things at a time. There is marked increase in planning, although there is decreased functional activity. The person is markedly social even with unknown people. Judgment is poor and this along with delusions of ideas or delusion of grandeur leads to *high risk activities* such as buying sprees, reckless driving, money distribution, foolish business investments and wearing of showy clothes. *Sleep is reduced* because it is not required. Insight is absent.

79. After an earthquake, a person recovered. Then he felt guilty about his survival. This reaction is an example of:
A. Post traumatic stress disorder **B.** Schizophrenia
C. Depression **D.** Mania *(AIIMS May 2002)*

Post traumatic stress disorder (PTSD) is seen after a catastrophic event in a person's or a close friend or relative's life which is usually life threatening or potentially fatal (war, robbery, accident, earthquake, riot etc.). It is essential for diagnosing the PTSD that symptoms must be of more than one month duration. 50% patients recover completely within 3 months while others may have symptoms for years. Features of PTSD are as under:

Avoidance	Intrusion	Hyper arousal
Detachment	Recurrent distressing dreams	Irritability
Survivor's guilt	"Flash backs"	Insomnia
Low interest in activities	Difficulty in recalling stressful events at will	Persistent anxiety
Inability to feel emotions		Poor coordination
Avoidance of reminder of events		

80. *Not* an anxiolytic drug:
A. Ketazolam
B. Diazepam
C. Buspirone
D. Fluoxetine

Antianxiety (Anxiolytic) Drugs

Benzodiazepines	Alprazolam; Bromazepam; Chlordiazepoxide; Clorazepate; Diazepam; Halazepam; Ketazolam; Lorazepam; Oxazepam; Prazepam.
Others	Meprobamate; Hydroxyzine; Buspirone.
Beta blockers	Propranolol.

81. Nightmares occur in which of the following stage of sleep:
A. REM
B. NREM-I
C. NREM-II
D. NREM–III & IV *(AI 2000)*

Nightmares (dream anxiety attacks) occur during **REM sleep** and cause full arousal, with memory for the dream-associated unpleasant episode.

82. *False* regarding obsession is:
A. May be treated with psychosurgery
B. Obsessive personality
C. Main treatment is ECT
D. May remits spontaneously *(UP 1996)*

ECT is *not* the first line treatment in OCD and may be used *only* in the presence of severe depression.

83. Simple schizophrenia is best characterized by:
A. Persistent hallucinations
B. Persistent delusions
C. Formal thought disorder
D. Predominant social withdrawal *(JIPMER 2002)*

Although termed "simple" it is one of the most difficult subtype of schizophrenia to diagnose. Onset is early and the progress is very insidious. The course is progressive and there is **marked social withdrawal**, shallow emotional response. The patient lives shabbily and wanders aimlessly with loss of initiative and drive. *Delusions and hallucinations are usually absent.* Prognosis is *very* poor.

84. "Punch drunk" syndrome is seen with:
A. Alcoholism
B. Boxing injury
C. Encephalitis
D. All of the above *(KERALA 1999)*

Recurrent head trauma in **professional boxers** may lead to dementia, sometimes called the "**punch drunk**" syndrome or **dementia pugilistica**.

85. Thanatophobia is fear of:
A. Closed spaces
B. Flights
C. High places
D. Death *(UP 1998)*

86. Claustrophobia means:
A. Fear of heights
B. Fear of lizards
C. Fear of closed spaces
D. Fear of open spaces *(JIPMER 1991)*

87. Agoraphobia is fear of:
A. Open space
B. Closed space
C. Flying
D. Blood

(PGI 1997)

Phobia	Fear from	Phobia	Fear from
• Acrophobia	Heights	• Homilophobia	Sermons
• Aerophobia	Flying	• Linonophobia	String
• Agoraphobia	Open spaces	• Monophobia	Being alone
• Aichmophobia	Sharp objects	• Musophobia	Mice
• Ailurophobia	Cats	• Mysophobia	Dirt and germs
• Amaxophobia	Vehicles, driving	• Nudophobia	Nudity
• Anthropophobia	People	• Numerophobia	Numbers
• Aquaphobia	Water	• Nyctophobia	Darkness, night
• Arachnephobia	Spiders	• Ochlophobia	Crowds
• Astraphobia	Lightning	• Ophidiophobia	Snakes
• Batrachophobia	Frogs, amphibians	• Ornithophobia	Birds
• Blennophobia	Slime	• Phasmophobia	Ghosts
• Brontophobia	Thunder	• Phobophobia	Phobias
• Carcinophobia	Cancer	• Pnigophobia	Choking
• Claustrophobia	Closed spaces	• Pogonophobia	Beards
• Clinophobia	Going to bed	• Pyrophobia	Fire
• Cynophobia	Dogs	• Siderodromophobia	Trains
• Dementophobia	Insanity	• Taphephobia	Being buried alive
• Dromophobia	Crossing streets	• Thanatophobia	Death
• Emetophobia	Vomiting	• Trichophobia	Hair
• Entomophobia	Insects	• Triskaidekaphobia	The number 13
• Genophobia	Sex	• Trypanophobia	Injections
• Gephyrophobia	Crossing bridges	• Xenophobia	Strangers
• Hematophobia	Blood	• Zoophobia	Animals
• Herpetophobia	Reptiles		

88. *Not* an ego defense mechanism:
A. Transference
B. Reaction formation
C. Conversion
D. Projection

(AI 1991)

Ego Defense Mechanisms

- Repression
- Displacement
- **Projection**
- **Reaction formation**
- Undoing
- Anticipation
- Schizoid fantasy
- Hypochondriasis
- Splitting
- **Conversion**
- Regression
- Isolation
- Distortion
- Sublimation
- Humor
- Retroflexion
- Inhibition
- Dissociation
- Denial
- Rationalization
- Intellectualization
- Suppression
- Acting on
- Introjection
- Compensation

89. Which of the following schizophrenia has early onset and poor prognosis?
A. Schizoaffective
B. Hebephrenic
C. Paranoid
D. Catatonic
(AI 1991, 1996)

Hebephrenic or disorganized schizophrenia is characterized by marked thought disorders. There is incoherence and severe loosening of associations. **Delusions and hallucinations are fragmentary and changeable. Onset is early (in 2nd decade) and recovery never occurs**. Course is progressive and downhill and severe deterioration without significant remission occurs over time.

90. All are *false* regarding Alzheimer's disease *except*:
A. Memory intact
B. A form of pre senile dementia
C. Lewy bodies seen
D. Increased incidence in Down syndrome
(PGI 1998)

91. Biochemical etiology of Alzheimer's disease is related to which of the following:
A. GABA
B. Acetylcholine
C. Dopamine
D. Serotonin

Alzheimer's disease is a progressive, neurodegenerative disease of unknown etiology which produces characteristic brain lesions and dementia. The *most common* genetic lesion producing Alzheimer's disease is lesion at chromosome 21 which is the site for *amyloid precursor protein*. **Alzheimer's disease is very common in patients of Down syndrome**. Abnormal amyloid precursor protein metabolism, tau protein, cholinergic neuronal dysfunction and aluminum have been implicated. Some authors suggest abnormal neuronal membrane phospholipid metabolism as the cause of Alzheimer's disease. *Research studies have indicated a general decrease in cerebrospinal fluid (CSF) acetylcholine and Aβ amyloid levels with an increase in tau protein.* The classical histopathological findings of Alzheimer's disease (AD) are neuronal loss, neurofibrillary tangles, neuritic plaques, granulovacuolar degeneration and amyloid angiopathy. The most seriously affected lobe is mediotemporal. **Dementia of Alzheimer type (DAT) is the *most common* cause of dementia and is responsible for 55% of cases.** Tacrine (reversible acetylcholine esterase inhibitor) causes transient reversing or slowing in cognitive decline in a small percentage of cases.

92. A patient of schizophrenia was treated for 5 years, and then he developed perioral movements. This is:
A. Malignant neuroleptic syndrome
B. Akathisia
C. Muscle dystonia
D. Tardive dyskinesia
(AI 1997)

Tardive dyskinesia or dystonia is a common complication of **long-term antipsychotic drug treatment** (with dopamine receptor antagonists). It is related to drug-induced super-sensitivity of striatal dopamine receptors. Clinical features include abnormal choreoathetoid movements, especially involving the face and mouth in adults and the limbs in children. Tardive dystonia may be focal, producing, for example, blepharospasm, torticollis, or oromandibular dystonia, or it may affect contiguous body parts (e.g. the face and neck or arm and trunk). Generalized dystonia is uncommon, especially in older patients.

93. Tardive dyskinesia is *not* seen with:

A. Clozapine
B. Flupenthixol
C. Fluoxetine
D. Reserpine
(UP 1999)

Tardive dyskinesia is a late side effect of treatment with antipsychotic drugs. *Fluoxetine* is *not* an antipsychotic drug but it is antidepressant.

94. *Not* a side effect of fluoxetine:

A. Diarrhea
B. Nervousness
C. Sweating
D. Weight gain
(AI 1994)

95. Fluoxetine is a:

A. Serotonin uptake inhibitor
B. Benzodiazepines antagonist
C. Nor adrenaline reuptake inhibitor
D. MAO–B inhibitor
(AI 1999)

Fluoxetine is a bicyclic, potent and **highly selective serotonin uptake inhibitor** largely devoid of anticholinergic, sedative and hypotensive side effects. It does not prolong cardiac conduction time. Nervousness, anxiety, insomnia, *anorexia,* increased sweating; diarrhea and headache are its side effects.

96. All are the features of Wernicke's encephalopathy *except*:

A. Ophthalmoplegia
B. Normal pupillary response
C. Disorientation
D. Retinal hemorrhage

Wernicke's encephalopathy is an acute reaction to severe thiamine deficiency and its *most common* cause is chronic alcohol abuse. The onset occurs after a period of persistent vomiting and important features are coarse nystagmus, ophthalmoplegia with bilateral external rectus paralysis, **pupillary irregularities**, retinal hemorrhage, and papilledema, impairment of vision, disorientation, and loss of recent memory, poor attention span, distractibility and apathy.

97. Drug *not* used in "akathesia" is:

A. Promethazine
B. Haloperidol
C. Diazepam
D. Trihexyphenidyl
(AI 1994)

98. Treatment of choice in akathesia is:

A. Haloperidol
B. Fluoxetine
C. Lithium
D. Propranolol
(JIPMER 2002)

99. Akathesia is:

A. Psychological restlessness
B. Cogwheel rigidity
C. Verbal restlessness
D. Motor restlessness
(JIPMER 2001)

Akathesia or **motor restlessness** may involve the entire body but is often *most obvious* in the patient's inability to keep her legs and feet still. It may be confused with anxiety or agitation. Akathesia may respond to **anti-parkinsonism drugs** (such as trihexyphenidyl or promethazine) but if the patient responds poorly a decrease in dose or change to another neuroleptic is indicated. In selected cases it can be successfully treated with **propranolol**, **benzodiazepines** or **vitamin E**.

100. Pavor nocturnus is:

A. Somnambulism
B. Sleep bruxism
C. Sleep apnea
D. Sleep terror
(PGI 1998)

• **Sleep walking**	Somnambulism
• **Sleep terrors or night terrors**	Pavor nocturnus
• **Sleep related enuresis**	Bed wetting
• **Bruxism**	Tooth grinding
• **Sleep talking**	Somniloquy

101. Irresistible urge to move about with inner restlessness is known as:
A. Dyskinesia
B. Hyperkinesia
C. Akinesia
D. Akathisia
(TN 1997, AI 1999)

Akathisia is an inability to sit down as the thought of doing so causes severe anxiety. The patient is restless, has an urgent need to move, and complains of muscular trembling. It may appear as a complication of therapy with antipsychotic drugs such as phenothiazines or reserpine.

102. Kleptomania is:
A. Irresistible desire to drink
B. Irresistible desire to steal things
C. Irresistible desire to set fire
D. Irresistible desire to tell lies
(AI 1999)

Kleptomania is the impulsive **stealing** and the motive not being in the intrinsic value of the article. The individual has enough money to pay for the stolen goods. The stealing is done without prior planning and without the assistance of others. There is increased tension before the theft and a sense of gratification while successfully committing the act.

103. In which of the following *tactile hallucinations* are seen:
A. Pentazocine
B. Cocaine
C. Heroin
D. Alcohol
(AI 1992)

Magnan's phenomenon is seen in chronic cocaine poisoning (cocainism). It consists of one of the following feelings:
- Grains of sands are lying under the skin.
- Small insects are creeping on the skin (**cocaine bugs**).
- These insects are biting and causing itching.

104. A 45-year-old man presented with waxy flexibility, negativism and decreased motor behavior. *Most likely* diagnosis is:
A. Simple schizophrenia
B. Paranoid schizophrenia
C. Catatonic schizophrenia
D. Hebephrenic schizophrenia
(AI 2001)

105. *Not* a feature of catatonia:
A. Negativism
B. Catalepsy
C. Mannerism
D. Automatic obedience
(JIPMER 1992)

Stuporous (retarded) catatonia is a type of **catatonic schizophrenia** characterized by extreme retardation of psychomotor function. There is **mutism**, maintenance of a rigid posture against efforts to be moved, motiveless resistance to all commands and attempts to be moved (**negativism**), voluntary assumption of inappropriate and bizarre postures for long periods (**posturing**), akinesis with mutism with preservation of conscious awareness (**stupor**), **echolalia**, **waxy flexibility**, tentative actions are made with no purposeful goal (**ambivalence**), e.g. when asked to show the tongue, the tongue is slightly protruded and then taken back, **mannerism**, the commands are followed irrespective of their nature (**automatic obedience**), and **verbigeration** (incomprehensible speech).

106. "Jargon aphasia" is seen in:
A. Wernicke's aphasia
B. Broca's aphasia
C. Conduction aphasia
D. Motor aphasia
(JIPMER 2001)

In **Wernicke's aphasia** comprehension is impaired for spoken and written language. Language output is fluent and maintains appropriate melody but is highly paraphasic and *circumlocutious*. The tendency for paraphasic errors may be so marked that it leads to strings of neologisms, which form the basis of "**jargon aphasia**."

*C**ircumlocution** means a roundabout, indirect, or lengthy way of expressing something.

107. Young lady presents with a history of excessive food intake following which she would induce vomiting. The *most likely* diagnosis is:

A. Binge eating disorder
B. Bulimia nervosa
C. Anorexia Nervosa
D. OCD *(AI 2002)*

108. Characteristic feature of bulimia nervosa is:

A. Common in middle aged woman
B. Excessive eating followed by *induced* vomiting
C. Excessive dieting
D. Loss of appetite *(UP 1998)*

109. All are *false* regarding anorexia nervosa *except*:

A. Hyperkalemia **B.** Amenorrhea
C. Lassitude and lethargy **D.** Exclusively in female *(UP 1994)*

Anorexia nervosa and bulimia nervosa are eating disorders in young, previously healthy women who develop a paralyzing fear of becoming fat.

	Anorexia Nervosa	**Bulimia**
Predominant sex	Female	Female
'Method' of weight control	Reduction of intake	Vomiting
Binge eating	Uncommon	Invariant
Weight at diagnosis	Markedly decreased	Near normal
Ritualized exercise	Usual	Rare
Amenorrhea	100%	50%
Other endocrine changes	Common	Uncommon
Antisocial behavior	Rare	Frequent
CVS changes (bradycardia, hypotension)	Common	Uncommon
Skin changes (hirsutism, dryness, carotenemia)	Usual	Rare
Hypothermia	Usual	Rare
Edema	Present or absent	Present or absent
Medical complications	Hypokalemia, cardiac arrhythmias	Hypokalemia, cardiac arrhythmias, aspiration of gastric contents, esophageal or gastric rupture

110. *False* regarding anorexia nervosa is:

A. Disturbed body image
B. Loss of appetitive
C. Amenorrhea
D. Loss of weight *(UP 1995)*

Signs and Symptoms of Anorexia Nervosa

Symptoms	Signs
1. **Weight loss** 2. Fatigue or weakness 3. **Appetite remains normal** 4. Morbid fear of fatness 5. **Disturbed body image** (Feel fat when thin) 6. Concern about weight leads to behavior changes • Dieting • Exercise • Diuretic or laxative abuse 7. Ritual behaviors (e.g. hand washing) 8. Hides disordered eating from others • Surreptitious mealtime behavior • Wearing of baggy clothes • Avoids food related behavior	1. Thinness (bone showing through) 2. Carotene pigment (yellow discoloration of skin) 3. Weight 15% below ideal weight 4. Lanugo hair (fine hair on back and cheeks) 5. Induced Vomiting signs • Calluses at Fingernails • Chipmunk cheeks (parotid hypertrophy) • Dental enamel erosion 6. Severe anorexia (starvation signs) • Edema • Bradycardia • Hypothermia
Major Criteria for diagnosis: • *Body weight maintained less than 85% of expected* • *Intense fear of fatness* • *Disturbed body self image* • ***Amenorrhea** for at least 3 consecutive months*	

111. Stealing, frequent lying and fire setting assault are:

A. Dissociated disorder　　**B.** Manic disorder
C. ADHD　　**D.** Conduct disorder *(PGI 1997)*

A persistent and significant pattern of conduct in which the basic rights of other individuals are violated or rules of society are not followed, characterize the **conduct disorders**. Disorder is 5-10 times more common in men and there are 4 types, viz. *under socialized aggressive type, under socialized non-aggressive type, socialized aggressive type and socialized non-aggressive type.* Characteristic clinical features are frequent lying, stealing or robbery, running away from home or school, violent acts like fire setting, use of weapons, assault and cruelty towards people and animals.

112. Ganser's syndrome is associated with which of the following:

A. Malinger　　**B.** Confabulation
C. Approximate answer　　**D.** Repeated lying

Hysterical pseudodementia or Ganser's syndrome is commonly seen in prison inmates and its characteristic feature is *vorbeireden* or "**approximate answers**". Although the answers are wrong but it is evident from the answers that the patient understands the nature of the question asked. For example when asked what 5 + 5 is the patient will tell 11 or when shown a blue pen the patient will call it red.

113. Identical mental disorder affecting 2 members of a family is:

A. Folie å quatre
B. Folie de porquoi
C. Folie å deux
D. Folie å trois *(PGI 1999)*

Folie å deux is a **shared paranoid disorder** in which there is "transfer" of delusions from one person to another. The second person is usually heavily dependent on the first and both persons have a closely knit emotional bond. On separation the dependent individual may give up his/her delusion. If more than two persons are involved then the condition is known as Folie å trois (3) or Folie å quatre (4).

114. Dissociative phenomenon is:

A. Lack of insight
B. Amnesia
C. Deafness
D. Fugue

115. A person missing from home, found to be wandering purposefully, well groomed and has some degree of amnesia. This condition is known as:

A. Acute anxiety
B. Schizophrenia
C. Dissociated amnesia
D. Dissociated fugue

(AI 2001)

Dissociative disorders or dissociative hysterias are characterized by disturbance in the normal integrated functions of *consciousness*, *identity*, and/or *memory*. Onset is *sudden*, disturbance is *temporary*, and recovery is *abrupt*. Often there is a *precipitating stress* before the onset and a *secondary gain* resulting from the symptoms may be found. Common types of dissociative disorders are *psychogenic amnesia, somnambulism, multiple personality,* **psychogenic fugues**, and *other dissociative states.* **Psychogenic amnesia is the most common clinical type of dissociative disorder** and is characterized by sudden inability to recall important personal information. **Psychogenic fugues** are characterized by episodes of wandering away from home and during this episode the person adopts a new identity with complete amnesia of earlier life. **The characteristic feature of fugues is assumption of a purposeful new identity with absence of awareness of amnesia.**

116. Phobia is a:

A. Psychosis
B. Fear of animal
C. Anxiety
D. Irrational fear

(AI 1998)

Phobia may be *defined* as **an irrational fear of an object, situation or activity leading to persistent avoidance of feared object, situation or activity.** Agoraphobia is the most common type of phobia seen in clinical practice.

117. *False* regarding malingering is:

A. Not caused by drugs
B. Unconsciously doing things
C. Done for some material gain
D. None of the above

(KERALA 1999)

Malingering is not a mental disorder or illness and the malingering individuals fully and **deliberately fakes or exaggerates illness with the conscious intent to deceive other people**. The reason for this may be monetary or legal and can be understood by examining the circumstances affecting these people. These people are often evasive or uncooperative for examination and there is marked discrepancy between their claimed disability and physical finding. This should be differentiated from **fictions disorders** in which the goals of the patients cannot be clearly understood even though the patient is voluntarily "causing" the symptoms of illness. No medical or psychiatric treatment is required.

118. Morbid jealousy is seen with which of the following:

A. Amphetamine
B. Cannabis
C. Alcohol
D. Opium

(AI 1994, JIPMER 2001)

Morbid jealousy is more common among alcoholics.

119. *Most common* age of depression is:

A. Old female
B. Old male
C. Adult female
D. Adult male

(AI 1996, 1998)

120. Endogenous depression is:

A. Schizophrenia
B. Anxiety
C. Hallucination
D. Worsening of early morning

(UP 1996)

"Emotions" are of two main types, viz. **affect** (feeling) and **mood.** Affect is a short lived emotional response to an event while mood is a lasting and dominant emotional response which *colors* the entire *psychic life* of a person. Therefore **depression and mania are mood disorders** and *not* affective disorders. The major mood disorders can be classified into 3 types, viz. **bipolar mood disorders (MDP), unipolar mood disorders and mild mood disorders.** Bipolar mood disorders are characterized by 1 or more episodes of mania and one or more episodes of depression while in unipolar mood disorders only one "pole" is present. Mild mood disorders include dysthymia and cyclothymia. The life time risk for development of major depression is 12% in males and 24% in females and a *typical* **depressive episode** is characterized by a depressed mood, depressive ideas, psychomotor activity, somatic symptoms, biological functions, psychotic features and suicide. The most important feature is **sadness of mood** or **loss of interest and pleasure in all activities.** Loss of interest results in *social withdrawal*, *decreased activity to function in occupation* and *decreased involvement in previously pleasurable activities.* The sadness of mood is associated with **pessimism** which results in hopelessness, helplessness and worthlessness. The "idea" of worthlessness leads to *feeling of guilt*. Thoughts of death and preoccupation with death are also common. **Suicidal ideas may be present and in severe cases delusion of nihilism** (ideas like *'there is no brain in skull or abdominal contents are rotting away'* or '*world is going to end soon*') **may occur.** In younger patients (< 40 years) retardation is common and in older patients agitation is common. Multiple somatic symptoms like vague body pain, heaviness of head are common. Insomnia, hypersomnia, loss of weight and appetite or sometimes hyperphagia and weight gain may occur. When the disturbance in biological functions become severe it is known as **melancholia** which is characterized by significant decrease in appetite and weight, early morning awakening, depression being worst in the morning, loss of reactivity to pleasurable stimuli and psychomotor agitation and retardation. Antidepressants are the treatment of choice for a majority of bipolar and unipolar depressive episodes.

121. Depression is *not* caused by:

A. Oral contraceptives
B. Methyldopa
C. Metyrapone
D. Bromocriptine *(JIPMER 1992)*

122. Depression is *not* caused by:

A. Clonazepam
B. Levodopa
C. Metronidazole
D. Corticosteroid *(UP 1999)*

Some Drugs Causing Depression

Acyclovir	Dapsone	Mefloquine
Amphetamines	Disopyramide	**Methyldopa**
Anticonvulsants	Disulfiram	Metoclopramide
Asparaginase	Estrogens	Metrizamide
Baclofen	Fluoroquinolones antibiotics	**Metronidazole**
Barbiturates	H2-receptor antagonists	Narcotics
Benzodiazepines	HMG-CoA reductase inhibitors	Pergolide
β adrenergic blockers	Interferon α	Phenylpropanolamine
Bromocriptine	Isotretinoin	**Progestins**
Ca^{++} channel blockers	**Levodopa**	Sulfonamides
Corticosteroids		Thiazide diuretics
Cycloserine		

123. Autism refers to:

A. Neuro-developmental delay
B. Condition seen following head injury
C. Deafness
D. Impaired reciprocal social and interpersonal interaction *(PGI Dec 2000, PGI May 2001)*

124. A 3-year-old boy keeps alone, does not mingle with others and is not attracted to toys. He gets irritable whenever he is slightly disturbed. The diagnosis is:

A. Hyperkinetic child
B. Autistic disorder
C. Attention deficit disorder
D. Schizophrenia *(AIIMS Nov 2001)*

Autism is the most important pervasive developmental disorder (PDD) of children and was first described by *Leo Kanner*, who gave the name **infantile autism**. This is 3-4 times more common in boys and onset is before 30 months of age. The child demonstrates **failure to make social contacts** and there is aloofness and **lack of eye contact**. Babbling, echolalia, poor articulation, pronominal reversal (you–I) are common. "The child shows no interest in his parents or other adults or children and does not speak voluntarily. He is fascinated with watching rotating objects and screams fiercely when his environment is altered in anyway". Some autistic children have isolated well developed skills such as musical ability, computation or memory (**Idiot savant syndrome**).

125. Mature defense mechanism is:
- **A.** Denial
- **B.** Anticipation
- **C.** Projection
- **D.** Reaction formation

(JIPMER 1991)

Mature Ego Defense Mechanism

• **Sublimation**	In this the unacceptable impulse is expressed in a socially acceptable way
• **Suppression**	Unacceptable emotions are "pushed" out of conscious awareness voluntarily
• **Anticipation**	Planning and thinking about future events in a realistic way
• **Humor**	To express unacceptable feelings without discomfort

126. Cognition means:
- **A.** Feeling
- **B.** Thought
- **C.** Behavior
- **D.** Perception

(UP 1995, AI 1997)

The psychiatric disturbances can be of 3 types, viz. that of **cognition** (*thought*), **connation** (*action*) and **affect** (*feeling*) or there may be disequilibrium between these three.

127. Tianeptine acts by:
- **A.** 5 HT antagonist
- **B.** Norepinephrine reuptake inhibitor
- **C.** Serotonin reuptake enhancer
- **D.** MAO inhibitor

Tianeptine increases 5 HT (serotonin) up take. It is *neither* sedative *nor* stimulant.

128. *Most common* postpartum psychosis is:
- **A.** Schizophrenia
- **B.** Dementia
- **C.** Depression
- **D.** Mania

(PGI 1999)

The ***most common*** type of postpartum psychosis is **major depression**.

129. Dysthymia is:
- **A.** Chronic mild depression
- **B.** Chronic severe depression
- **C.** Bipolar disorder
- **D.** Personality disorder

(JIPMER 2002)

Dysthymia is a mild form of depression lasting for 2 or more years while **cyclothymia** is mild form of bipolar disorder lasting for 2 or more years.

130. A patient presented to the casualty with a history of sudden palpitations, sensation of impending doom, and constriction in his chest. This lasted for about 10-15 minutes after which he became all right. The diagnosis is likely to be:
- **A.** Panic attack
- **B.** Generalized anxiety disorder
- **C.** Phobia
- **D.** Personality disorder

(AIIMS Nov 2001)

131. Treatment of panic attack includes:
- **A.** Carbamazepine
- **B.** Fluoxetine
- **C.** Imipramine
- **D.** Diazepam

(JIPMER 1995)

Unprovoked and sudden episodes of anxiety which usually reach their peak within a few minutes and subside in less than an hour are known as **panic attacks**. There is a sense of dread which is the most prominent psychological symptom. Physical symptoms seen in panic attacks are as under:

- Palpitation
- Sweating
- Dyspnea
- Chest pain
- Fainting
- Depersonalization
- Fear of dying
- Chills
- Tachycardia
- Tremors
- Feeling of choking
- Dizziness
- Derealization
- Feeling of going crazy
- Paresthesias
- Hot flushes

Benzodiazepines are the most effective anti anxiety drugs and are very useful in acute situational anxiety, anticipatory anxiety associated with panic attacks, generalized anxiety disorders and panic disorders.

132. Pseudodementia is commonly seen with:

A. Anxiety neurosis
B. Mania
C. Depression
D. Hysteria

(PGI 1997)

Psychiatric diseases may mimic dementia and **severely depressed individuals** may appear demented, a phenomenon known as **pseudodementia**.

133. Alexithymia is:

A. Inability to express one's own emotion
B. Motor restlessness
C. Sensory restlessness
D. Undue familiarity

(JIPMER 2001)

Alexithymia is a clinical feature common in post-traumatic stress disorder (PTSD) characterized by the inability to identify and articulate feelings.

134. Apraxia is a disorder of:

A. Cerebellum
B. Sensory system
C. Motor system
D. Initiating and planning movement

Apraxia is a disorder of initiating and planning movement. Unilateral apraxia of the right hand may be due to a lesion of the left frontal lobe (especially anterior or inferior), the left temporoparietal region (especially the supramarginal gyrus), or their connections. Left body apraxia is produced by lesions of these regions in the right hemisphere or by lesions in the corpus callosum that disconnect the right temporoparietal or frontal regions from those on the left. Bilateral apraxia is often due to bilateral frontal lobe lesions or a diffuse bilateral hemispheric disease.

135. A 50-year-old male complains of slowness of movements, postural instability, tremor and rigidity. *Most likely* diagnosis is:

A. Parkinsonism
B. Thyrotoxicosis
C. Multi-infarct dementia
D. Alzheimer's disease

(AI 2001)

Parkinson's disease is a chronic and progressive disorder in which idiopathic parkinsonism occurs without evidence of more widespread neurologic involvement. Parkinsonism is a syndrome of a *variable* combination of **tremor**, **rigidity**, **bradykinesia**, and a characteristic **disturbance of gait** and posture.

136. *False* perception without external stimulation is known as:

A. Obsession
B. Delusion
C. Illusion
D. Hallucination

(UP 1994, AI 1998)

Hallucination means perception *without* stimulus.

137. Disulfiram acts by:

A. Inhibiting aldehyde dehydrogenase
B. Inhibiting alcohol dehydrogenase
C. Both
D. None *(AI 1999)*

Disulfiram inhibits aldehyde dehydrogenase, causing very high levels of acetaldehyde to accumulate after alcohol is consumed.

138. In myoclonic seizures the drug of choice is:

A. Valproic acid
B. Clonazepam
C. Phenobarbitone
D. Lithium *(UP 1999)*

The **drug of choice for myoclonic seizures is valproic acid**. Clonazepam and acetazolamide are alternative drugs.

139. Neuroleptic malignant syndrome is characterized by:

A. Hypotonia
B. Hypothermia
C. Bradycardia
D. Labile blood pressure *(JIPMER 2002)*

Rigidity, *hyperthermia*, altered mental status resembling catatonia, *labile blood pressure*, and autonomic dysfunction characterize **neuroleptic malignant syndrome** which is a serious complication of treatment with antipsychotic (neuroleptic) agents, especially haloperidol. Associated clinical features include *tachycardia*, tachypnea, metabolic acidosis, and myoglobinuria that may be fatal.

140. *False* regarding dementia is:

A. Nootropics have limited role
B. Hallucination is not common
C. Often irreversible
D. Clouding of consciousness is common *(AI 1994)*

Dementia may be defined as a **chronic, organic psychiatric disorder** characterized by impairment of intellectual functions, memory (predominantly *recent* memory), abstract thinking, and judgment and impulse control. There is deterioration of personality with lack of personal care. All functions are impaired globally and interfere with day to day activities and interpersonal relationships. **There is no impairment of consciousness**. The disorder may have a progressive, stationary or reversible course. There is marked variation in emotional expression, *catastrophic reaction* (patient may go into a sudden rage when he is confronted with an assignment which is beyond the residual intellectual capacity). Thought abnormalities (delusion, preservation), urinary and fecal incontinence, disorientation in time, place and person may develop. Depending upon the underlying cause *the neurological signs may or may not be present.*

141. Wernicke-Korsakoff syndrome is due to the deficiency of which of the following:

A. Pyridoxine
B. Thiamine
C. Vitamin B_{12}
D. Riboflavin *(JIPMER 2000)*

Thiamine deficiency may involve the cardiovascular (wet beriberi) or nervous systems (dry beriberi and the **Wernicke-Korsakoff syndrome**).

142. In schizophrenia, drug of therapeutic benefit is:

A. Doxepin
B. Lithium
C. Imipramine
D. Fluphenazine *(AI 1993)*

In schizophrenia long-acting injectable preparations such as haloperidol decanoate and **fluphenazine** decanoate should be considered when noncompliance with oral therapy is a problem.

143. Delusions of nihilism and early morning insomnia are seen in:

A. Personality disorder
B. Mania
C. Schizophrenia
D. Major depression

(AI 1997)

The main feature of **mood disorders** is a disturbance of mood along "**happy-sad axis**". The DSM IV classifies "mood disorder" into major depressive disorder, bipolar I disorder, bipolar II disorder, dysthymia, cyclothymia, mood disorders due to general medical condition and substance induced mood disorder. The diagnosis of "mood disorders" requires the identification of "**mood episodes**" which may be major depressive episodes (MDE), manic episode, mixed episode and hypomanic episode. In order to level a certain mood episode an essential criterion is that the mood symptom should lead to serious distress or dysfunction and effect of drug, alcohol or medical condition should be ruled out. A patient of major depressive episodes (MDE) must exhibit *either* **depressed mood** *or* **a notable decrease in interest or pleasure (anhedonia).** The patient *typically* exhibits **neurovegetative symptoms of depression** such as changes in sleep and appetite. The sleep disturbance may involve trouble in falling asleep (**initial insomnia**), awakening during night (**middle insomnia**) or *early morning awakening* (**terminal insomnia**). Fatigue and impaired concentration are common and there is feeling of worthlessness and guilt. **Delusion of nihilism** (ideas like 'there is no brain in skull or abdominal contents are rotting away' or 'world is going to end soon') may occur.

144. In EEG, α wave is seen in:

A. Orthodox sleep
B. Paradoxical sleep
C. Mental work
D. Awake with eye open

(PGI 1997)

Nearly 33% of a person's life is spent in **sleep** and the EEG recordings show typical feature of sleep. The EEG recording during **waking state shows α waves of 8-10 Hz frequency.** Onset of the sleep is characterized by disappearance of α activity and **stage I** NREM is the first and lightest stage of sleep which is characterized by low voltage activity. **Stage II** NREM follows the stage I within a few minutes and is characterized by sleep spindles (regular spindle shaped waves of 13-15 Hz) and K complexes (high voltage spikes intermittently). **Stage III** NREM shows appearance of high voltage δ waves of 0.5-3 Hz frequency. **Stage IV** NREM shows predominant δ activity. NREM sleep is followed by **REM sleep** which is a light phase of sleep and EEG is characterized by **return of α waves.** Although REM stage is light stage of sleep, arousal is very difficult. The above mentioned stages occur regularly throughout the sleep and *first REM episode occurs typically after 90 minutes of onset of sleep*. In an 8-hour sleep usually 6 hours are spent in NREM sleep and 2 hours in REM sleep.

145. *True* regarding allodynia is:

A. Painful stimulus without stimulus
B. Painful stimulus to a normal nonpainful stimulus
C. Both
D. None

- **Allodynia** is the perception of a nonpainful stimulus as painful.
- **Hyperpathia** is an exaggerated pain response to a mildly painful stimulus.

146. Which of the following exclude painful stimuli from awareness:

A. Reaction formation
B. Rationalization
C. Projection
D. Repression

Repression is a primary ego defense mechanism in which the patient pushes unacceptable feelings into the unconscious mind.

147. In hashish the active substance is:

A. Tetrahydrocannabinol
B. Mescaline
C. LSD
D. Morphine

(AI 1991)

Hashish is prepared from concentrated resin of *Cannabis sativa* and contains a **δ-9-tetrahydrocannabinol** concentration of between 8 and 12 % by weight.

148. *True* about social phobia is:
- **A.** Fear of closed spaces
- **B.** Irrational fear of situation
- **C.** Irrational fear of activities
- **D.** Irrational fear of specified objects

(UP 2001)

In social phobia there is **"irrational" fear of activities** and is characterized by irrational fear of performing activities in presence of other people because the patient is afraid of his own actions being criticized by others resulting in his embarrassment or humiliation. There is marked distress and disturbance in daily functioning, e.g. there may be fear of eating in public, writing in public and fear of urinating in public lavatory.

149. Schizophrenia like syndrome is seen in drug abusers of:
- **A.** Pentazocine
- **B.** Opium
- **C.** Cocaine
- **D.** Amphetamine

(UP 1991)

Acute intoxication with **amphetamine** may present as a paranoid hallucinatory syndrome which closely **mimics paranoid schizophrenia**.

150. Lithium therapy may produce which of the following congenital anomaly:
- **A.** Renal agenesis
- **B.** Heart block (CVS malformation)
- **C.** Anencephaly
- **D.** Limb shortening

(AI 1993)

Data from lithium birth registers demonstrates an increased incidence of neonatal goiter and **congenital cardio-vascular malformations**, especially Ebstein's anomaly.

151. A 16-year-old girl was brought to the psychiatric emergency after she slashed her wrists to commit suicide. On enquiry her father revealed that she had made several such attempts of wrist slashing in the past, mostly in response to trivial fights in her house. Further she had marked fluctuations in her mood with a pervasive pattern of unstable interpersonal relationship. The most 'probable' diagnosis is:
- **A.** Borderline personality disorder
- **B.** Major depression
- **C.** Histrionic personality disorder
- **D.** Adjustment disorder

(AIIMS Nov 2002)

152. A female presenting with a prior history of slashed wrists and attempted suicide now presents with a similar history. The diagnosis is:
- **A.** Borderline personality
- **B.** Obsessive compulsive disorder
- **C.** Histrionic personality disorder
- **D.** Depression

(AIIMS Nov 2001)

Borderline personality disorder includes a pattern of instability in personal relationships, including frequent bouts of clinginess and affection and anger and resentment, often cycling between these 2 extremes at a rapid pace. These patients fear abandonment and this fear will often result in anger and aggressive behavior or acts that are used to 'make' others love them or stay with them. These acts include **pseudo-suicidal behavior**, **self-mutilating behavior such as cutting**, and instability of mood.

Further reading: *A Short Textbook of Psychiatry by Niraj Ahuja; 5th edition; page 122*

153. A 65-year-old male is brought to the outpatient clinic with one year illness characterized by marked forgetfulness, visual hallucinations, suspiciousness, personality decline, poor self-care and progressive deterioration in his condition. His mini-mental status examination (MMSE) score is 10. His *most likely* diagnosis:
- **A.** Dementia
- **B.** Schizophrenia
- **C.** Mania
- **D.** Depression

(AIIMS Nov 2002)

Dementia is a chronic organic mental disorder characterized by impairment of intellectual functions, impairment of memory (predominantly recent memory), and deterioration of personality with lack of personal care.

Further reading: *A Short Textbook of Psychiatry by Niraj Ahuja; 5th edition; page 24*

154. A 41-year-old woman presented with a history of aches and pains all over the body and cannot sleep because of the illness and has lost her appetite as well. She has lack of interest in work and doesn't like to meet friends and relatives. She denies feelings of sadness. Her *most likely* diagnosis is:

A. Somatoform pain disorder
B. Major depression
C. Somatization disorder
D. Dissociative disorder

(AIIMS Nov 2002)

Persistent somatoform pain disorder was previously called as psychogenic pain disorder. In this disorder, pain is the main feature, which is persistent, severe and distressing. Patient is commonly preoccupied with pain. Repeated change of physicians (doctor shopping) is very common with these patients. It is more common in females with an onset in 3rd or 4th decade of life.

Further reading: *A Short Textbook of Psychiatry by Niraj Ahuja; 5th edition; page 112 – 113*

155. A 41-year-old married female presented with headache for the last six month. She had several consultations. All her investigations were found to be within normal limits. She still insists that there is something wrong in her head and seeks another consultation. The *most likely* diagnosis is:

A. Phobia
B. Psychogenic headache
C. Hypochondriasis
D. Depression

(AI 2003)

156. A girl thinks her nose is ugly. Her idea is fixed and is not shared by anyone else. Next step in her management should be:

A. Do plastic surgery immediately
B. Reassure and send home
C. Refer to psychiatrist
D. Investigate and then operate

(AI 2001)

157. A patient came with complaints of having a deformed nose and also complained that nobody takes him seriously because of the deformity of his nose. He has visited several cosmetic surgeons, but they have sent him back saying that there is nothing wrong with his nose. He is probably suffering from:

A. Delusional disorder
B. Hypochondriasis
C. Obsessive compulsive disorder
D. Somatization

(AIIMS Nov 2001)

Hypochondriasis is defined as *a preoccupation with a fear or belief of having a serious disease, based on person's own interpretation of normal body function or a minor physical abnormality.* However, the complete physical examination and investigations do not show presence of any significant abnormality and the fear or belief persists despite assurance to the contrary by showing normal reports to the patient. Repeated change of physicians is common. *Treatment* is very difficult and consists of psychotherapy and treatment of underlying depression, if present.

158. A 15-year-old boy feels that the dirt has hung onto him whenever he passes through the dirty street. This repetitive thought causes much distress and anxiety. He knows that there is actually no such thing after he has cleaned once but he is not satisfied and is compelled to think so. This has led to social withdrawal. He spends much of his time thinking about the dirt and contamination. This has affected his studies also. The *most likely* diagnosis is:

A. Obsessive compulsive disorder
B. Conduct disorder
C. Agoraphobia
D. Adjustment disorder

(AI 2003)

Obsessive-compulsive disorder (OCD): An obsession may be defined as an "idea", "impulse", or an "image" which intrudes into the conscious awareness time and again. The idea is patient's own but is **ego alien,** i.e. foreign to the patient's personality and is **recognized as absurd and irrational by the patient** (**insight is present**) who tries to resist against it but is unable to do so. This failure to resist leads to marked distress. The "**obsession**" is associated with "**compulsion**" which is a form of *behavior* that *follows* the obsession. The aim of compulsion is to prevent or *neutralize* the distress or fear aroused by obsession. The behavior caused by compulsion is unrealistic and is *irrational* or *excessive*. As the insight is present the patient *also realizes the irrationality of compulsion.* In our country OCD is common in unmarried men of upper social strata with high intelligence and the average age of onset is in late twenties. **The *most common* type of patients of OCD are "washers".** There is obsession of *contamination* with dirt, germs, and body secretions and, naturally, the compulsion is *washing* of hands or whole body several times in a day.

159. Confabulation is:
- **A.** A state of confusion where patient is not able to describe the details
- **B.** Purposefully fabricating stories to project a certain image
- **C.** Filling up of gaps by fabrication to cover lapses in memory
- **D.** Seen in delirium

(SGPGI 2003)

Confabulation is a behavioral reaction to memory loss in which the patient fills in memory "gaps" with inappropriate words.

160. Parosmia is:
- **A.** Normal sense of odor
- **B.** Perversion about bad smell
- **C.** Perversion about sex
- **D.** Perceiving bad smell

(MANIPAL 2001)

Parosmia means any disorder or perversion of the sense of smell; a false sense of odors or perception of those that do not exist. Agreeable odors are considered offensive, and disagreeable ones pleasant.

161. *False* sense of perception without any external object or stimulus is known as:
- **A.** Illusion
- **B.** Impulse
- **C.** Hallucination
- **D.** Phobia

(AIIMS 11 May 2003)

162. All of the following are features of hallucinations, *except*:
- **A.** It is independent of the will of the observer
- **B.** Sensory organs are not involved
- **C.** It is as vivid as that in a true sense perception
- **D.** It occurs in the absence of perceptual stimulus

(AI 2003)

163. Hallucinations which occur at the 'start' of sleep is:
- **A.** Hypnagogic hallucinations
- **B.** Hypnopompic hallucinations
- **C.** Jactatio nocturna capitis
- **D.** Non-specific hallucination

(JIPMER 2002)

164. A patient presented with one-month history of abnormal hallucination, and delusion. The diagnosis is:
- **A.** Depression
- **B.** Paranoia
- **C.** Psychosis
- **D.** Schizophrenia

(AI 1997)

165. All are *true* regarding hallucinations *except*:
- **A.** It represents a state of inner mind's spatial orientation
- **B.** It is independent of the observer
- **C.** It is under voluntary control
- **D.** It is the perception which occurs in the absence of stimulus

(AI 2002)

166. Which of the following behavioral problems would suggest an organic brain lesion?
- **A.** Formal thought disorder
- **B.** Auditory hallucinations
- **C.** Visual hallucinations
- **D.** Depression

(AI 2002)

Hallucinations are false perception of a sensory stimulus. In hallucination, any sensory modality may be involved:
- **Auditory hallucinations** are found in psychosis and involve voices (not just sounds) which criticize, comment on the patient's action or may even give commands;
- **Visual hallucinations** are often found in 'organic' psychosis, especially toxic or drug related conditions;
- **Gustatory** (taste) and **olfactory** (smell) **hallucinations** should bring to the mind of physician a disorder of temporal lobe;
- **Tactile hallucinations** are also a feature of organic states such as alcohol withdrawal or cocaine and amphetamine abuse. Formication is the tactile hallucination of insects crawling over the skin;
- **Kinesthetic hallucination** is feeling of movement when none occurs;
- Hallucination of any type that occurs while falling a sleep (hypnagogic), or awakening (hypnopompic) is found in normal individuals and should not be considered pathologic.

Ref: *National Medical Series for Independent Study; Psychiatry; 3rd edition; page 4*

167. In narcolepsy, the *most common* symptom is?

A. Catalepsy
B. Hypnagogic hallucinations
C. Sleep paralysis
D. Snoring

(JHARKHAND 2003)

Narcolepsy is characterized by REM-onset sleep and the entire sleep cycle is affected, resulting in excessive day time drowsiness and sleep 'attacks'. Cataplexy is the loss of muscle tone and response to an emotion such as anger and excitement. On awakening the patient is transiently but completely paralyzed (sleep paralysis).

Symptom	Prevalence
• Excessive daytime sleep	100%
• Disturbed sleep	87%
• Cataplexy	76%
• Hypnagogic hallucinations	68%
• Sleep paralysis	64%
• Memory problems	50%

Ref: *Harrison's Textbook of Internal Medicine; 14th edition*

168. Sympathy towards captivator by captivated person is known as?

A. Cowden syndrome
B. Stockholm syndrome
C. Neurosis
D. Testamentary capacity

(CUPGME 2003)

Introjection is an ego defense mechanism in which there is unconscious internalization of the qualities of an object or person. Identification with the aggressor (e.g. sometimes seen in victims kidnapped by terrorists; also known as **Stockholm syndrome**) and grief reaction are examples in normal people.

Ref: *A Short Textbook of Psychiatry by Niraj Ahuja; 5th edition; page 214*

169. A 10-year-old boy presents with history of restlessness in class and inability to attend. He is quarrelling with classmates and does not take part in games. Which of the following is the *most likely* diagnosis?

A. Attention deficit hyperactivity disorder
B. Conduct disorder
C. Autism
D. Deafness

(AIIMS May 2002)

170. The *treatment of choice* in attention deficit hyperactivity disorder is:

A. Haloperidol
B. Imipramine
C. Methylphenidate
D. Alprazolam

(AIIMS 11 May 2003)

Attention-deficit / hyperactivity disorder (ADHD) is the *most common* neurobehavioral disorder of children. According to the fourth edition of diagnostic and statistical manual (DSM-IV), ADHD is characterized by inattention, including increased distractibility and difficulty in sustaining attention; poor impulse control and decreased self-inhibitory capacity; and motor overactivity and motor restlessness. These symptoms interfere with the individual's ability to function under normal circumstances. There are 3 types of ADHD, viz. predominantly hyperactive-impulse symptoms, predominantly inattentive symptoms, and combined type. Affected children commonly experience problem with academic under-achievement, interpersonal relationship with family members and peers, and low self-esteem. It frequently coexists with other emotional, behavioral, language and learning disorders. Stimulants are the most effective psychotropic agents in treating ADHD. Two main classes of stimulants are **methylphenidate** and its derivatives, and amphetamine and its derivatives.

Ref: *Nelson Textbook of Pediatrics; 17th edition; page 107 – 110*

171. Acrophobia is:

A. Getting caught in places from where escape would be difficult
B. Fear of heights
C. Fear of animals
D. Fear of closed spaces

(SGPGI 2003)

Acrophobia or hypsophobia is morbid **fear of high places.**

172. The following is a Schneider's first rank symptom:

A. Persecutory delusion
B. Voices commenting on actions
C. Delusion of guilt
D. Incoherence

(AIIMS 11 May 2003)

First Rank Symptoms (FRS) of Schizophrenia

- **Hallucinations of 3 types**: Audible thoughts or "thought echoes"; voices are heard arguing something, i.e. 2 or more hallucinatory voices discussing the subject in third person; and voices commenting on the patient's action.
- **Delusion of 6 types**: Thought withdrawal (thoughts stop and patient experiences them as being removed by some external force); thought insertion (patient experiences thoughts imposed by some external force on his passive mind); thought diffusion or "broadcasting" (patient experiences that his thoughts are escaping the confines of his self and are being known to others around him); "made" feelings (affect), impulses or volition of acts (patient experiences that feelings, impulses or actions are imposed by some external force and in "made" volition he thinks that his own acts are under the control of some external force and the subject is like a robot.
- **Delusional perception**
- **Somatic passivity** i.e. body sensation (sensory symptoms) imposed on body by external force.

Second rank symptoms (SRS) of schizophrenia

Other forms of hallucinations, affect disturbances and perplexity (to make a *person* uncertain, doubtful, or hesitant; confused; puzzled).

173. A 50-year-old man has presented with pain in back, lack of interest in recreational activities, low mood, lethargy, decreased sleep and appetite for 2 months. There was no history suggestive of delusions or hallucination. He did not suffer from any chronic medical illness. There was no family history of psychiatric illness. Routine investigations including hemogram, renal function tests, liver function tests, electrocardiogram did not reveal any abnormality. This patient should be treated with:

A. Haloperidol
B. Sertraline
C. Alprazolam
D. Olanzapine

(AI 2003)

174. Middle-aged man presented with pain in back, lack of interest in recreational activities, low mood, lethargy, decreased sleep and appetite for two months. There was no history suggestive of delusions or hallucinations. He did not suffer from any chronic medical illness. There was no family history of psychiatric illness. Routine investigations including hemogram, renal function tests, liver function tests, electrocardiogram did not reveal any abnormality. The patient should be treated with:

A. Haloperidol
B. Sertraline
C. Alprazolam
D. Olanzapine

(AIIMS 11 May 2003)

The lifetime risk for development of **major depression** is 12% in males and 24% in females and a typical depressive episode is characterized by a depressed mood, depressive ideas, psychomotor activity, somatic symptoms, biological functions, psychotic features and suicide. The most important feature is sadness of mood or loss of interest and pleasure in all activities. Loss of interest results in social withdrawal decreased activity to function in occupation and decreased involvement in previously pleasurable activities. The sadness of mood is associated with pessimism, which results in hopelessness, helplessness and worthlessness. The "idea" of worthlessness leads to feeling of guilt. Thoughts of death and preoccupation with death are also common. Suicidal ideas may be present and in severe cases delusion of nihilism (ideas like 'there is no brain in skull or abdominal contents are rotting away' or 'world is going to end soon') may occur. In younger patients (< 40 years) retardation is common and in older patients agitation is common. Multiple somatic symptoms like vague body pain, heaviness of head are common. Insomnia, hypersomnia, loss of weight and appetite or sometimes hyperphagia and weight gain may occur. When the disturbance in biological functions become severe it is known as melancholia which is characterized by significant decrease in appetite and weight, early morning awakening, depression being worst in the morning, loss of reactivity to pleasurable stimuli and psychomotor agitation and retardation. Antidepressants are the treatment of choice for a majority of bipolar and unipolar depressive episodes. **Sertraline** is indicated for the treatment of major depressive disorder.

175. Which of the following scientist propagated 'therapeutic-community' concept:

A. J B Watson
B. Maxwell Jones
C. Freud
D. Adler

(KARNATAKA 2000)

Maxwell Jones coined the term therapeutic-community.

Further reading: *A Short Textbook of Psychiatry by Niraj Ahuja; 5th edition; page 250*

176. Term catatonia was used by:

A. Karl Kahlbaum
B. Adolf Meyer
C. Leo Kanner
D. Karen Horney

(CUPGME 2003)

Catatonia is a mental state generally characterized by statuesque posturing, muscular immobility, mutism, and apparent stupor. The muscles are held in a pliant state called waxy flexibility, and the catatonic person obediently permits himself to be rearranged into awkward positions that he may subsequently hold for hours. Another form of catatonia involves continuous incoherent shouting, psychomotor agitation, and a violent destructiveness, which can lead to collapse and death if untreated. Loss of memory or intellect is not necessarily implied: catatonic patients often display excellent memory of their surroundings during the catatonic state. In recent years, drug therapy has been helpful in the avoidance of catatonic disturbances, and the appearance of catatonia is now quite rare. **Described by Karl Kahlbaum (1874) as catatonia**, the term was subsumed under Eugen Bleuler's concept of schizophrenia in 1911. The American Psychiatric Association has recently classified it as catatonic schizophrenia.

177. Among persons who successfully commit suicide, two most frequent psychiatric diagnoses are major depression and:

A. Somatization disorder
B. Schizophrenic disorder
C. Borderline personality disorder
D. Alcoholism

(KARNATAKA 1994)

178. *Most common* cause of suicide is:

A. Childhood depression
B. Depression in evolutional stage
C. Psychiatric depression
D. Reactive depression

(KARNATAKA 2000)

Suicide is the *most common* cause of death among psychiatric patients. It is type of *deliberate self-harm* (DSH) and is defined as a **human act of self-intentioned and self-inflicted death**. An attempted suicide is an unsuccessful suicidal act with a non-fatal outcome. Two to ten percent of all people who attempt suicide eventually successfully execute in next 10-years. Psychiatric illness is present in almost all people who commit suicide and co-morbidity (multiple psychiatric illnesses) is common. **Major depression is the *most common* disorder, and is present in about 50% of people who commit suicide. Alcohol is implicated in more than 25% of suicide.** About 5% of suicide victims have schizophrenia, whereas delirium, dementia, and other cognitive disorders constitute the 'primary' diagnosis in 4% of people who commit suicide. Diagnosis of 'panic-disorder' is statistically related to an increased incidence of suicide. Borderline and antisocial personality disorders occur in patients with suicidal behavior.

Ref: *National Medical Series for Independent Study; Psychiatry; 3rd edition; page 17*

179. Yawning is a common feature of:

A. Alcohol withdrawal
B. Cocaine withdrawal
C. Cannabis withdrawal
D. Opioid withdrawal

(AIIMS 11 May 2003)

The onset of **opioid withdrawal symptoms** occurs typically within 12 – 24 hours and subsides within 7 – 10 days. The characteristic symptoms include lacrimation, rhinorrhea, pupillary dilatation, sweating, diarrhea, **yawning**, tachycardia, mild hypertension, insomnia, raised body temperature, muscle cramps, generalized body ache, anxiety, piloerection, nausea, vomiting and anorexia.

Ref: *A Short Textbook of Psychiatry by Niraj Ahuja; 5th edition; page 45*

180. Flooding is the mode of treatment for which of the following:

A. Anxiety disorder
B. Depression
C. Fear
D. Mania

(MAHE 2001)

Flooding is a method used in treatment of **phobias**. In this kind of treatment, the patient is directly exposed to phobic stimulus and escape is made impossible. By prolonged contact with the phobic stimulus, therapist's guidance and encouragement and therapist's modeling behavior, anxiety decreases.

Ref: *A Short Textbook of Psychiatry by Niraj Ahuja; 5th edition; page 221*

181. Behavior therapy to change maladaptive behaviors using response as reinforcer uses the principles of:

A. Classical conditioning **B.** Modeling
C. Social learning **D.** Operant conditioning *(AI 2003)*

Operant is a designating conditioning in which the desired response, when it occurs, is reinforced by a stimulus. Operant conditioning is a common method for augmenting an adaptive behavior.

- In positive reinforcement, the desirable behavior is reinforced by a reward;
- In negative reinforcement, by performing the desirable behavior, punishment can be avoided;
- In modeling, the person is exposed to a model behavior and is induced to copy it

Ref: *A Short Textbook of Psychiatry by Niraj Ahuja; 5th edition; page 221*

182. An alcoholic is brought to the emergency OPD with the complaint of irrelevant talking. He had stopped using alcohol 3 days back. On examination, he is found to be disoriented to time, place and person. He also has visual illusions and hallucinations. There is no history of head injury. The *most likely* diagnosis is:

A. Dementia praecox **B.** Delirium tremens
C. Schizophrenia **D.** Korsakoff's psychosis *(AI 2003)*

183. Delirium tremens is characterized by confusion associated with:

A. Autonomic hyperactivity and tremors
B. Features of intoxication due to alcohol
C. Sixth nerve palsy
D. Korsakoff psychosis *(AI 2003)*

184. *False* regarding delirium tremens is:

A. Severe depression **B.** Disorientation
C. Excessive anxiety **D.** Perceptual defect *UP 1993*

185. Delirium tremens is seen in:

A. Alcohol withdrawal **B.** Alcohol overdoses
C. Morphine poisoning **D.** Atropine poisoning *(UP 1999)*

Delirium tremens is the *most severe* alcohol withdrawal syndrome, which occurs within 2 – 4 days of complete or significant abstinence from heavy drinking in 5% of patients. The course is short with recovery occurring within 3 – 7 days. It is an 'acute organic brain syndrome' with the following features:

- Clouding of consciousness with disorientation in time and place;
- Poor attention span and distractibility;
- Visual (and also auditory) hallucinations and illusions which are often vivid and frightening;
- Tactile hallucinations of insects crawling over body may occur;
- Marked autonomic disturbance with tachycardia, fever, sweating, hypertension and pupillary dilatation;
- Psychomotor agitation and ataxia;
- Insomnia with reversal of sleep-wake pattern; and
- Dehydration with electrolyte imbalance.

Ref: *A Short Textbook of Psychiatry by Niraj Ahuja; 5th edition; page 40*

186. An alcoholic presents with complaints of loss of memory of recent events, impaired insight, confabulation, and dementia of few months duration. The patient is suffering from:

A. Wernicke's encephalopathy **B.** Korsakoff's psychosis
C. Delirium tremens **D.** Binswanger's disease *(MAHE 2001)*

187. ***Not* seen in Korsakoff's syndrome:**

A. Clear consciousness
B. Inability to learn new things
C. Hallucinations
D. Confabulation

(JIPMER 2000)

Wernicke's encephalopathy is an acute reaction to severe thiamine deficiency and its *most common* cause is chronic alcohol use. Onset occurs after a period of persistent vomiting and its salient features are as under:

- **Ocular findings** consist of coarse nystagmus and ophthalmoplegia with bilateral external rectus muscle paralysis. Pupillary irregularities, retinal hemorrhages and papilledema may occur producing impairment of vision;
- **Higher mental function disturbances** present as disorientation, confusion, recent memory disturbances, poor attention span and distractibility. Apathy and ataxia are early symptoms.

Korsakoff's psychosis often follows Wernicke's encephalopathy and these together are known as **Wernicke-Korsakoff syndrome**. Korsakoff's psychosis presents as an **amnestic syndrome** characterized by gross memory disturbances with confabulation. Insight is often impaired. Neuropathological lesions are widespread but the most consistent changes are seen in bilateral dorsomedial nuclei of the thalamus and mammillary bodies. Changes are also seen in periventricular and periaquaductal gray matter, cerebellum and parts of brainstem. Its cause is severe, untreated thiamine deficiency secondary to chronic alcohol use.

Ref: *A Short Textbook of Psychiatry by Niraj Ahuja; 5th edition; page 40 – 41*

188. Psychological disorder *most commonly* associated with myxedema is:

A. Paranoid feeling
B. Phobia
C. Depression
D. Mania

(AI 1992)

189. Depression is a feature of which of the following condition:

A. Hypopituitarism
B. Hyperthyroidism
C. Hypothyroidism
D. Hypoglycemia

(UP 2001)

Psychiatric symptoms of hypothyroidism (myxedema)

- Apathy and lethargy
- Slow thinking
- Irritable mood
- Severe depressive episode
- Myxedema madness
- Memory impairment
- Poor attention span
- Paranoid ideation
- Dementia

Ref: *A Short Textbook of Psychiatry by Niraj Ahuja; 5th edition; page 156*

190. Which antipsychotic drug has prolonged action?

A. Fluphenazine
B. Penfluridol
C. Thioridazine
D. Triflupromazine

(AI 1993)

In schizophrenia **long-acting injectable preparations** (haloperidol decanoate and **fluphenazine decanoate**) are considered when noncompliance with oral therapy leads to relapses.

Ref: *Harrison's Principles of Internal Medicine; 14th edition*

191. Treatment is required in all of the following withdrawal symptoms *except*:

A. LSD use
B. Amphetamine
C. Alcohol
D. Cannabis

(AI 1996, 1998)

No withdrawal syndrome has been described with LSD use. However, sometimes, there is a spontaneous recurrence of LSD use 'experience' in a drug free state (**flashback**). Such episodes are usually induced by stress, fatigue, alcohol intake, and severe physical illness or marijuana intoxication.

Ref: *A Short Textbook of Psychiatry by Niraj Ahuja; 5th edition; page 52*

192. A 70-year-old patient was brought to the hospital with a 1-month history of auditory hallucinations with third person hallucinations. He has no history of similar problems previously. The diagnosis is *most likely* to be:

A. Dementia　　**B.** Schizophrenia
C. Pick's disease　　**D.** Multi-infarct dementia　　*(AIIMS Nov 2001)*

193. A 60-year-old male suffering from auditory hallucinations says that people staying upstairs are talking about him and conspiring against him. He dropped a police complaint against them but the allegations were proved to be wrong. The diagnosis is:

A. Schizophrenia　　**B.** Depression
C. Dementia　　**D.** Delusional disorder　　*(AIIMS MAY 2001)*

194. *Not* a characteristic feature of endogenous depression:

A. Loss of self-esteem　　**B.** Guilt psychosis
C. Third person hallucination　　**D.** Paranoid feeling　　*(AI 1992)*

195. *Most common* hallucination in schizophrenia is:

A. Auditory　　**B.** Visual
C. Olfactory　　**D.** Tactile　　*(JIPMER 1995)*

Hallucinations (perception without stimuli) are common in schizophrenia and **auditory hallucinations are by far the most common**. These can be of the following types:

- Elementary auditory hallucinations in which the patient 'hears' simple sounds rather than voices;
- Thought echo (audible thoughts); and
- Third party hallucinations (voices heard discussing and arguing about the patient in third person).

Only the third party hallucinations are 'characteristic' of schizophrenia.

Ref: *A Short Textbook of Psychiatry by Niraj Ahuja; 5th edition; page 57 – 58*

196. *False* regarding clozapine is:

A. Extrapyramidal side effect　　**B.** Agranulocytosis
C. Precipitates seizures　　**D.** Used in schizophrenia　　*(AI 1997)*

Clozapine is used only in the management of severely ill **schizophrenic** patients who do not respond to other neuroleptic agents or who cannot tolerate the adverse effects produced by those agents. Clozapine may produce a significant improvement in both the positive and negative symptoms of schizophrenia. Due to **significant risk of agranulocytosis and seizures** with clozapine, the patient should be given an adequate trial with at least 2 different standard antipsychotic medications before clozapine therapy is started.

Ref: *United States Pharmacopeial Convention*

197. All are antidepressants *except*:

A. Pimozide　　**B.** Fluoxetine
C. Amitriptyline　　**D.** Trazodone　　*(AI 1997)*

Pimozide is an **antidyskinetic** and **antipsychotic agent**. It is used for the suppression of motor and vocal tics in patients with Tourette's disorder whose symptoms are severe and who cannot tolerate or have failed to respond satisfactorily to haloperidol. It is used for maintenance therapy in the management of chronic schizophrenic patients without symptoms of excitement, agitation, or hyperactivity.

Ref: *United States Pharmacopeial Convention*

198. *False* regarding REM sleep is:

A. Dreaming sleep　　**B.** *Slow* eye movements present
C. Paradoxical sleep　　**D.** Alpha waves are seen　　*(UP 1999)*

One-third of our life is spent in sleep. This state occurs almost regularly and repetitively every day. EEG recording during the waking state shows alpha waves of 8 – 12 cycles/second. The onset of sleep is characterized by disappearance of this alpha activity. **Stage I, NREM sleep** is the first and the lightest stage of sleep characterized by an absence of alpha waves, and low voltage, predominantly theta activity. **Stage II, NREM sleep** follows stage I within a few minutes and is characterized by two typical EEG changes, viz. sleep spindles and K-complexes. **Stage III, NREM** sleep shows appearance of high voltage delta waves while **Stage IV, NREM** sleep shows predominantly delta activity in EEG. This **NREM sleep** is followed by **REM sleep,** which is a light phase of sleep. EEG is characterized by a return of alpha waves (alpha-wave sleep). One of the most characteristic features is REM or rapid (conjugate) eye movements. The first REM period occurs typically after 90 minutes of onset of sleep.

Ref: *A Short Textbook of Psychiatry by Niraj Ahuja; 5th edition; page 140 – 141*

199. Drug of choice for bipolar mood disorder:

A. Carbamazepine **B.** Lithium carbonate
C. Imipramine **D.** Buspirone *(MAHE 2001)*

Lithium is currently the drug of choice for treatment of manic episodes as well as for prevention of further episodes in bipolar mood disorder.

Ref: *A Short Textbook of Psychiatry by Niraj Ahuja; 5th edition; page 79*

200. Neurotransmitter, which is found in increased quantities in schizophrenia, is:

A. Noradrenaline **B.** Serotonin
C. Dopamine **D.** GABA *(AIIMS 1984, 1986, AI 1989)*

Schizophrenia is presently thought to be due to a **functional increase in dopamine** at the post-synaptic receptor sites, though other neurotransmitters like serotonin (especially 5-HT_2 receptors), GABA and acetylcholine are also probably involved.

Ref: *A Short Textbook of Psychiatry by Niraj Ahuja; 5th edition; page 65*

201. A 41-year-old woman working as an executive director is convinced that the management has denied her promotion by preparing false reports about her competence and has forged her signatures on sensitive documents so as to convict her. She files a complaint in the police station and requests for security. Despite all this she attends to her work and manages the household. She is suffering from:

A. Paranoid schizophrenia
B. Late onset psychosis
C. Persistent delusional disorder
D. Obsessive compulsive disorder *(AI 2004)*

The most common subtype of schizophrenia is paranoid schizophrenia, in which patient hold irrational beliefs that others are persecuting him/her or conspiring against him/her.

Paranoid type schizophrenia: More often than not, this is a misdiagnosed condition of prominent delusions or auditory hallucinations of persecution or grandeur, accompanied by a relative preservation of cognitive functioning. In reality, these are functionally normal individuals who have discovered the fact that some other individual or organization is conspiring or acting to torture, murder, or financially disable them, but are unable to produce legitimate evidence supporting their suspicions.

Ref: http://www.drleons.com/schizo/closet.htm

202. A 2-year-old girl child is brought to the Out Patient with features of hand wringing stereotype movements, impaired language and communication development, breath-holding spells, poor social skills, and deceleration of head growth after 6 months of age. The *most likely* diagnosis is:

A. Asperger's syndrome
B. Rett's syndrome
C. Fragile X syndrome
D. Cotard syndrome *(AIIMS Nov 2003)*

Rett's syndrome is a psychiatric disorder seen only in girls. After an apparent normal early development and normal head circumference at birth, there is a deceleration of head growth between the age of 5-months and 30-months. There is a loss of purposive hand movements and acquired fine motor manipulative skills with subsequent development of stereotyped hand movements. Later other movement disorders also develop and severe mental handicap is invariably present.

Ref: *A Short Textbook of Psychiatry by Niraj Ahuja; 5th edition; page 173*

203. A 30-year old male with history of alcohol abuse for 15 years is brought to the hospital emergency with complaints of fearfulness, mis-recognition, talking to self, aggressive behavior, tremulousness and seeing snakes and reptiles that are not visible to others around him. There is a history of drinking alcohol two days prior to the onset of the present complaints. He is *most likely* suffering from:

A. Delirium tremens
B. Alcoholic hallucinosis
C. Schizophrenia
D. Seizure disorder

(AIIMS Nov 2003)

Delirium tremens is the most severe alcohol withdrawal syndrome which occurs within 2 – 4 days of complete or significant abstinence from heavy alcohol drinking in 5% of patients. The course is short, with recovery occurring within 3 – 7 days. There is clouding of consciousness with disorientation in time and place, poor attention span and distractibility, visual and auditory hallucinations which are often vivid and frightening, marked autonomic disturbance such as tachycardia, fever, sweating, hypertension and papillary dilatation, psychomotor agitation and ataxia, insomnia and dehydration with electrolyte imbalance.

Ref: *A Short Textbook of Psychiatry by Niraj Ahuja; 5th edition; page 40*

204. A 16-year-old boy does not attend school because of the fear of being harmed by school mates. He thinks that his classmates laugh at and talk about him. He is even scared of going out to the market. He is *most likely* suffering from:

A. Adjustment reaction
B. Manic depressive psychosis
C. Anxiety neurosis
D. Schizophrenia

(AI 2004)

Adjustment disorders are one of the most common psychiatric disorders seen in clinical practice and are most frequently seen in adolescents and women.

Ref: *A Short Textbook of Psychiatry by Niraj Ahuja; 5th edition; page 116*

205. The Non- REM (NREM) sleep is commonly associated with:

A. Frequent dreaming
B. Frequent penile erections
C. Increased blood pressure
D. Night terrors

(AI 2004)

Night terrors occur early in the night and are a stage-4 NREM disorder. They are characterized by complete amnesia.

Ref: *A Short Textbook of Psychiatry by Niraj Ahuja; 5th edition; page 148*

206. A 30-year-old manic patient was prescribed haloperidol one week back. For last two days he has become restless and kept pacing in the room for a day. On examination he was found to have tremors of hand. He is *most likely* suffering from:

A. Anhedonia
B. Dystonia
C. Restless leg syndrome
D. Akathisia

(AIIMS Nov 2003)

Akathisia may appear within first 6 hours after dose; often indistinguishable from psychotic agitation; differentiation with benztropine may improve haloperidol-induced akathisia but not psychotic agitation.

207. Signs of organic brain damage are evident on:

A. Bender Gestalt test
B. Rorschach test
C. Sentence Completion test
D. Thematic Apperception test

(AI 2004)

The **Bender Visual Motor Gestalt test** (or Bender-Gestalt test) is a psychological assessment used to evaluate visual-motor functioning, visual-perceptual skills, neurological impairment, and emotional disturbances in children and adults ages three and older.
The Bender-Gestalt is used to evaluate visual-motor maturity and to screen children for developmental delays. **The test is also used to assess brain damage and neurological deficits**. Individuals who have suffered a traumatic brain injury may be given the Bender-Gestalt as part of a battery of neuropsychological measures, or tests.
The Bender-Gestalt is sometimes used in conjunction with other personality tests to determine the presence of emotional and psychiatric disturbances such as **schizophrenia**.

Ref: *http://www.healthatoz.com/healthatoz/Atoz/ency/bender-gestalt_test.html*

208. A 40-year-old male, with history of daily alcohol consumption for the last 7years, is brought to the hospital emergency room with acute onset of seeing snakes all around him in the room, not recognizing family members, violent behavior and tremulousness for few hours. There is history of his having missed the alcohol drink since 2-days. Examination reveals increased blood pressure, tremors, increased psychomotor activity, fearful affect, hallucinatory behavior, disorientation, impaired judgment and insight. He is *most likely* to be suffering from:

A. Alcoholic hallucinosis
B. Delirium tremens
C. Wernicke's encephalopathy
D. Korsakoff's psychosis *(AI 2005)*

Delirium tremens (DT) is the most severe alcohol 'withdrawal' syndrome. It occurs after 2 to 4 days of complete or significant abstinence from heavy alcohol drinking in 5% of patients. The course is short, with recovery occurring in 3 to 7 days. There is clouding of consciousness with disorientation in time and place, poor attention span and distractibility, **visual hallucinations which are often vivid and frightening**. Tactile hallucinations of insects crawling over body and auditory hallucinations may also occur. Marked autonomic disturbance such as tachycardia, fever, sweating, hypertension and papillary dilatation may occur. Psychomotor agitation, ataxia, insomnia, dehydration and electrolyte imbalance are other features. Sometimes death occurs due to cardiovascular collapse, infection, and hyperthermia or self-inflicted injury.

Ref: *A Short Textbook of Psychiatry by Niraj Ahuja; 5th edition; page 40*

209. A 45-year-male with a history of alcohol dependence presents with confusion, nystagmus and ataxia. Examination reveals 6th cranial nerve weakness. He is *most likely* to be suffering from:

A. Korsakoff's psychosis
B. Wernicke's encephalopathy
C. De Clearambault syndrome
D. Delirium tremens *(AI 2005)*

Wernicke's encephalopathy is a common and preventable disorder due to deficiency of thiamine. In the USA, alcoholics account for most cases, but patients are also at risk with malnutrition due to hyperemesis, starvation, renal dialysis, cancer, or AIDS. The characteristic **clinical triad is that of ophthalmoplegia, ataxia, and global confusion**. Ocular motor abnormalities include horizontal nystagmus on lateral gaze, lateral rectus palsy (usually bilateral), conjugate gaze palsies, and rarely ptosis. **Gait ataxia** results from a combination of polyneuropathy, cerebellar involvement, and vestibular paresis.

Ref: *Harrison's Principles of Internal Medicine; 14th edition*

210. A 25-year-old female presents with 2-year history of repetitive, irresistible thoughts of contamination with dirt associated with repetitive hand washing. She reports these thoughts to be her own and distressing, but is not able to overcome them along with medications. She is *most likely* to benefit from which of the following therapies?

A. Exposure and response prevention
B. Systematic desensitization
C. Assertiveness training
D. Sensate focusing *(AI 2005)*

Behavior therapy is an effective mode of therapy for OCD with a success rate of 80% especially for compulsive acts. The techniques used are:

- Thought-stopping (and its modifications);
- Response prevention;
- Systematic desensitization; and
- Modeling

Ref: *A Short Textbook of Psychiatry by Niraj Ahuja; 5th edition; page 100*

211. An 18-year-old boy came to the psychiatry OPD with a complaint of feeling changed from inside. He described himself as feeling strange as if he is different from his normal self. He was very tense and anxious yet could not point out the precise change in him. This phenomenon is *best* called as:

A. Delusional mood **B.** Depersonalization
C. Autochthonous delusion **D.** Over valued idea *(AI 2005)*

Depersonalization is characterized by alteration in the perception or experience of self so that the feeling of one's own reality is temporarily changed or lost.

Ref: *A Short Textbook of Psychiatry by Niraj Ahuja; 5th edition; page 113*

212. Dry mouth during antidepressant therapy is caused by blockade of:

A. Muscarinic acetylcholine receptors **B.** Serotonergic receptors
C. Dopaminergic receptors **D.** GABA receptors *(AI 2005)*

Dryness of mouth occurs due to blockade of *muscarinic acetylcholine receptors.*

Ref: *A Short Textbook of Psychiatry by Niraj Ahuja; 5th edition; page 193*

213. All of the following are hallucinogens, *except*:

A. LSD **B.** Phencyclidine
C. Mescaline **D.** Methylphenidate *(AI 2005)*

Hallucinogens

- Lysergic acid diethylamide
- Psilocybin
- Bufotenin
- Phencyclidine
- Lysergic acid amide
- Harmine
- Mescaline
- ^{9}Delta tetrahydrocannabinol

Ref: *Essentials of Medical Pharmacology by KD Tripathi; 4th edition; page 430*

214. Perseveration is:

A. Persistent and inappropriate repetition of the same thoughts
B. When a patient feels very distressed about it
C. Characteristic of schizophrenia
D. Characteristic of obsessive-compulsive disorder (OCD) *(AI 2005)*

Perseveration is persistent repetition of words beyond their relevance.

Ref: *A Short Textbook of Psychiatry by Niraj Ahuja; 5th edition; page 57*

215. A 50-year-old male presents with a 3-year history of irritability, low mood, lack of interest in surroundings and general dissatisfaction with everything. There is no significant disruption in his sleep or appetite. He is *likely* to be suffering from:

A. Major depression **B.** No psychiatric disorder
C. Dysthymia **D.** Chronic fatigue syndrome *(AIIMS May 2005)*

Persistent mood disorder is characterized by persistent mood symptoms which last for more than 2 years (one year in children and adolescents) but not severe enough to be labeled as even hypomanic or mild depressive episode. If the symptoms consist of persistent mild depression, the disorder is known as **dysthymia**; and if symptoms consist of persistent instability of mood between mild depression and mild elation, it is known as cyclothymia.

Ref: *A Short Textbook of Psychiatry by Niraj Ahuja; 5th edition; page 74*

216. A 25-year-old woman complains of intense depressed mood for 6 months with inability to enjoy previously pleasurable activities. This symptom is know as:

A. Anhedonia **B.** Avolition
C. Apathy **D.** Amotivation *(AIIMS May 2005)*

Anhedonia means inability to experience pleasure.

Ref: *A Short Textbook of Psychiatry by Niraj Ahuja; 5th edition; page 58*

217. Which of the following is an alternative to methadone for maintenance treatment of opiate dependence?

A. Diazepam
B. Chlordiazepoxide
C. Buprenorphine
D. Dextropropoxyphene

(AIIMS May 2005)

Methadone maintenance (agonist substitution therapy) is a very popular method used widely in the west. 20 to 25 mg/day of methadone is given to the patient to shift from hard drugs, thus decreasing IV use and criminal behavior. Other drugs like LAAM and *buprenorphine* can be used for maintenance treatment.

Ref: *A Short Textbook of Psychiatry by Niraj Ahuja; 5th edition; page 47*

218. A 31-year-old man with mood disorder, on 30 mg of *haloperidol* and 1000 mg of lithium, is brought to the hospital emergency room with history of acute onset of fever, excessive sweating, confusion, rigidity of limbs and decreased communication for a day. Examination reveals tachycardia and labile blood pressure and investigations reveal increased CPK enzyme levels and leukocytosis. He is *likely* to have developed:

A. Lithium toxicity
B. Tardive dyskinesia
C. Neuroleptic malignant syndrome
D. Hypertensive encephalopathy

(AIIMS May 2004)

The **neuroleptic malignant syndrome** can occur with phenothiazines and other drugs such as **haloperidol** and is characterized by muscle rigidity, autonomic dysregulation, and hyperthermia. This disorder is caused by the inhibition of central dopamine receptors in the hypothalamus, which results in increased heat production and decreased heat dissipation.

Ref: *Harrison's Principles of Internal Medicine; 14th edition*

219. A 34-year-old housewife reports a 3-month history of feeling low, lack of interest in activities, lethargy, multiple body aches, ideas of worthlessness, decreased appetite and disturbed sleep with early morning awakening. She is *likely* to benefit from:

A. Antipsychotics
B. Antidepressants
C. Anxiolytics
D. Hypnosedatives

(AIIMS May 2004)

Major depression is defined as *depressed mood on a daily basis for a minimum duration of 14 days*. An episode may be characterized by sadness, indifference or apathy, or irritability and is usually associated with change in a number of neurovegetative functions, including sleep patterns and **appetite** and weight, motor agitation or retardation, fatigue, impairment in concentration and decision making, feelings of shame or guilt, and thoughts of death or dying. Patients with endogenous depression have a profound **loss of pleasure in all enjoyable activities**, **exhibit early morning awakening**, feel that the dysphoric mood state is qualitatively different from sadness, and often notice a diurnal variation in mood. Paradoxically, these more severe features predict a good response to antidepressant treatment.

Ref: *Harrison's Principles of Internal Medicine; 14th edition*

220. A 23-year-old engineering student is brought by his family to the hospital with a history of gradual onset of suspiciousness, muttering and smiling without clear reason, decreased socialization, violent outbursts and lack of interest in studies for 8 months. Mental status examination revealed a blunt affect, thought broadcast, a relatively preserved cognition, impaired judgment and insight. He is *most likely* to be suffering from:

A. Delusional disorder
B. Depression
C. Schizophrenia
D. Anxiety disorder

(AIIMS May 2004)

Disorders of motor behavior in **schizophrenia** may manifest as either a decrease in psychomotor activity (stupor, inertia) or an increase (aggression, agitation, restlessness, excitement). Mannerisms, grimacing, stereotypes (repetitive strange behavior), reduced self care and poor grooming are common features. There is decreased functioning in work place, loss of ego boundaries (between self and environment), uncertainty about ones own identity and existence. Insight into the illness is absent but there is no disturbance of consciousness, orientation, attention, memory and intelligence.

221. A 30-year-old unmarried woman of average social-economic background believes that her boss is in secretly love with her. She rings him up at odd hours and writes love letters to him despite his serious warnings not to do so. She holds this belief despite contradiction from her family members and his denial. *However,* she is able to manage her daily activities as before. She is *most likely* to be suffering from:

A. Depression **B.** Schizophrenia
C. Delusional disorder **D.** No psychiatric treatment *(AIIMS Nov 2004)*

When the content of **delusions** is erotic (erotomanic), it is called as Clerambault's syndrome or erotomania. Occurring most often in women, there is an erotic conviction that a person with higher status is in love with the patient.

Ref: *A Short Textbook of Psychiatry by Niraj Ahuja; 5th edition; page 86*

ANSWERS

1 A	2 B	3 C	4 C	5 C	6 D	7 D	8 C	9 A	10 A
11 C	12 B	13 C	14 B	15 C	16 C	17 D	18 C	19 C	20 C
21 A	22 A	23 D	24 D	25 A	26 B	27 B	28 A	29 C	30 D
31 B	32 B	33 A	34 C	35 C	36 D	37 A	38 D	39 D	40 D
41 D	42 B	43 C	44 A	45 D	46 C	47 A	48 B	49 A	50 B
51 B	52 D	53 B	54 D	55 C	56 D	57 B	58 C	59 C	60 A
61 D	62 B	63 C	64 B	65 B	66 A	67 C	68 A	69 D	70 A
71 A	72 B	73 A	74 B	75 C	76 B	77 B	78 A	79 A	80 D
81 A	82 C	83 D	84 B	85 D	86 C	87 A	88 A	89 B	90 D
91 B	92 D	93 C	94 D	95 A	96 B	97 B	98 D	99 D	100 D
101 D	102 B	103 B	104 C	105 B	106 A	107 B	108 B	109 B	110 B
111 D	112 C	113 C	114 D	115 D	116 D	117 B	118 C	119 C	120 D
121 C	122 A	123 D	124 B	125 B	126 B	127 C	128 C	129 A	130 A
131 D	132 C	133 A	134 D	135 A	136 D	137 A	138 A	139 D	140 D
141 B	142 D	143 D	144 D	145 B	146 D	147 A	148 C	149 D	150 B
151 A	152 A	153 A	154 A	155 C	156 C	157 B	158 A	159 C	160 D
161 C	162 B	163 A	164 C	165 C	166 C	167 A	168 B	169 A	170 C
171 B	172 B	173 B	174 B	175 B	176 A	177 D	178 C	179 D	180 C
181 D	182 B	183 A	184 A	185 A	186 B	187 C	188 C	189 C	190 A
191 A	192 B	193 A	194 C	195 A	196 A	197 A	198 B	199 B	200 C
201 A	202 B	203 A	204 A	205 D	206 D	207 A	208 B	209 B	210 A
211 B	212 A	213 D	214 A	215 C	216 A	217 C	218 C	219 B	220 C
221 C